Y0-BXW-950

Diagnostic Neuroradiology

Diagnostic Neuroradiology

JUAN M. TAVERAS, M.D.

Professor of Radiology, College of Physicians and Surgeons, Columbia University; Attending Radiologist, Neurological Institute, Presbyterian Hospital of New York

ERNEST H. WOOD, M.D.

Professor and Chairman, Department of Radiology, School of Medicine, University of North Carolina; Director of Radiological Service, North Carolina Memorial Hospital; formerly Attending Radiologist, Neurological Institute, Presbyterian Hospital of New York

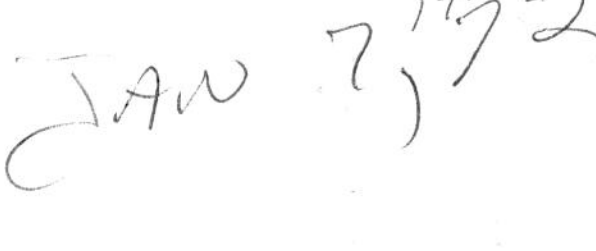

RC349
R3
T3
1964

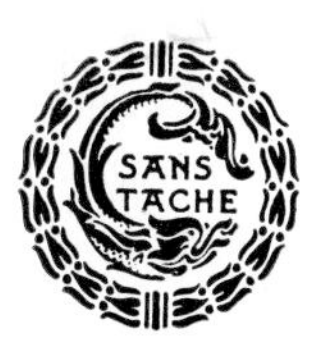

BALTIMORE / 1964

THE WILLIAMS & WILKINS COMPANY

167081

Copyright ©, 1964
The Williams & Wilkins Company
428 East Preston St., Baltimore 2, Md., U. S. A.
Made in the United States of America

Library of Congress Catalog
Card Number 64-19664

Reprinted from Golden's Diagnostic Roentgenology, where it forms Chapter I of the 1963-1964 renewal pages, and is there entitled Diseases of the Central Nervous System

Composed and printed at
Waverly Press, Inc.
Mt. Royal & Guilford Aves.
Baltimore Md. 21202, U. S. A.

To our wives

CONTENTS

The Skull

Intracranial Pneumography

Angiography

Selection of Diagnostic Procedure

Head Injuries and Their Complications

Diseases of the Spinal Cord

PREFACE

Neuroradiology has only recently celebrated its golden anniversary. The war of 1898. soon after Roentgen's discovery, saw radiologic methods employed extensively in the localization of foreign bodies, even intracranially. Not until the second decade of the twentieth century, however, were major accomplishments made. Early in this period Schüller, the father of neuroradiology, was at work, and his book of 1912 constituted the first publication of great significance on the subject. During the same period, Forssell and Stenvers also made important contributions to the plain film diagnosis of intracranial disease.

It was just a little more than half a century ago that Luckett and Stewart encountered their famous case of traumatic pneumocephalus, the prelude to Dandy's description of ventriculography and pneumoencephalography. Shortly afterward, Sicard and Forestier devised radiopaque myelography. Some years later Moniz reported his success, by perseverence, with cerebral angiography. In many countries angiography lay dormant, however, for many years until Torkildsen, Kristiansen and Engeset, through Engeset's report of 1944, described a hundred cases in which a water soluble substance was used rather than a colloidal mixture. They also revived Moniz's early method of percutaneous carotid puncture and paved the way for vertebral contrast study. Because of the inferior nature of contrast media available during World War II, the adoption of the angiographic method was retarded even then in many places, particularly in America. During the last fifteen years, angiography has arrived at its appropriate place of importance in diagnostic neuroradiology. Meanwhile, prior to the new angiographic era, many important refinements of pneumographic diagnosis were being worked out by Lysholm, Dyke, Twining, Robertson, Lindgren and others. All physicians involved in any aspect of radiologic or neurologic practice are deeply indebted to the pioneers, only a few of whom are mentioned above.

In recent years neuroradiology has extended greatly in scope. Many young physicians have specialized in clinical neurology and neurosurgery since the war of 1939–1945. Because of wider neurologic service, the demand for correlative roentgen diagnosis has spread into smaller communities. Many radiologists are called upon today to perform special procedures which, in years past, were carried out almost exclusively in neurologic centers.

The scope of neuroradiology has also been extended in depth. More accurate diagnosis of diseases of the central nervous system can now be attained through improved roentgen methods. As more minds devote more time to exploration of this still young subspecialty, many refinements of neuroradiologic diagnosis are evolving. The development is occurring, in part, through increases in knowledge and experience, allowing the radiologist to recognize variations from the normal and to localize abnormal shadows. The store of information being amassed in neurology, neuropathology, neurophysiology, and allied fields makes it possible for the radiologist to identify more frequently the abnormal processes that are found. This increasing knowledge puts greater demands on neuroradiology. The need will grow for radiologists especially trained in the diagnostic methods applicable to neural disease.

Also extending the depth of neuroradiology are the many examinations that currently are referred to as special procedures. Skill in instrumentation is now a requisite for the neuroradiologist, as well as ability in directing the making of films and the rendering of an interpretation. When faults of technique are committed by someone else, misinterpretation often follows. The head must always know what the hands have done. There is a strong trend away from a division of responsibilities, with every indication that this is proving beneficial for the patient.

The scope of neuroradiology now extends in length to both ends of the electromagnetic spectrum and into other media. The use of gamma rays from radioactive isotopes for scanning, and the use of heat waves in thermography, are now well-established procedures that are being incorporated in neuroradiologic clinical practice. The use of ultrasonic waves for echoencephalography also is widely accepted. Radiologists have made many important contributions to the development of these techniques and to other special methods of examination of the central nervous system. It cannot be foretold what future impact electronic devices will have in the diagnosis of neural disorders nor which of the newer procedures will fall within the province of the neuroradiologist. In the future, as in the past, a neuroradiologist with sufficient interest in the newer procedures can develop them to supplement the standard examinations.

Although many important books and monographs concerned with segments of neuroradiology have been published, only a few English language works dealing with the entire field have appeared. We have been led to believe, therefore, that it would be useful to bring together material which might serve as (1) a text for the student, (2) a handbook for those in the graduate study of radiology, and (3) a record of the working principles of neuroradiology found useful by the authors. The resulting volume is obviously incomplete. In the first place, our primary concern was roentgenology, rather than all of radiology. As a result we have not included detailed discussions of scintillation scanning and other newer procedures. Some reference, however, to their current importance is made in the section "Selection of Diagnostic Procedure." Second, even in the limited field of roentgenology the discussion of some subjects is not as detailed as some might like. Certainly no attempt has been made to include all of the controversial views that appear in the literature. Rather, we have tried to deal with the more commonly experienced diagnostic problems, as encountered in our daily practices, and to make available to the profession what we have learned about a variety of conditions. In our discussions of differential diagnosis we have sometimes gone afield, treating secondary subjects at considerable length despite the fact that they do not fit comfortably into the presentation. Third, we have limited our considerations to conditions of neurological importance insofar as possible. Extended descriptions of osseous lesions not primarily of neural significance have been omitted intentionally.

The work is divided into four major categories: (1) "The Skull," (2) "Intracranial Pneumography," (3) "Angiography," and (4) "Diseases of the Spinal Cord." Separately treated are two subjects that do not fit well into any of the four major categories: (1) "Selection of Diagnostic Procedure," and (2) "Head Injuries and Their Complications." The location of the former was chosen because it was felt that medical students and trainees in radiology could profit most from the considerations after exposure to the factual information presented in the first three sections of the work. The subject of trauma and its aftermath obviously spans all of the diagnostic categories.

We have, of course, drawn upon the experience of others as described in their writings and transmitted through personal communications. We have tried, even when only a concept or opinion has been borrowed, to make acknowledgment, and wherever possible to refer to the original work from which data were taken. When proper recognition has not been given, it certainly has not been the intent of the authors to minimize the importance of the works of others who have contributed to the field.

Dr. Ross Golden, who stimulated the undertaking of this work, has wisely pointed out that advancement of radiology is more easily achieved when a climate of cordial interdependence and mutual confidence between clinicians and radiologists pervades a medical institution. Such an atmosphere is exemplified by the Columbia Presbyterian Medical Center and is a particular heritage of the Neurological Institute of New York, from which the major portion of this work stems. The material is drawn from an experience now approaching a score of years during which we have served successively as attending radiologists to the Neurological Institute. In addition, we have been able to go back to the museum material collected by the late Dr. Cornelius G. Dyke, who preceded us in this post. We are most deeply indebted to all of the attending, visiting and house physicians and surgeons who have referred cases to us for radiologic examination, and have made their records so freely available over the years. Dr. H. Houston Merritt has unceasingly promoted the development of radiology at the Neurological Institute, and for his professional cooperation and personal interest we would like to take the opportunity to thank him most sincerely.

We would be most ungrateful if we failed to acknowledge with deep appreciation the aid given by the host of individuals concerned with the production of this work. We are deeply indebted to Dr. Laurence L. Robbins who read and criticized the manuscript, and to our associates, Dr. William B. Seaman and Dr. Charles A. Bream, who were helpful in many ways during its preparation. Important contributions have been made by Dr. D. Gordon Potts, Capt. Herbert F. Johnson, Dr. Luther E. Barnhardt, Mrs. Margery W. Westray, and many other individuals who assisted in assembling and checking various portions of the material. Our dedicated secretaries, who typed the manuscript, Mrs. Sallie J. Grenberg and Mrs. Winifred Sowa, deserve special recognition and thanks. Others who have helped are Miss Tod Dee Craig and Miss Adele Spiegler, who made the drawings, and Mr. Armand Diaz, who made almost all of the photographs. We also most sincerely appreciate the cooperation of those of our colleagues who have loaned material better suited for reproduction than that in our own files; individual recognition has been given with the illustrations.

We have been fortunate, indeed, to have The Williams and Wilkins Company undertake publication of this book. Mr. Francis E. Old, his scholarly editorial staff, and his highly skilled engravers and printers have made the final phases of preparation particularly easy for the authors. Mr. Old has been generous in his cooperation and personal attention to the work during its preparation and publication, and for his interest and many courtesies we are most sincerely grateful.

Juan M. Taveras
Ernest H. Wood

THE SKULL

Skull Radiography

Radiologic examination of the skull is an essential part of any investigation of patients suffering from neurologic conditions; its importance cannot be overemphasized. The examination should be thorough and geared to the particular problem; the films should be of the highest technical quality. At times special types of plain film examinations are required, such as laminagraphy. When the patient's history does not point to any specific area that requires special examination, the "routine views" are taken. These vary somewhat, depending on individual preferences, but certain basic films are always made. In dealing with any spherical object such as the skull, it is necessary to view the subject from more than one side. Because in radiographs a composite depiction of the right and left or front and back of the skull is obtained, at least right angle views must be made. Many prefer to take both right and left lateral views and posteroanterior and anteroposterior views in every instance. It is our custom routinely to take a single stereoscopic lateral view which permits us to have a three-dimensional view in every case without any additional expense. We consider it essential to obtain at least one stereoscopic lateral view because this view is helpful in detecting intracranial calcifications which might be obscured by the bones, in determining the position of an intracranial shadow, in defining the side where a given density is in relation to the bones, and in clarifying the relationship of the anterior clinoid processes, among other uses. This cannot be done when only right and left lateral views are made. For instance, it is not possible to tell from a lateral view which is the right and which is the left clinoid process, and whether a density not

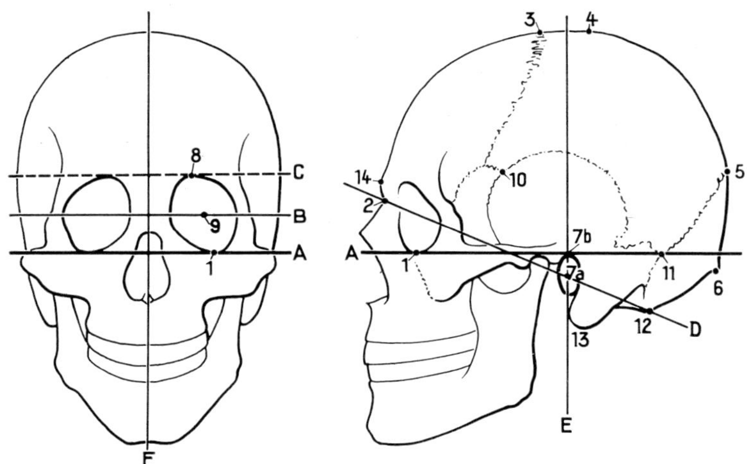

Fig. 1.—Reference Lines and Planes Used in Radiography of the Skull

(1) Infraorbital point. (2) nasion. (3) bregma. (4) vertex. (5) lambda. (6) inion. (7a) center of the external auditory canal or axis of the external auditory meatus. (7b) superior border of the meatus. (8) superior border of the orbit. (9) center of the orbit. (10) pterion. (11) asterion. (12) lowest point of the occiput. (13) mastoid tip. (14) glabella.

(A) The anthropologic basal line on lateral view; the infraorbital line on anteroposterior view. (B) the interorbital or interpupillary line. (C) the superior horizontal line. (D) the orbitomeatal basal line. (E) the auricular line.

(Revised 1963)

seen in the frontal views is to the right or to the left of the midline. On the other hand, in certain instances both lateral views are highly desirable, as in the case of suspected fractures, in dealing with young children, and in special clinical situations in which satisfactory stereoscopic films cannot be obtained. In the posteroanterior projection two films are usually made; one is the *straight posteroanterior view*, and the other is the *inclined posteroanterior view* (fig. 26). The third film in frontal projection is the *half axial view* (formerly called cerebellar, occipital, or Towne view) which may be made in the anteroposterior or posteroanterior projection.

The terminology and the reference lines or planes used throughout this text are in accordance with the recommendations of the International Commission on Neuroradiology of the World Federation of Neurology. Great confusion has existed up to the present in the methods used by the various authors in obtaining what are essentially the same results. This has brought with it a great variety of eponyms for the designation of the same views or minor variations thereof. Figure 1 represents the various reference lines and planes recommended by the Commission.

DEFINITIONS OF LINES, PLANES AND PROJECTIONS

Lines

1. *Anthropological basal line.* The line that joins the infraorbital point to the superior border of the external auditory meatus. Also known as Reid's base line.

2. *Orbitomeatal basal line,* which joins the center of the orbit (which usually, but not always, coincides with the outer canthus of the eye) to the center of the external auditory meatus.

The anthropological and the orbitomeatal basal lines meet at an angle of about 10°.

3. *Auricular line.* This line is perpendicular to the anthropological basal line and passes through the external auditory meatus.

4. *Interorbital or interpupillary line.* The line that joins the center of the two orbits or the two pupils. It is perpendicular to the median-sagittal plane.

5. *Infraorbital line,* which joins the two infraorbital points.

Planes

1. *Median sagittal plane.* The plane that divides the skull symmetrically in half.

2. *Horizontal plane of Frankfurt.* This plane contains the bilateral anthropological basal lines (anthropological plane).

3. *Orbitomeatal plane.* This plane contains the bilateral orbitomeatal basal lines.

4. *Frontal biauricular plane.* This plane is perpendicular to the horizontal plane of Frankfurt and passes through the center of the two external auditory meatuses.

Projections

1. *Lateral projection.* The median-sagittal plane is parallel to the film. The central ray is perpendicular to the median-sagittal plane and centered on the auricular line, 3.0 or 4.0 cm. above the external auditory meatus.

2. *Basal or axial projection.* The head is placed in hyperextension and the anthropological plane should be parallel to the film. The central ray is perpendicular to the anthropological plane and passes along the biauricular plane. This is a true axial projection. If the orbitomeatal plane is placed parallel to the film, the central ray must be angled 10 to 15° dorsorostrally.

3. *Subaxial projection.* The orbitomeatal plane is parallel to the film and the central ray is perpendicular to the orbitomeatal plane.

4. *Straight posteroanterior projection.* The orbitomeatal plane is perpendicular to the film; usually the forehead and nose touch the film; the median-sagittal plane is perpendicular to the film. The central ray is directed perpendicular to the film. The point of exit of the central ray is the nasion.

5. *Inclined posteroanterior projection.* Same position of the head as above, but the tube is angled 15° craniocaudally to form an angle of 15° with the orbitomeatal line (or about 25° to the anthropological basal line). The point of exit of the central ray is at the

nasion. This projection resembles the Caldwell's view.

6. *Anteroposterior half axial projection.* The head rests on the occiput. The median-sagittal plane is perpendicular to the film. The orbitomeatal plane is perpendicular to the film and the central ray makes an angle of 25 to 30° craniocaudally to the plane. If the anthropological plane is perpendicular to the film, the central ray makes an angle of 35 to 40° craniocaudally. The central ray passes through the external auditory meatus and through the median-sagittal plane.

7. *Posteroanterior half axial projection.* The orbitomeatal line is perpendicular to the film; the sagittal plane is perpendicular to the film; the tube is angled 25 to 30° caudocranially.

8. *Straight anteroposterior projection.* The same as the straight posteroanterior projection but with the occiput in contact with the film. The orbitomeatal line is perpendicular to the film; the central ray is parallel to the orbitomeatal line and is centered to the nasion.

9. *Inclined anteroposterior projection.* The same as the posteroanterior inclined projection but with the occiput in contact with the film. To obtain the same results, the tube is angled 15° caudocranially if the orbitomeatal line is perpendicular to the film; the central ray is centered to the nasion.

10. *Occipitozygomatic projection (Stenvers projection).* The face is rotated 45° to the opposite side of that being radiographed, the region of the zygoma is in contact with the film, the orbitomeatal line is perpendicular to the film. The central ray is angled 12° caudocranially and passes through the plane of the external auditory meatus.

The *optic foramen view* is also an occipitozygomatic projection but the tube is angled caudally about 15°. In a correctly positioned optic foramen view this structure is projected over the lower outer quadrant of the orbit. The exact position and angulation cannot be standardized because of great individual variability in skull shape and changes occurring with growth.

In patients who present special problems such as visual difficulties, diminished hearing, and involvement of cranial nerves, other views are necessary. The special views may be those of the optic foramina, the petrous pyramids, or the base of the skull. Films made in other projections, such as oblique views of the mastoid and views customarily employed in the examination of the sinuses, are also taken in some cases.

Without a thorough knowledge of the anatomy, it is not possible to make a proper interpretation of many of the shadows that are seen on the films as a result of all manners of distortions and projections that occur in x-ray examinations. In addition, considerable variation exists from patient to patient in the configuration of the various structures, in fact, *variation is the rule.* No anatomist, before the age of x-rays, was ever able to accumulate in a lifetime as many variations of the skull as are possible for the average interested radiologist who sees many thousands of skulls in just a few years.

In the following pages we will attempt to correlate the anatomy of the skull with that which is seen on the radiographs and to a limited extent to make specific comments about technique. In order to obtain the maximum amount of information, the radiographs should be of good quality. Films that are slightly overpenetrated are to be preferred in examining the skull because small but important calcium deposits in the brain could easily go undetected on lighter films, particularly in patients who have relatively thick cranial bones.

Anatomy

The skull is divided into two parts: (1) the *cranium*, which contains and protects the brain; and (2) the *skeleton of the face.* In the description to follow, the skeleton of the face will not be dealt with separately except for those portions that are near the base of the skull, to which reference must be made frequently.

LATERAL PROJECTION

A straight lateral view of the skull is made as described above. Another radiograph is immediately made without moving the head of the patient, after shifting the tube cephalad for a distance of 2.5 to 4 inches, depending on the distance between the tube and the film used to take the radiograph. The longer the distance between tube and film is, the longer the shift of the tube should be to obtain a good stereoscopic image. The tube shift used to take the stereoscopic film causes a slight separation of the floors of the anterior and middle fossae which is often advantageous. The lateral view has an appearance which simulates a sagittal section of the skull (fig. 2). A lateral view taken without turning the patient's head, usually made in the sitting position, is preferable.

In studying the lateral view of the skull, a method should be developed so that all of the anatomical structures are examined in an orderly fashion. The descriptions that follow will contain the usual sequence that has been our habit for many years. (1) Size and shape of the cranium. (2) Thickness and density of the bones. (3) The sutures. (4) The vascular markings. (5) The structures along the base. (6) The cranial cavity.

Size and Shape

Considerable variation exists in the size and shape of the skull of different individuals. Rather than to determine the absolute size, it is often more important to compare the approximate area occupied by the cranium with that occupied by the facial bones. The area occupied by the face is approximately half of the area of the cranium in an adult. In children, the facial area occupies less than 50 per cent that of the cranium, and the younger the child, the smaller the face is in relation to it. A skull that is longer than average is usually referred to as *dolichocephalic*; one that is shorter and broader than average is called *brachycephalic*; and one that is average in its relation between the length and the width is called *mesaticephalic*. These terms refer to the *cephalic index* obtained by the formula breadth × 100/length. A mesaticephalic skull has a cephalic index of 75 to 85. Over 85 is brachycephalic. Individuals with a dolichocephalic type of skull usually have a relatively shorter vertical diameter as measured from the basion to the bregma. On the other hand, those with a brachycephalic skull probably would have a greater vertical diameter. It is important to appreciate the shape of the skull when trying to estimate the relative positions of certain structures of the brain such as the pineal, the anterior cerebral artery, the deep cerebral veins, and the lateral ventricles. It is good practice, therefore, to pay attention to the cranial shape in every instance in order to develop a mental picture of the probable shape of the brain that would adapt to each skull. Such estimation must be made in every instance when one is trying to determine the correct position of the pineal calcification in the lateral projection. For further details see under "Pineal Localization," page 1.27.

Thickness and Density of the Bones

Great variations exist in the thickness of the bones of the *cranium* (also called calvaria and vault). On the average, the bones are thicker in the negro than in the white races, but this is by no means an infallible rule. Certain areas of the calvaria have a tendency to be thinner than others; a thin area is usually present in the frontoparietal region in the neighborhood of the coronal suture, and another, inferiorly above the roofs of the orbit. A thin area is usually present above the internal occipital protuberance. The most consistently radiolucent area of the skull is the temporal region, sometimes extremely so, because the temporal squamosa is usually thin. There is sometimes a band of increased density forming an arc at the upper portion of the temporal radiolucent area which represents perisutural density at the suture between the temporal squama and the parietal bone.

Convolutional markings. In addition to the normal areas of decreased density mentioned above, irregular areas of diminished density, called *convolutional impressions* or *digital markings*, are often seen spread

(*Revised 1963*)

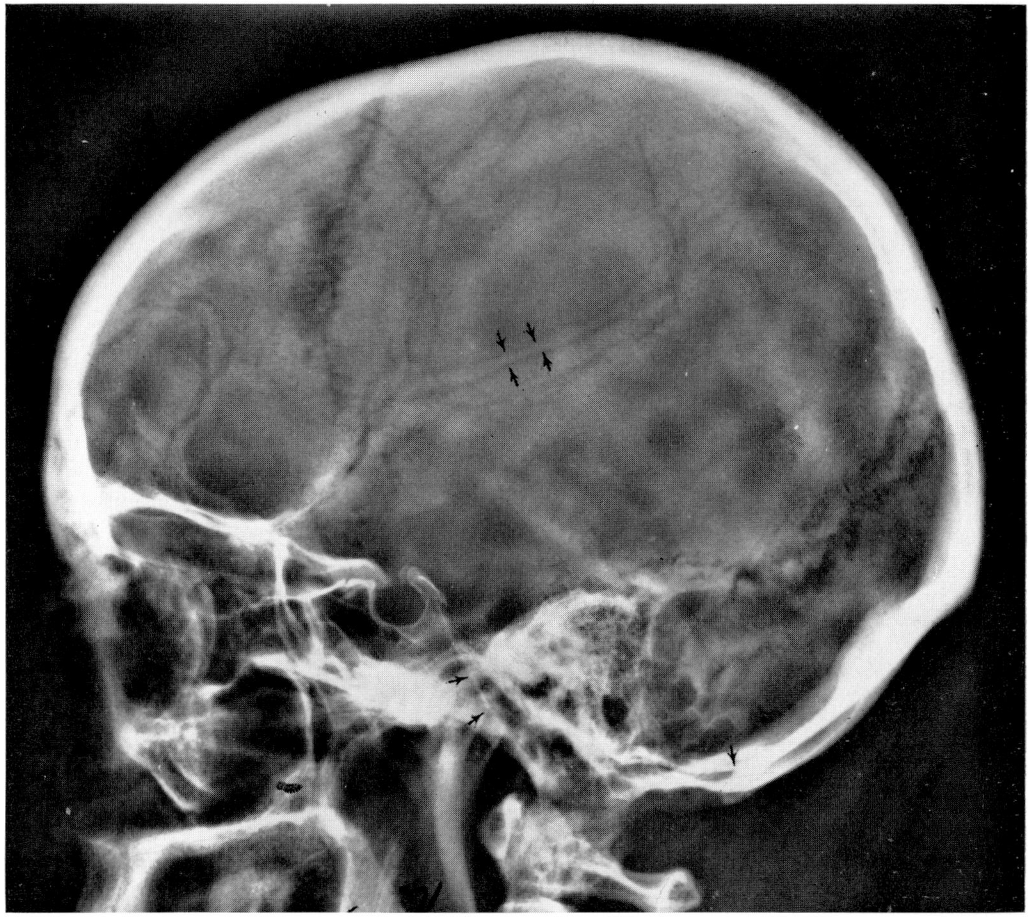

Fig. 2.—Normal Lateral View of Skull

The picture illustrates the normal appearance of the sutures and vascular markings as well as the normal appearance of the sella turcica and other basal structures. The middle meningeal channels are well shown and symmetrical (*arrows*) There are diploic venous channels in the frontal region which have their typical slightly irregular appearance. The appearance of the base of the skull is similar to that seen in Fig. 16. The clivus (*arrows*) is well shown, as is the lower margin of the foramen magnum (basion). The posterior margin of the foramen magnum (opisthion) can be easily found by following the line of the anterior margin of the posterior arch of the atlas upward and backward (*posterior arrow*).

throughout the bones of the skull. They represent depressions on the inner table of the skull undoubtedly related to pulsations of the brain and to the convolutions, although the depressions do not have the exact shape of the gyri of the brain. However, they must be related to the fact that there is a smaller cushion of cerebrospinal fluid over the convolutions than over the sulci and, therefore, pulsations of the convolutions would be transmitted readily to the inner table of the skull. For this reason, convolutional markings are frequently found in children, who have growing brains, but are less commonly found in adults. Convolutional markings tend to disappear after 12 or 13 years of age but are often found in young adults, particularly in females with relatively thin cranial bones. Sometimes the convolutional markings are not seen because the films are light, but if a darker film is made, at least some of them are seen. This is partly

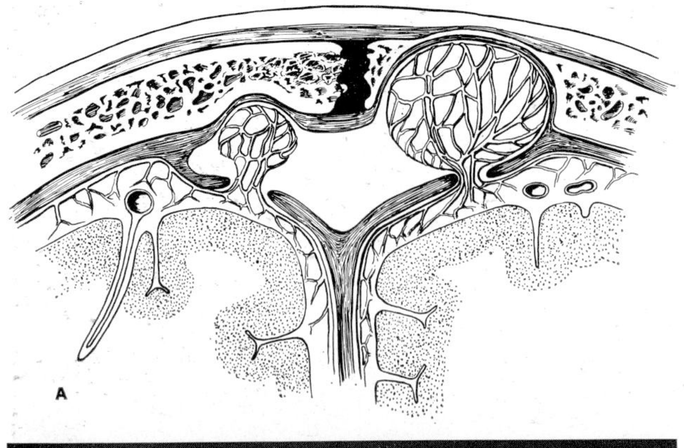

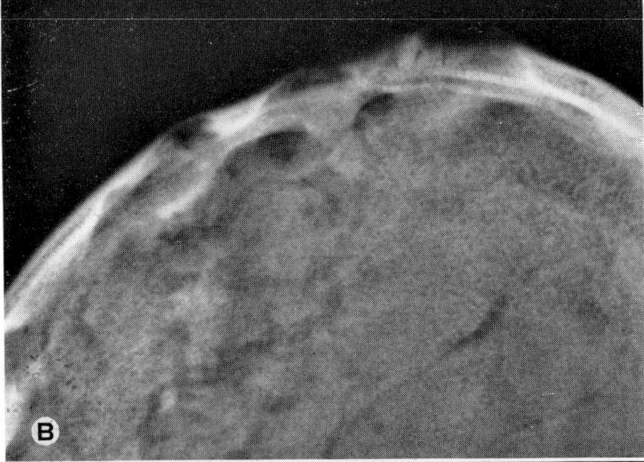

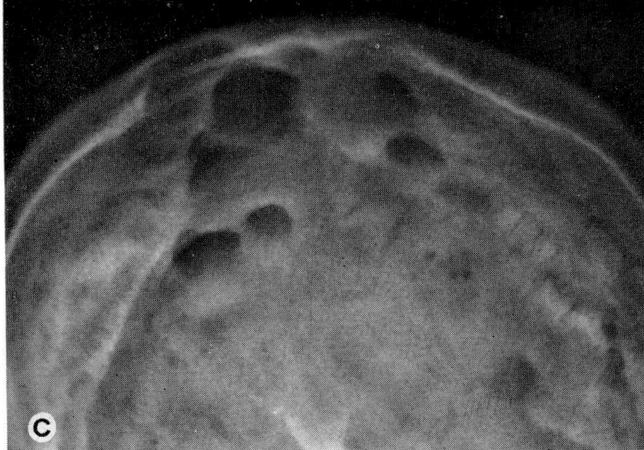

FIG. 3.—PACCHIONIAN GRANULATIONS

(A) Drawing of arachnoid granulations projecting into the superior longitudinal sinus and venous lakes. The Pacchionian granulations produce depressions on the inner table of the skull which sometimes become extremely prominent. In the case shown in (B) there was an extreme degree of prominence of these depressions which protruded beyond the outer table, displacing it outward, as shown on the diagram. At least one of these depressions protruded through the outer table and could be felt as a soft protrusion. All of these granulations are grouped along the longitudinal sinus and are usually within 2 to 3 cm. from the midline. The grouping around on each side of the middle is well shown in (C).

the reason why they are more commonly observed in young adults with thin cranial bones. In patients with premature synostosis who have some degree of craniostenosis, the convolutional markings become very prominent (fig. 45). Unless associated with other findings, the mere presence of prominent convolutional markings should not be interpreted as indicative of increased intracranial pressure. See page 1.79.

Pacchionian depressions. The superior longitudinal sinus communicates, through

(*Revised 1963*)

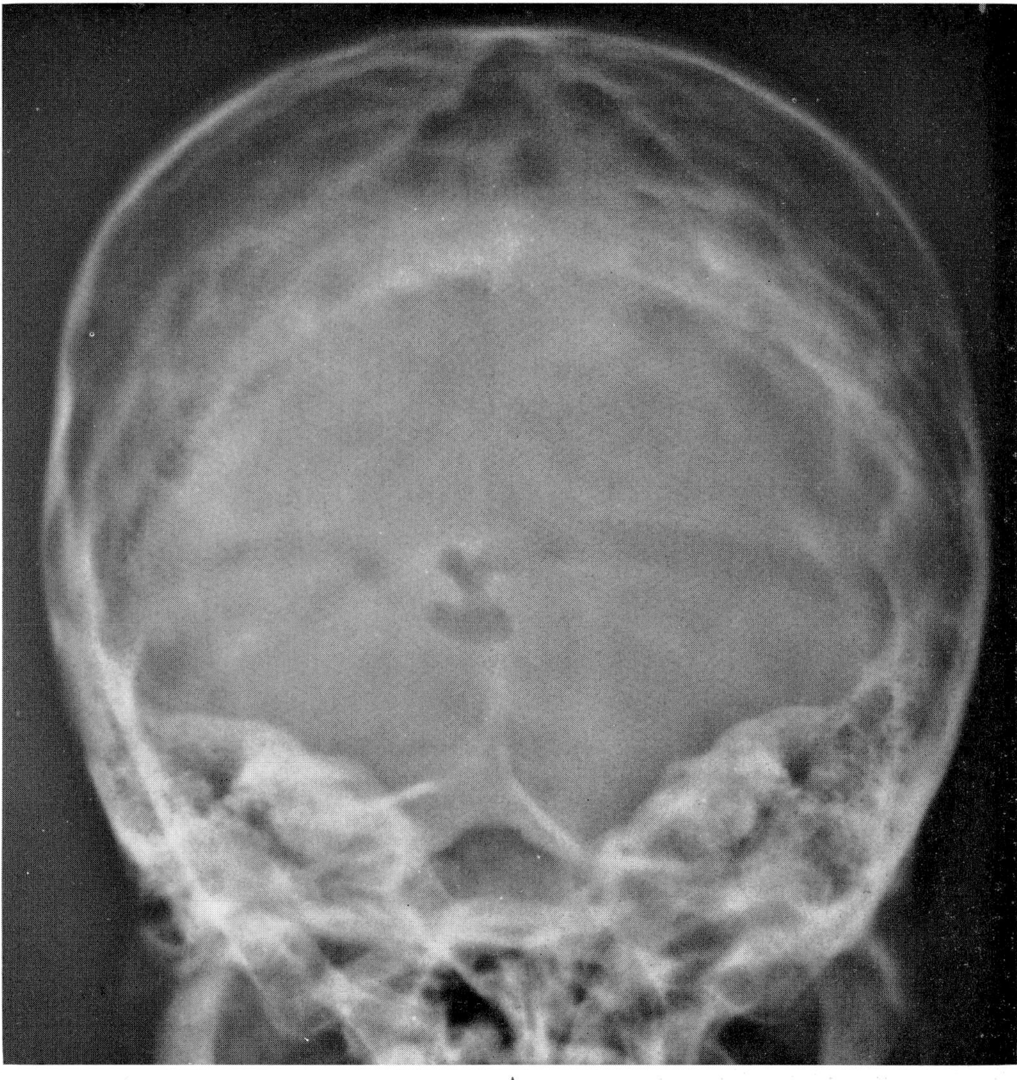

A

FIG. 4A.—PACCHIONIAN DEPRESSIONS IN THE REGION OF THE TORCULAR HEROPHILI

Pacchionian depressions are commonly found in the occipital region (A). The occipital emissary vein may have a similar configuration and may enlarge in cases of long-standing increased intracranial pressure. (See next page for Fig. 4B.)

small ostia, with the so-called *venous lacunae* which are situated in the posterior frontal, parietal, and superior occipital regions, usually three in number on each side. These are variable in size, the largest being the parietal venous lacuna. Several of the superficial superior cerebral veins along the outer surface of the cerebral hemisphere open into these lacunae. Arachnoid granulations or Pacchionian bodies project into them. They cause depressions on the inner table of the bone on each side of the superior longitudinal sinus which are usually referred to as Pacchionian depressions. The Pacchionian granulations are found not only in relation to the superior longitudinal sinus (fig. 3) but occasionally in the neighborhood of, or even projecting into, the lateral sinuses and the other sinuses, including the cavernous, superior petrosal, and the sphenoparietal

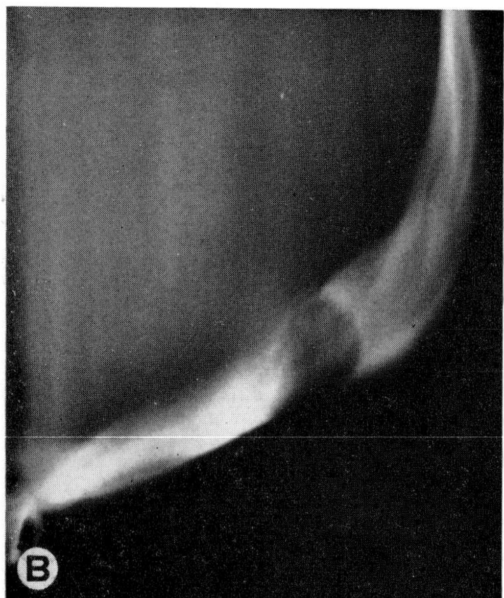

FIG. 4B.—The lateral view of another case shows the sharply outlined defect in the region of the torcular extending to but not necessarily through the outer table (B).

sinuses. The authors have seen a case where a large Pacchionian depression was present along the course of the bregmatic vein which, because of its unusual position, was mistaken for erosion produced by a superficial neoplasm of the brain or an epidermoid tumor. Sometimes the Pacchionian depressions may be very prominent and multiple such as in the case shown in Figure 3. Pacchionian depressions in the area around the torcular Herophili are found frequently (fig. 4). Erosions of the inner table of the skull produced by tumors may simulate those produced by Pacchionian granulations. It is usually possible to differentiate between the two because of the location. Pacchionian depressions are most frequently seen in the posterior frontal and anterior two-thirds of the parietal bones and are usually situated within 2.5 to 3.0 cm. of the midline, as seen in the frontal projection (fig. 3). They involve only the inner table, but sometimes they lift the outer table and the diploë disappears in this region, and occasionally the outer table is also defective (fig. 3). Only rarely is a Pacchionian depression seen more than 3 or 4 cm. from the midline, and in these cases it is not possible to differentiate between a Pacchionian depression and that produced by a superficially placed tumor (fig. 121). There is often a draining vein seen, starting at the Pacchionian depression.

Developmental thinness of the parietal bones. This condition may be considered as an anatomical variant that is apparently not hereditary (Pendergrass *et al.*, 1956). The area of thinness usually has an elongated oval shape, and is over the upper part of the parietal bone as seen in the lateral view. The diagnosis is usually made from the appearance in the frontal projection (fig. 5). The diploë disappears from this region, which is usually symmetrical on each side of the midline. The thinness takes place *at the expense of the diploë and the outer table of the skull.* The inner table is usually intact and has a normal shape over the area of thinning. Some patients present only a unilateral thinness (Camp and Nash, 1944).

Parietal foramina. The parietal foramina are two symmetrical openings on each side of the interparietal suture, situated in the posterior third near the upper edge of the parietal bone. These openings are usually very small and permit the passage of an emissary vein. In some individuals these foramina are large, and occasionally extremely large, measuring several centimeters in diameter. They are usually symmetrical and the bone tapers toward the defect at the expense of the outer table and diploë. The inner table usually remains in its normal position at the edge of the bone defect (fig. 6). This is a familial developmental defect and has no pathological significance (Pepper and Pendergrass, 1936).

Other defects. The following defects might be mentioned. (1) Defects in the region of the anterior fontanelle and upper portion of the frontal bone seen in cases of cleidocranial dysostosis. For more detail see under "Congenital Anomalies—Cranium Bifidum," page 1.71. (2) Defects in the skull associated with neurofibromatosis with radiologic absence of bone which may involve the base of the skull (usually the greater wing of the sphenoid) (fig. 55B), or it may

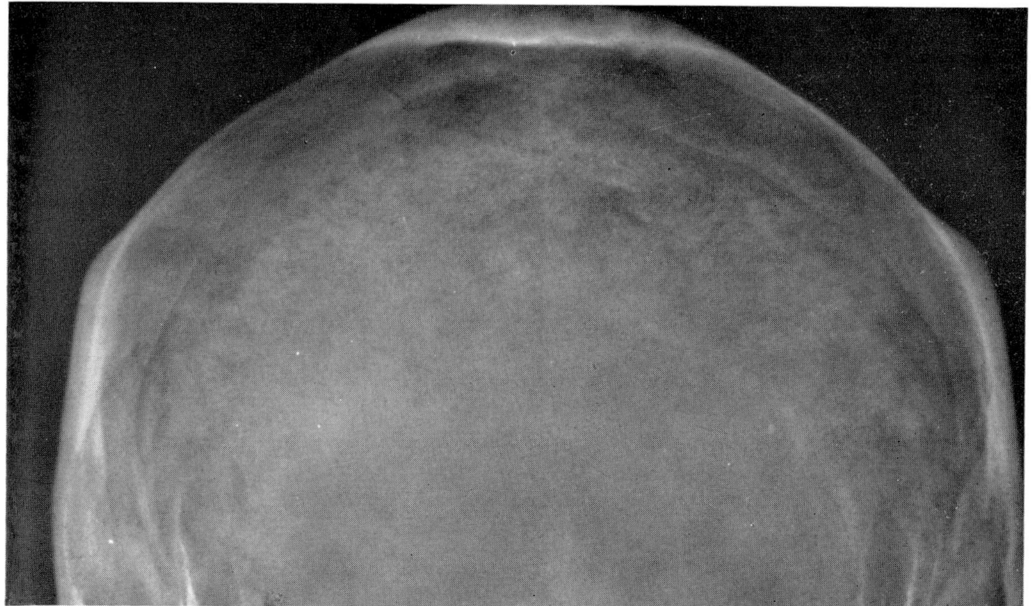

FIG. 5.—DEVELOPMENTAL THINNESS OF THE PARIETAL BONE, BILATERAL

The thinning takes place at the expense of the outer table and the inner table is usually normal; its contour is not interrupted.

involve the bones of the vault. (3) Skull defects associated with post-traumatic pulsating leptomeningeal cysts will be described under "Head Injuries and Their Complications," page 1.757. (4) The osseous defects representing destruction by benign or malignant neoplasms will be described under these conditions.

Localized thinning of bone may be associated with a superficially placed intracranial tumor (fig. 121) or it may be associated with subdural hematoma or hygroma. The last two are described under "Head Injuries and Their Complications." In addition thinning may occur with increased intracranial pressure.

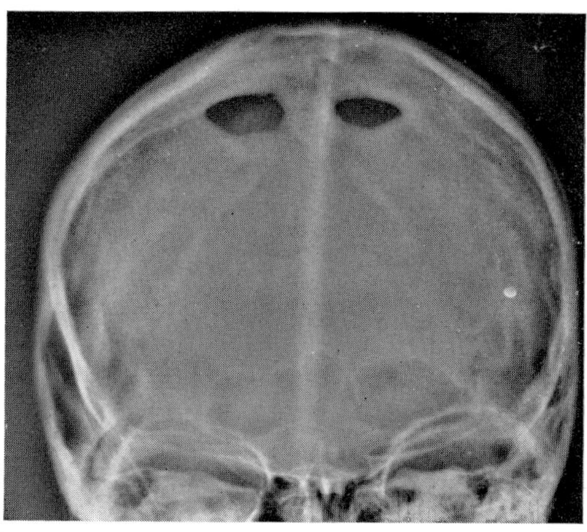

FIG. 6.—CONGENITALLY ENLARGED PARIETAL FORAMINA IN A 48-YEAR-OLD WOMAN WHO WAS OTHERWISE NORMAL

Diminished density. Diminished density of the skull in a diffuse manner occurs in senile osteoporosis. However, this is not clearly discernible in the vault and is more pronounced usually in the base of the skull, particularly in the sella turcica. It is often difficult to decide whether there is decrease in density of the sella turcica, particularly in the dorsum sellae, as a result of increased intracranial pressure or of simple osteoporosis. In osteoporosis the density of the dorsum sellae is less than usual, but there is no thinness of the dorsum and all its components are present. This is in contradistinction to increased intracranial pressure, which will usually cause thinning of the dorsum and destruction of its upper portion. See under "Increased Intracranial Pressure." The diminished density that is observed in hyperparathyroidism, Cushing's syndrome, and osteomalacia is usually clearly seen in the vault, contrary to that of generalized senile osteoporosis which, as mentioned above, is only clearly seen along the base of the skull but usually is not very pronounced on the vault.

Increased density. Increased density may be seen in conditions such as osteopetrosis (Albers-Schönberg disease), and in Englemann's disease (progressive diaphyseal dysplasia). In the latter instance the increase in density is usually associated with some increase in the thickness of the bones, involving also the base of the skull. The base of the skull is particularly dense in cases of osteopetrosis. In some instances the causes of the diffuse increase in density are unknown, particularly in young children.

Increased thickness. A simple increase in the thickness of the bones of the skull with normal inner and outer tables and a normal diploë is of no pathologic significance. If the increase in thickness is extreme, the possible presence of certain diseases should be considered. Among these are acromegaly, Cooley's anemia and sickle cell anemia, pseudo-hypoparathyroidism, craniometaphyseal dysplasia, and progressive diaphyseal dysplasia. Increase in thickness may also be seen in Paget's disease and fibrous dysplasia, but these are easily distinguishable. Occasionally iron deficiency anemia in children can cause diffuse increase in thickness.

Localized increase in thickness of the bones of the skull occurs commonly in *hyperostosis frontalis interna* found most often in women. It may be an even or an uneven increase in density and thickness involving the inner table only. It may also involve the parietal and temporal regions. Descriptive terms have been applied (by Moore) to the various localities and configurations observed on the roentgenograms (hyperostosis frontalis, frontoparietalis, calvaria diffusa, nebula frontalis). The authors feel that the term "hyperostosis of the inner table of the skull" is better because it avoids any possible error in considering Moore's various descriptive terms as having a different meaning. Although Moore considers these hyperostoses, which he calls metabolic craniopathy, as part of a syndrome associated with obesity, hypertension, virilism, and menstrual difficulties in the female and neuropsychiatric manifestations, it is probable that the hyperostoses are nothing more than an incidental finding in these cases because they are so frequently encountered in women without any of the symptoms noted above. The authors have seen hyperostosis frontalis as early as 16 years of age. Inner table hyperostoses is not rare in males, and except for its occurrence in association with acromegaly, it has no pathologic significance. An important characteristic of hyperostosis frontalis is that it stops just before reaching the midline (fig. 151) and that it tends to be bilateral. In some cases a single hyperostotic nodule of the inner table is present, which may be confusing, and differentiation from a meningioma is difficult (see p. 1.172).

In healed rickets it is possible to have thickening of the frontal bones, and sometimes of the parietal bones. The thickening of the skull in these cases is usually less around the coronal suture; the bones increase in thickness up to their midportion, as seen in the lateral view, and decrease as they approach the suture lines. The increased thickness may be limited to the parietal bones (Caffey, 1961).

Sutures

In the newborn, the sutures are difficult to visualize because the bones taper considerably and the ossified portion of the bone gradually disappears as it approaches the suture line (fig. 7). As the child gets older, the sutures approach the appearance of those of the adult. The normal sutures in the adult are surrounded by a narrow area of increased density (perisutural density), which is important to keep in mind when there is a question of whether a radiolucent line represents a suture or a fracture. The sutures that are clearly visible in the lateral view are the

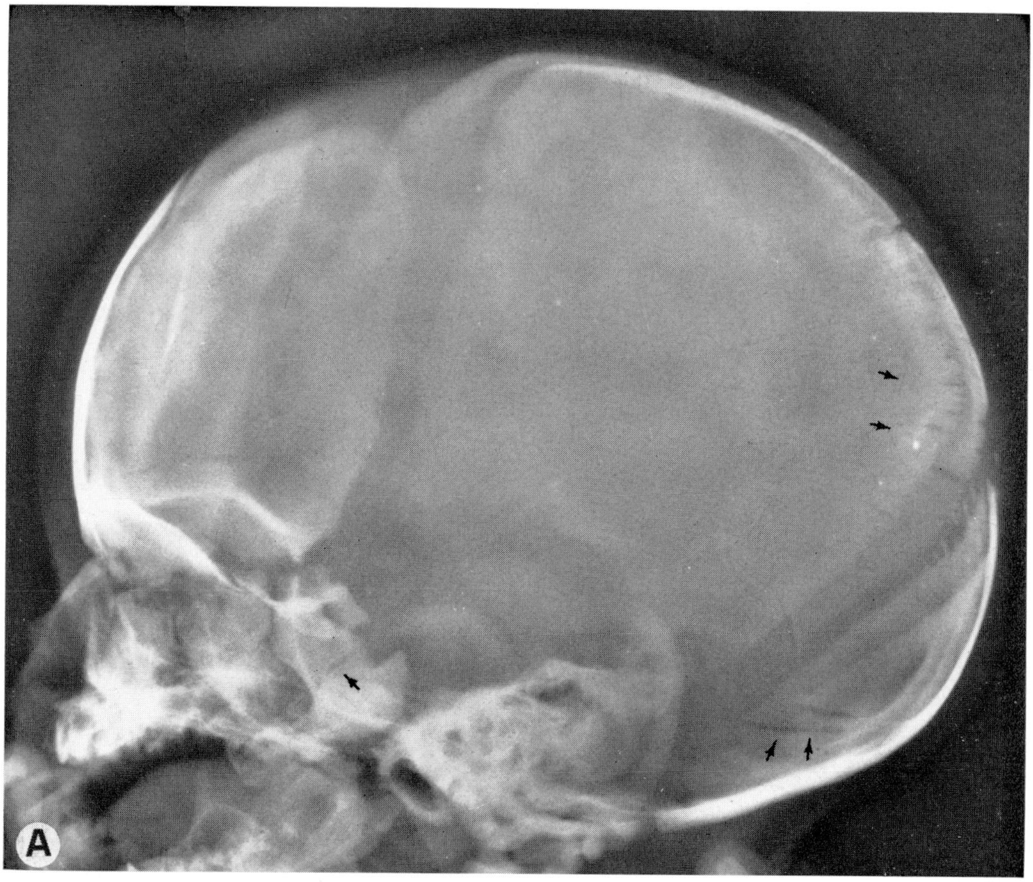

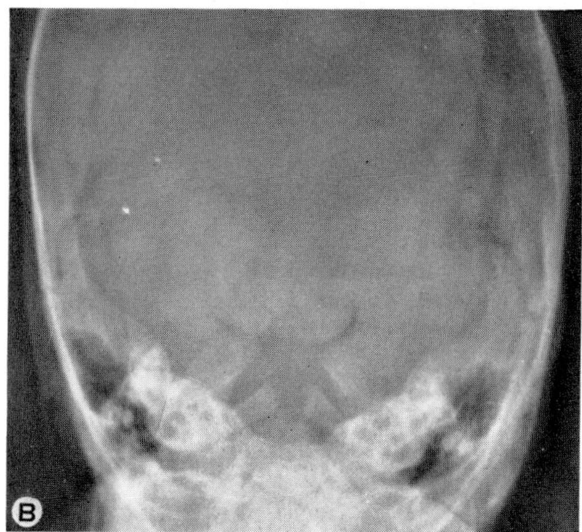

FIG. 7.—NORMAL ANTEROPOSTERIOR, HALF AXIAL, PROJECTION AND LATERAL VIEW OF INFANT

The suture lines are often difficult to visualize in newborn infants due to tapering of bone edge at the suture. In the lateral view (A), there are many small fissures in the parietal region, none of which goes very far off the edge (*arrows*). The mendosal suture which divides the occipital squama is visible (*lower arrows*). The craniopharyngeal duct is visible across the body of the sphenoid (*arrow*). The sella turcica is not well shown because the head was slightly rotated at the time that the film was made. (B) the frontal projection of another infant demonstrates some of the normal synchondroses in the occipital bone.

coronal and the lambdoidal sutures (fig. 8). Sometimes the pterion is well shown, but the configuration of this area is quite variable. To visualize the pterion with more detail, an off-lateral view may be taken by rotating the head along a vertical axis, plac-

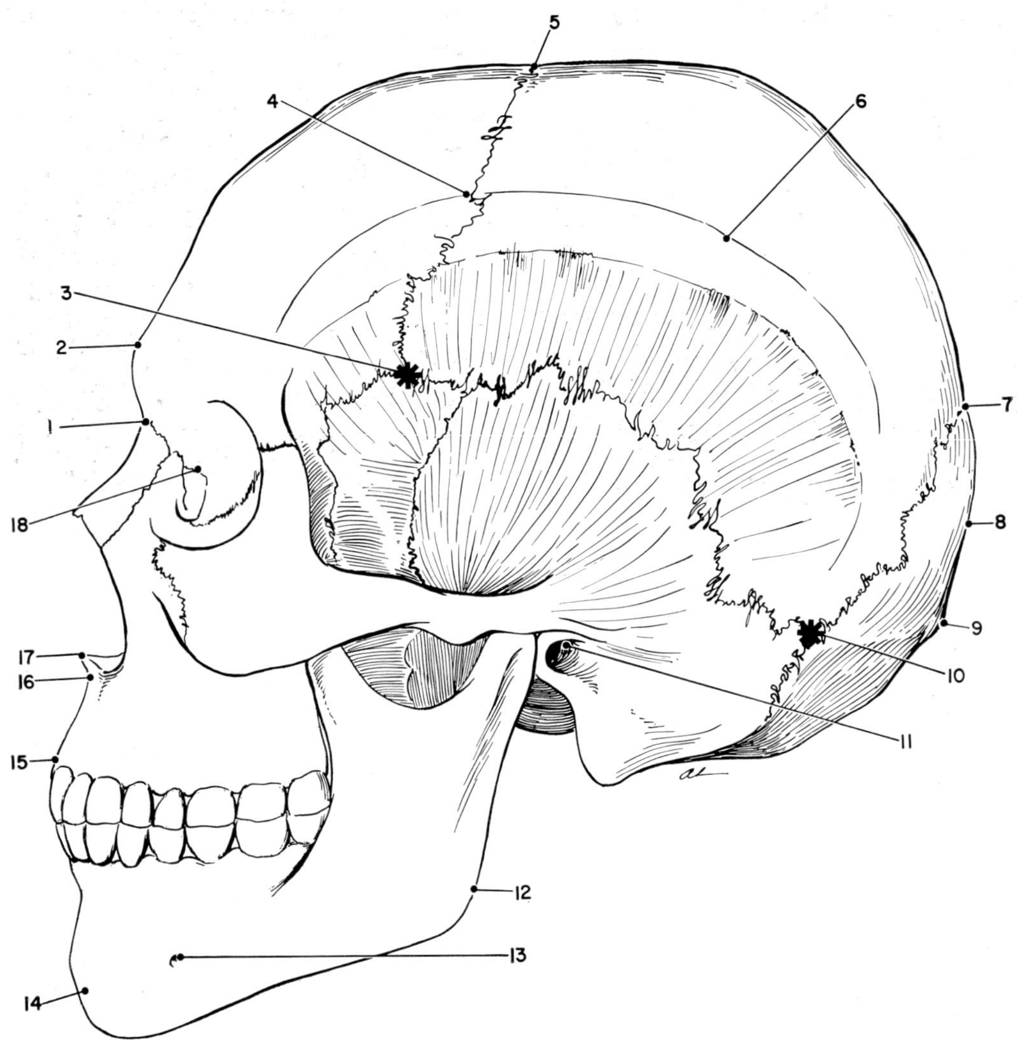

FIG. 8.—LATERAL ASPECT OF THE SKULL

(1) Nasion. (2) glabella. (3) pterion. (4) stephanion. (5) bregma. (6) euryon. (7) lambda. (8) occipital point. (9) inion. (10) asterion. (11) porion (external auditory meatus). (12) gonion. (13) mental foramen. (14) mental point (gnathion). (15) alveolar point (prosthion). (16) base of the nasal spine. (17) subnasal point. (18) dacryon (midorbital point in lateral view).

ing the face on the side being radiographed closer to the film. The parietomastoid suture is usually also seen in the lateral projection, but because of its tapering configuration, the temporal squamous suture is not usually seen unless there is the thickening sometimes found along the inner side of the suture. The upper portion of the coronal suture is at times sharply and distinctly visualized because of its lack of digitation, which has led to its being confused with a fracture, particularly if there has been trauma to this portion of the skull (fig. 9). The increase in density on each side of the radiolucent line serves to differentiate this condition from a fracture.

(Revised 1963)

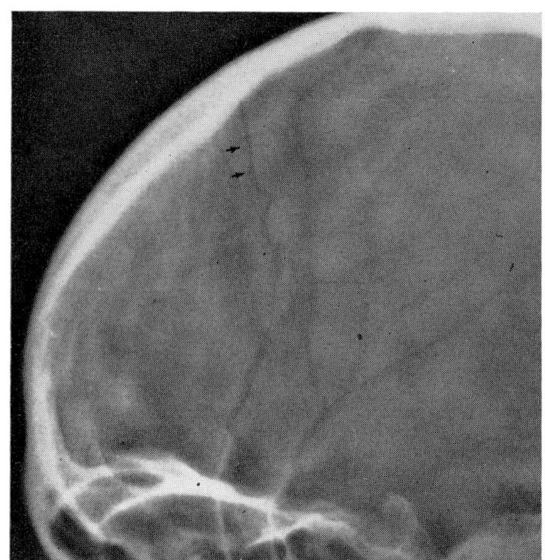

FIG. 9.—NORMAL LATERAL VIEW OF THE SKULL SHOWING THE UPPER PORTION OF THE CORONAL SUTURE WHICH SIMULATES A FRACTURE

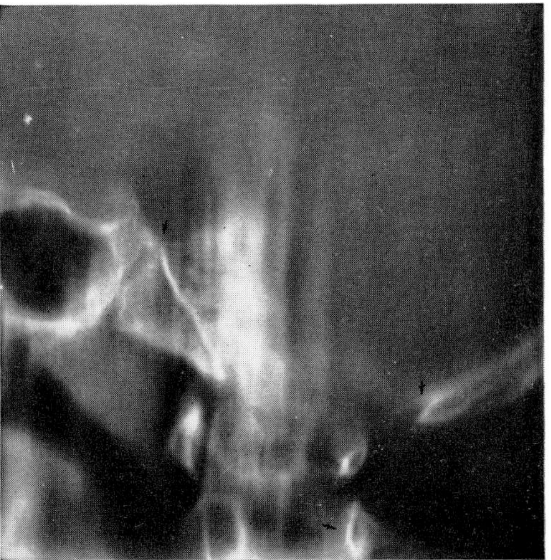

FIG. 10.—LATERAL LAMINAGRAM OF THE SKULL IN A BOY 12 YEARS AND 9 MONTHS OF AGE, SHOWING BEGINNING FUSION OF THE SPHENO-OCCIPITAL SYNCHONDROSIS AT THE UPPER MARGIN OF THE CARTILAGINOUS SPACE

The posterior margin of the foramen magnum is further back than the anterior margin of the posterior arch of the atlas would indicate. This individual has a posterior arch of the atlas which is slightly further forward than is usually the case. It is also slightly in front of C2.

In estimating the width of the suture line in children, the top of the coronal suture, as seen in the lateral view, has been found to be the most reliable. In children older than 3 years of age it should be less than 2 mm. See under "Increased Intracranial Pressure." The parietomastoid suture often gives the impression of being a fracture line. During the development of the skull certain synchondroses are seen which eventually disappear when ossification takes place. These are shown in Figures 7 and 10.

The remaining sutures are seen in the frontal and in the half axial projections. These include the sagittal suture (interparietal) and the lower portion of the lambdoidal suture on either side.

Variations of the suture lines. The *metopic suture* exists during fetal development between the two halves of the frontal bone and extends from the anterior fontanelle down to the horizontal portion of the frontal bone. In 5 to 10 per cent of all individuals there is partial or complete persistence of this suture (fig. 11). It can be distinguished from a fracture by means of its slight digitations and, in the absence of these, through the perisutural density which is usually present. When the suture line extends all the way down to the lower portion of the frontal bone, the frontal sinuses do not reach the midline.

(Revised 1963)

The development of secondary ossification centers resulting in separate bones within the suture lines is common, particularly in the lambdoidal suture. These are called sutural or Wormian bones and occur in the region of the lambda or all along the lambdoidal suture down to the occipitomastoid portion of this suture. Occasionally they occur in the region of the coronal suture and in the pterion. The largest of the sutural bones is the interparietal bone which is triangular in shape and represents the interparietal portion of the occipital bone above the mendosal suture.

A rare finding is a suture line that extends horizontally across the parietal bone and divides it into a superior and an inferior portion.

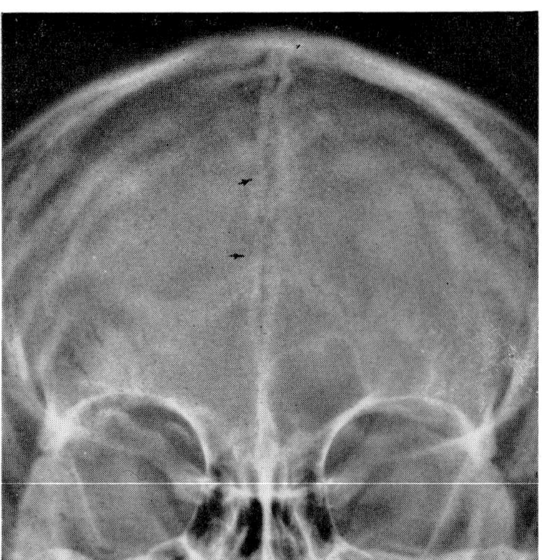

FIG. 11.—PERSISTENT METOPIC SUTURE

The suture persisted from the anterior fontanelle down to the horizontal plate of the frontal bone (*arrows*) and is surrounded by a thin band of increased density (perisutural density). The frontal sinus is developed only to the left of the suture.

Radiographic closure of the sutures is often seen in older individuals. At least partial closure (bridging) of some of the sutures begins at about age 22 and at least some of the sutures are completely fused in the later decades of life. The inner aspect of the suture may complete its closure before the outer aspect. There is considerable individual variation (Todd and Lyon, 1925). The term *double suture line* applies to the appearance of a straight radiolucent line produced by the inner aspect of a suture which is superimposed upon the shadow of the outer aspect of the same suture, which presents normal digitations. This appearance may on occasion be erroneously interpreted as a fracture. In general the suture digitations are less conspicuous or altogether absent on the inside of the skull.

Vascular Markings

The vascular markings which are most prominently seen on the lateral view are of two types: (1) vascular grooves, usually on the inner table of the skull but occasionally on the outer table, and (2) the diploic vascular channels.

The vascular grooves usually seen on the inner table of the skull are depressions produced by the meningeal arteries and veins and their branches as they course along the surface of the dura (fig. 2). There are an anterior group and a posterior group of middle meningeal arterial branches. The middle meningeal artery penetrates the skull through the foramen spinosum and from here it is directed forward and laterally. Shortly thereafter it divides into an anterior branch and a posterior branch. The anterior branch continues its course forward and laterally to become visible in the lateral view as a groove at the lateral aspect of the sphenoid ridge. The artery actually produces a groove on the greater wing of the sphenoid in its horizontal portion before ascending, but this is not usually visible on films unless an oblique view is obtained by rotating the skull on an anteroposterior axis; even then it may not be seen clearly. The trunk of the anterior subdivision of the middle meningeal artery ascends in a groove which is almost always situated at or very near the coronal suture. The groove is usually wider than the middle meningeal artery because this vessel is usually accompanied by veins (fig. 12). Sometimes a groove becomes partly closed on the inner table and forms a tunnel. At other times a larger vein is present in this groove which ends below in the sphenoparietal sinus. The groove or channel may be very wide, extending up to the coronal suture or a little behind it. It has also been called the bregmatic vein (Lindblom, 1936). The arterial grooves become smaller as they go distally. They are usually surrounded by a slight halo of increased density which tends to differentiate them from fracture lines. Also, the arterial grooves are not as radiolucent as fracture lines because they do not involve the entire thickness of the skull, as a fracture does. The posterior branch of the middle meningeal as it ascends upwards and posteriorly over the inner table of the temporal bone sometimes casts a very straight shadow which simulates a fracture (fig. 13).

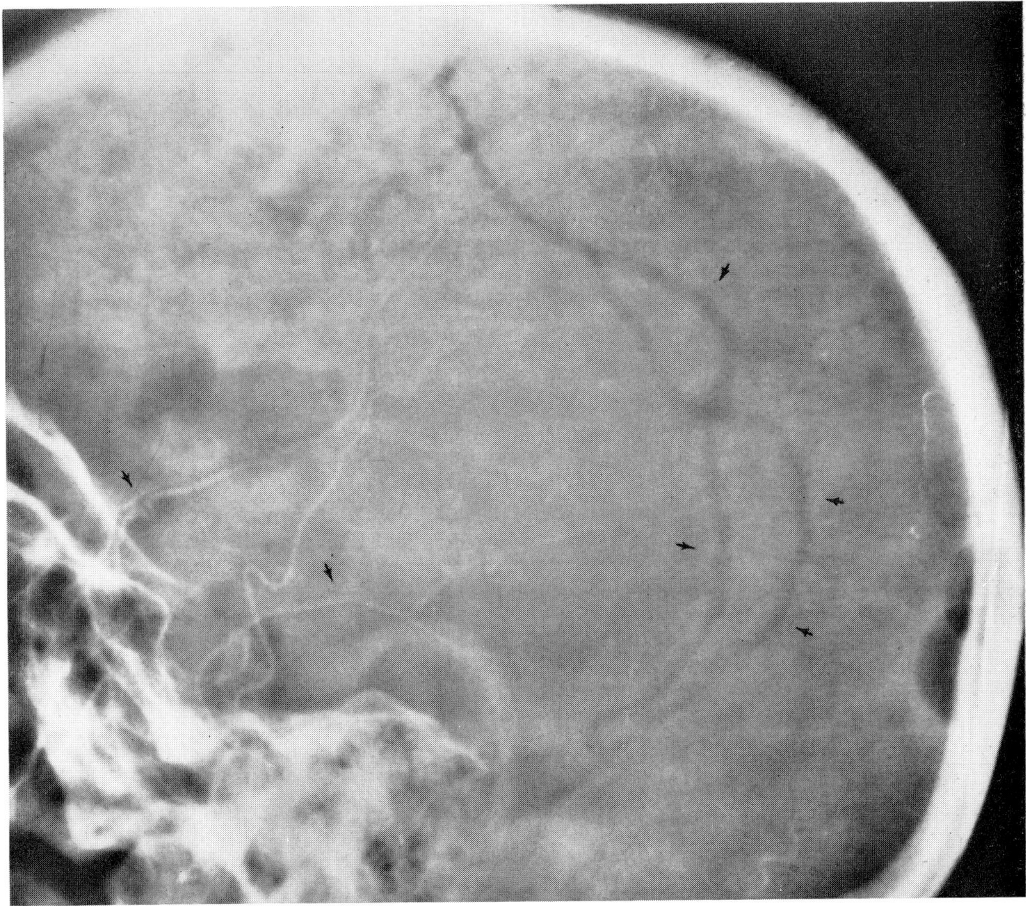

FIG. 12.—MIDDLE MENINGEAL ARTERY BRANCHES SHOWN BY EXTERNAL CAROTID ANGIOGRAM

The anterior branch is emerging at the usual point, the anterior margin of the greater wing of the sphenoid (*arrow*). Actually, the arterial channel does not fill the entire vascular groove as seen on the plain films because there are usually accompanying veins. The posterior branch is fairly straight and produces a slightly curved groove, but not as straight as shown on Fig. 13. The posterior temporal emissary veins are very clearly shown (*arrows*). These veins sometimes become enlarged in patients who have meningiomas in the parasagittal region or that arise from the falx.

Schunk and Maruyama have recently stated that similar straight grooves simulating fractures can be produced by a branch of the superficial temporal artery on the outer table of the temporal bone. These can be easily differentiated from fractures if they are bilateral and symmetrical. Differentiation is more difficult when they are unilateral. If the radiolucent line is surrounded by a slight halo of increased density and if it branches out in its upper portion, the diagnosis of fracture should not be made. These arterial grooves can look as radiolucent as a fracture line because the temporal bone is often extremely thin in this region.

(Revised 1963)

Diploic venous channels or veins of Breschet. These are venous channels that are present in extremely variable positions, chiefly in the frontal and parietal bones. These venous channels have very thin walls formed of endothelium resting upon a layer

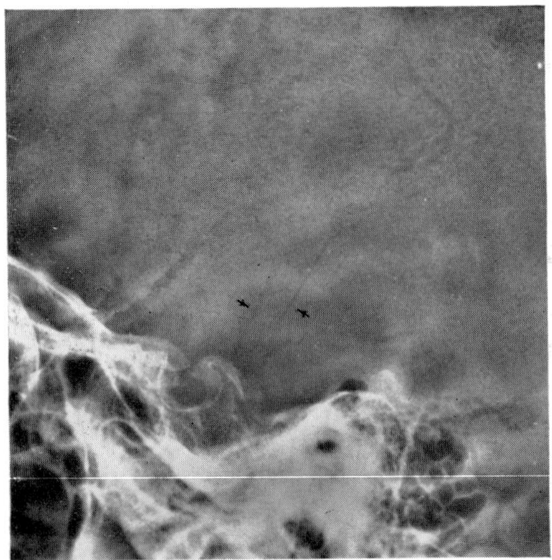

FIG. 13.—POSTERIOR MIDDLE MENINGEAL CHANNELS SIMULATING FRACTURE OF THE TEMPORAL BONE

In this instance, the grooves are bilateral and symmetrical and confusion with a fracture is, therefore, less likely (*arrows*).

of elastic tissue. They present areas of dilatation that are called venous lakes. A venous lake may exist without a radiologically visible diploic venous channel leading to it. These venous channels communicate with the meningeal veins and the sinuses of the dura mater, and with the veins of the pericranium. Therefore, under certain circumstances, they can be of considerable importance as anastomotic channels, such as may happen in sinus thromboses. In spite of their extreme variability, four major systems may be described: (1) the *frontal*, which is usually inconspicuous and opens into the superior sagittal sinus or into the supraorbital vein; (2) the *anterior temporal*, which opens into the sphenoparietal sinus and into one of the deep temporal veins; (3) the *posterior temporal*, which is situated in the parietal bone and is often distinctly seen on films (fig. 12), and which usually ends in the transverse sinus through an emissary foramen present in the lower angle of the parietal bone or in the mastoid bone; and (4) the *occipital diploic vein*, which opens into the transverse sinus or into the torcular Herophili.

Venous lakes, because of their round or oval configuration, are often difficult to distinguish from a destructive lesion of bone. The following characteristics may help in differentiation: (1) a diploic venous channel can usually be traced to the area of radiolucency; (2) the diploic venous channel is usually less radiolucent than a destructive lesion of bone of the same size, because the venous lake does not destroy the inner or the outer table; (3) stereoscopically it may be possible to see that the venous lake is situated between the two tables of the skull; (4) if a tangential view of the area in question can be obtained, it is possible to show that the venous lake is situated between the two tables; the same illustration may be accomplished by laminagraphy; (5) a venous lake usually has a slightly ragged configuration and a poorly defined margin at least in some portion of its contour.

Venous lakes and venous channels apparently become more prominent in older age. This is not necessarily the result of an increase in the size or in the number of these spaces, but may result from a relative degree of osteoporosis which tends to bring out the diploic defects produced by the veins. In one instance, shown in Figure 14, there were numerous venous lakes and venous channels which became more prominent with the passage of time.

Enlargement of the arterial grooves takes place in those cases that are associated with increased blood flow through these vessels. These include the meningiomas, and the arteriovenous malformations of the brain which have some blood supply by way of the external carotid branches. Some cases of fibrous dysplasia and Paget's disease present evidence of increase in the size of the meningeal arterial channels. The relative size of these arterial grooves should be noted; if one of the branches of the middle meningeal artery produces a wider groove than other adjacent branches, the possibility of an abnormal increase in blood flow through this branch should be suspected; this is commonly due to meningioma (fig. 506). When the skull is reexamined after an interval of time it is important to compare the size of the vascular grooves. The importance of this is ex-

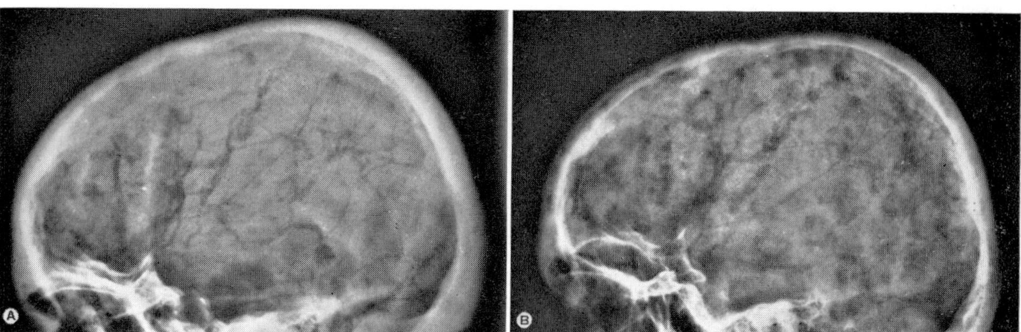

FIG. 14.—PROMINENT DIPLOIC VENOUS CHANNELS AND LAKES BECOMING MORE PROMINENT WITH THE PASSAGE OF TIME

The original examination (A) revealed the prominent vascular markings and lakes. An examination performed 12 years later (B) demonstrated an apparent increase in the size and in the number of vascular channels and lakes. It is probable that the increase in prominence may be due to increased osteoporosis with the passage of time in this elderly lady. Exhaustive clinical tests and further follow-up of three years beyond the second examination, a total follow-up of 15 years, have failed to turn up any disease that would produce diffuse bone destruction. The patient, when last seen, was in a good state of health.

emplified in the case shown in Figure 15, where, if the second set of films, taken at a later date, were read without reference to previous films, the skull would have been called normal, but because a previous examination was available, the increase in the size of the vascular channels and grooves was apparent. Further details on this subject are given under "Meningiomas" and in the section on cerebral angiography under "Diagnosis of Intracranial Masses by Abnormal Circulation."

In normal patients, the arterial grooves of the middle meningeal artery are symmetrical when the right side is compared with the left although occasionally one side may be slightly larger than the other. It might be mentioned that in lateral views, magnification causes the middle meningeal grooves situated on the side against the film to appear smaller than those on the opposite side. If there is a question, on a given lateral view, whether the grooves are larger on one side, it is necessary to take stereoscopic lateral views with the other side against the film. When the middle meningeal grooves become enlarged, they usually become tortuous in their proximal portion. Slight tortuosity is sometimes seen in normal cases but if the tortuosity extends up for several centimeters or if it is accompanied by an increase in the width of the grooves, enlargement should be suspected (fig. 503).

Some patients have extremely marked development of the diploic venous channels, particularly in the parietal bone, and unless it is accompanied by enlargement of arterial channels, it should be regarded as of no clinical significance. Sometimes the venous channels in the parietal region develop in a radiating pattern. In some patients an extremely marked degree of development of the venous channels takes place; in these cases one might speak of "congenital phlebectasia" of the skull, which is of no diagnostic significance, although in these cases the bone may bleed excessively at the time of surgical intervention for intracranial disease.

Enlargement of the arterial branches of the middle meningeal artery was seen in a case of cephalohematoma deformans, in a case where the meningeal arteries supplied the intracranial circulation through the rete mirabile following thrombosis of both inter-

(Revised 1963)

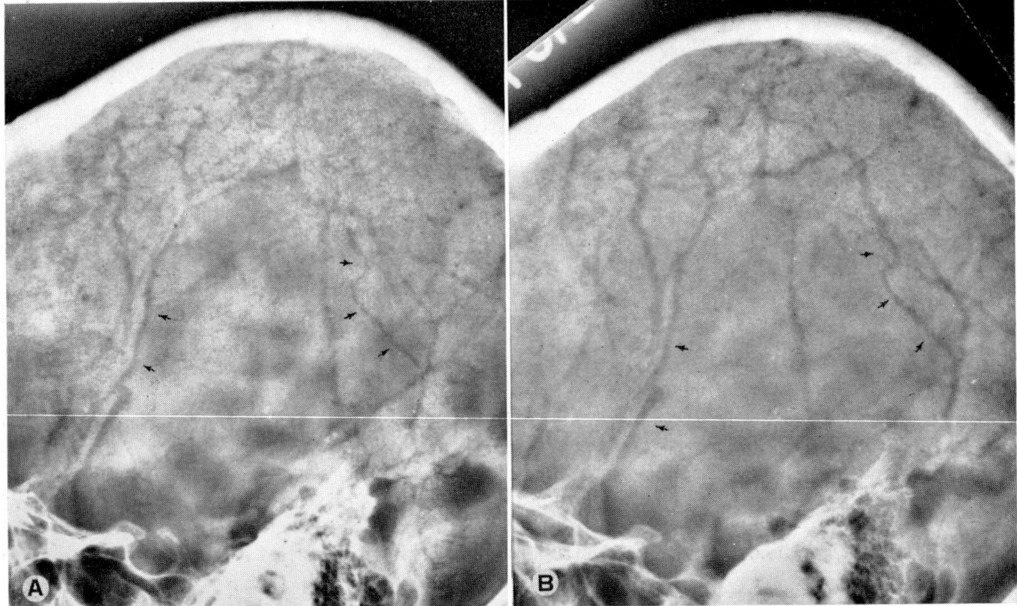

FIG. 15.—INCREASED VASCULARITY OF SKULL DUE TO PARASAGITTAL MENINGIOMA OVER 18-MONTH PERIOD

(A) Original film; (B) film made 18 months later. The increase in the size of the middle meningeal channels (*anterior arrows*) and of the posterior temporal diploic channels (*posterior arrows*) is evident.

nal carotid arteries (fig. 562), and in some cases of fibrous dysplasia (fig. 127).

In addition to the arterial grooves and the diploic venous channels, we have to consider the grooves on the inner table of the skull produced by the dural sinuses. The most prominent of these is the lateral sinus, the groove of which starts at the torcular Herophili on the internal occipital protuberance and extends almost horizontally forward to the mastoid region where it turns downward to become the sigmoid sinus. The depth of the groove determines the clarity of the radiographic demonstration. The grooves are usually asymmetrical; the right is larger than the left. However, in many instances they are equal and sometimes the left is larger than the right. The relative size of these grooves may be seen in the half axial projection and will be mentioned later when this view is discussed. The superior longitudinal sinus makes a groove of variable depth in the inner table of the skull along the sagittal suture and in the frontal and occipital bones. These are shown almost exclusively in the frontal projections and will be mentioned when these views are discussed. The dural sinuses are illustrated in Figure 404.

Structures Along the Base

Anterior fossa. Anteriorly, the two tables of the skull become separated by an air space, the frontal sinuses. The frontal sinuses are of variable size, and whereas in most patients they extend into the vertical portion of the frontal bone, in some patients they are too small to do so. The frontal sinuses may extend along the horizontal plate of the frontal bone as far back as the anterior clinoid process. In the usual normal case, seen in the lateral view, there are three lines representing the floor of the anterior fossa. The upper two lines are formed by the roofs of the orbit on each side which, in a perfectly straight lateral view, could be superimposed but usually are not (fig. 16). These lines represent the highest point of the roofs of the orbit. In the midline there is a depression representing the olfactory groove. In the center of this depression is the crista galli.

(*Revised 1963*)

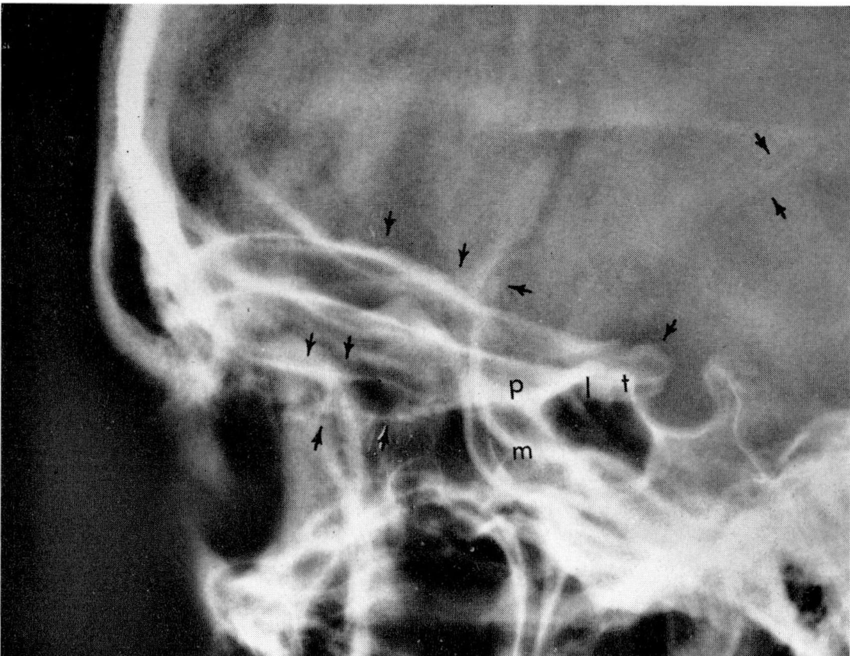

Fig. 16.—Normal Lateral Radiograph of the Skull

The grooves of the middle meningeal artery (*arrows*) are not very conspicuous in this instance. The structures along the base are well shown. One side of the floor of the anterior fossa (*upper vertical arrows*) can be traced backward and ends at the anterior clinoid process (*arrow*). The two anterior clinoid processes are well shown. The line below the one marked with the arrows represents the opposite side. The third line in the anterior portion (*double arrow*) represents the upper margin of the ethmoid cells. The cribriform plate is below that and is shown by the lower anterior arrows. The cribriform plate can be traced back where it is continuous with the planum sphenoidale (*p*) which, more posteriorly, becomes the limbus (*l*). Behind the limbus is the chiasmatic groove, not very well defined in this patient, and immediately behind it is the tuberculum sellae (*t*). The curved shadows of the greater wings of the sphenoid (middle fossa) are well seen (*m*). They end superiorly on the density formed by the lateral aspect of the greater wing and the lateral aspect of the horizontal plate of the frontal bone (*horizontal arrow*) where the middle meningeal groove usually becomes visible.

The crista galli per se is not usually visualized on lateral views unless laminagrams are made; it is too thin to cast a shadow. Posteriorly the lower line is formed by the planum sphenoidale (fig. 16). As the planum extends forward, it is continuous with the cribriform plate of the ethmoid bone. The cribriform plate is actually at a lower level than the planum and is visible in some cases (fig. 16). Quite often what seems to continue the shadow of the planum sphenoidale in a forward direction is nothing but the superior margin of the frontoethmoidal cells. Other times the upper margin of the frontoethmoidal cells is distinct from the shadow of the planum sphenoidale (fig. 16). The two shadows that are cast by the uppermost portions of the roofs of the orbits are seen on the radiograph to end posteriorly on the anterior clinoid process on each side, whereas the lower shadow—the planum sphenoidale—ends at the tuberculum sellae. Just in front of the tuberculum sellae, however, the planum sphenoidale is seen to bend upward and then downward, and sometimes presents a slight concavity. This flattened and sometimes grooved segment just anterior to the tuberculum sellae is called the *chiasmatic groove*.

Sella turcica. The anterior clinoic processes are of variable size and one may be larger than the other in the same individual. Underneath the anterior clinoid processes and slightly medial to them are the optic foramina. These will be studied in detail later because they are not visible in the lateral projections. The tuberculum sellae is continuous with the anterior wall of the sella turcica (fig. 16).

On its anterior aspect, the sella turcica sometimes presents a small projection which represents the middle clinoid processes. These usually are not visible in the lateral radiograph, although a rudimentary middle clinoid process may be visible in the dry specimen in most instances. Sometimes there is a calcified portion of the dura extending from the middle clinoid to the tip of the anterior clinoid process completing a foramen, the carotid foramen, through which normally passes the internal carotid artery. This foramen, when present, may be best demonstrated in views of the optic foramen (fig. 115).

On the anterior aspect and also below the floor of the sella turcica is the sphenoid sinus, the development of which shows considerable variation. The contour of the sella turcica is usually distinct and quite dense and smooth. Sometimes a "double contour" is seen; in the latter case two lines are seen, one very close to the other. This results from the presence of a slight depression in the central portion of the sella turcica, where the pituitary gland actually lies, and is normal. On each side of the sella turcica immediately lateral to the contour of the floor shown on the lateral view, there is a depression in the form of a shallow groove. This depression is produced by the cavernous sinus and the internal carotid arteries and is called the *carotid groove* (fig. 76). Sometimes the carotid groove is apparent in the lateral view and is one of the causes of a "false double floor." Another reason for the production of a false double floor is uneven development of the sphenoid sinuses; if one sinus extends beyond the midline, its upper margin will produce a shadow that follows the same contour as that of the sella turcica. In that case the upper margin of the smaller sinus will be slightly below the floor (fig. 76). A false double floor can be differentiated from a true double floor because it does not follow the entire contour of the sella turcica but only part of it; for example, it may not extend into the dorsum sellae or into the tuberculum sellae. For greater details see under "Local Bone Erosions—the Sella Turcica" (p. 1.95).

The dorsum sellae is, like the other portions of the sella turcica and in fact of all of the skull, quite variable. It varies in height, in thickness, and in shape. Its upper portion ends on the posterior clinoid processes, which are two small projections, one on each corner of the dorsum sellae (figs. 2 and 32). The dorsum sellae may extend upward and slightly forward, producing a "closed type" of sella, or it may be more vertical, producing what is termed an "open type" of sella. The medial attachment of the tentorium takes place partly on the posterior clinoid process but the main attachment is on the anterior clinoid process. This portion of the tentorium is called the interclinoid ligament, which often calcifies and "closes" the outline of the sells turcica radiographically.

The estimation of the size of the sella turcica is intimately related to the study of sellar enlargement due to intrasellar masses, and will be discussed under that subheading (p. 1.100).

Floor of the middle fossa. The next important structure to be seen along the base in the lateral projection is the floor of the middle fossa or greater wing of the sphenoid on each side. These structures produce regular, curvilinear, sharply outlined shadows concave upward (fig. 16). One contour of the floor of the middle fossa is always in front of or above the one on the other side, depending on a slight degree of rotation of the head which is usually present, and on the fact that the central x-ray beam does not go through the floor of the middle fossa but is usually placed above this point. The contour of the middle fossa that is situated in front is usually that on the side away from the film. This is almost always the case, but to be certain, stereoscopic lateral views are required. Because of a slight degree of magnification which is usually present, the floor of

(Revised 1963)

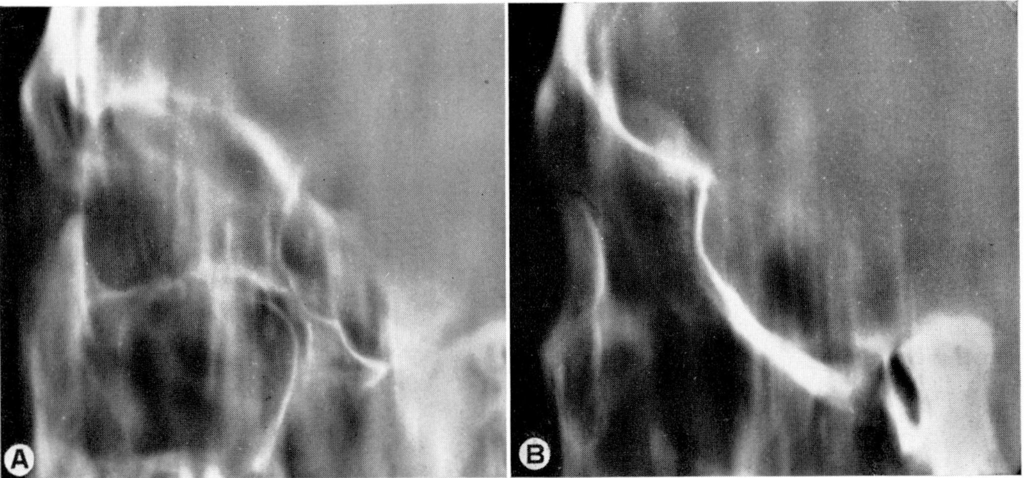

FIG. 17.—ASYMMETRICAL MIDDLE FOSSAE SHOWN BY LAMINAGRAPHY

On the right side (A) there is a slightly scalloped configuration to the greater wing of the sphenoid whereas on the left side (B) the appearance is smooth. The middle fossa is also slightly larger on this side although there is a slightly greater degree of magnification of the left middle fossa than on the right because the laminagrams were made with the patient lying on the right side. There was no history or sign that might suggest cerebral hemiatrophy in this patient. Additional laminagraphic cuts at different levels on the same side as that shown in (B) revealed a similar configuration.

the middle fossa away from the film usually appears to be larger than the other. To be sure, when in doubt about the presence of enlargement of one middle fossa, a stereoscopic lateral view of the opposite side should be made. In the cases of true enlargement of the middle fossa, the discrepancy will persist.

The floor of the middle fossa represents the temporal fossa of the skull, and the tip of the temporal lobe of the brain reaches a point quite close to the most anterior aspect of this dense line. In trying to estimate the position of the tip of the temporal lobe, therefore, this line can serve as a fairly accurate point of reference. The outline of the floor of the middle fossa can be traced posteriorly, where it gets lost in the dense shadow of the remainder of the base of the skull. The curve of the shadow of the middle fossa can increase when there is enlargement of the middle fossa, as in temporal fossa subdural hygromas or chronic subdural hematomas in childhood, and in some cases with slowly growing temporal lobe tumors. The size may also decrease; smallness of the middle fossa may be seen in patients with atrophy of the temporal lobe or of the entire hemisphere such as may be seen in cerebral hemiatrophy, usually associated with cranial hemihypertrophy. However, a small middle fossa may be present in these cases, without cranial hemihypertrophy. Asymmetrical middle fossae are sometimes found in normal individuals (fig. 17). On its anterior aspect the shadow produced by the middle fossa or greater wing of the sphenoid is continuous with a dense line directed upward and slightly backward. This line is produced by the lateral aspect of the horizontal plate of the frontal bone and the greater wing of the sphenoid. It represents on the dry skeleton an actual crest that is present on the inner table associated with an increase in the thickness of the bone in this region. Behind this dense line is where the middle meningeal groove usually appears (fig. 16).

Clivus. The clivus is the continuation of the dorsum sellae and the sphenoid bone with the occipital bone ending at the anterior aspect of the foramen magnum. Early there is a spheno-occipital synchondrosis which fuses at approximately 20 years of age, but fusion may start earlier (Irwin, 1960). The shadow of the clivus extends downward and backward and is usually partly or completely obscured by the dense shadows of the petrous pyramids and mastoids. In underpenetrated films the shadow of the clivus cannot be seen at all, but in films adequately or overpenetrated, this shadow is always visible. The clivus ends at the anterior margin of the foramen magnum. Its tip normally lies at a point directly above the tip of the odontoid process of the axis. The clivus is usually slightly concave backward or straight in normal cases. In patients with basilar impression the clivus may become slightly convex backward. Radiolucent shadows that overlie this area of the skull are from the mastoid cells and the shadows of the external auditory canals.

Basal angle. Welcker (1862) defines the basal angle as that formed by two lines having the apex at the tuberculum sellae. The anterior line extends from the nasion to the tuberculum sellae and the second starts at the tuberculum and goes to the basion (anterior margin of the foramen magnum). The average size of this angle in the adult is 134°. It ranges between 123 and 143° according to Welcker. When the basal angle is greater than 143°, the skull is considered to be *platybasic* and if the angle is much less than 123° it is considered to be kyphotic. More details about this and other reference points are given under "Platybasia" (p. 1.64).

Foramen magnum. The actual shadow of the foramen magnum cannot be seen in the lateral view, but the exact anteroposterior diameter of the foramen can be ascertained. Usually, the lower end of the clivus is visible. The posterior margin of the foramen magnum can be found by tracing the inner table of the occipital bone downward and forward and finding the point where it seems to merge with the outer table. The point where this happens usually corresponds to the prolongation of the line of the posterior margin of the cervical spinal canal as it curves upward and backward (fig. 2). There is usually a separation between the lower margin of the skull at the foramen magnum and the upper surface of the arches of the atlas. This distance varies depending on the state of flexion or extension of the head. In extension the distance between the occipital bone and the posterior arch of the atlas decreases; in flexion, this distance increases. Anomalies in the region of the foramen magnum are common and will be discussed under this subheading. It is important to learn to recognize the plane of the foramen magnum as seen in the lateral view because it is the point of reference for measurement of pineal displacement in the vertical plane.

Cranial Cavity

In concluding the examination of the lateral view of the skull, we should look for the presence of intracranial calcification, which can be normal or abnormal.

The nonpathologic calcifications are listed below.

Calcifications in the dura mater. These calcifications are usually of no clinical significance. They are not associated with trauma and are the result of a degenerative process involving the collagen. The most frequent locations for calcifications in the dura are the petroclinoid ligaments behind the dorsum sellae (fig. 156); the calcifications in the falx cerebri; the calcifications in the wall of the superior longitudinal sinus; and the calcifications in the tentorium, which may occur at the junction of the falx and tentorium, sometimes simulating pineal calcification, or over the edge of the tentorium (fig. 156). Calcifications may also occur in the dura over the frontal, parietal, and temporal regions.

Calcification in the pineal body. This occurs in approximately 55 per cent of adults over 20 years of age (Vastine and Kinney, 1927). The calcification is usually irregular and occurs in a speckled manner. The area of calcification of the pineal body usually measures 3 to 4 mm. in depth and 6 to 8 mm. in length. However, sometimes the pineal calcification occupies a larger area and occasionally it presents a shell of calcium. This is due to the development of a small cyst within the pineal and is a normal variant. The largest *cystic pineal* that the authors have seen measured 14 mm. in diameter. In these cases it is necessary sometimes to perform a pneumoencephalogram in order to rule out

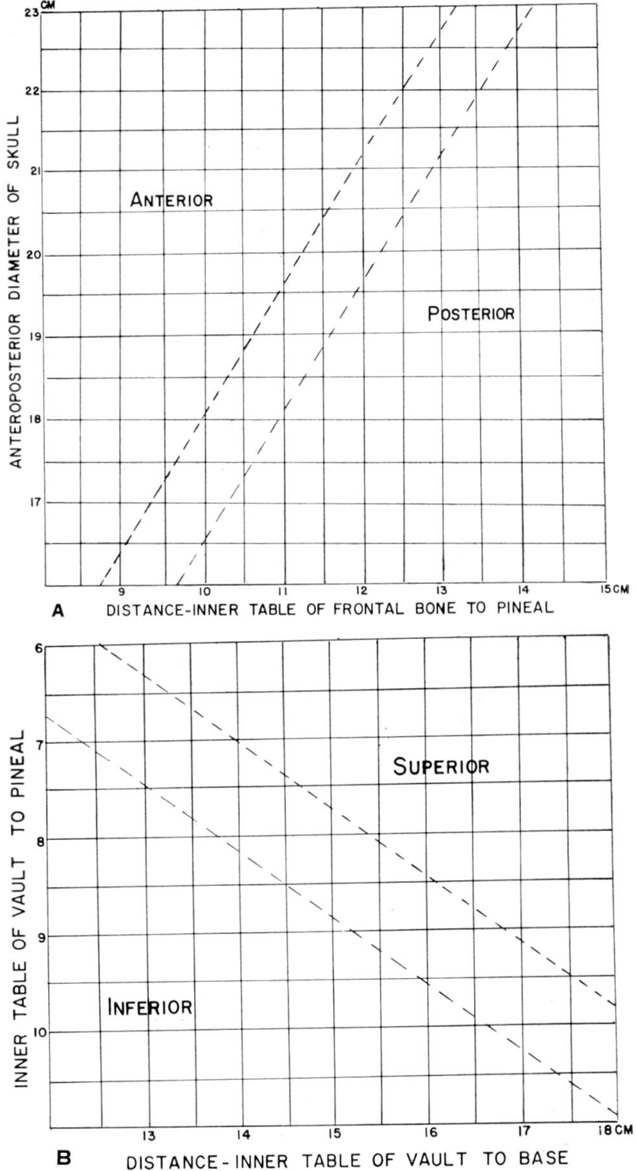

Fig. 18.—Vastine-Kinney Method of Measuring the Pineal Calcification to Determine Displacement in the Anteroposterior Diameter (A), and in the Vertical Diameter (B)

the possible presence of a true tumor of the pineal, a pinealoma.

Methods for determining the normal position of the pineal in the lateral projection have been devised by Vastine and Kinney (fig. 18), and by Fray. Modifications of the Vastine-Kinney method have been suggested by Dyke (1930).

Measurement of the position of the pineal calcification. In the method devised by Vastine and Kinney the measurement of the total length of the skull from the inner table in the frontal bone to the inner table in the occipital bone is related to the distance from the inner table of the frontal bone to the center of the pineal calcification (fig. 18). For vertical displacement of the pineal, the distance from the vertex (inner table) of the skull to the plane of the foramen magnum and from the inner table of the vertex *to the*

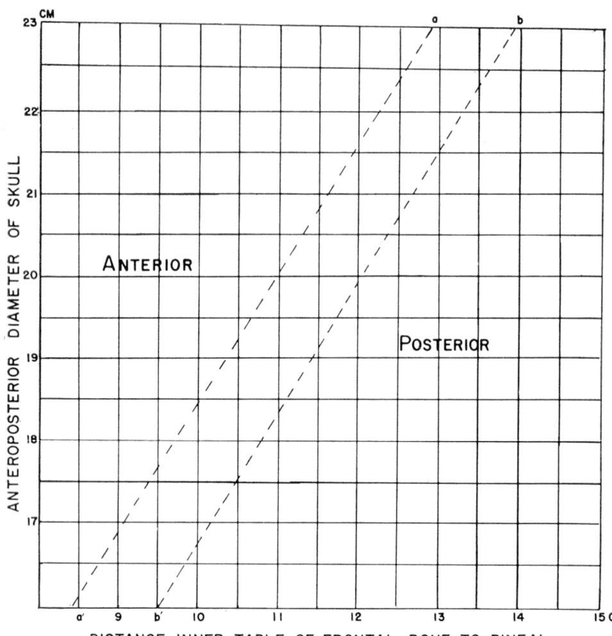

FIG. 19.—DYKE MODIFICATION OF VASTINE-KINNEY CHART FOR DETERMINING PINEAL DISPLACEMENTS IN THE ANTEROPOSTERIOR DIAMETER

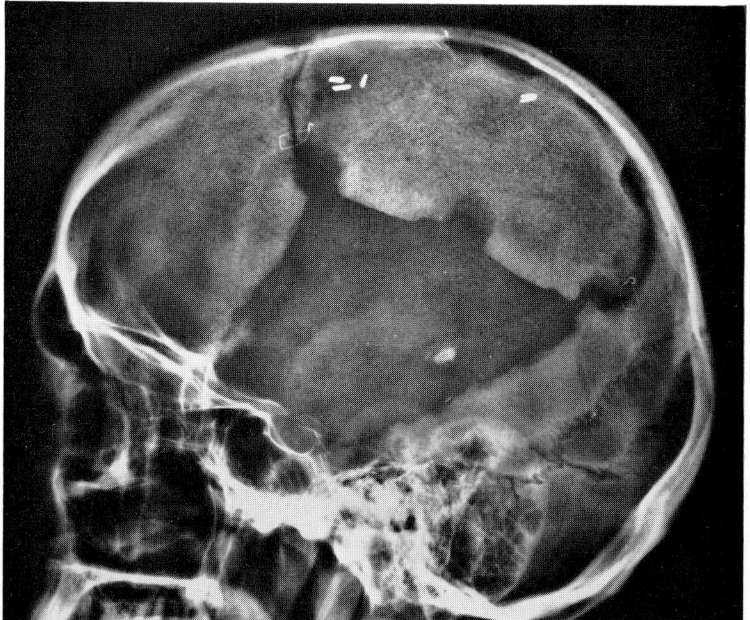

FIG. 20.—NORMAL LATERAL VIEW OF THE SKULL SHOWING CALCIFICATION IN PINEAL AND HABENULAR COMMISSURE

The pineal is in normal position and the absence of bone permits unusually good visualization of the pineal for illustration. The posterior aspect of the head is relatively flat in this patient, and in these cases there is a tendency for the pineal to fall either at the posterior limit of normal or slightly behind the normal zone, even though it is normal.

(Revised 1963)

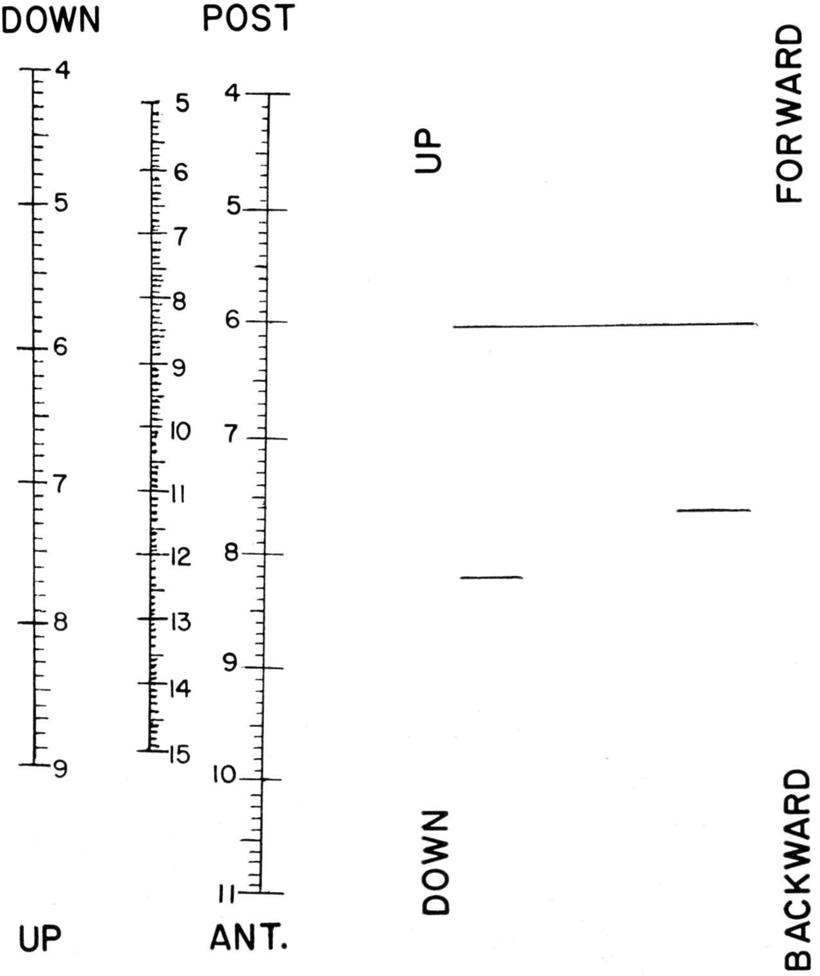

FIG. 21.—RULER FOR CALCULATION OF PINEAL DISPLACEMENT IN THE ANTEROPOSTERIOR AND IN THE VERTICAL DIAMETERS

The proportions, as shown on this figure, are correct and may be transferred to another paper photographically. The right side of the picture can be transferred to transparent x-ray film. When placed over the ruler, it will indicate the direction of the displacement if it falls outside the normal zone. The long transverse line is used for the distance from the inner table of the frontal bone to the pineal calcification on the center portion of the ruler. If the pineal does not fall between the long and the short line it is displaced in the direction indicated by the ruler.

center of the pineal calcification is used (fig. 23). Dyke (1930), on the basis of the examination of 3000 roentgenograms of the skull, substantiated the work of Vastine and Kinney and modified the chart they devised to determine the anteroposterior position of the pineal body by moving the normal zone forward 4 mm. (fig. 19). This became necessary because it was found that a good percentage of pineal shadows (14 per cent), when plotted, were outside the normal zone and most of these were anterior to it. Since this occurred in patients without a verified intracranial mass or clinical indications of it, it was considered advisable to move the anterior limit 4 mm. so as to decrease the number of false positives. However, this has caused a certain number of pineal calcifica-

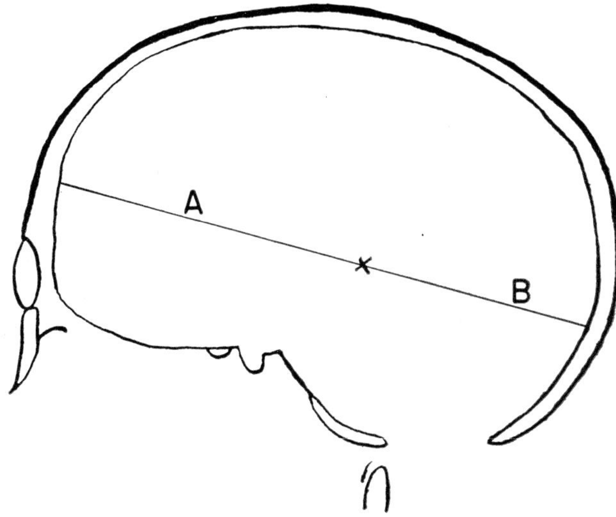

FIG. 22.—FORMULA FOR THE CALCULATION OF PINEAL DISPLACEMENT IN AN ANTEROPOSTERIOR DIRECTION

$$\frac{2(A + B)}{3} = A \pm 0.5\,\text{cm}$$

tions to fall behind the normal zone, suggesting posterior displacement. This is particularly true when the patient has a relatively flat posterior aspect of the skull such as that shown in Figure 20. The converse is true when using the Vastine-Kinney charts; that is, if the patient has a relatively long posterior portion of the head, the pineal is going to be anterior to the normal zone in a certain percentage of the cases, as indicated above.

At the Neurological Institute the modification proposed by Dyke has been in use for the last three decades. For ease of handling, the chart has been transferred to a ruler which incorporates both the anteroposterior and the vertical pineal displacements (fig. 21). This ruler can be further simplified by the use of a mathematical formula for the anteroposterior displacement; $2(A + B)/3 =$ Distance of pineal from frontal inner table to center of pineal calcification ± 5 mm. (Pousner, 1961). In practice, it is our custom to use the anterior aspect of the pineal calcification as a routine because if this places the pineal behind the normal zone, it is considered to be displaced posteriorly. This is particularly important if the patient has a flat posterior aspect of the head, as mentioned above. On the other hand, if the head is long with a relatively long occipital region, which is readily apparent upon inspection of the film, the center of the pineal calcification should be measured. When measuring the posterior end of the cranial cavity, it is often found that there is a double contour which may be produced by the midline elevation for the superior longitudinal sinus at the cruciate eminence. Therefore, the most posterior margin should be used. If the skull shows too much rotation along the vertical axis, which may be checked by noting the relative positions of the ascending rami of the mandible, it may be that the two margins posteriorly may represent the right and the left sides of the occipital bone. In this case another lateral view should be used. Sometimes only the habenular commissure is calcified and this should be recognized. If the measurement is applied to the habenular commissure, it could place the pineal anterior to the normal zone.

Posterior and downward displacement of the pineal are much more common than anterior and upward displacement.

It has been found that, if the pineal falls

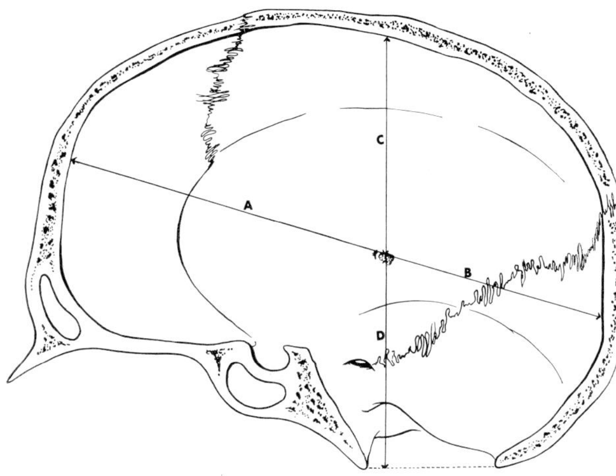

Fig. 23.—Manner in Which Pineal Measurements are Usually Made in the Anteroposterior and in the Vertical Direction

In determining displacement in the vertical direction, the center of the pineal calcification should be used. The lower measurement is taken from the center of the pineal to the plane of the foramen magnum.

above or below the normal zone, it is usually truly displaced, whereas the pineal calcification sometimes falls slightly behind the normal zone in the anteroposterior direction in a patient who does not have an intracranial mass, as explained above. Of course, any separation from the normal involving more than 2 or 3 mm. in the anteroposterior direction should be regarded as strong evidence for posterior displacement. Posterior displacement as well as downward displacement is not always due to an intracranial mass lesion and may result from ventricular dilatation sometimes associated with aqueduct stenosis.

Habenular calcification. Calcification on the anterior margin of the habenular commissure is fairly common. It may be encountered in association with pineal calcification or may be seen in the absence of any pineal calcification. Stauffer *et al.* (1953) identified calcification in the habenula in 89 out of 187 normal skull examinations. The habenular calcification is usually situated an average of 5.8 mm. anterior to the center of the pineal calcification.

Calcification in the glomus of the choroid plexus. This may be unilateral or bilateral. The calcium deposits may be very faint or may be more distinctly shown. Sometimes one calcified area in the glomus may be situated lower or higher than the one on the oppostie side, but this is not necessarily significant.

Greater details on intracranial calcifications are given elsewhere (see p. 1.182).

FRONTAL PROJECTIONS

It is our custom to make at least three radiographs of the skull in frontal projection; two may be made in posteroanterior and one in anteroposterior projection or vice versa.

Straight Posteroanterior and Inclined Posteroanterior Views

The two posteroanterior projections are made one with the orbitomeatal line perpendicular to the film and without angling the tube. The other is made with the orbitomeatal line perpendicular to the film and the tube angled at 15° (instead of 23° as in Caldwell projection) craniocaudally. In the first view the petrous pyramids are projected through the orbits, and in the second, the petrous pyramids are projected at the lower portion of the orbit, thus bringing out the superior orbital fissure and the greater and lesser wings of the sphenoid (figs. 24, 26, and 27). These views are necessary for a routine examination of the skull; otherwise, the examination cannot be considered as supplying sufficient information. It is understood, of course, that in special situations, other films may be required in addition. The

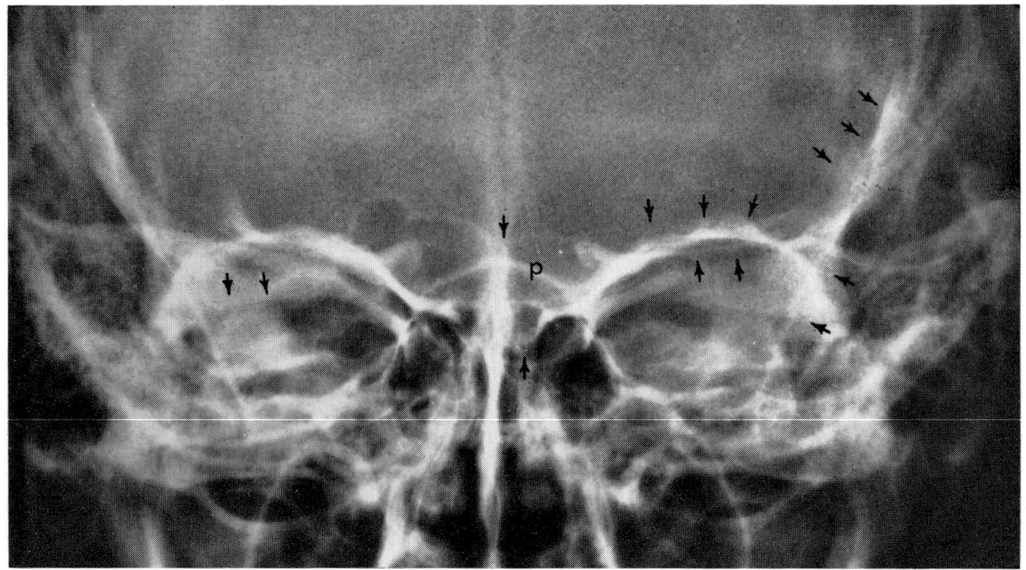

FIG. 24.—STRAIGHT POSTEROANTERIOR VIEW OF THE SKULL

The petrous pyramids are projected through the orbits and obscure the details of the orbital structures. The internal acoustic meati are fairly well shown (*arrows*). The curvilinear shadow demarcating the highest point of the roof of the orbit (*three vertical arrows*) is superimposed on the shadow of the posterior margin of the floor of the anterior fossa (*two arrows*) and, although on the left side they can be followed individually, they are partly obscured because of the superimposition. The outer aspect of the posterior margin of the floor of the anterior fossa joins the upper aspect of the oblique line of the orbit and contributes to the formation of the heavy line in the temporal area of the skull (*three oblique arrows*). The cribriform plate and crista galli are also seen (*upper and lower midline arrows*). (*p*) indicates the tuberculum sellae and upper margin of sphenoid sinus. This figure should be studied at the same time as Fig. 27.

anatomy depicted in these views is best explained on a series of radiographs and drawings (figs. 24, 25, 26, and 27).

In examining the frontal projections, a system similar to that followed in the lateral projection is advisable. The shape of the skull and the symmetry of the two sides should be ascertained. It is difficult to emphasize the importance of comparing the two sides for symmetry. The thickness of the bones of the calvaria should be compared in the two sides; the sutures and the vascular markings are looked for and any asymmetries noted. A slight degree of asymmetry of the skull is present in every individual (Thibaut, 1961). The right side, therefore, is not strictly comparable to the left, but the asymmetry is usually slight and not systematized. That is, the parietal bone may be slightly thicker over one side, but there would not be, on the same side, evidence of elevation of the petrous pyramid and enlargement of the sinuses such as is found in cerebral hemiatrophy. According to Thibaut, some of the asymmetries in patients with epilepsy described by McRae may be within normal limits.

In looking at the region of the base of the skull and the orbits in these projections, it is well to keep in mind the normal anatomical configuration already described in the lateral projection. The upper portion of the orbit presents *three lines* (1) the superior border of the orbit, the one that can be felt by palpation, which is anterior in location and often rather inconspicuous on the roentgenogram; (2) the highest point of the roofs of the orbit, which describes a curvilinear shadow concave downward, sometimes presenting irregularities due to the convolu-

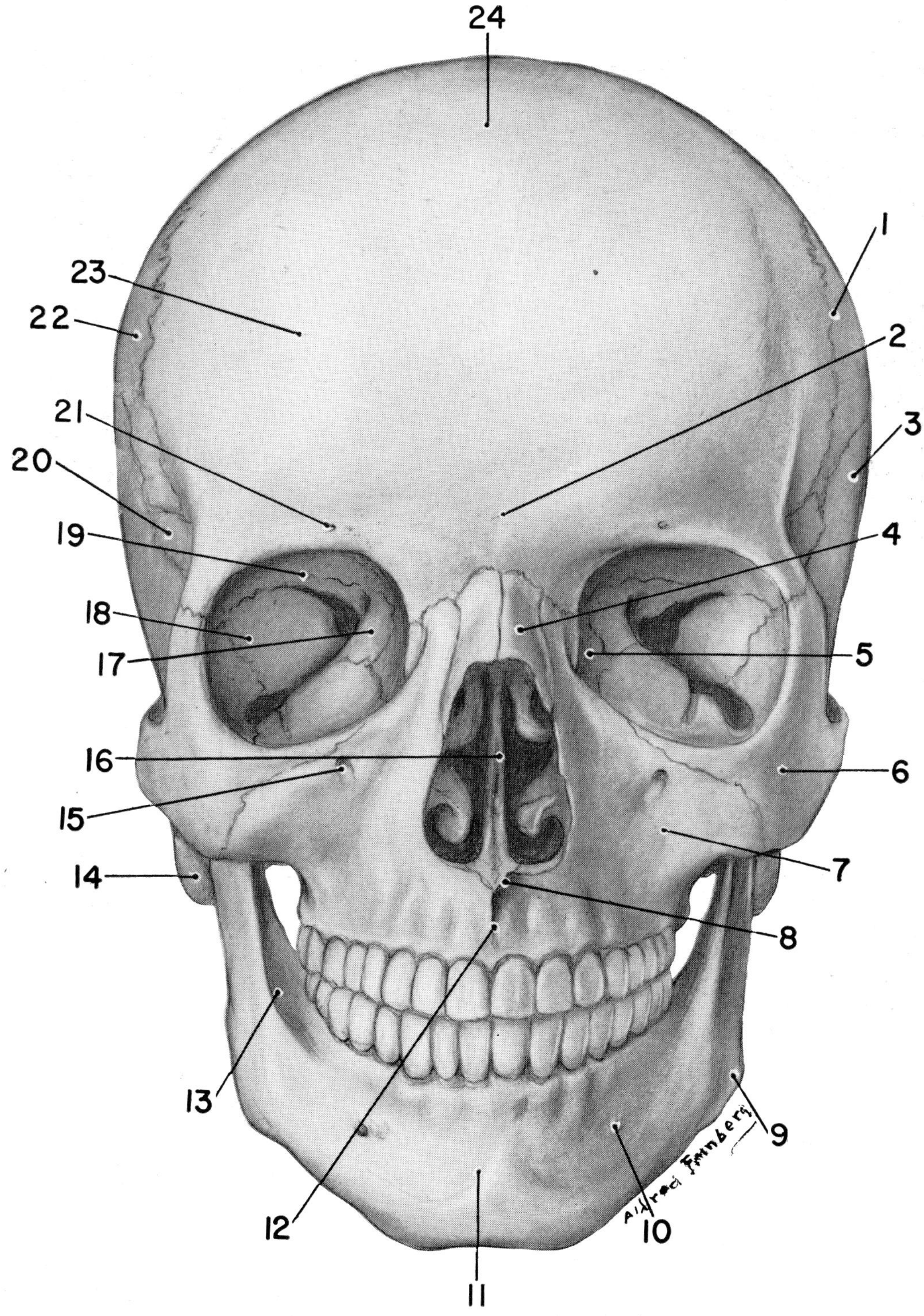

FIG. 25.—DRAWING OF FRONTAL VIEW OF THE SKULL

(1) coronal suture. (2) glabella. (3) temporal. (4) nasal. (5) lacrimal. (6) zygomatic. (7) maxilla. (8) anterior nasal spine. (9) angle of mandible. (10) mental foramen. (11) mandible. (12) intermaxillary suture. (13) ramus of mandible. (14) mastoid process. (15) infra-orbital foramen. (16) osseous nasal septum (17) ethmoid. (18) great wing of sphenoid. (19) frontal. (20) great wing of sphenoid. (21) supra-orbital foramen. (22) parietal. (23) frontal eminence. (24) frontal.

(Revised 1963)

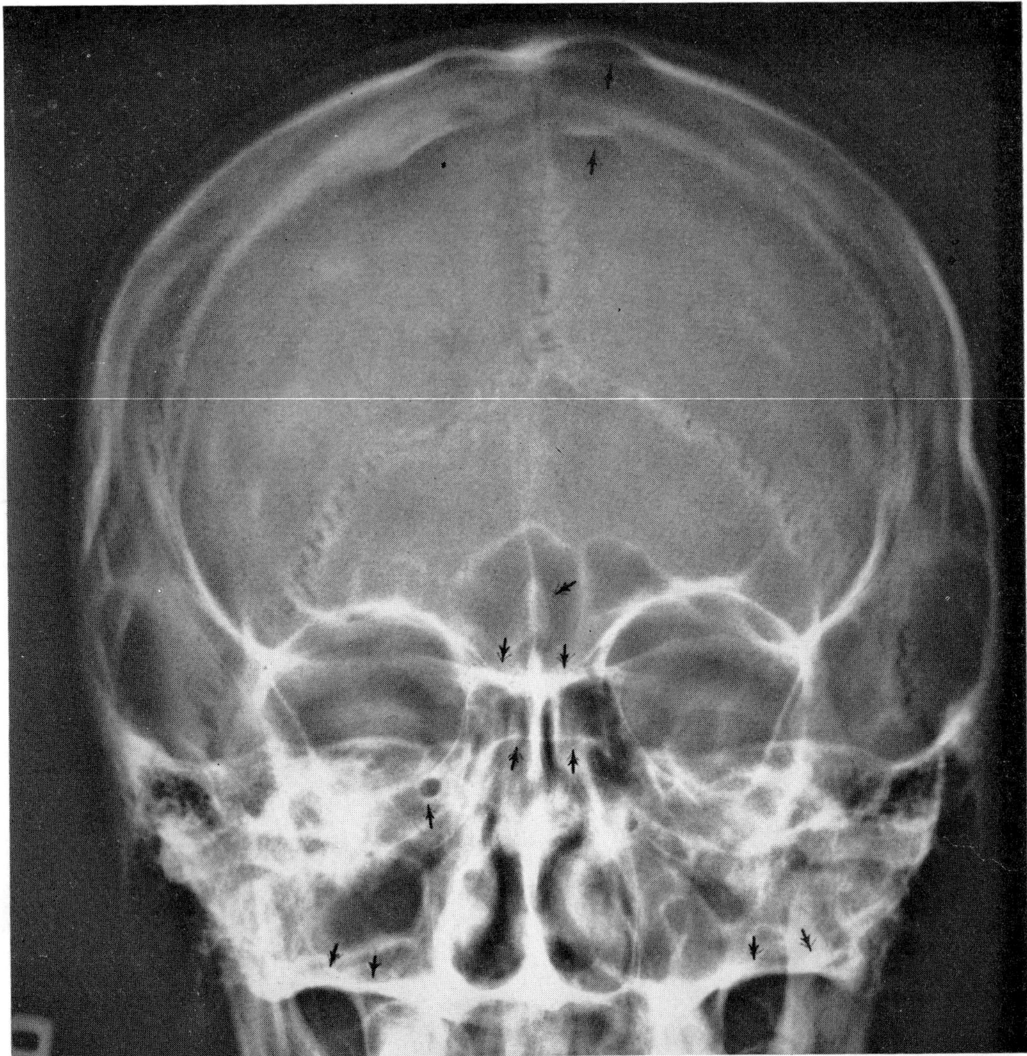

Fig. 26.—Normal Inclined Posteroanterior View of the Skull

The structures around the orbits should be compared with those shown in Fig. 27. The midline arrow points at the crista galli. The crista galli is perpendicular to the planum sphenoidale (*arrows*). The planum sphenoidale joins the two lesser wings of the sphenoid. The lower midline arrows point at the floor of the sella turcica. The foramen rotundum is seen on the reader's left (*arrow*) and is partly obscured on the right. The shadow of the floor of the posterior fossa on each side is shown by the lower arrows. Shallow Pacchionian depressions are seen at the upper portion of the skull just off the midline (*arrows*).

tional markings of the floor of the anterior fossa; and (3) the posterior aspect of the floor of the anterior fossa which is formed by the posterior portion of the horizontal plate of the frontal bone and the wings of the sphenoid (figs. 26 and 27).

The two lines seen on the lateral superior aspect of the orbit on each side are as follows. One is the oblique line of the orbit. The lower two-thirds of the oblique line of the orbit are formed by the outer surface of the greater wing of the sphenoid. The upper

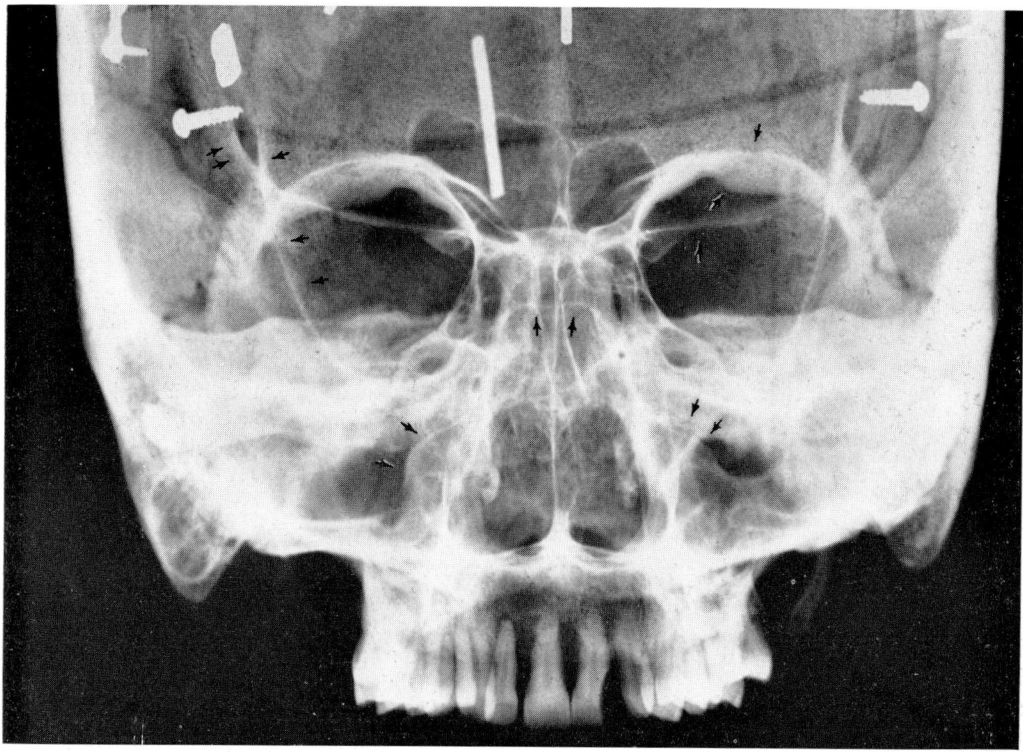

FIG. 27.—INCLINED POSTEROANTERIOR VIEW OF DRY SKULL

The palpable border of the orbit is clearly shown with its supra-orbital notch on each side (*arrow*). The superior margin of the orbit representing the highest point of the floor of the anterior fossa is always clearly visible in inclined posteroanterior projections (*upper right arrow*). The posterior margin of the floor of the anterior fossa, usually called sphenoid ridge on radiographs, is clearly shown (*lower right arrow*). On its medial end on each side is the thicker portion of the lesser wing of the sphenoid which ends at the anterior clinoid process. The superior orbital fissures are asymmetrical in this skull. The oblique line of the orbit is well shown (*arrows*). As it moves upward and outward, it crosses the base of the zygomatic process of the frontal bone. The heavy line produced mostly by the lateral aspect of the greater wing of the sphenoid, and partly by the superimposed shadow of the heavy bone of the temporal crest of the frontal bone, is shown by the double arrow. The lines marked by arrows in this illustration should be compared with those in Figs. 24 and 26. The lines shown by the lower double arrows on each side represent the inner aspect of the occipital bone above the condyles. The floor of the sella is shown by the two midline arrows.

portion is produced by the temporal surface of the frontal bone. The portion of the frontal bone that produces this shadow is the outer or temporal surface of the frontal bone immediately behind the zygomatic process; the line crosses the base of the zygomatic process of the frontal bone (figs. 26 and 27). The second line (mentioned above) is a rather heavy, roughly horizontal line that is produced almost totally by the lateral aspect of the posterior portion of the floor of the anterior fossa and the greater wing of the sphenoid, and by the heavy bone at the temporal line of the frontal bone which contributes most of the density. The two lines are superimposed in straight posteroanterior projections (fig. 24) and can be separated in the views where the tube is angled caudally (figs. 11, 26, and 27).

The relative position of the three lines described above at the upper margin of the orbit would depend upon the projection that

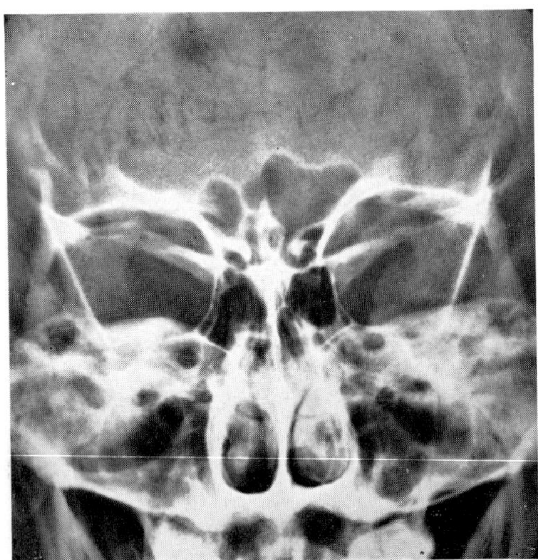

FIG. 28.—ASYMMETRICAL SPHENOID FISSURES (SUPERIOR ORBITAL FISSURES) AND LESSER WINGS OF THE SPHENOID IN NORMAL PATIENT

is used. For instance, the shadow produced by the posterior aspect of the floor of the anterior fossa and lesser and greater wings of the sphenoid is lower than the roof of the orbit in the inclined posteroanterior projection, whereas in a straight posteroanterior view it may be slightly higher or overlying the upper surface of the orbit. What is usually termed *sphenoid ridge* refers to the lesser wing of the sphenoid and the dense horizontal line described above (fig. 27). Between the lesser and the greater wings of the sphenoid is the *superior orbital* or *sphenoid fissure* on each side. The sphenoid fissures are often asymmetrical; sometimes extreme degrees of asymmetry are found in normal patients (fig. 28). When the asymmetry is marked, it may be difficult to decide whether or not there is any bone erosion present. No special rules can be given to differentiate between asymmetry and a pathologic process producing bone destruction. However, if a sharp margin is seen, this should suggest bone destruction; if there is a change in the texture of the trabeculae of the bone when compared with the other side the possibility of an invasive lesion of bone such as meningioma should be explored.

The same appearance to the structures described above may be obtained in an anteroposterior view, but the orbits will be relatively magnified.

The shadow of the anterior clinoid process is shown in the straight posteroanterior film projecting slightly upward and medially from the superior medial surface of the orbit (fig. 24). In the inclined posteroanterior projection, the anterior clinoid processes are the most medial portion of the lesser wings of the sphenoid.

The petrous pyramids are projected through the orbits in the straight posteroanterior projection. This is a different view of the petrous pyramid from that obtained in the half axial and in the Stenvers projection which will be described later. The internal acoustic canal is often clearly visible in this view but usually is not as well seen as in the half axial or in the Stenvers projection. An area suggestive of a canal is often seen medial to the internal acoustic meatus which is formed by the upper border of the petrous pyramid and the upper margin of the carotid canal. This appearance should not be confused with the shadow of the internal acoustic canal. The straight posteroanterior view is useful to show the tip of the petrous pyramid through the orbits. It is worthwhile to point out here that a slight degree of rotation causes an apparent asymmetry in the appearance of the petrous tips; it makes one side look more radiolucent than the other, often giving the impression of bone destruction. This error is a common one. In these projections there is often a deep notch along the superior border of the petrous pyramids laterally. This notch is produced by a large sigmoid sinus, and when present, it is more conspicuous in these views than it is in the half axial projection described below. Medial to the superior margin of the petrous pyramid there is often a dense line which represents calcification in the petroclinoid ligament as seen in the frontal projection. The shadow of the calcified intracavernous portion of the internal carotid artery is seen as a circle which overlies the lower margin of the anterior clinoid process (fig. 161); the calcified supracavernous portion of the internal carotid artery shows up as a circle which overlies the anterior clinoid process or is slightly above it.

(Revised 1963)

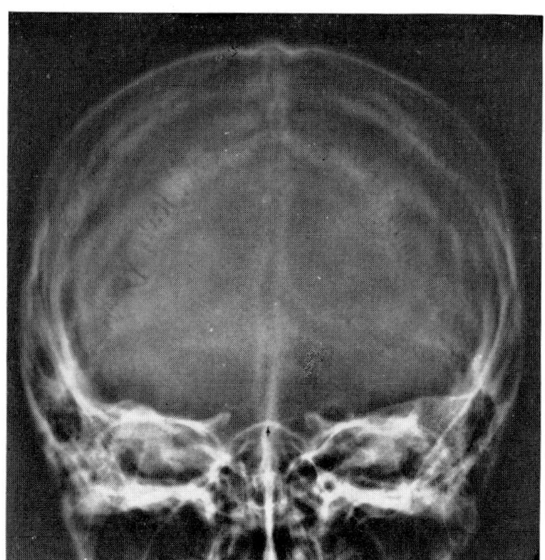

FIG. 29.—GRANGER VIEW OF THE SKULL
This projection may be used to bring out the anterior clinoid processes and the top of the dorsum sellae. The tuberculum sellae is shown at the midline arrow. The upper margin of the petrous pyramids projects above the roof of the orbit.

In the midline between the two orbits, the most conspicuous shadow, in the inclined posteroanterior projection, is the horizontal line produced by the *planum sphenoidale* (fig. 26). In the straight posteroanterior projection, the region of the tuberculum sella is seen instead; the shadow of the olfactory groove and cribriform plate are seen further down, and the crista galli is also visible in this projection (fig. 24). On the other hand, in the inclined posteroanterior projection, the shadow of the olfactory groove is not seen, but the crista galli is usually well shown (fig. 26).

Another posteroanterior view of the skull which is rarely used is the Granger view, obtained by placing the orbitomeatal line perpendicular to the film and angling the central beam 10° cephalad. In this view the superior margin of the petrous pyramids projects just above the upper surface of the orbits; the upper margin of the sphenoid sinus is projected between the roofs of the orbit (fig. 29).

In the frontal projection, the floor of the sella turcica is often visible (figs. 24 and 26). It is easier to find it when the sphenoid sinuses extend under the floor of the sella turcica, which can be ascertained in the lateral projection. Frontal laminagrams will demonstrate the floor of the sella turcica to better advantage (fig. 83), but this is usually not necessary because the frontal projection, particularly taken stereoscopically, may also clearly show it. Slight slanting of the floor of the sella turcica is sometimes seen in normal subjects. This is the reason for the production of a slight double floor as seen in the lateral view in some normal cases. Sometimes a slight depression to the central portion of the floor of the sella turcica is clearly visible in some individuals. The ethmoid sinuses tend to obscure the outlines of the sella turcica. The dorsum sellae is almost never visible in routine posteroanterior projection unless it projects above the planum sphenoidale, such as in the Granger view or in reversed half axial view. The shadow of the *middle fossa* is partly obscured by the petrous pyramids and by the structures of the lower margin of the orbit, but it can be seen if looked for (fig. 26); laminagrams are usually necessary for this purpose. The shadow of the floor of the posterior fossa is usually clearly visible in both the straight and the inclined posteroanterior views.

In the straight as well as the inclined posteroanterior projections, the groove produced by the superior longitudinal sinus along the inner table in the midline is visible in most individuals. The depth of the groove is variable. The Pacchionian depressions described above appear as a radiolucent shadow along the upper aspect of the convexity of the calvaria. As previously mentioned, these Pacchionian depressions are not usually more than 2.5 to 3 cm. away from the midline. If they are further away from the midline, they should be regarded as possibly of pathologic significance. The Pacchionian depressions can be distinguished from destructive lesions of the skull because the outer table may be thinned out but is usually intact. Occasionally the outer table bulges outward (fig. 3). Because they represent a depression, these radiolucent shadows, which are sometimes very conspicuous, only show superior and lateral margins on the films; the inferior margin always fades so that no sharp outline can ever be seen on the inferior aspect except in the occipital bone where it is seen *en face* (fig. 4). This would indicate that it is not an area of destruction but an area of depression on the inner table. The same applies to depressions on the inner table produced by superficially placed tumors (fig. 121).

The visible sutures in the frontal projections are the sagittal, coronal, and lamboidal sutures. Which one is more conspicuous depends on the projection. The coronal suture can be identified, even though the digitations of the sutures are not visible, because of the perisutural density that is usually present. The metopic suture between the two halves of the frontal bone is often visible. It is estimated that between 5 and 10 per cent of all individuals have either partial or complete persistence of the metopic suture, which is of no clinical significance. This suture often has no digitations and its straight appearance may, at times, raise the question of fracture. The presence of perisutural density should indicate that it is not a fracture (fig. 11).

The vascular channels are fairly symmetrical when the right is compared with the left. Sometimes there is a predominance of diploic channels on one side or the other. If excessive asymmetry is present, the possibility of abnormal vascularity of the skull, as may be seen in meningiomas, or arteriovenous malformations supplied by the external carotid artery should be suspected.

In addition to the parietal foramen which serves for passage of an emissary vein, there are other small foramina which may serve for the passage of anastomosing veins between the intracranial and the extracranial circulation. One of these veins is the *occipital emissary* which is seen in the region of the torcular Herophili. This vein is usually small and may be seen to grow in size in cases of longstanding increased intracranial pressure. In the region of the torcular Herophili there are often sharp areas of radiolucency projecting outward from the inner table and almost reaching the outer table, which is made extremely thin as a result. These areas may also be encountered along the course of the lateral sinus and represent Pacchionian depressions similar to those already described. They are not abnormal and are not associated with increased intracranial pressure. Sometimes they are extremely conspicuous and raise the question of a destructive process. Their characteristic location in the region of the torcular should serve as the chief differential diagnostic point. In addition, they are observed to come from the inner table and to extend to the outer table, occasionally pushing the intact, though thin, outer table outward. Sometimes laminagrams in the lateral projection are necessary to clarify this point (fig. 4B).

Sinus pericranii. Communication between the intracranial and the extracranial circulation through emissary veins is sometimes found in the frontal region. In some cases, the abnormal communication becomes annoying in that every time that the patient leans down, such as to tie his shoes, the area becomes engorged and an actual lump may be felt on palpation. This will also occur when a Valsalva maneuver (forced expiration against a closed glottis) is performed which increases the intracranial venous pressure. The abnormality has been termed *sinus pericranii.* The communication with the intracranial circulation may be demonstrated by the direct injection of a contrast substance subcutaneously after aspiration of some blood. The puncture may be done with the head in the dependent position, and after blood has been aspirated, the patient may be placed in the supine position and the injection made. Occasionally, lesions that behave somewhat like sinus pericranii turn out to have some arterial elements in them (fig. 30). The defect in the bone is usually quite inconspicuous and requires stereoscopic films of good quality to be detected in many instances. Laminagraphy will sometimes be of help in demonstrating the venous channels through the skull.

Half Axial View (Anteroposterior Towne, Occipital, or Cerebellar View)

The next view of the skull to be discussed is the occipital view or half axial view. This view is obtained by placing the occiput in contact with the film and angling the tube 35° caudally from the orbitomeatal line.

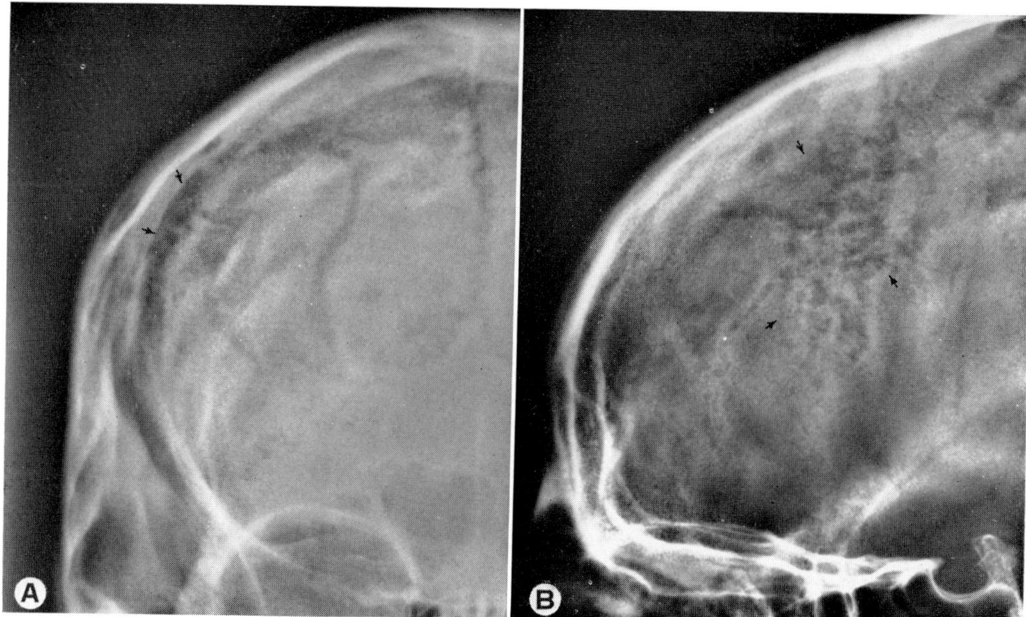

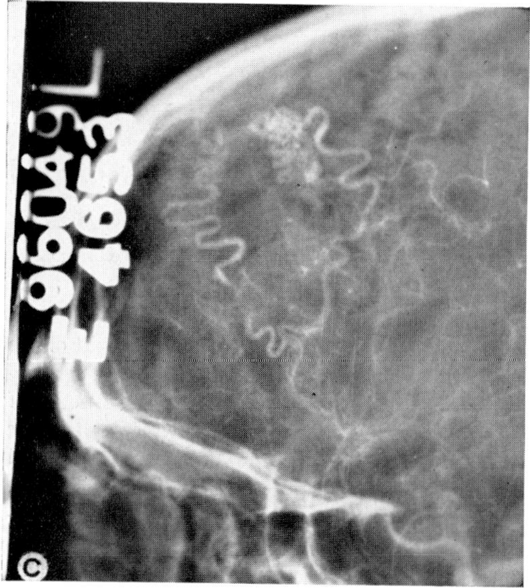

FIG. 30.—ARTERIOVENOUS ANGIOMA OF THE SCALP SIMULATING SINUS PERICRANII

The patient complained clinically of a soft compressible mass in the left frontal region which became worse with straining or when the head was leaned forward, as to tie his shoes. Clinical diagnosis of sinus pericranii was made but because of certain features (slight pulsation of the mass), an angiogram was performed. The common carotid angiogram demonstrated, in the late arterial phase of the intracranial structures, the presence of enlarged convoluted external carotid vessels, branches of the superficial temporal artery leading to an angiomatous lesion. Venous drainage was fairly brisk from this region, although slower than in arteriovenous angiomas involving the internal carotid branches. The plain films demonstrated local increased vascularity of the bone, such as is seen in sinus pericranii (*arrows*). (A) and (B) are plain films. (C) is an angiogram. The lesion was surgically removed.

This projection shows the occipital bone well. The dorsum sellae usually projects through the foramen magnum. The petrous pyramids are fairly well shown. However, it is felt that a view made with a 25° caudal angulation above the canthomeatal line is more satisfactory to visualize the petrous pyramids. In fact, it is our custom to use this modified projection routinely and only in those cases where it is desirable to visualize the foramen magnum do we use the classical projection. In the modified half axial view, the foramen magnum is not visualized (figs. 31 and 32). The modified half axial view is probably the best film to study the petrous pyramids. The internal acoustic canals are well shown; they are projected as a radiolucent band parallel to the bottom of the film. The two portions

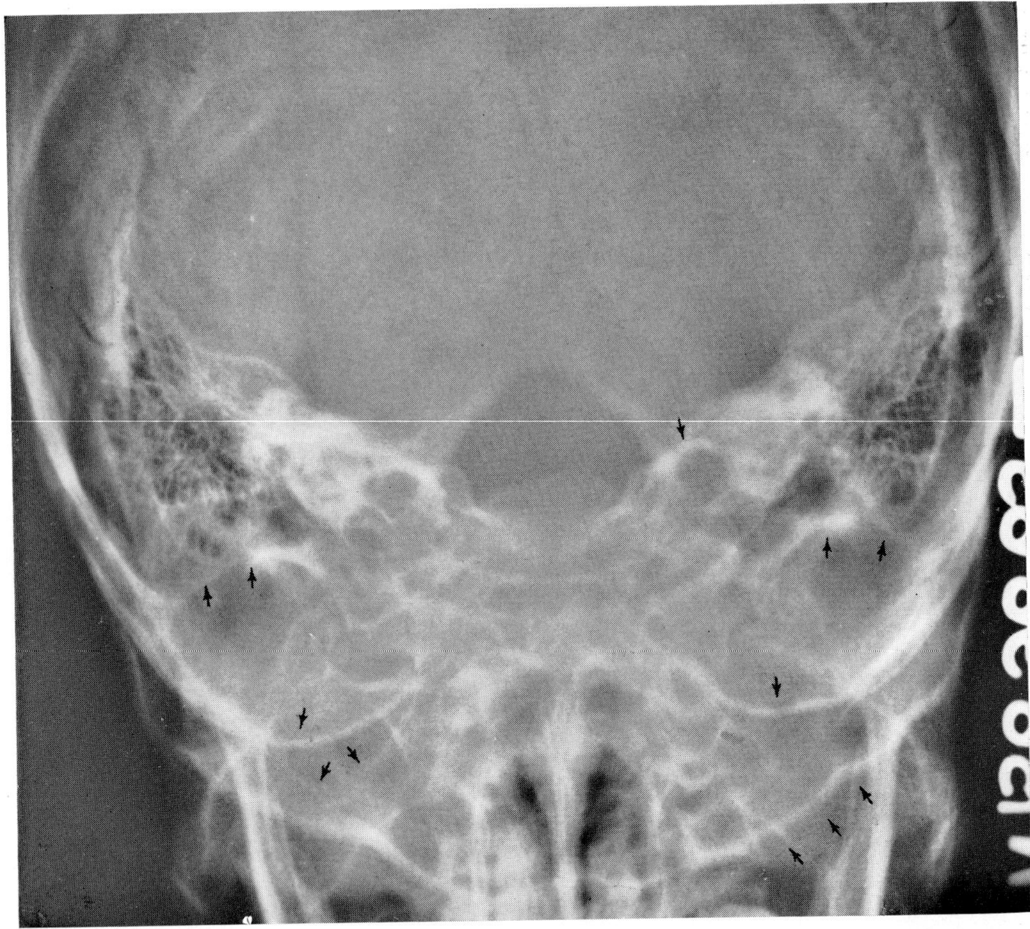

Fig. 31.—Half Axial View of the Skull

The posterior half of the foramen magnum is visible in this projection (A). The arrow to the right of the foramen magnum points at the condylar foramen and fossa. The two arrows on each side mark the glenoid fossa. The internal acoustic meati are not nearly as well shown in this view as in the modified half axial view shown in Fig. 32. The symmetrical shadows of the middle fossae are well shown (*single arrow on each side*). The angular shadow of the infratemporal crest of the greater wing of the sphenoid and the posterior margin of the inferior orbital fissure are shown in this case but not as clearly as in Fig. 32 (*arrows*). The heavy line on the right marked by the lower three arrows represents the anterior inferior aspect of the floor of the anterior fossa which is projected downward.

of the porus acousticus internus, the canal portion and the meatus or entrance of the canal, are well shown here (figs. 32 and 96). For greater detail, see page 1.118. The modified half axial projection is also an excellent view to study the mastoids; the mastoid antrum is clearly visualized (fig. 32). The petrous tips are seen well in this view but not as clearly as in the straight postero-anterior view.

The half axial view is also useful to visualize the floor of the middle fossa on each side and to compare the two sides of the middle fossa when looking for asymmetry (figs. 31 and 32). Enlargement of the middle fossa is readily seen in half axial projections (fig. 31A). This is more accurate than the lateral projection, which is subject to error resulting from magnification of the side away from the film. An angular shadow

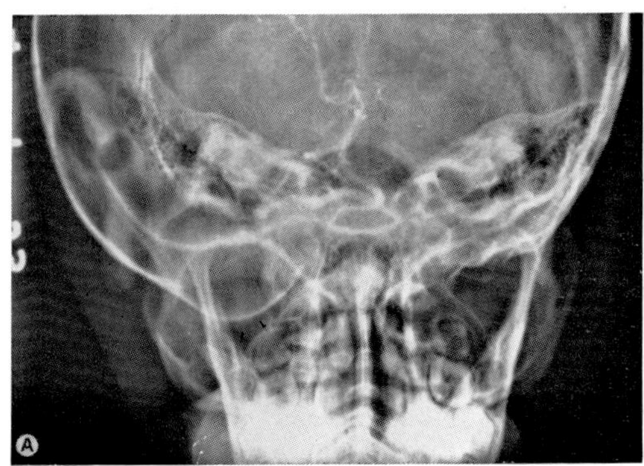

FIG. 31A (*cont'd.*).—ENLARGED MIDDLE FOSSA IN PATIENT WITH CHRONIC SUBDURAL HYGROMA
The asymmetry on the two sides (A) is readily appreciated (*arrows*).

is seen just below the floor of the middle fossa which represents the infratemporal ridge and the sphenomaxillary surface of the greater wing of the sphenoid (fig. 31). The medial portion of this angular shadow represents the posterior surface of the inferior orbital fissure (figs. 31 and 32). These two lines are several millimeters away from the inner surface of the greater wing of the sphenoid which represents the most anterior portion of the floor of the middle fossa.

The occipital bone usually presents a slight elevation along the course of the superior longitudinal sinus and on the lateral sinuses, which join together at the midline in the region of the torcular Herophili. Below the torcular Herophili there is another, narrower, elevation or crest along the inner table which serves for the insertion of the falx cerebelli. A small sinus, the occipital sinus, is situated at the base of the falx cerebelli. The falx cerebelli is quite narrow; that is, it does not penetrate deeply. To the left of the midline above and below the ridges of the venous sinuses, the occipital bone is quite thin. The thin area above the transverse sinus is usually called the *cerebral fossa* of the occipital bone; below the transverse sinus it is referred to as *cerebellar fossa* on each side of the midline. The elevations or ridges for the sinuses form a cross in the midline which is named the *occipital cruciate eminence.*

The lambdoidal suture usually shows well in the half axial projection. The occipitomastoid portion of the suture is often straight and lacks digitations, which sometimes suggests a fracture line, particularly if there is slight rotation of the head so that one side is not seen whereas the other is clearly visible.

Multiple Wormian bones are often present in the region of the lambda. Sometimes a suture is seen extending straight across the upper portion of the occipital squama between the exoccipital and the supraoccipital. The suture isolates the upper portion of the occipital squama which is triangular in configuration and is called the interparietal bone. The coronal suture projects across the occipital bone; the height at which it projects depends on the angulation of the tube used to make the radiograph. This is the best view to study the actual configuration of the upper two-thirds of the coronal suture, the lower portion of which is best studied by stereoscopic lateral views. Further details about suture lines are found on pages 1.14 and 1.758.

As mentioned above, the foramen magnum is not seen in the modified half axial projection except for its posterior margin. In the half axial projection or one taken with greater caudal angulation of the tube (35°), the foramen magnum shadow is quite conspicuous. Usually only its posterior two-thirds are well outlined; its anterior one-third is partly obscured by the dense bone of the clivus and by other overlying structures (fig. 31). Through the shadow of the foramen magnum the posterior arch of the atlas can be seen, which sometimes presents a spina bifida occulta. The shadow of the dorsum sellae usually projects through or slightly above the shadow of the foramen magnum. The dorsum sellae is more satisfactorily shown in films taken with less angulation of the tube but this is variable. If too much angulation is used, the x-ray beam is parallel to the clivus and the dorsum is projected over the shadow of the clivus. Lateral to the margin of the foramen magnum there is a radiolucent space which is sometimes a foramen and at other times is only a depression. This is the condyloid fossa (some times condyloid foramen) which gives passage to an emissary vein connecting with the transverse sinus (fig. 33). The fossa is on the

(*Revised 1963*)

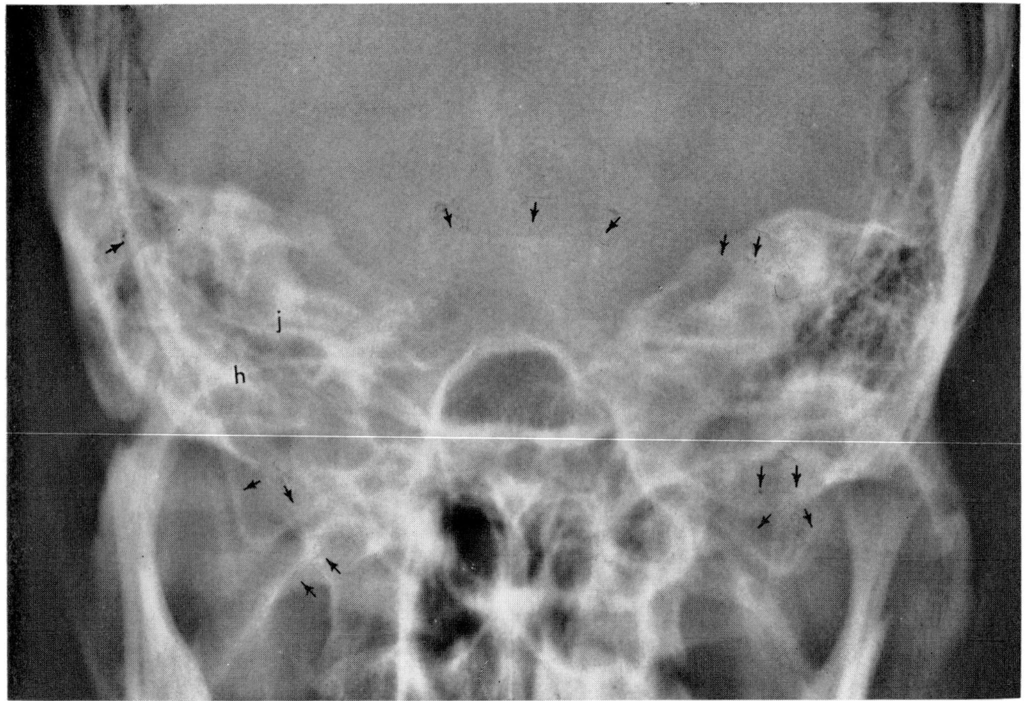

FIG. 32.—MODIFIED HALF AXIAL PROJECTION

The foramen magnum is not visible. The dorsum sellae is projected over the lower portion of the occipital bone (*midline upper arrows*). The internal acoustic canal is usually well shown on both sides in well penetrated films. The medial of the two arrows over the porus acousticus internus is over the meatus portion, and the more lateral one is over the canal portion. The posterior wall of the canal presents a medial margin which is inclined downward and medially. The mastoid antrum is well shown (*left upper arrow*). The curve of the middle fossa is well seen on both sides (*lower right arrows*). The angular lines seen just below the middle fossa represent the infratemporal ridge of the greater wing of the sphenoid and its sphenomaxillary surface on the outer aspect, and the posterior aspect of the inferior orbital fissure on its medial side (*arrows*). The anterior margin of the inferior orbital fissure is marked by the two lower arrows on the left. The upper margin of the sphenoid sinus is seen between the two petrous pyramids. (h) indicates the superior margin of the orbit and (j) indicates the posterior margin of the jugular foramen.

posterior margin of the occipital condyle on each side, where the posterior margin of the superior articular facet of the atlas comes to rest when the head is bent backward. Except for the posterior margin, the shadows of the condyles themselves are not usually seen in the half axial projection, but may be visualized in base views, which will be described later; in the lateral view they are superimposed. Laminagrams may be necessary to visualize them to better advantage. The condyles can be seen through the facial bones in the straight posteroanterior views and in the inclined posteroanterior views described above, but the confusing shadows of the sinuses and facial bones often make identification of these structures difficult without laminagraphy. The hypoglossal foramen is situated at the base of the condyle of the occipital bone. It gives passage to the hypoglossal or 12th cranial nerve, to a meningeal branch of the ascending pharyngeal artery, and to a thin plexus of emissary veins communicating the transverse sinus with the vertebral vein and the deep veins of the neck. This foramen is sometimes visible in half axial projection, but it is usually obscured by the shadow of the petrous tips.

(*Revised 1963*)

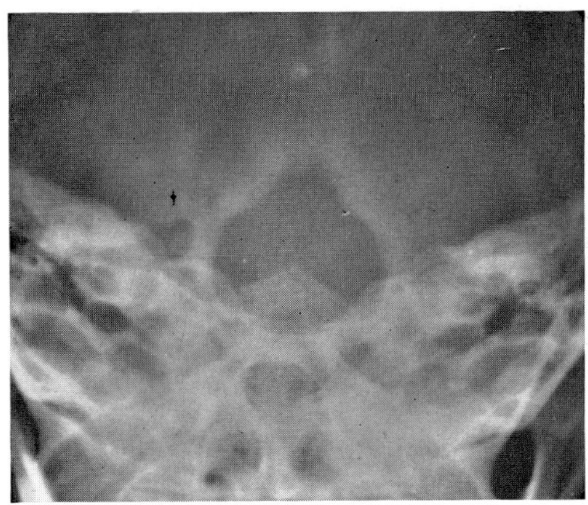

FIG. 33.—HALF AXIAL VIEW OF THE SKULL
A complete condyloid foramen is present on one side but not on the other. The petrous pyramids do not show a clear detail of the structures around the internal acoustic meatus in this projection. Compare with Fig. 32.

The *jugular foramen* and the fossa that bears the same name are sometimes clearly visible in the half axial projection along the irregular inferior aspect of the petrous pyramid (fig. 32). It is often obscured by other overlying structures, however. Through the jugular foramen pass, in its posterior portion, the transverse sinus, and in its anterior portion, the inferior petrosal sinus, the glossopharyngeal, vagus, and spinal accessory (11th) nerves. The inferior petrosal and lateral sinuses join in the jugular fossa to form the jugular vein.

The half axial projection also shows the roof of the sphenoid sinuses which are more or less conspicuous depending on the degree of pneumatization (fig. 32).

Laterally the shadows of the glenoid fossa on each side and of the condyles of the mandible are clearly visible. This view permits a comparison of the two sides and asymmetries are easily detected not only in the condyles, but also in the width of the joint space (fig. 31). Fractures and deformities of the mandibular condyles are readily visible in these views.

The petrous ridge is the superior border of the petrous pyramid. This border is not straight but slightly undulated, and the degree of irregularity is variable. For greater detail see "Petrous Pyramids" in the section on "Local Bone Erosions" (p. 1.118).

(Revised 1963)

Base Views

The base view, axial or submentovertical view, is extremely useful to visualize the structures of the base of the skull. The film is made usually by placing the top of the skull against the film and having the central ray travel in a caudocephalad direction. Occasionally, if the patient is unable to cooperate, the extended chin may be placed against the film and the central ray directed caudally. It is our custom to place the canthomeatal line parallel with the film and to angle the x-ray beam 15° rostrally. If the anthropological (Reid's) base line can be placed parallel to the film, the central ray is perpendicular to the film. The central ray is centered on the biauricular plane. This projection places the horseshoe of the mandible a little behind the frontal sinuses. More structures become visible in this manner, particularly the pterygoid process and the posterior ethmoid cells as well as the basal foramina. The latter structures are often covered by the mandible if the central ray is made to pass perpendicular to the orbitomeatal line. During the film exposure, the patient is asked not to move and *to continue to breathe through his nose* in order to prevent contraction of the nasopharyngeal muscles which would cause encroachment on the air shadow.

Two sets of structures are to be carefully studied in the base view: the first one (and the one that usually receives the most attention) is the osseous structure of the base of the skull. The second is the soft tissue and the air shadows of the nasopharynx. The latter are too often neglected.

It is our custom to take stereoscopic views at any time that examination of the base of the skull is indicated on clinical grounds, in order to visualize the bony structures and the air shadows of the nasopharynx to best advantage. By taking a single radiograph of the base, it is often difficult to determine what a given shadow represents. It is also possible to have venous channels and arterial grooves as well as venous lakes of the cal-

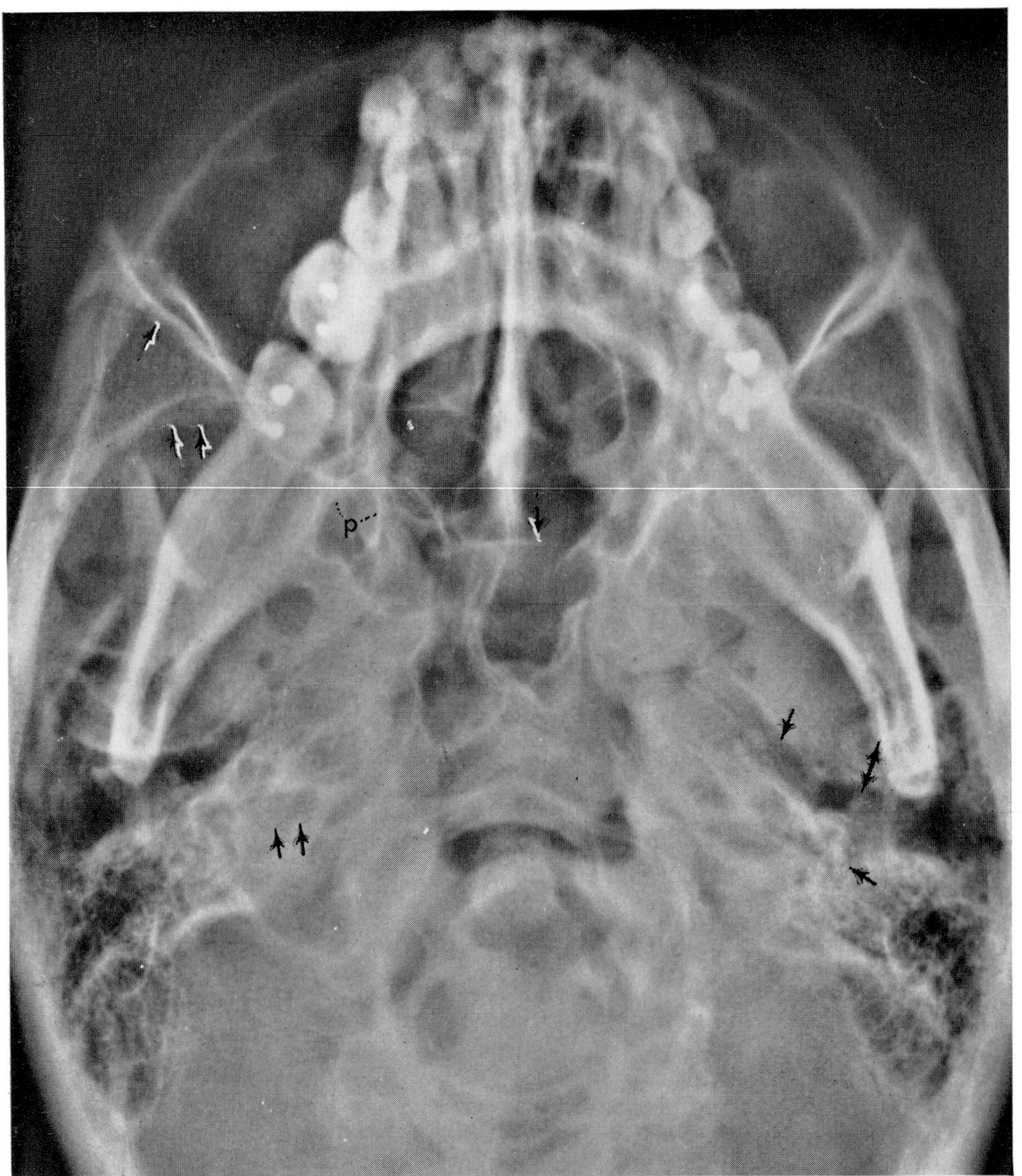

Fig. 34.—Normal Full Axial View of the Skull

The upper arrow points at the posterolateral wall of the orbit (and posterior margin of the inferior orbital fissure). This line crosses the lateral wall of the maxillary antrum forming an "X" with this line. Behind the arrow the arched anterior margin of the middle fossa is shown. The posterior margin of the lesser wing of the sphenoid is actually behind the denser anterior margin of the middle fossa and is shown by double arrows. The arrow pointing downward in the center of the skull indicates the transverse outline of the anterior margin of the sella turcica. This should not be confused with the sinus plate of the sphenoid and ethmoid sinuses. The foramen ovale on the patient's left side is crossed by a radiolucent line that simulates a fracture. It actually represents a vascular groove on the vault projected over the foramen. Stereoscopic views demonstrated a shift of this line in relation to the foramen ovale. The arrow behind the foramen spinosum points out the radiolucency of the eustachian tube. The external auditory canal is well shown just behind the condyle of the mandible and the middle ear ossicles are partially visualized (*crossed arrow*). The internal acoustic canal is shown on both sides, but as is usually the case, its shadow is not very conspicuous (*double posterior arrows*). (p) points at the wings of the pterygoid process. The most posterior arrow on the left side points to the inner ear structures, the semicircular canals.

(Revised 1963)

varia superimposed on the shadows of the base, which can be confusing and could be mistaken for a pathologic process. Stereoscopically, these shadows can easily be resolved (fig. 34).

Bony structures and the shadows of the paranasal sinuses. These can be studied best by examining the picture in Figure 34. However, several structures, listed below, should receive special scrutiny in every instance.

1. The septa of the ethmoid cells and the medial walls of the maxillary sinuses.

2. The inferior orbital fissure. Two lines are seen here which are partly superimposed on each other; the more anterior one is usually S-shaped and represents the maxillary antrum, and the more posterior represents the orbital surface of the greater wing of the sphenoid and the posterior margin of the inferior orbital fissure (fig. 34).

3. The sphenoid ridge. Behind the inferior orbital fissure on each side, a curvilinear shadow concave backward can be seen which is the lesser wing of the sphenoid in its medial two-thirds, and the greater wing in its lateral one-third. Actually the lateral aspect of the horizontal plate of the frontal bone joins the greater wing laterally, but most of this portion of the shadow (*i.e.*, the outer third) is produced by the greater wing of the sphenoid as proved by the fact that it disappears when the sphenoid bone is removed (Etter, 1955). The curvilinear posterior margin of the sphenoid ridge ends medially in the anterior clinoid processes. The anterior clinoid processes usually are not visible because they are mostly obscured by the sphenoid sinuses and the pterygoid processes. A transverse dense line is usually seen in most cases in the midline corresponding to the anterior margin of the sella turcica. This is more conspicuous when the sella is round in configuration, as seen in lateral view. If the anterior portion of the floor of the sella turcica slopes backwards, it would not produce a shadow such as that shown in Figures 34 and 38. The importance of getting used to looking at this shadow is that in patients where there is enlargement of the sella turcica resulting from an intrasellar mass, this shadow is almost always well seen and longer (fig. 84).

(Revised 1963)

4. Sphenoid sinuses. The outline of the dense sinus plate of the sphenoid sinuses should be carefully scrutinized in all cases. This is particularly important when one is trying to detect early bone destruction in patients who have a nasopharyngeal or sphenoid sinus carcinoma. Like all sinuses, the size and shape of the sphenoid sinuses are extremely variable; the main septum, which always separates the right from the left sphenoid sinus, may be considerably deviated to one side.

5. The pterygoid processes are projected over the medial portion of the sphenoid ridge and partly obscure the shadows of the anterior clinoid processes. The short medial and the larger lateral pterygoid laminae are sometimes clearly visible and at other times cannot be adequately visualized; however, the general density produced by the base of the pterygoid process is usually visible. It should be remembered that the base of the pterygoid process makes a small "U," whereas the laminae, particularly the lateral lamina, flare lateralward (figs. 34, 35, and 37).

6. Foramen ovale. Behind and slightly lateral to the base of the pterygoid process is the foramen ovale. The size and shape of this foramen varies among individuals and may vary from right to left in the same individual. Sometimes the bone at the edge of the foramen ovale becomes so thin as it approaches the foramen that it does not cast a shadow on the film. In these instances stereoscopic base views usually will show the foramen and demonstrate that the bone around it is thin but intact. Laminagrams of the base are sometimes necessary to establish this point. Occasionally the foramen ovale is divided into two sections by a calcified pterygo-alar ligament. The importance of this anomaly is that, when present, it will impede the performance of a puncture through the foramen ovale to anesthetize the Gasserian ganglion used in the treatment of trigeminal neuralgia. The possibility of a coincidence of these two conditions is rare. Through the foramen ovale passes the third division of the trigeminal nerve, and, in addition, an accessory meningeal artery and sometimes the lesser superficial petrosal nerve.

Behind and slightly lateral to the foramen

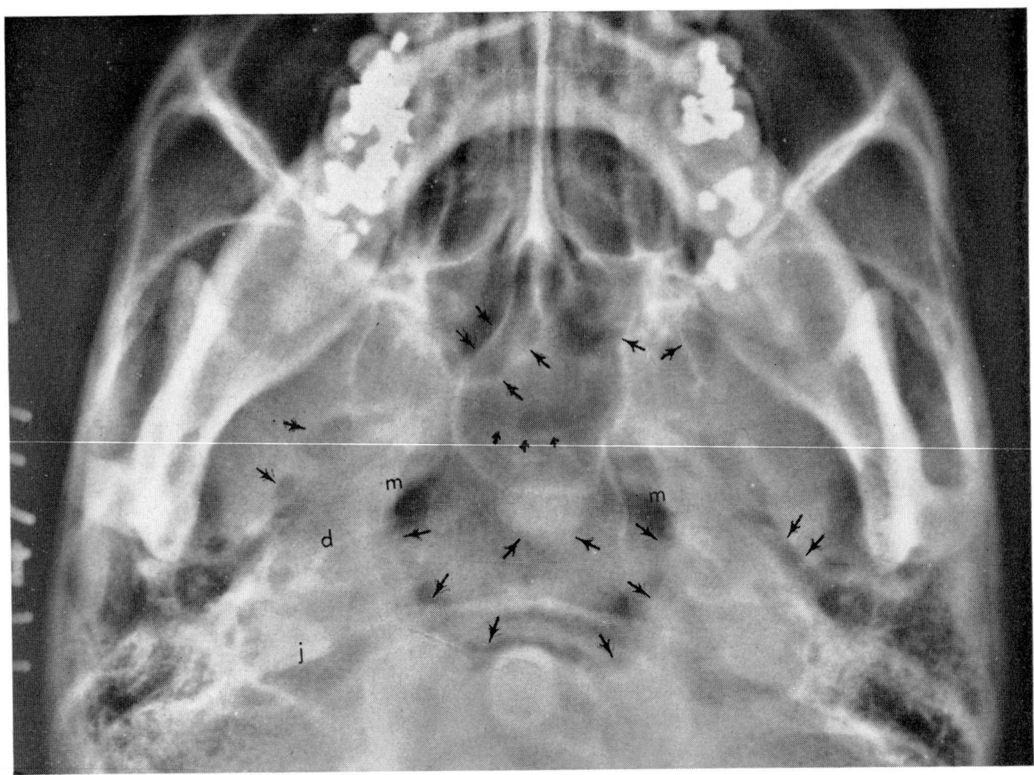

FIG. 35.—NORMAL AXIAL VIEW OF THE SKULL

The U-shaped configuration of the pterygoid process is shown (*arrows*). The foramen ovale and spinosum are seen on the reader's left side, but on the right side they are not well shown, probably due to slanting edges of the foramina on this side. The shadow of the lateral margin of the Eustachian tube is well shown (*two arrows*). The soft tissue shadow of the nasopharynx is relatively round in configuration and symmetrical (*multiple arrows*). In the middle of the air shadow of the nasopharynx, there is a rounded density representing the uvula (*two arrows*). The median septum of the sphenoid sinus is much more deviated in this case than on the preceding figure. Two contours are seen at the median septum owing to slanting of this septum where the right and the left sinuses come together so that the superior as well as the inferior margin form a separate line (*arrows*). The three vertical arrows point at the posterior margin of the pituitary fossa.

The letter (m) is at the anterolateral edge of the foramen lacerum; (d) marks the anterior margin of the external orifice of carotid canal; (j) indicates the anterior aspect of jugular foramen and also indicates the triangular posterior wall of the porus acousticus internus.

ovale is the foramen spinosum which transmits the middle meningeal artery. The foramen spinosum is usually fairly symmetrical from side to side, but sometimes one is larger than the other (fig. 84). Enlargement of the foramen spinosum is encountered when there is an increase in the size of the middle meningeal artery such as is seen in meningiomas. However, because of the fact that normally one foramen can be larger than the other, this sign is not too reliable, unless it is accompanied by enlargement of the middle meningeal grooves on the inner table of the skull. The spine of the sphenoid is posterior to the foramen spinosum and usually produces an area of increased density (fig. 35); sometimes the spine is clearly visible.

Behind the foramen spinosum an inconspicuous but clear, dense line is seen extending obliquely backward and lateralward. This represents the anterolateral margin of the Eustachian canal through which passes

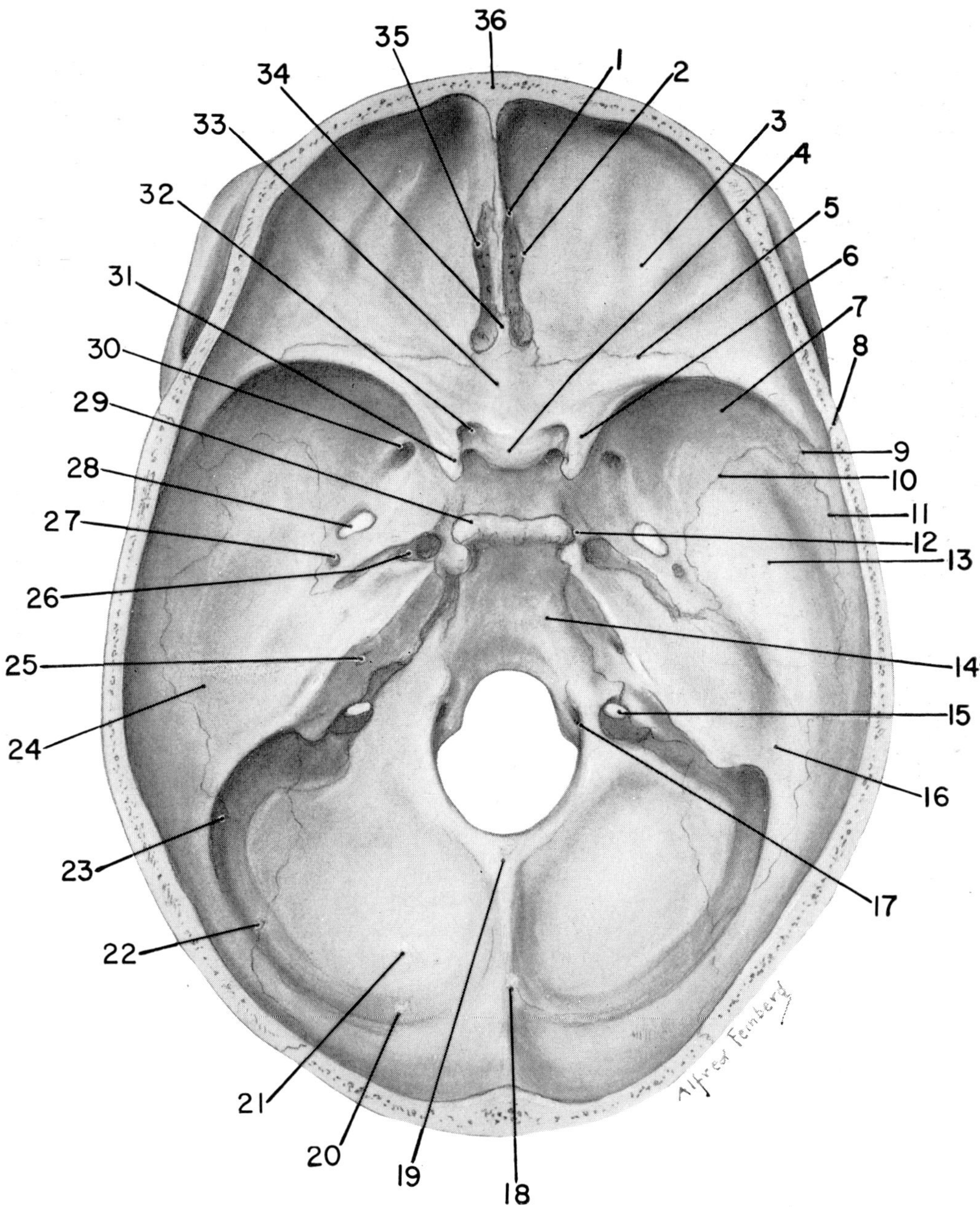

Fig. 36.—Drawing of Base of Skull, Inner Aspect

(1) crista galli. (2) fronto-ethmoidal suture. (3) frontal bone (orbital plate). (4) olivary eminence (tuberculum sellae). In front of it is the chiasmatic groove and anterior to the chiasmatic groove is the limbus sphenoidalis. (5) sphenofrontal suture. (6) lesser wing of sphenoid. (7) greater wing of sphenoid. (8) coronal suture. (9) sphenoparietal suture. (10) sphenosquamosal suture. (11) squamosal suture. (12) carotid groove. (13) squamous portion of temporal bone. (14) clivus. (15) jugular foramen. (16) petrous portion of temporal bone. (17) hypoglossal canal. (18) internal occipital protruberance. (19) internal occipital crest. (20) groove of transverse sinus. (21) occipital bone. (22) lambdoid suture. (23) sigmoid sinus groove. (24) temporal bone. (25) internal auditory meatus. (26) foramen lacerum. (27) foramen spinosum. (28) foramen ovale. (29) dorsum sellae. (30) foramen rotundum. (31) anterior clinoid process. (32) optic foramen. (33) sphenoid bone (planum sphenoidale). (34) ethmoid spine. (35) cribriform plate. (36) frontal crest.

(Revised 1963)

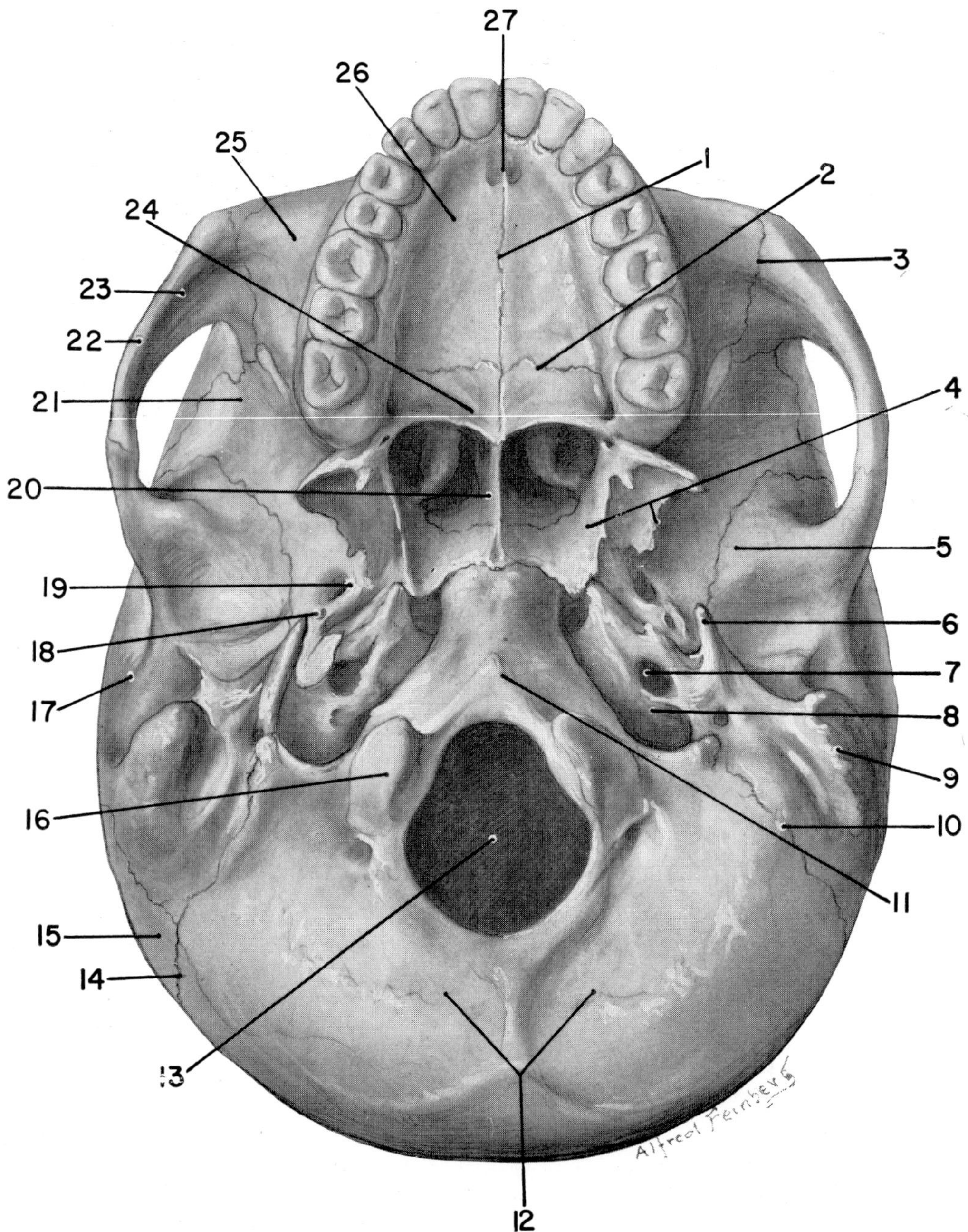

FIG. 37.—DRAWING OF BASE OF SKULL, OUTER ASPECT

(1) Median palatine suture. (2) transverse palatine suture. (3) zygomatic maxillary suture. (4) medial and lateral laminae (pyterygoid process). (5) sphenosquamosal suture. (6) styloid process. (7) external carotid foramen. (8) jugular fossa. (9) mastoid process. (10) occipitomastoid suture. (11) pars basilaris occipital bone. (12) occipital bone. (13) foramen magnum. (14) lambdoid suture. (15) parietal bone. (16) occipital condyle. (17) temporal bone. (18) foramen spinosum. (19) foramen ovale. (20) vomer. (21) sphenoid bone. (22) zygomatic arch. (23) zygomatic bone. (24) palatine bone. (25) maxilla. (26) palatine process of maxilla. (27) incisive fossa and foramen.

(Revised 1963)

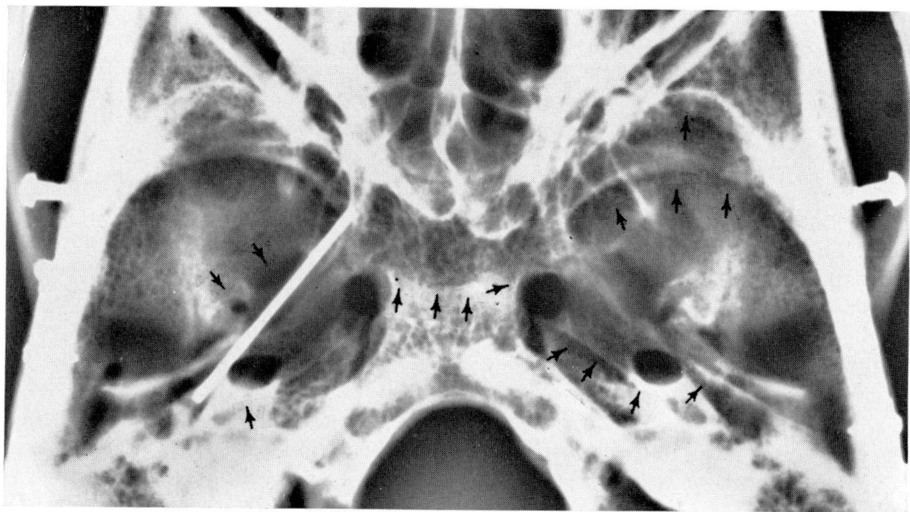

FIG. 38.—AXIAL VIEW OF SKELETON HEAD

The metal probe was put through the Eustachian canal, the counterpart of which can be seen on the opposite side (*arrow*). Because this skull has slanted margins to the foramen ovale, this structure is only faintly visualized (*arrow*). On one side the foramen spinosum is well shown and on the other side it has a slightly unusual configuration and orientation and is not shown well in this particular projection. On the actual skeleton, it is about half the size of the one on the opposite side. The outer orifice of the carotid canal is well shown on both sides (*posterior arrow*) and the carotid canal itself can be followed to the region of the foramen lacerum (*arrows*). The edge of the sphenoid ridge (3 *arrows*) is visible behind the most anterior aspect of the middle fossa (*forward arrow*). The three vertical arrows in the center point at the posterior aspect of the pituitary fossa.

the Eustachian tube in going from the tympanic cavity to the nasopharynx (figs. 34, 35, and 38).

7. *The foramen lacerum* is not clearly outlined in many instances except for its medial portion, which often presents a very sharp, punched-out, margin produced by the internal carotid artery as it curves to enter the cavernous sinus (fig. 38). It should be remembered that the internal carotid artery does not pass through the foramen lacerum, but it only passes over it on the endocranial aspect. The carotid canal of the petrous bone is usually not clearly seen on ordinary radiographs unless looked for carefully. Its location can be approximated by following it along the long axis of the petrous tip starting at the medial margin of the foramen lacerum if the latter is visible.

8. *The clivus and foramen magnum.* The lateral margin of the clivus sometimes is well shown on the films (fig. 35). The clivus ends posteriorly in the anterior margin of the foramen magnum. The base view is usually not very satisfactory for study of the foramen magnum because its outlines are covered by the first and second cervical vertebrae. However, a view of the approximate relationship of the atlas and the odontoid process of the second cervical vertebra with the foramen magnum is obtained. The shadow of the anterior arch of the atlas usually overlies the anterior margin of the foramen magnum (fig. 34). Attention is called to a shadow that often simulates that of the anterior arch of the atlas but is slightly thinner than it. This shadow represents the body of the hyoid bone; sometimes the calcified thyroid cartilage will be projected in this region.

9. *Jugular fossa.* The jugular fossa and jugular foramen on each side are situated at the junction of the petrous portion of the temporal bone and the occipital bone. They are usually poorly delineated in this view, but the general location of these structures is usually visible because a radiolucent area is

(*Revised 1963*)

present (fig. 35). Asymmetry in the sizes of the jugular fossae is occasionally present, which may lead to an erroneous diagnosis of a mass lesion eroding the bone (Shapiro and Janzen, 1960). Behind and slightly lateral to the jugular foramen is the groove of the lateral sinus which in some instances is very conspicuous and in others is not seen (figs. 36 and 38). The jugular foramen is studied in greater detail elsewhere (p. 1.131).

10. Some variants of the basal foramina. As mentioned previously, the *foramen ovale* can be larger on one side than on the other and its margins can be indistinct throughout or only on one side. Sometimes stereoscopic views will show the foramen well in these cases and at other times a film made with slight tilt of the head or of the central ray (usually accomplished by the stereoscopic shift of the tube), will show the foramen. The foramen ovale cannot be considered as showing erosion unless it is clearly enlarged, has become rounded in configuration, and its bony margins have become ragged. The so-called double foramen ovale may be essentially produced by an overlying calcified pterygospinous ligament, but at other times an actual bony ridge is seen through it which does not have the appearance of a calcified ligament.

The *foramen spinosum* can be asymmetrical in size in normal cases, as mentioned previously; it may lie at the edge of the posterior margin of the greater wing of the sphenoid so that its posterior margin is incomplete; or it could be absent occasionally. Occasionally it may not be separated from the foramen ovale.

The *foramen rotundum* is not usually visualized on base views of the skull because it forms an angle of approximately 70° with the plane of the base. For this reason it is visible in an inclined posteroanterior view or in a modified Waters view (see below for definition of this view), as demonstrated in Figure 26. The authors have seen at least one case in which the foramen rotundum was much larger on one side than on the other, and surgical exploration did not show evidence of a tumor. Nevertheless, clinically the patient had symptoms compatible with a lesion involving the second division of the trigeminal nerve. Because of failure to reveal a causative factor for the enlargement of the foramen it was considered to be a congenital anomaly, although the possibility of a small meningocele, which could have been overlooked at the time of surgery, cannot be excluded.

The inconstant *condyloid foramen* situated behind the condyle of the occipital bone is sometimes seen in the base view but is more easily shown in half axial projection.

The shadows connected with the petrous pyramid and other temporal bone structures will be studied together under "Local Bone Erosions—The Petrous Pyramids" (p. 1.118).

Nasopharyngeal soft tissue shadow. The second set of structures to be studied in the base view is the soft tissues and the air shadows of the nasopharynx. A careful study of these shadows and an understanding of the physiology of the muscles of the nasopharynx are helpful in the interpretation of the base views of the skull. The soft tissues of the nasopharynx are affected early in malignant lesions, namely, carcinomas of the nasopharynx. The pharyngeal constrictor muscles tend to narrow the air shadow of the nasopharynx when they are in a state of contraction. When they are relaxed, the nasopharyngeal shadow is wider. If a patient is asked to stop breathing, he will usually constrict the glottis and may or may not do a slight Valsalva maneuver subconsciously, but will probably also constrict his pharyngeal muscles. The same applies when the patient is asked to breathe through the mouth. Breathing through the mouth entails movement of the soft palate backward against the posterior pharyngeal wall. This movement usually causes a simultaneous contraction of the pharyngeal constrictors so that the air is deviated toward the mouth. On the other hand, if the patient is asked to breathe through his nose, he will relax his soft palate, which will drop forward; and the pharnygeal constrictors and the shadows of the nasopharynx filled with air will be shown in their relaxed state. In order to ascertain whether or not pharyngeal asymmetry is pathologic, it is sometimes necessary to place the naso-

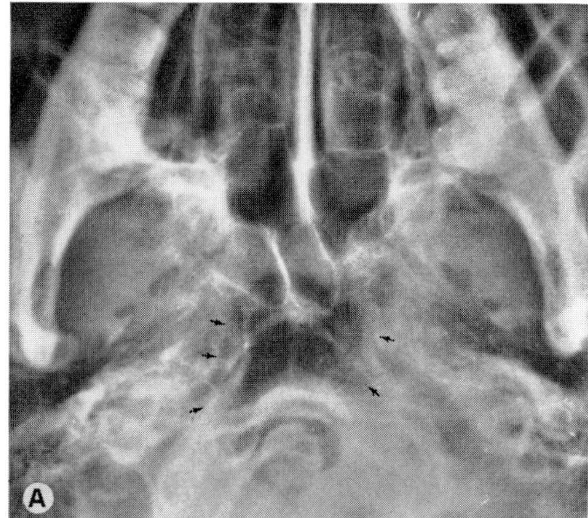

FIG. 39.—APPEARANCE OF THE NASOPHARYNGEAL SOFT TISSUE SHADOW IN VARIOUS PHASES OF RESPIRATION

(A) Patient was holding breath. (B) Patient was breathing through the nose. (C) Patient was performing "nose Valsalva." In the last film the patient was holding his nose with his fingers and blowing some air out to assure that the glottis was not closed involuntarily. The transverse soft tissue shadow in (C) represents the base of the tongue

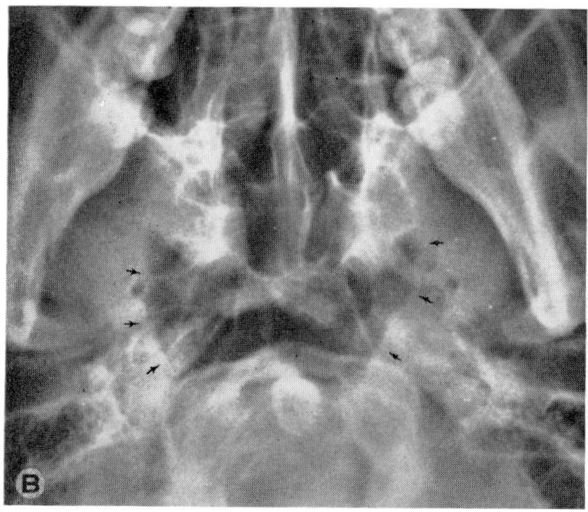

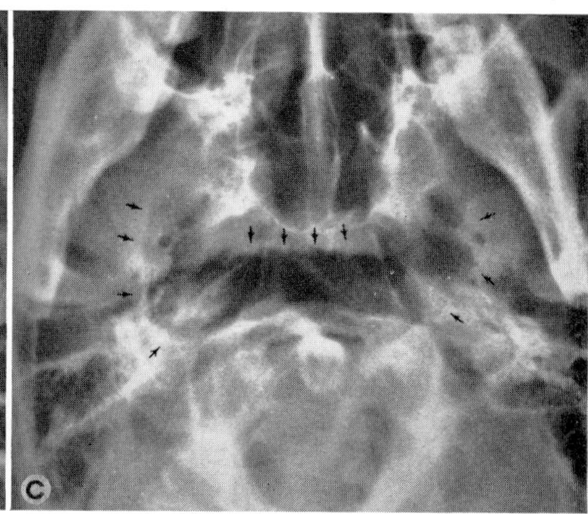

pharynx in a state of overdistention. To accomplish this state one must have the patient do a "nose Valsalva," which is performed by having the patient hold his own nose and blow out through the nose. In order to make sure that this has been accomplished, the patient should actually let air escape slowly through his nose by relaxing partially the pressure from his own fingers.

The different configurations of the nasopharyngeal soft tissue shadow visualized under these various conditions are shown in Figure 39. It will be noted that the film made during "nose breathing" and that made with "nose Valsalva" show the nasopharyngeal soft tissue shadow best. In the "nose Valsalva" there is a forward extension of the air shadow lateral to the posterior tonsillar pillars which is also present sometimes in the "nose breathing" films (fig. 39C).

(Revised 1963)

The diagnosis of nasopharyngeal carcinoma can be made in many instances before bone destruction takes place or, at least, before bone destruction is visible on the roentgenogram. It may also help in directing the position from which an attempt at taking a biopsy can be made. Biopsy of nasopharyngeal tumors is always difficult in that so many cases that are clear-cut clinically, radiologically show negative results. Treatment had to be administered in the absence of a positive biopsy in over 30 per cent of the cases in our experience.

The subaxial view (central beam perpendicular to orbitomeatal line) is used mainly to show the foramen magnum re-

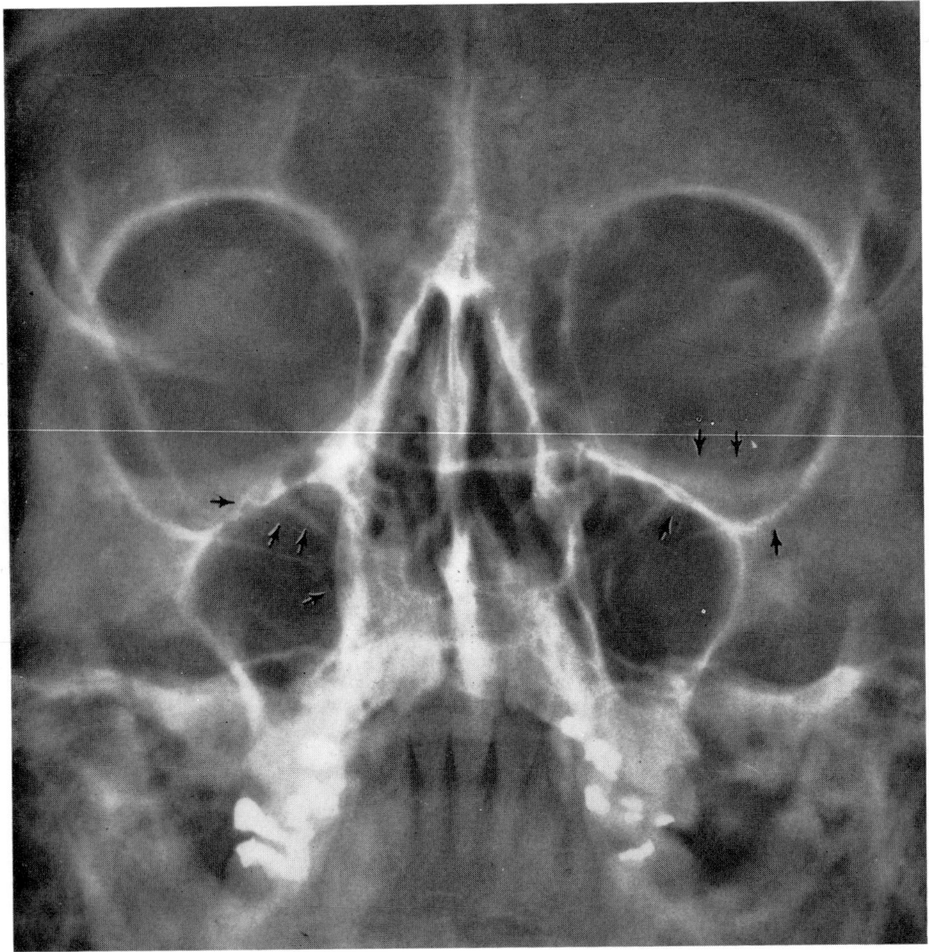

FIG. 40.—WATERS VIEW OF SKULL

In this projection the outline of the orbits are unusually well shown. The superior border of the orbit is superimposed on the orbital roof almost completely, but the lower (palpable) border (*arrows*) is well shown and distinct from the floor of the orbit which represents the roof of the maxillary antrum (*lower arrows*). The Waters view is the standard film for the maxillary sinuses. The infraorbital foramen is shown well and an elevation on the roof of the maxillary antrum is also well shown behind this foramen (*arrows*). The foramen rotundum is not usually well shown in Waters views and may be shown better on inclined posteroanterior views or in a Waters view taken with a 30° inclination of the orbitomeatal line.

gion and the atlas. Similar results may be obtained by a Waters view made at a 45° angle (fig. 41).

Waters View

The anatomy of the facial bones and sinuses will be described only briefly because it is not considered to be within the scope of this work. However, one of the standard views that are used to study the sinuses, the Waters view, is sometimes useful in studying certain lesions involving particularly the base of the skull and the floor of the anterior fossa.

The Waters view is made by placing the orbitomeatal line at an angle of 37° with the plane of the film. Usually the chin touches the film and the tip of the nose is a variable distance away from the film, depending upon the configuration of the patient's face (fig.

(*Revised 1963*)

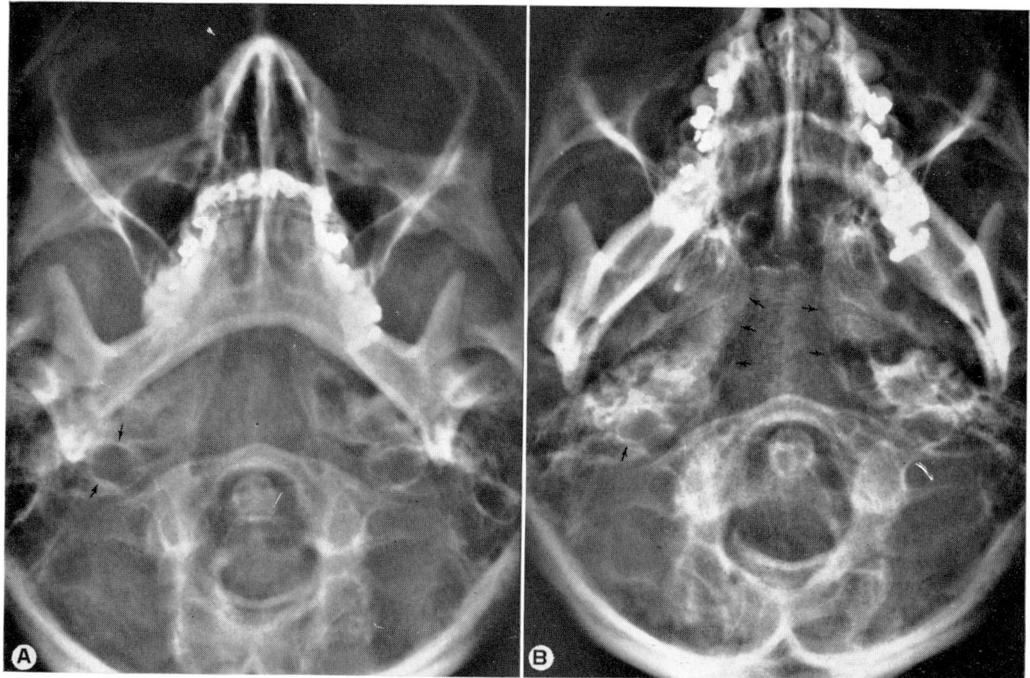

FIG. 41.—EXAGGERATED WATERS PROJECTION (45° ANGULATION OF ORBITOMEATAL LINE), AND SUBAXIAL VIEWS OF SKULL

These films are usually made to study the posterior aspect of the base of the skull, the atlas, the foramen magnum region, and the jugular foramen on each side. Compare with appearance noted in Fig. 34 where the posterior aspect of the base of the skull is not well shown. In (A), an exaggerated Waters projection, the atlas is unusually well shown, and the jugular foramen is clearly demarcated on both sides (*arrows*). (B) is a subaxial view of the skull which is somewhat similar to (A) but made in the anteroposterior direction. This view brings out the margins of the clivus much more clearly than the full axial view because the x-ray beam is almost perpendicular to the clivus. At the medial margin of the foramen lacerum, there is an indentation produced by the internal carotid artery (*anterior arrows*) The jugular foramen is also well shown in this projection.

40). The Waters view gives an unusually clear picture of the roofs of the orbits, but because the bone here is rather thin, it does not cast much of a shadow since it is superimposed on the bones of the vault. However, when there is bone destruction in the roof of the orbit, such as may be seen in mucoceles of the frontal sinuses, in carcinomas of the lacrimal gland, and in some cases of meningiomas and epidermoids, it will be clearly shown in this view. These findings may also be shown in other views, particularly in those taken in an inclined posteroanterior projection. The lower margin of the orbit is usually very well shown in this view (fig. 40). The superior orbital fissure is not well shown because it is partly obscured by the inferior orbital border. The foramen rotundum is often shown in Waters projection but it is more frequently seen in a modified Waters view which is made by decreasing the angle of the orbitomeatal line to about 25°; this frequently may be accomplished by having the nose and the chin touch the film without angling the tube. In the modified Waters projection, the petrous pyramids obscure the lower third of the maxillary antrum whereas in the Waters projection, the petrous pyramids are just below the lowest portion of the maxillary antrum.

An exaggerated Waters view is made by using an angle of about 45° of the orbitomeatal line with the plane of the film. In this way the mandible clears the posterior portion of the base of the skull more completely and it is a good way to study, anatomically, the atlas and its relation with the foramen magnum as well as the jugular foramen and fossa (fig. 41).

In order to visualize the sphenoid sinuses, an open-mouth Waters view is often taken, which usually results in an exaggerated Waters projection. The exaggerated Waters is closer to a base view and will demonstrate some of the structures that are shown in these projections.

Congenital Anomalies

PREMATURE CRANIOSYNOSTOSIS

Premature craniosynostosis refers to a fusion across the suture line that occurs in infancy or early childhood. Normally the sutures remain open until adult life, but partial closure (bridging) of some of the sutures begins at about age 22 so that some or all of the sutures are completely fused in the later decades of life. The inner aspect of the suture may complete its closure before the outer aspect. There is considerable individual variation (Todd and Lyon, 1924, 1925).

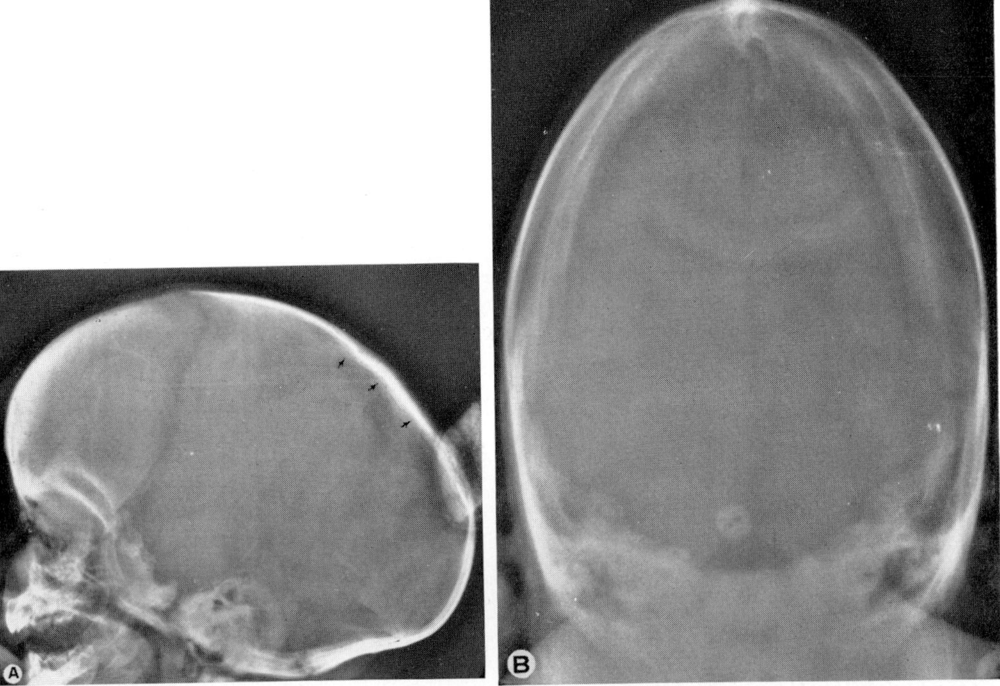

FIG. 42.—PREMATURE CLOSURE OF THE SAGITTAL SUTURE

The lateral view (A) demonstrates the abnormal dolichocephaly. The thickened bone along the parietal bone particularly in its posterior half (*arrows*) indicate that that was the last portion of the suture to close. The thinner portion of the bone is usually at the site where the earliest closure took place. The frontal projection (B) shows a ridge of bone along the sagittal suture. The sagittal suture appeared to be completely closed at the time of the examination.

R621-S871

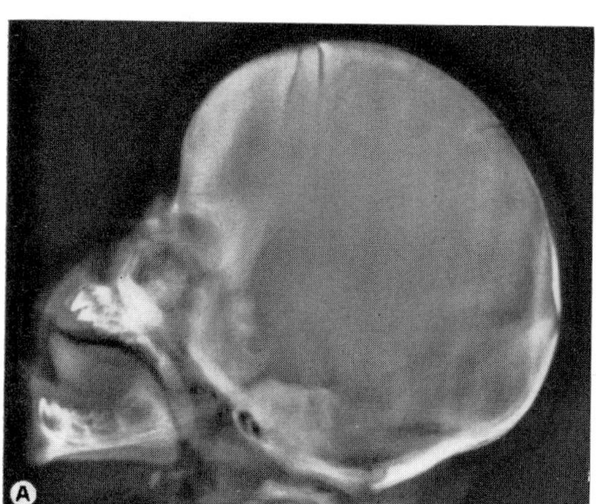

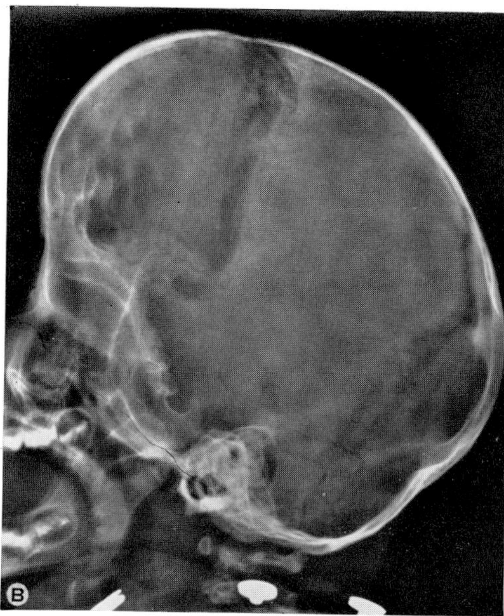

Fig. 43.—Premature Closure of the Coronal Suture in an 8-day-old Infant

The lower portion of the coronal suture is closed on both sides, but the upper portion is still open. The head is small, but because of the age of the child, this is not necessarily abnormal. The basal angle measured 159° in (A). A film made at 17 months of age (B) postoperatively, shows the growth of the head with little change in the general shape, which is often the case in coronal suture craniosynostosis. The basal angle at this time measured 146°.

Craniosynostosis is usually present at birth or, less commonly, it occurs after birth. Only one suture may be closed, but in other cases all of the sutures may be prematurely fused. Premature closure of the cranial sutures occurs more commonly in males than in females; the proportion has been stated to be as high as 5 to 1. In the group of cases reported by Ingraham and Matson (1954) there were 76 male and 44 female patients.

The suture that closes prematurely determines the shape that the head will acquire. Premature closure of the sagittal (interparietal) suture, termed the *dolichocephalic type* of craniostenosis, causes an elongated head, because the skull cannot grow in a direction perpendicular to the closed suture and the missing area of growth must be compensated for by the other sutures in order to maintain the skull volume required by the growing brain. Premature closure of the coronal or of the lambdoidal sutures causes a short head, the *brachycephalic type* of craniostenosis. In the latter cases the head is short and also high (turricephaly) (figs. 43 and 48). In the *generalized type* of craniostenosis, the shape will depend on which suture or sutures close first. If the coronal suture is the first to close, the head will have a brachycephalic configuration with a high vertical diameter of the skull. On the other hand, if all of the sutures close at the same time, the head will have a normal shape (fig. 45). Plagiocephaly, that is, an irregularly shaped skull, is common in the generalized croniostenoses because not all the sutures close at the same time. Plagiocephaly is also often due to premature closure of one-half of either the coronal or the lambdoidal sutures (figs. 44, 46, and 47).

The classification of premature synostoses proposed by Simmons and Peyton (1947) is as follows.

Complete early premature synostosis of the cranial sutures (oxycephaly, turricephaly, and Turmschadël). This includes (1) oxycephaly without facial deformity; (2) craniofacial dysostosis of Crouzon; (3) acro-

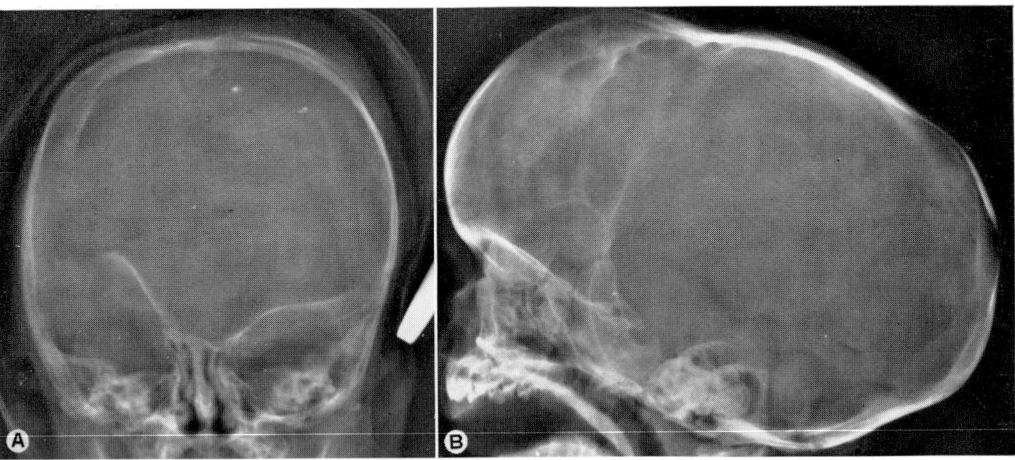

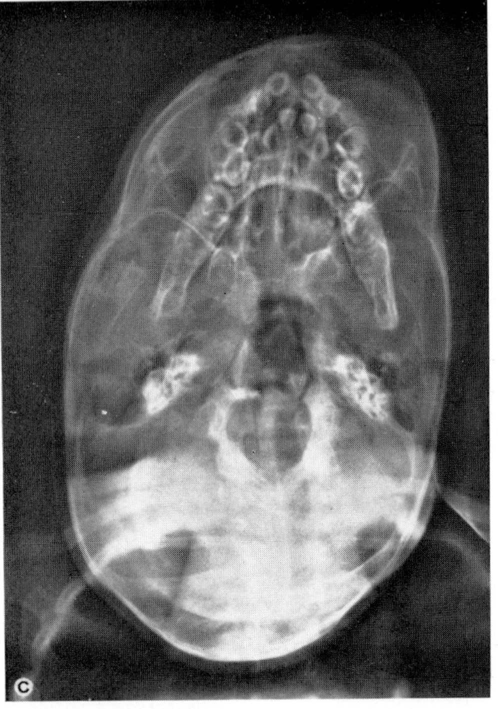

FIG. 44.—PREMATURE CLOSURE OF ONE-HALF OF THE CORONAL SUTURE AND OF THE SAGITTAL SUTURE IN A 3-MONTH-OLD GIRL

The posteroanterior film (A) reveals the typical elevation of the supraorbital ridge which is usually associated with early premature synostosis of the coronal suture. The sagittal suture is fused across. The lateral view (B) demonstrates abnormal dolichocephaly due to the premature closure of the sagittal suture. Her twin sister also had premature closure of the sutures but not in the same locations as these. It is probable that if left alone, the child may well develop generalized premature craniosynostosis. However, following surgical intervention, a follow-up revealed no further closure of the sutures at least for a few years. The base view (C) demonstrates a marked degree of asymmetry which was not shown in the frontal film.

cephalosyndactylism; and (4) delayed oxycephaly (onset after birth).

Incomplete early synostosis of the cranial sutures. This includes (1) scaphocephaly, premature closure of the sagittal suture (this may also be called dolichocephalic craniostenosis); (2) brachycephaly, premature closure of the coronal suture or of the coronal and lambdoidal sutures (brachycephalic craniostenosis); (3) plagiocephaly, asymmetrical premature closure of the sutures, usually the coronal or the lambdoidal, more frequently the former; (4) mixed.

Late premature synostosis of the cranial sutures occurs after the skull has reached adult or nearly adult size so that no deformities and no symptoms result. This condition is usually of no clinical significance.

(*Revised 1963*)

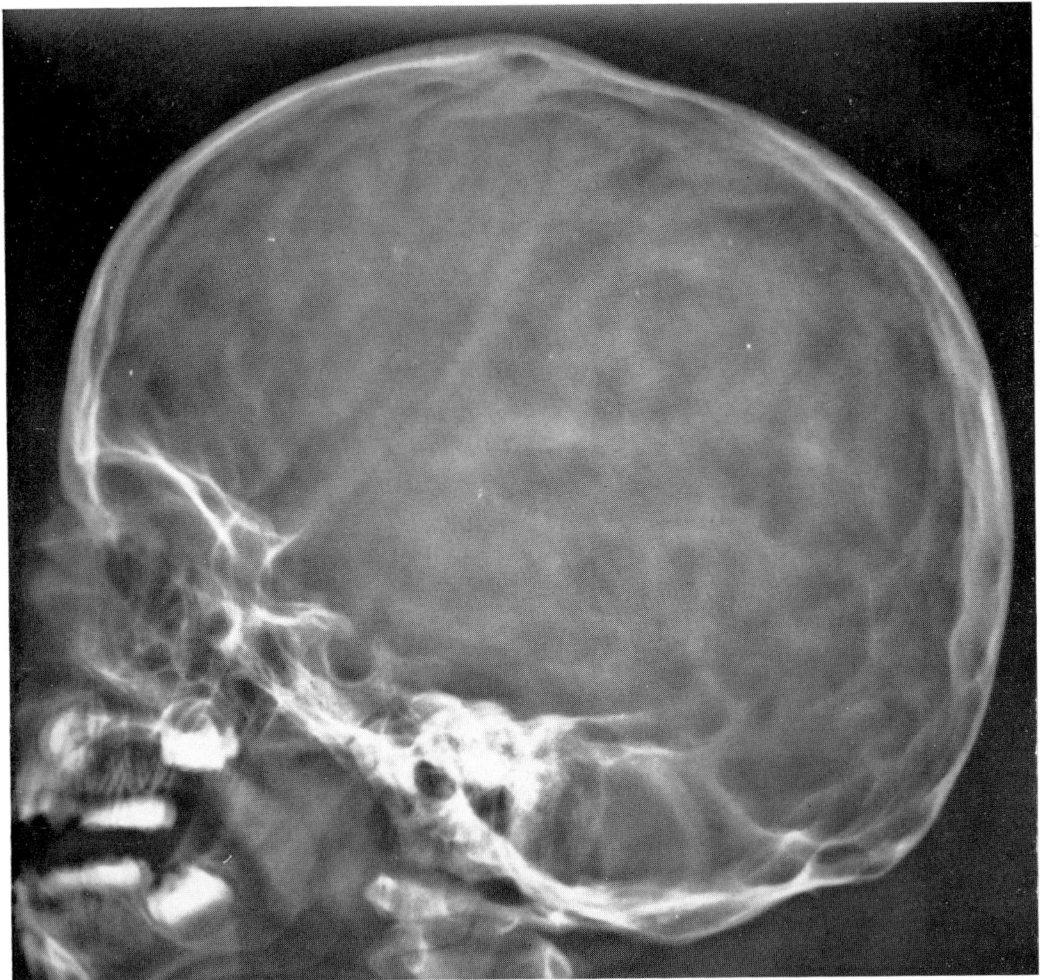

FIG. 45.—GENERALIZED CRANIOSYNOSTOSIS WITH FAIRLY GOOD PRESERVATION OF NORMAL SHAPE OF HEAD IN 2-YEAR-OLD CHILD

No suture lines are visualized. There is evidence of exaggerated convolutional markings due to a relative degree of craniostenosis.

Early premature synostosis. It is probable that untreated premature synostosis, particularly of the generalized type, occurring in the prenatal or immediate postnatal period, may hamper the normal growth of the brain sufficiently to produce mental retardation. It is well known that cranial nerve symptoms may appear as a result of abnormal growth, particularly diminished vision or even blindness. In the operated group of cases reported by Mount (1961), at least 90 per cent had an average intelligence followed for a period up to 10 years of age, longer in some cases. Therefore, surgical intervention may be indicated early not only to prevent the deformity and to improve the appearance of the child but also to prevent damage to the brain. The best time for surgical intervention is not agreed upon by all workers, but it would appear that no later than 4 to 5 months of age is the best, and some advocate operation as soon as the diagnosis is made and the child is over two months of age. This can easily be understood

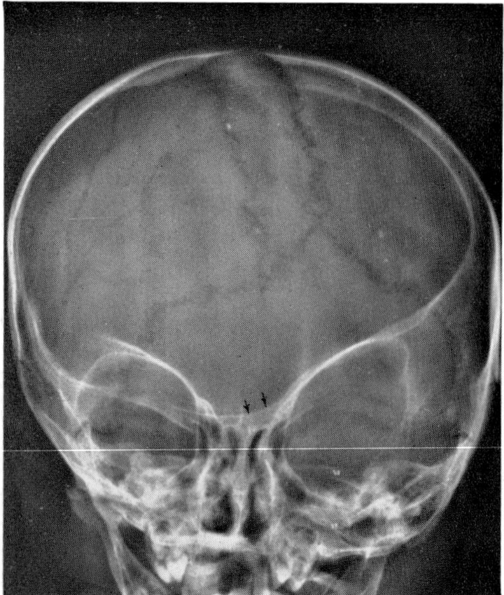

FIG. 46.—PLAGIOCEPHALY DUE TO PREMATURE CLOSURE OF ONE-HALF OF THE CORONAL SUTURE

There is elevation of the superior margin of the orbit and of the sphenoid ridge on the occluded side. On this side the child presented a flattened portion of the forehead. The planum sphenoidale (*arrow*) is also elevated on the occluded side.

if one remembers that the brain doubles its weight in the first seven or eight months of life and triples its weight by the age of two and one-half years, according to Copolletta and Wolbach (1933).

The etiology of this condition is evidently the result of an embryologic disturbance. The most accepted theory is that of a displacement of the ossification centers, which come closer to the suture line and fuse across at one point in the suture, which later leads to closure of the entire suture. However, this theory does not explain the generalized premature closure of the sutures. Moss (1959) suggests that generalized premature synostosis may be due to abnormal attachments of the dura mater at the base of the skull during embryologic development owing to malformed lesser wings of the sphenoid and crista galli. Craniosynostosis occurs in children with hypophosphatasia (Currarino *et al.*, 1957), which suggests that there may be various etiologic factors (fig. 48).

In Crouzon's disease, there is usually a generalized craniosynostosis and hypoplasia of the facial bones. The term acrocephalosyndactylism is applied to the cases where craniosynostosis is associated with anomalies of the fingers and toes; other anomalies may also be encountered (figs. 48D, E and F).

Radiologic findings. The radiologic findings are those of abnormal shapes which are obvious at first glance. Attention is called to the fact that the prematurely closed suture may appear to be open on the films and that only a very small segment of it may be fused across. It is therefore necessary to visualize the entire extent of all of the sutures when a search is being made for premature synostosis (fig. 43). The portion of the suture that has not fused will continue to grow and to pile up bone adjacent to the suture line, which will give the bone edge a "squared" appearance instead of the tapering configuration of the bone in the normally growing suture. The suture will eventually close throughout its length. Sometimes the overgrowth is quite pronounced and an actual ridge can be palpated by the examining finger along the closing or closed suture (fig. 42). Once the suture is closed, the tendency is for the bone to smooth out and the ridge to disappear. In examining the patient for possible premature synostosis, the standard anteroposterior and lateral projections should be made, and in addition, oblique views in the anteroposterior projection and oblique base views may be necessary in order to visualize the sutures throughout their entire extent. In microcephaly resulting from a hypoplastic brain, the sutures do not usually taper as they do in the normal growing skull, and various views will demonstrate the normal shape of the head and the absence of closed sutures. In some cases actual suture fusion may take place (see below).

Plagiocephaly, when resulting from a premature synostosis of one-half of the coronal suture, must be differentiated from other conditions such as a large subdural hematoma or hygroma in the middle fossa, particularly in older children. The appearance shown in Figures 44 and 46 may be compared with that demonstrated in Figures 55B and 605. As may be noted, in premature

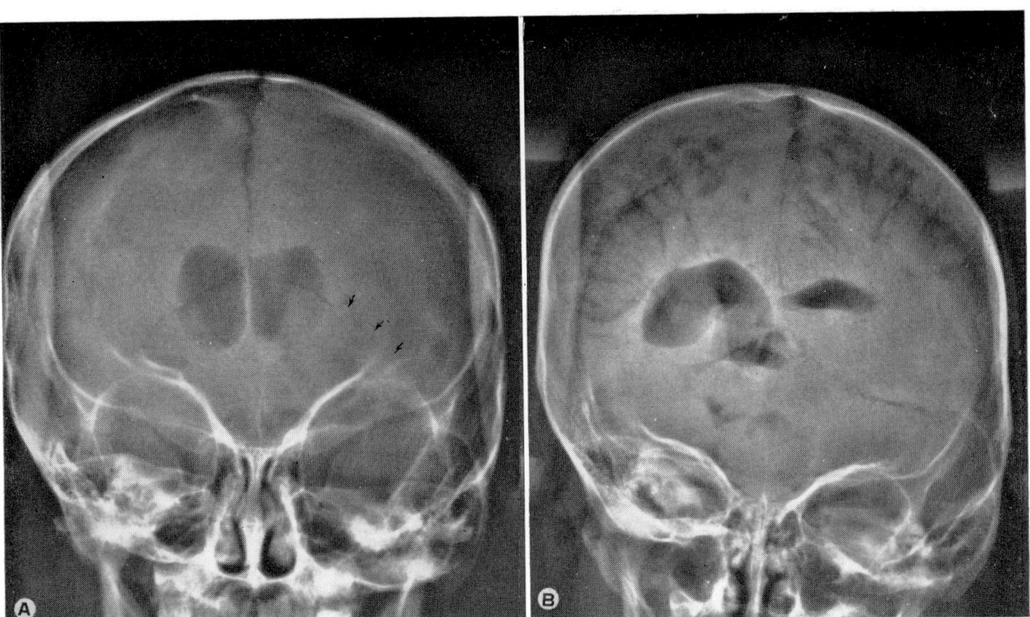

Fig. 47.—Plagiocephaly Due to Premature Synostosis of One-half of the Lambdoidal Suture

In the anteroposterior projection, the closed portion of the suture is seen (*arrows*). Although only a portion of the suture is closed, it nevertheless cannot grow. There is depression of the petrous pyramid and of the floor of the posterior fossa on this side (*arrows*). The child had a flat portion of the skull over the left occipital region. A posteroanterior projection taken in a slightly different position shows the marked asymmetry (B). Because the posterolateral aspect of the skull is unable to grow, the brain then grows downward toward the posterior fossa to compensate for the loss of space. The pneumoencephalogram was normal; it was performed because, in the presence of idiopathic convulsive seizures, cerebral hemiatrophy could not be excluded in the differential diagnosis.

synostosis of the coronal suture there is elevation of the superior lateral aspect of the orbit as well as depression of the floor of the middle fossa and the petrous pyramid. In the subdural hematomas of childhood, the sphenoid ridge is elevated but the superior and lateral aspects of the orbit are not. In addition, the suture is normal. Premature closure of one-half of the lambdoidal suture produces a plagiocephaly which should be differentiated from the cases of cranial hemihypertrophy secondary to cerebral hemiatrophy. On the side of the premature closure, the posterior aspect of the head would be flat, and on the same side there is a depression of the floor of the posterior fossa and of the petrous pyramid. This appearance may be mistaken for elevation of the petrous pyramid on the opposite side (fig. 47). It is a well known fact that cranial asymmetries are sometimes very obvious clinically and yet the radiographs will show no apparent deformity. This is particularly true in deformities localized to either the anterior or the posterior aspect of the skull, for in these cases the normal portion of the skull situated in front or behind the deformed area, whichever is the case, will tend to make the skull symmetrical. Asymmetries, however, can be very well shown on base views and on exaggerated Waters views (fig. 44).

Trigonocephaly is presumed to be a premature synostosis of the metopic suture. The presence of hypotelorism in these patients would be in favor of this hypothesis. Although Riemenschneider has reported one case of open metopic suture in a patient with trigonocephaly, it is quite possible that although the upper segment was open, the lower segment may have closed prematurely and this is sufficient to prevent growth of the entire suture. A bony ridge with increased

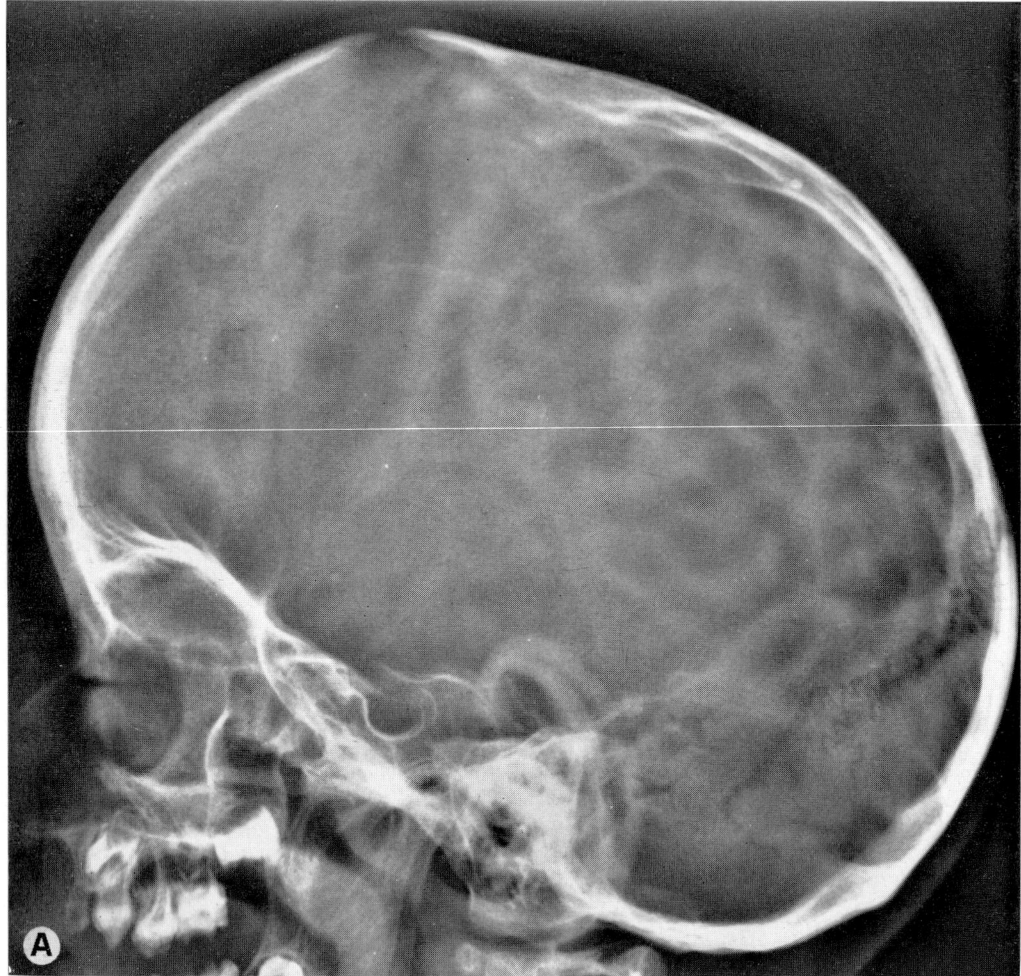

FIG. 48.—PREMATURE CRANIOSYNOSTOSIS IN A 2-YEAR-OLD CHILD WITH HYPOPHOSPHATASIA
The lateral view (A) shows closure of the coronal suture with elevation in the region of the anterior fontanelle which is still not completely closed. The frontal projection (B) shows the complete closure of the sagittal suture. A film of the knees and ankles (C) demonstrates the generalized bone changes associated with this condition.

thickness of the area of the metopic suture is seen in these cases in a manner similar to that seen in premature synostoses elsewhere (fig. 49). Welcker thought that trigonocephaly is secondary to hypoplasia of the frontal lobes, but this is not always true because patients with trigonocephaly are often normal. Moreover, trigonocephaly in milder cases may regress spontaneously. Of four cases seen by the authors, one resolved spontaneously and the others were operated upon for cosmetic reasons. At least three of these children were considered to have normal intelligence on psychological testing.

As mentioned above, in the generalized premature craniosynostosis the shape of the skull varies, probably according to which suture closes first; the head may be long and narrow, high and broad with hypertelorism, or perfectly normal in shape although small.

In the premature closure of the coronal sutures there is also an abnormality of the

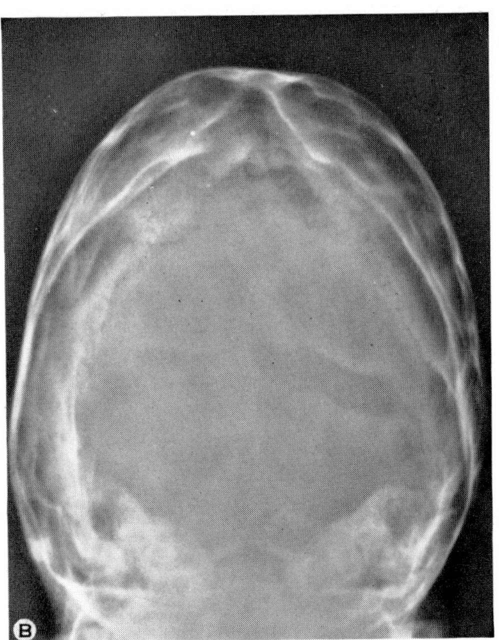

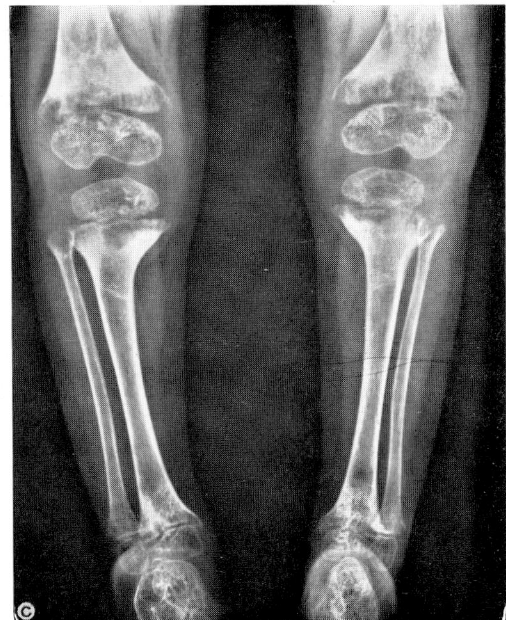

FIG. 48 B and C

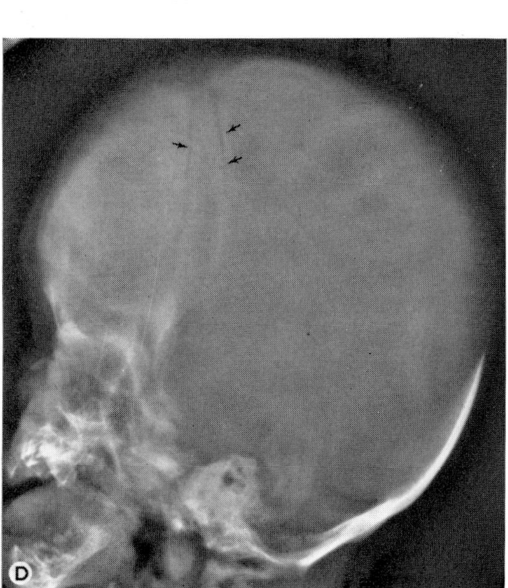

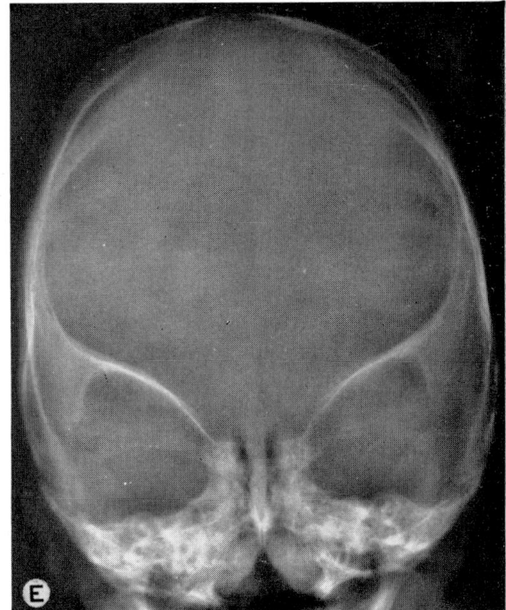

FIG. 48 (*Cont.*).—PREMATURE SYNOSTOSIS OF THE CORONAL SUTURE IN CHILD WITH ANOMALIES OF THE FINGERS AND TOES (ACROCEPHALOSYNDACTYLISM)

The lateral view (D) shows a rounded head which could be confused with hydrocephalus. However, the coronal suture is visible in its upper half and is actually denser and more prominent than usual, which is the opposite of hydrocephalus (*arrows*). The frontal projection (E) shows the typical appearance of bilateral closure of the coronal suture (compare with Fig. 46). The sagittal suture is open and its margins show tapering, growing edges. The film of the hands (F) shows the anomalies of the various fingers with bilateral syndactylism.

(Revised 1963)

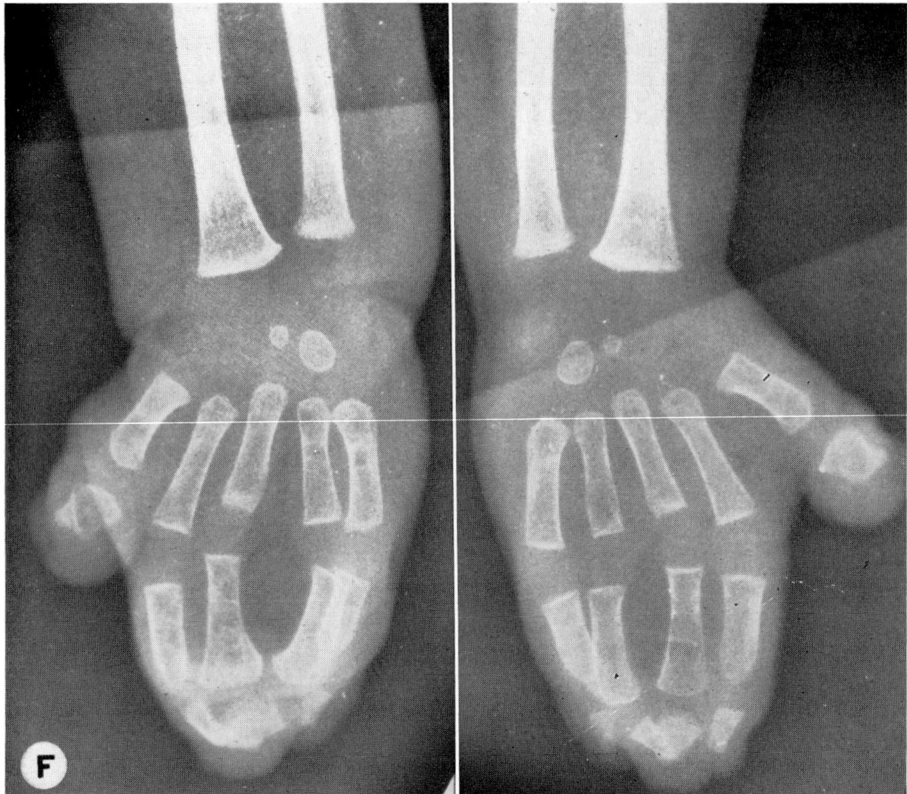

FIG. 48F

base of the skull, probably due to premature synostosis between the frontal bone and the sphenoid bones, which results in a short base of the skull; a relative degree of platybasia may be present in these cases.

The most benign form of premature synostosis is that of the sagittal or interparietal suture, and the best surgical results are seen in this type. The basal angle may be normal, it may be in the lower ranges or even below the lower limit of normal of 125°.

Evidence of long standing, increased intracranial pressure is often present in the children with generalized craniosynostosis as evidenced by exaggerated digital markings or a hammered silver appearance. Some of these patients may have a normal sella or they may have a deep or even enlarged sella turcica secondary to increased pressure.

Delayed premature synostosis. Delayed premature synostosis is not of any clinical significance. It may cause some variations in the shape of the skull which are sometimes expressive of a familial trait, and sometimes it may be a racial characteristic. For example, the tendency to premature synostosis of the lambdoidal suture in late childhood is frequently seen among inhabitants of the Middle East, who exhibit a relatively flat posterior portion of the skull with a relatively higher head posteriorly.

Secondary craniosynostosis. It is important to segregate the primary from the secondary example of premature craniosynostosis. The latter is caused by varying degrees of microcephaly which differ radiologically from those usually seen, in which the sutures become bridged. In these instances the cranial shape is always normal or may exhibit slight posterior flattening from prolonged occupation of the supine position. The head is always small. Increased convolutional markings denoting increased intracranial pressure do not develop in these cases. If surgery is

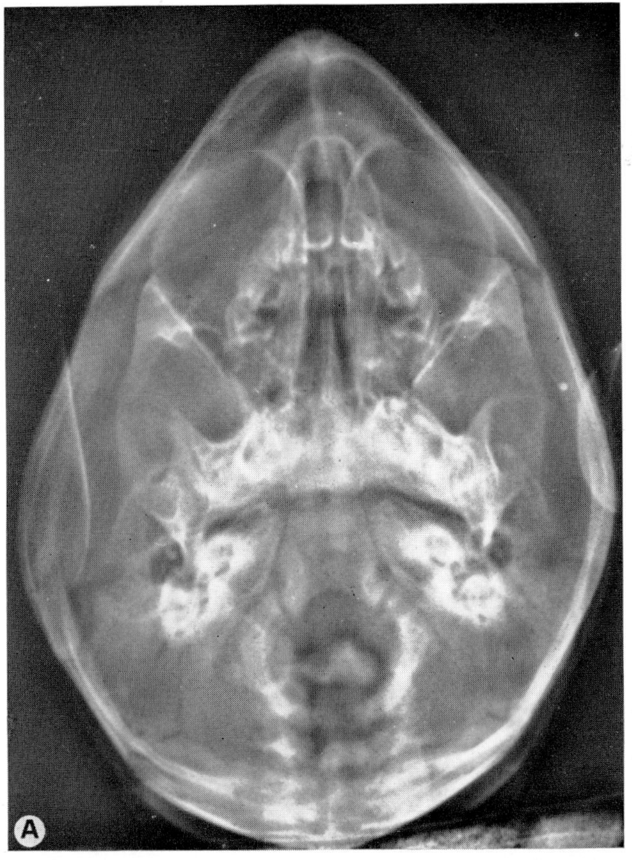

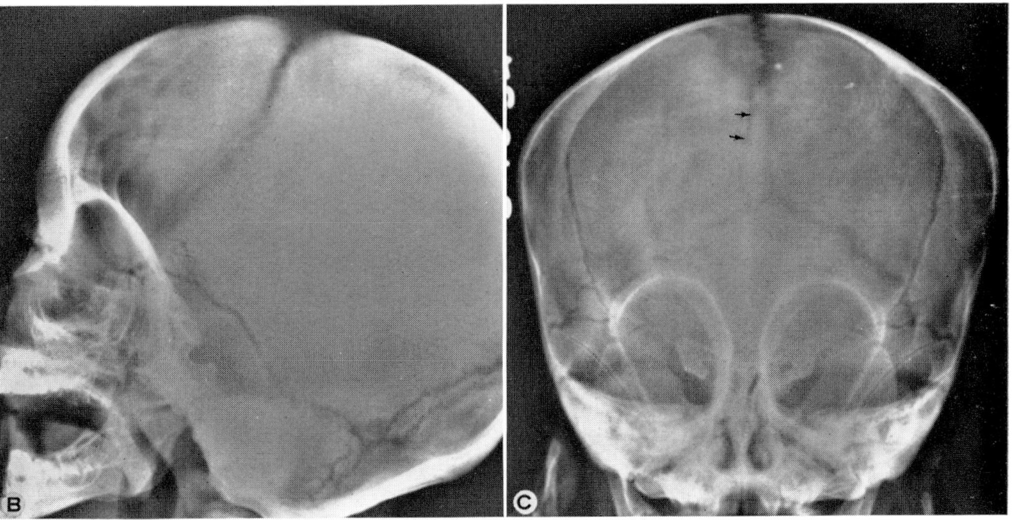

FIG. 49.—TRYGONOCEPHALY

The deformity can best be demonstrated in films made in exaggerated Waters projection (A). The increase in thickness of the bone at the metopic suture is apparent in this film in a manner similar to that seen in other premature synostoses. The lateral projection (B) demonstrates the thickening of the bone in the frontal region with relative elevation of the orbital roofs. The other sutures are normal. The frontal projection (C) shows the marked degree of hypotelorism which is presumably due to premature closure of the lower portion of the metopic suture. The upper portion of the metopic suture (*arrows*) is still open. The child had average intelligence on testing up to the age of 2 years.

(*Revised 1963*)

performed, early recurrence of bridging often takes place with no essential change in the size of the head and no improvement in the patient's condition.

PLATYBASIA

Strictly speaking, the term "platybasia" indicates a flat base of the skull. Using Welcker's basal angle, which is obtained by tracing a line from the nasion to the tuberculum sella and from here to the basion (anterior margin of the foramen magnum), a skull is called platybasic when this angle measures more than 143°. The normal limits are between 125 and 143°. However, in practice, platybasia has come to indicate the group of abnormalities encountered in the region of the foramen magnum which includes basilar impression and basilar invagination as well as other anomalies in this area, such as narrowing of the foramen magnum associated with congenital fusions of the atlas and occipital bone. *Basilar invagination* may exist without platybasia; it is found in patients who have Paget's disease, in osteogenesis imperfecta, in osteomalacia, and occasionally in patients with hyperparathyroidism, that is, in conditions that are associated with softening of the bones of the skull.

The term *basilar impression* is used to indicate an elevation of the floor of the posterior fossa of the skull, usually associated with platybasia. This anomaly is almost always associated with partial or complete atlanto-occipital fusion and often with a deformity of the foramen magnum. The upward displacement of the base of the skull can be simply evaluated in practice by using Chamberlain's line. This line extends from the hard palate to the posterior margin of the foramen magnum (fig. 50). Normally up to one-third of the odontoid process of the axis projects above this line. When there is basilar impression or basilar invagination, one-half or more of the odontoid process projects above this line. McGregor (1948) proposes the use of a line drawn from the posterior margin of the hard palate to the inferior margin of the occipital squama. According to McGregor, the tip of the odontoid process should not rise more than 4 to 5 mm. above this line. Hinck and co-authors (1961) found differences between the female and male groups in the relationship of the odontoid to this reference line, and also encountered discrepancies when their own measurements were compared with those of McGregor. Fischgold and Brégeat (1952) suggest the use of the digastric line as the plane of reference. This line is determined in the frontal projection by tracing a line from the digastric groove on one side to the digastric groove on the other side (fig. 51). It is relatively easy to find the digastric groove by taking a point medial to the base of the mastoid process. Normally this line is 11 mm. with a standard deviation of ±4 mm. (Hinck *et al.*) above the middle of the atlanto-occipital joints. In the presence of basilar impression or basilar invagination, the atlanto-occipital joint is closer to the line or it may actually lie above this line (fig. 53). If necessary, the exact anatomical landmarks may be very well outlined by means of frontal laminagrams (fig. 52). McRae (1953) traces a line from the anterior to the posterior margin of the foramen magnum. If the upper margin of the occipital squama on each side of the foramen magnum is convex upward or if it lies above the line of the foramen magnum or if the condyles are above the foramen magnum, basilar impression is present, according to McRae.

Platybasia *per se* is not necessarily associated with symptoms. When symptoms are present they are usually of a varied nature suggesting multiple sclerosis or a degenerative disease of the central nervous system such as syringomyelia. The presence of symptoms is usually associated with downward displacement of the cerebellar tonsils through the foramen magnum with consequent difficulties in the circulation of cerebrospinal fluid and long-standing pressure on the medulla and upper cervical spinal cord (Arnold-Chiari malformation). At other times there is no evidence of tonsillar herniation but there is compression of these struc-

(Revised 1963)

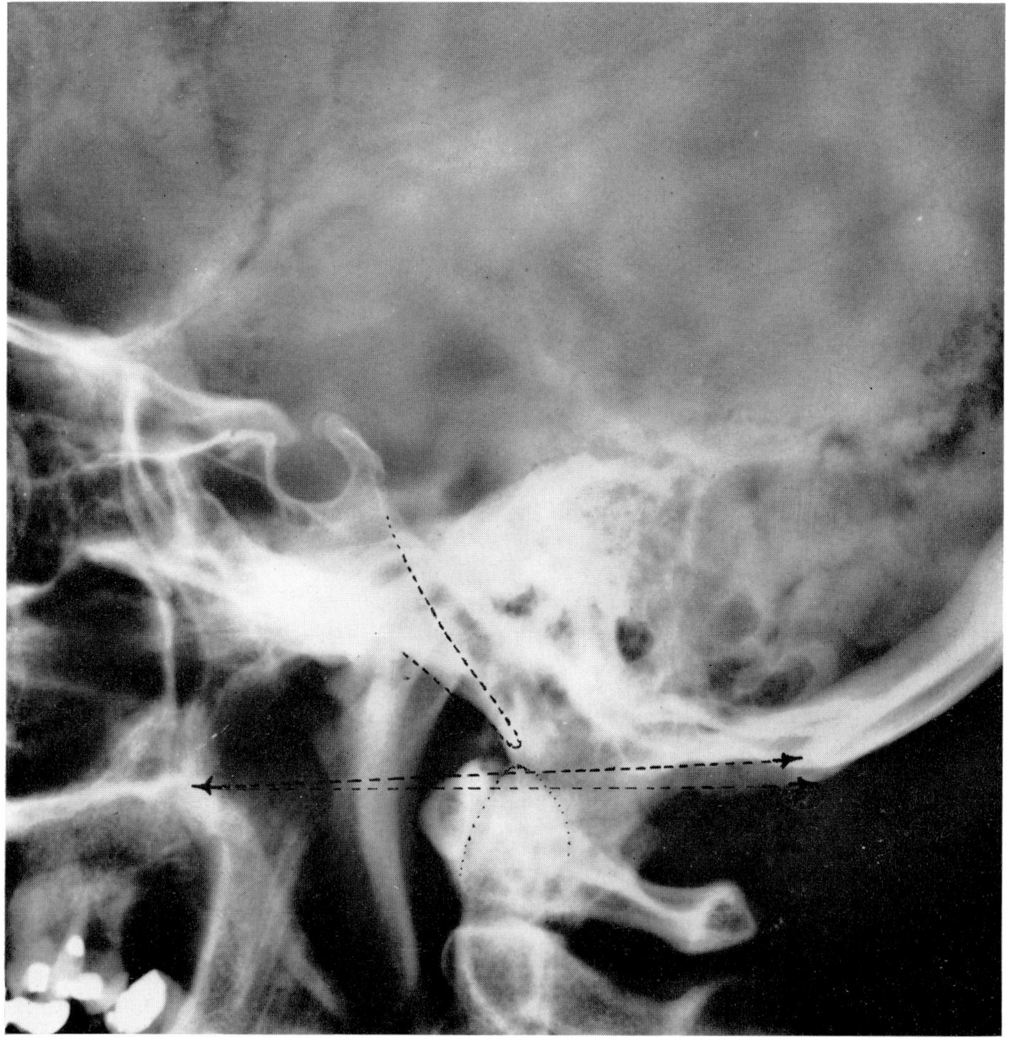

FIG. 50.—CHAMBERLAIN'S LINE AND McGREGOR'S LINE
Chamberlain's line extends from the posterior margin of the hard palate to the posterior margin of the foramen magnum. McGregor's line extends from the posterior margin of the hard palate to the lower margin of the occipital squama. In this particular case, McGregor's line would lie only a few millimeters below Chamberlain's line, but in cases that have a low position of the occipital squama with an upward sweep to its more anterior portion, McGregor's line could be separated from Chamberlain's line by a relatively large distance.

tures by the odontoid process, by fibrous bands, or a tight dura mater in the region of the foramen magnum. The presence of tonsillar herniation may be best demonstrated by pneumographic examination of the foramen magnum; the air is injected with the patient in the sitting position with his head in a marked degree of flexion, which will prevent the air from entering the cranial cavity (figs. 53C and D). This condition may be demonstrated also by Pantopaque myelography (fig. 52). Some of the associated anomalies of the upper cervical spine may also produce symptoms. Among these anomalies the following should be considered: deformity and asymmetry of the foramen

(*Revised 1963*)

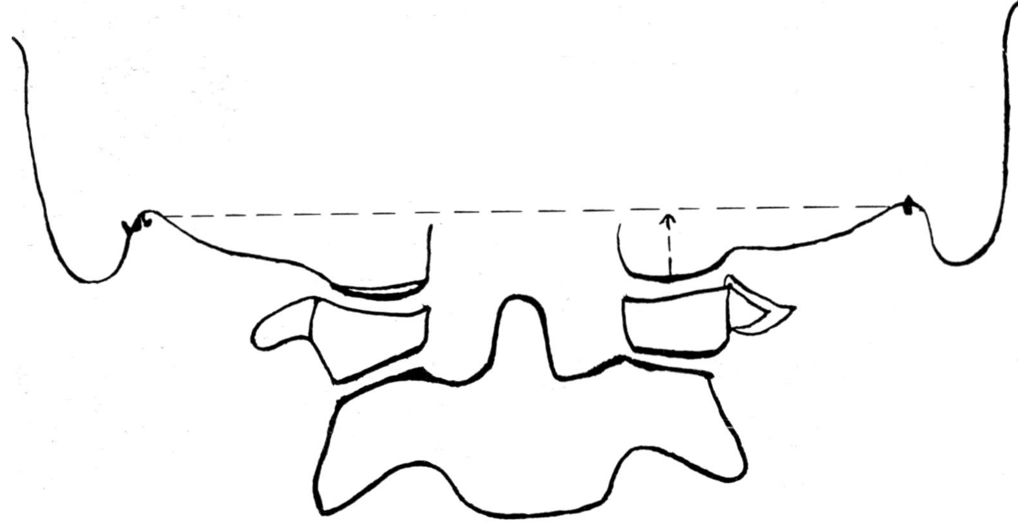

FIG. 51.—DIGASTRIC LINE OF FISCHGOLD

The line is traced from one side of the digastric groove to the other. The distance from the atlanto-axial articulation to this line averages 1.1 cm. with a standard deviation of ±0.4 cm.

magnum associated with partial or complete assimilation of the atlas; hypoplastic odontoid process permitting intermittent luxation of the odontoid process under the transverse ligament of the atlas; ununited odontoid process; and Klippel-Feil malformation or congenital failure of segmentation of the upper cervical vertebrae.

In general it is easy to understand that platybasia *per se* causes the angle subtended by the spinal cord and medulla as it goes through the foramen magnum to be more acute than is ordinarily the case. The acuteness of the angle is a mechanically poor arrangement for these very important structures. Thickening of the dura or arachnoidal adhesions may occur as a result of the poor mechanical arrangement or on a congenital or inflammatory basis which may cause difficulties in the circulation of cerebrospinal fluid. The case shown in Figure 53 had platybasia with basilar impression, without chronic tonsillar herniation, but with some thickening of the meninges in the region of the foramen magnum. In this case there was a rather marked degree of ventricular dilatation for which no cause other than the mechanical difficulties apparently caused by the platybasia was found at autopsy. It is rare to find any symptoms secondary to basilar impression in children before the age of 12. The patient shown in Figure 53C and D was a 15-year-old Negro boy.

The true basilar invagination seen in

FIG. 52.—BASILAR IMPRESSION WITH ANOMALIES IN THE REGION OF THE FORAMEN MAGNUM AND TONSILLAR HERNIATION

The frontal laminagram (A) demonstrates an anomalous 2d cervical vertebra. The joints between the atlas and the occipital bone as well as between the atlas and the 2d cervical are not shown because the atlas was fused to the occipital bone. It is clear that the atlanto-occipital joints would lie well above the digastric line of Fischgold. The lateral projection taken during myelography (B) with Pantopaque demonstrates the extreme degree of upward protrusion of the anomalous odontoid process which actually lies behind and well above the lower tip of the clivus (*arrow*). The radiolucent area at the posterior aspect of the column of oil just below the foramen magnum (*arrows*) represents tonsillar herniation. Another film taken during Pantopaque myelography (C) shows the extreme degree of deformity with some of the Pantopaque now going over the high odontoid process.

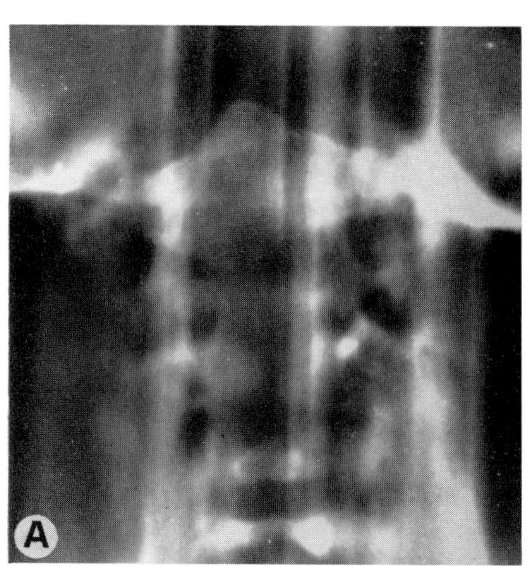

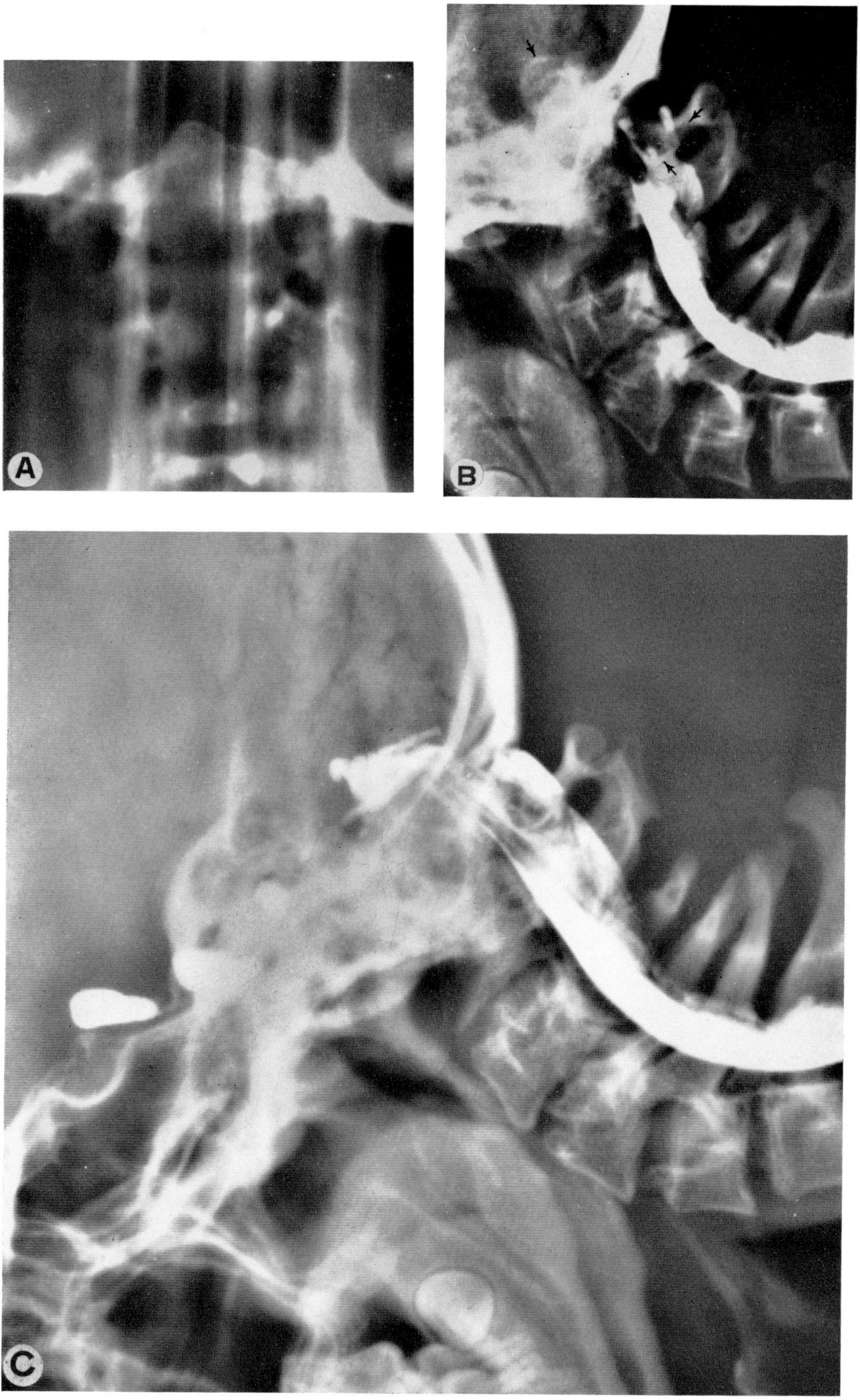

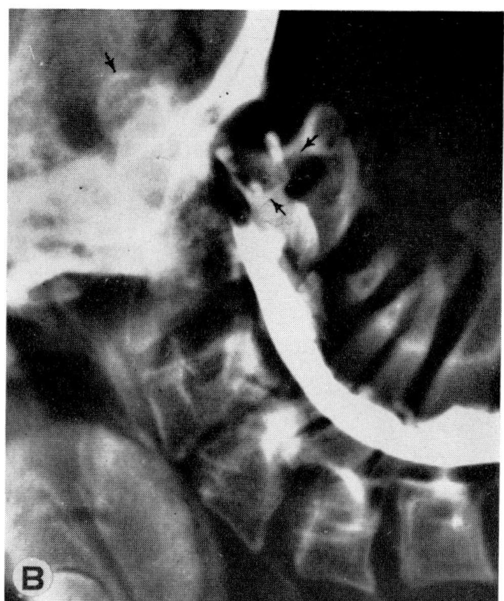

Fig. 52

(*Revised 1963*)

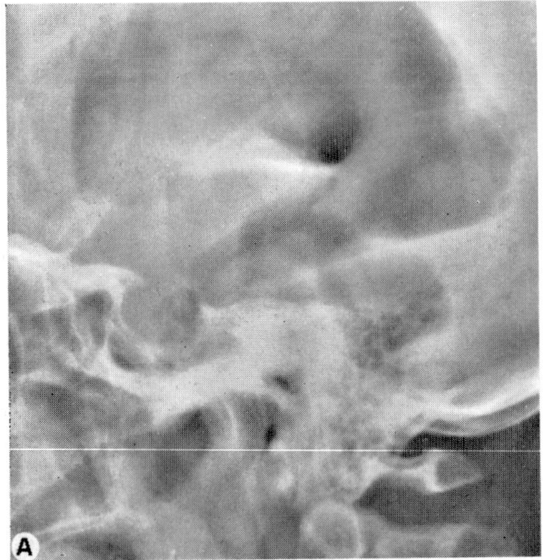

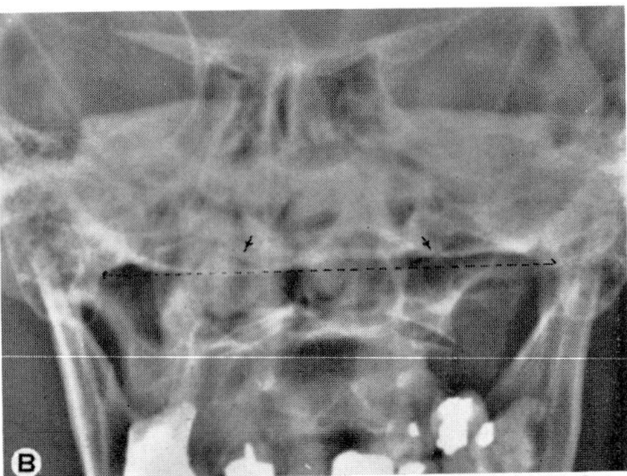

FIG. 53.—PLATYBASIA WITH THICKENING OF THE BASAL MENINGES AND HYDROCEPHALUS

The patient was a 50-year-old woman who gradually developed symptoms of increased intracranial pressure without definite localizing signs. Ventriculography (A) demonstrates marked ventricular dilatation with obstruction of the outlet of the 4th ventricle. The sella turcica is enlarged due to a pituitary cyst. The frontal projection (B) demonstrates a mild degree of basilar impression. The atlanto-occipital joint (*arrows*) lies at or slightly above the digastric line.

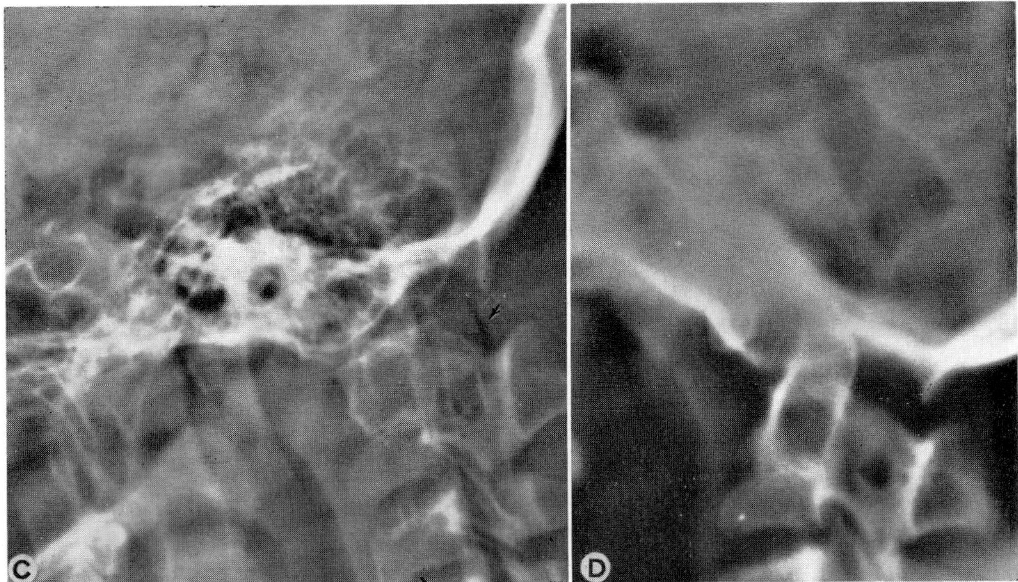

FIG. 53. (*Cont.*)—PLATYBASIA WITH ANOMALIES IN THE FORAMEN MAGNUM AND TONSILLAR HERNIATION IN A 15-YEAR-OLD NEGRO BOY

The pneumoencephalogram (C) demonstrated the tonsils to go down to the level of C2 (*arrow*). The laminagram taken during pneumoencephalography (D) showed the low position of the 4th ventricle, which was enlarged. There is a very narrow anteroposterior diameter to the foramen magnum, from the posterior margin of the odontoid process to the posterior margin of the foramen magnum, which is formed by the fused posterior arch of the atlas with the occipital bone. The odontoid process is displaced backward in relation to the lower end of the clivus. Symptoms had appeared in this patient several months before this examination was performed.

(Revised 1963)

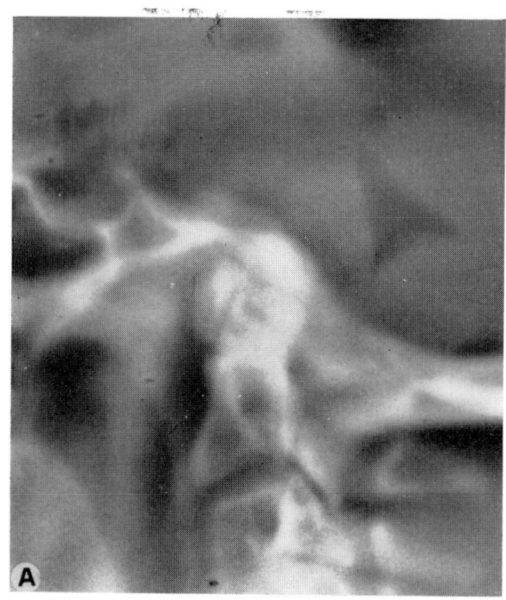

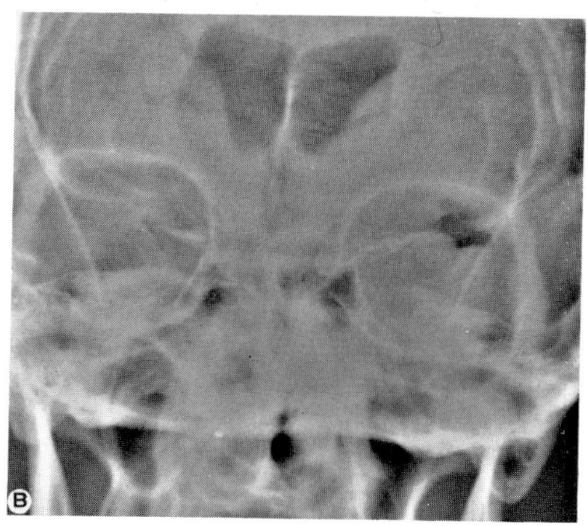

Fig. 54.—Basilar Impression in a 32-year-old Negro Male

There is marked elevation of the odontoid process in relation to Chamberlain's and McGregor's line. There is assimilation of the atlas with the occipital bone. The clivus has assumed an almost horizontal position as seen in the lateral view. A pneumoencephalogram (A) was performed which showed a moderate degree of ventricular dilatation. The tomograph with air in the 4th ventricle demonstrates the relationship of the lower aspect of the 4th with the lower end of the clivus. A thickening is noted at the lower end of the clivus which is one of the manifestations of the occipital vertebra. The frontal projection (B) demonstrates the upward direction of the upper margin of the petrous pyramids which is usually encountered in patients with moderate or severe degree of basilar impression or invagination.

Paget's disease (more commonly than in hyperparathyroidism and in the rare disease known as osteogenesis imperfecta) may be asymptomatic although not always so. Apparently the reason for this is that although there is an indentation of the base of the skull, it is on the side at the level of the condyles, and the angle of the upper cervical spine and medulla as it goes through the foramen magnum is undisturbed.

Radiologically, the presence of basilar impression should be suspected in any patient who presents an anomaly in the region of the foramen magnum with partial or complete fusion of the atlas to the occipital bone. Symptomatic cases usually have an upward displacement of the odontoid process which may encroach on the anterior aspect of the foramen magnum; that is, instead of the lower tip of the clivus being just above the tip of the odontoid process, the latter lies behind the tip of the clivus, which is more horizontal in position than usual (fig. 52). According to McRae (1953), the most significant finding in cases of assimilation of the atlas *with neurological symptoms* was an odontoid process of abnormal size, in abnormal position, or with abnormal mobility. The exact relationship can easily be determined by means of laminagraphy. In some cases the occipital bone posterior to the foramen magnum is slanted upward and forward instead of horizontally or slightly downward as is usually the case (fig. 54). Chamberlain's line will show that the entire odontoid process lies above it.

In the frontal projection, the petrous pyramids are directed upward and medially instead of slightly downward and medially as in the normal (fig. 54). This finding may be more pronounced in patients with basilar invagination due to softening of the skull, but may also be seen in congenital platybasia.

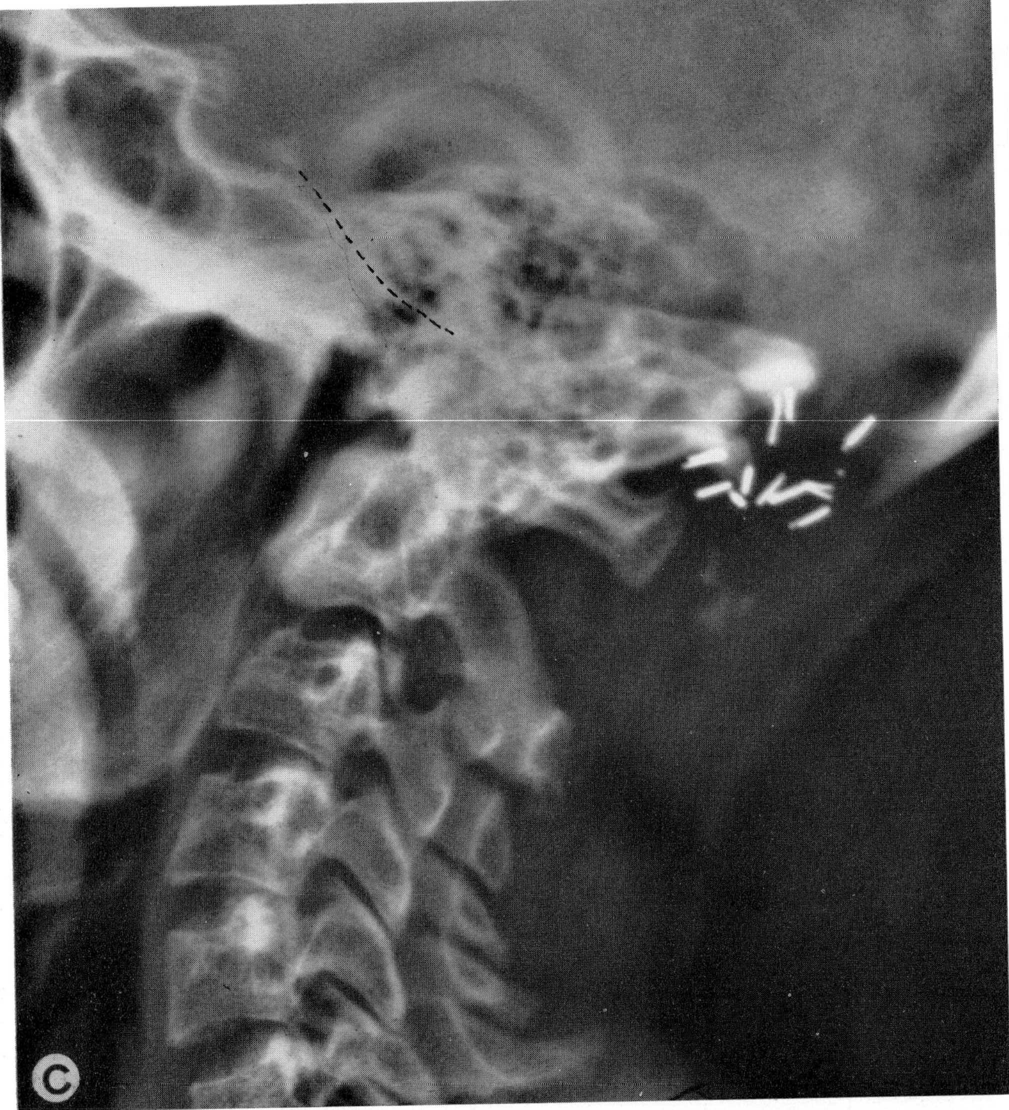

FIG. 54. (*Cont.*)—ACQUIRED PLATYBASIA DUE TO SUBOCCIPITAL CRANIECTOMY EARLY IN CHILDHOOD (C). The basal angle now measures over 155°. An examination done 12 years before this had shown the basal angle to be 148°.

The digastric line traced as a reference point will show that the atlanto-occipital joints lie at the level of or above this line instead of over 0.7 cm. below it as is normal.

Bull, Nixon, and Pratt (1959) have proposed the use of the angle between a line following the plane of the hard palate and a line traced through the center of the anterior and posterior arches of the atlas as a reference. If the angle measures more than 13°, these authors believe that basilar impression is present. However, this angle is apt to vary with changes in position and the above named authors recommend that these reference planes be used in films made in the prone position with the head turned. The authors prefer to use a method for determining basilar impression in which the films are taken with the head and the neck unturned, that is, in a true lateral position for both the skull and the cervical spine.

A wide basal angle (over 143°) is usually present in the brachycephalic type of craniosynostosis but not in the dolichocephalic type of craniosynostosis. A wide basal angle was also reported by Pendergrass and coauthors (1956) in the postural type of turricephalic skull in children maintained in a hyperextended position on the Bradford frame for the treatment of tuberculosis of the spine. It is possible that the hanging weight of the brain on the vault of the skull may have caused the platybasia in these cases. Platybasia may be acquired and is often seen following suboccipital craniotomies early in childhood (fig. 54C).

CRANIUM BIFIDUM

This term applies to an abnormal opening in the skull, usually in the midline, through which the meninges herniate (meningocele); sometimes the meninges as well as a portion of the brain may herniate through the opening (meningoencephalocele). The anomaly is more common in the parieto-occipital and in the frontal regions. It is much less common in the midparietal region. Clinically the meningoceles present as a soft lump on the skull, usually in the midline, which becomes harder when the child cries. Meningoceles are occasionally observed in the frontonasal region where they may protrude into the nasal cavity and produce nasal obstruction in an infant. These defects are

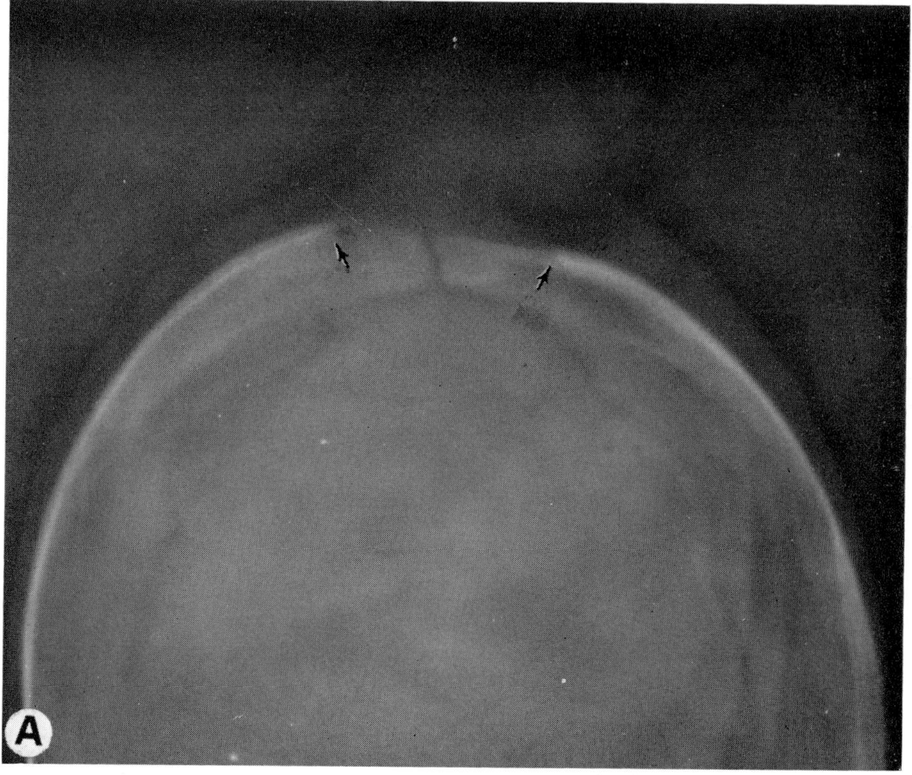

Fig. 55A.—Congenital Meningocele in a 2-month-old Infant

The defect is in the parieto-occipital region and the edges of the bone are seen to taper at the expense of the inner table (A). This type of tapering is typical of meningoceles and, in general, of any mass which protrudes outward from the intracranial contents.

(Revised 1963)

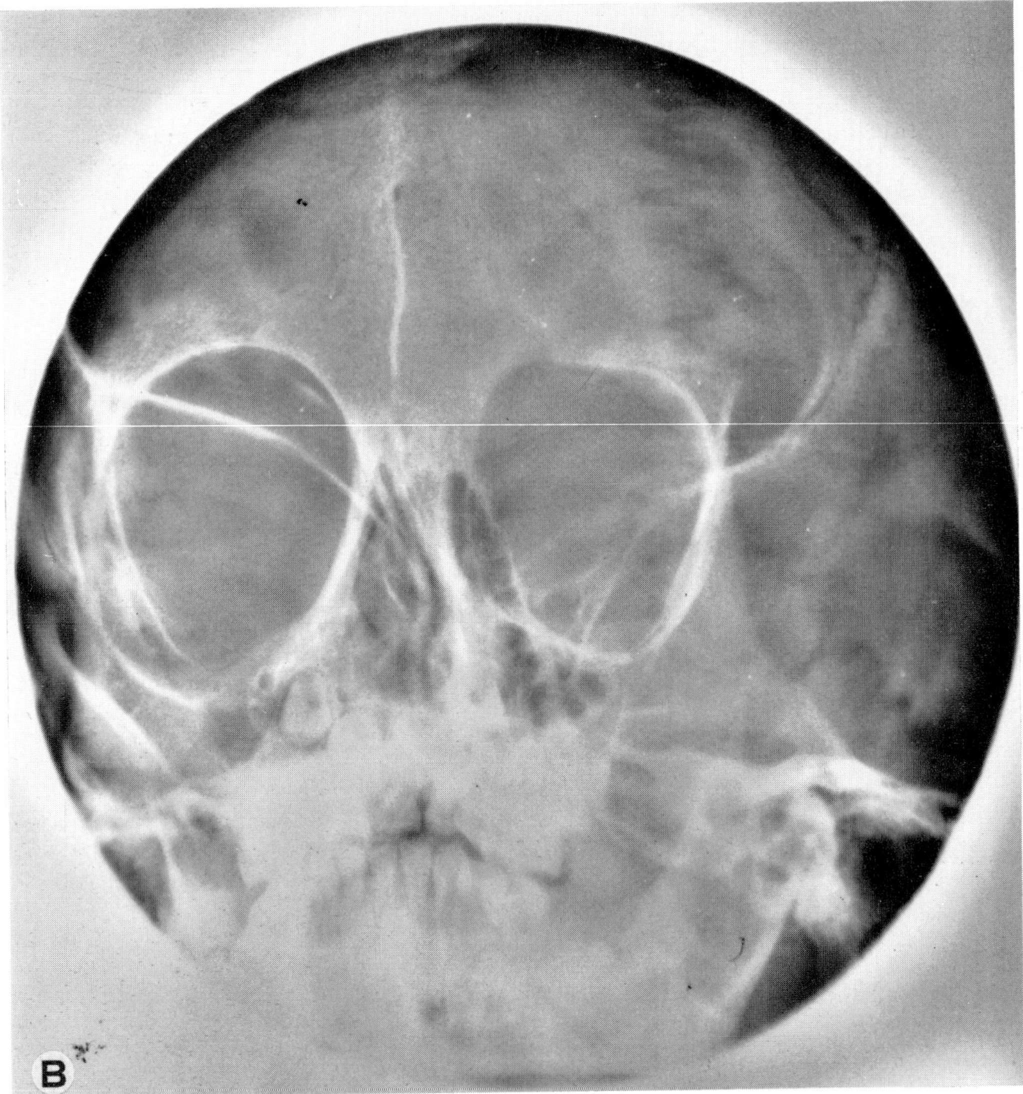

Fig. 55B.—Congenital Absence of Greater Wing of Sphenoid in Child with Neurofibromatosis
The defect includes not only the greater wing but there is elevation of the sphenoid ridge, part of which may also be absent (B). The appearance is rather typical for this condition.

sometimes associated with a cleft palate. Meningoceles are sometimes seen to protrude through the orbit leading to exophthalmus. These are often associated with congenital defects in the greater wing of the sphenoid in patients with neurofibromatosis; the result is usually a rather marked protrusion of the eye forward. This protrusion does not have to be a pulsating exophthalmus and in rare instances exophthalmus is found.

Radiographically, the findings are those of a small defect in the bone, usually in the midline, and characteristic tapering of the bone is seen as it nears the defect at the expense of the inner table. That is, the inner table curves outward to meet the outer table (fig. 55). This curvature tends to distinguish this condition from a lesion that destroys bone, in which both tables would be equally involved or, if the inner table is more involved than the outer table, it cannot be followed out to meet the edge of the outer table but rather it stops at some distance. The latter appearance is sometimes seen in patients with healing eosinophilic granuloma and xanthoma.

In the differential diagnosis one should consider the benign destructive lesions of the skull described above. However, these lesions are rarely in the midline whereas meningoceles are practically always in the midline. The congenital dermal sinuses usually found in the occipital region present a typical dimple on the scalp over the defect in the bone. This is the opposite of a meningocele. Usually diagnostic procedures such as pneumoencephalography should be carried out before operation on suspected meningoceles in order to exclude the presence of other anomalies.

The congenital defects in the greater wing of the sphenoid are often seen in association with neurofibromatosis. In these cases there is usually marked elevation of the sphenoid ridge as seen in the orbital views of the skull (fig. 55B).

The term *cranium bifidum occultum frontalis* is used to indicate defects in the skull encountered usually in the region of the anterior fontanelle in patients with cleidocranial dysostosis. It is due to a nonossified portion of the skull in this region associated with an abnormally large and irregular anterior fontanelle. Sometimes it may be present without the other manifestations of cleidocranial dysostosis.

HYDROCEPHALUS

The diagnosis of hydrocephalus should be made on the basis of special studies and on clinical examination rather than on radiologic investigation by means of plain films alone. It is well known that the hydrocephalic infant has a larger head than normal at birth. The head tends to be round with a high forehead. The fontanelles are wide open and the skull is generally soft on palpation due to the widening of all of the fontanelles. When increased intracranial pressure is present, the fontanelles tend to bulge outward. Radiographically the appearance is that of wide sutures and fontanelles with extremely thin bone in the neighborhood of these sutures. The tapering of the bones toward the suture is an indication of the rate of growth. The faster the head grows, the thinner the bone in the neighborhood of the suture is apt to be. In young infants, widening of the fissures normally present in the bones (particularly the parietal bones) may also be seen.

However, it is not possible to differentiate, on the basis of plain films, which type of hydrocephalus we are dealing with or, indeed, whether we may be dealing with an intracranial mass lesion or with sub-dural hematoma. Although some patients with the Dandy-Walker syndrome (inperforate foramina of Luschka and Magendie) have an enlargement of the posterior fossa with relative elevation of the internal occipital protuberance, it is also true that one cannot depend on the relative size of the posterior fossa to make a certain diagnosis. A small posterior fossa is supposed to be present in the infant with aqueduct stenosis but this is not always the case, or at least it is difficult to evaluate on the radiograph.

If hydrocephalus is arrested spontaneously or after surgical procedures, the suture becomes narrower, and the fontanelles tend to close. When the hydrocephalus disappears relatively suddenly as a result of a short-circuiting procedure, the skull contents become smaller and the fontanelles and sutures are depressed. Under these circumstances, bone continues to be laid down at a rapid rate along the suture line, which becomes dense. Details on congenital hydrocephalus are given on page 1.348.

(*Revised 1963*)

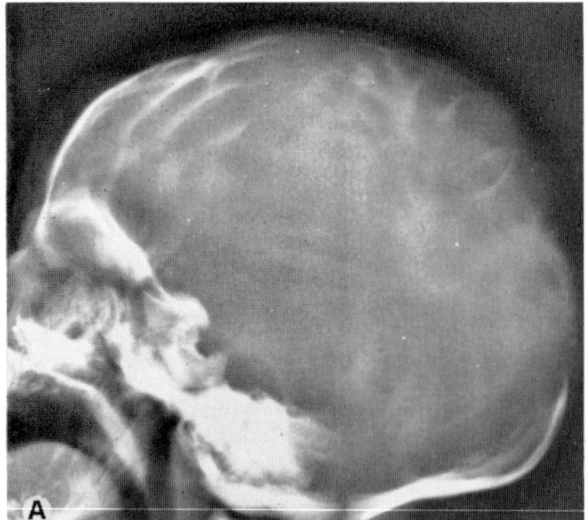

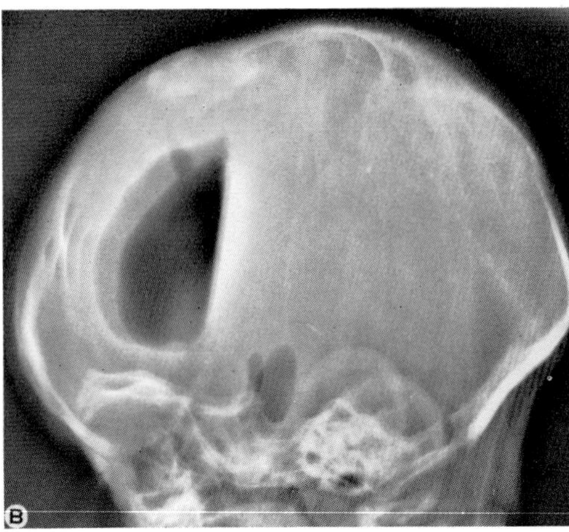

FIG. 56.—*Craniolacunia (Lückenschädel)*

There is an appearance which is suggestive of exaggerated convolutional markings (A). The infant had a meningocele. A film made six weeks later (B) during ventriculography shows growth of the head with almost complete disappearance of the bony ridges characteristic of craniolacunia. This would tend to reinforce the theory that at least some of the cases of craniolacunia are associated with increased intracranial pressure *in utero*.

CRANIOLACUNIA (Lückenschädel)

This term is applied to a peculiar congenital abnormality of the skull in which an irregular honeycomblike configuration of the bones of the skull is seen on the radiograph. Dense bony ridges are separated by radiolucent areas in which the bone may actually be absent (fig. 56). Since the radiolucent areas do not correspond to the convolutions of the brain, it is thought that the abnormality is due to a disturbance in ossification. However, craniolacunia is often associated with meningoceles and meningoencephaloceles, and it is possible that at least some of the cases are associated with increased intracranial pressure *in utero*. This possibility is confirmed by the fact that the bone changes tend to disappear after birth and at the same time hydrocephalus develops and the head grows larger.

MICROCEPHALY

The term microcephaly is used clinically to indicate simply a small head. This may be associated with microencephaly and mental retardation. Some cases of microcephaly may be secondary to premature craniosynostosis and for this reason x-ray examination of the skull is recommended to differentiate between the two, although it is possible in some cases clinically to determine whether or not the bones move at the sutures. In microcephaly the area occupied by the skull in relation to the face is relatively smaller than normal. Radiographic examination of the skull usually reveals that all the sutures are normal and the fontanelles are closed. The sutures are very well seen in infants with microcephaly contrary to those of the normal infant which are less conspicuous. Secondary premature synostosis may occur in some of these cases. With the passage of time, the bones themselves become thicker.

Cerebral hypoplasia with cranial hemihypertrophy. This condition is usually due to vascular occlusions or trauma early in life, but may also result from primary hypoplasia of the brain. See page 1.339.

(Revised 1963)

Miscellaneous Anomalies

Third occipital condyle (condylus tertius). According to Davis (1867), this was first described by Meckel. It is a tubercle in the middle of the anterior edge of the foramen magnum. It articulates with the odontoid process and can be well demonstrated by laminagraphy of the skull made in the lateral projection.

Bathrocephaly. This applies to an overlap of the upper aspect of the occipital bone which is more posterior than the parietal bones as seen in the lateral view in the region of the lambda. This condition is of no clinical significance and should not be confused with a depressed fracture (see p. 1.759).

Persistent craniopharyngeal canal. The craniopharyngeal canal is the opening in the sphenoid bone through which the craniopharyngeal duct (Rathke's pouch) passes during fetal life. Normally this opening becomes obliterated, but it may persist throughout life in a rudimentary manner. The canal may be only 1 mm. in size but occasionally it is wider, measuring several millimeters in diameter. It may be seen in the base view and sometimes in the lateral view, particularly in midline laminagraphy.

Increased Intracranial Pressure

Increased intracranial pressure may result from a disturbance of cerebrospinal fluid dynamics or from increased intracranial mass due to the bulk of a new growth. There may be an overproduction of cerebrospinal fluid or an underabsorption or an obstruction to its circulation between its site of formation and the site of absorption. In many instances, more than one of these mechanisms is active, as occurs frequently when a sizable tumor obstructs some portion of the ventricular system. In the great majority of instances, particularly in adult life, increased intracranial pressure is caused by a brain tumor.

Radiologic evidence of increased intracranial pressure is present on plain films of the majority of patients harboring tumors and frequently is found in patients with increased pressure of non-neoplastic origin, providing that films of superior quality are available and sufficient attention is given to the study of details. The changes may be generalized, affecting the whole skull, or they may be localized and involve exclusively or predominantly one bone. Whether or not radiologic changes develop as a result of increased intracranial pressure depends on both the height of the pressure and its duration. There has been general disagreement regarding the length of time required in the average case for radiologic changes to develop. It is usually impossible to determine by history or clinical findings exactly when the elevated pressure began. It was felt by Dyke (1941) that a period of three to four months of continued high intracranial pressure is required to produce radiologic changes in the average case of brain tumor. In an instance in which the earliest possible time of onset could be established precisely, a patient who developed a brain abscess as a complication of gunshot wound, Camp (1923) found pressure atrophy of the sella turcica at necropsy 37 days after the injury. On the basis of this case, Camp made the conservative estimate that sellar changes may be found within one month of onset of abnormal pressure.

The authors have seen a case in which changes were present 30 days after an injury resulting in subdural hematoma. With a high grade of increased intracranial pressure, it may take four to ten weeks for radiologic changes to develop. With a low grade of pressure, it may take years for film changes to occur or they may never develop. On the other hand, in a young child, signs of pressure may become manifest within a few days as widening of the sutures. In general, it may be stated that clinical signs of increased intracranial pressure are present in a very high percentage of cases in the first weeks or months of the disease and tend to decrease or disappear altogether as time goes on. In contrast, radiographic signs are

FIG. 57.—TABLE I

NORMAL SKULL MEASUREMENTS AT VARIOUS AGES. The measurements are made from outer table to outer table, unless obvious asymmetry of thickness exists on frontal view.

Age	Length	Breadth
years	*cm.*	*cm.*
Birth	13.8	11.0
.25	15.9	12.3
.50	16.1	13.6
.75	17.0	14.6
1	17.5	14.6
1.50	17.9	14.3
2	18.8	14.7
3	19.6	15.3
4	19.8	15.2
5	20.0	15.4
6	20.2	15.9
7	20.0	16.1
8	20.4	16.3
9	20.4	16.3
10	20.8	16.5
11	20.7	16.6
12	20.7	16.6
Adult	21–22	17–18

absent initially (except in the young child) but tend to increase in frequency of occurrence and in severity with time.

Radiologic Manifestations

Cranial enlargement. The simplest manifestation of generalized increased intracranial pressure is enlargement of the head, or megacephaly. Enlargement of the head may be detected readily and early clinically and a table of normal radiographic measurements also has been worked out (Table I, fig. 57). The infantile brain grows quite rapidly. At birth, the brain weighs, on the average, 335 grams (Coppoletta and Wolbach, 1933). At eight months the brain has more than doubled its weight at birth, at two and one-half years the size is tripled, and at 12 years the weight is quadrupled. At this time, the weight closely approximates that of the adult which, in the average male, is 1400 grams. Weights up to 300 grams greater or less than the average are considered the limits of normal. At all ages the capacity of the cranial cavity exceeds the brain size only very slightly, and any significant increase will be reflected in expansion of the cranium if this is possible or a pressure effect if enlargement cannot occur.

Megacephaly usually is seen in children. Enlargement of the cranial bones without a disturbance at their sutural junction occasionally occurs as an isolated finding. This is seen frequently in patients who have a mild degree of hydrocephalus which becomes spontaneously arrested. The authors have also encountered instances of cerebellar neoplasm in children in which enlargement of the cranium by measurement was the only radiologic manifestation of increased intracranial pressure. When seen beyond childhood it denotes a long standing process that started early in life. Megacephaly can sometimes be the result of megalencephalon in which the brain is unusually large without hydrocephalus.

Suture widening. Much more often bone growth cannot keep up with the intracranial expansion and there is widening of the major sutures and often bulging of the soft tissues through the anterior fontanelle. The latter is helpful for early diagnosis in infancy, particularly during the first year of life. The posterior fontanelle is closed at or shortly after birth. By the middle of the second year of life, the anterior fontanelle is narrowed to fingertip size and usually is closed radiologically by the end of the second year. The coronal and sagittal sutures are affected by pressure most often, and in more severe cases there also is widening of the lambdoidal suture. During early life the portions of the coronal and lambdoidal sutures adjacent to the fontanelles are wider than the rest of the sutures and this should be taken into account when interpreting films (fig. 58).

After three years of age, the same general rule may be applied to the definition of suture widening in children as is used later in this text to establish the absolute widening of diastasis, namely that a separation of the normal interdigitating portions of more than two millimeters is excessive. In some normal individuals the major sutures will remain quite prominent throughout life but

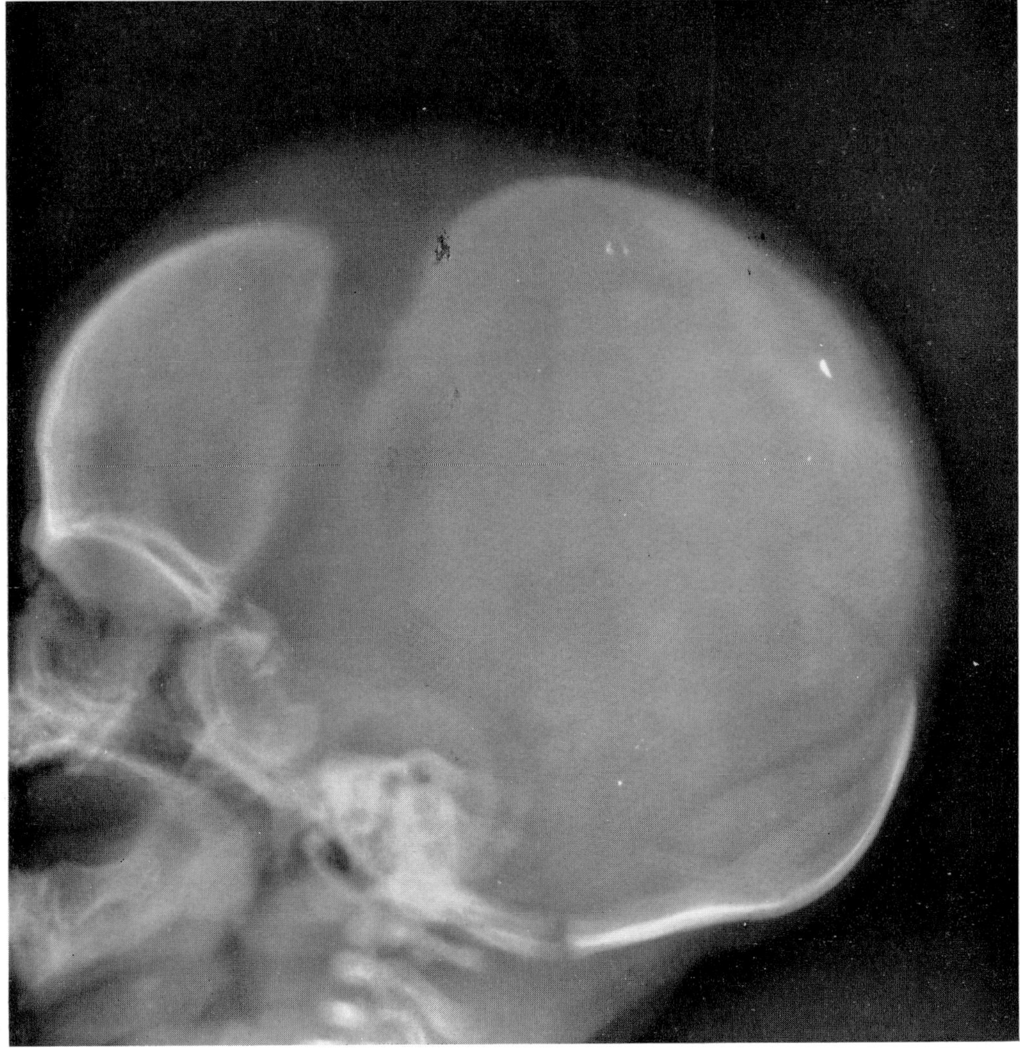

Fig. 58.—Increased Intracranial Pressure in Infancy

Megacephalous is present and the sutures are abnormally wide, even for the patient's age. The soft tissues overlying the anterior fontanelle are bowed outward by pressure beneath. Bulging at the fontanelle, when the infant is not crying or struggling, is indicative of increased intracranial pressure.

usually at no point is there a suture width of more than one millimeter measurable on the films. Although suture widening that results from abnormal pressure is seen most frequently below the age of 12 years, the authors have encountered a number of patients 16 years of age who exhibited widened sutures, either as a result of tumor or aqueduct stenosis. Rarely, a patient older than 16 years may exhibit suture widening as a result of increased intracranial pressure, but for the most part, widened sutures after this age may be assumed to be the result of traumatic diastasis, unless other changes of advanced, long standing increased pressure also are present.

The degree of suture widening with brain tumor varies considerably. Both the chronicity of the process and the age of the patient are important factors. The importance of age

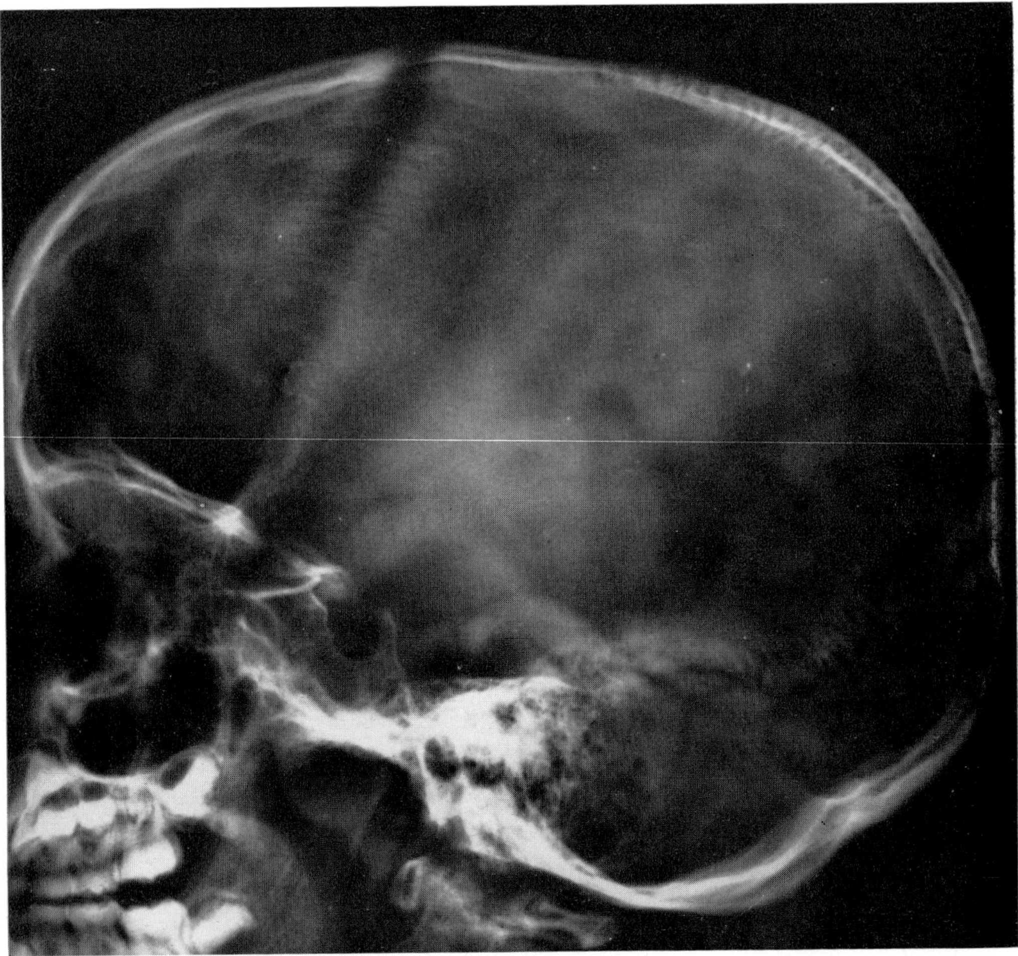

Fig. 59.—Increased Intracranial Pressure in Childhood

Prominent widening of the coronal, sagittal, and lambdoidal sutures is present in an 8-year-old child who had a cerebellar tumor. There is generalized prominence of the convolutional markings throughout the skull, and an area of diffuse demineralization is present in the posterior parietal region. Despite prolonged increased intracranial pressure, the boundaries of the sella turcica are well mineralized owing to the decompression afforded by the suture widening. The tuberculum and planum of the anterior portion of the sphenoid bone, although well mineralized, are not well developed.

is illustrated by the fact that younger patients present a much higher degree of suture widening. While the height of the increased pressure is important, as illustrated by the case described by Camp (1923), the chronicity is undoubtedly a very important factor in most cases, as described by Schreiber (1930). As noted elsewhere, the more benign, slowly progressive lesions more often result in roentgen changes over a long period of time than rapidly growing invasive tumors (fig. 59).

As a result of the spontaneous decompression that results from cranial enlargement in young patients, either bone growth or suture widening, the ordinary reflections of increased pressure seen in the adult in the region of the sella turcica and along other basal bones usually are not found. Excepted are lesions which prominently enlarge the third ventricle, the anterior portion of which may exert direct pressure upon the sellar region. During the middle years of the second decade of life, it is frequent to find sphenoid bone changes in association with suture widening and diffuse changes of the cranial bones.

Convolutional markings. The convolutional markings of the inner table of the skull are perhaps the most difficult to evaluate objectively of any of the commonly seen manifestations of increased intracranial pressure. The markings appear as generally rounded areas of diminished density separated by areas of normal bone density or low ridges of bone. The general appearance and size of the markings suggest that they may be areas of bone thinning resulting from local pressure from the underlying pulsating convolutions of the brain, and it is from this hypothesis that the markings derive their name. It has been shown, however, that the pattern of the markings does not fit well with the arrangement of cerebral convolutions. Nevertheless, circumstantial evidence is strong that expanding cerebral convolutions in some way play a role in the development of the markings. The term digital markings is used by some writers. The markings are most often found during the years when the brain is growing, and they are rarely marked in cases of cerebral hypoplasia or when there is a buffer between the brain surface and the inner table of the skull, such as occurs with subdural hematoma.

Through the examination of a large number of skull films, Davidoff and Gass (1949) found that convolutional markings rarely begin to appear in the normal skull before one and one-half to two years of age, the time of closure of the anterior fontanelle. The incidence of occurrence of convolutional markings increases rapidly from this age until four years, when their presence continues to be observed in a high percentage of normal children until the age of approximately eight years. Following this, there is a decline in the frequency with which convolutional impressions are normally encountered. In some individuals, however, convolutional markings may be conspicuous well into adult life and they are more prominent in persons having relatively thin cranial bones.

Convolutional markings of the normal skull are found most often in the frontal and occipital regions. They occur normally also in the temporal and parietal areas, although they are less numerous. The occurrence of prominent markings in the parietal area, therefore, may be considered of more significance than numerous deep markings of the occipital and frontal poles. It is very difficult to define, however, the borderline between normality and abnormality, particularly in children. Nevertheless, an increase in the number, depth, and visible prominence of the markings in skull roentgenograms is a well recognized result of increased intracranial pressure. If their prominence can be used as a measure of any parameter of intracranial tension, perhaps the appearance of these markings gives a better clue to the duration of convolutional imprint rather than the height of pressure or even the existence of abnormal pressure. It is a safe rule to say that a radiologic diagnosis of increased intracranial pressure should not be made on the basis of prominent convolutional markings alone. A conspicuous appearance may be considered additional evidence of disease when one or several of the more commonly encountered changes of increased pressure are present, such as atrophy of the sella turcica or widening of the cranial sutures. An exception to this statement may be found in the case of craniostenosis and occasionally under other circumstances.

Increased vascularity. A relatively uncommon change resulting from increased intracranial pressure is a generalized or a localized increase in vascularity. A localized increase in vascularity, particularly an increase in the number and size of arterial channels in one specific part of the skull, is found fairly frequently with certain tumors, especially meningiomas. In these instances, the term *neovascularity* might better be applied. Similar changes are found with certain vascular lesions, of which arteriovenous malformation is a noteworthy example. An increase in the size of Pacchionian granulations and of draining veins frequently is seen in young patients with compensated hydrocephalus. Perhaps in these instances the vascular enlargements are more an indication of the specific type of lesion present than of increased intracranial pressure, since it has been suggested that the dilatation of these channels is in response to an inadequate number of Pacchionian bodies in communicating hydrocephalus.

Attention was called to enlargement of the bony channel carrying the occipital emissary vein as a result of elevated intracranial pressure more than a quarter century ago by Lindblom (1936). The vein is vertically directed along the midline of the occipital bone below the torcular. Lindblom established the upper limit of normal size for the foramen as 2 mm. He found it to be enlarged above this diameter only in patients with elevated intracranial pressure but considered it a relatively common finding under these circumstances. Lindblom considered the enlargement to result from pressure internally interfering with drainage of external soft tissue vascular structures into the dural sinus. Other emissary veins and their apertures may enlarge as a generalized manifestation of increased intracranial pressure.

Atrophy. Cranial bones may become *diffusely atrophic* or locally destroyed as a result of intracranial hypertension. Diffuse atrophy of the vault may occur after a prolonged high degree of increased intracranial pressure. The bony architecture becomes indistinct and there may be actual thinning with the result that there is reduced bone—soft tissue contrast in the radiograph. Diffuse atrophy of the vault is most commonly seen in infants with hydrocephalus, but may be seen in the adult.

Atrophy of individual cranial bones as well as local erosion of portions of bones may result from generalized increased intracranial pressure. Individual bony structures of the skull base are much more frequently involved than the bones of the vault. Multiple structures may exhibit erosions in some instances, and the demonstration of atrophy of structures in certain combinations may give a good indication of the location of the disease process. The *sphenoid bone* is the most common cranial osseous component to be affected by the atrophy of increased intracranial pressure. The superior portion, and particularly the sella turcica because of its vulnerable intracranial extension and ease of radiographic visibility, is the most important single structure involved in the detection of increased intracranial pressure after the age of 12 years. Because increased pressure in the adult is most often caused by brain tumor, pressure atrophy of the sella turcica becomes the most common and the most important evidence of brain tumor in plain skull radiographs.

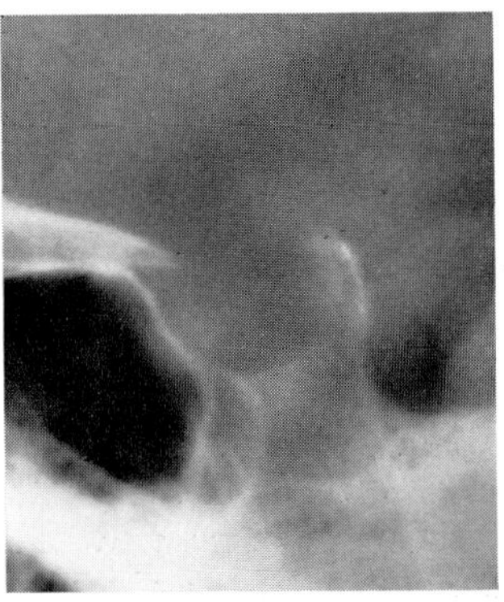

FIG. 60.—EARLY PRESSURE ATROPHY OF THE SELLA TURCICA

Erosion of the cortical bone bounding the interior of the sella turcica along the anterior aspect of the dorsum is present. Normal mineral content of the other bony structures is preserved.

Sella turcica. It is not within the scope of this work to discuss in detail the mechanisms involved in various manifestations of sphenoid bone atrophy. This has been the subject of a monograph by Mahmoud (1958). It may be pointed out, however, that normally the interior of the sella turcica is bounded by smooth compact cortical bone which, in lateral radiographs, appears as a continuous white line. Anteriorly, this plate of cortical bone is reflected over the tuberculum onto the anterior and middle clinoid processes and onto the planum sphenoidale. Anteriorly and inferiorly, the sphenoid sinus usually extends to the wall of the sella

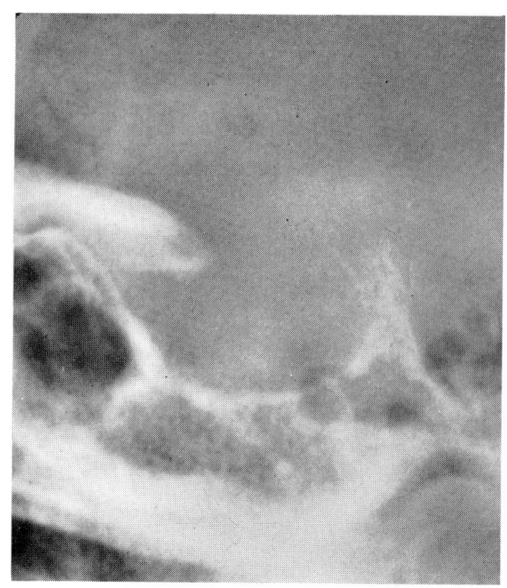

FIG. 61.—EROSION OF THE POSTERIOR CLINOID PROCESSES

The superior cortex of the posterior clinoid processes has disappeared. The cortex bounding the dorsum, both anteriorly and posteriorly, is discontinuous. The cancellous bone of the upper dorsum sellae and of the remaining elements of the clinoid processes is markedly demineralized. The changes occurred in a patient who had mild intracranial hypertension of prolonged duration owing to a slowly growing frontal tumor.

turcica with only the plate of cortical bone separating the pituitary fossa from the air-filled sphenoid sinus. Inferiorly and posteriorly, the cortical sellar boundary is usually abutted by cancellous bone, but in many instances the spenoid sinus develops in this area and may even extend into the dorsum sellae. The cortical bone plate forms the posterior sellar wall where it covers the dorsum and, after being reflected over the posterior clinoid processes, it also bounds the posterior aspect of the dorsum of the sella above the clivus.

The earliest detectable radiologic evidence of increased intracranial pressure in this area is erosion of the *cortical bone bounding the interior of the sella turcica along the anterior aspect of the dorsum sellae.* In lateral radiographs, the cortical bone is seen to be indistinct and discontinuous rather than sharply and densely outlined. With almost equal frequency, atrophy of the superior and anterior cortical margin of the *posterior clinoid processes* is found. If the elevated pressure continues, atrophy of the compact cortical bone along the posterior aspect of the clinoid processes and dorsum sellae often occurs. In time, the dorsum and clinoid processes may become very thin and finally become invisible with the result that the dorsum appears shortened and often pointed (figs. 60 and 61).

Concomitant with the changes of the dorsum sellae and clinoid processes, thinning of the rim of cortical bone forming the floor of the sella turcica begins. By the time the dorsum appears thin and shortened, there are usually discernible atrophic changes of the floor of the sella turcica, particularly posteriorly. With continued elevation of intracranial pressure, particularly of high degree, similar changes take place further forward in the sella turcica. Eventually, not only the sella turcica but even other bony structures may be affected. The changes in various bony elements are best described radiologically as atrophy or erosion of cortical bone rather than decalcification or destruction. Erosion and atrophy are considered essentially synonymous for the purpose of the present discussion. Both imply an interference in bone metabolism involving concomitantly excessive wearing away of existing bone and failure of normal replacement. Decalcification and destruction are seen most often in the presence of lesions immediately adjacent to the sella turcica. The former results from the hyperemia associated with inflammatory processes or a vascular tumor. The latter is produced by direct invasion of bone by tumor, such as occurs in the case of meningioma and chordoma. The intimate relation of the various basic changes was emphasized by Camp (1949). After surgical relief of increased intracranial pressure, the bony structures frequently return to normal density within a relatively short period of time, although occasionally with slight alteration of configuration.

The greatest difficulty in radiologic diagnosis appears to arise in the positive iden-

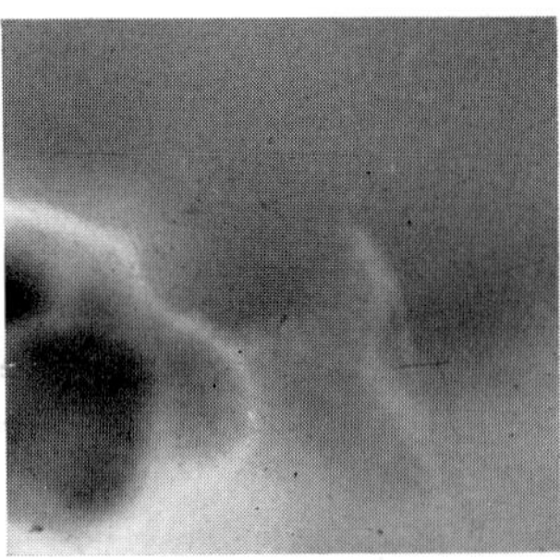

FIG. 62.—ATROPHY OF THE FLOOR OF THE SELLA TURCICA

A midsagittal tomogram reveals absence of a cortical boundary along the anterior aspect of the dorsum sellae and along the posterior half of the floor of the sella turcica. The subcortical bone of the posterior inferior aspect of the sella is demineralized and irregular.

tification of early changes of pressure atrophy of the posterior clinoid processes and dorsum sellae, particularly in patients with thin skulls and in older individuals in whom background changes of generalized skeletal degeneration are present. In the older patients, there may be marked osteoporosis or demineralization of the dorsum sellae and clinoid processes and also along the posterior aspect of the sellar floor, if the sphenoid sinus has not extended into this area. However, even in the presence of generalized decalcification, the compact bone forming the cortical lining of the interior of the sella turcica is intact with simple aging. Similarly, the continuation of this cortex over the posterior clinoid tips and along the posterior aspect of the dorsum sellae can be traced. Sometimes differentiation is extremely difficult. It has been our experience that most radiologists, in their eagerness not to overlook evidence of brain tumor in skull films, "overcall" atrophy of the sella turcica, but this high index of suspicion is commendable.

Many factors must be taken into consideration in arriving at an opinion of atrophy of the posterior clinoid processes or dorsum sellae, including simple technical variations such as overpenetration, particularly in the presence of the decalcified skull of advancing age, and also scattering of radiation. Our policy is to first try to relate the calcium content of the sella turcica to that of the vault and other areas, such as the jaw, as viewed in routine lateral stereoscopic projections. If there is then any question concerning a disproportionate decalcification of the sella turcica, either a well coned lateral spot film of the sella turcica is obtained in as straight lateral projection as possible or we go directly to the use of midsagittal laminagrams. Three sections usually are made, one through the midline and one section on each side of the midline. In the majority of instances, these additional films will, with experience, serve to remove doubt concerning the presence or absence of pressure atrophy.

With continued increased intracranial pressure, atrophy of the floor of the sella turcica frequently occurs, but in the average case changes in the posterior clinoid processes and dorsum sellae usually are well marked by this time. The sharp white line of the sellar floor, as seen in the lateral skull film, may be generally thin and at several points discontinuity is evident (fig. 62). The gas shadow of the sphenoid sinus is no longer completely separated from the soft tissue shadow of the pituitary fossa contents by a bony barrier, and the sellar contents may appear to bulge slightly into the sphenoid sinus area. However, there is hardly ever the frank break through the floor of the sella turcica, particularly posteriorly and inferiorly, such as occurs with pituitary adenoma. At this stage, with absence of calcific boundaries in the region of the clinoids, along the dorsum and along the sellar floor, the sella may appear enlarged and in some instances it does actually enlarge, not only by bulging into the sphenoid area but also through elongation. Occasionally, it is difficult to differentiate between such deformity of the sella turcica resulting from pressure and that produced by a relatively small pituitary adenoma. In these instances, some of the minor changes mentioned elsewhere in connection with the diagnosis of pituitary tumors may be of considerable help in differentiating an extrasellar tumor producing generalized

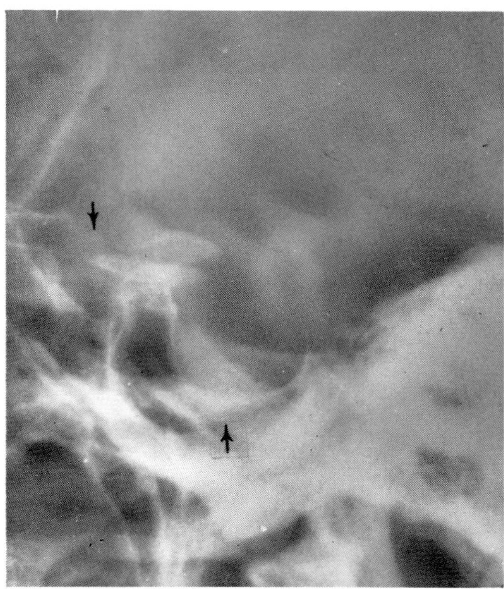

Fig. 63.—Late Sella Turcica Changes of Increased Intracranial Pressure

The posterior clinoid processes and dorsum sellae are absent. The residual bone at the base of the dorsum is pointed. The floor of the sella turcica is thin anteriorly as well as posteriorly with bulging of the soft tissues of the pituitary fossa into the sphenoid sinus (*lower arrow*). There is also discontinuity along the superior surface of the sphenoid bone anterior to the sella in the region of the planum (*upper arrow*).

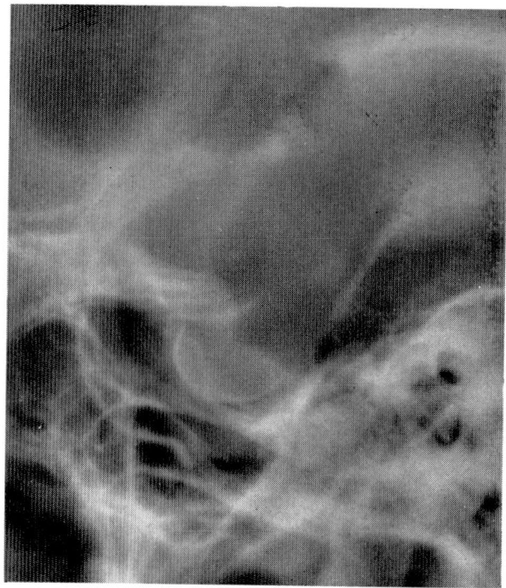

Fig. 64.—Sella Turcica Erosion by a Large Third Ventricle

Dilatation of the hypothalamic portion of the 3d ventricle is present owing to ventricular obstruction by a posterior fossa tumor. The infundibular recess is markedly dilated and projects downward not only on to the area formerly occupied by the dorsum, which is absent, but projects into the pituitary fossa (see also Fig. 244).

increased intracranial pressure from an intrasellar mass (fig. 63).

The tuberculum sellae and the anterior clinoid processes do not reflect evidence of increased intracranial pressure nearly as often as the posterior portion of the sella and the sellar floor. When sellar changes result predominantly from enlargement of the third ventricle, however, the tuberculum sellae may be affected and this pressure may extend even further forward to the posterior margin of the planum (fig. 64). When changes in the anterior portion of the sella are associated with unmistakable changes of increased intracranial pressure further posteriorly, then they may properly be interpreted as evidence of high pressure of long standing and probably with obstruction distal to the outlet of the third ventricle (fig. 65). On the other hand, when changes anteriorly are isolated, then it is more probable that these atrophies result from local erosions. Thus, atrophy and depression of the tuberculum sellae are most often seen with optic chiasm glioma, suprasellar meningioma, and occasionally with other mass lesions in the immediately adjacent suprasellar region and, in addition, pituitary adenoma. As has been noted elsewhere, the anterior clinoid processes are most often affected by carotid artery aneurysm which may produce unilateral changes of erosion, shortening, or "pointing" and thinning. Thinning and erosion of the inferior aspect of one or both anterior clinoid processes with apparent elevation is almost surely reliable evidence of a pituitary adenoma. This change ordinarily is not seen unless there is already enlargement of the sella turcica in length and depth and, in addition, rounding anteriorly and ventrally

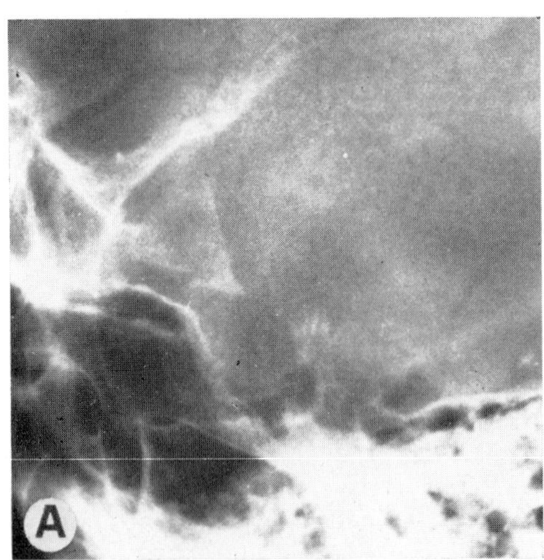

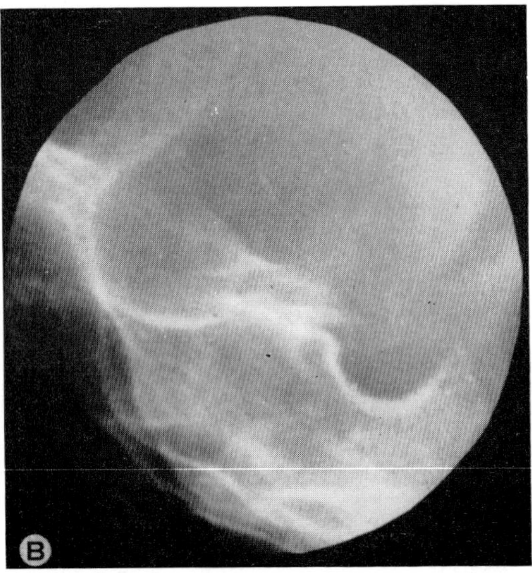

FIG. 65.—TWO TYPES OF SELLA DAMAGE FROM POSTERIOR FOSSA TUMORS

The entire interior cortex of the sella turcica is atrophic and the floor of the sella depressed (A). One anterior clinoid process is indistinctly visible and the other pointed, owing to the pressure of an enlarged third ventricle in a patient who had a cerebellar medulloblastoma. A patient with a slowly growing posterior fossa tumor suffered from intracranial hypertension over a period of years (B). The posterior clinoid processes are absent and the remaining portion of the dorsum is pointed and the cortical boundary thin. The anterior clinoid processes also appear thin. The tuberculum and floor of the sella turcica are well mineralized. Along the forward portion and just anterior to the planum sphenoidale there is a large scalloped depression in the superior portion of the sphenoid bone owing to prolonged pressure by a markedly enlarged third ventricle. Such changes are more conspicuous and may develop more easily when the sphenoid sinus is not developed, as in this case. In (A), implants may have been present.

where the prominence of the tuberculum sellae formerly was present.

In summary, the changes of increased intracranial pressure reflected in the sella turcica enumerated above are: (1) and (2) atrophy of the posterior clinoid processes and dorsum sellae; (3) demineralization, thinning, intermittent discontinuity or complete loss of outline of the bony floor of the sella; (4) enlargement of the sella turcica resulting from continuing pressure upon the decalcified sellar floor and posterior wall, most frequently recognized by bulging of the pituitary fossa contents into the sphenoid air sinus; (5) atrophy of the tuberculum sellae, which is evident in cases of long standing, increased intracranial pressure or those in which the third ventricle, pulsating upon the anterior portion of the sella and into its cavity, often plays a large role; (6) atrophy of the anterior clinoids, deformities of which are much more commonly the result of focal erosion by local lesions.

In general, pressure changes in the adult occur most frequently in the order just given and they can be recognized in routine lateral films. Occasionally, however, sella turcica changes may be appreciated in straight frontal views, in a basal mentovertical projection, and quite frequently in the half axial projection. The sella is perhaps best visualized in the frontal view when it is enlarged and it is frequently possible to appreciate asymmetrical depression of the sellar floor in this manner, although little is added to lateral stereoscopic study in most instances. On the other hand, the half axial projection often provides clear appreciation of changes in the region of the posterior clinoids which are too minimal even to be seen well in stereoscopic lateral view. Such changes include marginal beveling and even demineralization of one lateral aspect of the dorsum which may be seen as the result of generalized increased pressure, erosion by aneurysm, or a point of greatest expansion in the case of pituitary tumor. In this projection the dorsum flaring outward as it extends downward from the clinoids is less dense centrally than on the sides. Occasionally, one may see an oval, window-like area of thinness in the central portion of the mid-dorsum; when this occurs under normal circumstances it is quite smooth, while with disease, irregular thinness may be detected.

Other sphenoid bone structures. The sella turcica is not the only portion of the sphenoid bone that may be affected by the atrophy of intracranial hypertension. There may be erosion and thinning of the planum sphenoidale. The lesser and greater wings of the sphenoid on one or both sides also may exhibit thinning. There is so much variation in connection with the appearance of the sphenoid wings and ridges that minor degrees of asymmetry frequently result from technical factors. These variations usually are, however, in the region of the wing plates, as seen in frontal view. The superior and inferior orbital fissures usually are well marginated, as are the optic foramina in the average case. Slight enlargement of the optic canal may be seen in unusual cases. Pressure changes may result in marginal atrophy and apparent erosion, when one side is compared with the other, or with a normal case in the instance of bilateral atrophy.

Ordinarily, lesser and greater sphenoid wing atrophic changes occur late, and by this time there is usually confirmatory evidence in the region of the sella turcica. However, it is important to recognize that sphenoidal changes are of hypertensive origin when they occur in this manner and to avoid attaching incorrect localizing significance to them. Local erosion may be found owing to expanding lesions of the middle cranial fossa or tumors of the orbit. The sphenoid wings are also sites of frequently occurring congenital defects. In the basisphenoid area, pressure changes may be found rarely in the region of the clivus, perhaps from the effect of the basilar artery which is displaced forward against it in the case of posterior fossa tumors.

Anterior fossa. In the anterior fossa, the ethmoid and frontal bones exhibit generalized pressure changes relatively frequently. Along the cribriform plate of the ethmoid, the bone is rather spongy and there are frequently orbital and paranasal sinus shadows closely adjacent or superimposed which may make the cortical boundary of this medial area difficult to trace. Tumors occurring in the frontal region, particularly in the subfrontal area along the olfactory groove, notoriously cause demineralization of the ethmoid plate and often a downward depression. In the lateral roentgenogram, this appears as an inferior convexity out of proportion to the normal slope in this region, often with encroachment upon the air sinus area.

Not only frontal tumors, however, will produce anterior fossa changes. Posterior tumors of long standing with ventricular obstruction and marked dilatation of the anterior horns of the lateral ventricles will cause atrophy and depression of the ethmoid plate. Similarly, the supraorbital ridges may show decalcification and thinning not only with frontal tumors but with posterior obstructing lesions, again best visualized in stereoscopic lateral skull roentgenograms. The vertical portion of the frontal bone exhibits generalized pressure changes less frequently. It may share in the diffuse thinning of the bones of the vault previously described. In cases of severe, long standing, increased intracranial pressure, the vertical portion of the frontal bone is vulnerable to the anterior horn distention of internal hydrocephalus. An instance is illustrated (fig. 66) in which such severe pressure was generated in the case of a fourth ventricular ependymoma that the brain substance thinned the meninges and broke through the dura at multiple points. The roentgenograms revealed many small spotty areas of radiolucency which resulted from erosion of the inner table of the skull by herniated brain substance imbedded in the diploic space.

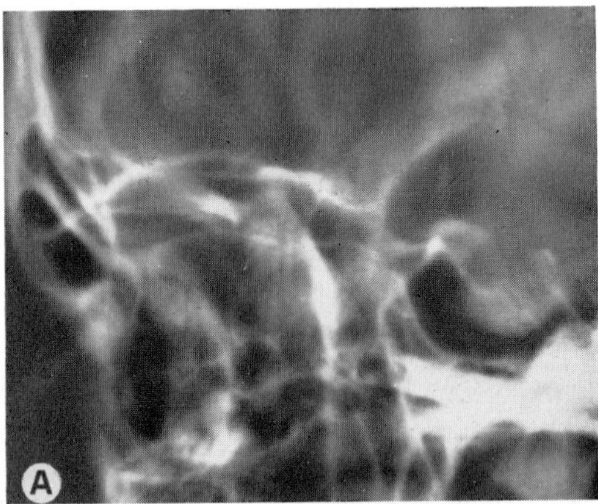

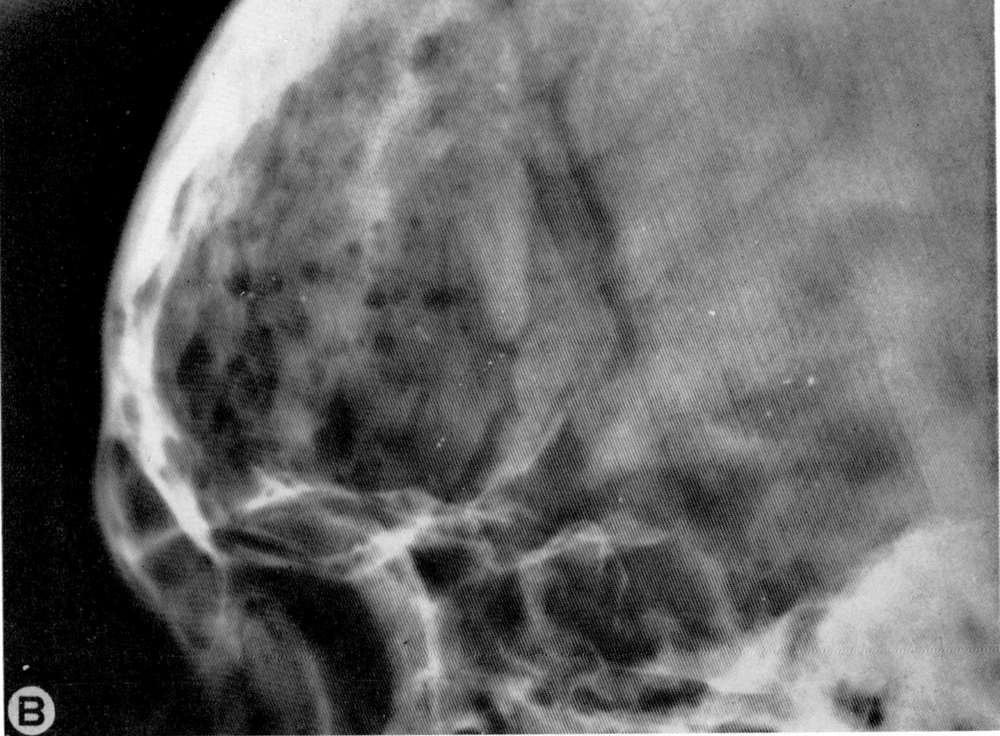

FIG. 66.—PRESSURE CHANGES IN THE FRONTAL REGION

The medial portion of the floor of the anterior fossa is grossly demineralized and the supraorbital ridges are thin (A). The lines of the compact bone edges at the cribiform plate are not visible and there is depression of anterior fossa soft tissues into the ethmoid sinuses. Similarly, bulging of the pituitary into the sphenoid air space is shown.

Numerous small rounded areas of bone destruction are present in the vertical portion of the frontal bone, involving the inner table and diploic space (B). There also is depression and inferior convexity of the cribiform plate margins and bone thinning in the ethmoid and supraorbital areas. The sella turcica, planum sphenoidale, and lateral aspects of the sphenoid bone exhibit severe damage by pressure erosion. The findings occurred in a middle-aged woman with an ependymoma of the fourth ventricle of many years duration. An extreme degree of hydrocephalus had caused marked thinning of the frontal dura mater; herniation of the cerebral cortex through the dura and the inner skull table had occurred, with embedment of brain tissue in the diploic space at many points.

(Revised 1963)

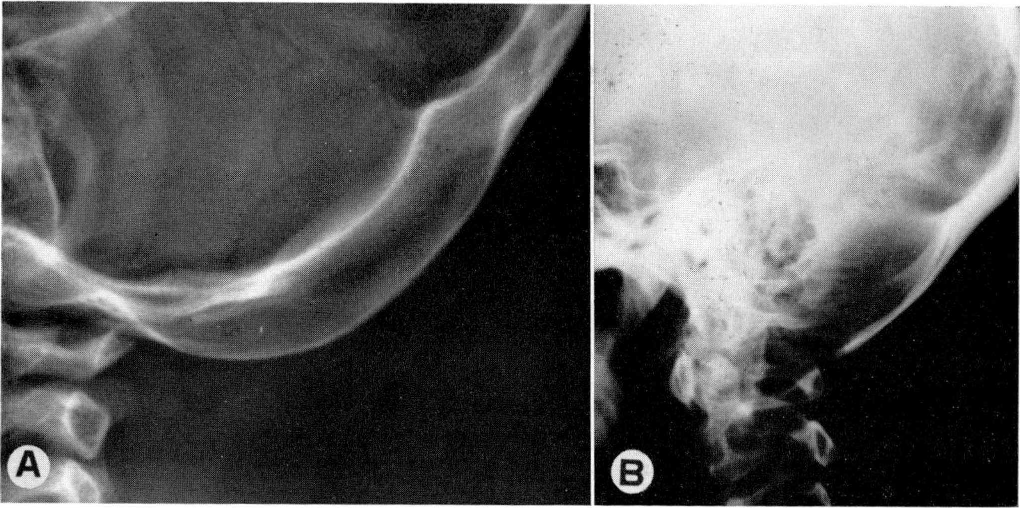

FIG. 67.—CEREBELLAR ASTROCYTOMA WITH OCCIPITAL BONE ASYMMETRY
A child with generalized increased intracranial pressure from a hemispheric astrocytoma of the cerebellum exhibited suture widening, increased convolutional markings, and asymmetry of the occipital bone (A). On the side of the tumor, the occipital squama is thin from a point just behind the rim of the foramen magnum to the inion. Some outward bulging is present, and the lateral sinus groove on the side of the tumor is higher than on the contralateral side. In some instances, such bony changes can be closely correlated with a localized expanding lesion; technical causes of an asymmetrical posterior fossa must always be excluded (see text). In another case (B), the slope of the occipital bone was sharp on one side; the occipital squama was thin and tapered toward the rim of the foramen magnum, which was low on one side.

The herniated substance was anchored so tightly that it was extremely difficult to remove the brain at the time of necropsy.

Temporal bone. The temporal bone is affected more often by lesions producing local erosion than by changes of generalized increased intracranial pressure. The latter, however, should not be mistaken as being of localizing value. It is not rare, in instances of continued intracranial hypertension, for the petrous pyramids and particularly the tips to exhibit decalcification. Careful observation, however, will reveal that the ghost-like outline of the atrophic petrous tips remains. Even though calcium content has been reduced considerably, it may remain highest along the line outlining the internal auditory canal. It is conceivable that long standing increased intracranial pressure could cause slight enlargement of both canals. Quite the reverse is true in the case of acoustic neurinoma. The squamous portion of the temporal bone seldom exhibits evidence of atrophy, except in those instances where diffuse atrophy of the vault occurs. The bone here is normally thin and devoid of convolutional markings, but digital impressions may appear with prolonged increased pressure. The portion of the floor of the middle fossa formed by the temporal bones frequently is deformed by local erosions but changes of generalized pressure are difficult to appreciate here.

Occipital bone. In the occipital area, posterior fossa enlargement sometimes is seen with posterior fossa tumor, Dandy-Walker syndrome, and certain other lesions. These changes consist of an altered slope of the lower half or the supraoccipital portion of the occipital bone which becomes more horizontal. This may be associated with a high position of the lateral sinus grooves and occipital protuberance, asymmetry and irregularity of the margins of the foramen magnum, and atrophy in the region of the clivus (fig. 67). With all of these alterations, usually the results of increased pressure in the posterior fossa and neighborhood pres-

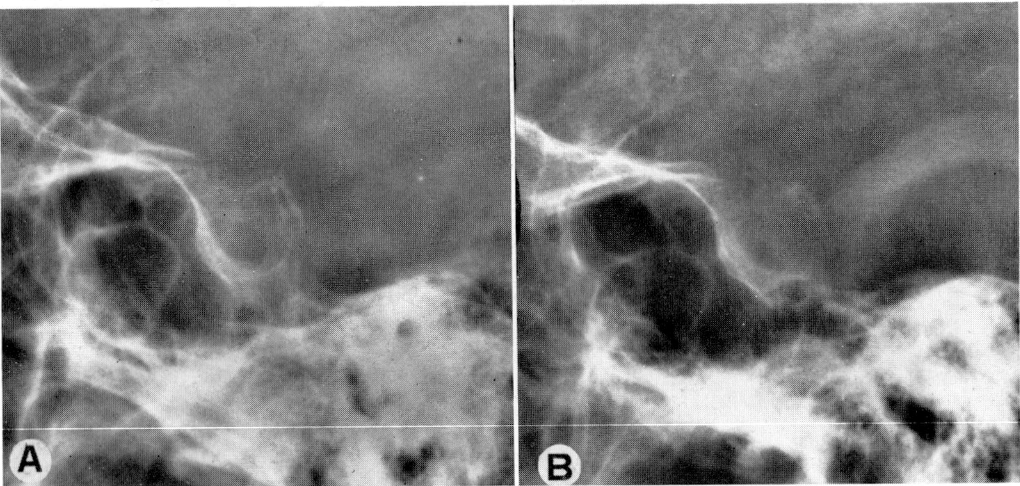

Fig. 68.—Sella Turcica Changes with Aging

A man of late middle age had generalized osteoporosis of the skeleton, including the sella turcica, when first examined (A). When re-examined five years later (B), there had been advancement of the process of demineralization which might be mistaken for the atrophy of increased intracranial pressure. In most instances of osteoporosis, the posterior clinoid processes and dorsum sellae, although radiolucent, will exhibit a faintly detectable remnant of the cortical boundary.

sure effects, there is often an element of generalized decalcification or atrophy which can be striking. It is important to recognize that such widespread changes can occur on the basis of intracranial hypertension alone and to be cautious in attributing localizing significance to atrophic changes.

Differential Diagnosis

Systemic disease. There are a number of systemic diseases in which intracranial hypertension occurs or in which changes are found which clinically mimic increased intracranial pressure. The plain-film changes, therefore, may simulate those of brain tumor and the fact that atrophy of the sella turcica occurs most often in the adult as a result of brain tumor has been emphasized elsewhere. The occurrence of benign lesions simulating tumor is being recognized with increasing frequency, and one can no longer assume that an expanding intracranial lesion is a neoplasm or even that plain-film changes are the result of a localized mass lesion of benign nature. The difficulties encountered in connection with attempts to diagnose the significance of changes in the sella turcica early are encountered with such frequency that the term "pseudoerosion" of the sella turcica has appeared in the medical vocabulary.

The most common systemic condition to cause diagnostic difficulty is the normal process of *aging*. The sella turcica shares in the generalized mineral loss of the skull, and because of the thinness of the structures concerned there is frequently an apparent disproportionate demineralization of the clinoid processes and dorsum sellae and even the sellar floor. Some allowance in appearance of the sella turcica must be made for aging changes, and it is not possible in our experience to define an age below which this allowance is not applicable. The majority of patients above 60 years, particularly women, exhibit calcium loss and it is not rare to find such changes below the age of 40 years. It is quite probable that many patients with brain tumor cannot be diagnosed early because of this limitation of the radiologic diagnostic method (fig. 68).

The changes in the sella turcica associated with *increased adrenal cortical activity* or the administration of steroid compounds have been long recognized and were described by Cushing (1932) in conjunction with the

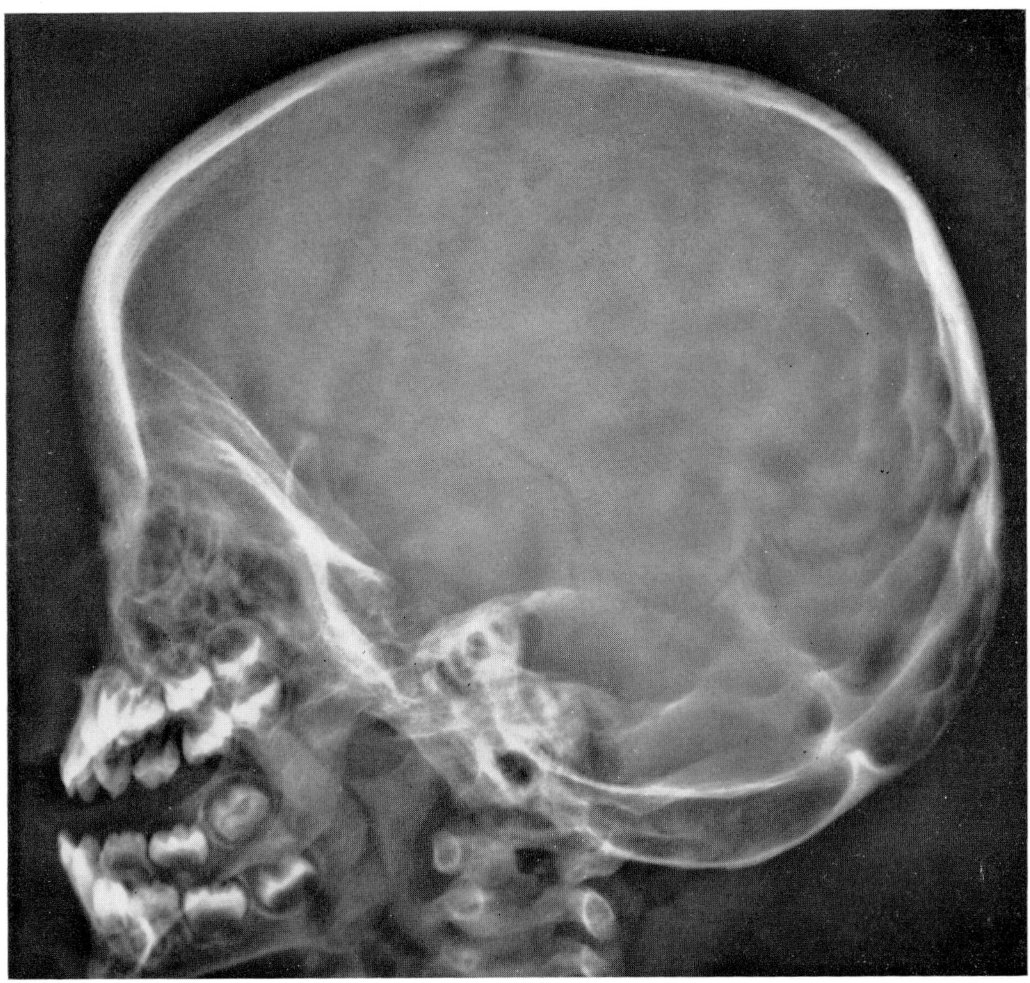

Fig. 69.—Increased Intracranial Pressure in Hypoparathyroidism

A 21-month-old child was admitted because of generalized convulsions recurring during a 2-week period. The serum calcium was found to be 7.4 mg. per 100 ml., and the phosphorus was 9.0 mg. per 100 ml. An abnormal rise in urinary phosphorus excretion was found on testing (Elsworth-Howard method). Clinical and radiologic evidence of increased intracranial pressure was present, the latter showing widening of the major sutures and prominent digital markings posteriorly. (Courtesy of Dr. John Caffey, Primary Children's Hospital, Salt Lake City, Utah.)

condition he called pituitary basophilism. The changes result from marked mineral loss from the entire sella turcica, particularly the thin dorsum and sellar floor with the occasional impression that the sellar cavity is absolutely enlarged. It was noted earlier, however, that the great majority of basophilic adenomas are microscopic lesions which, in themselves, are incapable of producing an increase in size of the bony sella.

In both the naturally occurring and induced forms of the Cushingoid state, the clinical and other general radiologic changes are so apparent that the question of sellar atrophy due to increased intracranial pressure does not arise frequently.

Similarly, *hyperparathyroidism* results in a generalized demineralization of the skeleton, including the skull, which is usually prominently involved. There may or may not be a

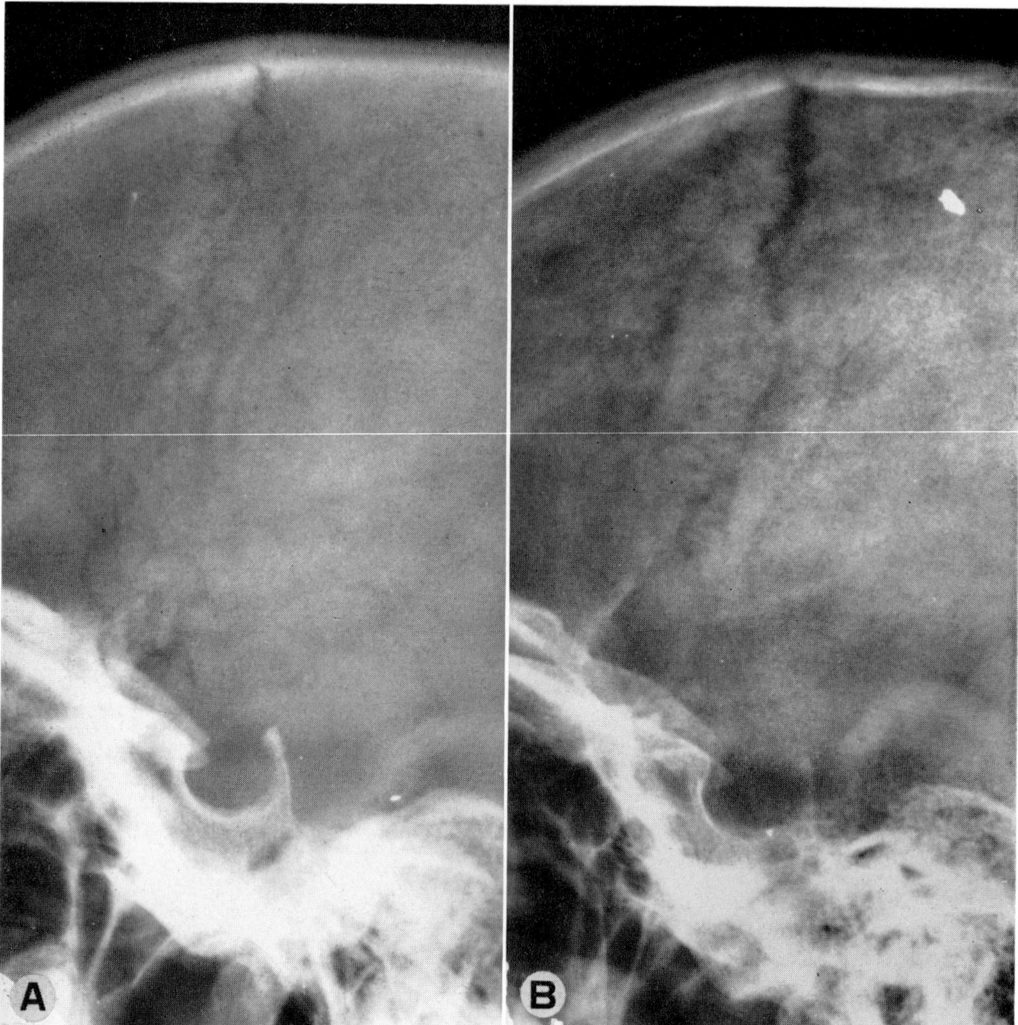

FIG. 70.—JUVENILE HYPOTHYROIDISM UNDER SUBSTITUTION THERAPY

The rounded and slightly enlarged (88 sq. mm.) sella turcica of a 13-year-old female cretin is shown (A). The patient became euthyroid in a short period of time under heavy triiodothyronine therapy. A film made five months later, with the patient still under treatment, reveals widening of the coronal suture (B), considered to be the result of rapid brain growth paralleling an increase in general stature. The patient had papilledema at this time.

correspondingly striking change in the sella turcica, but in some instances the boundaries of the pituitary fossa are indistinguishable due to mineral loss. The changes usually are more pronounced in primary hyperparathyroidism than in secondary hyperparathyroidism, and therefore, sellar changes are more often seen in adults than in children. Since the cranial vault has a characteristic granular decalcification, and there are associated changes in other bones, such as the mandible, it is usually possible to suspect the true nature of the pathologic process and appreciate that the findings are apparent rather then real indications of increased intracranial pressure. Metastatic calcification in the meningeal and cerebral blood vessels may occur in long standing increased activity of the parathyroid glands (fig. 165).

On the other hand, *decreased parathyroid*

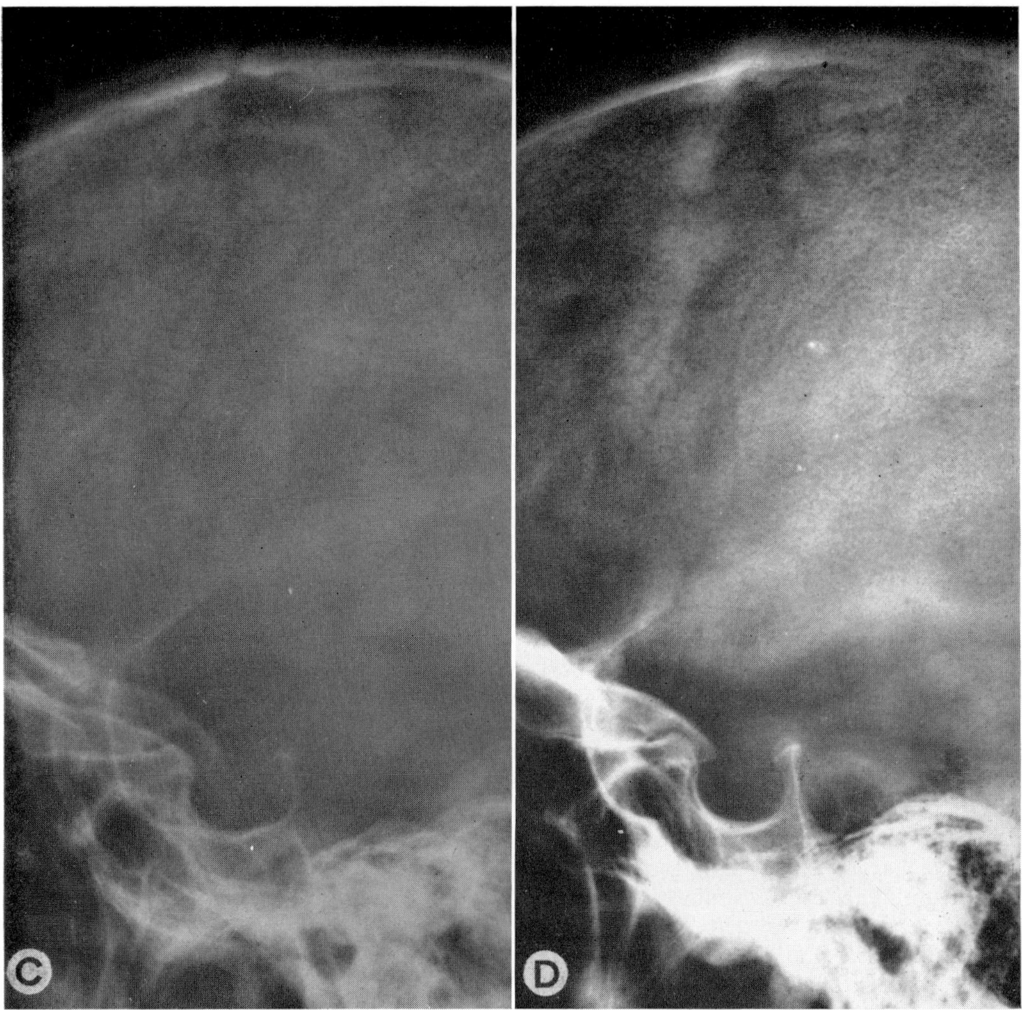

Fig. 70

The medication was changed to desiccated thyroid extract in moderate dosage and the increased intracranial pressure promptly disappeared. Examination six months later (C) revealed the coronal suture to be normal, but there had been continued enlargement of the pituitary fossa (94 sq. mm.) and deformity suggesting the presence of an adenoma (the clinical and laboratory findings also suggested a pituitary adenoma). Upon examination one and a half years later (D), when the patient had regained normal pituitary function clinically and by laboratory findings, the sella turcica was smaller (81 sq. mm.) and the boundaries were well mineralized (see text).

activity may result in true increased intracranial pressure and real rather than apparent radiologic changes may be present in some instances. The increased pressure is explained as the result of an alteration of intra- and intercellular fluid and electrolytes, a process which also is supposed to be involved in the deposition of calcium in the basal ganglia and gray nuclei. Papilledema is a well known occurrence in surgical hypoparathyroidism and was found by Steinberg and Waldron (1952) in 7 of 52 patients with idiopathic hypoparathyroidism. Of the seven patients with calcification in the basal ganglia studied by Steinberg and Waldron, two had increased intracranial pressure. The detection of nuclear calcification is helpful in making a correct radiologic diagnosis since there are no other distinctive features of the pressure manifestations. In the example illustrated in Figure 69, increased intracranial pressure occurring in a three-year-old child with idiopathic hypoparathyroidism was manifested by widening of the major sutures and abnormal prominence of the convolutional markings.

Hyperthyroidism may result either in apparent or real changes of increased intracranial pressure. The former is not a common finding and not one of particular clinical importance, although it has been described by some writers for many years. A general slight decalcification of the skeleton may occur with hyperthyroidism, including the bones of the vault and base of the skull. The bony architecture may have a delicate, finely reticular pattern, and the skull often is thin and frequently the diploic space is not prominently depicted. The findings may resemble, to some extent, the diffuse atrophy of the vault which in some instances accompanies increased intracranial pressure.

Of greater interest, however, are a small group of hypothyroid children recently encountered who have been treated with thyroid hormone, sometimes in large doses. In these cretins, the chief cause of the radiologic changes of increased pressure which result is rapid brain growth plus alterations in fluid balance. The changes in the skull also parallel a rapid growth in stature under substitution treatment, which further suggests that the former is the result of rapid growth of an underdeveloped brain. The patients exhibit distinct widening of the sutures and there may be changes in the sella turcica as well. In the patient shown in Figure 70, the radiologic changes of increased intracranial pressure developed in a period of five months. Disappearance of the suture widening can be demonstrated if the quantity of thyroid hormone administered is reduced. A latent effect, however, may be an increase in diameter of the sella turcica and a change in its configuration to resemble that seen with pituitary adenoma. At this stage, increased pituitary activity may be evidenced by end organ changes in several modalities (Van Wyk and M. M. Grumbach, 1960). In some of these patients, with the passage of time, normal adolescent hormonal activity may supervene with a return of the patient's clinical picture to normal and reversal of the sella turcica to a normal radiologic appearance.

The Cushingoid skull and also the skull of hyperparathyroidism may be simulated to some extent by diseases affecting the hematopoietic system generally. *Leukemia* with infiltration of the bone marrow of the skull may result in an appearance simulating generalized osteoporosis, prior to or instead of the development of spotty or confluent areas of diminished density which can more readily be recognized as osteolytic disease. Likewise, in some cases of *myelomatosis* there may be a generalized demineralization rather than the more typical occurrence of discrete, well-defined, rounded areas of bone destruction. In leukemia, it is not unusual to have true increased intracranial pressure as a result of meningeal and brain infiltration. With neuroblastoma, *diffuse metastasis* is common and the intracranial contents have a predilection for such metastatic deposits. The cranial bones also frequently contain skeletal metastases and the combination of changes of increased intracranial pressure with osteolytic lesions of the cranium, occurring in a young child, should always suggest neuroblastoma as a prime diagnostic possibility. *Lead poisoning* in children produces an encephalopathy with increased intracranial pressure and frequently with marked widening of the major sutures (fig. 71). A high index of suspicion or good clinical information may lead the radiologist to the correct diagnosis through the demonstration of zones of heavily increased density caused by profound growth disturbances at the ends of long bones.

Dysplasia of bone. Certain disease processes, such as *neurofibromatosis*, may mimic not only the localized changes of general pressure but also may resemble local erosion by adjacent focal lesions even though no tumor is present. Developmental abnormalities of many mesenchymal tissues may be involved without the presence of nerve sheath tumors in the areas of malformation.

(Revised 1963)

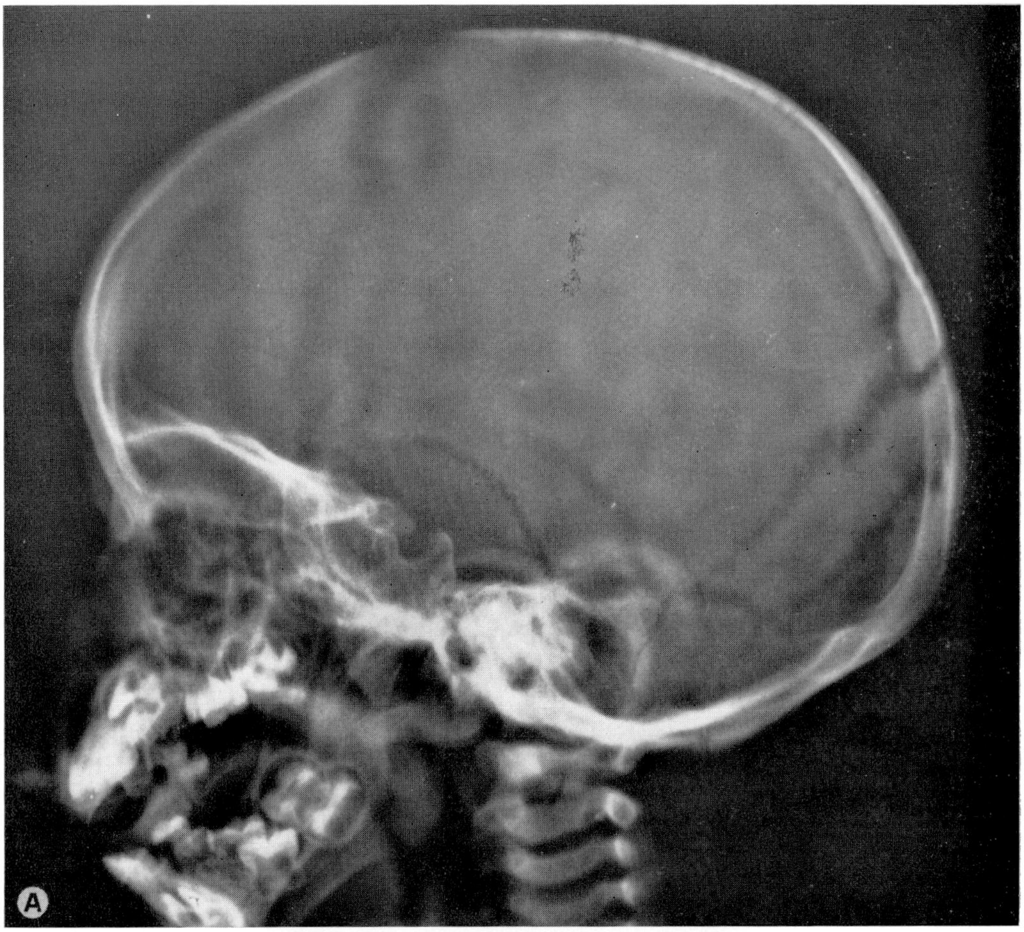

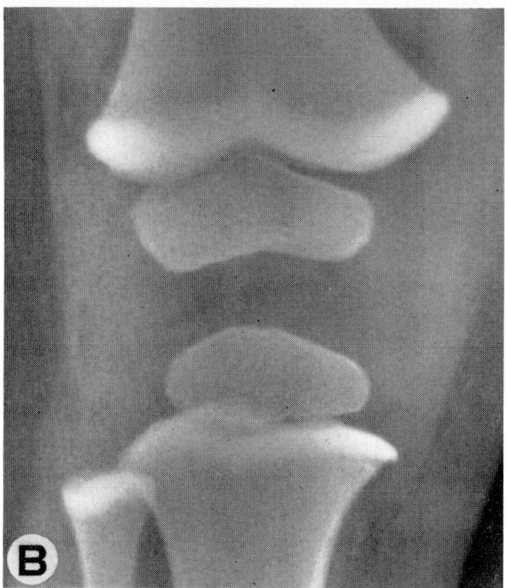

FIG. 71.—LEAD ENCEPHALOPATHY

Lead intoxication with encephalopathy may occur following the inhalation of the fumes from burning storage batteries. The skull film of a child who acquired plumbism in this way exhibits widening of all of the major cranial sutures (A). If the exposure is chronic, as in this case, a wide band of heavy density will develop at the ends of the shafts of rapidly growing long bones (B).

(Revised 1963)

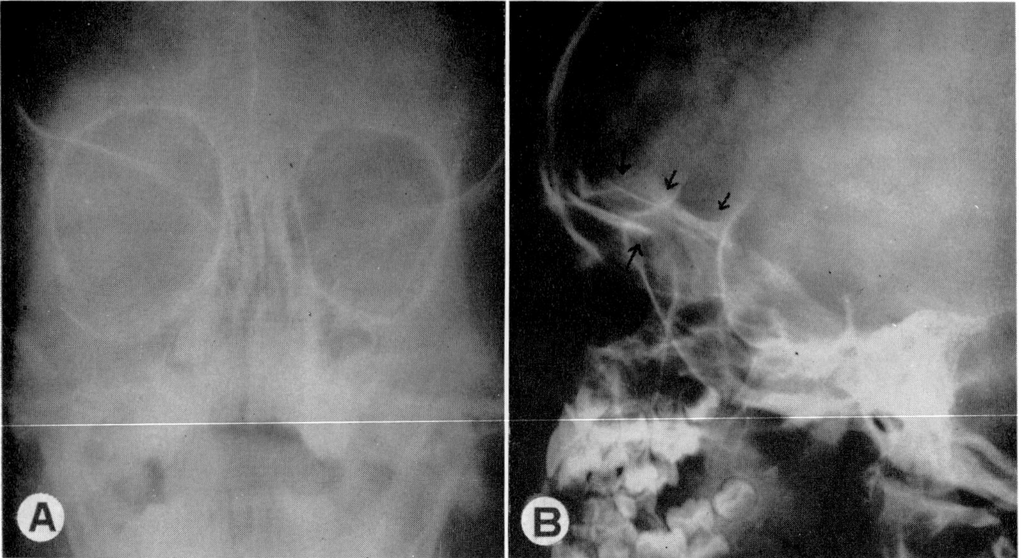

FIG. 72.—NEUROFIBROMATOSIS WITH BONE DEFECTS RESEMBLING PRESSURE CHANGES

Areas of bony dysplasia are found in neurofibromatosis which may simulate pressure erosion; the sphenoid bone is frequently affected in the skull and the changes may be mistaken for those of a middle fossa mass, such as subdural hematoma (A). The greater wing of the sphenoid often is high and very thin; the posterior bony wall of the orbit may be absent. The superior orbital fissure frequently is poorly defined. The inferior and lateral orbital walls also may be poorly formed. If the posterior bony wall of the orbit is absent, exophthalmus may occur and the involved orbital cavity may be denser than usual. When sphenoid wing changes develop owing to erosion by middle fossa hematoma, the bony margins and fissures usually are preserved (see Fig. 605).

In lateral view (B), the abnormal slope of the sphenoid wing on one side is associated with an ipsilateral shortening of the anterior fossa and defective formation of the superior orbital plate (*arrows*). A large sella turcica is a common associated finding as in this case; a large sella with anterior deformity, associated with other manifestations of defective formation of the sphenoid bone, should suggest the possibility of neurofibromatosis.

Therefore, the bone defects are not the result of erosion by an adjacent tumor or by a neoplastic process developing within bone.

The sphenoid bone frequently displays evidence of the osseous dysplasia. Changes in the anterior portion of the sella turcica in the region of the dorsum and the planum sphenoidale may occur, resulting in a long, shallow sella turcica with flattening of the tuberculum. The result may be a sella turcica which, in the lateral roentgenogram, resembles the letter J lying on its side, which can be associated with a tumor in the immediate vicinity, such as optic gliomas and other suprasellar lesions. A sella turcica of this type occasionally may be found in normal children, and it is very commonly encountered in patients with neurofibromatosis without the implication of pressure erosion by tumor in this region. On other occasions, a large sella turcica is found associated with neurofibromatosis. The enlargement usually is mild, and the sellar margins ordinarily are distinct and of normal density. In some instances, however, the appearance may closely simulate either a pituitary adenoma or the mild, generalized enlargement of the sella turcica which may result from generalized increased intracranial pressure.

The sphenoid wings may be defectively formed in neurofibromatosis to such an extent that one or both wings appear very thin or absent in frontal projection (fig. 72). The structure of the sphenoid wing, particularly its thickness, is so variable, however, that in many normal patients it may appear quite asymmetrical in roentgenograms. However, such changes may occasionally be seen in instances of long standing pressure resulting from tumor, particularly masses of the middle fossa. Without other stigmata of von Recklinghausen's disease, it may be difficult to be certain that one is dealing with bone dysplasia rather than bone destruction. In the usual case of sphenoid wing thinning resulting from increased intracranial pressure, there is other radiologic evidence of pressure atrophy involving cranial structures. Defective formation of the posterior orbital wall may be so extensive that pulsating exophthalmos may be present. Even middle fossa hematomas, tumors, dural cysts, and porencephalic cysts do not result in erosion of a magnitude simulating absence of the sphenoid wing in neurofibromatosis. Furthermore, the space-occupying lesions usually produce bulging and thinning along the side wall or floor of the middle fossa which indicate their erosive nature (fig. 605).

The clinically silent intrasellar pituitary adenoma and the normally large sella turcica remain as difficult problems in differentiation from the sellar enlargement of increased intracranial pressure. Instances frequently are encountered in which, in lateral view, the sella turcica definitely exceeds in length and depth the usual upper limits of normal, especially in women, and explanations for this are discussed in the section to follow. It is to be remembered, however, that the measurements in general use were obtained by examination of a significant number of clinically normal individuals, from the standpoint of sellar disease, and that random exceptions to the accepted range are to be expected. When doubt exists about whether or not one is dealing with evidence of increased intracranial pressure, an expanding pituitary lesion or a normal case, a contrast study should be carried out if clinically indicated. In borderline instances, and if there is no clinical support for the diagnosis of disease, the radiologist has little alternative but to request follow-up examinations at three-month intervals until it is possible to be certain whether an abnormality in the form of a progressively expanding lesion is present.

Local Bone Erosions

In this section the following will be considered: sella turcica, petrous pyramids, optic foramen, jugular foramen, and erosions of the inner table of the skull. In each instance the study of local erosions will be preceded by a discussion of the normal anatomy. In addition, the tumors of the cranial vault and the destructive lesions of the base of the skull that are more commonly encountered in neuroradiologic practice will be considered.

THE SELLA TURCICA

Anatomy

A detailed study of the anatomy of the sella turcica is justified here because of the great importance that the sella has in diagnosis of intracranial conditions from plain roentgenograms. We will consider (1) the anterior aspect which comprises several important structures; (2) the floor; and (3) the dorsum. The pituitary fossa is that portion of the sella that contains the pituitary gland.

1. Anterior aspect. The forward portion comprises (*a*) the posterior extremity of the planum sphenoidale, (*b*) the limbus sphenoidalis, (*c*) the chiasmatic groove, (*d*) the tuberculum sellae, (*e*) the anterior clinoid processes, and (*f*) the middle clinoid processes.

(*a*) The *planum sphenoidale* represents the posterior portion of the floor of the anterior fossa in the midline. This is usually formed by a sharp dense plate of bone variable in thickness. It is usually quite thin. At other times, in normal individuals, it is slightly thicker

(*Revised 1963*)

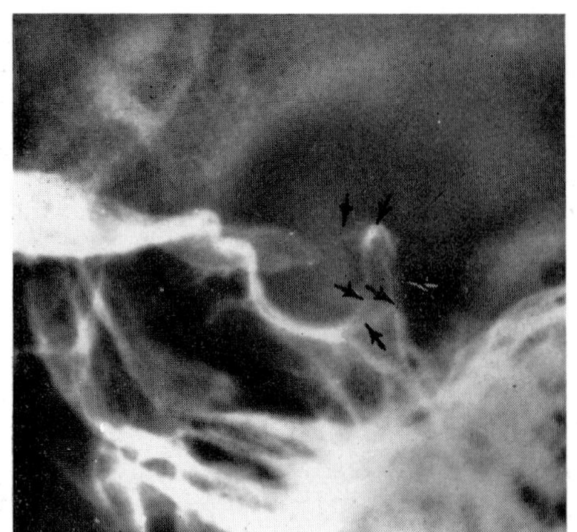

FIG. 73.—NORMAL SELLA TURCICA WITH WELL DEFINED LIMBUS SPHENOIDALIS AND TUBERCULUM SELLAE

The dense straight shadow of the planum ends posteriorly in the limbus sphenoidalis (*arrow*). Behind this there is another elevation, the tuberculum sellae, and between the two is a depression which is called the chiasmatic groove. The dorsum sellae presents three lines: the anterior line (*forward arrow*) represents the lateral margins of the dorsum sellae, the dense line in the middle (*middle arrow*) represents the posterior margin of the pituitary fossa at the center of the dorsum, and the posterior margin (*posterior arrow*) represents the posterior margin of the dorsum. The posterior clinoid processes are visible (*arrow*), and the upper border of the central portion of the dorsum presents a rounded top (*arrow*).

(fig. 16) and the outlines are quite sharp in contradistinction to abnormal thickening, which usually gives it a spongy appearance (fig. 424). Sometimes the planum ends posteriorly in an even denser and heavier area of bone which represents the limbus sphenoidalis.

(*b*) The *limbus sphenoidalis* is an inconstant elevation which limits the planum sphenoidale posteriorly. In some patients it is very clearly defined (fig. 16), but usually it is rather inconspicuous. At other times it is limited posteriorly by a deep narrow groove visible in the lateral projection (fig. 73).

(*c*) The *chiasmatic groove* is of variable depth; it is usually very shallow, well demarcated in some individuals and not present in others. The chiasmatic groove ends laterally in the optic foramen on each side. In some patients the optic chiasm is very close to the bone, whereas in other individuals there is a variable distance present which is sometimes as long as 1.5 cm. The chiasmatic groove may be extremely prominent in some patients, resulting in flattening of the region of the tuberculum sellae. This may be of pathologic significance and is seen in patients with optic gliomas, hydrocephalus, and other conditions (see below).

(*d*) The *tuberculum sellae* represents the actual anterior boundary of the pituitary fossa in the midline. It is usually well demarcated and easy to pinpoint on the films; it represents the point at which the horizontal portion of the presellar area just described is continuous with the vertical or sloping anterior boundary of the pituitary fossa. When seen from above, in the dry skull, the tuberculum sellae represents an elevation that has also been called the *olivary eminence* but when seen in lateral roentgenograms, it simply represents the angle at the superior portion of the pituitary fossa. On each side and slightly anterior to the tuberculum sellae is the optic foramen, which will be described later (fig. 36). The diaphragma sellae inserts in the tuberculum sellae anteriorly and in the upper margin of the dorsum posteriorly.

(*e*) *Anterior clinoid processes.* These are not actually part of the pituitary fossa because they are situated on each side of the tuberculum sellae. However, roentgenographically, they are always projected over and slightly above the tuberculum sellae in lateral view. On films made with sufficient penetration, the tuberculum sellae is always visible through the shadows of the anterior clinoid processes. The anterior clinoid processes seem to be the posterior prolongation of the roofs of the orbits as seen on the lateral roentgenograms (fig. 16). The anterior clinoid processes are quite variable in size and shape. Sometimes they are voluminous and partly or completely pneumatized, and at other times they are extremely thin, in normal individuals. The latter appearance always suggests possible increased intracranial pressure or erosion. However, in the absence of other findings indicative of ero-

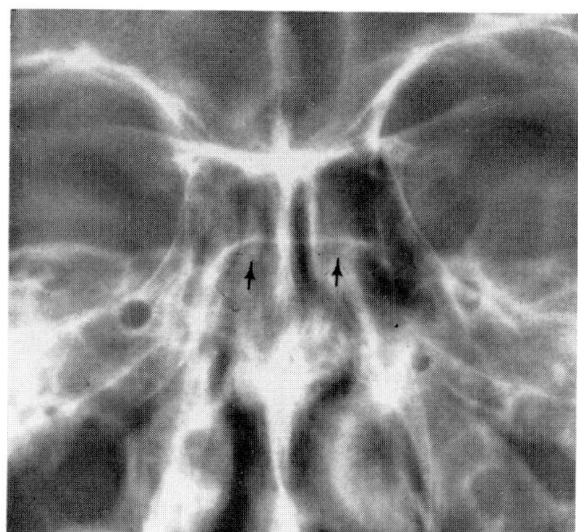

FIG. 74.—NORMAL FLOOR OF SELLA TURCICA

In the frontal projection the floor of the sella turcica is usually visible (*arrows*) although it is often difficult to find without laminagraphy.

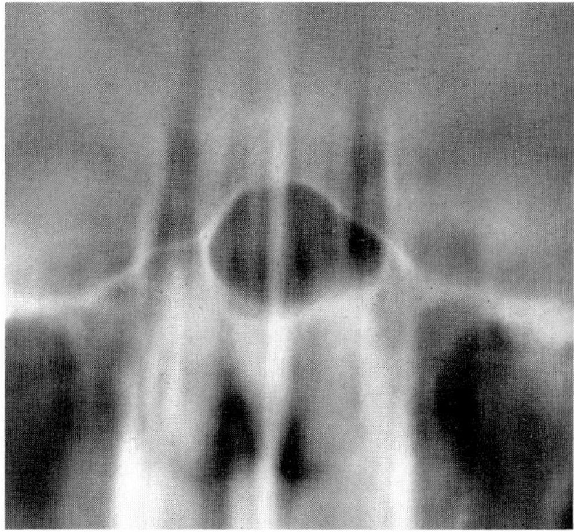

FIG. 75.—FRONTAL LAMINAGRAM OF THE SELLA TURCICA SHOWING A SLANTED FLOOR

In this case a lateral view of the sella would show a slight degree of double floor, but the transverse diameter of the sella turcica is normal and there is no real depression or concavity of the sella.

sion or increased pressure, the presence of thin anterior clinoid processes is usually a normal finding. One anterior clinoid process may be eroded or appear elevated in unilateral parasellar or intrasellar lesions (figs. 85 and 89). The interclinoid ligaments insert on each side in the anterior clinoid processes (see below).

(*f*) The *middle clinoid processes* are two small inconstant elevations situated on each side of the anterior portion of the floor of the sella turcica below the anterior clinoid processes. The internal carotid arteries pass anterolateral to the middle clinoid processes when emerging from the cavernous sinuses curving upward to pass medial to the anterior clinoid processes. The dura of the cavernous sinuses inserts in the middle clinoid process and extends from there to the tip of the anterior clinoid process. When this dural fold ossifies, it produces a foramen which is called the *caroticoclinoid foramen.* This foramen may be seen sometimes in lateral views; in other cases, it is visible on optic foramen views and should not be confused with the optic foramen (fig. 115).

2. Floor. The floor of the sella turcica is always formed by a thin, dense plate of bone which is continuous throughout the extent of the sella but is most pronounced in the floor portion. It is usually thinner in the dorsum. The sphenoid sinuses extend under the floor of the sella turcica to a variable extent. The sinuses usually are under the anterior portion, but they may occupy the entire floor with the exclusion of the dorsum sellae, or they may pneumatize the dorsum sellae completely.

In most instances the floor of the sella turcica is composed of a single dense line, but sometimes two lines are seen. The latter configuration is called a *double floor.* A double floor of the sella turcica is usually considered as an abnormal finding and is seen most frequently in intrasellar tumors, particularly pituitary adenomas. However, in some instances a normal double floor, which could be called pseudodouble floor, is encountered. The appearance of a pseudodouble floor may be produced by any of four anatomical conditions. (*a*) There may be a slight depression of the central portion of the sella turcica. This depression is usually smooth and the double floor that this anatomical variation produces is characterized by the fact that the separation between the two contours is small. This could be proved beyond doubt by the taking of a frontal

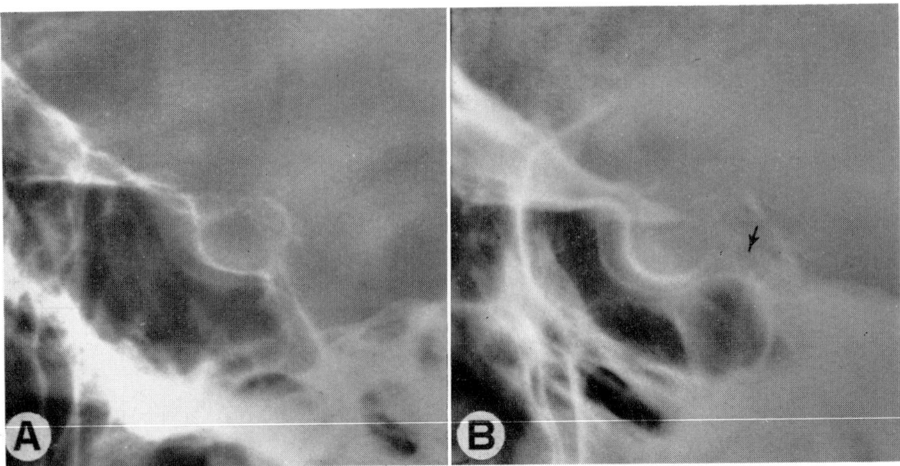

FIG. 76.—DOUBLE FLOOR OF SELLA TURCICA PRODUCED BY THE CAROTID GROOVE

(A) Two contours are seen on the inferior aspect of the sella turcica; the lower contour is produced by the groove on each side of the sella turcica caused by the cavernous sinus which has within it the internal carotid artery. This is differentiated from a true double floor in that it does not extend into the dorsum sellae but curves downward as it reaches the posterior aspect of the dorsum sellae.

(B) shows another case of false double floor probably produced by uneven development of the sphenoid sinuses. Again, the lower level does not extend into the dorsum sellae but curves downward. It is noted that one side of the sphenoid sinus extends higher than the lower contour (*arrow*) and represents the larger sphenoid sinus. The lower contour represents the upper margin of the smaller sphenoid sinus. This can be demonstrated in the frontal projection, particularly if laminagraphy is used.

laminagram of the sella. (*b*) Asymmetrical development of the floor of the sella turcica; one side is higher than the other which may be seen in simple frontal films of the skull. If necessary, this condition may also be demonstrated by laminagraphy, which would ordinarily show without question that one side of the floor is lower than the other. A slightly slanted floor is usually a normal finding but it could conceivably be associated with enlargement of one side of the pituitary fossa contents. In the latter cases, the sellar floor becomes more concave and thin (fig. 75). (*c*) Uneven development of the sphenoid sinuses. If one side of the sphenoid sinuses is much larger than the other and the septum between the two sides of the sphenoid sinuses is off the midline, it is possible to get a double floor image because one side of the sphenoid sinus goes all the way up to the floor of the sella, but the other side has a segment of bone between its roof and the floor of the sella turcica. The upper contour of the smaller sinus will then cast a shadow which will give an appearance of a double floor (fig. 76). This can be demonstrated also if necessary in frontal laminagrams of the sella turcica. In these cases, the lower of the two lines forming the sellar floor does not join the anterior contour of the dorsum sellae posteriorly but rather, with the sphenoid sinus, it will curve downward upon reaching the posterior portion. (*d*) On each side of the floor of the sella turcica there is usually a small depression or groove produced by the cavernous sinus and the intracavernous portion of the internal carotid artery. The latter lies close to or actually against the medial wall of the cavernous sinus. This depression is called the *carotid groove* and is often the cause of a false double floor of the sella turcica. Again its contour can be followed backward and instead of curving upward to follow the dorsum sellae, it will curve downward to follow the internal carotid artery as it bends caudally towards the foramen lacerum (fig. 76).

3. Dorsum sellae. The dorsum sellae is, like the other portions of the sella turcica, variable in thickness and height. Its anterior surface is usually distinctly shown and is continuous with the dense plate forming the floor. Its cortex is slightly thinner than that of the floor of the sella just described. Mahmoud (1958) has determined by means of microradiographs of sagittal sections of the sella turcica that the thickness of the cortical dense bone in the dorsum is slightly less than that of the floor. Therefore, when there is increased intracranial pressure developing, it is possible that the inner aspect of the dorsum will show signs of demineralization earlier than the floor. The posterior surface of the dorsum is often irregular, particularly in older individuals. The irregularity is partly produced by the presence of the basilar venous plexus which may erode it, and by the presence of calcifications of the dura over the dorsum and of the petroclinoid ligaments. The dorsum is usually inclined forward, tending to give the pituitary fossa a round or oval configuration, but sometimes it is more vertical, producing what is termed by some an "open sella." In the presence of an "open sella" configuration, the possibility of posterior displacement by a lesion should always be considered before regarding it as normal. In the abnormal cases, the dorsum is apt to be thin or demineralized.

The *posterior clinoid processes* are the upper angles of the dorsum; they project slightly laterally upward and forward. On a roentgenogram they are projected slightly in front of the dorsum sellae. This is distinctly visible in some individuals, particularly in children, and in these cases it is possible to determine the exact position of the upper margin of the dorsum sellae as separate from that of the posterior clinoid processes (fig. 73). The dorsum sellae sometimes presents a slanted configuration; one posterior clinoid process may be absent and occasionally both clinoid processes are absent. In these cases, the top of the dorsum sellae assumes a somewhat rounded configuration, as seen in the half axial projection. At the lower portion of the lateral margin of the dorsum sellae there is sometimes a sharp notch which is produced by the internal carotid artery. Pneumatization of the dorsum sellae is quite variable. Sometimes it is completely pneumatized, whereas at other times it is pneumatized only in its lower portion; in these cases the upper portion, which presents no pneumatization, is much thinner than the lower portion.

Posteriorly, the dorsum sellae and adjacent portion of the sphenoid unite with the occipital bone to form the clivus. Between the sphenoid and the occipital bone there is a synchondrosis which disappears by fusion at about the 20th year. Fusion may occur as late as the 25th year and occasionally it never occurs, in which case a suture line results in its place. Fusion may start as early as the 12th year (Irwin, 1960).

Calcification in the petroclinoid ligaments and in the dura behind the dorsum sellae is common, and in some cases the calcified dura is more conspicuous than the cortex of the posterior margin of the dorsum sellae. This condition is particularly frequent in older individuals with evidence of osteoporosis. When osteoporosis is present, the calcified dura will be actually more dense, sometimes considerably more dense, than the dorsum sellae itself (fig. 77). A demineralized dorsum sellae in an older individual is not considered the result of increased intracranial pressure unless it is associated with thinning of the dorsum. Loss of calcium without a decrease in the thickness of the dorsum is usually secondary to osteoporosis in the same age group.

The *interclinoid ligaments* are bands of dura between the anterior and posterior clinoids on each side; they represent the forward extension of the tentorium which actually inserts on the anterior clinoid processes. Between them is the diaphragma sellae. The diaphragma sellae and the ligaments can become completely calcified together or independently. Calcification of the interclinoid ligaments produces the so-called bridging of the clinoid processes, which is of no clinical significance. Camp (1923) found a 5 per cent incidence of unilateral calcification and 1 out of 110 specimens in which there was bilateral interclinoid calcification. Bridging of the clinoid processes

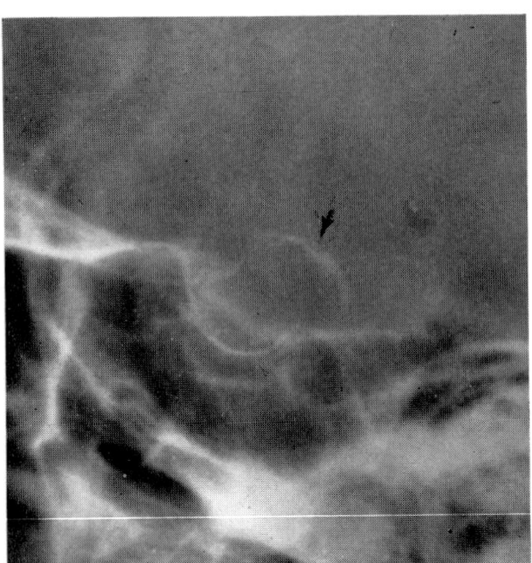

FIG. 77.—OSTEOPOROSIS OF THE DORSUM SELLAE WITH CALCIFIED PETROCLINOID LIGAMENT SIMULATING THE DORSUM

There was a marked degree of osteoporosis of the dorsum; the petroclinoid ligament, which is calcified (*arrow*), simulates the dorsum sellae, which is actually anterior to it. In these cases it is always difficult to rule out increased intracranial pressure if the shadow of the dorsum sellae is not visible, but the calcified petroclinoid ligament should not be confused with a thin posteriorly displaced dorsum.

makes the sella turcica look smaller. It is probable that a previously calcified interclinoid ligament loses its calcium if the sella becomes enlarged, for it is unusual to see an association of calcified interclinoid ligaments and sellar enlargement.

The *diaphragma sellae* is a fold of dura extending between the two interclinoid ligaments. It has a central opening for the passage of the infundibulum or pituitary stalk. The size of this opening is quite variable; in some instances it is very small, just enough for the passage of the pituitary stalk, and in other instances it is very large. It is probable that the "competence" of the diaphragma sellae is a determining factor in the way in which an intrasellar tumor will behave. If the diaphragma sellae has a large opening, it will permit early upward, suprasellar, extension of the tumor and the sella turcica may not become enlarged. On the other hand, when only a small opening is present, the chances are that the tumor will first grow intrasellarly, causing sellar enlargement, and the suprasellar extension will occur later.

Development

The entire base of the skull develops in cartilage. The sphenoid bone, around the sella turcica, ossifies by two paired centers of ossification, the basisphenoid and the presphenoid. These centers meet and become united in the region of the tuberculum sellae. In the newborn the sella turcica is shallow, the dorsum presents only a stump, the rest of the dorsum does not show any ossification. By about 4 years of age, the dorsum sellae begins to show ossification and the future shape of the structure is visible. The sella does remain relatively flat for several years; the posterior clinoid processes do not become ossified until after 5 years of age. As the dorsum sellae continues to increase in width and height, it causes the sella turcica to become gradually deeper. The general outline of the sella turcica changes slowly from the 4th to the 11th year, and after that it increases in size at about the rate of 0.5 to 1 mm. per year. The maximum size of the sella turcica is reached slightly earlier in girls than in boys (Silverman, 1957).

Size

Much has been written on the estimation of the size of the sella turcica from skull roentgenograms. It varies extremely from individual to individual and there is a wide range of normal. The sella turcica can be classified into three basic shapes: (*a*) oval (58 per cent); (*b*) round (25 per cent); (*c*) flat (17 per cent), according to Camp (1924). In children, Gordon and Bell (1922) found the round type in 70 per cent of cases. The sella may acquire a rounded configuration when there is calcification in the interclinoid ligaments.

Smallness of the sella turcica has no pathologic significance in spite of the fact that an occasional case with primary pituitary insufficiency will have a small sella turcica. In these cases the coincidence might be considered significant, but this is extremely rare.

(*Revised 1963*)

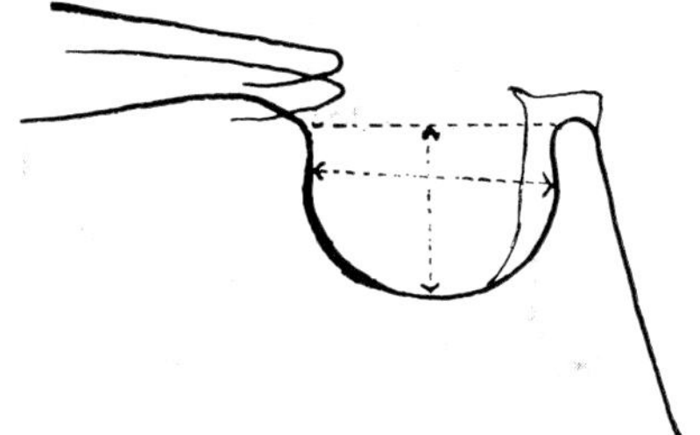

FIG. 78.—METHOD TO OBTAIN LINEAR MEASUREMENTS OF THE SELLA TURCICA, ANTEROPOSTERIOR AND VERTICAL DIAMETER

The anteroposterior diameter is taken from the most anterior to the most posterior margin of the pituitary fossa. Care should be taken to measure to the anterior margin of the midportion of the dorsum and not to the lateral edges, as shown. See Fig. 73. The vertical diameter is taken from the lowest point in the pituitary fossa to a line extending from the top of the dorsum sellae to the tuberculum sellae.

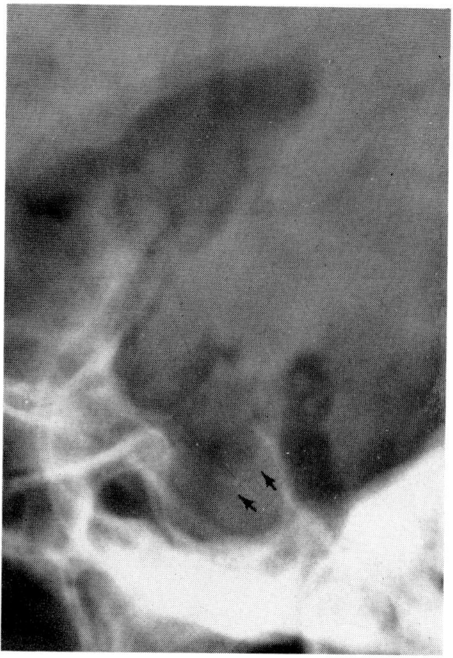

FIG. 79.—AIR GOING INTO AREA OF SELLA TURCICA IN PATIENT WITH SLIGHT ENLARGEMENT OF THIS STRUCTURE

This middle-aged woman complained of nonspecific neurologic symptoms, including headache. Because the sella turcica was found to measure 16 mm. in length by 15 mm. in depth and, therefore, was absolutely enlarged, it was recommended that a pneumoencephalogram be performed. Pneumoencephalography demonstrated air going into the sella turcica (*arrows*). To rule out the possibility that this was air projected over the sella, tomograms were made which demonstrated the air shadow to be within the sella. Therefore, there was no evidence of enlargement of the contents of the pituitary fossa.

On the other hand, enlargement of the sella turcica is most important and therefore it is necessary to establish criteria to determine the possible presence of enlargement. Two basic methods may be employed. The first is used daily by practically everyone and consists in the use of linear measurements for the length and the depth of the sella turcica; the other is based on the area of the pituitary fossa. According to Camp (1924), the anteroposterior diameter of the sella measured from the tuberculum sellae to the most distant point in the dorsum sellae varies from 5 to 16 mm. (average 10.5 mm.). The depth varies from 4 to 12 mm. (average 8.1 mm.).

All of our films are made at a 40-inch target-film distance where the head is placed on the Bucky table, which is 2 inches from the Bucky tray. When a head machine is used, such as the Schonander or the Franklin units, a target-film distance of 36 inches is used and the head is about 1 inch from the Bucky tray.

It is our custom to use the *greatest anteroposterior diameter* of the pituitary fossa. This diameter is measured sometimes at the level of the tuberculum sellae and sometimes below this structure, whichever is furthest forward, depending on the shape. We consider this important because if a line is traced from the tuberculum sellae to the most posterior portion of the dorsum, one may be measuring an oblique diameter of the sella rather than the straight anteroposterior diameter. In addition, in the cases where there is a forward extension of the sella turcica underneath the tuberculum sellae, the actual anteroposterior diameter is larger than the measurement from the tuberculum to the dorsum would indicate (fig. 84). Using the greatest anteroposterior linear measurement of the pituitary fossa

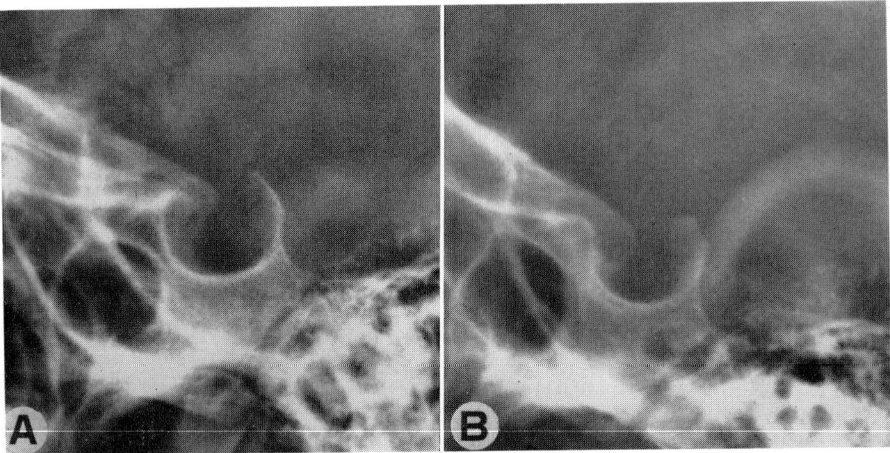

Fig. 80.—Enlargement of the Sella in Patient with Primary Hypothyroidism Showing Decrease in Size after Institution of Appropriate Therapy

In the original examination (A) the sella turcica measured almost 15 mm. in anteroposterior diameter and 11 mm. in depth. Re-examination only 7 months after the institution of therapy showed that the sella measures approximately 12 mm. in length and under 10 mm. in depth. The patient was a 7-year-old girl with precocious puberty who was found to have primary hypothyroidism. The configuration of the sella turcica actually changed in the interim. In (A) there is slight undermining of the tuberculum sellae which is a typical appearance in an enlarged or enlarging sella turcica due to an intrasellar mass. In (B), on the contrary, the anterior aspect of the sella turcica has a slanted configuration.

proper, we rely on the figure of 17 mm. as the upper limit of normal. A figure greater than 17 mm. is practically always abnormal, whereas frequently a measurement of up to 17 mm. is found in patients who have no symptoms or findings of pituitary tumors, or of any lesion that would cause enlargement of the sella turcica. This is an experience based on many thousands of examinations of the skull. On the other hand, a sella may be considered abnormal, although not enlarged according to these measurements (see below). The *depth* of the pituitary fossa is measured as explained in Figure 78. The depth is the greatest distance downward to the floor, perpendicular to a line traced between the tuberculum sellae and the top of the dorsum sellae. An upper limit of 13 mm. seems to be satisfactory in that it is not common to find a normal sella that surpasses this figure. The finding of a deep sella turcica, measuring 14 mm. or more, is not rare however. In these cases, if the anteroposterior diameter is near the upper limit of normal, one would have to consider the sella as presenting absolute enlargement and, depending on the clinical findings, further diagnostic procedures such as pneumoencephalography may have to be carried out. Pneumoencephalography will show, in the normal cases, that the air in the suprasellar cisterns *extends actually inside the sella turcica* (fig. 79). Air along the sides in the parasellar region, however, may simulate gas penetrating into the area of the sella turcica and stereoscopic films or laminagraphy may be required to ascertain this fact. On the other hand, in the presence of a pituitary or other type of intrasellar tumor, air will not enter the sella turcica and the intrasellar soft tissue contents may bulge upward. A careful scrutiny of this air and multiple films as well as stereoscopy and laminagraphy may be necessary to establish a very small suprasellar soft tissue bulge. In the normal cases the pituitary gland does not usually occupy the entire sella turcica, particularly if the sella is large. Indeed, there is no absolute correlation between the size of the sella turcica and the actual volume of the pituitary gland (Rasmussen, 1924). Some of the space, as much as 25 per cent by

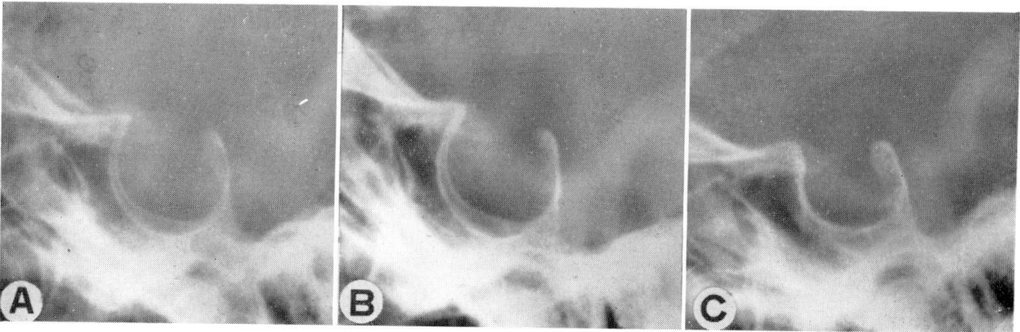

FIG. 81.—PITUITARY ADENOMA SHOWING DECREASE IN SIZE OF SELLA TURCICA FOLLOWING RADIATION THERAPY

The original film (A) showed typical round enlargement of the sella turcica; the sella measured 17 mm. in length by 16 to 17 mm. in depth and presented a slight double floor. The patient then received radiotherapy for a pituitary adenoma, and re-examination 4 months later showed that the sella turcica was not smaller; if anything it was very slightly larger (B). Re-examination 5 years later (C) shows that the sella turcica is essentially normal in appearance, measuring 14 mm. in length by 12 mm. in depth. The patient was a 23-year-old woman who had clinical manifestations compatible with those of a pituitary adenoma. Such marked decrease in the size of the sella turcica in adults following surgical removal or radiation therapy is unusual, but decrease in size following removal of an intracranial mass or shrinkage by radiotherapy is the rule in children or young teenagers.

weight, may be made up by the dural coverings that surround the gland. But in addition there may be a free space—subarachnoid space—between the gland and the diaphragma sellae. The average weight of the pituitary gland is greater in pregnant and in multiparous women than in men (Rasmussen). In spite of previous statements to the contrary (Wislocki, 1937), the subarachnoid space which surrounds the infundibulum of the pituitary gland does not stop at the diaphragma sellae but frequently extends below it. The size of this intrasellar extension varies, but in some patients it is sufficiently large to hold air that can be shown on a pneumoencephalogram (fig. 79). This seems to be more frequent in patients who have relatively large sellas. Conceivably, in these individuals, the pituitary gland enlarges during the period of active growth, causing the sella to enlarge with it. Later the gland may decrease in size but the sella remains unchanged. Otherwise it would be difficult to explain how the pituitary fossa would enlarge beyond the size necessary to contain the gland. Indeed, in children the pituitary fossa enlarges with the gland and becomes smaller if the gland decreases in size. This is well demonstrated in the case of primary hypothyroidism shown in Figure 80. We believe that in adults, the sella usually does not decrease in size if the gland shrinks. An exception is shown in Figure 81. It is therefore possible, after the gland caused enlargement of the sella turcica, to have an increase in the "free space" within the pituitary fossa. Recalcification of the floor of the sella may sometimes give the impression of diminution in size.

The linear measurements are fairly satisfactory in practice; however, measurements based on the area of the sella turcica, as recommended by some authors, are probably more accurate. Hare *et al.* (1949) suggest a figure of 130 square millimeters as the maximum size of the sella turcica, beyond which it should be considered enlarged. Hurxthal (1947) has constructed a chart, which he calls "sella meter," that contains the various sizes and shapes of the sella turcica which can be superimposed on the roentgenogram; the area in square millimeters is indicated on a series of models. Whichever one of the diagrams corresponds to the sella in question will contain the number of square millimeters for the particular shape and size. For abso-

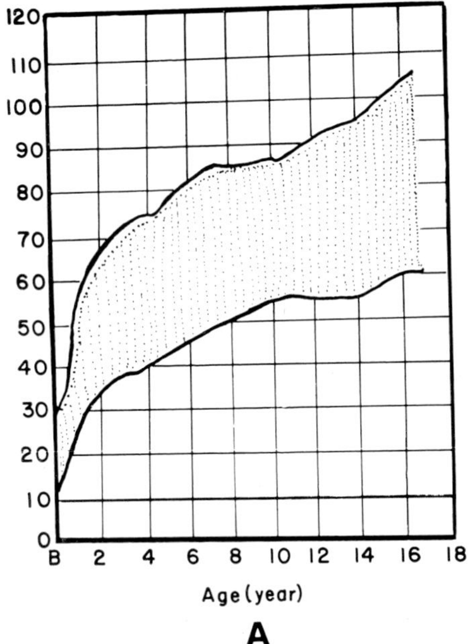

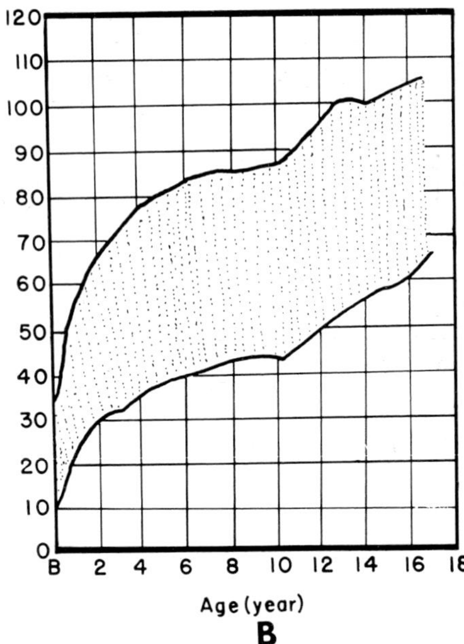

Fig. 82.—Variations in Sella Area in Children, Males and Females, According to Silverman

Maximum sella size is achieved slightly earlier in girls than in boys. (A) Fifth and ninety-fifth percentiles of pituitary fossa area in sq. mm.—males, birth to 17 years. (B) Fifth and ninety-fifth percentiles of pituitary fossa area in sq. mm.—females, birth to 17 years.

lute accuracy in determining the area of the pituitary fossa it is necessary to use a compensating planimeter.

Silverman published a series of curves representing the area of the sella turcica in boys and girls. He related the area to age and to stature. The diagrams in Figure 82 are according to Silverman and relate sella area to age, in boys and girls. The upper and lower limits at each age represent the 5th and the 95th percentile.

The *width of the sella turcica* is visible on skull films made in frontal projection. It is possible to see it in many instances on plain films, but in some cases laminagraphy is necessary for this purpose. The floor is visible as a plateau about 1.0 cm. below the lower margin of the anterior clinoid processes or it may be slightly concave (fig. 83). In order to find the floor of the pituitary fossa in the frontal projection, the anterior clinoid processes are used as a reference. On each side of the sella there is a sharp downward slope representing the medial side of the floor of the middle fossa (fig. 75). The shape of the floor of the sella as seen in this projection is variable, but it conforms to a few patterns: it may be slightly concave in its central portion; it may be completely flat and horizontal; or one side may be a little higher than the other with either a flat or a slightly concave configuration (fig. 75). The normal width of the sella, as measured on roentgenograms, varies from 10 to 15 mm. In one case the sellar width measured 18 mm. and in one case it measured 9 mm. out of 100 "normal" subjects (Di Chiro, 1960).

When the sella is normal, the angle at the sloping edges of the sella as seen in frontal projection are rounded (figs. 26, 27, 74). When the sella is enlarged, the edges of the plateau are sharp and angled (see below).

Di Chiro (1960) has suggested that it is possible to calculate the volume of the pituitary fossa (which does not necessarily represent the exact size of the pituitary gland) by applying the mathematical formula for the volume of an ellipsoid. A simplified formula given by him is as follows:

Volume (in cu. cm.)

$$= \frac{\frac{1}{2}(\text{Length} \times \text{Width} \times \text{Height in mm.})}{1000}$$

(Revised 1963)

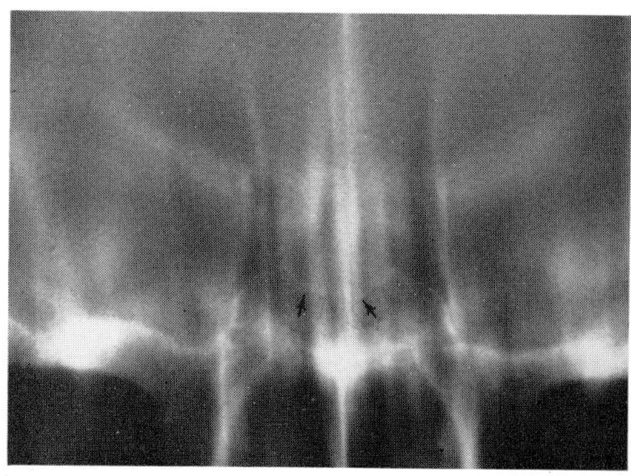

FIG. 83.—LAMINAGRAM OF SELLA TURCICA, NORMAL

In the anteroposterior projection there is a concave configuration to the floor of the sella turcica (*arrows*). The sloping sides of the medial portion of the middle fossa are well shown. See Fig. 74.

The mean value was 594 cu. mm. and the maximum was 1092 cu. mm. in 173 adults (Di Chiro and Nelson, 1962).

The width in frontal films is the distance between the two angles delimiting the horizontal plateau of the sellar floor.

The average volume of the pituitary gland is 0.6 cc. In estimating the width of the pituitary fossa, the *base view* may sometimes be useful because the anterior aspect of the sella is usually visible (fig. 34). If the sella becomes enlarged, the length of its anterior aspect will increase (fig. 84). It is frequent to see a relative increase in density over the area of the sphenoid sinuses overlaid by the enlarged sella (figs. 34 and 35).

Enlargement

The intrasellar lesions that produce enlargement of the pituitary fossa are enlargement of the sellar contents, most commonly due to a pituitary adenoma, less commonly to craniopharyngiomas, and more rarely to intrasellar extension of suprasellar or tuberculum sellae meningiomas. Intracavernous aneurysms of the internal carotid artery may produce unilateral enlargement of the sella turcica. Increased intracranial pressure, particularly those cases in which there is dilatation of the 3d ventricle, also causes enlargement of the sella.

(*Revised 1963*)

How to determine the presence of pituitary fossa enlargement was described in the discussion of size of the sella turcica. Linear measurements are found to be easiest to apply in practice, but area measurements and even volumetric estimations may be used, as explained above. It is not uncommon to find a sella which presents an increase in its anteroposterior diameter, beyond the upper limit of 17 mm., when the depth is within normal limits, that is, under 14 mm. At other times, the depth is increased beyond the upper limit of normal, but the length is within normal limits. In these cases, measurements of the area of the sella may be used as a guide, and if it is beyond 130 sq. mm., the sella is considered as *absolutely enlarged*. Even in the absence of other roentgenological findings suggestive of an intrasellar tumor our experience has been that it is impossible to rule out an intrasellar mass in these cases and a pneumoencephalogram is usually recommended unless the clinical findings are not in any way related to the sella turcica region. Indeed, in these borderline cases, particularly if the clinical findings do not indicate a lesion in this area, further studies usually reveal that there is no tumor. Air may extend into the pituitary fossa into what might be called an enlarged intrasellar subarachnoid space (fig. 79). It is possible, as discussed above under "Size," that in these patients, the pituitary gland enlarged either during puberty or, perhaps, during gestation, which caused enlargement of the sella turcica. Later, the gland decreased in size but the pituitary fossa remained enlarged. The space is taken over by an enlargement of the usually very small subarachnoid space which accompanies the pituitary stalk. In our experience, the patients with enlargement of the sella turcica without a tumor are usually females (fig. 79). In one case in which the sella turcica was enlarged, autopsy revealed a cyst of the pituitary gland (fig. 53).

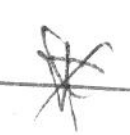

When the sella becomes enlarged as a result of an intrasellar tumor there is usually ballooning of the sella turcica; that is, it becomes rounded and extends forward underneath the anterior clinoid processes or tuberculum sellae. This is called *under-*

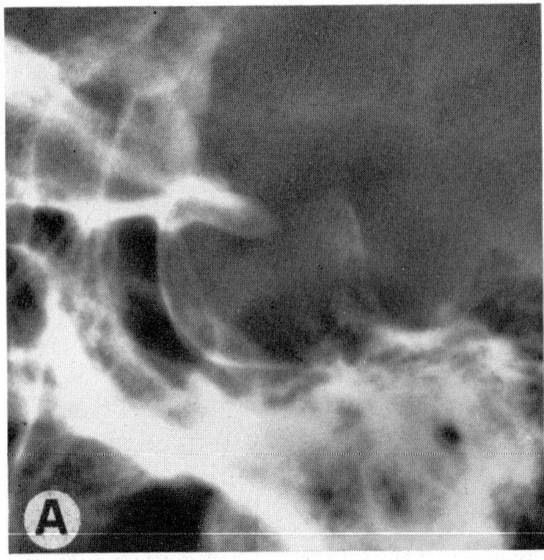

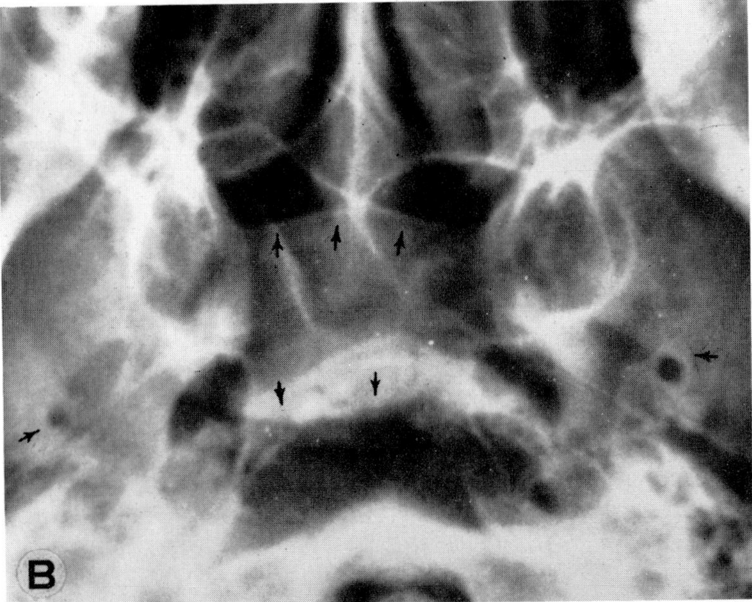

FIG. 84.—TYPICAL ENLARGEMENT OF THE SELLA TURCICA IN A PATIENT WITH A CHROMOPHOBIC PITUITARY ADENOMA

(A) There is rounding of the sella turcica, undermining of the anterior clinoid processes and tuberculum sellae, and thinning of the dorsum sellae with preserved posterior clinoid processes.

In the base view (B) it is possible to visualize the increase in the width of the anterior aspect of the sella turcica (*arrows*) which is not seen in the lateral view. The posterior margin is also visible (*two arrows*). The frontal projection may also be of help. This patient demonstrates asymmetry of the foramen spinosum; the left side is much larger than the right, but there was no evidence of meningioma in this instance.

mining of the clinoid processes or of the tuberculum sellae, which is good evidence for an intrasellar mass. In some instances the tuberculum sellae is obliterated. The lower portion of the dorsum sellae is displaced posteriorly, but the posterior clinoid processes which are held by the interclinoid ligaments usually remain in their normal position or are displaced posteriorly only slightly. This also tends to give the sella a rounded

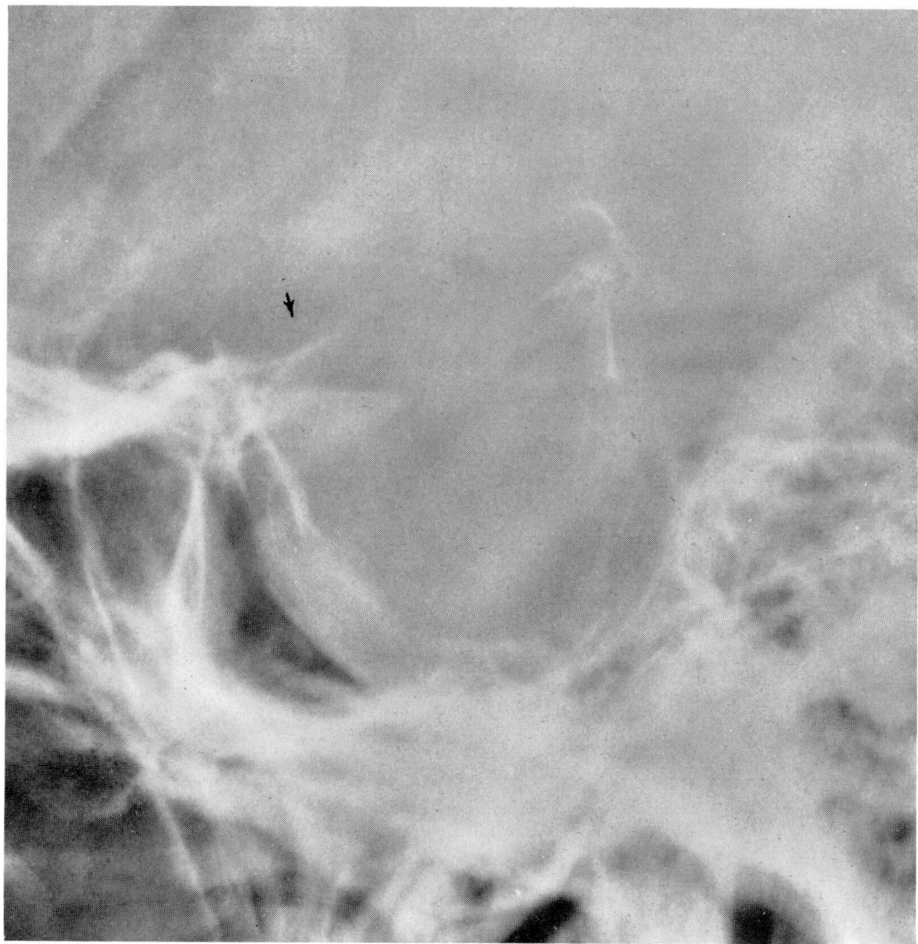

Fig. 85.—Pituitary Adenoma Causing Elevation of the Anterior Clinoid Process and Destruction of the Dorsum Sellae with Preservation of the Posterior Clinoid Processes

There is destruction of the dorsum of the sella turcica with preservation of the posterior clinoid processes. One anterior clinoid process is elevated and thinned (*arrow*). In our experience this is seen more commonly in patients with pituitary adenomas than in those with intracavernous aneurysms of the internal carotid artery. The floor of the sella turcica has lost most of its density due to the fact that this is an active tumor at this time.

configuration. The portion of the sella which presents the earliest signs of involvement by an intrasellar mass is the area of junction of the dorsum and floor. There is, first, a loss of density of this portion of the inner contour of the sella turcica and, later, backward displacement of the dorsum will be noted. As the enlargement progresses, the dorsum is progressively displaced dorsally and becomes thinner; complete disappearance of the shadow of the lower two-thirds of the dorsum may take place (figs. 84 and 85). The upper portion of the dorsum tends to remain calcified, particularly the area immediately adjacent to the posterior clinoid processes (fig. 85). The rate of disappearance of the shadow of the dorsum and floor of the sella turcica is related to the activity of the growth of the intrasellar contents. In a rapidly growing intrasellar lesion, the entire cortex of the

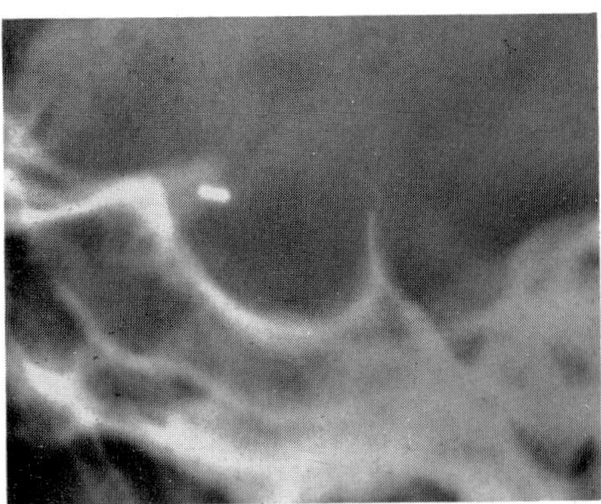

Fig. 86.—Dense Sella Turcica in Patient with Craniopharyngioma

There is a marked degree of increase in density of the contour of the sella turcica. The dorsum sellae is thin and the posterior clinoid processes are demineralized. The sella is of the "open type," This film was made immediately postoperatively, and a silver clip is seen in the area of the sella turcica.

floor and dorsum sellae is apt to disappear. On the other hand, in a process that is expanding very slowly, the cortical bone of the sella has time to reossify. The density of the sellar contour is directly proportional to the activity of the growth process, and when the growth process ceases, the sellar outline is apt to reappear in the course of time. This is well shown in treated pituitary adenomas where, with rare exceptions, the sella turcica does not actually become smaller but simply reossifies after having been destroyed. Later, if activity of the process recurs, the sella will become demineralized again, but will not enlarge unless the mass cannot extend upward. Approximately 10 per cent of patients with craniopharyngiomas show an increase in the density of the sella turcica, sometimes quite marked, as reported by Barnett (1959) in a review of 62 patients with this condition seen at the Neurological Institute (fig. 86).

Double floor. A double contour to the floor of the sella turcica is frequently seen in patients who have intrasellar lesions (fig. 87). In our experience it is much more common in patients with pituitary adenomas. A double floor is produced by an uneven growth of the intrasellar tumor, which will enlarge one side of the sella turcica more than the other. It may, in some cases, be due to depression of the central portion of the sella turcica (fig. 88), but in most instances it is due to depression of one side, as can be well demonstrated by laminagrams made in frontal projection (fig. 87). Sometimes a double floor can be produced by a parasellar lesion such as an aneurysm of the intracavernous portion of the internal carotid artery and an occasional meningioma of the middle fossa. The causes of a *pseudo-double floor*, as a normal finding, have been discussed on page 1.97. Attention should be paid to slight but significant changes producing a double floor (figs. 88C and D).

Elevation of the anterior clinoid process. Large intrasellar tumors produce apparent elevation and pointing of both anterior clinoid processes. The tumor may erode the undersurface of the clinoid process at its base, and occasionally it will completely erode it so that its tip hangs free. In cases of asymmetrical sellar enlargement, only one process may be elevated (fig. 85). In the latter cases, the possibility of an intracavernous aneurysm of the internal carotid artery should be considered because this lesion usually produces changes only on one side and is an indication for the performance of a carotid angiogram as the first diagnostic procedure. Bilateral intracavernous aneurysms are not rare, however. The anterior clinoid processes are often thin in normal individuals and care should be taken not to call these cases abnormal due to an intrasellar tumor or to increased intracranial pressure. In fact, the great majority of sharp anterior clinoid processes are normal; only a very small percentage of these is directly related to an existing abnormal condition. In the case of an intracavernous aneurysm of the internal carotid artery, the anterior clinoid process may be completely eroded and a characteristic picture is seen in the inclined posteroanterior projection; the shadow of the anterior clinoid process disappears, which is easily ascertained by following the lesser wing of the sphenoid toward its medial portion (fig. 89). Larger aneurysms may produce erosion of the adjacent portion of the lesser wing of the sphenoid. Calcifica-

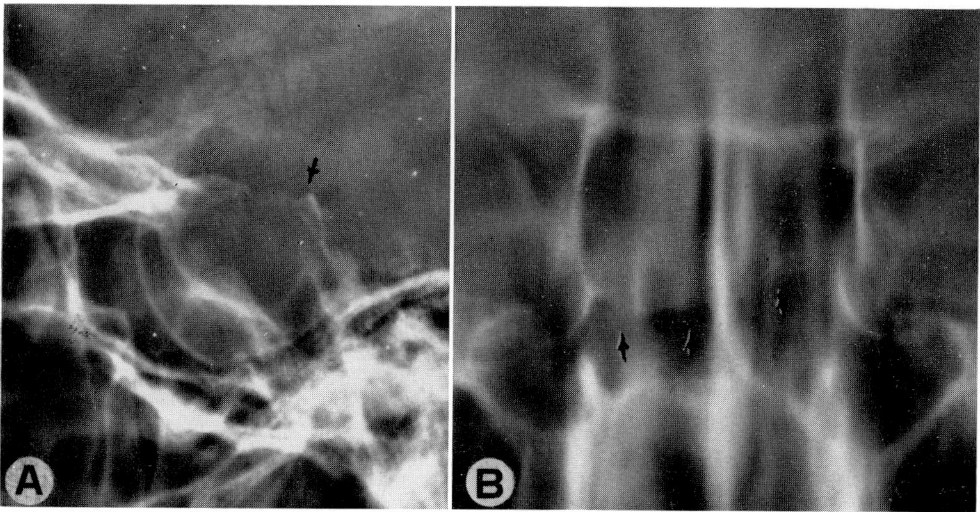

Fig. 87.—Double Floor of Sella Turcica in Patient with Pituitary Adenoma

The lateral view (A) demonstrates a typical double contour of the sella turcica; one side is almost normal whereas the other side shows marked enlargement with undermining of the anterior clinoid process and tuberculum sellae and posterior displacement of the dorsum sellae. There is only very slight posterior displacement of the posterior clinoid process, however, because this portion of the sella is fixed by the interclinoid ligaments. A frontal laminagram (B) demonstrates the depression of the sella involving only one side of the pituitary fossa (*arrows*). There is marked increase in width of the floor of the sella turcica, which measured a total of 30 mm.

tion in the wall of these aneurysms is relatively common. The elevation and erosion of the anterior clinoid process can be produced equally by a pituitary adenoma (fig. 85).

Causes of Enlargement

Pituitary adenomas. Pituitary adenomas are extremely rare in children under 14 years of age. Only one case has been seen at the Neurological Institute out of approximately 400 cases. The pituitary gland is divided into an anterior and a posterior lobe separated by a thin, cleft-like portion called the "pars intermedia." Adenomas usually arise from the anterior lobe which contains the three types of cells: chromophobic, eosinophilic, and basophilic.

Chromophobic pituitary adenomas. Chromophobic pituitary adenomas are by far the most common. They are characterized by enlargement of the sella turcica, sometimes extremely marked, without any other roentgenologically evident metabolic bone changes in the skull or elsewhere in the body. They are the type of tumor which most commonly breaks through the diaphragma sellae and projects in the suprasellar region, producing compression of the optic nerve and chiasm. It is probable that the size of the diaphragmatic opening in an individual case determines how early the pituitary adenoma will extend suprasellarly. Indeed, in some patients, the pituitary adenoma extends to the suprasellar region before causing any significant sellar enlargement, but usually causing some thinning of the dorsum sellae and the floor of the sella turcica. Approximately 5 to 10 per cent of chromophobic pituitary adenomas fail to produce any sellar enlargement, although, as mentioned above, slight sellar changes indicative of a possible tumor may be present (fig. 90). In other patients, it is possible that the diaphragma sellae is well formed, with a very small opening for the entrance of the pituitary stalk, hindering upward extension of the tumor and causing it to extend downward. In these cases the tumor will displace the floor of the sella turcica encroaching

(*Revised 1963*)

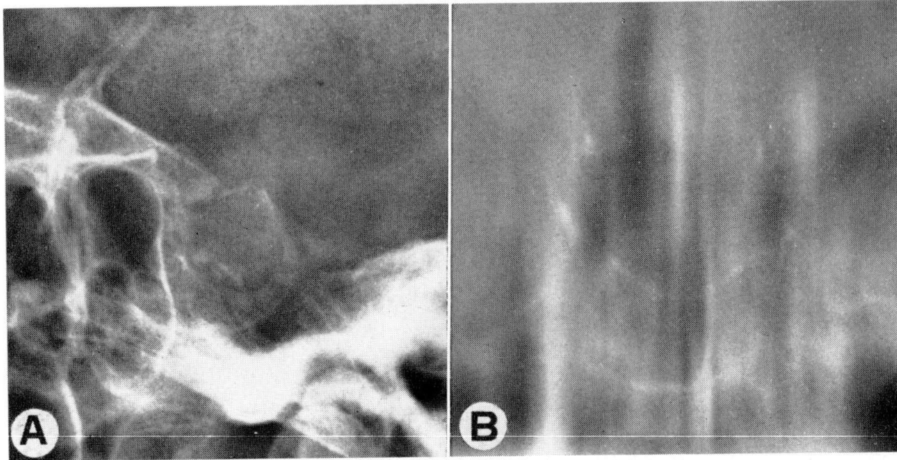

FIG. 88.—ENLARGEMENT OF SELLA TURCICA WITH DOUBLE FLOOR

The lateral projection (A) shows the double contour of the sella turcica. There is calcification overlying the sella turcica due to calcium in the walls of the internal carotid arteries. The posterior clinoid processes appear to be intact, but the dorsum is thin. Laminagrams in frontal projection (B) demonstrate that the depression is in the center of the sella turcica (*arrows*). Compare with Fig. 87.

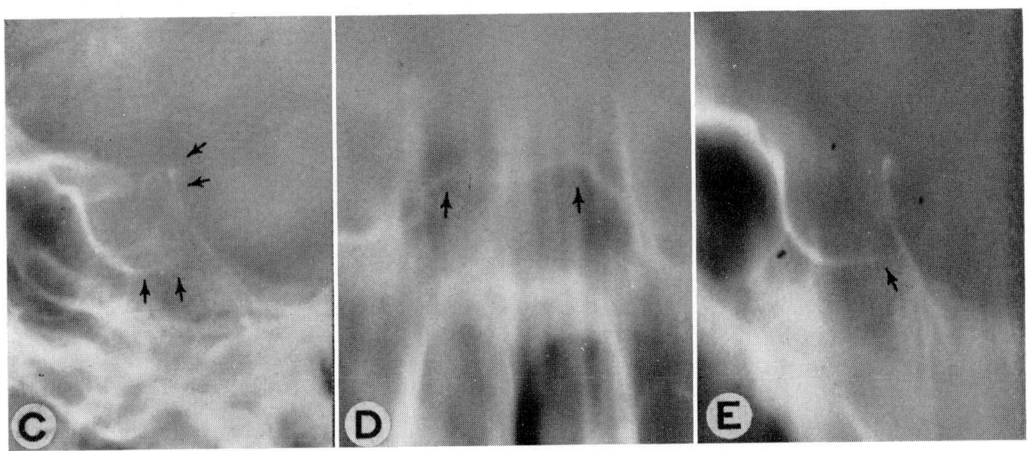

FIG. 88 (*Cont.*)—SMALL INTRASELLAR MASS PRODUCING ONLY SLIGHT ENLARGEMENT OF PITUITARY FOSSA

(C) The sella presents a double contour only on its posterior aspect (*arrows*). It is noted that the lower of the two contours in this region can be traced upward to end at the posterior clinoid process which is also displaced backward (*upper two arrows*). In the frontal laminagram (D), there is noted a depression of one side of the sella turcica which is enlarged; the transverse diameter of the sella measures 20 mm. Laminagram (E) shows the sella turcica passing through the area of the larger side of the sella. The beginning destruction at the angle between the dorsum and the posterior portion of the floor is evident.

(*Revised 1963*)

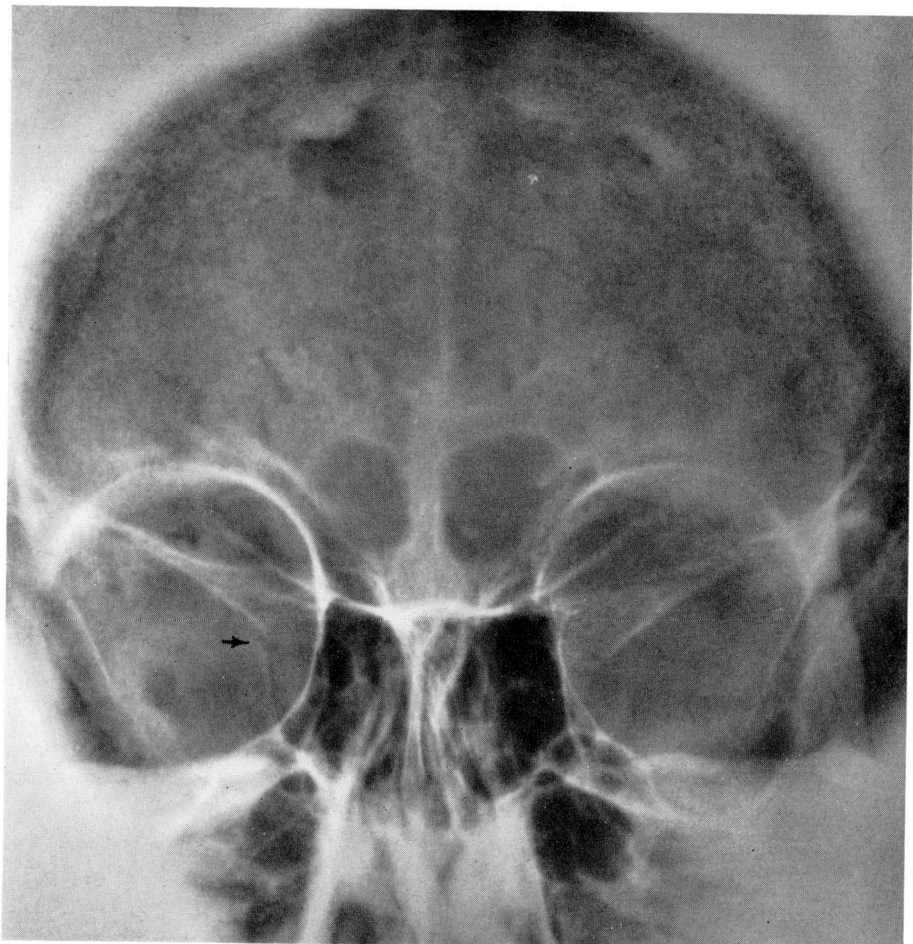

Fig. 89.—Erosion of Anterior Clinoid Process Due to Intracavernous Aneurysm
The erosion is seen on the right side (*arrow*), and is easily ascertained in comparison with the appearance on the opposite side.

upon the sphenoid sinuses. Occasionally the capsule may break and allow actual extension of the tumor into the sphenoid sinus.

In some cases, growth of the pituitary adenoma may be extreme and there is an area of erosion 6 to 7 cm. in diameter that is centered at the sella turcica and involves the medial portion of the floors of the middle fossae on each side, the upper portion of the clivus, and the petrous tips on both sides, and extends forward to involve the posterior ethmoid cells (fig. 91). The latter changes are best demonstrated on base views. Base views are often of value in differentiating lesions which produce diffuse destruction in this region, for they will usually demonstrate that the process is exactly localized to the center and extends symmetrically in all directions. This is characteristic of pituitary adenomas as against other destructive lesions involving the floor of the skull which do not destroy bone concentrically in relation to the sella turcica. Some of the patients with the greatest degree of destruction of the base of the skull produced by pituitary adenomas have no evidence of suprasellar extension of the mass, which again tends to confirm the probable role of the diaphragma

(Revised 1963)

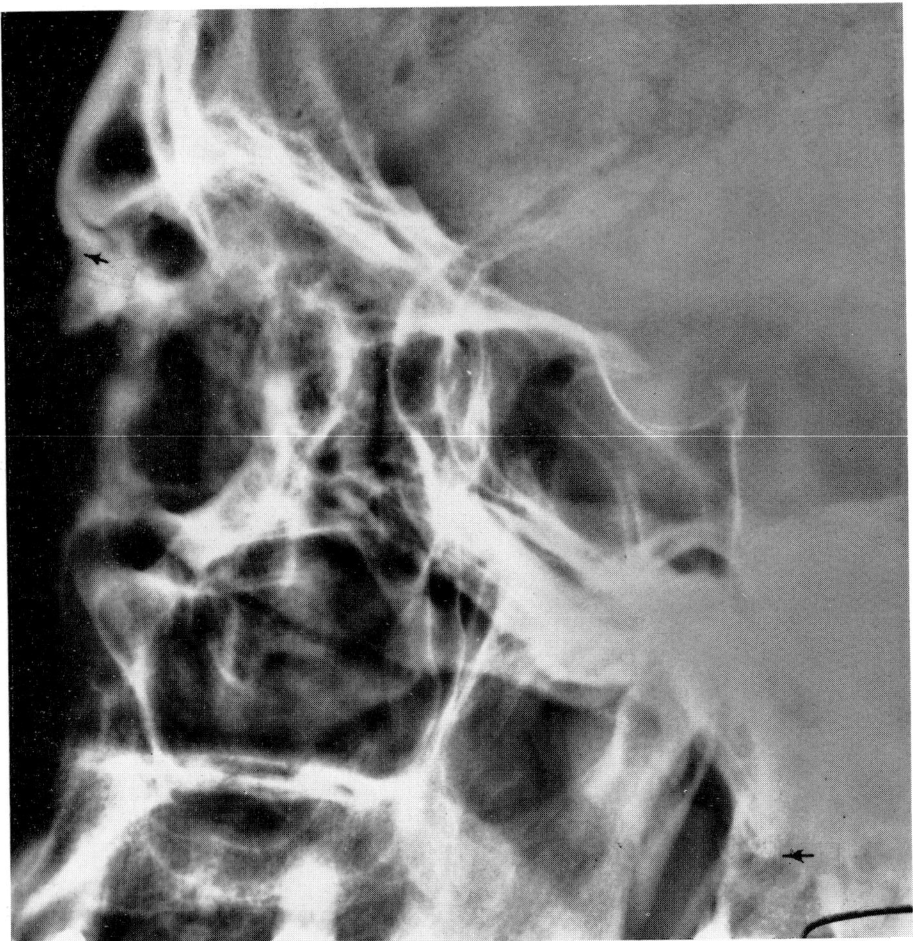

FIG. 90.—PITUITARY ADENOMA IN A PATIENT WITH A NORMAL SIZED SELLA

The sella is shallow, but its anteroposterior diameter is 17 mm. The sphenoid sinus is large and extends into the dorsum sellae. This is the type of case that often does not show significant sella enlargement in the presence of a pituitary adenoma. It has been stated that this could be due to a more resistant bone at the floor in these cases, but it may also have something to do with the configuration of the sella turcica, with a wider opening for the diaphragma sellae. The patient had a moderate degree of basal kyposis; the basal angle measures 118°. The clivus and the nasion are indicated by *arrows*.

sellae in determining the direction of the main growth of the pituitary tumor.

Chromophobic pituitary adenomas rarely calcify. Sometimes a rim of calcification may be seen in some portions of the tumor, probably in the walls of cysts (fig. 159). Calcification probably occurs in less than 5 per cent of cases.

Occasionally a pituitary adenoma which destroys the wall of the sphenoid sinus will be the cause of a cerebrospinal fluid rhinorrhea which occurs spontaneously. Sometimes a leak follows surgery, particularly if the transnasal route is used.

Eosinophilic adenomas. The eosinophilic cells of the anterior lobe of the pituitary are probably concerned with growth. Overactivity of these cells produces gigantism in youth and acromegaly in adults. Eosinophilic pituitary adenomas usually cause only slight enlargement of the pituitary fossa, although some cases will show a greater degree of

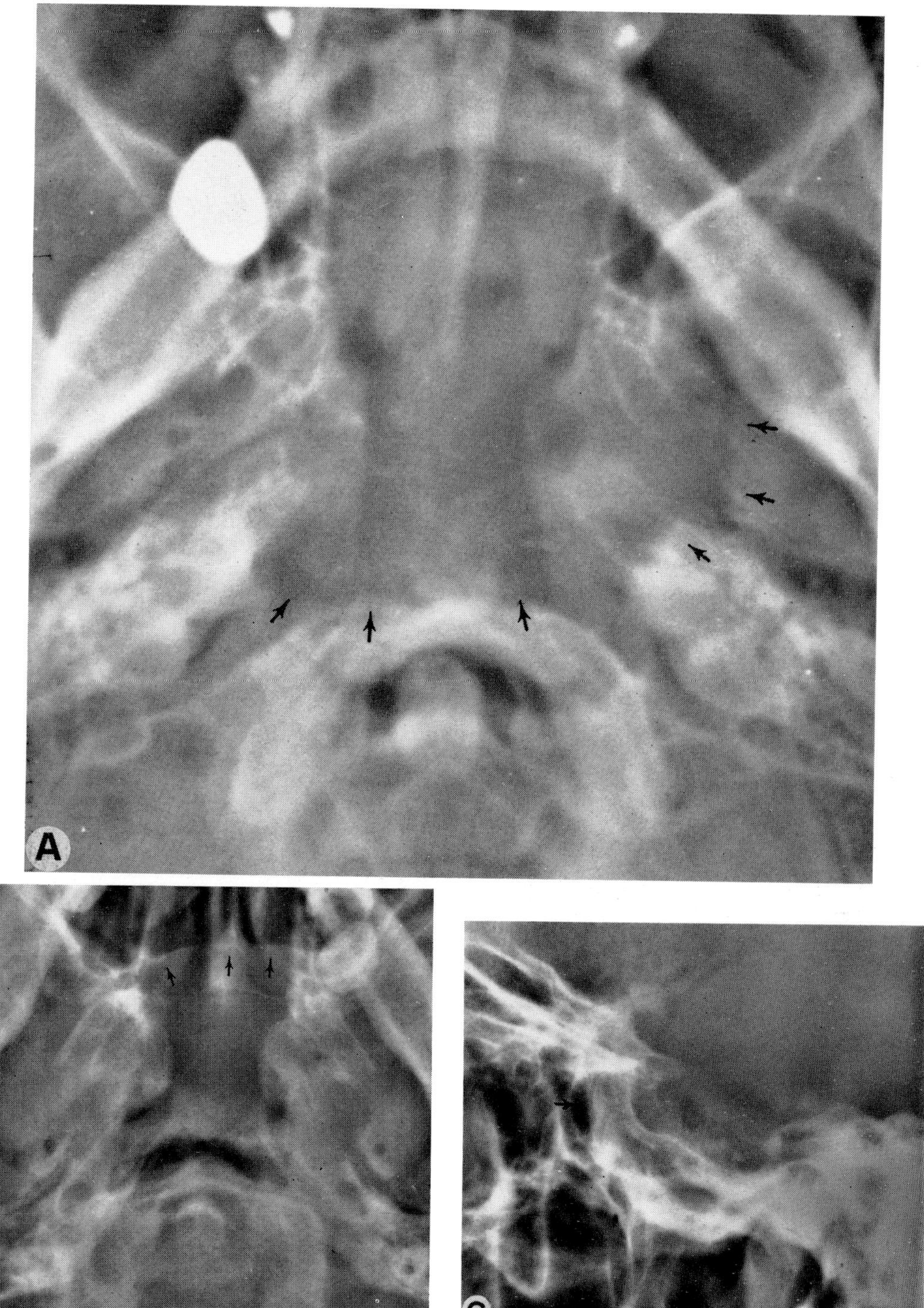

FIG. 91.—PITUITARY ADENOMA PRODUCING WIDE AREA OF DESTRUCTION IN THE BASE OF THE SKULL

In (A), the anterior margin of the tumor cannot be seen, but there is no evidence of the normal septations of the posterior ethmoid cells and no evidence of an outline for the sphenoid sinuses. There is radiolucency on the left side of the middle fossa (*arrows*) and destruction of the petrous tip on both sides, more marked on the left (*arrows*), as well as destruction of the clivus. The patient had a pituitary adenoma of the chromophobic type, nonmalignant. In (B), there is a clear outline to the anterior margin of the sella turcica (*arrows*) indicating the forward extension of the tumor. The sphenoid sinuses have been obliterated by tumor, and the adjacent portion of the clivus has been destroyed, but the destruction has not extended to involve the petrous tips. In (C), the lateral view of the case shown in (B), the sella turcica is completely destroyed, and the anterior margin of the ballooned sella is visible in this view as well (*arrow*).

(*Revised 1963*)

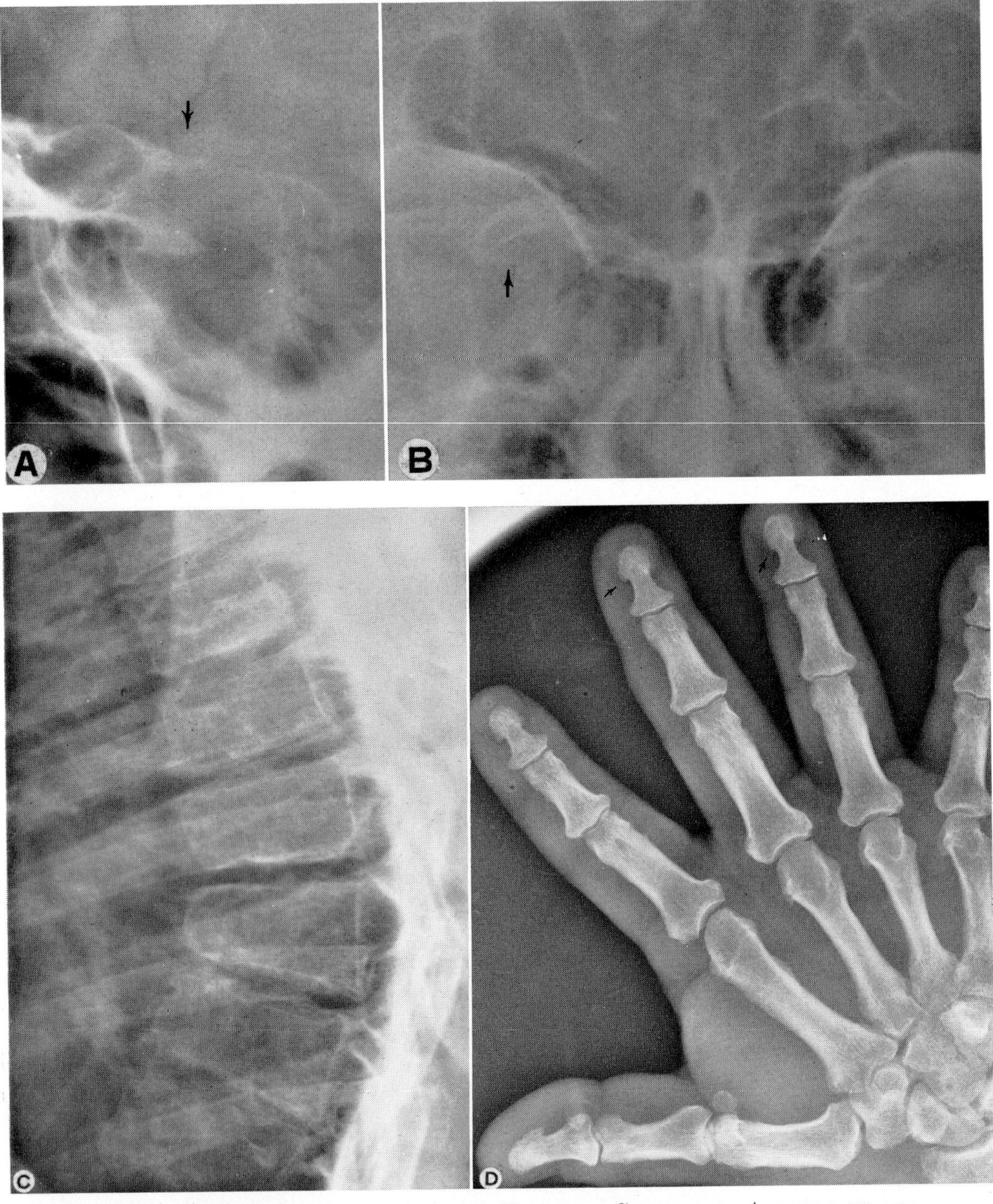

FIG. 92.—EOSINOPHILIC ADENOMA OF THE PITUITARY GLAND WITH ACROMEGALY AND SPINE CHANGES

The lateral view (A) demonstrates enlargement of the sella turcica; one anterior clinoid process is markedly elevated. There is marked enlargement of the sinuses and increase in the thickness of the skull with hyperostosis of the inner table. The frontal film (B) shows the changes in the anterior clinoid process due to the elevation and erosion of this structure similar to that seen in intracavernous aneurysms (*arrow*). A lateral view of the thoracic spine (C) demonstrates the marked widening of the anteroposterior diameter of the thoracic vertebral bodies associated with the acromegaly. A radiograph of the hand (D) demonstrates the marked increase in the thickness of the soft tissues in relation to the size of the bone, which is the most significant feature. There is enlargement of the ungual tuft (*arrows*).

(*Revised 1963*)

enlargement. The outlines of the sella turcica are usually well defined and the margins are well calcified in the majority of cases. Only an occasional case will extend above the sella turcica to cause compression of the optic chiasm. In addition to enlargement of the sella turcica, eosinophilic adenomas will be accompanied by other features of acromegaly, such as enlargement of the sinuses, increase in the thickness of the bones of the skull, and enlargement and elongation of the mandible, which leads to prognathism. Enlargement of the hands is easier to appreciate clinically than roentgenographically. Radiography of the hands usually shows an increase in the thickness of the soft tissues around the fingers and enlargement of the ungual tuft of the terminal phalanges. Another finding is an increase in the anteroposterior diameter of the thoracic vertebral bodies associated with the kyphosis which these patients often acquire (fig. 92). In our experience, this is a rare occurrence. Roentgenologically, it is difficult to determine whether or not there is an increase in activity of the tumor at a given time. Growth of tumor, as explained above, is usually accompanied by loss of density in the outline of the sella turcica, but this is frequently absent in eosinophilic adenomas. Some eosinophilic adenomas may well be inactive when first discovered. Arrested adenomas occasionally exhibit calcification (fig. 160).

Multiple endocrine adenomatosis is a syndrome (Wermer syndrome) in which adenomata of the hypophysis, of the parathyroid, pancreas, and adrenal cortex may be encountered. The condition is hereditary. The presenting symptom is, not uncommonly, recurrent gastric ulcers. The presence of other endocrine adenomata complicates the management of these cases (Wermer, 1954).

Basophilic adenomas. These are usually tiny adenomas and only very rarely do they acquire sufficient size to produce enlargement of the sella turcica. Two cases with enlargement of the sella have been seen at the Presbyterian Hospital; one was a pure basophilic adenoma in a patient who had Cushing's disease, and the other had a mixed

(Revised 1963)

basophilic and chromophobic adenoma, also in a patient with Cushing's syndrome. The usual finding in Cushing's syndrome is that of a normal sized sella turcica with generalized loss of density of the surroundings of the sella turcica and of the skull and, indeed, of the entire skeleton. The process of deossification is thought to be due to a negative protein balance found in patients with Cushing's syndrome which causes insufficient bone matrix replacement necessary in the daily process of bone repair. In the case of pure basophilic adenoma, which was producing enlargement of the sella turcica, there was suprasellar extension and clinical evidence of compression of the optic chiasm necessitating surgical intervention.

Mixed pituitary adenomas. Some pituitary adenomas show histological evidence of a chromophobic tumor with many eosinophilic elements in them. It is not uncommon to find a patient who has no evidence of acromegaly clinically while radiologically exhibiting an enlarged sella without significant increase in density around the base of the skull and region of the sella turcica, but with considerable increase in the thickness of the skull bones such as is seen in patients with eosinophilic adenomas. These cases might be referred to radiologically as mixed pituitary adenomas.

Craniopharyngiomas. These tumors arise from remnants of the craniopharyngeal duct or Rathke's pouch. As is well known, the anterior lobe of the pituitary gland has an ectodermal origin and comes from a pouchlike extension of the oral cavity occurring at about the third month of gestation. The pouch elongates and then becomes constricted forming the craniopharyngeal duct. It gives origin to the anterior lobe, the pars intermedia, and the pars tuberalis which is fused to the anterior aspect of the infundibulum. The infundibulum is a downward extension of the hypothalamus connecting it with the posterior lobe of the pituitary gland. The infundibulum and posterior lobe are embryologically originated from a downward diverticulumlike extension of the 3d ventricle. It is from the pars tuberalis which, as mentioned above, is

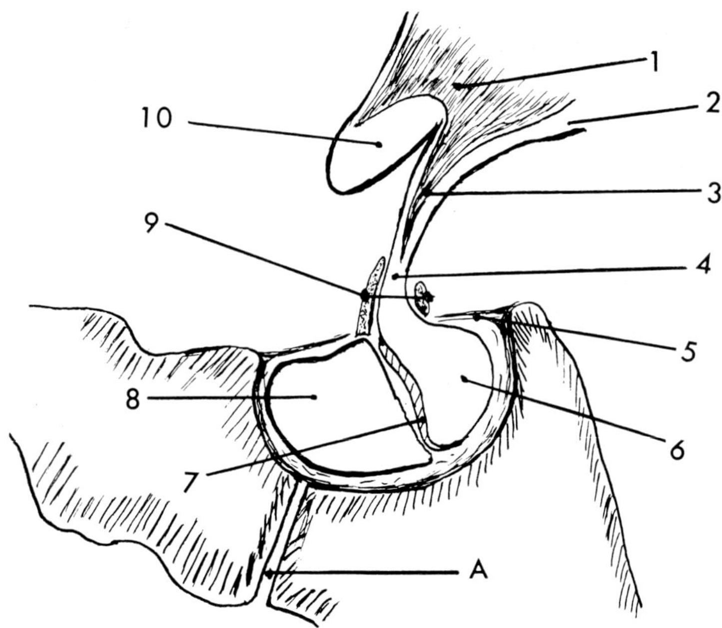

Fig. 93.—Diagram of Sagittal Section of the Hypophyseal Region of Embryo of Approximately 3 Months

(1) Third ventricle. (2) wall of hypothalamus. (3) infundibular recess. (4) infundibular stalk. (5) diaphragma sellae. (6) pars neuralis. (7) pars intermedia. (8) pars distalis (anterior lobe). (9) pars tuberalis. (10) optic chiasm. (A) craniopharyngeal duct.

attached to the anterior aspect of the infundibulum (fig. 93), that craniopharyngiomas arise.

In a review of 62 patients with craniopharyngiomas seen at the Neurological Institute, Barnett (1959) found that the sella turcica was slightly or moderately and sometimes markedly enlarged in 46 (74 per cent). In the rest of the cases the sella was normal in size, and in a good number of those where it was enlarged, the enlargement was only slight. In this group of cases, 28 were from 0 to 20 years of age and the rest were 21 years or older. The oldest patient was 67 years old. Eight patients were over 50 years of age and the youngest patient was 2 years of age. Various types of changes around the sella turcica including erosion, most frequently involving the dorsum sellae, sometimes the anterior clinoid processes or the floor, was present in 50 patients (81 per cent). An *increase in the density of the floor* of the sella turcica and sometimes of the clinoid processes was present in approximately 11 per cent of the patients (fig. 86); in one patient there was a marked increase in density of the contours of the sella turcica without other significant findings around the sella. Calcification of various types was present in 43 cases (69 per cent). It has been stated that an "open type sella" is more frequently seen in craniopharyngiomas than in pituitary adenomas. That is, the dorsum tends to be more vertical in these cases. Although this is true in many instances of craniopharyngiomas, it is also seen in patients with pituitary adenomas and is not always reliable as a differential point unless it is accompanied by other signs, such as diffuse increase in density or calcifications (fig. 94).

Other causes of enlargement. Unilateral enlargement of the sella turcica is occasionally seen in patients with intracavernous aneurysm of the internal carotid artery. In these patients there is usually erosion of one anterior clinoid which may be

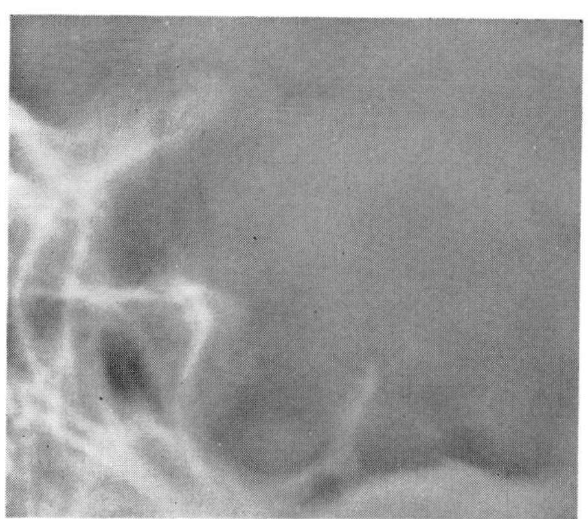

FIG. 94.—OPEN-TYPE SELLA IN CHILD WITH CRANIOPHARYNGIOMA

The dorsum sellae goes vertically upward, and the sella itself is enlarged. The floor is moderately dense. Inasmuch as pituitary adenomas are rare in children, the diagnosis of craniopharyngioma is justifiable wherever an intrasellar tumor is suspected.

completely absent or it may be elevated and thinned (fig. 89). Calcification in the wall of the aneurysm is common. The appearance may produce a double floor and in these cases the opposite side of the sella is completely normal which is not usually the case in pituitary adenomas. Occasionally, however, a pituitary adenoma may produce a strictly unilateral enlargement (fig. 87). The erosion of the anterior clinoid process is best shown in a posteroanterior view made in inclined posteroanterior projection (figs. 89 and 92). Sometimes there is erosion of the adjacent portions of the lesser and greater wings of the sphenoid producing an enlargement of the medial portion of the superior orbital fissure.

An occasional suprasellar meningioma will actually extend into the sella turcica and cause enlargement of this structure. At times, a meningioma of the medial portion of the temporal fossa or other parasellar tumors will also cause enlargement.

The most frequent cause of enlargement of the sella turcica, other than pituitary adenomas and craniopharyngiomas, is enlargement of the anterior portion of the 3d ventricle which actually projects into the sella turcica. In these cases there is usually a long standing obstruction of the posterior portion of the 3d ventricle or of the aqueduct which causes the gradual enlargement. It is conceivable that in these cases the dorsum sellae was originally destroyed and then it recalcified in a more posterior position, which would suggest certain intermittency of the pressure effect. Otherwise, the chances are that the dorsum sellae would be completely destroyed and the appearance of enlargement of the sella would be obscured. In some of these patients, the sella takes on a ballooned appearance suggestive of an intrasellar mass. The differential diagnosis is sometimes difficult but can be readily made by pneumographic studies. Usually the posterior clinoid and top of the dorsum sellae are demineralized or eroded and have completely disappeared, whereas in intrasellar tumors producing ballooning of the sella turcica the lower and middle portions of the dorsum are more involved or have completely disappeared whereas the top of the dorsum and the posterior clinoid processes may still be visible.

Sometimes, in patients with arrested hydrocephalus the sella takes on an elongated appearance. The anteroposterior diameter is markedly increased whereas the vertical diameter is within normal limits. In a less pronounced way, this is occasionally seen in normal patients.

Optic gliomas may produce enlargement of the sella turcica. For further details on optic gliomas, see under this subheading below.

As mentioned above, the pituitary fossa may become enlarged in children with *primary hypothyroidism* probably due to overactivity of the pituitary gland (VanWyk and Grumbach, 1960). The enlargement in these cases may not go beyond the upper limits of normal, but can be ascertained by seeing the decrease in the size of the sella turcica following the appropriate therapeutic measures (fig. 80).

In Cushing's syndrome, enlargement of the pituitary fossa following *bilateral adrenalectomy* is sometimes seen; this may be due to hypertrophy of the gland or it may be associated with enlargement of a pre-existing small basophilic adenoma. Out of 12 patients reported by Salassa *et al.* (1959), enlargement of the sella turcica following bilateral adrenalectomy was encountered in 3. The other 9 patients had some evidence of a pre-existing pituitary tumor prior to adrenalectomy. The 12 cases in which enlargement of the sella occurred in association with Cushing's syndrome were from a group of 122 patients reviewed by these authors.

THE PETROUS PYRAMIDS

The petrous pyramids must be examined very frequently to detect the presence of enlargement or erosion of the petrous tip and internal acoustic meatus and to detect destruction in the region of the middle ear, the jugular foramen, etc. It is, therefore, crucial to learn to do an orderly and complete examination of this structure based on the clinical findings in a given patient. If the symptoms are those of a tumor of the cerebellopontine angle, the examination should be concentrated on the petrous tip and on the internal acoustic canal region. On the other hand, if the clinical findings indicate that the involvement is in the posterior cranial nerves (9th through 12th, etc.) the examination should be concentrated on the posterior portion of the cranial fossa, and special views of the jugular foramen and condylar foramen should be made as explained under this subheading (p. 1.131).

However, regardless of the history which would point to an individual area in the posterior cranial fossa, a certain number of films should be taken to show the petrous pyramid in various projections in every case. These include the modified half axial projection (using a 25° angulation of the tube); two posteroanterior views, one where the petrous pyramid projects through the orbits and one where the petrous pyramid projects at the lower portion of the orbits (inclined posteroanterior projection); lateral views, base views of the skull, and Stenvers views. These are routine views used on every patient who is referred for an examination of the skull with the addition of the base views and the Stenvers views of the petrous pyramids which are not usually made routinely in every patient. The importance of obtaining these routine views is emphasized by the case shown in Figure 114.

Anatomy

The petrous pyramid is inclined at an angle of approximately 45° with the long axis of the skull. Its anatomical shape is usually compared with a three-sided truncated pyramid where one border is uppermost. The superior border of the petrous pyramid is called the "petrous ridge" and gives attachment to the tentorium which separates the middle from the posterior cranial fossa. The slope forward from the upper border is the anterior surface, and behind is the posterior surface. The inferior surface is rough and irregular. The anterior border is continuous with the squamosal portion of the temporal bone. The medial extremity articulates with the greater wing of the sphenoid. The posterior border articulates with the occipital bone and with the basisphenoid. Along this border is the jugular foramen and jugular fossae which are described separately. A film made in modified half axial projection will show the petrous ridge or superior border of the petrous pyramid to best advantage. In the inclined posteroanterior projection, the x-ray beam is nearly tangential to the anterior surface of the petrous pyramid, but in this projection the petrous pyramid is not as clearly shown as in other views because of overlying facial bones. In spite of it, this projection is important because it may bring out some details not clearly shown in other views.

Superior border. Along the superior border of the petrous pyramid are encountered, starting at its lateral aspect: (1) the groove of the lateral sinus; (2) a relatively flat surface which is formed by the tegmen tympani and corresponds to the thin plate of bone situated above the attic portion of the tympanic cavity; (3) the arcuate eminence which, contrary to usual opinion, does not always correspond to the position of the

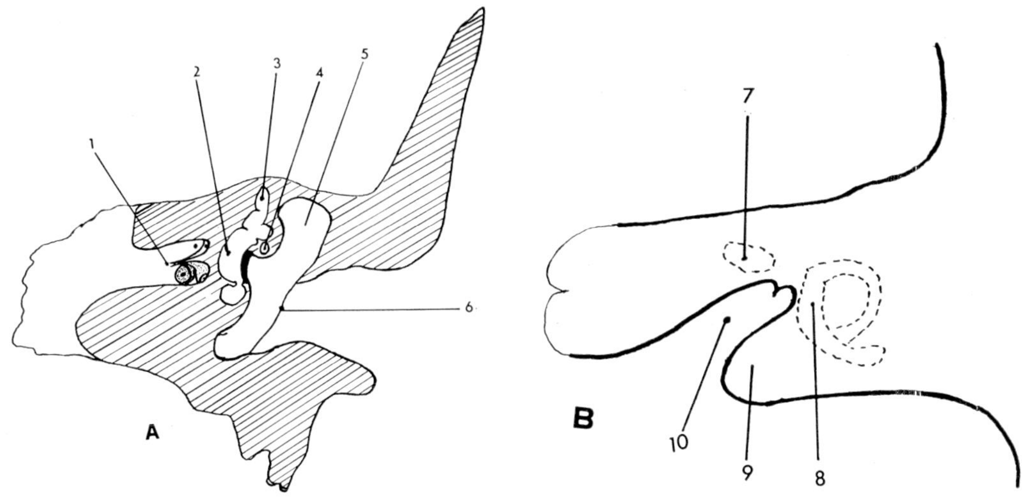

FIG. 95.—DIAGRAMS OF PETROUS PYRAMID

(A) represents a cross section following the longitudinal axis of the petrous pyramid. (B) shows a diagram of horizontal cross section of petrous pyramids seen from above. (1) Falciform crest of internal acoustic canal. (2) vestibule. (3) superior semicircular canal. (4) facial canal. (5) attic portion of middle ear cavity. (6) ear drum. (7) cochlea. (8) vestibule and horizontal semicircular canal. (9) posterior wall of internal acoustic canal. (10) internal acoustic canal.

superior semicircular canal, which may be medial to this eminence (the tegmen tympani and the arcuate eminence are more conspicuous on the anterosuperior surface of the petrous pyramid but here they are not shown on the roentgenogram); (4) medial to the arcuate eminence there is a slight depression followed by another elevation usually above the entrance of the internal auditory canal (in the depressed portion there is a small orifice termed the canalis facialis for the passage of the superior petrosal nerve which is on the anterior surface and not on the border); (5) medial to the elevation over the internal acoustic meatus there is another depression which corresponds to the notch where the trigeminal nerve lies. The superior margin of the petrous pyramid is actually grooved by the superior petrosal sinus and gives attachment to the tentorium. (fig. 36).

Internal auditory canal (Porus acusticus internus). It is extremely important to study in detail the internal auditory canal because of the frequency with which we must deal with this structure radiologically. The internal acoustic canal is in the posterior wall of the petrous pyramid. Its long axis forms an angle with the superior border of the petrous pyramid so that, in the modified half axial projection, the acoustic canal is approximately parallel with the bottom of the film whereas the superior border of the petrous pyramid is always directed obliquely downward and medially (fig. 96). When one looks at the internal acoustic canal from above, as in a base view or mentovertical view of the skull, the acoustic canal forms an angle with the long axis of the petrous pyramid of about 45°. For this reason, the internal acoustic canal is also approximately parallel with the bottom edge of the film in the base view of the skull (figs. 34 and 35).

The internal acoustic canal (porus acusticus internus) will be divided into two portions: the canal and the meatus.

Canal portion. The canal portion has an anterior and posterior wall, and a superior and inferior wall. In addition, the fundus or lateral wall should be considered. The anterior wall merges with the posterior surface of the petrous pyramid on the medial side.

The posterior wall of the canal is variable in length; sometimes it is very short, repre-

(*Revised 1963*)

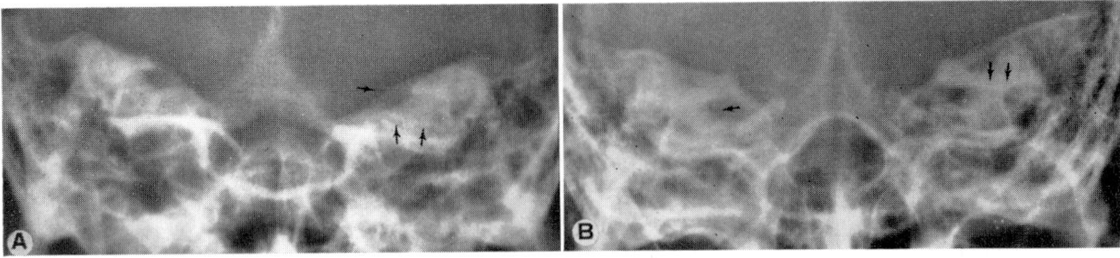

Fig. 96.—Normal Petrous Pyramids as Seen in Modified Half Axial Projection

In (A), the shadow of the canal portion is seen as a slightly radiolucent band which is approximately horizontal (*arrows*). The meatus portion is seen as a radiolucent area medial to the canal portion (*medial arrow*). The medial margin of the posterior wall of the canal delimits the lateral aspect of the meatus and is fairly symmetrical when the right side is compared with the left. In (B), another normal case, the configuration is slightly different, but also easy to identify. The medial margin of the posterior wall (*arrow*) is slightly different in configuration when the right is compared with the left. In this case, the suprameatal portion is much wider than in (A). The irregular shadows of the inner ear structures are seen to overlie the lateral aspect of the canal portion in both (A) and (B). However, the anatomy cannot be evaluated as clearly as in Stenvers projection.

senting merely a rim of bone as seen on the films, whereas at other times it is longer and measures as much as 10 mm. (fig. 95). However, the posterior wall tends to be relatively symmetrical when the right side is compared with the left side on the same patient (fig. 96). A film made with slight penetration will bring out the posterior wall, whereas an overpenetrated, darker film will burn through the posterior wall which may become invisible (fig. 97). As seen on a base view or in a horizontal cross section, the posterior wall has a triangular shape (figs. 95 and 35).

The inferior and superior walls are usually shown on the radiographs as a line delimiting the superior and inferior aspects of the canal. It is common to see these borders appear to continue medially for a certain distance forming a "pseudocanal." This is often a source of confusion leading to erroneous placement of the acoustic canal and will be discussed below. The fundus or *lateral wall* of the canal is divided into an upper and a lower portion by a horizontal ridge, the falciform crest (figs. 95 and 98). Another less conspicuous vertical crest divides it into an anterior and a posterior portion, so that there are actually four portions.

Meatus. Through the internal acoustic meatus pass the 7th or facial nerve, the nervus intermedius which is part of the facial nerve, and the 8th or acoustic nerve as well as the internal auditory branch of the basilar artery. As these nerves reach the fundus of the canal, the 7th nerve goes through the anterosuperior portion of the fundus of the

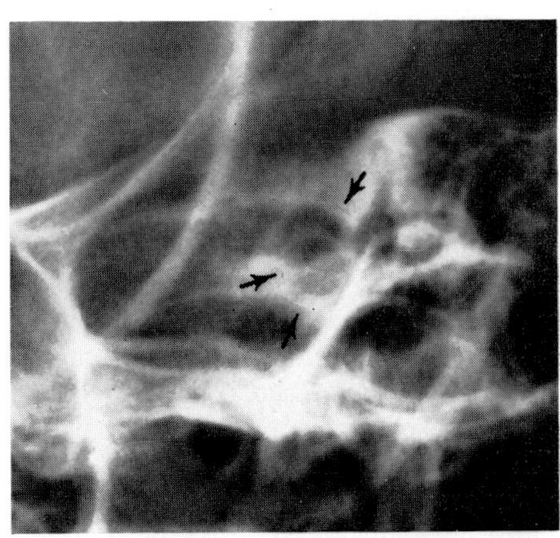

Fig. 97.—Normal Petrous Pyramid in Stenvers Projection

The internal acoustic canal is well shown, but the posterior wall is not well demonstrated because a higher degree of penetration was used. The vestibule is seen just lateral to the lateral wall of the acoustic canal, and from it the superior and the horizontal semicircular canals are seen to arise. Overlying the lower half of the lateral aspect of the acoustic canal is a rounded radiolucency representing the cochlea (*arrows*). The meatus portion cannot be separated from the canal portion in this case and with this degree of penetration.

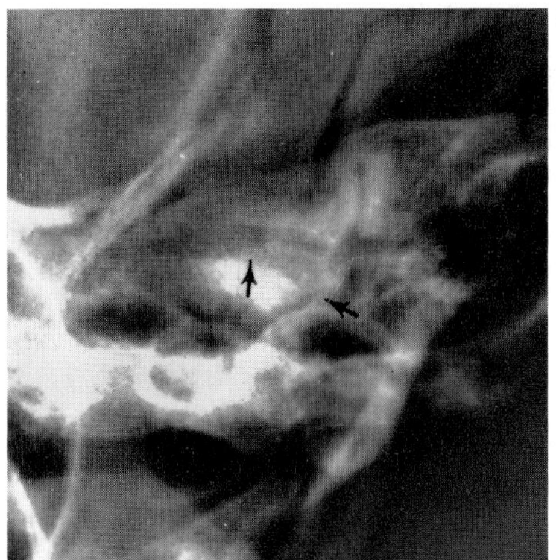

FIG. 98.—NORMAL PETROUS PYRAMID, STENVERS VIEW

The relation of the lateral aspect of the internal acoustic canal with the vestibule is again clearly shown. The falciform crest is well defined. The medial portion of the posterior wall (*arrow*) delimiting the lateral margin of the meatal portion is well seen. The meatal portion is slightly narrower in vertical diameter than the canal portion. The radiolucency of the cochlea is well shown (*arrow*).

canal and the 8th nerve goes through the inferior portion as well as through the posterosuperior aspect of the fundus. On the anterior inferior portion is the tractus spiralis foraminosus which is superimposed on the cochlea (fig. 95). The fundus of the canal is best shown in Stenvers views (fig. 97).

The *suprameatal segment* is above the superior margin of the canal. This space is variable and serves to separate the canal from the superior border of the petrous pyramid. This space tends to be symmetrical (although not absolutely symmetrical) when both sides are compared. Attention should be paid to the size of the suprameatal space, because when there is erosion of the internal acoustic canal produced by 8th nerve tumors, the first portion that will show changes will be the superior margin which will eventually encroach on the suprameatal space (figs. 103 and 106). This is not always so, however.

(*Revised 1963*)

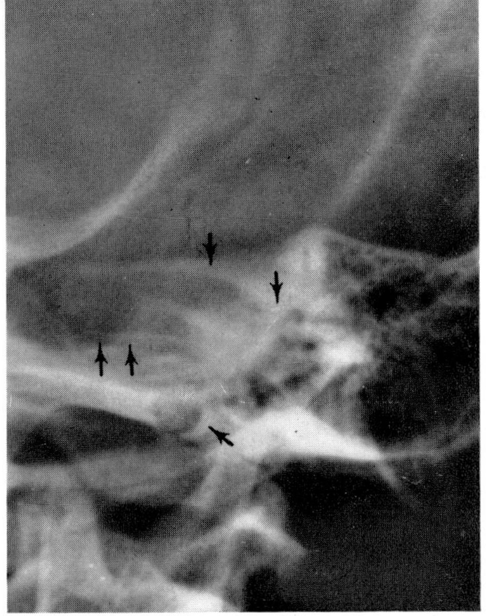

FIG. 99.—NORMAL PETROUS PYRAMID, STENVERS PROJECTION

The internal acoustic meatus is well shown and delimited laterally by the medial margin of the posterior wall (*arrow*). The canal portion is seen to extend almost to the shadow of the vestibule (*arrow*). The shadow of the meatus seems to continue medially because its upper margin joins the upper margin of the petrous pyramid. The superior wall of the carotid canal is well shown (*arrows*), and between the upper margin of the petrous pyramid and the carotid canal there is a wide space which simulates an internal acoustic canal. The lower arrow points at the hypoglossal foramen.

Radiologic Anatomy

It is important to learn to recognize the correct shadow or shadows that represent the internal acoustic canal on the films. It is easy to confuse the canal with other densities in the petrous pyramid. Films of best quality facilitate the correct identification of all the structures.

The *Stenvers view* is made by rotating the head 45° toward the side being examined with the face against the film. The canthomeatal line is placed perpendicular to the film and the central beam is angled cephalad 12°. The central beam is approximately perpendicular to the long axis of the petrous pyramid. There are several modifications of

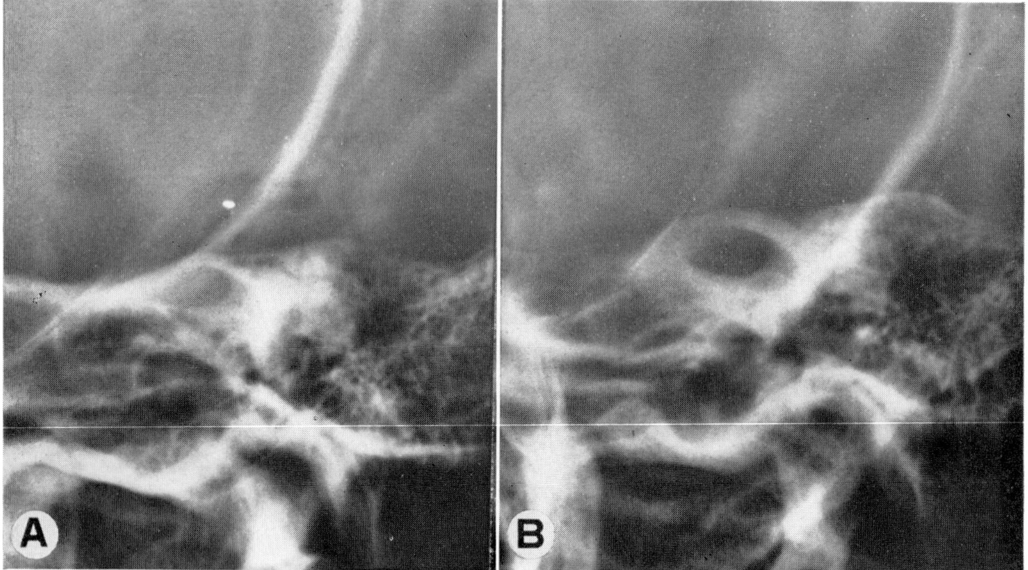

FIG. 100.—VARIATION IN THE SIZE OF THE INTERNAL ACOUSTIC MEATUS

The meatus portion is larger on one side than on the other in this patient. The posterior wall is relatively small. There is a 2-mm. difference in the vertical diameter of the canal portion as well as the meatus portion when one side is compared with the other. It is probable that both meati and canals are slightly wide in this patient, who had long-standing increased intracranial pressure due to a cerebellar tumor. There was no evidence, upon surgical intervention and on follow-up examinations, of any tumor involving the 8th nerve.

this basic position. The films could be made in an anteroposterior projection by reversing the landmarks and the angulation of the tube. Other variations have been proposed (Merrill, 1949). All of these films show the anatomy in approximately the same manner. We prefer the basic Stenvers position.

The first structure that should be identified is the labyrinth. The vestibule and the superior and lateral semicircular canals should be found. The vestibule marks the lateral wall of the internal auditory canal, in fact, the deepest portion of the lateral wall is situated about 1 to 2 mm. medial to the vestibule (fig. 97). After identifying the lateral wall of the canal, it is easy to relate the remainder of the canal to this point without fear of error. The direction of the acoustic canal is very slightly upward and medial, forming an angle with the upper border of the petrous pyramid (fig. 99). The *posterior wall of the canal,* as mentioned above, is variable in length and its medial margin is seen to better advantage in films that are not overpenetrated (lighter) as against those that are darker (figs. 97 and 98). Sometimes the posterior wall is but a rim of density just medial to the lateral wall of the canal, whereas at other times it measures as much as 1.0 cm. The appearance of a short posterior wall is exaggerated in Stenvers projection owing to foreshortening. The superior and inferior walls are usually easy to identify once the position of the canal portion is determined. The superior margin of the canal is sometimes prolonged medially by a dense line which is not part of the porus acusticus internus but medial to it (fig. 99). The inferior margin of the canal is usually clearly visible. Sometimes, it is superimposed on the upper margin of the carotid canal of the petrous pyramid so that the inferior wall appears to be continued toward the petrous apex for a considerable distance (fig. 99). This confusion can be avoided by realizing that the inferior wall should stop at the meatus. The vertical diameter of the canal portion is often slightly

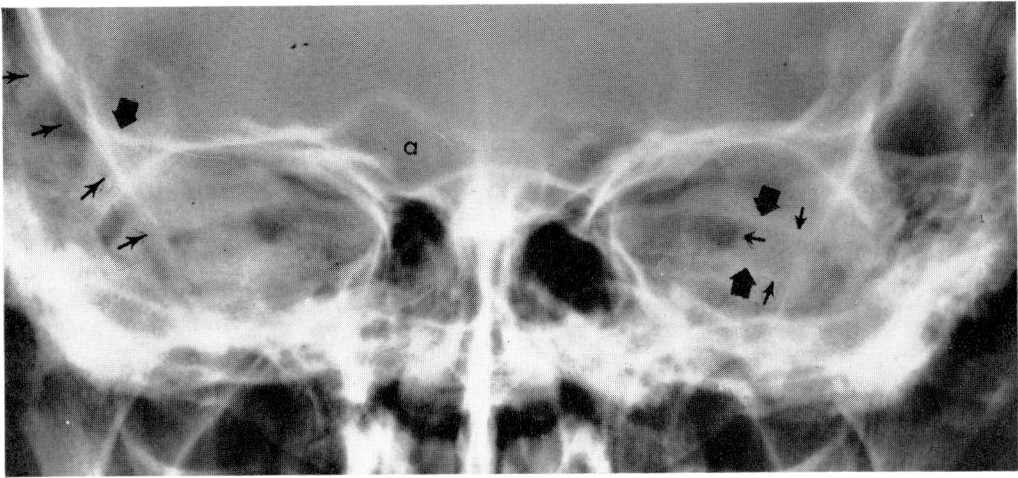

FIG. 101.—STRAIGHT POSTEROANTERIOR VIEW OF THE SKULL

The petrous pyramids are projected through the orbits. The internal acoustic meati are fairly well shown (*arrows*). The medial margin of the posterior wall can be seen demarcating the lateral margin of the meatus which shows up as a darker shadow (*horizontal arrow*). The outer aspect of the posterior margin of the floor of the anterior fossa joins the upper aspect of the oblique line of the orbit and contributes to the formation of the heavy line in the temporal area of the skull (*arrows*). (a) indicates the anterior clinoid process.

larger, as much as 2 mm., than the meatus or entrance of the porus acusticus internus. Camp and Cilley (1939) found the canals to be slightly asymmetrical in about 60 per cent of the cases. In roughly 50 per cent of the skulls, the difference varied between 0.5 to 1.5 mm. In about 8 to 10 per cent the difference was between 1.5 and 2.5 mm. when the right was compared with the left side (fig. 100).

The *meatus portion* is actually the entrance to the canal and it is usually well defined in the cases where the posterior wall is visualized (figs. 96 and 99). Its vertical diameter is usually slightly smaller than that of the canal. In an overpenetrated film the actual shape of the meatus cannot be ascertained. Because of the variation in the length of the posterior wall there is great variation in the size of the meatus and its relationship with the canal (figs. 98 and 100). The most important is the vertical dimension of the meatus, however.

The *suprameatal segment* is the portion of the petrous pyramid situated between the upper margin of the canal and the upper margin of the petrous pyramid. This space is variable from individual to individual but tends to be relatively symmetrical when the right is compared with the left in the same patient. Sometimes this space is pneumatized with tiny cells or, occasionally, with relatively large petrous cells. Whenever there is pneumatization of this portion of the petrous pyramid, the relative density of the compact bone forming the upper margin of the canal is enhanced. When there is pneumatization by tiny cells, the suprameatal space could mimic the acoustic canal if the landmarks for identification of the latter structure are not used. Pneumatization of the petrous pyramid also enhances the dense bone around the labyrinth. When air cells are slightly larger, they should be seen distinctly surrounded by dense bone. Occasionally, erosion produced by an acoustic neurinoma will mimic a petrous cell, but in these instances, the outline of the cell cannot be traced completely (fig. 108). The upper margin of the petrous pyramid near the apex together with the upper margin of the carotid canal often delimit a radiolucent band which simulates the internal acoustic canal (fig. 99).

The modified half axial films are obtained

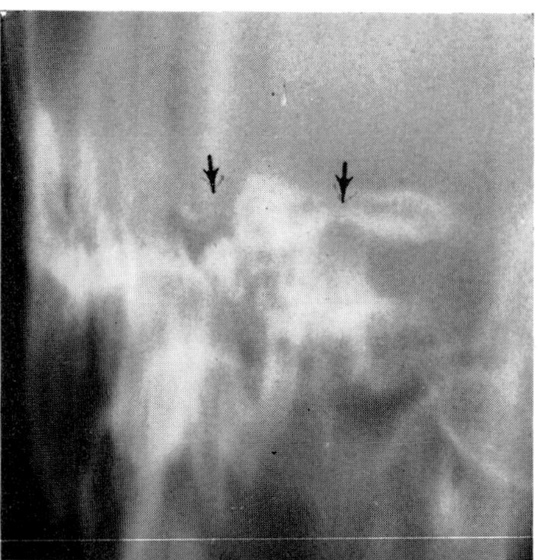

FIG. 102.—ANTEROPOSTERIOR LAMINAGRAM OF THE PETROUS PYRAMID

The laminagraphic section was made at the level of the internal acoustic canal and the posterior wall is visible, delimiting the lateral margin of the meatus. It can clearly be shown that the canal portion (*arrow*) is wider than the meatus. Lateral to the canal, and partly superimposed on the lateral wall of the canal, can be seen some of the inner ear structures, but not very clearly. They were shown better in laminagraphic cuts taken within a few millimeters anterior and posterior to this section. More laterally, the cavity of the middle ear is visible. The lateral arrow points at the upper margin of the attic underneath which can be seen the ossicles. The external auditory canal is also clearly shown.

by using a 25° caudal angulation of the tube from the canthomeatal line. A slightly different angulation may be required, depending on the shape of the patient's head. Less angulation tends to obscure part of the petrous pyramids and more angulation tends to obscure the outline of the canal as shown in Figure 31. In the modified half axial projection, the x-ray beam is approximately perpendicular to the long axis of the internal acoustic canal. The meatal portion is usually well shown and the length of the posterior wall of the canal is longer in this projection than it is in Stenvers projection, where it is foreshortened. The long axis of the canal is usually parallel with the bottom of the film. In this view, the structures of the inner ear (semicircular canals, cochlea, and vestibule) are not as easily identified as in Stenvers projection, described above. However, at least some of these structures can be seen. The meatus (or entrance) of the canal is usually visible as a radiolucent shadow with its long axis directed obliquely from above downward and medially, although occasionally it is round (fig. 96). The canal portion is usually clearly visible lateral to this radiolucent area and, depending upon the penetration of the film, the posterior wall may be more or less well shown. The suprameatal segment is clearly visible, and it is usually easy to compare the two sides on the same film. It is essential to obtain the correct projection to visualize the internal acoustic canals for if the wrong angulation and positioning are used, considerable difficulty is encountered in identifying these structures correctly. The findings are illustrated in Figure 96.

In the straight posteroanterior projection, the petrous pyramids are well shown; the internal acoustic canal and meatus are often well seen (fig. 101). However, the authors prefer the Stenvers and half axial projections.

Laminagraphy may also be used and is advantageous in certain cases. The films are usually made in straight anteroposterior projection (fig. 102).

Diseases Involving the Internal Acoustic Canal

The most important of the lesions that affect the internal acoustic canal is the tumor of the 8th nerve. These tumors may be partly outside and partly inside the canal. They occur unilaterally but are sometimes encountered bilaterally, usually in patients with neurofibromatosis. The neoplasm may not involve the intracanalicular portion, but swelling of the nerve could still cause changes in the bone. The changes observed on the radiographs are those of erosion produced by continued locally increased pressure and pulsations due to enlargement of the nerve. Inasmuch as the majority of these tumors start outside of the internal acoustic canal, it is logical to assume that the changes are more often noted in the meatus portion,

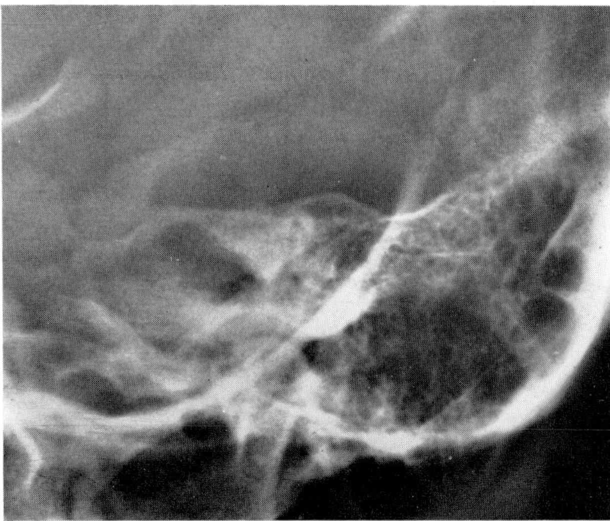

FIG. 103.—ACOUSTIC NEURINOMA PRODUCING AN EROSION OF THE SUPERIOR WALL OF THE CANAL AND MEATUS

It is clear that the suprameatal space is much thinner than would be expected from the position of the upper margin of the lateral aspect of the canal, and the greatest degree of thinning of this segment is above the meatal portion.

that is, at the entrance of the canal which becomes widened. If the tumor or the swelling extends to the distal end of the undivided nerve, the entire canal would then be involved. If the tumor starts in the portion of the nerve situated within the internal acoustic canal, the enlargement would involve first this portion and not the meatal portion. This variety may be termed the *intracanalicular type*, but the tumor may eventually grow outside the canal and the entire structure will be disrupted (fig. 110).

When the meatus is enlarged, the canal acquires a *funnel configuration* (fig. 111). The enlargement of both the meatus and canal takes place usually at the expense of the superior wall, and this results in a narrowing of the suprameatal segment (figs. 103 and 106). The reverse is true with tumors of the glomus jugulare, in the case of which the inferior wall and other structures are frequently significantly destroyed (Rice and Holman, 1962).

In addition to the actual enlargement of the meatus or canal, there is a *loss of sharpness of the superior margin*. In borderline cases, the loss of sharpness of the canal is the most prominent feature (fig. 104). A slight degree of asymmetry in the vertical diameter of the canal, when the right is compared with the left, commonly is present in normal patients. Up to 2 mm. difference is considered within normal limits by most authors. A difference of more than 2 mm. is considered indicative of enlargement. Therefore, the presence of slight widening, without any other change, is not in itself diagnostic of an acoustic neurinoma. On the contrary, if there is indistinctness of the superior margin and a decrease in size of the suprameatal space on the presumably abnormal side, the possibility of the findings being abnormal is very strong. In some instances, the superior margin of the canal acquires a superiorly curved configuration owing to ballooning of the canal by the tumor (fig. 106). Such a finding, however, should be evaluated with caution and other findings sought because curvature may be found in normal cases. Enlargement of the meatus is easier to visualize in many instances in modified half axial projection than in other views (fig. 104). *Destruction of the posterior wall* is a fairly common

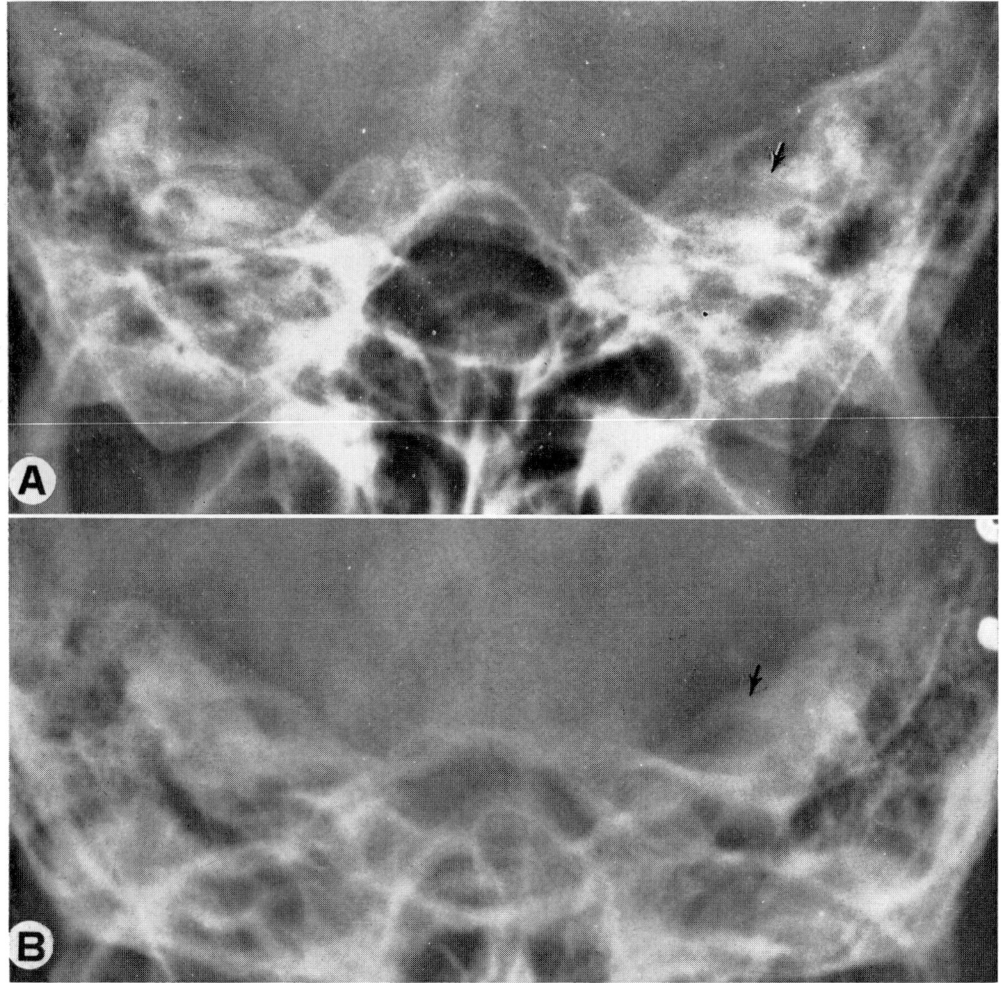

FIG. 104.—(A) ACOUSTIC NEURINOMA SHOWING ONLY DECREASE IN THE SHARPNESS OF THE SUPERIOR MARGIN OF THE CANAL; (B) FUNNEL CONFIGURATION

The superior margin of the canal on the left side (*arrow*) has lost its normal sharp outline in comparison to the other side. In addition, the meatus is not well defined and the normally slightly narrower portion at the meatus in comparison to the canal portion has disappeared. (B) represents another instance of 8th nerve tumor. The abnormal side (*arrow*) has a clear cut funnel configuration as compared to the other side. The medial border of the posterior wall of the canal is not visible. These appearances were not well shown in the Stenvers projection but were very clearly discernible in the modified half axial view and, in this instance, this projection was superior to the Stenvers projection.

finding and can be evaluated by taking a film with less than the usual penetration. Ordinarily, the lighter film should show the posterior wall, if present. The posterior wall can be rather short particularly in Stenvers projection, but the two are usually symmetrical when the right is compared with the left side (fig. 107).

A tumor can produce a depression just medial to the meatus which may be confused with a petrous air cell (fig. 108), but in these cases usually the meatal portion of the bone also will be enlarged. Differentiation of normal from abnormal may be difficult. An area of erosion does not have the usual very sharp outline of an air cell

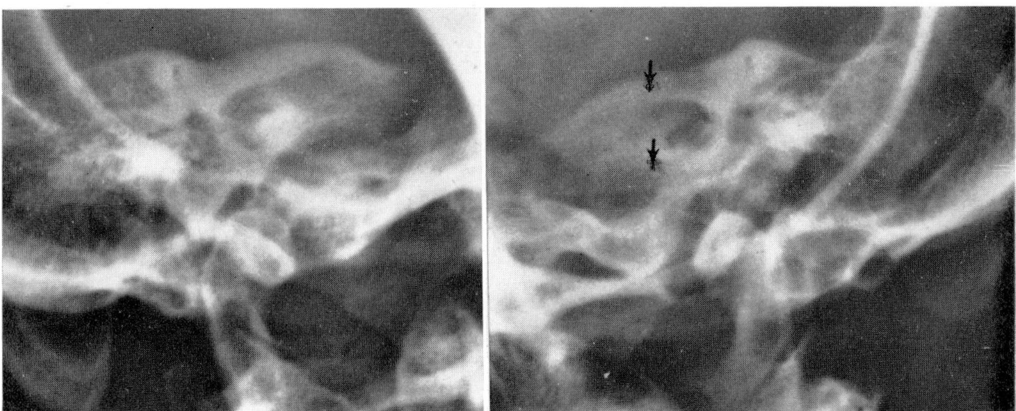

FIG. 105.—ENLARGEMENT OF INTERNAL ACOUSTIC MEATUS AND CANAL DUE TO ACOUSTIC NEURINOMA

On the reader's right, there is evidence of widening of the meatal portion as compared with the opposite normal side (*arrows*). The canal portion is also wider in its vertical diameter than the one on the opposite side. The canal, on the abnormal side, has acquired a slightly funnel-shaped configuration, but in this instance the sharpness of the superior wall has been fairly well preserved.

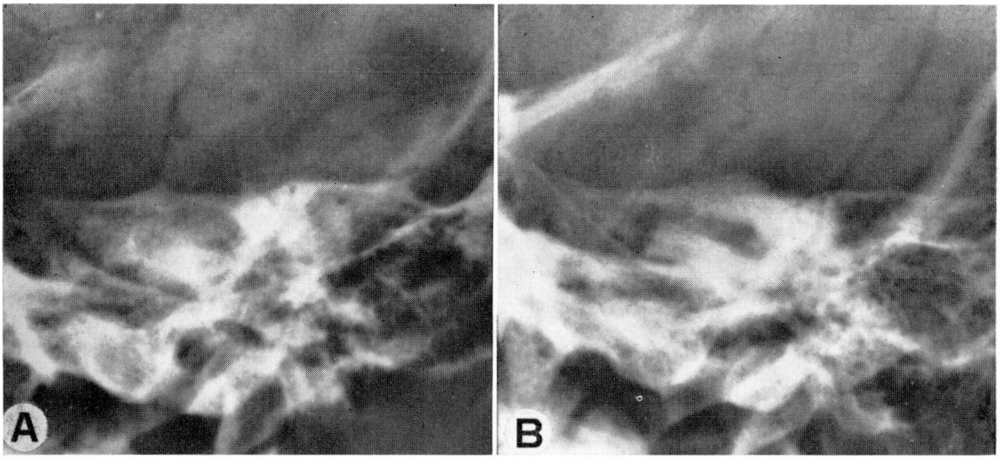

FIG. 106.—ACOUSTIC NEURINOMA PRODUCING EROSION OF INTERNAL ACOUSTIC CANAL

The abnormal side (A) demonstrates a curved upper margin of the canal portion with the meatus portion still apparently well defined. The lower wall, however, of the meatal portion cannot be seen on these films. The posterior wall must be extremely short and can be seen as a very thin rim of bone just medial to the deepest portion of the canal. The falciform crest is still visible. The appearance here would be difficult to interpret were it not for the opposite side (B) which shows an entirelydifferent configuration to the internal acoustic canal and meatus in this patient. Inasmuch as the porus acusticus internus tends to have a relatively symmetrical configuration in the same patient, the lack of symmetry is often the only indication of the presence of a tumor which, however, cannot be diagnosed on that basis alone. The suprameatal space on the involved side is extremely thin in comparison to the normal side.

which should be completely surrounded by a dense layer of bone. As destruction continues, the findings become much more obvious and the entire petrous tip may be eroded.

In summary, the radiologic findings of

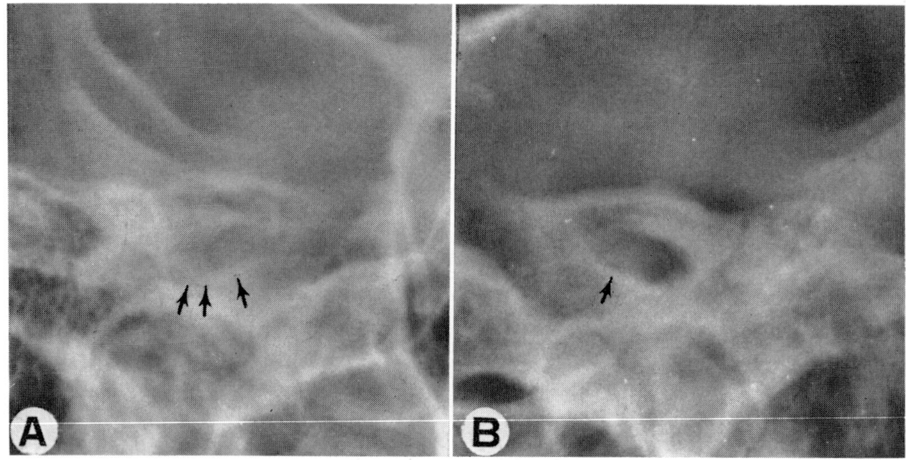

Fig. 107.—Acoustic Neurinoma Producing Destruction of Posterior Wall of Acoustic Canal

The normal side (A) shows a normal canal and meatus portion (*arrows*). On the abnormal side (B) there is greater radiolucency because of the lack of posterior wall, and the meatus portion is as wide as the canal portion. The posterior wall is almost completely absent on this side and, therefore, the lateral margin of the meatus cannot be seen. In general, it is easier to visualize the posterior wall and the lateral margin of the meatus in the modified half axial projection than in the Stenvers projection because of foreshortening.

neurinomas of the 8th nerve are: (1) enlargement of the meatal portion of the canal (a vertical measurement greater than 8 mm. should be regarded with suspicion); (2) indistinctness of the superior canal margin; (3) a funnel-shaped configuration with the wider portion medially; (4) decrease in the size of the suprameatal segment; (5) destruction of the posterior canal wall; (6) enlargement of one canal in excess of 2 mm. when compared to the opposite side; (7) erosion of the petrous tip in addition to involvement of the internal auditory canal (fig. 109).

With careful attention to anatomical and technical details it is possible to diagnose approximately 65 per cent of acoustic schwannomas by plain films alone. In an additional small percentage of cases some findings may be present which can be interpreted as the result of bone erosion retrospectively, but they are not sufficient to allow a definite diagnosis from plain films alone. If the clinical findings are fairly typical of an 8th nerve tumor and the plain films show positive findings, surgical intervention should be performed without further radiologic study. The same applies to cases with an atypical clinical picture, but with characteristic radiographic findings. The cases without radiographic evidence of typical erosion of the auditory canal probably should undergo further examination such as pneumoencephalography or vertebral angiography. Special studies are particularly advisable in cases which present an atypical or incomplete angle tumor syndrome. It is important to remember that angle meningiomas also may occur and that they may produce a clinical picture similar to that of acoustic schwannomas. Moreover, it is essential to try to differentiate these two tumors before surgical intervention because a meningioma may require a different surgical approach from that used for an 8th nerve tumor.

The sella turcica shows evidence of increased intracranial pressure in a small percentage of the cases of acoustic neurinoma. The sella turcica actually can be enlarged in 8th nerve tumors and this may lead to an erroneous diagnosis of pituitary tumor. In one case seen at the Neurological Institute, the patient had received treat-

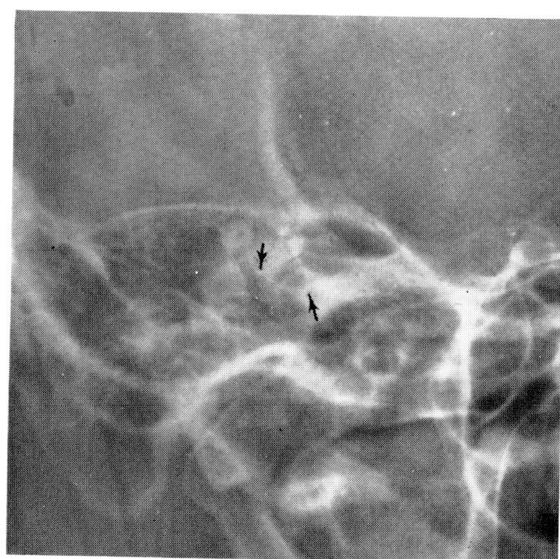

Fig. 108.—Neurinoma of the 8th Nerve Producing Erosion Adjacent to Internal Acoustic Meatus

A radiolucency is seen on the medial aspect of the petrous pyramid which does not have the exact characteristics of petrous air cells. Also, the walls of the acoustic canal and meatus are not seen through the area of the air cells, as is normally the case. Because of the position of the vestibule (upper *arrow*) and the superior semicircular canal, it is easy to determine the lateral aspect of the canal and it can, therefore, be seen that the medial portion of this structure is disrupted.

ment for a presumed pituitary adenoma some time prior to admission.

Slight enlargement of the internal auditory canal may occur in patients with increased intracranial pressure (see p. 1.87). The authors have noted this more frequently in children. In one case of brain stem glioma with unilateral cranial nerve involvement there was moderate enlargement of the acoustic canal on the ipsilateral side. Surgical intervention revealed a brain stem glioma and the 8th nerve appeared swollen to the surgeon. All symptoms disappeared following radiation therapy.

Differential diagnosis. Erosion of the petrous tip may be encountered in neurinomas of the 5th nerve as described by Holman (1961) (fig. 112). However, because of their greater frequency, it is common to see petrous tip erosion in extremely large pituitary adenomas. In both conditions, the erosion starts at the petrous tip and extends laterally but may not reach the internal acoustic canal. Differentiation usually is easy in pituitary adenomas because of the symmetrical involvement of both sides and because of enlargement of the sella turcica (fig. 91). With neurinomas of the

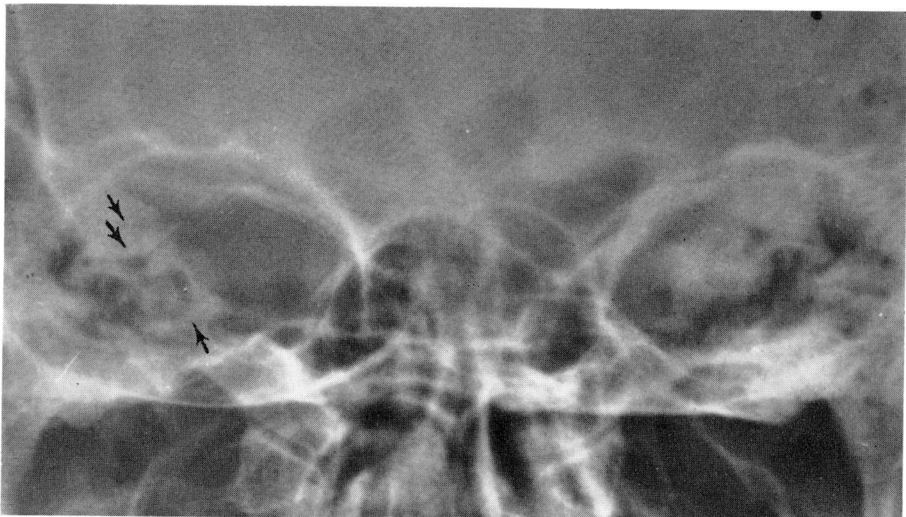

Fig. 109.—Acoustic Neurinoma Producing Wide Area of Erosion of Petrous Tip

The straight anteroposterior projection demonstrates the wide area of erosion of the petrous tip which involves the upper half of the petrous pyramid, including the upper margin. The lateral aspect of the canal is also completely destroyed. The expected position of the canal can be easily ascertained by the position of the cochlea and semicircular canals (*arrows*). Destruction in this position is usually associated with neurinomas of the 8th nerve.

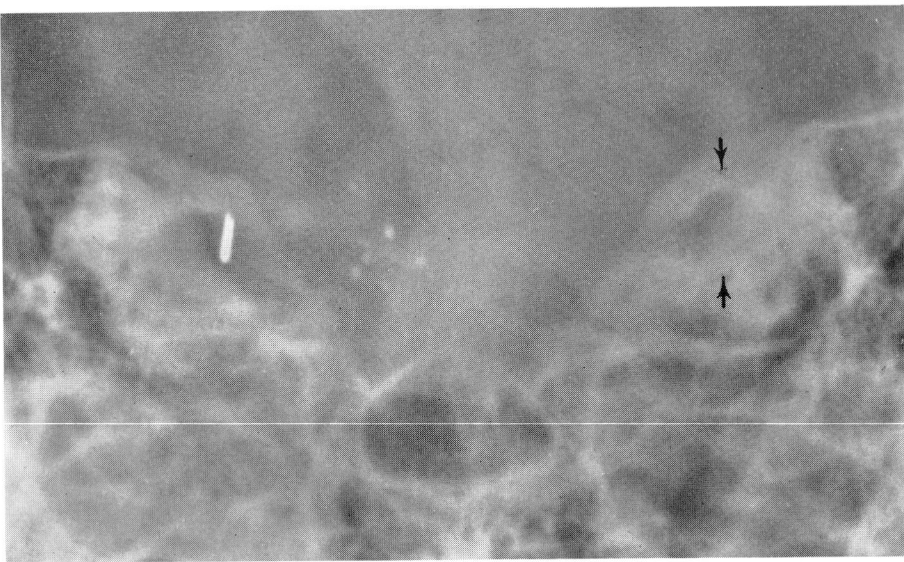

FIG. 110.—8TH NERVE TUMOR, NEURINOMA, INTRACANALICULAR VARIETY

This patient, who had neurofibromatosis, had had a previous 8th nerve tumor removed on the opposite side. He later developed decreased hearing on the left side and examination revealed ballooning of the canal portion of the porus acusticus internus without widening of the meatus (*arrows*). This presumably indicates that the tumor is localized within the canal at this time.

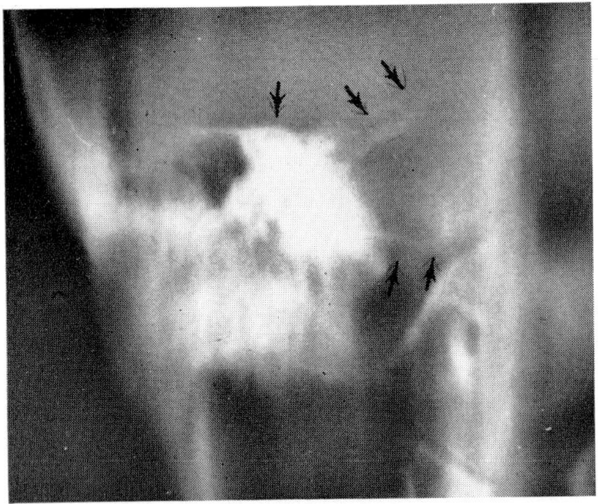

FIG. 111.—ACOUSTIC NEURINOMA PRODUCING FUNNEL-SHAPED DEFORMITY OF INTERNAL ACOUSTIC CANAL, LAMINAGRAM

The laminagram passing though the internal acoustic canal shows a funnel-shaped configuration with a wider end medially assumed by the internal acoustic canal. The lateral arrow points at the superior semicircular canal.

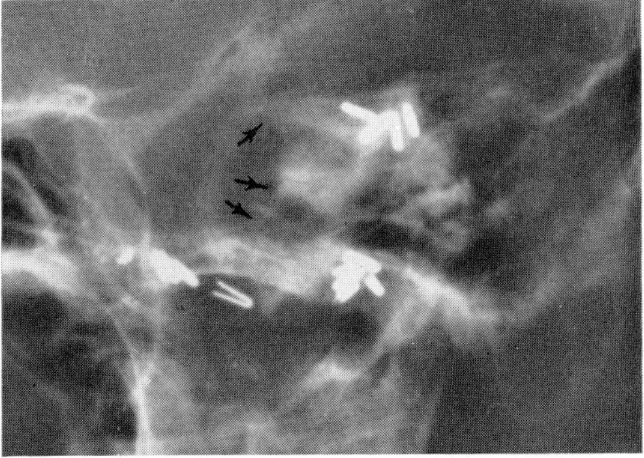

FIG. 112.—EROSION OF PETROUS TIP PRODUCED BY 5TH NERVE NEUROMA

There is a sharp margin to the area of erosion without widening of the internal acoustic canal. The erosion extends to involve part of the meatal portion of the porus.

5th nerve, there is often concomitant bone erosion in the region of the middle fossa.

Meningiomas of the cerebellopontine angle frequently are attached to the petrous pyramid as well as to the adjacent portion of the tentorium. They may produce diffuse changes including a loss of definition of the osseous structures and, at times, even some bone destruction. In actuality, the majority

(*Revised 1963*)

of meningiomas in this region do not produce any identifiable bone changes.

Destruction of the petrous pyramid by malignant disease usually is obvious. Sometimes congenital tumors, such as cholesteatomas, are found which involve only the medial portion of the petrous pyramid and not the mastoid antrum. These are probably developmental and not associated with chronic inflammatory disease of the middle ear. Air study may be necessary to arrive at a correct interpretation and evaluation of the clinical significance of such lesions. While there may be evidence of destruction in the region of the internal acoustic canal, the pneumoencephalogram reveals a normal cerebellopontine cistern.

JUGULAR FORAMEN AND JUGULAR FOSSA

It is common to have patients admitted to a neurological service who have multiple cranial nerves involved. One of the most difficult tasks in plain-film diagnosis or even in pneumoencephalography and angiography is to find the etiology of the cranial nerve paralyses. After all studies are completed, it is not uncommon to fail to demonstrate the cause of the paralyses which, in many instances, are found later to be due to malignant involvement with bone destruction. It is possible that in the earlier stages there was no evidence of bone destruction and that the cranial nerve involvement was due to perineural infiltration by neoplastic cells which extended through the foramina at the base of the skull into the epidural space. It is equally true, however, that in some of these cases bone destruction could be found if a careful plain-film and laminagraphic examination is carried out. It is not uncommon, therefore, to fail to apply the proper treatment (adequate radiation therapy) in some of these patients until it is too late to affect a satisfactory result. With supervoltage equipment it is now possible to obtain a fairly high percentage of five-year survivals in malignant nasopharyngeal tumors, even in the presence of bone destruction. It is, therefore, essential to carry out a complete examination of the base of the skull in patients presenting multiple cranial nerve involvement to detect bone erosion or destruction.

The base views of the skull already described (p. 1.43) will show some of the basal foramina and will, ordinarily, give a fairly satisfactory view of the middle fossa structures. However, the region of the petrous pyramids and the posterior fossa are not well shown on the ordinary base views because the position in which the film is made causes the incident ray to be oblique to the plane of the posterior structures. In addition, there is obliteration of the posterior structures by the soft tissues of the neck and by the cervical vertebrae. In order to visualize the posterior structures to best advantage, the base views should be modified so that instead of having the canthomeatal line parallel with the film and angling the central beam 15° rostrally, the central beam should be perpendicular to it. This will throw the horseshoe of the mandible backward and will give a much better picture of the jugular foramen on each side (fig. 41). The atlas will also be better visualized in this projection. The advantage of the latter view over other special individual views of the jugular area is that it will permit comparison of the right and the left jugular foramina and fossae. An easy way to effect the same modified base view is by using an exaggerated Waters position; that is, (1) the chin is placed on the film, (2) the tip of the nose is placed away from the film so that the canthomeatal line makes a 37° angle with the plane of the film, (3) the central beam is angled 15° caudad. An equivalent view will be made by lifting the nose off the film further so that the canthomeatal line makes an angle of approximately 45 to 55° with the plane of the film (fig. 41). This may be made in the prone as well as in the sitting positions.

To obtain a view of the jugular foramen

(Revised 1963)

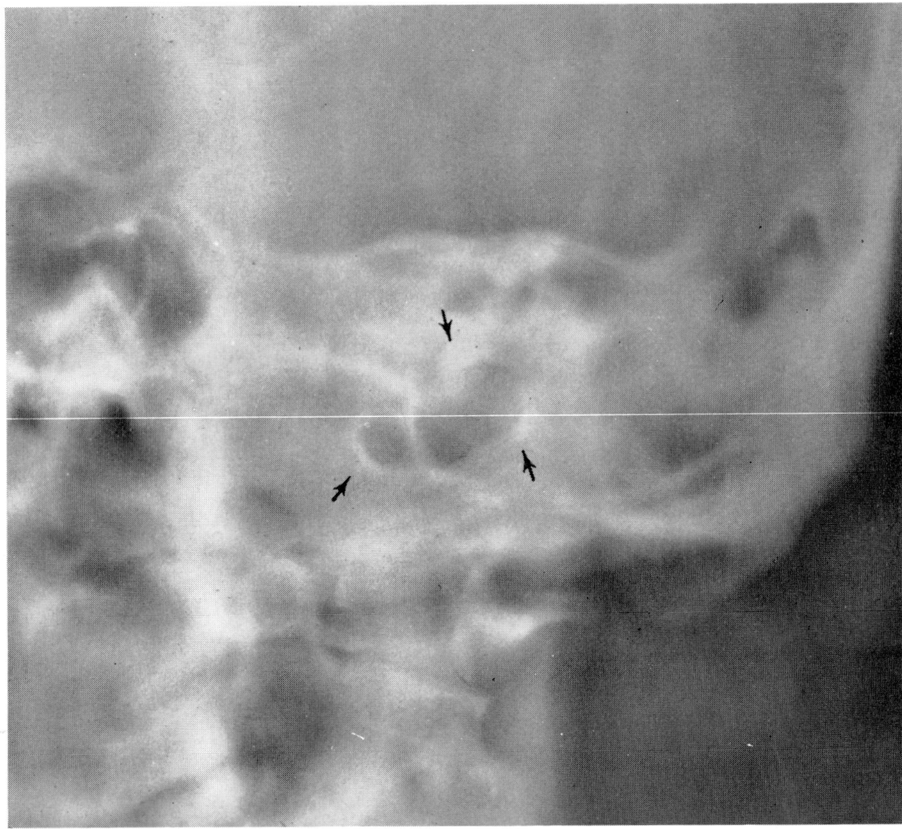

FIG. 113.—LAMINAGRAM OF THE JUGULAR FORAMEN MADE IN THE OCCIPITO-ZYGOMATIC PROJECTION
The jugular foramen and fossa are well shown (*arrows*). In addition, the foramen hypoglossum is shown in a position slightly medial and at the inferior aspect of the jugular foramen (*lower arrow*).

in which the x-ray beam is perpendicular to its axis, a position very similar to that used to take the optic foramen is used. The head is rotated 45° toward the side being examined. With the canthomeatal line perpendicular to the film, the central beam is angled 15° caudad, but instead of centering the beam with the orbit, it will be centered to emerge at the notch below the malar bone as recommended by Giraud *et al.* (1961). Laminagraphy may be performed in the same position. Fischgold *et al.* (1952) recommend tomography of this region, rotating the head only 30° toward the opposite side in the anteroposterior projection. The canthomeatal line is placed at an angle of 10° from the vertical by lifting the chin slightly; otherwise Reid's base line is placed perpendicular to the film. In addition to the jugular foramen, these views demonstrate the hypoglossal foramen for the passage of the 12th nerve which projects slightly anterior and inferior to the midportion of the jugular foramen. Laminagraphy in the same position may be advantageous (fig. 113).

Erosion of the jugular foramen may develop slowly. The fossa becomes enlarged, but the outline remains sharp, as in neuromas of the 9th, 10th, or 11th nerves. In rapidly progressing erosion due to malignant lesions, the outlines are usually irregular. The hypoglossal foramen also may be eroded and enlarged by neurinomas of the 12th nerve or may be destroyed by an

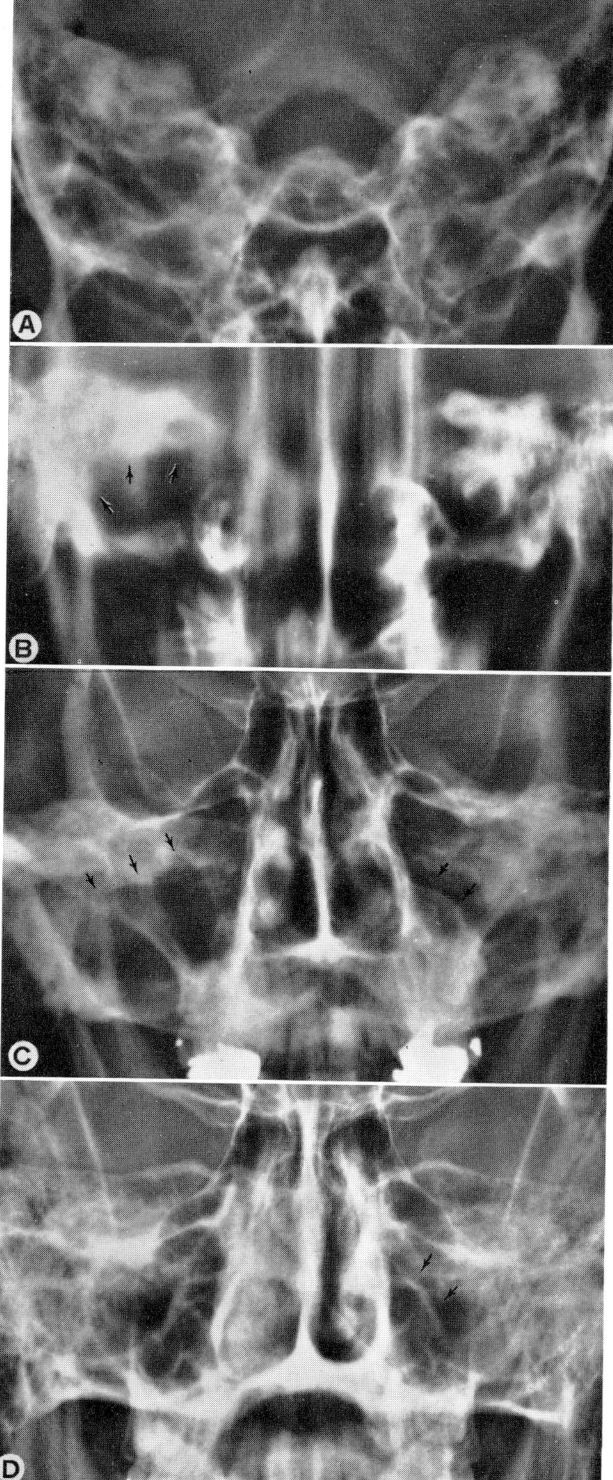

Fig. 114.—Glomus Jugulare Tumor Producing Erosion of Lower Aspect of Petrous Pyramid

The half axial projection (A) does not demonstrate the erosion very clearly. A laminagram of this region made in the frontal projection (B) demonstrates wide area of erosion in the region of the jugular foramen and involving also the medial aspect of the petrous pyramid (*arrows*). A film made in inclined posteroanterior projection (C) demonstrates the area of erosion very clearly, and it is also seen that the inner aspect of the occipital bone above the occipital condyle is eroded as demonstrated by the fact that the line, shown by the two arrows on the opposite side, is absent on the side of the lesion. This appearance should be compared with that of a normal case shown in (D), in the same projection. The case emphasizes the importance of studying the petrous pyramids in all possible projections. The wide area of destruction was overlooked on the original routine radiographs before the laminagraphic examination was carried out.

infiltrating malignant lesion, usually arising from the nasopharynx, or by glomus jugulare tumors. Considerable destruction of bone in this region may be present which can be overlooked on films made during conventional radiography of the skull unless careful attention is paid to all details (fig. 114).

OPTIC FORAMEN

Anatomy

The name optic foramen is a misnomer for this structure is actually a canal through which passes the optic nerve and the ophthalmic artery. The optic canal measures 5 to 7 mm. in length. For this reason it is often difficult to obtain optic foramen views in which this structure is shown to best advantage. If the central beam of radiation is not parallel with the long axis of the foramen, this will appear elongated or narrow in one diameter or it might have a biconvex configuration which is artifactual. Normally, in obtaining views of the optic foramen the head is rotated 45° toward the side being examined and the orbit is against the film. The chin is dropped in order that the canthomeatal line makes an angle of 15° with the vertical; the central beam is anglde 15° caudad. The reason for this is that the canal is inclined about 40 to 45° medially and 30° caudally.

The optic foramen is bounded medially by the body of the sphenoid. The sphenoid sinus is usually developed in this portion of the sphenoid. The inferolateral aspect is formed by a bridge of bone called the *sphenoidal strut*, which separates the foramen from the superior orbital or sphenoidal fissure. The superolateral aspect is formed by the base of the anterior clinoid process and the superior margin by the superior root of the lesser wing of the sphenoid. By using the Pfeiffer board it is possible to obtain comparable symmetrical views of both optic foramina in almost every patient.

The optic canal reaches its full size on the 3d year of life. On radiographs made using 36- to 40-inch target-film distance, the optic foramen measures up to 6.5 mm. in its maximum diameter. This is considered by us as the upper limit of normal. Only rarely is a normal optic foramen found to be larger. Slight asymmetry in the size of the foramina is common, since only one-half of patients have symmetrical foramina. The others show a slight difference in size, ranging up to 1.5 mm. A difference of 2 mm. between the two sides should be considered as grounds for suspicion of an abnormality. The abnormality could be due to enlargement of one optic foramen such as may be encountered in tumors of the optic nerve and in certain other conditions, or it may be due to shrinkage of the smaller foramen which is seen after enucleation of an eye and atrophy of the optic nerve, with meningioma or with fibrous dysplasia. Actually, the optic canal is rather ovoid in configuration with its upper outer aspect slightly narrower than its lower inner aspect. Therefore, the vertical or the oblique diameter is usually greater than the transverse diameter. Artifacts may be produced by projection as explained above. Inasmuch as the length of the canal is variable, a longer canal is more likely to obtain an unusual shape in films made so that the central beam is not parallel with the long axis of the foramen.

The ophthalmic artery enters the orbit through the optic canal below and lateral to the optic nerve. At times the ophthalmic artery produces a groove on the inferolateral aspect of the optic canal and rarely it may pass through a separate foramen.

Sometimes a "double foramen" is seen on the films. This is produced by the optic canal and the "caroticoclinoid foramen." The latter is formed when the dural fold, which extends from the middle clinoid to the tip of the anterior clinoid process at the point of emergence of the internal carotid artery from the cavernous sinus becomes calcified (fig. 115). The caroticoclinoid foramen is projected infralaterally to the optic canal, but is not visible on the usual optic foramen views where the optic canal is ideally projected on the lower outer quad-

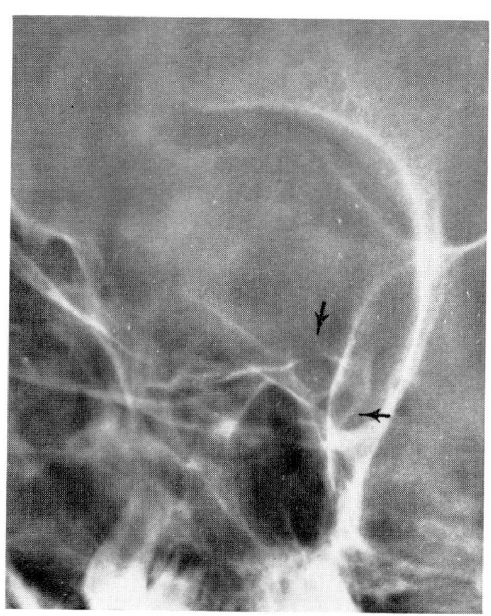

FIG. 115.—NORMAL OPTIC FORAMEN VIEW SHOWING CAROTICO-CLINOID FORAMEN

The upper larger foramen is the optic foramen (*arrow*) and the lower, more lateral foramen, is the caroticoclinoid foramen (*horizontal arrow*).

rant of the orbit. When sufficient rotation is used and in some cases on films made in correct position, the caroticoclinoid foramen may be visible. The caroticoclinoid foramen is sometimes well seen on rotated lateral views. In a series of 2187 skulls, Keyes found a complete or an incomplete caroticoclinoid foramen in 35 per cent of the cases, and in two-thirds of these it was bilateral.

The anterior clinoid process may sometimes produce a confusing round shadow lateral to the optic foramen if it is pneumatized or when it is large and has sufficient cancellous bone surrounded by cortex (fig. 116).

Enlargement

An optic foramen is considered to be enlarged if it measures over 6.5 mm. in diameter or if it measures 2 mm. more than the one on the opposite side. The latter does not apply when there is a condition which may cause shrinkage of the optic foramen, such as may follow enucleation in children. Decrease in size of the optic canal after enucleation does not usually occur in adults.

The enlargement of the optic foramen may be associated with erosion. In this case it may be produced by lesions which invade the optic canal, such as meningiomas, or rarely by an aneurysm of the ophthalmic artery. It is more common to find pure enlargement of the optic canal without erosion. If the margins are sharp and without diminished density, it is likely that we are dealing with a glioma of the optic nerve. The reason for the absence of erosion, loss of sharpness or diminished density in the entire margin or part of the margin of the foramen in optic gliomas is apparently that these tumors grow very slowly. In more rapidly developing conditions or in those associated with hyperemia of the bone or invasion of bone, diminished density or destruction is the rule. However, in some cases of meningioma, no erosion is found and the entire foramen may be surrounded by an area of increased bone density im-

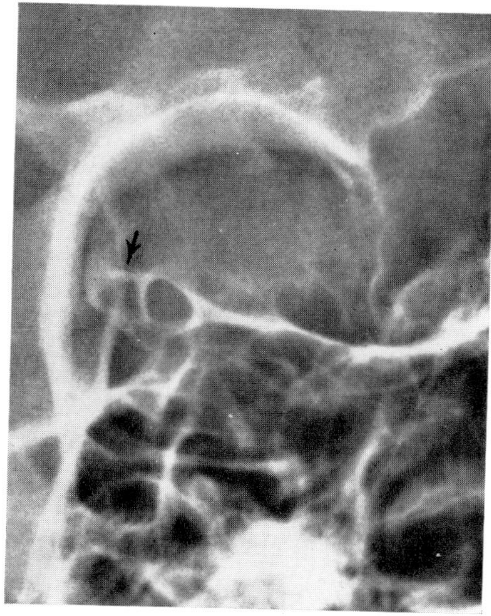

FIG. 116.—ANTERIOR CLINOID PROCESS SIMULATING OPTIC FORAMEN

The optic foramen is well shown; it clearly demonstrates the slightly greater oblique diameter than the vertical diameter. Another oval shadow is seen lateral to the optic foramen (*arrow*) which is the anterior clinoid process, seen end-on.

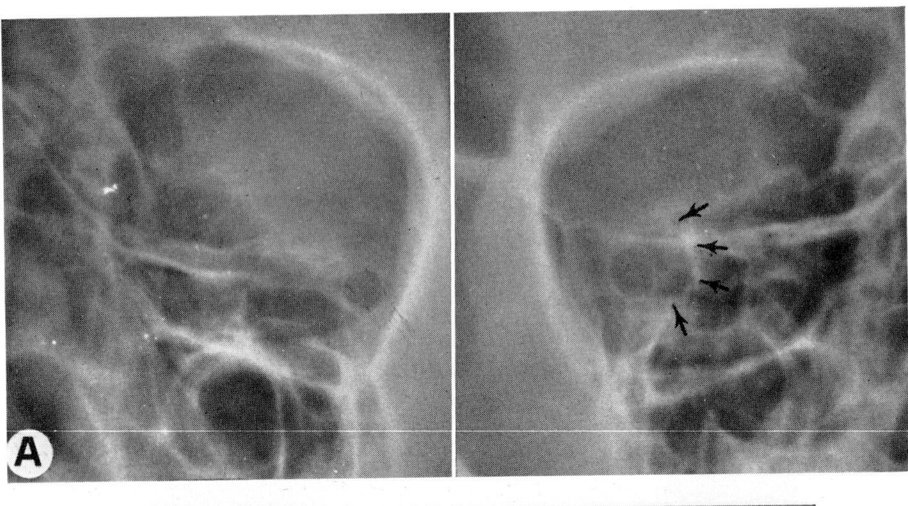

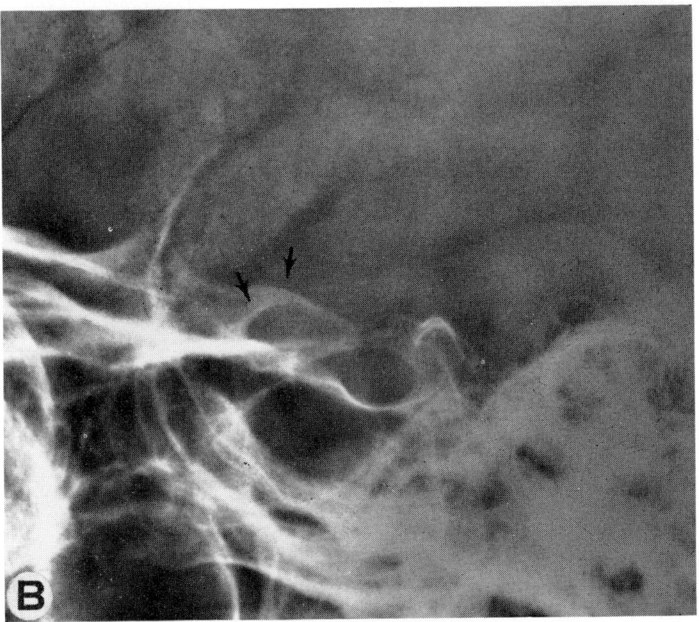

FIG. 117.—OPTIC GLIOMA INVOLVING THE INTRACRANIAL PORTION OF THE NERVE WITH FUNNEL-SHAPED DEFORMITY OF OPTIC CANAL

The optic foramen views (A) show that the left foramen is slightly larger and presents, on the medial side of the optic canal, another radiolucent area which represents, stereoscopically, funnel-shaped enlargement on the intracranial side. The lateral view (B) demonstrates the enlargement of the optic canal with elevation of the superior aspect of the anterior clinoid process which has actually become larger than the one on the opposite side. In addition, the region of the tuberculum sellae and the chiasmatic groove have become flat, giving the sella the typical appearance of J shape or pear shape. The patient was a 20-year-old man who had only intracranial optic glioma extending into the 3d ventricle but no evidence of exophthalmus.

mediately adjacent to the margin. In other cases of perioptical meningiomas, no changes are discernible in the films.

Enlargement of the optic foramen without erosion may be seen in cases of neurofibromatosis. It apparently is due to enlargement

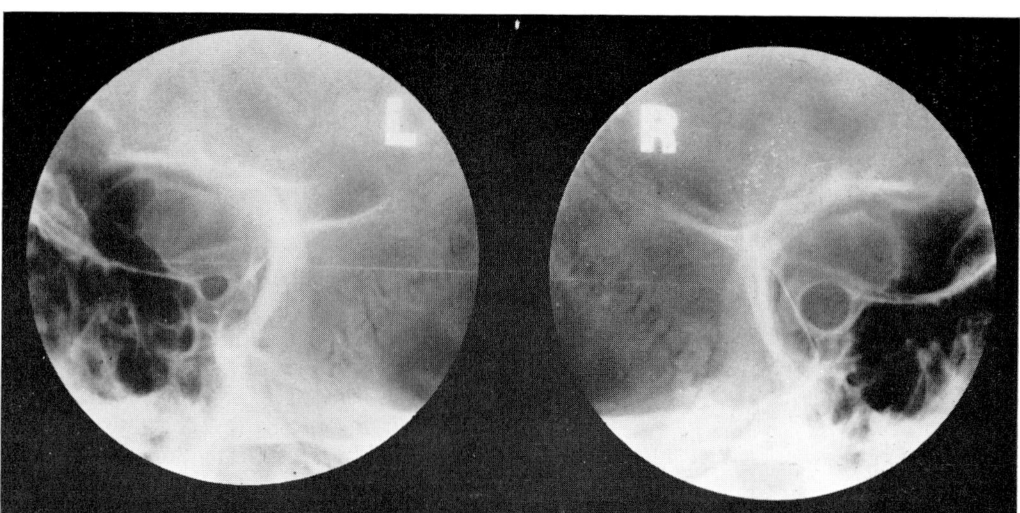

FIG. 118.—TYPICAL ENLARGEMENT OF THE OPTIC FORAMEN PRODUCED BY GLIOMA OF THE OPTIC NERVE

The enlargement is uniform, and there is no evidence of erosion of the margins of the canal. The films, made on a Pfeiffer board, illustrate the correct projection of the optic canals in the outer lower quadrant of the orbit.

of the optic nerve and unless it is associated with impairment of vision, the diagnosis of optic glioma is not justified. It is, however, well known that optic gliomas are much more frequent statistically in patients with fragmentary manifestations of neurofibromatosis

Roentgenographic features of optic gliomas. Optic gliomas are tumors most frequently encountered in childhood. As mentioned above, they are more frequent in patients with evidence of neurofibromatosis. However, they are seen in patients without any manifestations or without a family background of this condition. Such tumors may be seen in adults. Of the 34 cases reported by Taveras, Mount, and Wood (1956), 8 were in adults and the rest in children under 15. The average age was 13 years. There were 19 females and 15 males. In the group described above, 13 (38 per cent) had exophthalmus. The presence of exophthalmus usually means that the bulk or all of the tumor is in the orbital cavity. On the other hand, in the group of cases seen at the Neurological Institute, the majority (21 cases) had no exophthalmus and the major site of the tumor was in the chiasm and in the intracranial portion of the optic nerves. Enlargement of the optic canal without marginal atrophy was present in 24 cases (70 per cent). The presence of optic canal enlargement indicates that the tumor has extended to involve the intracranial portion of the nerve. Funnel-shaped deformity may be seen in some cases; the intraorbital portion of the canal is then wider than the cranial end. The opposite may also occur (fig. 117). The optic canal usually is not atrophic, apparently because these tumors grow rather slowly (fig. 118). Arrest in the growth of the tumor due to radiation treatment or surgical intervention with regression in size of the tumor and of the optic nerve may later lead to a diminution in the size of the foramen. The fact that the optic canal can decrease in size following surgical or radiation treatment indicates that the enlargement of the canal is not congenital, but is directly related to the tumor.

In addition to enlargement of the optic canal, the intracranial optic gliomas produce a flattening or actually a depression on the anterior aspect of the sella turcica. The tuberculum sellae is flattened due to deep-

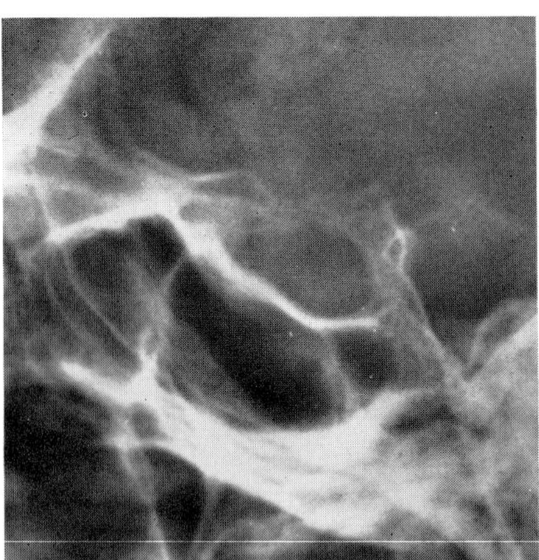

FIG. 119.—ELONGATED, J-SHAPED SELLA IN PATIENT WITH OPTIC GLIOMA

There is a flattening in the region of the tuberculum sellae and chiasmatic groove which gives the sella the typical elongated configuration. The description "pear-shaped" may also be applied to this appearance.

ening and lengthening of the chiasmatic groove (fig. 119). This causes an elongation which has been called the J-shaped sella. The term pear-shaped sella appears to be more accurate. Sometimes an actual depression in the region of the chiasmatic groove is seen which produces a W-shaped sella. It has been stated by some that the changes in the chiasmatic groove region indicate that the tumor had to be present before birth. However, this is not necessarily the case and any slowly growing tumor can produce depressions which, at the time of the examination, may show a good cortical bone edge. Even in adults, cases are found in which a slowly developing pressure erosion will allow the preservation of good cortical bone as exemplified by the intrasellar lesions.

If the tumor is more unilateral, it may produce a depression only on one side of the anterior aspect of the sella turcica (fig. 120).

If the tumor extends into both optic nerves, bilateral enlargement of the optic foramina may be present. Some cases of optic chiasm gliomas will not present any findings on the plain films.

Histologically, gliomas of the optic nerve most often are piloid astrocytomas. The cells are elongated, probably because they are growing among tight nerve fibers. Some of the optic chiasm gliomas may extend directly into the hypothalamus and later may grow into the third ventricle and into the thalamus. It is sometimes difficult to determine in the latter cases, even at autopsy, whether they arose primarily in the hypothalamus and extended into the optic chiasm or vice versa. The tumors can grow to be quite bulky and may produce blockage of the foramen of Monro, even though they may not actually grow into the 3d ventricle. At other times the block at the foramen of Monro and hydrocephalus are due to growth of the tumor into the 3d ventricle.

In the *differential diagnosis* one should consider the "perioptical meningiomas." These are sheathlike meningiomas wrapped around the optic nerve which go through the optic foramen and extend into the orbit. There may or may not be exophthalmus. Impairment of vision is common. In one of our cases there was actually an increase in the density of the optic foramen at the same time that it was enlarged. The age at which meningiomas occur is different from that at which the majority of optic gliomas occur. Meningiomas frequently are seen, however, in relatively young adults, usually young females around the third decade of life.

Another type of meningioma that may produce impairment of vision and visual field defects due to pressure on the chiasm is the group arising from the tuberculum sellae. These also tend to occur in relatively young individuals, usually females. The appearance may be that of sclerosis in the region of the tuberculum sellae and adjacent portion of the planum sphenoidale. A curious phenomenon seen in some of these cases is the apparent increase in the size of the ethmoid and sphenoid sinuses under the tuberculum sellae and planum sphenoidale. They tend to bulge upward. This has been called "blistering reaction." Apparently, the mechanism of the increase in the size of the

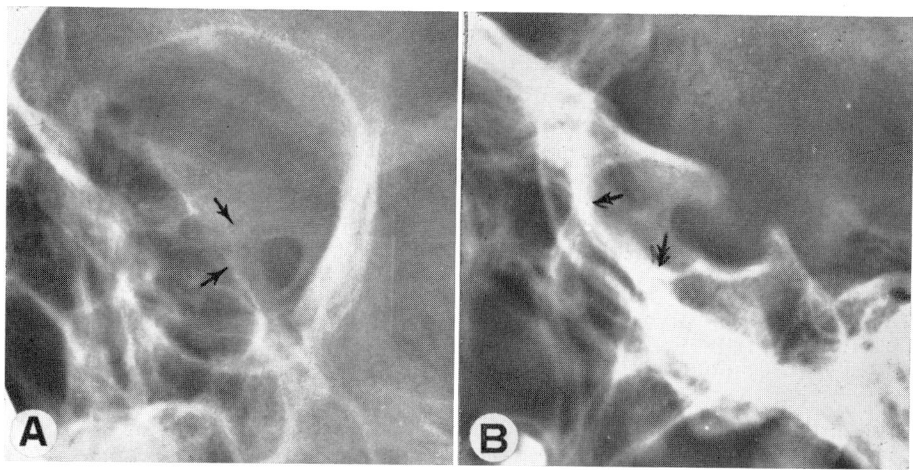

FIG. 120.—OPTIC CHIASM AND NERVE GLIOMA PRODUCING A UNILATERAL EROSION IN THE ANTERIOR ASPECT OF THE SELLA

The optic foramen view (A) shows no evidence of enlargement or erosion of the foramen. The lateral view of the skull (B) demonstrates the presence of an erosion on one side of the sella turcica (*arrows*). The opposite side is normal and does not present erosion. Upon surgical exploration it was found that the tumor involved the optic chiasm and extended into one optic nerve, on the right side. Upon careful observation of the optic foramina, it may be seen that on the right side there is a slight double contour which represents a funnel-shaped enlargement (*arrows*).

sinuses is that the meningioma extends to involve the sinus plate and bone over the sinus which is usually quite thin, and as the plate reforms, the sinus becomes larger since the meningioma usually does not grow into the sinuses. Over a period of time as the sinus plate reforms, perhaps several times, the result is a much larger sinus which bulges intracranially (fig. 144). Only rarely, meningiomas may be invasive and appear as a soft tissue mass within the sinuses.

A pear-shaped or J-shaped sella may be seen in congenital internal hydrocephalus and in patients with gargoylism. Occasionally it may be seen in infants, a condition for which no explanation is found. However, in the absence of hydrocephalus and gargoylism, *a pear- or J-shaped sella should be regarded as an abnormal finding until it can be explained otherwise.* Since diagnosis of an optic glioma should not be made in the absence of impairment of vision or visual field changes or both, the mere presence of a pear-shaped or J-shaped sella, or for that matter, of enlargement of the optic canals, should not lead to the diagnosis of optic glioma. Enlargement of the optic canal and a "J" sella can be found in some cases with neurofibromatosis, probably due to a bulky optic nerve, but without impairment of vision. Attention should be called to the fact that in infants, impairment of vision may be difficult to evaluate.

EROSIONS OF THE INNER TABLE OF THE SKULL

Superficially placed gliomas and cysts occurring in the brain cortex can produce localized erosion of the inner table of the skull. Only slowly growing lesions (chiefly oligodendrogliomas and cystic astrocytomas) are capable of producing these areas of local thinning. The mechanism is that of transmitted pulsations of a hardened area of brain cortex not surrounded by a cerebrospinal fluid cushion to diffuse the pulsation over a larger area. The case shown in Figure 121 demonstrates a very sharply circum-

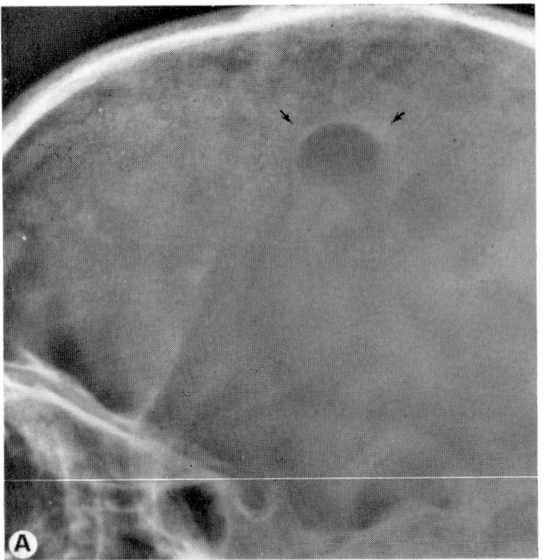

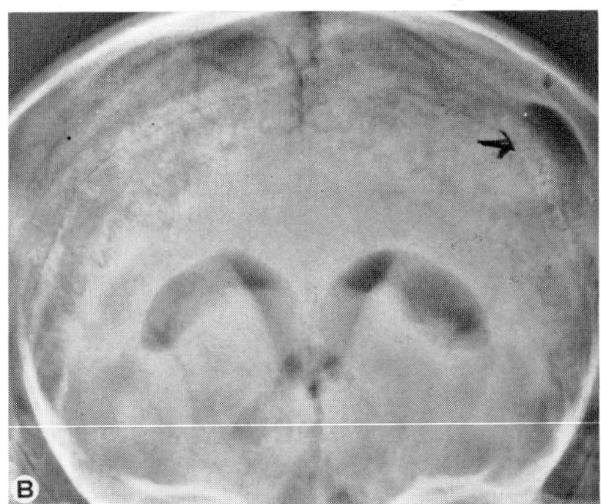

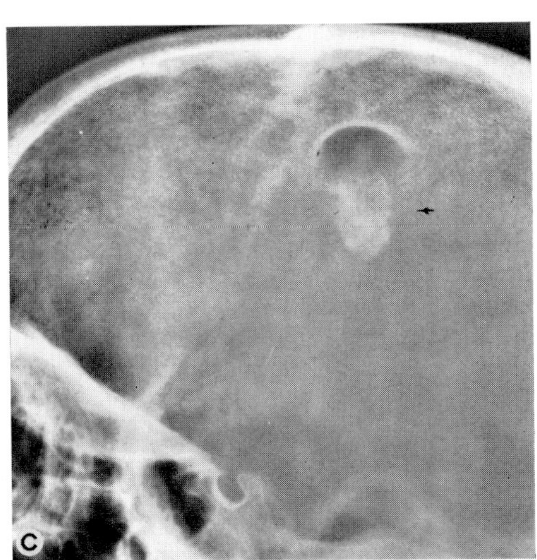

Fig. 121.—Erosion of Inner Table Produced by Superficially Placed Oligodendroglioma

An area of erosion is shown in the lateral view (A) with a sharp upper margin and a fading lower margin typical of inner table depressions. A penumoencephalogram (B) demonstrates the position of the erosion in the frontal projection and the absence of any shift or deformity of the ventricular system. In fact, there was a slight degree of enlargement of the corresponding lateral ventricle. Re-examination three years later (C) shows the area of erosion has become larger and there is calcification underneath it. The diagnosis of tumor is obvious. The patient was an 8-year-old child.

scribed area of bone erosion which was thought originally to represent an aberrant Pacchionian depression, although this was considered most unusual in its location—too far away from the midline. Pneumoencephalography and angiography were entirely normal. Later, calcification appeared, making the diagnosis of tumor obvious.

In our experience such lesions are most frequently encountered in children. Pneumographic studies and angiography are often normal or show only minimal findings because these are usually very slowly growing lesions which cause no significant edema of the surrounding brain tissue.

Thinning of the middle fossa as well as diminished density of the sphenoid ridge may be seen in slowly growing temporal tumors and in chronic juvenile subdural hematomas. In the latter case there is usually enlargement of the middle fossa and elevation of the sphenoid ridge (see under "Head Injuries and Their Complications").

Thinning and bulging in the occipital region may be produced by anomalous development of the cisterna magna (fig. 122).

(Revised 1963)

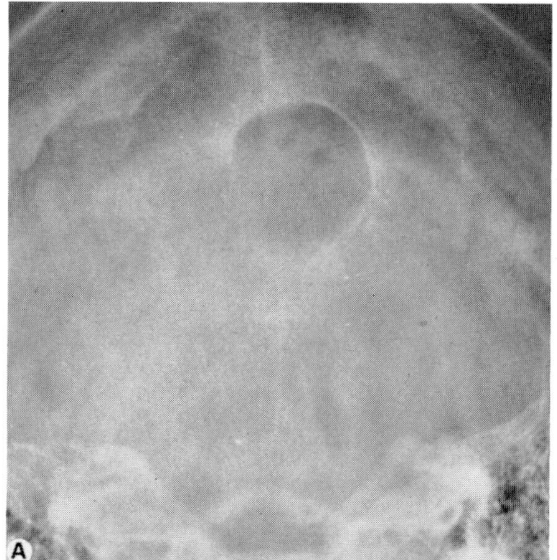

FIG. 122.—THINNING AND BULGING OF OCCIPITAL BONE PRODUCED BY ANOMALOUS CISTERNA MAGNA

In the frontal projection (A) there is a rounded area of erosion which extends further to the left than the right of the midline. A pneumoencephalogram (B) demonstrates a very large cisterna magna which extends into the supratentorial region, evidently through a defect in the tentorium, and produces the erosion of the inner table of the occipital bone. The frontal projection taken during pneumoencephalography (C) demonstrates the fluid level and the perfect adaptation of the anomalous cisterna magna to the area of bone erosion. Courtesy of Dr. Robert Hochstim, Long Island, N.Y.

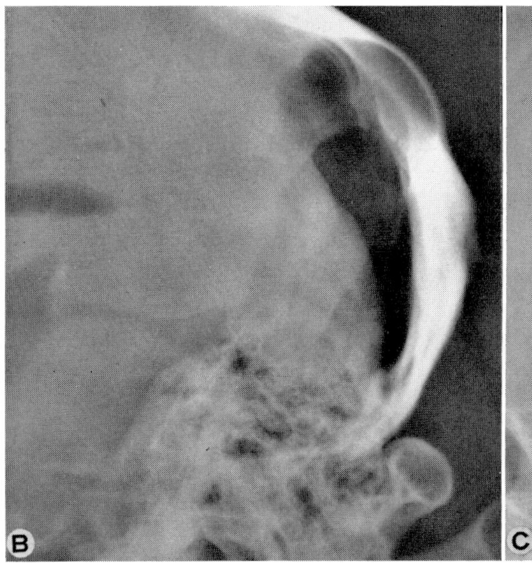

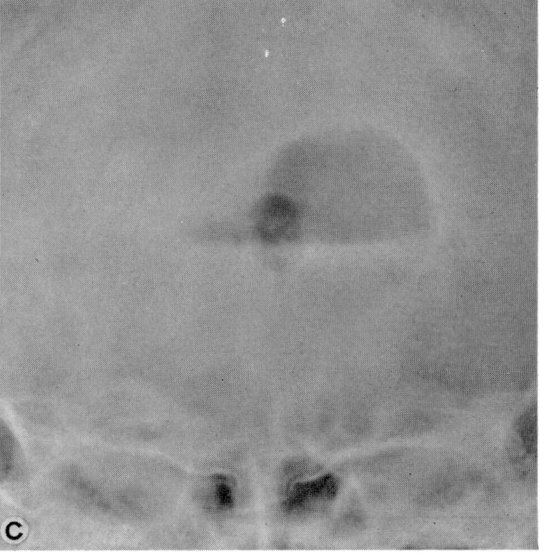

TUMORS OF THE CRANIAL VAULT

Benign tumors of the cranial vault are not rare. They are usually easy to recognize on the radiographs and a preoperative histological diagnosis is possible in the majority of them.

Epidermoid tumors. Epidermoidomas or cholesteatomas of the skull are characterized by the fact that they produce a clear area of bone destruction which is surrounded by a very sharply delimited margin of increased density. The shape may be slightly lobulated. These tumors arise from a remnant of dermal tissues within the skull which usually is congenital but can result from a penetrating wound. Bone destruction takes place because the cells grow and desquamate in the same manner as the skin. This forms a cystic space filled with sebaceous material. The bone is not invaded but growth compresses

(Revised 1963)

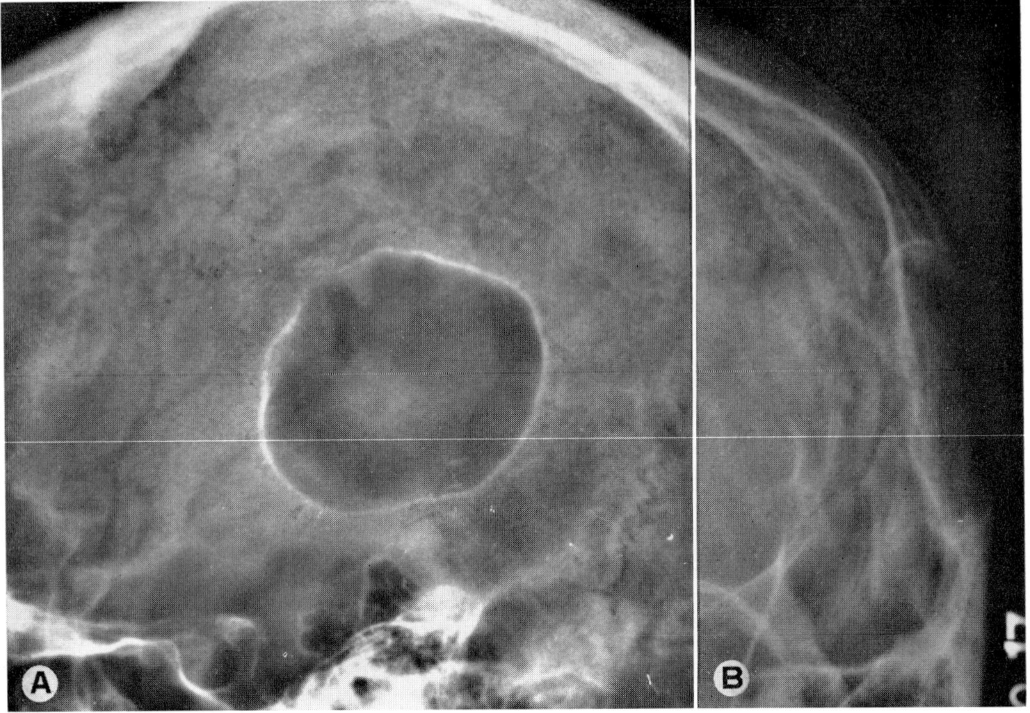

FIG. 123.—DIPLOIC EPIDERMOID TUMOR EXTENDING MORE INTRACRANIALLY THAN EXTRACRANIALLY

The lateral view (A) shows the typical appearance of the water-clear defect in the bone with very sharp, dense, slightly lobulated, margins. If remnants of bone still persist within the area of bone destruction, these will cast irregular plaque-like shadows of increased density which are different from those in cavernous hemangioma of bone. The frontal projection (B) demonstrates the location of the tumor within the diploë and extending more intracranially.

the bone peripherally and leads to the formation of the sharply delimited compact layer around the clear density. These cholesteatomas occur most frequently in the vault, but may also occur in the orbital region, usually in the roof of the orbit, and also in the occipital bone, sometimes near the midline. Most frequently, they arise in the diploë, and as they grow, they may protrude intracranially without actually extending significantly extracranially. This is one of the reasons why epidermoid tumors should be removed surgically when diagnosed, since it is not possible to tell the degree of intracranial protrusion of the mass (fig. 123). The epidermoids in the occipital region should be differentiated from the dermoid tumors which are usually seen in children and which are accompanied by a cystic mass in the posterior fossa or in the occipital region. The defect in the occipital bone in the latter cases is usually small.

Cavernous hemangioma of the skull. These tumors are usually found in the vault. They are characterized by an area of irregularly diminished density with many bony spicules within the area of bone destruction. The margin surrounding the hemangioma is usually well circumscribed, sometimes sclerotic, but may merge with the surrounding bone (fig. 124). Characteristically, these tumors have radiating spicules which on tangential views taken with soft tissue technique will have an appearance reminiscent of meningiomas. Differentiation from the epidermoid tumors is easy because hemangiomas contain many areas of increased density within the area of

(Revised 1963)

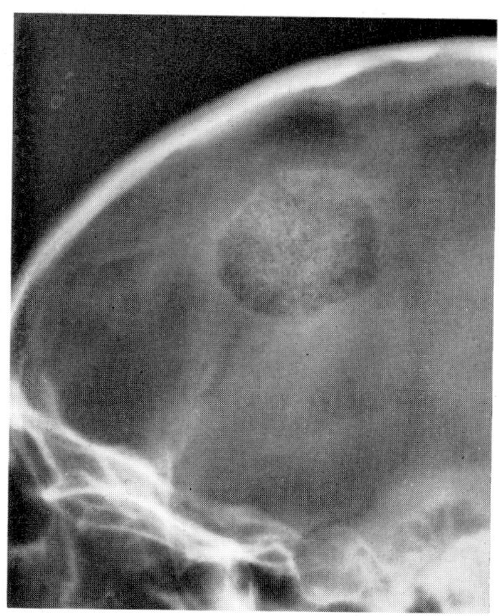

Fig. 124.—Cavernous Hemangioma of Bone

There is a fairly well circumscribed, slightly lobulated, area of decreased density in the frontal region with many speck-like areas of increased density within the radiolucency, which represent spicules of bone remaining between the cavernous spaces of the hemangioma.

destruction, which is not the case with the great majority of epidermoid tumors. Some epidermoid tumors of the vault may destroy one table more than the other and thus leave some of the bony density of the remaining plate. However, they have an entirely different appearance from the cavernous hemangiomas. Cavernous hemangiomas of the skull may grow over a long period of time. Trauma may cause them to bleed and form a large hematoma. If they continue to grow under observation, surgical removal is usually recommended. Angiography may demonstrate its arterial supply and a homogeneous tumor stain.

Eosinophilic granuloma and xanthoma. These tumors are seen more frequently in younger individuals or in children, but they may also occur in adults. Characteristically, they represent an area of bone destruction which is surrounded by a poorly circumscribed but clear margin. A slight "halo of increased density" may be seen immediately adjacent to the margin, particularly when the lesions are regressing. The margins are irregularly lobulated and some uninvolved areas of bone may remain in the center of destruction, giving it an irregular configuration (fig. 125). It is not uncommon to see that one of the tables is involved to a greater degree than the other table of the skull, especially in the healing stage. The lesions tend to be solitary but may be multiple. When they are multiple, it is probable that the patient either has or will develop Hand-Schüller-Christian disease or some other form of xanthomatosis. These lesions need not be removed surgically except when the diagnosis cannot be made without a biopsy, and they respond to small doses of radiation.

Localized fibrous dysplasia. The lesions of fibrous dysplasia in the vault may produce an irregular area of decreased density surrounded by an irregularly dense margin and, therefore, they have to be differentiated from the above described lesions. The shape is usually unevenly oval or lobulated, and areas of increased density are present within

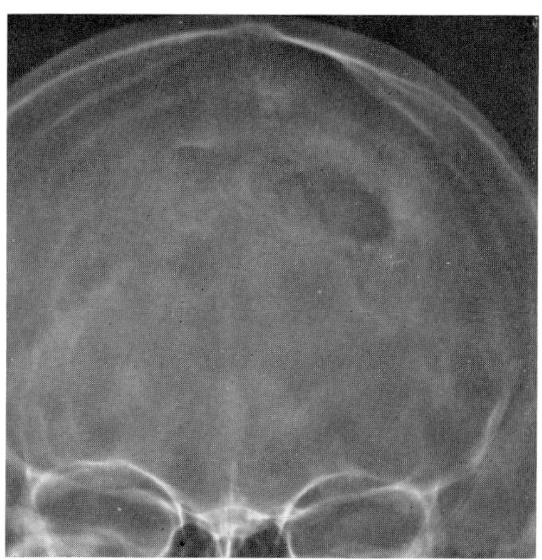

Fig. 125.—Eosinophilic Granuloma in a 12-Year-Old Boy

The destructive lesion presents some typical characteristics. The margin is not very sharp and there is suggestive double contour on the inferior aspect of the destructive area, indicating that one table is more involved than the other. There is also a slight halo of increased density around the lesion.

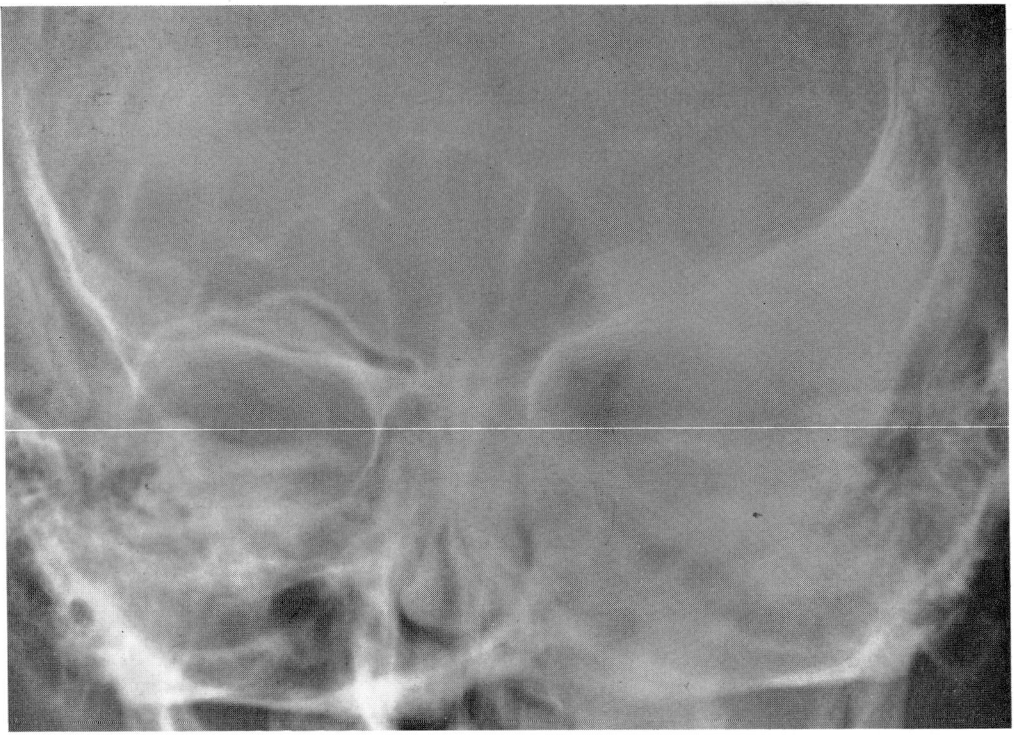

FIG. 126.—FIBROUS DYSPLASIA OF THE SKULL INVOLVING THE ORBITAL REGION
There is an area of increased density with some distortion of the anatomical outline in the lateral and superior aspect of the orbit involving the greater wing of the sphenoid as well. In addition, there is flattening of the lateral aspect of the orbit on the involved side as compared with the opposite side. The latter usually indicates that the lesion dates back to the growing years.

the radiolucency. These characteristics are typical of fibrous dysplasia of the localized type, but several varieties may be observed in the vault and in the base of the skull. In a series of 46 cases of fibrous dysplasia of the skull, Leeds and Seaman encountered the following types: (1) the *cystic type* is often best shown on a tangential view which will demonstrate the radiolucent center with outward bulging but no inward protrusion; (2) the *sclerotic type*, which is rare in the vault and cannot be differentiated from meningiomas; (3) the *mixed sclerotic and radiolucent type*, which is the most common in the vault. Fibrous dysplasia often involves the orbits and the base of the skull and in these areas it is often purely sclerotic, although in most cases some areas of radiolucency may be observed. The flattening of the superolateral aspect of the involved orbit is a frequent finding in fibrous dysplasia and is a helpful differential point, indicating that the lesion probably dates back to childhood (fig. 126). In the more localized sclerotic lesions of the base and sphenoid ridge, it is impossible to differentiate this type from meningioma on roentgenological grounds, unless involvement of the extracranial (facial) bones can be recognized. Some cases may even present an increase in size of middle meningeal arterial grooves (fig. 127). In some patients the skull manifestations are only part of a generalized process (polyostotic fibrous dysplasia).

Sinus pericranii

A soft tissue lump may occur in the scalp, usually in the frontal region, as the result of an enlarged communication be-

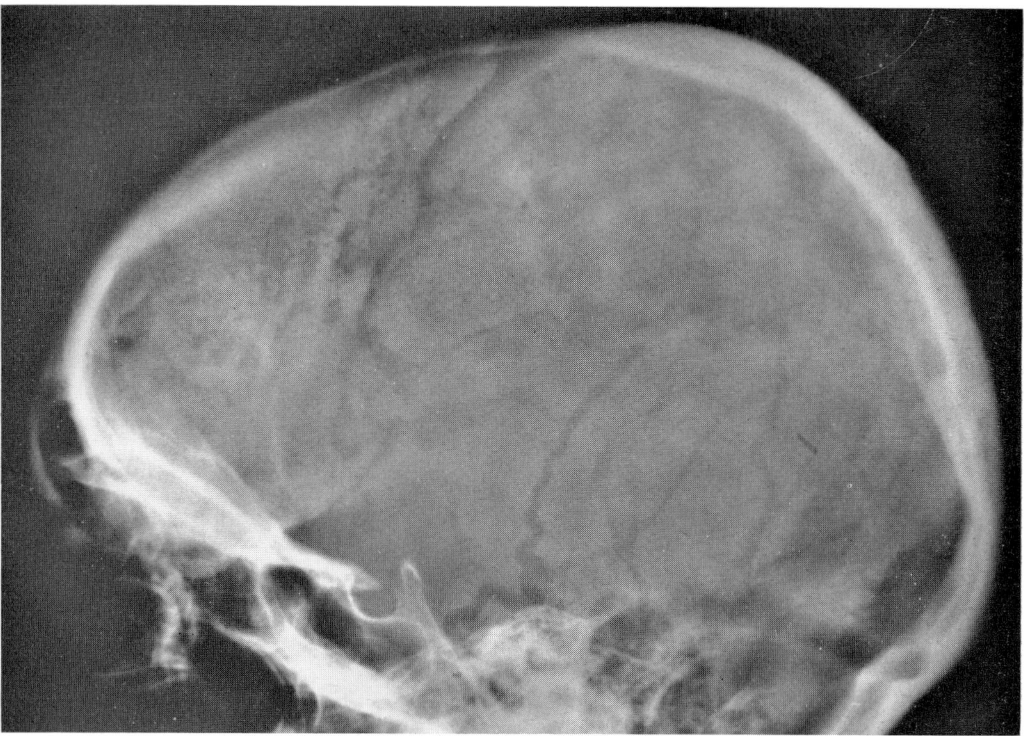

FIG. 127.—FIBROUS DYSPLASIA OF THE SKULL WITH ENLARGEMENT OF THE MENINGEAL CHANNELS
Two areas of patchy increase and decrease in density are seen in the parietal and frontal regions and there is evidence of increase in the size and tortuosity of the meningeal arterial channels. It is evident that some cases of fibrous dysplasia are associated with increased vascularity of the skull and others are not.

tween the intracranial and the extracranial venous circulation through emissary channels. The emissary channels may be demonstrable on stereoscopic films of the area and sometimes laminagraphy may be required. Characteristically, these lesions bulge when the patient leans down, as to tie his shoes, and flatten out when the head is lifted. Some of these lesions contain arterial elements and are evidently not of the same type as the one just described (fig. 30). Angiography of the external carotid artery will demonstrate the latter group. In addition, a small needle may be inserted directly into the lump in the recumbent position or during a Valsalva maneuver, and the injection of contrast substance will demonstrate the tangle of veins and the drainage by way of the dural intracranial sinuses.

(Revised 1963)

Differentiation by roentgenologic methods between the lesions described above usually is possible. Epidermoidoma and eosinophilic granuloma may have an atypical configuration, and in these instances, only biopsy can determine the histological diagnosis. The most frequent difficulty encountered is in distinguishing between venous lakes and the destructive lesions of bone. It is easy to distinguish venous lakes if one can obtain a tangential view of the area which shows that the radiolucency is situated between the two tables of the skull (fig. 128). Stereoscopically it may be possible to determine that the radiolucency does not involve the inner table by visualizing the fine arterial grooves of the meningeal vessels crossing the inner table. In addition, the relative radiolucency of a venous lake is usually less than that of a destructive bone

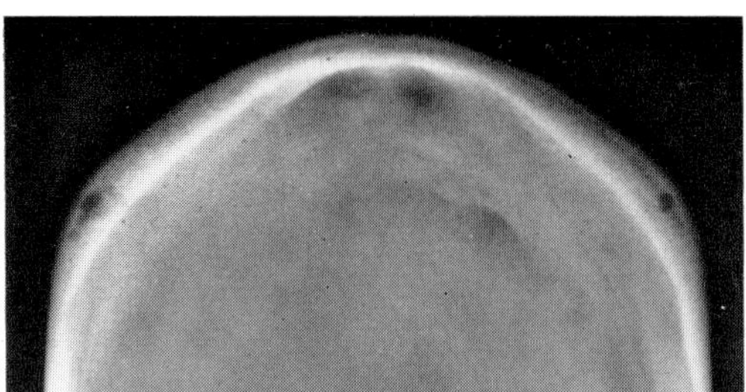

Fig. 128.—Venous Lakes in Diploic Regions Seen in Tangential View

A large venous lake was present in this patient and tangential view demonstrated the lesion to be entirely within the diploë and did not involve the inner or the outer table. This is typical of venous lakes.

lesion of the same size because a destructive lesion would ordinarily involve both tables, particularly the malignant lesions, whereas the diploic venous lake will not involve either of the tables. Nevertheless, occasionally it is difficult to differentiate a venous lake from a destructive bone lesion unless a diploic vein can be traced to the area.

Osteoma. Osteomas in the skull usually involve the outer table. They produce a hard lump outside of the skull and tangential films show that the osteoma is separated, at least in part of its extent, from the outer table of the skull by a very thin radiolucent space (fig. 129). Characteristically, osteomas do not extend into the diploë and if they involve the inner table, they cannot be differentiated from meningiomas. Osteomas can result from trauma with a subperiostial hemorrhage that later ossifies.

Malignant lesions (metastatic). Almost any tumor which metastasizes to bone may metastasize to the skull. There are no characteristic features except that the lesions usually are purely destructive and involve both the outer and inner table in addition to the diploic portion. The outlines may be ragged or irregular and not sharply circumscribed except in the smaller lesions. It is the smaller lesions of multiple myeloma and of carcinomatous metastases which offer difficulties in their differentiation from multiple venous lakes. As mentioned under "Normal Anatomy," multiple venous lakes can be quite prominent, but usually veins can be traced into most of them. Overpenetrated films and stereoscopic views may demonstrate these diploic venous channels in instances where they were not discernible in the routine films. Rarely, metastatic lesions of the skull may result in an osteoblastic reaction. This type of change is seen almost exclusively with secondary deposits from the breast. Even when metastases elsewhere in the skeleton are osteoblastic, those in the skull usually are osteolytic.

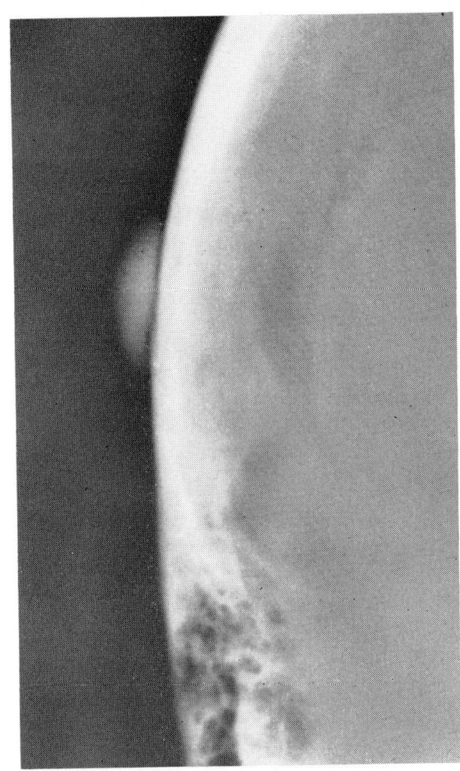

Fig. 129.—Osteoma of Skull

Hard lump could be palpated in the parietotemporal region in this patient. A tangential view demonstrates that the lesion is separated from the outer table of the skull by a radiolucent line. This is typical of benign osteomas of the skull.

EROSION OF THE BASE OF THE SKULL

Carcinoma. The most frequent cause of erosion of the basal structures is squamous cell carcinoma of the base of the skull which may arise in the nasopharynx, in the sphenoid sinuses, or in the other paranasal sinuses. These neoplasms are usually lumped together under the term nasopharyngeal carcinomas. How often carcinomas start in the *sphenoid sinus* and extend to the other structures is difficult to state. The experience at the Neurological Institute indicates that carcinomas that start in the sphenoid sinus and secondarily extend to the adjacent structures are fairly common. These patients often present with symptoms of cranial nerve involvement, often diplopia, and pain or numbness as the earliest signs. Roentgenologic examination at this stage may only disclose evidence of a mass lesion in the sphenoid sinus without evidence of increased thickening of the nasopharyngeal soft tissues, and repeated nasopharyngeal biopsies often are negative. At other times, the lesion appears first in the soft tissues of the nasopharynx and pain or cranial nerve involvement may be present without any demonstrable evidence of bone destruction in the base of the skull.

Other lesions that may produce bone destruction in this region are the glomus jugulare tumors and the chordomas. Meningiomas arising in the base of the skull may sometimes be invasive and may extend into the nasopharynx after filling the sphenoid and ethmoid sinuses. Mucoceles of the sphenoid sinuses are capable of producing bone destruction here, and some pituitary adenomas also produce extensive destruction in this region (even though they are not malignant) by virtue of their size, as was described in the section on pituitary adenomas. In addition, secondary deposits from carcinoma of the breast, the lung, the prostate, and occasionally other primary sites may produce bone destruction in the base. Before studying the bone changes and the changes in the soft tissues visible on the base of the skull, the reader should consult the section on "Normal Anatomy, Base View of the Skull," page 1.43.

Bone destruction in the base of the skull is often difficult to discern, while frequently it is clearly shown as a complete disappearance of the structures of the foramen ovale and spinosum and adjacent portions of the clivus and sphenoid sinuses, at other times the changes are more subtle. In the authors' experience, the most useful shadow in the base to detect early bone destruction is the wall of the sphenoid sinuses. The sinus plate should be carefully followed all the way around for evidence of a break in its continuity (fig. 130). A mere diminished density of the sinus plate without disappearance of it should not be taken as evidence of bone destruction. Diminished density may be seen in the presence of chronic hyperemia without bone destruction and may be associated with inflammatory sinus disease. The presence of soft tissue shadows within the sphenoid sinuses should be evaluated carefully. Polyps and mucoceles are sometimes seen in the sphenoid sinuses but they are seen here less frequently than in the other sinuses.

Care should be taken in evaluating the foramen ovale region which occasionally gives the impression of bone destruction when none is present. In any questionable case multiple projections should be made with slightly different angulation of the tube. It is the authors' custom to take stereoscopic base views in all cases in which examination of the base is indicated on clinical grounds. When bone destruction is present, the foramen ovale usually tends to become round and the margin of the destroyed bone is usually clearly visible but has an irregular outline. The presence of bone destruction in other structures of the base may be present without any evidence of bone involvement in the region of the sphenoid sinuses or foramen ovale. For example, the pterygoid process may be involved, or only the posterior ethmoid cells, without bone destruction more posteriorly. There may be destruction of the inferior aspect of the petrous pyramid and the adjacent portion of the clivus or the greater wing of the sphenoid. This area is often the earliest to be destroyed in patients with glomus jugulare tumors (fig. 114).

In general, when looking for bone destruction along the base, it is important to look for the detail and relative density of the various structures which usually stand out in the base on each side. These are: the wall of the sphenoid sinuses, the septa of the ethmoid cells, the base of the pterygoid process and the pterygoid laminae, the foramen ovale, the foramen spinosum, the spine of the sphenoid, the margins of the

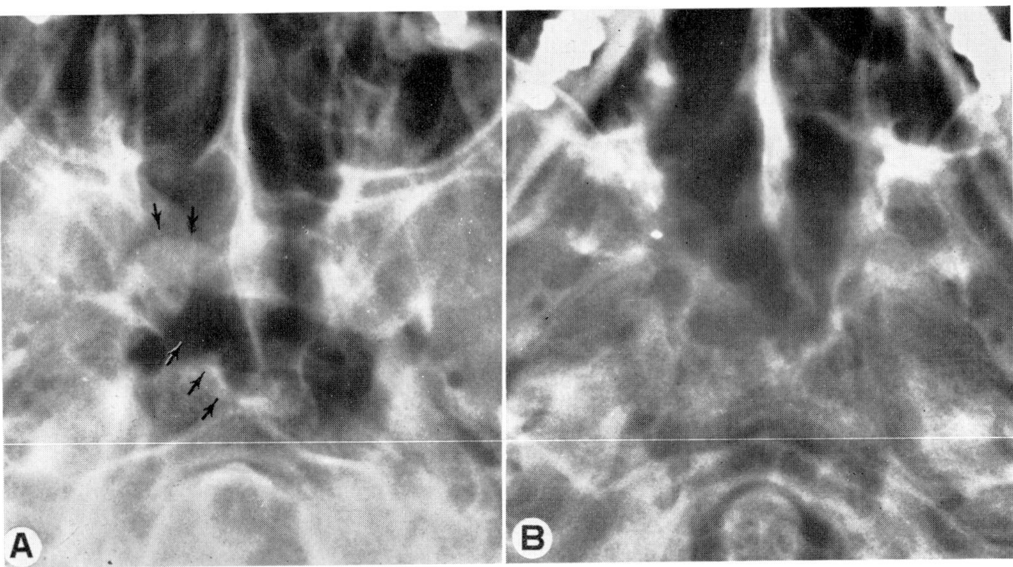

Fig. 130.—Carcinoma of Sphenoid Sinus, Early, Producing Involvement of Sinus Plate

The original film (A) reveals a loss of definition of the sinus plate of the right sphenoid sinus over a relatively short segment (*arrows*). A small soft tissue mass is present in the sphenoid sinus, the anterior aspect of which can be visualized (*arrows*). The air shadow of the nasopharynx is not distorted. The medial aspect of the foramen lacerum is prominent in this patient on both sides, which is a normal variant. Biopsy revealed squamous cell carcinoma. Reexamination 2 months later revealed an extension of the involvement of the wall of the sphenoid sinus which has now extended to involve the septum. This film was made following radiation therapy. It should be noted that at this time, the outline of the medial aspect of the foramen lacerum has become blurred on each side, but more on the original side of involvement. It is likely that this area was involved at the time of the original examination, but the involvement was not clear enough to show on the x-ray films. The lesion has never extended to involve the floor of the middle fossa on either side, and this has not occurred in a 7 year follow-up on this patient.

Eustachian tube, the margin of the clivus (the latter is sometimes not visible in normal cases), and the foramen lacerum. In addition, the petrous pyramid with the various structures of the inner and middle ear should be scrutinized.

Some patients present with a syndrome of multiple cranial nerve involvement without any demonstrable evidence of bone destruction in radiographs. This is a fairly frequent situation in practice. Some of these patients have no actual bone destruction and the involvement is due to tumor growth through the foramina of the skull and spread of the cancer cells in the epidural tissues. On the other hand, some patients actually have bone involvement which is not detected by radiography. We cannot emphasize sufficiently the importance of studying these patients thoroughly and of obtaining stereoscopic radiographs in multiple projections. Sometimes laminagraphy may show a lesion which is not evident otherwise. It is also unfortunate that in many of these patients, pneumoencephalography is of no help. Sometimes cerebral angiography will show evidence of displacement or narrowing of the internal carotid artery in its intracavernous and, particularly in its precavernous, segment (fig. 492). This is possible because the internal carotid artery is extradural in this segment. On the other hand, in the posterior fossa, there are no extradural vessels and unless there is a bulky mass in the epidural space which may displace the vessels or the pre-pontine gas shadow in pneumoencephalography, no abnormal findings may be present either in the angiogram or in the pneumoencephalogram. It is for this reason that we must depend on

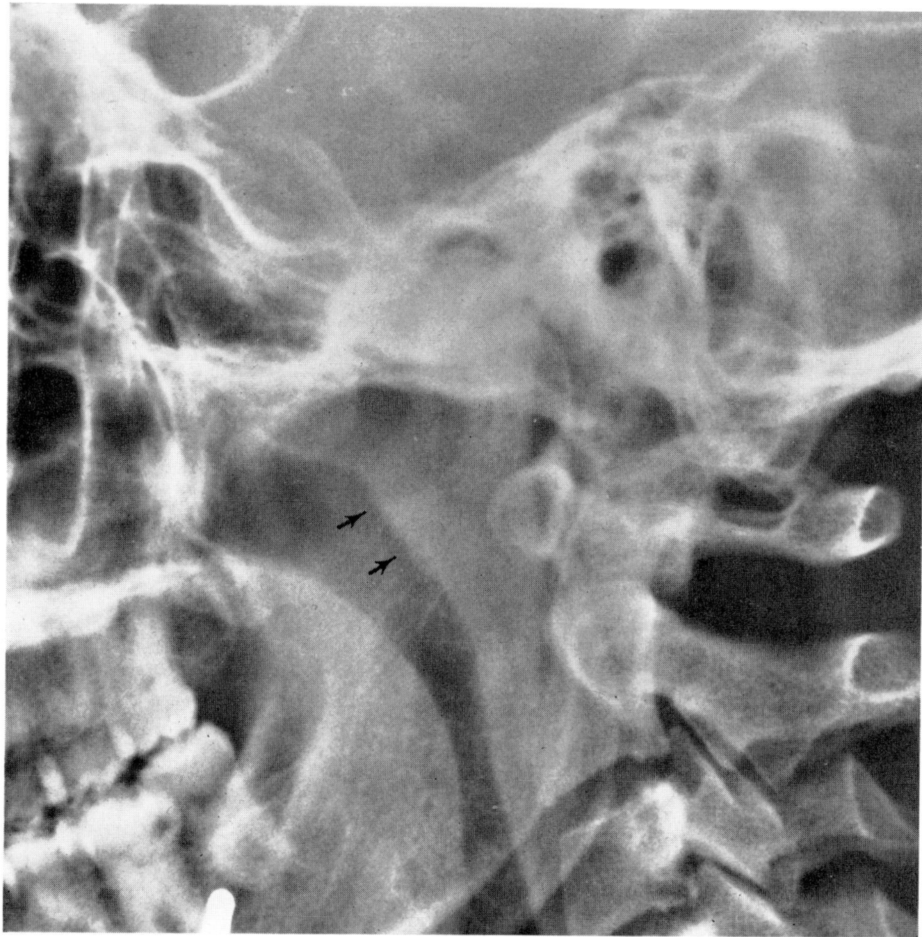

FIG. 131.—NASOPHARYNGEAL SOFT TISSUE SWELLING IN PATIENT WITH A CARCINOMA OF THE NASOPHARYNX

The lateral view of the neck including the base of the skull shows the presence of increase in the thickness of the nasopharyngeal (prevertebral) soft tissue space (*arrows*). A slight degree of irregularity is present. This appearance could be normal in a young person or child. The patient was a 45-year-old man.

plain films to arrive at a radiographic diagnosis.

The *soft tissues of the nasopharynx* are an important clue to the presence of malignant disease in this region. In the lateral projection, the prevertebral soft tissues may be widened. Normally, the prevertebral soft tissues are about one-fourth to one-third of the anteroposterior diameter of the 4th cervical vertebral body as seen in the lateral view. When it reaches the base of the skull, the soft tissue space becomes slightly thicker as it curves smoothly forward. In younger individuals, however, particularly in children, the lymphoid tissue of the nasopharynx will produce a convex shadow at the base of the skull. In adults over 30, this lymphoid shadow, if present, is small. The nasopharyngeal contour tends to become flatter in time or it may become concave. It is often difficult to determine whether the soft tissue shadow of the nasopharynx at the base of the skull is or is not increased in thickness because rules cannot be estab-

(Revised 1963)

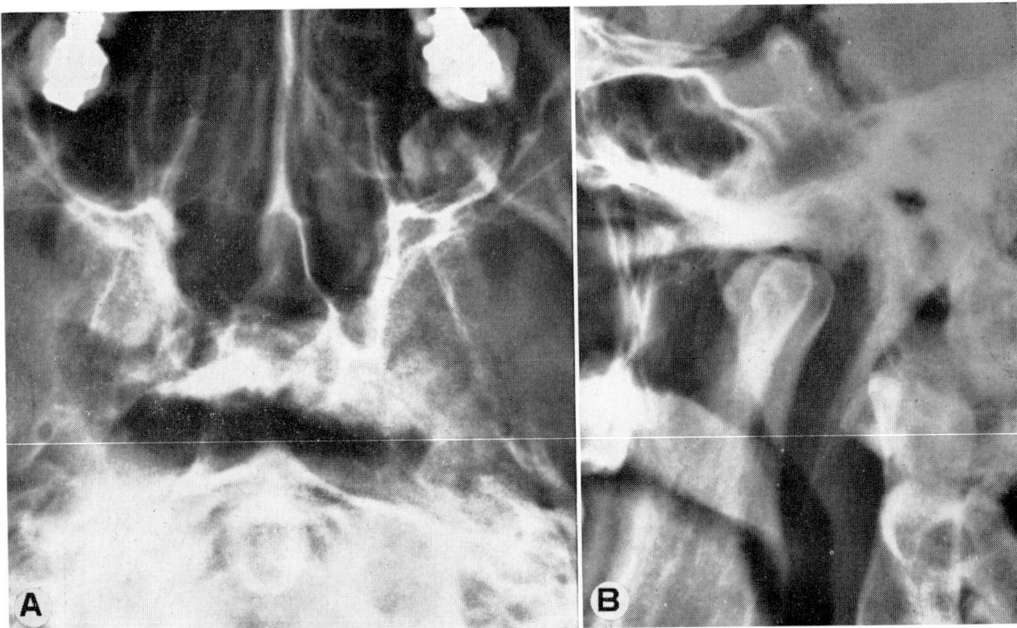

FIG. 132.—NASOPHARYNGEAL CARCINOMA

The base view (A) shows asymmetry in the soft tissue shadow of the nasopharynx. On the reader's left side the air shadow is normal, whereas on the other, it is encroached upon. There is also some indistinctness in the outline of the bone structures in the floor of the middle fossa, but the foramen ovale is not visible on the normal side either and this could, therefore, be normal. The lateral view (B) demonstrates a prevertebral soft tissue mass at the nasopharynx. The air in the suprasellar cisterns is normal, even though this patient had evidence of multiple cranial nerve involvement.

lished. If the shadow is irregular in its outine in an adult over 30 and if, at the same time, it is increased in thickness it probably is abnormal (fig. 131). On the other hand, this appearance will be perfectly normal in children or teenagers and even in young adults.

In order to evaluate the nasopharyngeal soft tissues in the lateral projection, a straight lateral view of the skull and of the neck without any rotation of the head is needed. Evaluation of these shadows in a lateral projection where the cervical spine is in an oblique projection and the head has been turned, should not be attempted.

The other film in which nasopharyngeal soft tissues can be evaluated is the base view of the skull. A discussion of the normal anatomy of this area depending on the degree of distention of the nasopharynx, was given under "Normal Anatomy" (p. 1.50). If the films are taken during nasal breathing and during a Valsalva's test, the distention of the nasopharynx should be symmetrical when the right side is compared with the left. Lack of symmetry may indicate either swelling or neoplastic invasion of one wall of the nasopharynx (fig. 132). Sometimes an actual mass can be seen bulging into one side of the air shadow of the nasopharynx which cannot be made out on the lateral projection. Stereoscopic base views may be necessary, and in some cases laminagraphy may be of help. The laminagram should be made while the patient breathes through his nose.

Tumors of the glomus jugulare. Glomus jugulare tumors usually produce bone destruction at the base of the petrous pyramid and later may extend widely and invade most of the bones of the base. Because these tumors are so vascular, a bruit may be heard by the patient and also by the physician through auscultation. A small

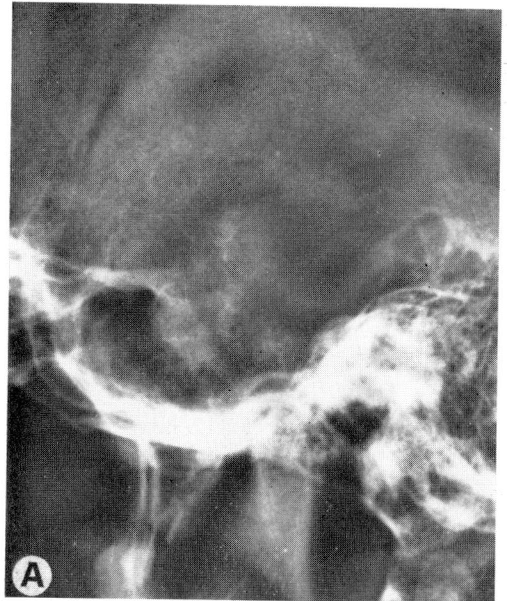

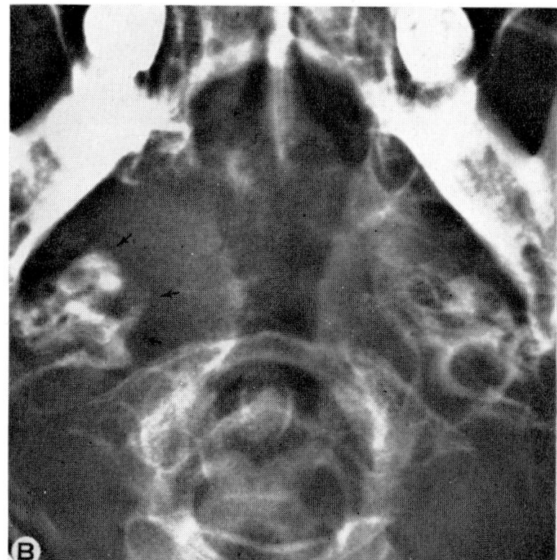

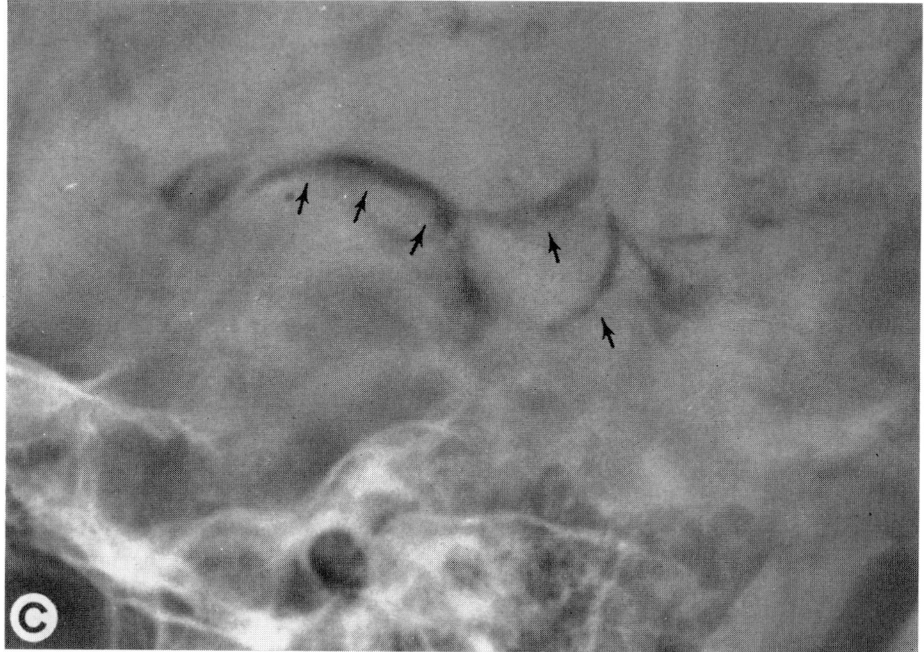

Fig. 133.—Chordoma in 23-Year-old Girl Producing Marked Destruction and Intracranial Mass

The plain film lateral view (A) shows the area of destruction involving the upper portion of the clivus and the sella turcica with area of sclerosis within the area of destruction. The base view (B) shows extensive destruction also involving the petrous tip on one side and extending into the middle fossa (*arrows*). A pneumoencephalogram (C) demonstrates lack of filling of the lateral ventricles. A prominent air shadow is seen around the mass (*arrows*). Epidural masses almost always allow the passage of air between the brain structures and the mass, whereas intradural tumors such as meningiomas often do not. One retrothalamic cistern is markedly elevated in comparison to the other (*single arrows*). This indicates extension laterally on one side.

(*Revised 1963*)

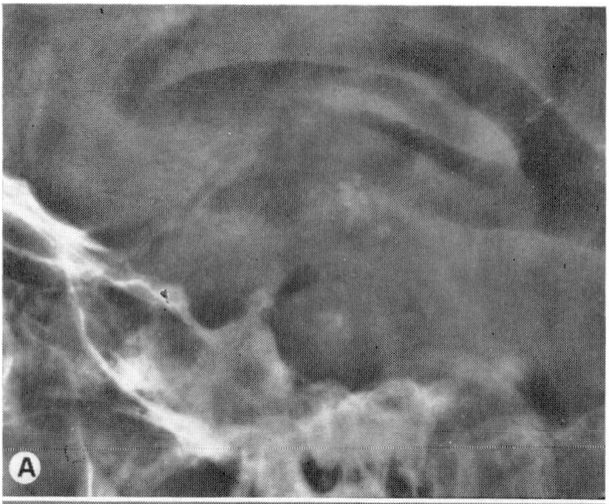

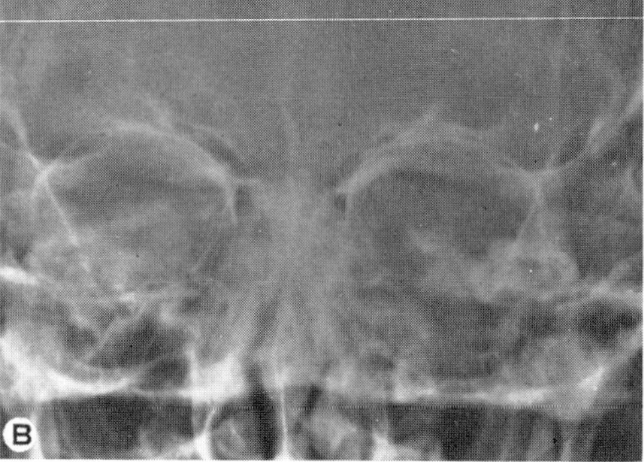

FIG. 134.—CHORDOMA THAT PRODUCES SCLEROTIC CHANGES IN THE CLIVUS EXTENDING LATERALLY

The lateral view (A) shows a diffuse increase in density of the clivus and floor of the sella turcica and dorsum as well as extension into the sphenoid sinus. There is evidence of calcification in the area posterior to and above the dorsum sellae. There is marked elevation of the temporal horn indicating lateral extension. The frontal projection (B) demonstrates the involvement of the medial aspect of the petrous pyramid which is irregularly destroyed in its upper and lower aspects.

bloody tumor may present at the ear drum. Laminagraphy may be of help in detecting early destruction of the base of the petrous pyramid, and for this purpose, films in coronal planes with the head in a straight anteroposterior projection are preferable (fig. 114). Cerebral angiography of the external carotid artery may show the blood supply of these tumors (fig. 532).

Chordoma. Chordomas arise from remnants of the notochord which originally extended from the dorsum sellae down to the last coccygeal segment. The nucleus pulposus of the intervertebral discs is the remnant of the original notochord. Notochordal remnants may also be present just anterior to the clivus, in the nasopharyngeal soft tissues, and in the epidural space dorsal to the clivus intracranially. Chordomas are relatively slowly growing and may occur at any age but are more frequently seen in young individuals; the youngest of our patients was a 5-year-old child. Most chordomas produce a mass intracranially or intraspinally, but in some instances they may produce a mass which projects forward exclusively without any intracranial or intraspinal component. The latter cases are difficult to differentiate from other types of lesions. The location of the masses and their epidural position as demonstrated by pneumoencephalography is characteristic. Pneumoencephalography will show a layer of air in the subarachnoid space which separates the tumor from the intracranial structures (fig. 133). The wide subarachnoid space as demonstrated by air differentiates these extradural masses from other extracerebral but intradural tumors which have either a very thin cleavage line or no air is seen between the tumor and the surrounding brain.

Chordomas are usually seen first at the clivus, and from here they may extend further laterally (fig. 134). Occasionally, a chordoma will start eccentrically and the clivus may be intact until the area of bone destruction grows to considerable size. In these cases the diagnosis of chordoma may not be made originally because of the location of the lesion in the floor of the middle fossa or in the cerebellopontine angle. Another location is the foramen magnum region involving the lower portion of the clivus and the upper cervical vertebrae.

Chordomas may exhibit areas of calcific density. Calcium deposits in the tumor or sequestrated bony fragments were found in one-third of the cases reviewed by Wood and Himadi (1950) (fig. 134). Some chordomas involve the upper cervical vertebrae. Indeed, some of them originate in the region of the odontoid process or in the body of the second cervical vertebra and produce bone destruction above and below this region.

Erosion of the base, particularly of the region of the foramen ovale and the tip of the petrous pyramid may be produced by *neurinomas of the 5th nerve*. The erosion of the petrous tip is characteristic in these lesions (fig. 112). The erosion of the floor of the middle fossa is not always characteristic, but may be produced by meningiomas or other destructive bone lesions. The tumors of the 5th nerve may lie almost entirely anterior to the petrous pyramid, but usually are situated both in the middle fossa and in the posterior fossa extending through the incisura and eroding the tip of the petrous pyramid. Jefferson has emphasized the hourglass configuration of these 5th nerve tumors which have to be attacked surgically through the middle fossa and through a lateral suboccipital craniectomy.

Inflammatory conditions producing destruction are quite rare today, but it is still possible to have bone destruction secondary to osteomyelitis starting in the ethmoid, sphenoid, or mastoid sinuses. *Mucoceles* of the sphenoid sinus may be confused with chordomas because they produce an area of bone destruction that centers here and also involves the entire sella turcica. They are very rare and unless this entity is considered in the differential diagnosis, the correct interpretation will not be made preoperatively.

Mucor mycosis is a fungal disease which may involve the orbital area and also cause destruction of the base of the skull. Wegener's granuloma should also be included in the differential diagnosis.

MENINGIOMAS

GENERAL CONSIDERATIONS

The most common tumor of the meninges, which is now most often referred to as the meningioma, has been known to medicine for more than three centuries. According to Netsky and Lapresle (1956), the first account of a meningioma was given by a Swiss physician, Felix Plater, in 1614. This report antedates by more than a century the report of Kaufman in 1743 and the first review of a group of cases by Antoine Louis in his famous "memoir" on fungating tumors of the dura mater (1774). During the last century, there was considerable interest in these tumors among pathologists, and Cruveilhier (1856) and others described the gross pathologic features of numerous cases. Virchow (1864) directed attention to the histologic structure of the tumors, and because he was impressed by the deposition of lime salts in the tumors, he designated them as "psammomas of the dura mater" in his text published in 1864.

Until 1922 these tumors were principally referred to as dural endotheliomas because of their dural attachment and their cellular resemblance to the endothelial lining of the dura. In this year Cushing, in reviewing the largest collection of such tumors studied until that time, suggested the term meningioma because he felt some uncertainty existed concerning their histologic nature. Subsequently, Cushing and Eisenhardt (1938), in their correlative study, described in detail their extensive experience with almost 300 patients with meningioma, and it is upon this classic work that most present day thinking regarding meningiomas is based.

According to Traub (1961), the earliest radiologic demonstration of a meningioma was by Obici and Bollici in 1897. A relatively early discussion, based on modern radiologic concepts, was given by Sosman and Putnam in 1925. Subsequently, numerous valuable additional contributions were made by Dyke, Pendergrass, and many other investigators. More recently, numerous writers have discussed the angiographic diagnosis of meningiomas.

For the most part, tumors arising from the meninges belong to the ordinarily benign, localized type of growth now commonly called meningioma. Although the term is noncommittal, other tumors of meningeal origin, such as meningeal sarcomatosis, meningeal melanoblastosis, and tumors of the teratoma group, ordinarily are not included when the term meningioma is used. Meningiomas occur in two general gross forms: (1) globular and (2) flat. The globular tumors may be further subdivided into the sessile growths, pedunculated tumors, and tumors without dural attachment. The sessile tumors arise by a wide dural attachment, often almost as broad as the diameter of the spherical tumor mass. The sessile tumor is the most commonly encountered type of meningioma. The pedunculated tumors and meningiomas without dural attachment are relatively uncommon; the former are confined chiefly to the parasagittal area, while the latter are found in the ventricles or in the fissures of the brain. Globular tumors usually are smoothly lobulated and well encapsulated with the result that characteristically, the adjacent brain is not invaded and an intact pial covering usually is present. Since the tumors grow slowly, cerebral tissue is displaced by the tumor, then indented as the tumor grows, and finally, when large size is attained, the tumor may be found deeply seated in compressed cerebral substance. The flat tumors, on the other hand, which are commonly referred to as meningioma *en plaque*, are less well encapsulated, with involvement of the pia as well as almost universal invasion of overlying bony structures.

The histologic classification of meningiomas has received extensive attention by pathologists, and some considerations are quite intricate. It is now generally agreed that meningiomas arise from arachnoid cells imbedded in the dura, usually in the form of arachnoid granulations or arachnoid cell nests as described by Aoyagi and Kyunō (1912). Different cells, however, play a varying role of dominance with the result that meningiomas actually constitute a family of tumors of variable histologic structure. A relatively simple and radiologically useful classification has been evolved by Courville and Abbott (1941) who described three basic cell types: (1) syncytial, (2) fibrous, and (3) angioblastic. In addition, they described a transitional or mixed type and, as is agreed by most investigators, placed the sarcomatous meningiomas aside as a specific type.

The syncytial group comprises the tumors that are quite cellular, with the cells supported by a fine fibrillary stroma. The syncytial tumors contain small blood vessels and degenerative changes are infrequent, psammoma bodies being found only occasionally. The fibrous meningiomas, on the contrary, have a heavy connective tissue stroma and a prominent feature is whorl formation. The tumor is moderately vascular, and psammoma bodies are frequently found, occasionally to an extensive degree, forming the basis for psammomatous meningiomas, as described by Virchow. Angioblastic meningiomas are the most variable, and several subtypes have been described. Mixed meningiomas are found in which both lobules of cells and whorl formation are prominent. In addition, combined types are encountered in which syncytial, fibrous, and angioblastic areas of varying size are present. Sarcomatous meningiomas constitute a distinct tissue type which are encapsulated and have a dural attachment but which are highly cellular and malignant throughout their course. The tumors are to be differentiated from other meningiomas which undergo malignant metaplasia and become invasive. Approximately two-thirds of meningiomas are of the fibrous type, and they are encountered three times as often as syncytial tumors. Mixed tumors and angioblastic meningiomas form the minority of the histologic varieties.

The high incidence of meningioma in relation to other intracranial tumors attests to its clinical significance and the importance of radiologic diagnosis. That meningiomas constitute approximately 15 per cent of all intracranial neoplasms is generally accepted. It appears significant, however, that more recent reports, particularly those of the last decade, conclude an even higher incidence. In the largest series of intracranial tumors, totaling over 5,000, de-

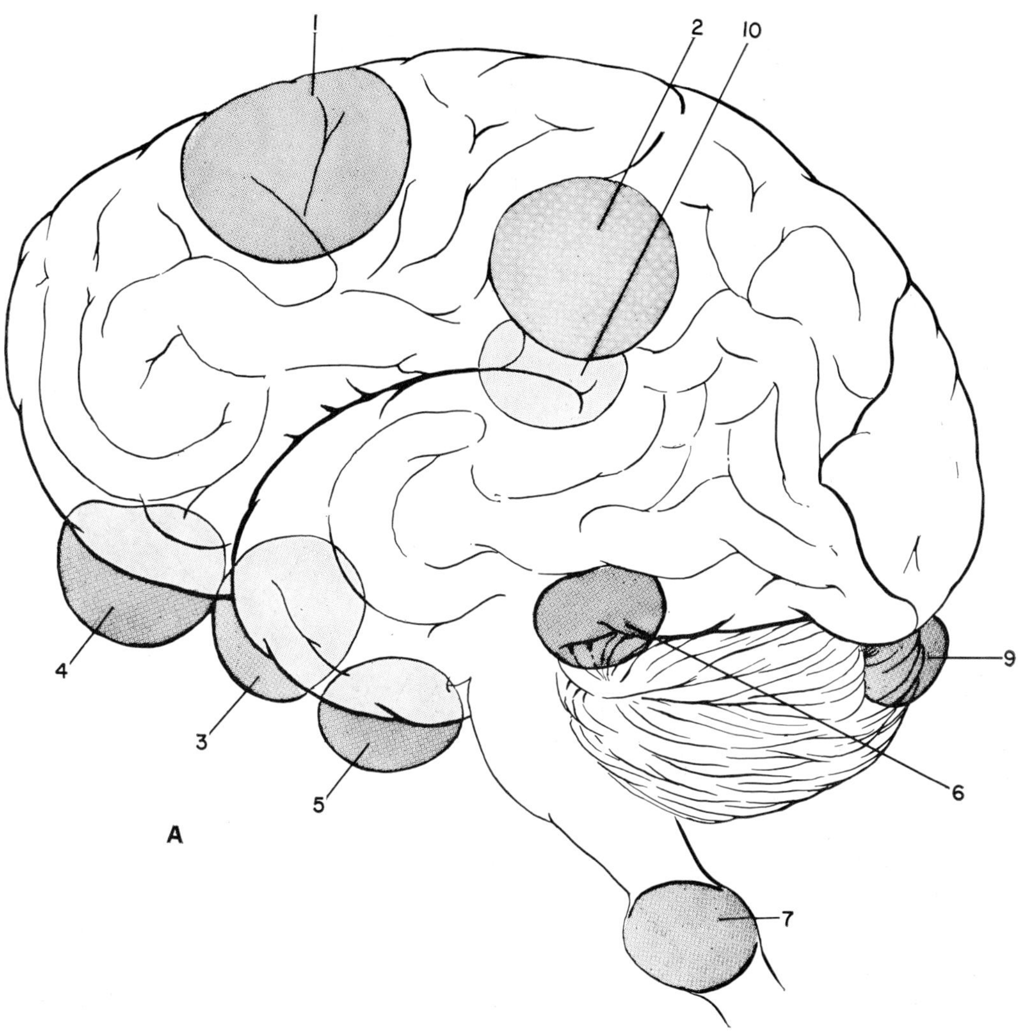

FIG. 135.—THE COMMON SITES OF OCCURRENCE OF MENINGIOMAS OF THE CENTRAL NERVOUS SYSTEM, IN ORDER OF FREQUENCY

scribed by Hoessly and Olivecrona (1955), there were more than 1,000 meningiomas for an incidence of more than 19 per cent. If tumors only above the tentorium are considered, meningiomas constitute well over one-fifth of all brain tumors. For the most part, the meningioma is a tumor of middle-aged adult life, and an even higher incidence pertains in patients over 40 years of age. The tumors are more commonly encountered in women than in men, and in certain locations, particularly in the region of the sphenoid ridge and middle fossa, the tumors are much more frequently encountered in women. A disproportionately high ratio of women to men also exists in relation to tumors of the suprasellar region and posterior fossa.

The occurrence of meningiomas in certain specific intracranial sites is of interest and of considerable diagnostic importance. The relative frequency of meningiomas by location in a diminishing order of incidence from one to ten is shown in Figure 135. The relationship of basal meningiomas, in particular in relation to the anatomic location of

(Revised 1963)

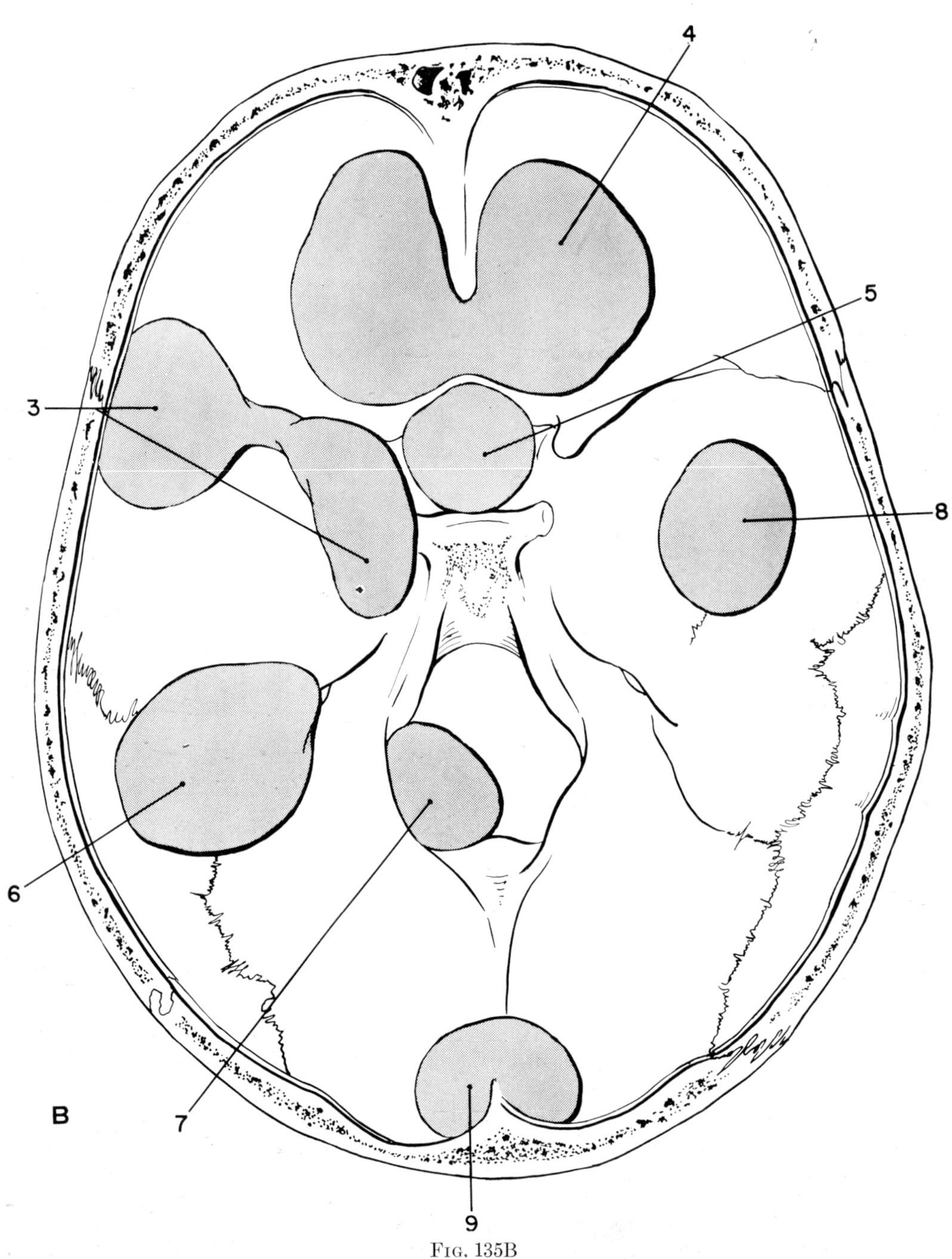

Fig. 135B

Fig. 136.—Extracerebral Meningioma

A 53-year-old woman complained of frontal headache and a slowly progressive swelling of the right forehead. The frontal skull film (A) reveals a 2.5-cm. rounded osteolytic defect, with well defined margins laterally, in the right supraorbital region. The lateral view (B) reveals minimum evidence of hyperostosis along the posterior and superior aspects of the demineralized zone. Two small vascular channels (*anterior arrows*) extend forward from an anterior branch (*posterior arrow*) of the middle meningeal artery toward the lesion. At the time of operation, an extradural meningioma was found in the frontal bone. Microscopic examination revealed the lesion to be largely syncytial in type, with only loose connected tissue and an occasional psammoma body.

(*Revised 1963*)

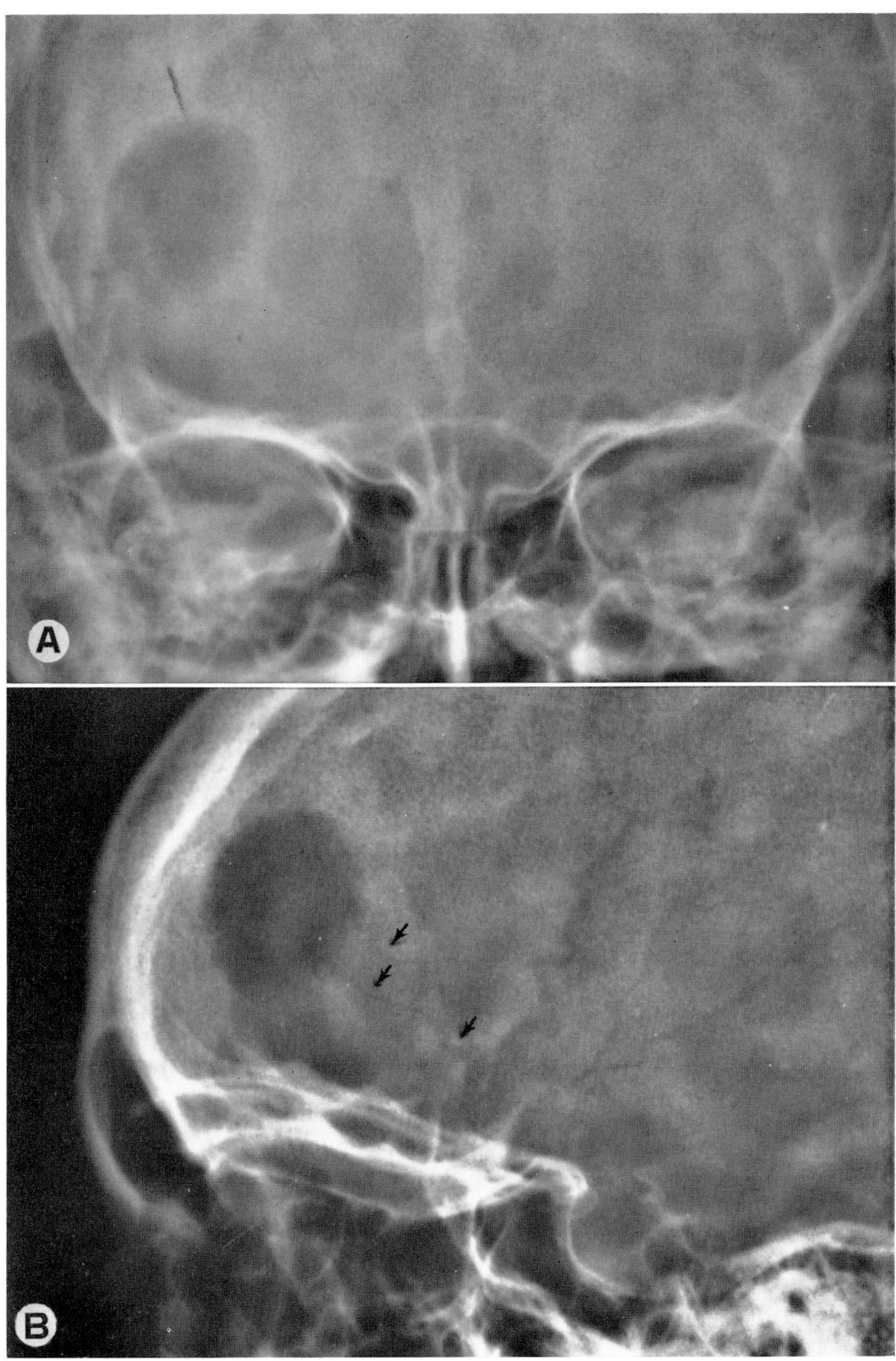

Fig. 136

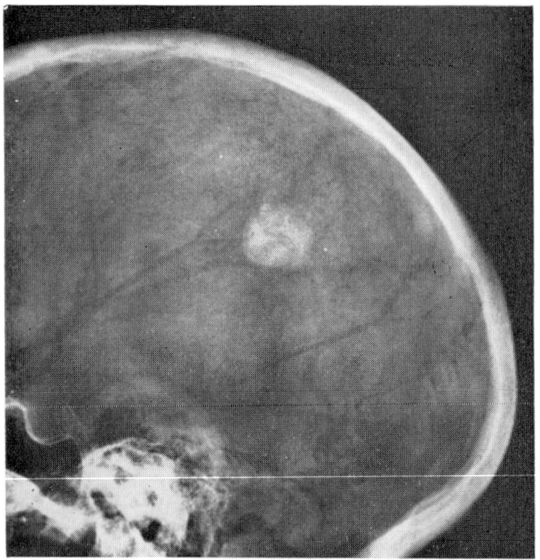

Fig. 137.—Convexity Meningioma

A 2-cm. rounded area of localized hyperostosis is present on the parietal convexity. The margins are well defined, particularly along the anterior and inferior aspects. Several prominent posterior branches of the middle meningeal artery are shown extending to the area of the mass, and one of the branches extends directly to the lesion. At the time of operation, a small meningioma corresponding closely in size to the calcific density was found. The patient also was found to have a meningioma of the spinal cord.

clusters of arachnoid cells over the basal dura of the skull, as described by Aoyagi and Kyunō (1912), is noteworthy. The relationship of meningioma growth to the anatomic location of Pacchionian bodies on the superior surface of the brain is even more evident from the radiologic standpoint. Between one-third and one-half of all meningiomas arise in the parasagittal region, attached either to the falx or the superior longitudinal sinus. The next more common location is the cerebral convexity. When tumors of the sphenoid ridge and posterior fossa are added to the lesions of the cerebral convexity and parasagittal area, it is found that these four locations account for approximately 80 per cent of meningiomas. Tumors occurring at other sites of predilection along the midline anteriorly in the region of the olfactory groove and tuberculum sellae account for more than 10 per cent of all meningiomas and most of the remaining lesions. This leaves only a small percentage to be divided among the other various scattered locations, with the intraventricular tumors least frequent in almost all series, except for the rare and unusual types not ordinarily categorized. Examples of the latter type of lesion are those which occur extradurally as cranial or extracranial tumors (fig. 136). Presumably such tumors arise from ectopic arachnoid cells which are incorporated in the bony skull during its growth or which protrude between bones in early life and are trapped extracranially.

Approximately 2 per cent of patients who have a meningioma will harbor a second or multiple lesions. Simultaneous involvement of the brain and spinal cord is not rare (fig. 137). Of the patients with more than one meningioma, approximately one-half will have true multiple tumors, while in the other half, a meningioma or meningiomas may occur in connection with von Recklinghausen's disease. Multiple meningiomas occurring in von Recklinghausen's disease often are very numerous, located chiefly in the parasagittal area, and the number may be sufficiently great for use of the term meningiomatosis. Cushing and Eisenhardt (1938) described true multiple meningiomas as "more than one meningioma and something less than a diffusion of them." In addition, it is not unusual for gliomas, particularly glioblastoma multiforme, to occur in association with a meningioma.

Meningiomas rarely may be found in distant organs, presumably the result of blood-borne metastasis. Because of the close relationship of many meningiomas to large vascular channels, such as dural sinuses which they frequently invade, and the extreme vascularity of many tumors themselves, seeding of tumor cells into the blood stream must occur frequently, but the majority of deposits fail to thrive. The lung is the most common organ in which metastatic meningiomas are found, and the authors have observed three patients in whom secondary pulmonary deposits of benign intracranial meningioma were found.

(Revised 1963)

RADIOLOGIC FINDINGS

In the diagnosis of meningioma, radiologic methods play a key role. The careful analysis of simple skull films is as important in the detection and identification of meningioma as in any other aspect of neuroradiology, since the yield of positive findings from plain skull films is much higher with meningioma than with almost any other type of intracranial mass lesion. The great majority of patients with meningioma will exhibit either indirect or direct evidence of an intracranial tumor. In a high percentage of instances, it is possible not only to confirm the presence of an expanding intracranial lesion but to determine its location and its identity as a tumor of meningeal origin. In the experience of Dyke (1941), approximately 50 per cent of meningiomas can be diagnosed from plain skull roentgenograms.

Indirect Evidence of Tumor

The generalized radiographic evidences of meningioma are those resulting from increased intracranial pressure and such changes are found in more than one-half of patients when first examined. Widening of the sutures occurs but is encountered infrequently since meningiomas are found predominantly during the middle years of adult life. Similarly, prominent convolutional markings are encountered infrequently, but occasionally there may be diffuse atrophy of the bones of the vault. In these cases, however, intracranial pressure usually has been abnormal for a considerable period of time and other radiologic manifestations of elevated intracranial pressure usually are apparent.

The majority of patients with meningioma exhibit pressure atrophy of the sella turcica, most commonly in the region of the dorsum, at the clinoid tips and along the floor of the sella turcica. The pressure changes occurring in the region of the sella turcica do not differ from those occurring with other types of intracranial tumor except that the atrophy frequently is more pronounced because of the chronic course of these slowly growing neoplasms (figs. 140 and 147). Sella turcica changes are found most often with tumors which block the ventricular pathways, such as posterior fossa and intraventricular meningiomas, or with tumors growing adjacent to the sella turcica in the region of the tuberculum, which also may produce third ventricular obstruction. The bulky tumors of the cerebral convexity, of the olfactory groove, and of the floor of the middle fossa produce pressure changes in the great majority of patients. Only about one-third of patients with parasagittal meningiomas exhibit plain-film changes of increased intracranial pressure, but in a high incidence of patients, these tumors produce convulsive seizures. This suggests that because of the location of the tumors, irritative phenomena signal the tumor's presence when it is still small and before there is sufficient bulk or blockage to produce pressure changes. The flat tumors of the sphenoid ridge also have a low incidence of pressure atrophy of the sella turcica.

The occurrence of sellar atrophy found radiologically can be correlated with the presence of papilledema found funduscopically in a high percentage of patients with meningioma. In some patients harboring meningiomas, papilledema will be present and sella turcica atrophy absent, and the reverse also may be true. The former is not surprising since papilledema, on the average, develops more rapidly than radiologic changes. In the latter group, the discrepancy is found chiefly in the case of meningiomas of the sphenoid ridge and tuberculum sellae, and in these instances the location of the tumor presumably interferes with development of edema of the optic nerve head. Tumors in these locations and occasionally tumors arising further forward in the region of the olfactory groove and extending backward may result in the Foster Kennedy syndrome (1911), one of the features of which is optic atrophy on the side of the tumor, or ipsilateral to its principal growth, associated with papilledema on the contralateral side.

A second finding of considerable importance in the diagnosis of meningioma is dis-

(Revised 1963)

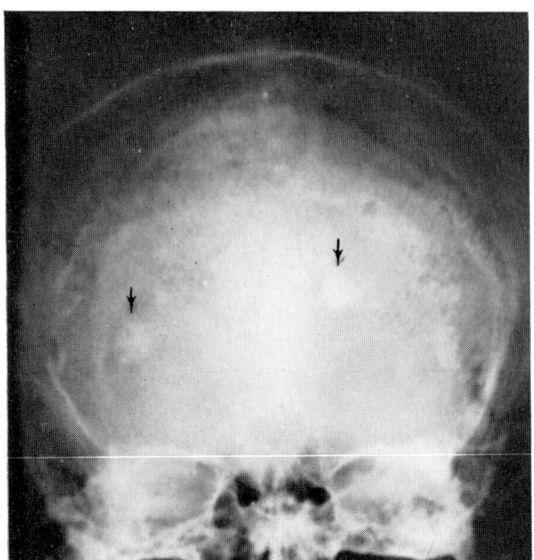

Fig. 138.—Tentorial Meningioma

The glomus of the chorioid plexus on the left is markedly elevated and displaced medially, owing to a large meningioma arising from the superior surface of the tentorium. Displacement of a calcified chorioid glomus is most commonly the result of masses behind and beneath the atrium of the ventricle.

placement of physiologically calcified intracranial structures. While displacement of such a structure does not serve to differentiate between meningiomas and other intracranial mass lesions, it may be of considerable localizing value in the absence of specific changes of meningioma. The most common structure to be visibly displaced is the pineal body because of its high frequency of calcification, which is demonstrable radiologically in more than half of all adult patients. Approximately two-thirds of patients with meningioma who have pineal calcification visible in frontal radiographs will exhibit lateral displacement of the pineal.

Displacement of the calcified pineal body in lateral projection outside of the normal zone as revised by Dyke (1930) is found somewhat less frequently than lateral displacement in the frontal view. Meningiomas of the cerebral convexity are those which most often produce a pronounced lateral pineal shift. Parasagittal tumors more often result in displacement in the lateral projection than tumors of other loci and the displacement usually is downward. Tumors arising in the region of the tuberculum sellae and in the posterior fossa least frequently result in shift of the pineal body either to the side, as seen in frontal view, or in any direction in the sagittal plane, as seen in the lateral projection.

Calcification in the glomus of the choroid plexus unfortunately is demonstrable radiologically in only between 10 and 15 per cent of patients, and occasionally only unilateral calcification may be present. While the calcified choroid glomus may be displaced in any direction, it can most readily be appreciated radiologically and appears to be of more definite localizing value when the dislocation is forward, medialward, or upward. Such displacements occur most often with posterior tumors and particularly meningiomas which are attached to the superior surface of the tentorium (fig. 138). Meningiomas of the floor of the middle fossa also may result in a choroid displacement in one or more directions. It may be worthwhile to point out here that the glomus may appear displaced when actually it is not, because the structure may be pedunculated and calcification may occur ectopically. For this reason, care should be taken not to overemphasize the significance of asymmetrical choroid calcification if it is an isolated finding.

Calcifications in other structures, such as the falx cerebri and the walls of the superior longitudinal sinus, and calcification of the falx cerebelli, of the tentorium cerebelli, and the diaphragma sellae are not often observed displaced either by meningiomas or other tumors, although the former would appear to have a better opportunity to dislocate and deform these structures since they are often directly attached. The falx cerebri, however, is not infrequently observed to be angulated in contrast studies, and when calcified, displacement of a few millimeters may be observed. Interpretation is made more difficult, however, by the frequent presence of uneven and asymmetrical calcification in this structure.

(Revised 1963)

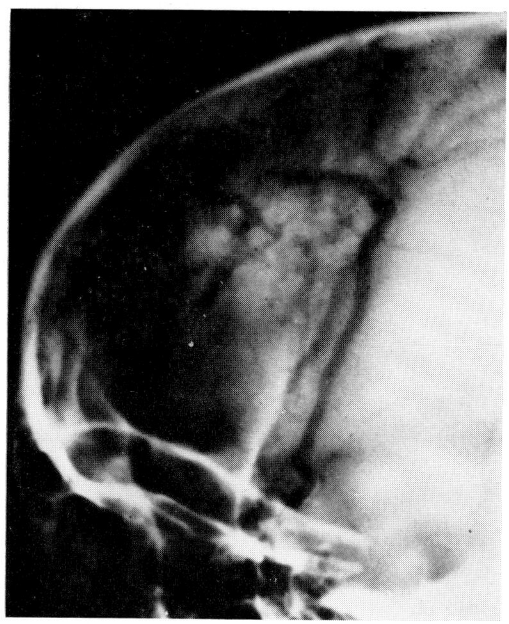

FIG. 139.—A LARGE FRONTAL MENINGIOMA

The lateral portion of the frontal bone exhibits extensive hyperostosis over a wide area, which crosses the suture line to extend into the anterior parietal region. Very large meningeal vascular channels are present and numerous new channels have developed, some of which are quite sizable. One very large anterior branch of the main middle meningeal trunk is shown extending forward over the superior portion of the hyperostotic area. Forward turning of middle meningeal branches, even of normal size, very often is abnormal (see text).

Direct evidence of meningioma may be discerned from plain skull films in a remarkably high percentage of patients. Dyke (1941) stated that in one-half of patients harboring meningioma the diagnosis could be made radiologically, while Traub (1961) stated that a radiologic diagnosis was possible in one-third of the cases that he reviewed. It is our impression that the percentage of cases in which plain film diagnosis is possible has been decreasing in recent years owing to earlier clinical diagnosis and treatment. The cardinal signs of meningioma are: (1) hyperostosis, (2) increased vascularity, and (3) tumor calcification. It is our belief that the presence of any one of these cardinal signs properly observed and evaluated can be adequate for the diagnosis of meningioma. Any two in combination or any one together with evidence of increased intracranial pressure or displacement of a calcified physiologic structure should form the basis for a firm diagnosis of meningioma.

(Revised 1963)

Hyperostosis

The first and most frequent direct evidence of meningioma is hyperostosis of the skull, although increased vascularity is seen nearly as frequently. The new bone formation occurring in the neighborhood of a meningioma is a reactive change in the skull and not an integral part of the tumor (Rowbotham, 1939). The exact mechanism of hyperostosis is not well understood and there is considerable lack of agreement among writers with extensive experience. Cushing and Eisenhardt (1938) described eight varieties of bone involvement by underlying meningiomas. Rowbotham (1939) believed that the nature of the hyperostosis depends not only on the properties of the tumor but also on the bone of the host that is affected. The fact that tumor cells cannot always be found in areas of hyperostosis would support this opinion. While in all probability it is necessary for some tumor cells to invade the overlying bone to invoke hyperostosis, the density of the change found in some cases and the difficulty of identifying tumor cells in the densely hyperostotic area denote a bone reaction out of proportion to the quantity of invading tumor. Conversely, bone destruction may be a prominent feature in some instances, as will be mentioned later.

The inner table of the skull, the diploic space, and the outer table all may be involved in the hyperostotic process. In any given case, any one alone of these portions of the skull may be most conspicuously involved or multiple areas may be implicated. *The inner table*, however, is by far the most common cranial layer to be affected. The hyperostotic process takes place through the laying down of bone in multiple sheets parallel to the plane of the tabular cortex. In radiographs, the changes involving the inner table will appear as an area of extra

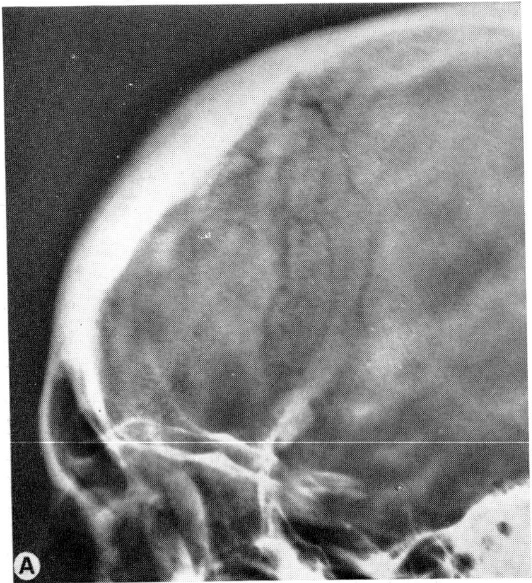

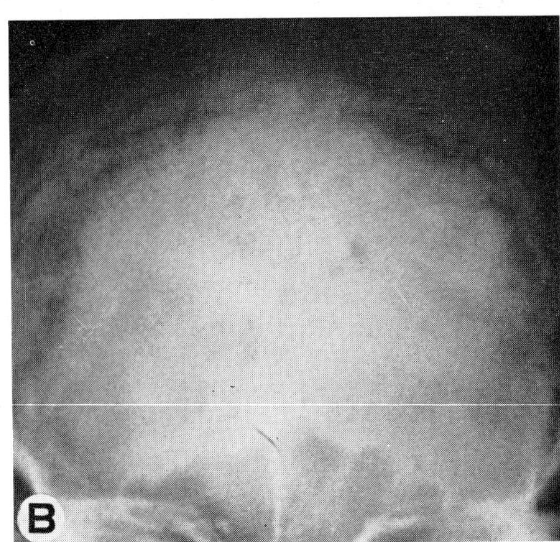

FIG. 140.—BIFRONTAL MENINGIOMA

The lateral film (A) shows tangentially marked hyperostosis of the inner table of the vertical portion of the frontal bone anteriorly. There is also hyperostosis involving the diploic space, and the outer table is thickened and elevated. A number of prominent forward-extending branches of the middle meningeal arteries are shown. The sella turcica exhibits increased intracranial pressure. The frontal film (B) shows, face on, the area of bony thickening in the frontal region, together with some of the abnormal vascular channels. It is noteworthy that the greatest thickening and increased density is midline in position, and there is no cleft in the hyperostotic area, as occurs with benign frontal hyperostosis (compare with Fig. 151).

density when viewed face on, while in tangential view the change will present as an enostosis. The *en face* projection will obscure normal bony architecture in the area of thickening, while the tangential view will demonstrate the intact nature of the diploic space and outer table if the hyperostosis is isolated. Isolated hyperostosis of the inner table of the skull is most common in the presence of meningioma of the cerebral convexity and parasagittal areas.

True alteration of bony architecture usually occurs with involvement of the *diploic space*. It may become only hypertrophied with preservation of the spongy architecture. More often, however, obliteration of the spongy appearance takes place through the deposition of large amounts of compact bone within the diploic area. Hypertrophy of the diploë may be related to increased vascularity within it, while sclerosis may be related to the infiltration of the Haversian system.

Involvement of the *outer table* with the production of an external mound of bony tissue and often a clinically detectable mass may be seen under various circumstances but is most common in the thin portions of the skull where the inner and outer tables are in close approximation. Thus, while it is uncommon for a palpable mass to be present in the case of convexity meningiomas, exophthalmos is an expected finding in patients with meningioma of the sphenoid ridge. Such flat tumors, lying along the sphenoid ridge where there is essentially no diploic space, result in a marked bony thickening along both the inner and outer tables, usually easily appreciated in either frontal or lateral view (fig. 142). Tumors of the alar and clinoidal portions of the sphenoid ridge particularly invoke a dense hyperostosis, and a similar change is found in patients suffering from meningioma of the tuberculum sellae.

In connection with hyperostosis, two par-

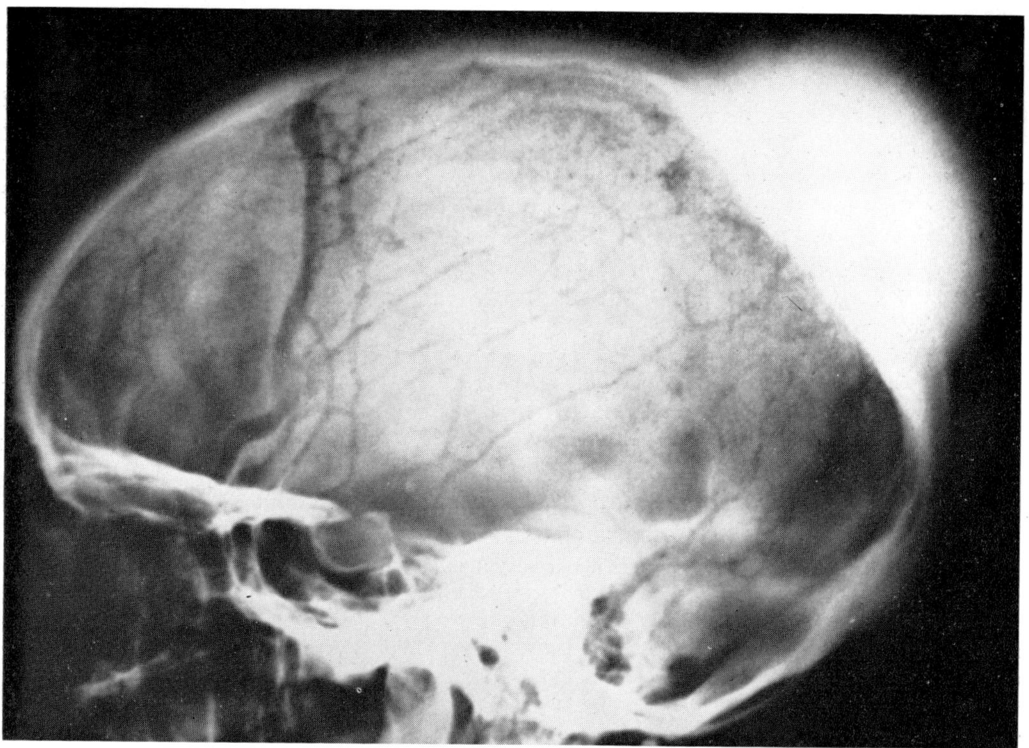

FIG. 141.—CLASSICAL MENINGIOMA

An unusually large area of hyperostosis is present in the posterior parietal region, bridging the usual concavity of the inner margin of the cranial vault. In addition, the tumor has grown through the skull, and a large extracranial mass presented when the patient was first seen. Extending over the parietal convexity are extensive vascular changes with many extrameningeal vessels extending to and from the tumor to the base of the skull. Numerous rounded areas of diminished density are present, including some measuring more than 1 cm. (compare with Fig. 152). One main meningeal vascular trunk is enormously dilated.

ticular variations deserve special mention. While in the majority of instances the new bone formation is parallel to the inner or outer table of the skull, occasionally perpendicular changes are present resulting in "spicule" formation. In these instances, there appears to be a propensity for the tumor to extend extracranially, usually with mild or even absent radiologic evidence of involvement of the inner table. This extension may result in what Cushing called a "pancake" of tumor between the bone and the galea. For the most part, the laying down of bone at right angles to the plane of the skull, or spicule formation, occurs with tumors of the cerebral convexity or of the parasagittal area (fig. 143).

(Revised 1963)

A somewhat related bony change is seen in connection with tumors of the *tuberculum sellae.* Here a brushlike area of hyperostosis may develop internally, perhaps more a calcification in the attachment of the tumor than a true bony reaction. A unique change found in this region is upward bulging of the bony cortex forming the posterior boundary of the ethmoid cells and the anterior portion of the sphenoid sinus. This change was referred to by Dyke (1941) as "blistering" and it is considered a specific sign of meningioma. There may be an associated area of hyperostosis in the region of the planum sphenoidale and tuberculum or the perpendicular brushlike change may be found in some instances. In lateral films, an upward bowing

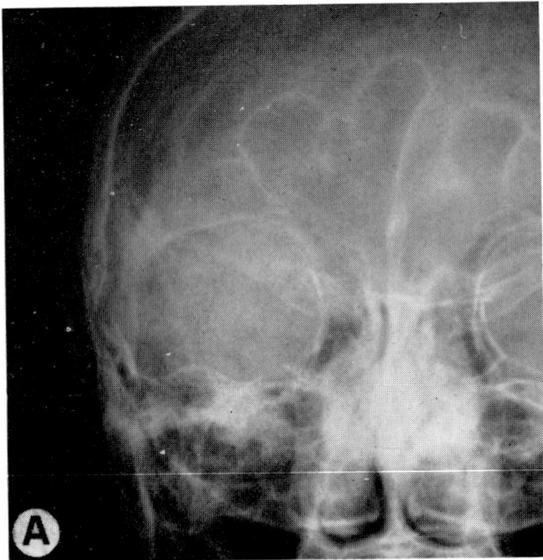

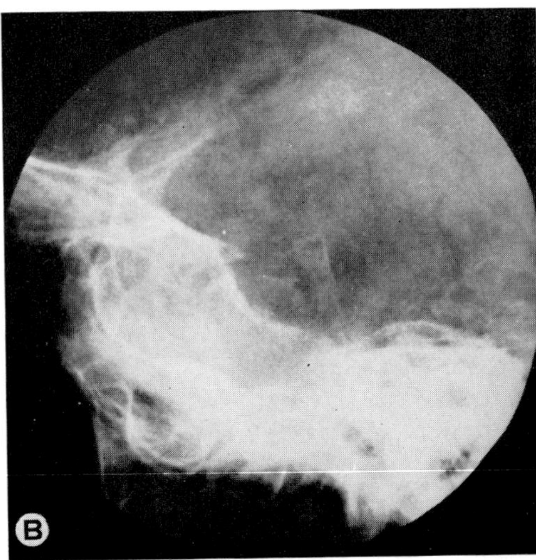

Fig. 142.—Meningioma of the Sphenoid Ridge

The right sphenoid wing exhibits increased density and lack of good definition of the anatomic structures of the wing (A). Both the lesser and greater wings are poorly defined, the posterior orbital wall is thickened, and the margins of the superior orbital fissure are indistinct. Asymmetry of the orbits in frontal view often is one of the earliest radiologic changes and may be due in part to exophthalmos in addition to hyperostosis.

In another case (B), hyperostosis of the sphenoid wing and obliteration of the sphenoid sinus is shown.

of the posterior cortex of the ethmoid area or a similar change in the anterior sphenoid region should direct attention to the tuberculum and planum for the possibility of related evidence of hyperostosis (fig. 144).

Increased Vascularity

The second of the cardinal manifestations of meningioma is increased vascularity. This change occurs essentially as frequently as hyperostosis and, when properly evaluated, its significance can be just as important. The increase in vascularity takes two different forms: (1) an area of localized increased vascularity, hypervascularity or neovascularity of the bone in the area of the tumor, and (2) enlargement of the vascular channels either supplying or draining the tumor area. The latter occurs more commonly than the former, but neovascularity is considered a much more specific change. Statistics regarding altered vascularity occurring in plain skull films are of little significance, however, since, for the most part, only those tumors occurring in distal areas provide the opportunity for such changes to be visualized. Thus, the great majority of tumors exhibiting abnormal vascularity are those of the cerebral convexity and parasagittal areas. With basal tumors, visualization of the blood supply of the tumor in plain films is infrequent, even though it may be as great as in the case of tumors of the vault.

Neovascularity may occur in only a small area beneath the tumor and be significant, but when encountered, the hypervascularity usually is in a rounded or oval pattern, measuring several centimeters, in the vault. The basic gross pathologic change is the perforation of the skull by many small arteries and veins extending to and from the tumor. The development of this neovascularity results in the presence of a multitude of small punctate radiolucent areas, a condition that is often referred to as *stippling* (fig. 145). Occasionally, stippling alone will be present beneath the tumor, and for all practical purposes it may be considered a diagnostic sign of meningioma. In the great majority of cases, however, other changes

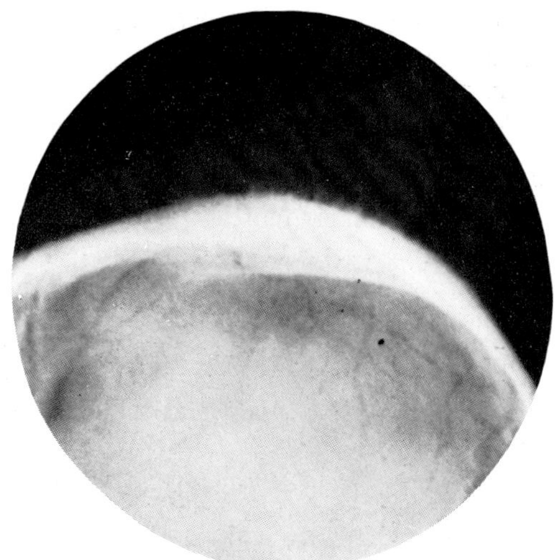

Fig. 143.—Parietal Parasagittal Meningioma

A tangential film shows hyperostosis involving all layers of the skull. Perpendicular bony spicules are present, extending outward from the external table. The patient had a palpable mass in the scalp.

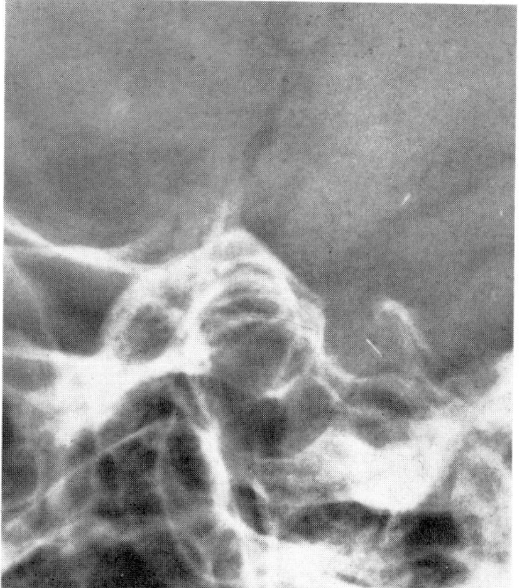

Fig. 144.—Meningioma of the Planum Sphenoidale

Meningiomas arising in relation to air sinuses of the skull, particularly the sphenoid sinus, often produce a characteristic reaction which has been called blistering. The portion of the sinus beneath the tumor becomes enlarged and projects intracranially. In most instances, hyperostosis also is present to varying degrees.

will be found in the general vascular pattern, and it is common to find hyperostosis in association with a localized patch of neovascularity.

Enlargement of the meningeal vascular channels occurs even more often than stippling, and in the majority of instances when stippling is found, enlargement of the meningeal vascular channels is present also. The most frequent and important changes occur along the course of the middle meningeal artery; the anterior and posterior meningeal arterial pathways are less conspicuous radiologically. The two basic changes that occur in the middle meningeal groove, which carries both the meningeal artery and veins, are: (1) unilateral enlargement of the main vascular channel, and (2) abnormal branching. Evidence of enlargement may be found at the point where the middle meningeal artery enters the skull through the *foramen spinosum*. The importance of study of the foramen spinosum was investigated by Lindblom (1936). Since the foramen can be oval as well as round, he established a range of normal for the shorter diameter of the foramen spinosum. The range established is between 1.5 and 3 mm., with an average of 2 mm., as seen in basal radiographs of the skull. However, considerable variation on the two sides is observed and it is not uncommon to find a larger foramen spinosum even on the side opposite the tumor. By itself, therefore, the presence of a large foramen spinosum cannot be considered a reliable diagnostic finding. It would be interesting, however, to have more data concerning this subject, since basal views ordinarily are not made as a routine part of the examination and the possibility of foraminal changes of significance being present in the case of basal lesions deserves further exploration.

Much more importance may be attached to the appearance of the main middle meningeal channel as it courses upward and backward over the vault of the skull. An enlarged channel may maintain a straight course, but in other instances it may be un-

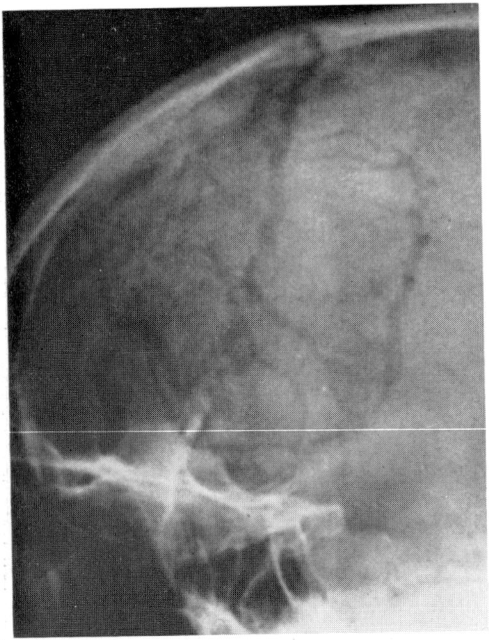

FIG. 145.—FRONTAL MENINGIOMA

Increased vascularity occasionally may be found with meningioma without hyperostosis. In the case illustrated, the main meningeal channels are markedly enlarged, many abnormal new channels have developed, and a number of abnormal branches of the middle meningeal artery extend forward into the tumor area. The sella turcica exhibits pressure atrophy and enlargement.

usually tortuous. Tortuosity of the vascular groove is an important radiologic appearance found often in patients with meningioma, and it usually denotes enlargement of the artery. A slight degree of tortuosity of the middle meningeal groove is not uncommon in normal cases, but only in the initial portion of the trunk of this artery as it begins its ascent in the region of the greater wing of the sphenoid. In the normal case, the tortuous segment is short, 1 to 2 cm. in length, and in the majority of instances is not associated with any suspicious increase in the width or prominence of the groove. In the lateral skull view, an enlarged channel appears as a wider, deeper (and therefore darker) shadow, and more sharply marginated than under normal circumstances. The enlarged channel often remains of evenly increased diameter until the level of the tumor on the vault is reached rather than tapering, as in normal arborization.

The most important feature of enlargement of the middle meningeal channel itself is unilaterality. Whenever there is a discrepancy in appearance, with one middle meningeal channel more conspicuous in either the frontal or stereoscopic lateral radiographs, the case must be regarded with high suspicion. Some normal variation does occur, but unfortunately, the absolute limits of normal and the normal range of dissimilarity of the middle meningeal channels on the two sides is not well defined. When only the main channel is prominent on one side, it is to be expected that in a fairly sizable group of patients no clinical or other evidence of intracranial disease will be found. However, whenever asymmetry exists, it is incumbent upon the radiologist to make a very careful search for other evidence of intracranial disease, routinely through the careful study of the ordinary projections and also through study of additional views as required, particularly additional stereoscopic pairs of films. It must also be kept in mind that both middle meningeal vascular grooves may be enlarged, and under these circumstances, both may be quite conspicuous but relatively symmetrical. Meningiomas of the falx and of the parasagittal areas are the most frequent to invoke such a bilateral change (fig. 147), and bifrontal tumors may also result in symmetrical enlargement (fig. 140).

Another significant alteration in the middle meningeal vascular channel that favors the diagnosis of meningioma is abnormal arborization. As visualized radiologically, the main channel of the middle meningeal artery courses upward and slightly backward posterior to the coronal suture, and the great majority of normal branches seen are posterior ones which course upward and backward over the surface of the parietal bone. While some normal anterior branches are present, they usually do not cause conspicuous markings or grooves in radiographs. Whenever anterior branches of a middle meningeal artery are found extending forward over one side of the

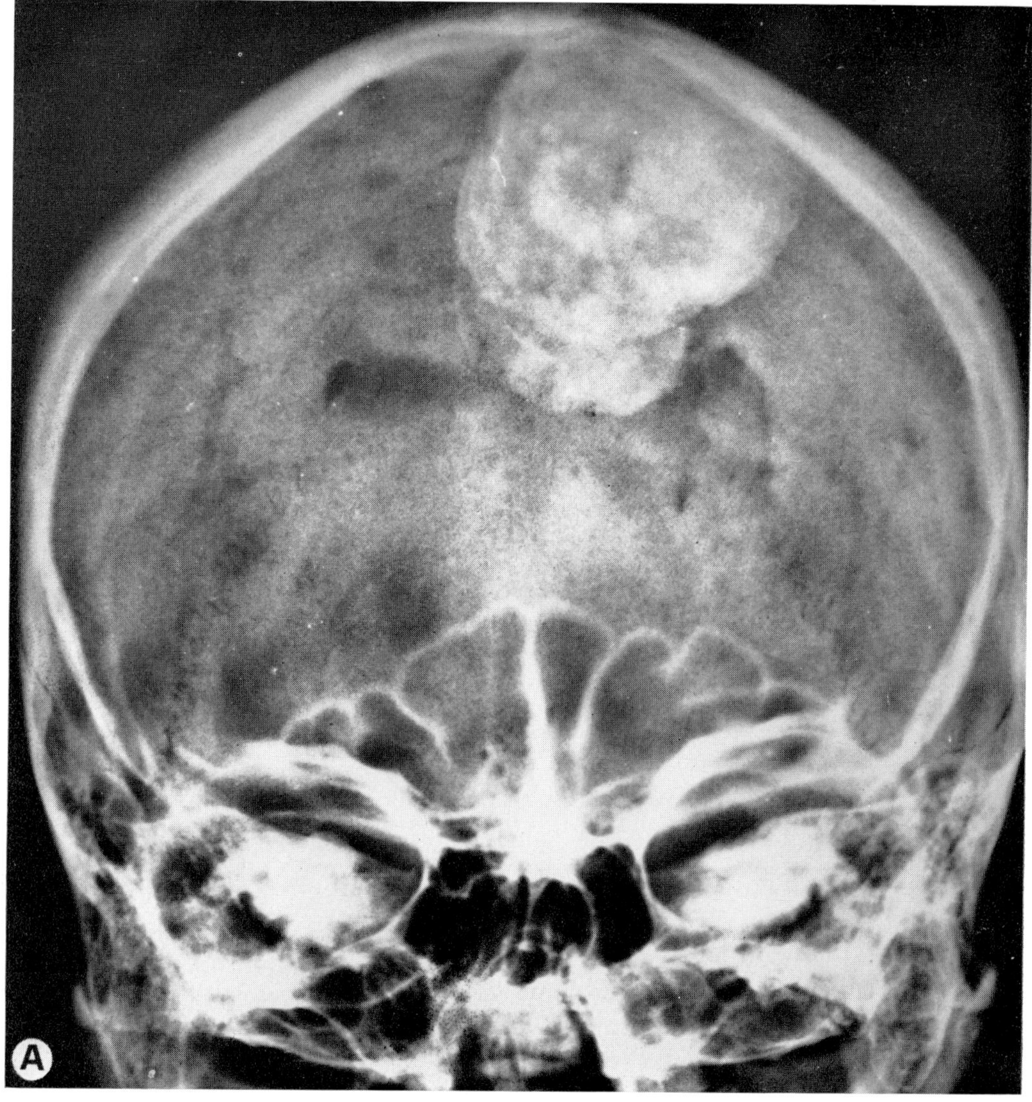

FIG. 146.—CALCIFIED MENINGIOMA

A large globular mass of calcium is present in the left parasagittal area, attached to the vault by a wide base measuring 5 cm. The tumor extends intracranially 6 cm. The frontal film (A) shows the tumor to be attached entirely on the left but to have grown across the midline. The lateral film (B) exhibits a number of abnormal bony vascular channels in relation to the tumor. At the time of operation, the lesion was found to be a completely calcified psammomatous meningioma, identical in size to the area of the calcium cloud shown radiologically.

vertical portion of the frontal bone, we tend to regard them with suspicion (fig. 145). In these cases, a careful search should be made at the termination of the rostral meningeal branch for evidence of other local changes such as stippling or hyperostosis which might confirm the suspicion of meningeal tumor or for evidence of increased intracranial pressure. In general, it may be stated that whenever a branch is conspicuously

(Revised 1963)

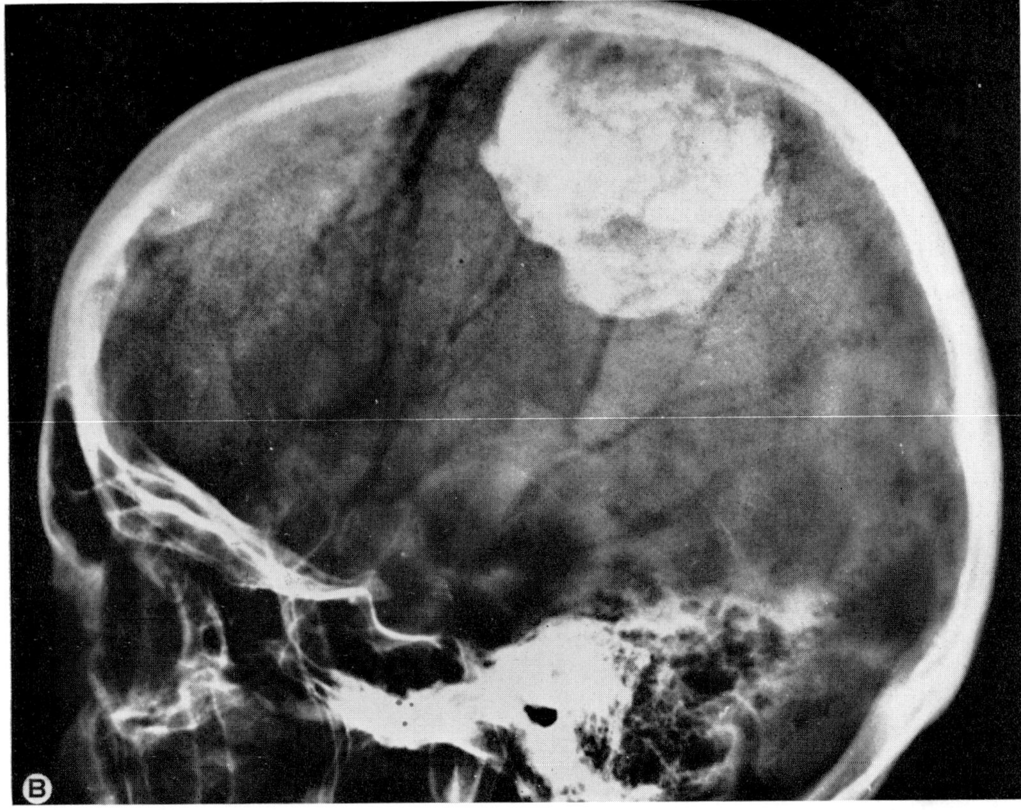

FIG. 146B

larger than an adjacent groove from the same parent vessel, it should be regarded as highly suspicious of an abnormality.

Posterior branches of unusual size also are to be regarded with suspicion. For the most part, such abnormal vessels arise from the main middle meningeal trunk and extend to the parietal convexity or the parietal parasagittal region (fig. 141). The chief normal posterior branch of the middle meningeal usually arises from the main vessel along the base of the skull. Its groove frequently can be seen coursing upward across the temporal squama and then curving backward to spread out over the posterior half of the parietal bone and even into the occipital area. However, the secondary and tertiary subdivisions of the posterior branch of the middle meningeal artery are not ordinarily as conspicuous in radiographs as are the branches of the main trunk. The posterior branch may be enlarged with meningioma and also with certain other vascular lesions of the posterior region.

Venous enlargement in the diploic space often is a more difficult finding to evaluate than changes in the meningeal channels. The diploic veins form a generally constant pattern anatomically, extending downward over the vault and communicating freely with intracranial venous structures as well as extracranial ones through emissary foramina. Radiologically, however, the veins appear less constant and there is considerable variation between patients as regards the prominence or conspicuous nature of various diploic trunks. The diploic veins have been a popular subject of study for many years and there is considerable radiologic literature concerning their appearance. Generalized prominence of the diploic veins usually is not of pathologic significance. Some skulls are extremely vascular to the extent that the term "phlebectasia" has been

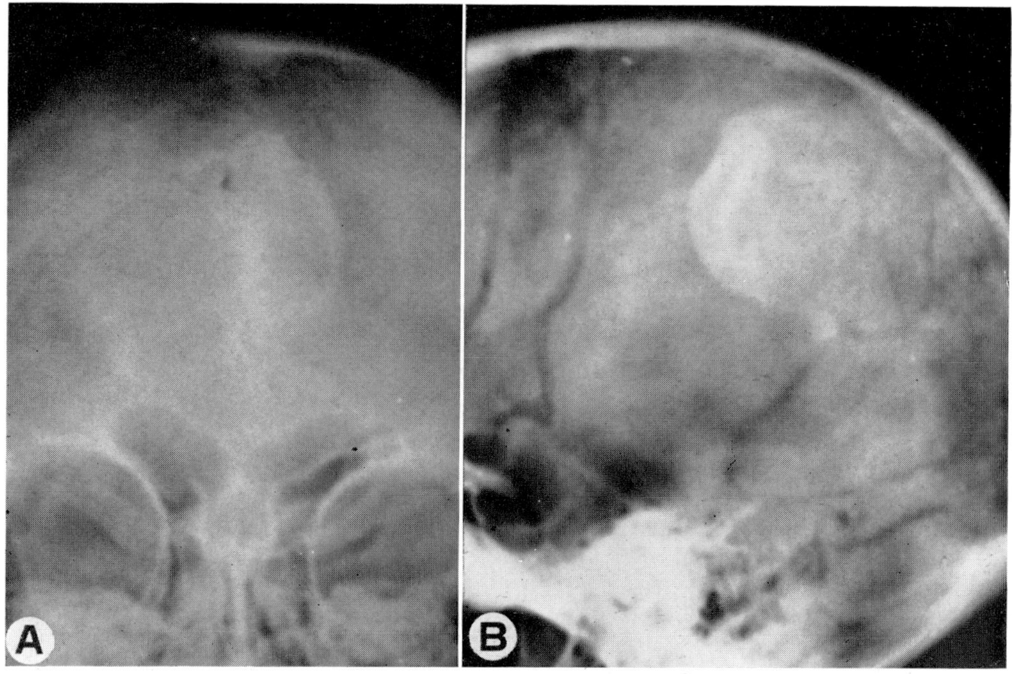

FIG. 147.—CALCIFIED MENINGIOMA

A meningioma of the falx is present in the parietal area, its calcific rim extending predominantly to the left (A). The calcified portion of the lesion is largely peripheral. The lateral view (B) shows a crescentic area of conglomerate calcification along the anterior margin of the tumor. Increased vascularity and increased intracranial pressure also are shown.

coined to describe them. The main clinical significance of such a finding is troublesome bleeding that may develop with intracranial surgery in such cases. However, localized enlargement of diploic veins or a very conspicuous appearance of a regional trunk may occur in connection with meningioma. Such localized prominence may be found in connection with the frontal diploic vein along one side of the vertical portion of the frontal bone (fig. 145). In the case of parasagittal meningioma, enlargement of the anterior temporal or posterior temporal draining diploic trunks may be found. Usually, however, there are other findings to support the diagnosis of meningioma, often some other change in vascularity. Enlargement of diploic veins and trunks, even regional enlargement, may be encountered in the presence of lesions other than meningioma (fig. 152).

(Revised 1963)

Calcification

The third cardinal finding for the diagnosis of meningioma is tumor calcification. Its occurrence has been reported variously. Camp (1950) described tumor calcification as occurring in as high as 18 per cent of patients. Most other observers have described an incidence of something less than 10 per cent.

The extent of calcification shows marked variation radiologically, just as it does pathologically. The most common type of calcification evident is a cloudlike, globular shadow of increased density resulting from the conglomeration of multitudes of psammoma bodies. In some instances, the entire tumor may be fairly evenly opacified (fig. 146). In other instances, the calcification appears to occur predominantly about the tumor margin or in one quadrant of the tumor (fig. 147). Thus, the plain films may reveal not only the identity of the tumor

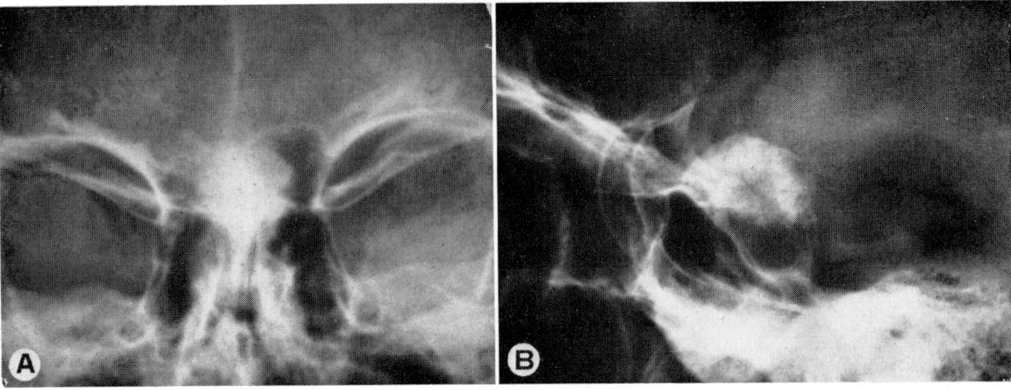

Fig. 148.—Meningioma of the Tuberculum Sellae

A calcified meningioma is shown, measuring 2.5 cm. in length and 2 cm. in width and covering the area of the tuberculum sellae and of the diaphragm sellae. The calcific mass extends upward 1.5 cm. above the sella turcica as seen in both the frontal (A) and the lateral (B) views. The structures of the superior surface of the sphenoid bone are remarkably well preserved, although encompassed in the bony mass.

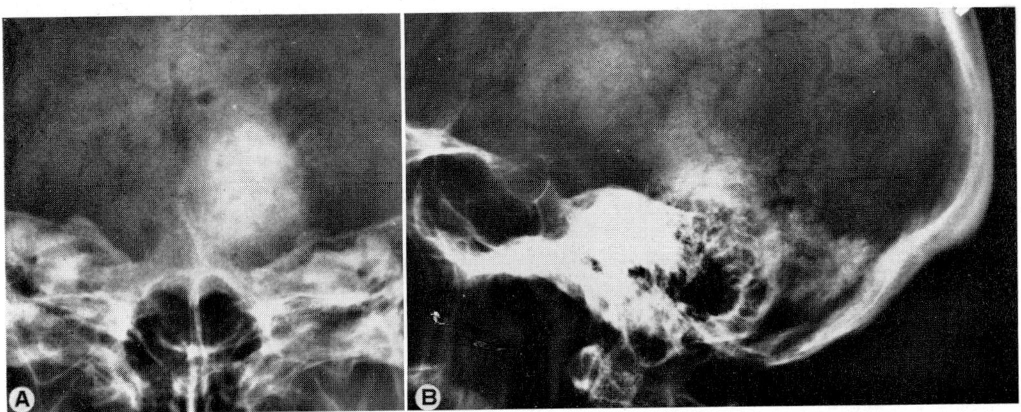

Fig. 149.—Peritorcular Meningioma

A largely calcified meningioma of the torcular herophili is shown to extend predominantly to the left of the midline (A) and downward (B) in relation to the falx cerebelli and the tentorium, respectively. The anterior extent of the calcified portion of the tumor, poorly defined because of superimposed mastoid air cells, is marked by arrows. Hyperostosis of the inner table of the skull extends into the area of the torcular itself, and above, the depression of the sinus confluence being poorly defined. Prominent and abnormal vascular channels also are present in the area.

but its extent without the necessity of contrast study. A radiograph of the pathologic specimen often will allow superimposition of the tumor shadow on the radiograph of the living subject.

In some tumors, unfortunately, the calcification is of nonspecific type rather than a homogeneous conglomerate collection of psammoma bodies. Branching plaques of calcium may be present which resemble calcification in granulomas or glial tumors. In other instances, true bone may be formed, as may occur with other degenerative changes. In our experience, conglomerate psammoma calcification is the type encountered in the majority of instances, and there appears to be no significant site of predilection for the development of fibrous menin-

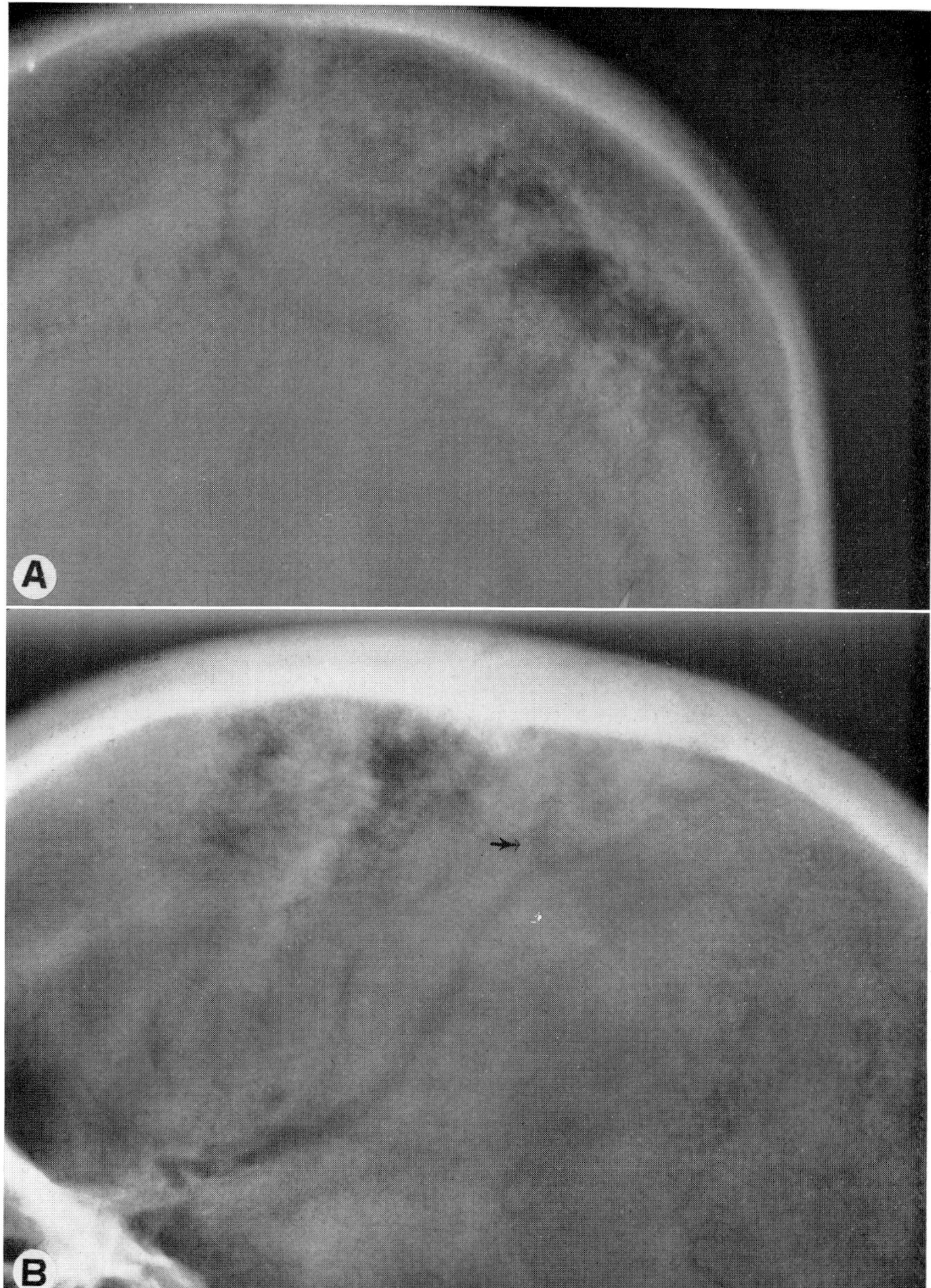

FIG. 150.—PREDOMINANTLY DESTRUCTIVE MENINGIOMA

A poorly defined osteolytic process is present which extends from the high frontal convexity (A) laterally and downward, following the general course of the coronal suture which is bridged by the destructive process (B). The posterior portion of the lesion exhibits hyperostosis with changes along the inner table and in the diploic space. The middle meningeal channel on the side of the lesion is larger than on the normal side, and there is branching below the area of hyperostosis; the anterior branch extending upward appears larger than the parent vessel (*arrow*). The margins of the area of bone destruction are very irregular in outline, and at some points the osteolvtic process extends through both tables of the skull.

(*Revised 1963*)

giomas exhibiting this type of change. Such tumors are encountered arising along the vault, particularly parasagittally, in the region of the tuberculum sellae and in the floor of the middle fossa (figs. 146, 148, and 283). It is doubtful that the limited number of calcified tumors available to any one observer would contradict the general incidence of global, fibrous tumors arising in various sites.

Other Direct Evidence of Meningioma

Aside from the cardinal findings of meningioma, two other plain film changes are worthy of mention. *Bone destruction* may occur in a small percentage of patients, and this may develop alone or in connection with hyperostotic changes. It is thought by some that the presence of destruction with meningioma may be only quantitative and associated with heavy infiltration of bone by tumor (Cushing and Eisenhardt). In the absence of associated hyperostosis, calcification, or vascular changes, differentiation of these purely destructive meningiomas from malignant tumors may be difficult. The presence of bone destruction with meningioma is not indicative of a malignant type of neoplasm if associated with hyperostosis (fig. 150). Pure osteolytic or destructive changes, however, are more often associated with meningiomas which are primarily sarcomatous.

A second and less common type of bony abnormality resulting from meningioma is *pressure erosion* and bone thinning. This type of change occurs with tumors that have not extended through the dura but which, because of their position contiguous to the inner table of the skull, cause an area of erosion owing to pressure through the intact dura. This type of radiologic abnormality is uncommon and, unless there is other plain film evidence of meningioma, it may be difficult to differentiate this type of shallow erosion of the inner table and diploic space from that secondary to subdural hematoma of long standing, porencephalic cysts, and other erosions, described elsewhere.

DIFFERENTIAL DIAGNOSIS

A wide variety of conditions may mimic meningioma, some closely while others are only remotely similar. The pathologic processes may be systemic in nature or they may be localized. In addition, as previously noted, certain intracranial processes, chiefly gliomas which calcify, may on occasion be indistinguishable from meningioma.

Systemic Disease. Hyperostosis

Hyperostosis frontalis interna (Morgagni-Stewart-Morel) is a very common occurrence; occasionally, the bony thickening may simulate the hyperostosis of a meningioma. More often, a bifrontal meningioma is mistaken for benign hyperostosis. The incidence of hyperostosis frontalis interna is particularly high in women; a significant degree of hyperostosis probably occurs in 15 per cent of women 40 years of age or older. Hyperostosis frontalis interna is uncommon in men except those suffering from pituitary adenomas of the eosinophilic type. The presence of such hyperostosis in men should prompt a careful search for hormonal changes or some other evidence of an eosinophilic pituitary new growth; the diagnosis of benign hyperostosis should be accepted in men only after exclusion of more significant systemic processes.

Hyperostosis frontalis interna appears to be a disturbance of endocrine origin, but the exact causal relationship has not been clearly established (Moore, 1955). A fairly high percentage of patients complain of headache which often is the reason for the radiologic examination. It is thought by many, however, that the occurrence of headaches and hyperostosis are purely coincidental. Similarly, obesity, which frequently is present in these cases, is not thought to be related to hyperostosis; in the true hypopituitary states of chromophobic pituitary adenoma and craniopharyngioma, such hyperostosis is not seen. On the contrary, hyperostosis occurring in association

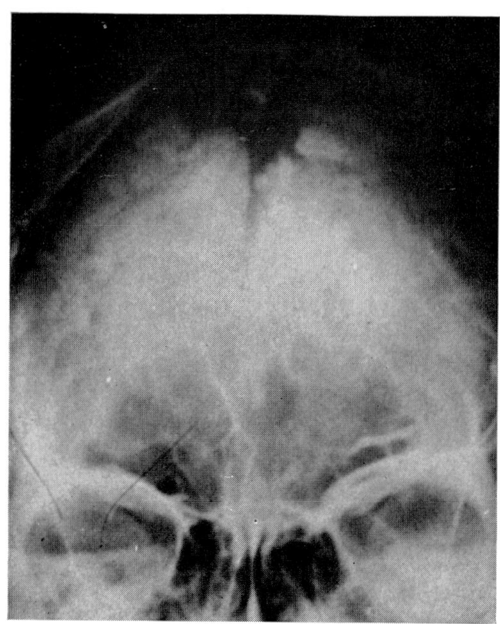

Fig. 151.—Hyperostosis Frontalis Interna

Even very extensive hyperostosis of the frontal bone, extending into other areas, does not produce an intracranial mass of clinical consequence and rarely is there difficulty in radiologic interpretation. In cases of benign hyperostosis, a midline cleft of absence of reaction usually is present beside the falx. In addition, isolated nodular areas of hyperostosis away from the principal reaction are seen, and increased vascularity does not occur.

with acromegaly suggests that increased pituitary activity may play a part in the bone production.

Radiologically, thickening may occur along either the vertical or horizontal portion of the frontal bone alone, or there may be thickening in both portions of similar or different degree. Typically, the inner table is greatly increased in thickness, usually along the vertical portion of the frontal bone; the thickening is fairly symmetrical, as seen in frontal view. The thickening of the inner table may encroach upon the diploic space. Usually, however, some frontal diploë is left, and the outer table is spared. The inner table thickening is at the expense of the intracranial cavity for the most part; instances are seen in which the thickness reaches sizable proportions, frequently more than 1 cm. and sometimes approaching 2 cm.

(Revised 1963)

As seen in lateral view, the bony thickening is characterized by deep ribs or areas of less marked thickening. In frontal view, these areas of sparing are seen to be near the midline and are rather symmetrical in location. The defects in the hyperostosis widen medially, and presumably these symmetrical changes are related to blood vessels draining into the superior longitudinal sinus. Typically, there is a midline cleft in the hyperostosis, with shading off of the thickened area toward the midline in a smoothly rounded manner. The midsagittal line of normal thickness is along the usual point of attachment of the falx cerebri carrying the superior longitudinal sinus (fig. 151). Demonstration of a midline cleft may be of importance in some instances to differentiate hyperostosis frontalis interna from bifrontal meningioma (fig. 140). In the latter, the hyperostosis bridges the midline; neither the vertical sparing for the superior longitudinal sinus and falx nor the transverse sparing for tributary vessels is seen. On the contrary, extension beyond a suture line may occur with benign hyperostosis and does not indicate an invasive process. It is not unusual to demonstrate such benign hyperostosis extending far posteriorly along the vault, even to the mid or occasionally posterior parietal areas.

The thickening of hyperostosis frontalis interna which occurs along the horizontal portion of the frontal bone may present more of a problem when olfactory groove meningioma is suspected. In the former, the thickening is even and usually diffuse over the supraorbital plates but even extends into the cribriform region. In some instances, far lateral extension of the hyperostosis is present, involving the sphenoid wing and causing thickening in the region of the pterion which may be mistaken for meningioma. Usually, the hyperostosis of the horizontal portion of the frontal bone is fairly symmetrical, as seen in frontal stereoscopic films, although isolated benign hyperostosis may occur which can present a diagnostic problem. Such localized thickening in the region of the pterion, often asymmetrical, frequently is found; caution should be exercised in attaching significance to minimal thickening and asymmetry in this region unless other changes of meningioma are present, such as increased vascularity or increased intracranial pressure.

Rickets causes hyperostosis in a high percentage of instances, but in the average case, the changes are symmetrical and readily recognized. There is usually generalized thickening of the frontal bones, of the parietal bones, or both. In addition, the base of the skull occasionally is thicker and denser than usual, but the base is less frequently involved than the vault. The greatest thickening is in the region of the frontal and parietal convexities, with tapering toward the bone edges. In young patients, this may be quite pronounced since there is a tendency for the anterior fontanelle to be delayed in closure. Often there is a change in shape of the skull which assists in diagnosis, such as where the over-all configuration is brachycephalic with the occiput flattened, and the bone posteriorly often is thin.

In other instances, however, and particularly in renal rickets, there may be marked thickening of the vault and extreme stippling. Both tables of the skull and the diploic space may be affected, as with meningioma. When the changes are localized, diagnostic difficulty may be encountered; differentiation of rachitic changes from Paget's disease or certain cases of hyperparathyroidism is more often a problem than differentiation from meningioma.

In *osteitis deformans* (Paget's disease), the skull may be involved relatively early in life; the authors have seen several cases of involvement during the second decade. The outer table and the diploic space usually are involved first, and even in advanced cases the changes are greater in these portions than along the inner table. Thickening of the skull results from widening of the diploic space, which exhibits irregular rounded or oval areas of increased density, separated by patches of decreased density, the latter representing uncalcified osteoid tissue. The onset of the more typical patchy increased density of Paget's disease may be preceded by a phase of decalcification known as *osteoporosis circumscripta.* The osteolytic changes begin either in the frontal or occipital areas and extend toward the vertex (Kasabach and Dyke, 1932). Rather sizable areas of mineral loss may be present which simulate bone destruction. The margins of the calcified areas are usually sharp but irregular in outline, and they are not confined by suture lines. The base of the skull is commonly affected in Paget's disease. As a result of the softening of bone during the early stages of the process, there is indentation of the base from the weight of the head, often with compromising in the region of the posterior fossa.

Commonly a distinct increase in vascularity of the skull is present in Paget's disease. It is unusual, however, for vascular channels to develop in a manner which may simulate meningioma, even though, at certain stages of development, the bony thickening of osteitis deformans may simulate the hyperostosis of meningioma. The earlier concept of *osteitis fibrosa localisata* (juvenile Paget's disease), in which the bones of the skull and even of the face become markedly increased in density and thickness, has been discarded since it is apparent that in the majority of such patients the pathologic process is fibrous dysplasia. Likewise, *leontiasis ossea* of Virchow is now considered to be only a descriptive term since the pathologic and radiologic changes are the result of a variety of disease processes. It would appear, however, that many of these patients also are afflicted with an adult or arrested form of fibrous dysplasia since in the "generalized" type, other portions of the skeleton, particularly the long bones, are affected.

Chronic *anemias* invoke marrow hyperplasia in the skull, which in turn causes hyperostosis and sclerosis of the cranial structures. Again, the greatest change is in the outer table of the skull and the diploic space; for this reason, confusion with meningioma is unlikely. Frequently the outer table cannot be detected as a distinct shadow, and striations occur perpendicular to the inner table of the skull as seen in profile. Certain en face views may exhibit a localized spongy appearance, with a suggestion of tabular defects, owing to hyperplasia of the bone marrow in the diploic space.

When asymmetrical changes of hyperostosis and sclerosis develop owing to marrow hyperplasia, or when apparent bony defects appear, there may be a problem in differentiating these lesions from those of meningioma. For the most part, however, the changes of the anemias are readily recognized because of the generalized nature of cranial involvement, and the inclusion even of facial bone structures, as well as many other portions of the skeleton in the process. The same basic changes are present in connection with erythroblastic anemia, congenital hemolytic anemia, sickle cell disease, and the secondary polycythemia of cyanotic congenital heart disease. In children, iron deficiency anemia may result in similar bony changes.

As in the case of increased intracranial pressure, parathyroid disease may provide a problem in diagnosis. In *hyperparathyroidism,* patches of sclerosis may occur in the vault of the skull, possibly simulating meningioma. The increase in thickness of the skull occurs owing to obliteration of the diploic space and increased density along the inner and outer tables, often with a mottling in the area of bony change (fig. 165). Such increases in density are seen most often in the quiescent state of hyperparathyroid disease, or after treatment, such as following the surgical removal of a parathyroid adenoma. Secondary renal failure also may result in such skull thickening. *Pseudohypoparathyroidism* likewise may cause a localized thickening of the skull owing to an increased thickness and density of the diploic space. Occasionally, localized areas of bony thickening may be seen in the skull in cases of *progressive diaphysial dysplasia and familial metaphysial dysplasia.* How such cranial changes fit into the over-all picture of "long bone disease" is not clear. *Osteopetrosis* (marble bones, Albers-Schoenberg disease) ordinarily presents in such a manner that there is no question concerning the nature of the bony thickening and extra density that occurs. Even in this condition, however, atypical cases have been described in which there was confusion with fibrous dysplasia; ordinarily, consideration of the possibility of meningioma does not arise, although the skull may be disproportionately affected (Alexander, 1923).

Polyostotic *fibrous dysplasia* (Albright's disease) in its full blown form consists of a triad of abnormalities: (1) bone lesions that tend to be unilateral, (2) nonelevated brown-pigmented areas of skin on the same side as the bone lesions, (3) endocrine dysfunction in the female resulting in precocious puberty. The bizarre syndrome was described by Albright, Butler, Hampton, and Smith in 1937 and later more fully discussed by Albright and Reifenstein (1948). The work of these investigators has provided considerable understanding of radiologically demonstrable skeletal lesions which previously were obscure in nature. While the most severe cases usually present all three features of the syndrome, it is not unusual to find instances in which one or two of the characteristic abnormalities are missing. Typical bone lesions frequently are found without skin lesions or precocity in the female. In the typical case, there is disseminated (not generalized) osteitis fibrosa involving multiple bones of the skeleton, predominantly unilaterally. However, similar histologic lesions may be found isolated in one bone, or in a group of neighboring bones. The frequent involvement of the skull, particularly about its base, is a prominent feature of the condition; it is not unusual to find apparent isolated involvement of cranial bones.

The bony lesions of osteitis fibrosa pathologically are found to be both hyperostotic and hypostotic. The presence of fibrous tissue is seen, on histologic examination, between ossified areas, about which many osteoblasts and osteoclasts are located. Islands of cartilage frequently occur and, as pointed out by Albright and Reifenstein, the condition has some of the features of dyschondroplasia. The latter does not appear to be a complete explanation, however, since the vault of the skull, derived from membranous bone, is frequently involved. There

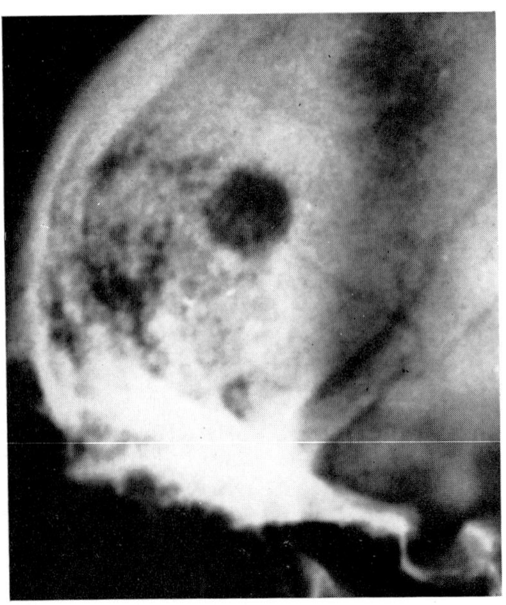

Fig. 152.—Fibrous Dysplasia

The lateral portion of the frontal bone on one side is extensively involved by fibrous dysplasia. The bony thickening extends into the horizontal portion of the frontal bone as well. In addition to the calcified elements of the lesion, numerous nodular and conglomerate noncalcified areas are shown. Large rounded areas frequently may be found simulating those associated with large meningiomas. In the case illustrated, an anterior branch of the middle meningeal artery extends directly forward to the lesion. The changes of fibrous dysplasia frequently involve extracranial bones of the facial area.

may be an elevation of serum phosphatase in fibrous dysplasia, but other blood chemical studies usually are normal. The various pathologic and clinical findings do not point clearly to a simple etiology of the disease. The distribution of the bone and skin lesions, when multiple, exclude an endocrine or metabolic cause but suggest a neurologic or embryologic basis of development. Since the precocity may be on a "neuro-humeral" basis, the one common denominator of the full blown syndrome could be a widespread neurologic disturbance.

Radiologically, the lesions of fibrous dysplasia may fall into one of three general categories: (1) cystic, (2) sclerotic, (3) mixed. The cystic lesions are found in the vault of the skull, situated in the diploic space, which may be markedly expanded over an area not infrequently measuring as much as 10 cm. in length. The outer table may be markedly thinned and may bulge outward, often to a striking degree; a clinically palpable mass may be present. The inner table usually is spared. Such cystlike lesions may resemble cholesteatomas when the bony structure is largely replaced by fibrous tissue; more often, some radiologically visible elements remain in the cystlike area. Cartilage, portions of which exhibit calcification, may be present even in the lesions of the vault, as previously noted.

The sclerotic lesions are most typical and are found with greatest frequency involving the bones of the base of the skull. The frontal and sphenoid bones often are affected. The involvement of the occipital bone with bulging of the suboccipital region apparently impressed Albright. In some instances, therefore, a bandlike zone of change, extending from the supraorbital to the suboccipital region, is encountered. Extension of the process across the midline of the skull may occur. In these cases, a broad zone of basal extension several centimeters in width and of heavy density may be seen with the result that normal basal architecture is obscured.

The mixed lesions involve frequently the vertical portions of the frontal and occipital bones. There is a gross increase in thickness of the skull in the area of which are scattered radiolucent areas, usually rounded (fig. 152). It is in connection with these latter lesions that the problem of differentiation from meningioma arises occasionally; the predominantly sclerotic lesions of the base may rarely simulate the dense hyperostosis of meningioma arising in the sphenoid area. The rounded radiolucencies may resemble the larger areas of increased vascularity seen with meningioma.

Clinically, as well as radiologically, a similarity between meningioma and fibrous dysplasia may be present in some cases. Proptosis, which occurs in a high percentage of patients with fibrous dysplasia, may suggest meningioma and often the occular changes are among the most serious aspects of the cranial changes. Foraminal narrowing, including constriction of the optic foramen, may be present in some patients to cause difficulty in differentiation. It has been the experience of the authors, however, that a significant progression of the process of fibrous dysplasia after it is first diagnosed is uncommon, an observation conforming with the experience of Albright and Reifenstein. The present authors have observed radiologically demonstrable progression in two young patients but no appreciable radiologic evidence of advancement in older patients, even when neurologic deficits developed or advanced. The fact that fibrous dysplasia is a disease of early life, while meningiomas occur more frequently during the later decades, also helps in differentiating the two conditions.

Tuberous sclerosis may provide the basis for the development of sclerotic plaques along the inner table of the skull and thickening of the diploic space. Only occasionally do the changes simulate meningioma sufficiently to be an important consideration in differential diagnosis. In the average case, other manifestations of tuberous sclerosis, either clinical or radiologic, provide clues to the proper diagnosis.

Local Bone Changes

In addition to the various systemic conditions in which changes in thickness and density of the skull may occur, localized changes frequently are seen, which apparently are isolated reactions. In addition, changes in vascularity over a limited area may be found, some of which are normal variations while others are related to pathologic processes other than meningioma. Bone destruction also may be encountered; in these instances, it may be difficult or impossible to differentiate an osseous osteolytic lesion from the occasional meningioma which exhibits pure bone destruction or mixed productive and destructive changes.

Localized hyperostosis. This condition may be even more difficult to differentiate from meningioma than the generalized and frequently symmetrical variety. Anatomic variations in thickness occur throughout various portions of the same skull, and there is tremendous variation in skull thickness from individual to individual. In addition to the thinness seen in many normal patients along the greater wing of the sphenoid, there is frequently thickening at the outer end of the sphenoid ridge in the region of the pterion; this may be an isolated finding on only one side and not related to hyperostosis frontalis interna. In perfectly straight lateral films, there is often an apparent increase in density in this region. Stereoscopic study will allow a more satisfactory evaluation of the bony appearance on the two sides. When only a normal pterional asymmetry exists, the bone in this region may appear more compact on one side than the other, but there is no stippling or other evidence of increased vascularity; increased intracranial pressure is absent. Frontal views which are rotated, *even slightly*, may cause the outer third of one sphenoid wing to appear relatively more dense than the corresponding area on the opposite side. In the absence of any other variation or abnormality, it is usually safe to disregard such an isolated finding of minimal asymmetry; follow-up skull films should be obtained.

In addition to the lateral sphenoid regions, asymmetrical thickness and density of the skull may occur in the vault. In children, a trabecular arrangement perpendicular to the inner and outer tables of the skull in the diploic space often is found. In these cases, the outer table is thin; an erroneous impression of the perpendicular proliferative changes of meningioma may be gained, unless the film is carefully examined under a bright light.

Osteomas and *osteochondromas* are observed arising from the skull relatively frequently. Osteomas often are small, measuring in the neighborhood of 1 cm. in diameter; they may attain a size of 2 to 3 cm. or even more. Frequently, only the outer table is involved. Occasionally, a rounded or oval area of compact bone is found in the diploic space without the tables being appreciably af-

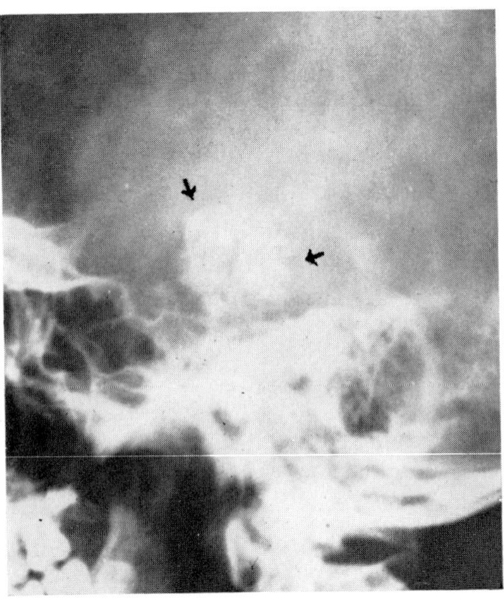

FIG. 153.—OSTEOCHONDROMA OF THE TEMPORAL BONE

A large area of bony overgrowth is present, projecting intracranially from the temporal squama. The margins are irregular but sharply defined, and the calcification of the tumor is quite dense. No unusual vessels are present, and there is no evidence of increased intracranial pressure. Osteomas may grow either extracranially or intracranially, and may be found almost anywhere in the skull, although they are more commonly seen near the skull base; tumors containing cartilage are found almost exclusively in the basal areas.

fected. In these instances, the appearance may resemble a bone island occurring elsewhere in the skeleton. Osteomas which involve the inner table provide the greatest difficulty in differentiation from the hyperostosis of a meningioma. Frequently, such small rounded proliferations of the inner table are present in the frontal region and along the temporal squama. Because of the thinness of the diploic space in the latter area, both tables may be involved.

In radiographs, the smoothness of contour and uniformity of density are good clues to the true nature of an osteoma. Often, the change from normal bone to the osteoma is abrupt, although occasionally a marginal gradation will be found. Stereoscopically, the area of extra density will exhibit no internal structure, and in the typical case there are no unusual blood vessels in the vicinity of the lesion (fig. 153). Occasionally, such a lesion is surgically removed because of concern regarding the possibility of meningioma. The small tumors are found to be made up of mature lamellar bone which is densely packed, accounting for the eburnated appearance in the films and the similar appearance of the gross specimen. No soft tissue element is associated with such pure osteomas. If an opportunity is provided to observe such a lesion radiologically over a period of time, very slow growth may be found, often extending over a period of years. Osteomas arising in the paranasal sinuses are commonly seen, and rarely they may grow sufficiently to erode the inner sinus wall (Cushing, 1927).

Osteochondromas are found along the base of the skull in the areas derived from cartilage. The majority are found near the midline in the anterior fossa, along the floor of the middle fossa, and in the basioccipital regions. Two general types are encountered—in the first, there is a dense sclerotic form somewhat resembling an osteoma, and in other instances, the tumors may be large and globular in outline. In the latter type, spotty areas of decreased density are frequently present among the areas of calcification and ossification. The tumors may attain appreciable size, and those that occur along the floor of the middle fossa may simulate closely a meningioma of this region. On other occasions, the cartilaginous new growth may cause destruction of basal structures, simulating a malignant lesion. Surgical intervention, if incomplete, may be followed by recurrence, and the growth rate of the recurrence often is more rapid than that of the original tumor. In one instance encountered, an osteochondroma which remained histologically benign became aggressive after incomplete removal; it involved a large portion of the middle and posterior fossa on one side with extensive neural damage and eventual death of the patient.

Calcified hematomas, either subperiosteal or epidural, may resemble meningiomas in some instances. The former occur commonly in the newborn; calcification may be clearly visible beginning along the periphery of the hematoma within a few days of birth (fig. 604). The changes are found most frequently in the parietal areas, although occipital and frontal location is not unusual. The hematoma contracts as it undergoes organization and ossification, and the end result ordinarily is an area of localized thickening of one of the bones of the skull. The outer table may be preserved but also may become indistinct in the ossification process. Such deformities, which persist into adult life, have been referred to as cephalhematoma deformans. While such a process has no pathologic significance later in life, the possibility of confusion with the hyperostosis of meningioma and also with the bony thickening of several systemic and infectious diseases exists.

Epidural hematoma results from hemorrhage between the inner table of the skull and the dura mater. Such a hemorrhage usually occurs owing to a tear of the middle meningeal artery, or one of the larger veins or dural sinuses by trauma. Fractures with wide separation of the bone edges are particularly prone to produce such a vascular tear; meningeal vessels which are situated in deep grooves are more likely to be involved by fracture than vessels which run in shallow troughs. In some instances, epidural hematoma, particularly of the frontal region, may occur as a complication of ventriculography owing to collapse of the ventricles and brain when a large quantity of fluid is removed in hydrocephalus. Epidural hematomas may calcify and, because these changes are along the inner table of the skull, the possibility of meningioma may be suggested in some instances (fig. 157). Evidence of old trauma, either an old fracture or a deformity from previous surgical treatment, will indicate the true nature of the process. In any event, when maturely organized and calcified, there is no evidence of adjacent increased vascularity or of increased intracranial pressure.

Infectious diseases involving the bony skull are encountered infrequently under modern methods of medical management. Pyogenic osteomyelitis as well as tuberculous and luetic osteitis have been rare since the beginning of the antibiotic era. Secondary localized osteomyelitis is still seen occasionally as a result of contaminated wounds. Paranasal sinus infection may result in marked sclerosis of adjacent bone, and occasionally in a degree of increased vascularity sufficient to cause bone absorption. The basal structures, particularly in the region of the sphenoid sinus, are more commonly affected than other areas. Occasionally, the chronic thickening and increase in density of basal bones, following osteitis secondary to sinus infection, will result in an appearance simulating the flat hyperostosis of a meningioma. Similar changes may be found in the frontal regions in connection with frontal sinus infection. In these instances, a marked sclerosis of the diploic space may occur; in addition, there may be heavy proliferation of the inner table of the skull, on occasions measuring 1 to 2 cm. thickness, extending as far back as the parietal region. Evidences of chronic sinus disease, as seen in the same radiographs, are the best indication of the true nature of the pathologic process. In addition, as with the other local bony hyperostoses described above, there is absence of increased vascularity and increased intracranial pressure. In the middle fossa, however, differentiation may be more difficult than in the frontal region because flat meningiomas of the sphenoid wing may not be associated with demonstrable increased vascularity in plain films. *Petrositis* may be a complication of infection of the mastoid sinuses. Usually the infection is of low virulence resulting in a sclerosing osteitis, especially when this portion of the temporal bone is poorly pneumatized.

Increased vascularity. Attention has been given earlier to the differentiation between normal and abnormal vascular patterns of the skull in connection with the diagnosis of meningioma. The importance of localized increased vascularity as contrasted with generalized prominence of the vascular channels has been emphasized. Generalized prominence of the diploic veins (phlebec-

(Revised 1963)

tasia) is not of clinical significance, except possibly in connection with excessive bone bleeding when intracranial surgery is necessitated.

While there is usually no great difficulty in recognizing the prominent depressions produced by large Pacchionian granulations, in some instances a problem may arise. Occasionally, a group of unusually large Pacchionian impressions may be found along the midsagittal plane of the skull and even extending for a considerable distance out from the midline. It has been postulated that such Pacchionian body enlargement may be the result of a deficiency in number of these structures with compensatory hypertrophy. In some instances, an indentation of the inner table of the skull which measures 2 cm. in diameter may be found, and occasionally there may be erosion of the entire thickness of the vault with subgaleal presentation of the vascular bodies. More often, however, the enlarged Pacchionian bodies remain covered by a layer of the outer table which may be very thin and bowed outward to such an extent that it may be clinically palpable. Somewhat similar changes may be found in instances of arrested hydrocephalus, again presumably a deficiency of the absorptive structures; compensatory enlargement of certain of the functioning Pacchionian bodies takes place. In some instances, large veins may be demonstrated in connection with these deep impressions, suggesting the possibility of a meningioma.

Similarly, the increased vascularity associated with arteriovenous malformations may provide the basis for considering the diagnosis of meningioma. With these lesions, however, the prominent vascular markings ordinarily are quite long, often traversing one-half of the length of the skull. Small amorphous and granular calcium deposits superficially situated along the course of such vascular channels, often near their termination, suggest the true nature of the pathologic process.

The increased vascularity which may develop as a result of *collateral circulation* may present more of a problem than many other conditions, especially when the increased flow is in the external carotid system. The increase in size of vessels connecting the venous system of the brain with the external system, which occurs as a result of increased intracranial pressure, has been described earlier. Such changes usually involve enlargement of the emissary foramina, and ordinarily the question of true increased vascularity of meningioma is not raised. In some cases of sinus thrombosis, the collateral circulation which develops may cause an alteration of vascular markings of unusual appearance. More significant, however, are the changes resulting from collateral circulation on the arterial side owing to occlusion, particularly of the internal carotid artery or middle cerebral artery. Under such conditions, there may be circulation from the external carotid artery system to the internal carotid system through the dura mater. This may take place largely by way of an arterial plexus, the rete mirabile. In these instances, the perforating vessels may give an appearance of stippling which may simulate meningioma. The absence of any detectable hyperostosis in such instances may be the best plain film clue to the diagnosis. Angiography will give a definitive indication of the true nature of the underlying process and demonstrate the collateral changes.

Certain vascular bone tumors may occasionally simulate meningioma. Benign hemangiomas of cavernous type ordinarily are easily recognized by their well defined margins and well organized internal architecture. Such hemangiomas may be 2 to 3 cm. in diameter but usually are smoothly rounded and often exhibit a radial arrangement of coarse trabeculae within the central portion of the vascular tumor. Prominent vascular channels may be present in connection with such hemangiomas, and marginal stippling frequently is seen.

More bizarre and confusing appearances may be encountered in the presence of vascular metastatic lesions involving the bony skull. A metastasis from thyroid may involve an area of the vault several centimeters in diameter and cause an enlargement of the diploic space with perpendicular striations and bony spicules similar to those found with meningioma. Occasional metastases from neuroblastoma will expand the diploic space in a fusiform manner with erosion of the inner and outer tables in a striated fashion; the majority of such metastatic lesions occur in early life.

Bone destruction. Since purely destructive changes are caused by meningioma only infrequently, differentiation from the wide variety of conditions producing radiolucent defects is not often a problem. As noted above, meningiomas may occasionally produce pressure erosion of the skull through the dura without actual bone destruction. Some other slowly growing tumors, such as astrocytomas, may invoke similar effects; such changes are encountered more often, however, in connection with subdural hematoma and porencephaly.

The bone destruction which may be encountered with myeloma, Hodgkin's disease, primary sarcomas, and metastatic carcinoma may simulate a purely destructive type of meningioma which aggressively invades and destroys bone (figs. 136 and 150). Localized areas of involvement by eosinophilic granuloma may cause more difficulty in diagnosis on occasion than the malignant lesions just mentioned. Fortunately, the necessity of differentiating a purely osteolytic meningioma from a truly destructive bone process does not occur very often since, in the majority of instances, the destructive changes of meningioma are accompanied by proliferative changes and increased vascularity.

Calcification

The difficulty in differentiating the calcification occurring in the minority of meningiomas is described above. In the majority of cases, the calcification of meningioma is cloudlike and rather homogeneous. Typically, a part of the smoothly lobulated margin of the calcified tumor is interrupted by the bony skull to provide its wide base of attachment. In some instances, however, only atypical calcium deposits may be found in the globular mass of a meningioma.

(Revised 1963)

Under such circumstances, the appearance of the calcium may suggest an astrocytoma, ependymoma, or other glial neoplasm.

Aneurysms of the suprasellar region may simulate a tuberculum sellae meningioma clinically, and both may calcify. Although the mass associated with each type of lesion may be relatively similar in size, the nature of the calcification may serve to differentiate the two. The calcification of meningioma is more homogeneous throughout while the calcification of aneurysm is ringlike (compare fig. 148 with fig. 163). In one example illustrated, there was complete peripheral calcification of the aneurysm; the calcification of the wall often is not as complete and the calcium lines may appear as curvilinear arcs rather than complete rings. The differential diagnosis of suprasellar masses in general pertains in these cases since craniopharyngiomas and pituitary adenomas also may contain calcium deposits; this has been discussed in detail earlier.

Similarly, calcifications occurring distal to the circle of Willis may have calcified walls with a ringlike shadow visible in the radiograph. In most instances, these lesions are clearly deeply seated, but occasionally a peripheral calcification may be found in a location where meningioma is commonly seen (figs. 154 and 162). In these instances, differentiation from true intracerebral calcification of glial tumor, old inflammatory lesions, and other calcific residues is apt to be more of a problem than differentiation from meningioma. Again, the ringlike nature of calcification occurring with aneurysm suggests the correct diagnosis.

It is apparent, therefore, that when typical changes are present, the diagnosis of meningioma should be made without difficulty and with a high degree of certainty. Atypical changes are frequent, however, and a host of conditions may simulate meningioma to varying degrees, some closely, others remotely. In some instances, cranial changes simulating meningioma may provide the best clue to the diagnosis of systemic disease. Since the meningioma is a benign tumor in the general sense, every

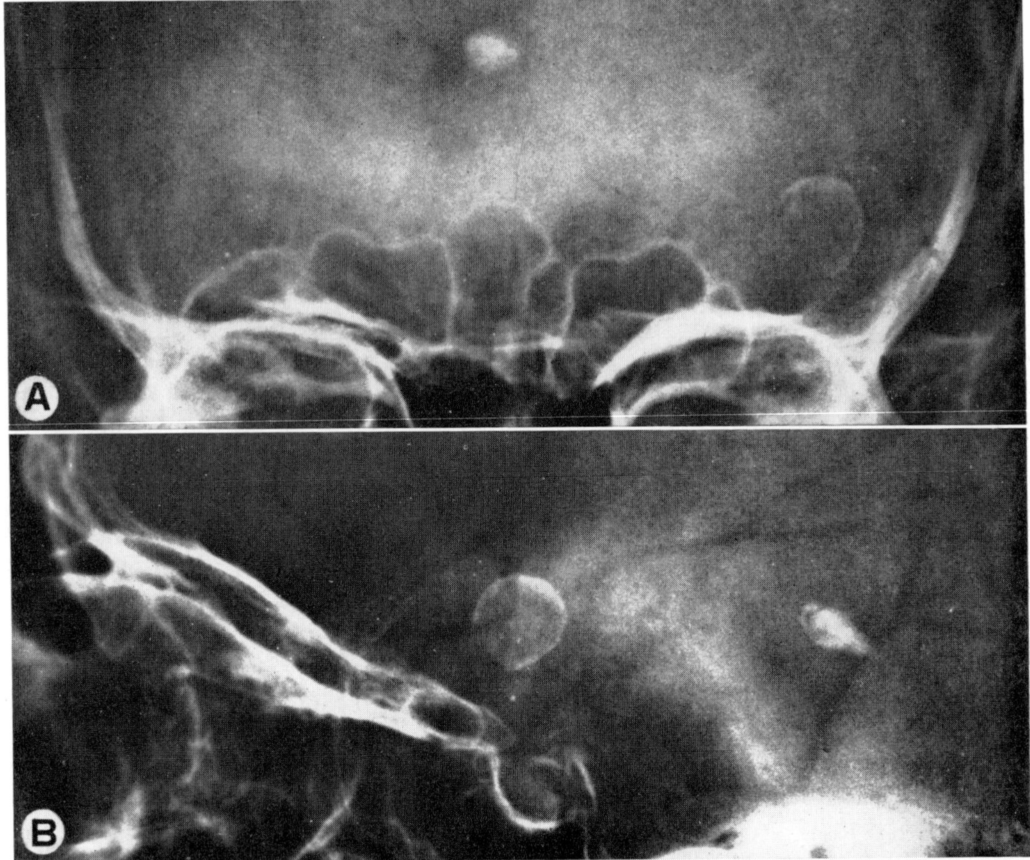

FIG. 154.—ANEURYSM OF THE MIDDLE CEREBRAL ARTERY

A rounded 1.5-cm. calcific shadow is present projected through the region of the pterion in lateral view (B) but from the frontal projection (A) is seen not to have bony attachment. The calcification is ringlike, characteristic of an aneurysm.

effort should be made to detect its presence from the various plain-film manifestations which it produces, however minimum. While in many instances a contrast examination, either pneumography or angiography, will be recommended to determine the size and vascular supply of the lesion, the detection and identification of meningiomas should rest on the careful evaluation of plain skull films.

INTRACRANIAL CALCIFICATION

General Considerations

The deposition of calcium salts in tissues other than bone is a pathologic process and is known as calcification. In calcification the same salts concerned with ossification are deposited in tissue which is either dying or dead and from which cell structure has disappeared. In the presence of hypercalcemia, degeneration on the part of the tissues is not involved and lime salts are deposited in living cells. It is much more common, however, for calcium to be laid down in dead tissue without reference to blood calcium.

Necrosis and hyalin changes are the two chief antecedents of calcification. Physical rather than chemical structure appears to be

TABLE II

A. Surface (Extracerebral)	B. Deep (Intracerebral)
1. Membranous	1. Localized
a. Physiologic	a. Physiologic
(1) Falx cerebri and superior longitudinal sinus	(1) Pineal
(2) Falx cerebelli	(2) Habenular
(3) Tentorium cerebelli and petroclinoid ligaments	(3) Chorioid
(4) Diaphragm sellae, bridged clinoids	b. Pathologic
(5) Dural plaques	(1) Brain abscess
(6) Arachnoid granulations	(2) Granuloma (tuberculoma, etc.)
b. Pathologic	(3) Hematoma
(1) Subdural hematoma	(4) Glioma
(2) Psammomatous meningioma	(5) Teratoma (dermoid and cholesteatoma)
(3) Tuberculous meningitis	(6) Angioma
2. Hypophysial	2. Multiple Scattered
a. Craniopharyngioma	a. Tuberous sclerosis
b. Pituitary adenoma	b. Encephalitis
c. Cranial tumors of the basisphenoid	(1) Toxic
(1) Chordoma	(2) Viral (cytomegalic inclusion disease)
(2) Osteochondroma	(3) Parasitic
3. Vascular	(a) Toxoplasmosis
a. Arterial calcification	(b) Cysticercosis
(1) Arteriosclerosis	c. Metastatic neoplasm
(2) Arterial aneurysm	d. Endarteritis calcificans
(3) Metastatic	3. Multiple Symmetrical
b. Angiomatous malformations	a. Neoplastic (lipoma)
(1) Venous angioma (Sturge-Weber)	b. Basal ganglia
(2) Arteriovenous malformation	c. Dentate nucleus
	d. Cortical

FIG. 155.—COMMON CAUSES OF INTRACRANIAL CALCIFICATION

the important factor in determining the deposition of calcium (Wells, 1910). Tissue inactivity results in a low carbon dioxide tension and by diffusion the phosphate and carbonate calcium salts are absorbed by the hyalinized substance from the accessible body fluids of surrounding living tissue.

Another method of calcification, thought to occur less frequently, takes place through fatty degeneration (Klotz, 1905). Through hydrolysis of fat, a fatty acid is liberated and calcium is first deposited through union with the acid to form a calcium soap. The fatty acid radical later is replaced by carbonate and phosphate. Such a mechanism probably occurs in fat necrosis and may be seen in a degenerating lipoma.

It is of interest that the calcification with which we ordinarily concern ourselves in clinical work does not occur in neural tissue. Some calcium salts may be deposited in dead ganglion cells of the brain and in the corpora amylacea of glial origin, and perhaps under other circumstances at the cellular or cellular aggregate level. The calcifications in which the radiologist is interested, however, are large enough to be visible to the unaided eye and are of sufficient size and density to cast visible shadows in radiographs. Essentially all such calcifications develop through degenerative changes in fibrous tissue (Table II, fig. 155).

The diagnosis of intracranial calcification may be divided into two parts: the detection of calcification in the cranial cavity of the living subject by radiologic methods and, once detected, identification of the pathologic process involved. Of the technical aids, stereoscopy is considered the most valuable. The advantages gained by such a method of procedure can only be appreciated fully when it is consistently followed. In no other way can intracranial calcification even be detected in a reasonable percentage of cases, and in the identification of intracranial calcification, stereoscopy is invaluable. Through three-dimensional study it should be possible to determine whether a calcium shadow is located on or arises from the surface of the brain, or whether it is situated deep in the cerebral substance. Some calcifications, particularly the membranous and vascular ones, are situated in major fissures, but still are considered calcifications of the cerebral surface. Laminagraphy may also be of value in certain cases.

Radiologic Findings

Membranous Calcification

Most of the membranous calcifications lie in the processes of the cranial dura mater, which project into the cavity of the skull. The dura is composed of two layers, an outer or endosteal constituting the periosteum of the inner surface of the cranial bones, and an inner or meningeal layer. Processes are formed by duplication of the inner layer of the membrane and are four in number: the falx cerebri, the falx cerebelli, the tentorium cerebelli, and the diaphragma sellae.

The dura mater is composed of white fibrous tissue and elastic fibers, and like all collagenous connective tissue, it often undergoes hyalin degeneration and calcification. Just why calcification occurs so frequently in this cerebral membrane is not clear. While it transports an abundant vascular supply for other structures, it is not particularly vascular itself, and this may be the principal cause. Trauma, particularly birth injury, has been suggested often as an explanation for the extensive calcifications sometimes found, but correlation of a history of very remote trauma and the discovery of extensive dural calcification is difficult to establish.

Physiologic calcification. Some form of membranous calcification occurs in approximately 10 per cent of normal individuals. In many persons, more than one form is present. In a study of almost 3,000 skull films of patients of all ages, Dyke (1941) found that calcification in the *falx cerebri* is most common, being present in 7 per cent of individuals. The falx calcium deposits usually are found along the superior longitudinal fissure. Single or multiple deposits may be present. Most often the calcification is oval and flat in form, with the long axis oriented in the sagittal plane. Occasionally, this plaquelike deposit may be tented on one or both lateral aspects. Along the vertex, a falx deposit may divide and pass laterally over the superior longitudinal sinus to form the shape of the letter Y as seen in frontal view. If calcium is present only in the dural walls of the superior longitudinal sinus, the calcium may appear as an oblique linear shadow or, if bilateral, in the shape of the letter V. The margins of a falx calcium plaque usually are smooth. Falx calcification is homogeneous in appearance and devoid of visible internal architecture. Even small deposits usually are visible in frontal view, but in lateral projection the calcification appears faint because of its thinness.

Calcification in the *falx cerebelli* is seen less commonly than in the falx cerebri. An incidence in adults of 5 per cent was reported by Dyke (1941). The plaquelike configuration and the homogeneous appearance characteristic of falx cerebri calcification is also typical of the posterior fossa membranous deposits.

The *petroclinoid* reflection of the tentorium is particularly subject to the development of calcification, although it may occur in the tentorial apex or in any one of its reflections. The extent of petroclinoid calcification is quite variable and may be heavy. In lateral view, the shadows are linear and are disposed in an oblique plane forming an angle with the clivus. Calcification is more often seen at the clinoid end of the dural reflection and it extends backward and downward toward the porus acousticus. Frontal, basal, or half axial views may allow visualization of the calcification as bilateral paired calcium deposits diverging as they pass laterally as well as posteriorly and downward from the posterior clinoid processes to the petrous tips of the temporal bones. The clinical importance of petroclinoid calcification is that it may be mis-

(Revised 1963)

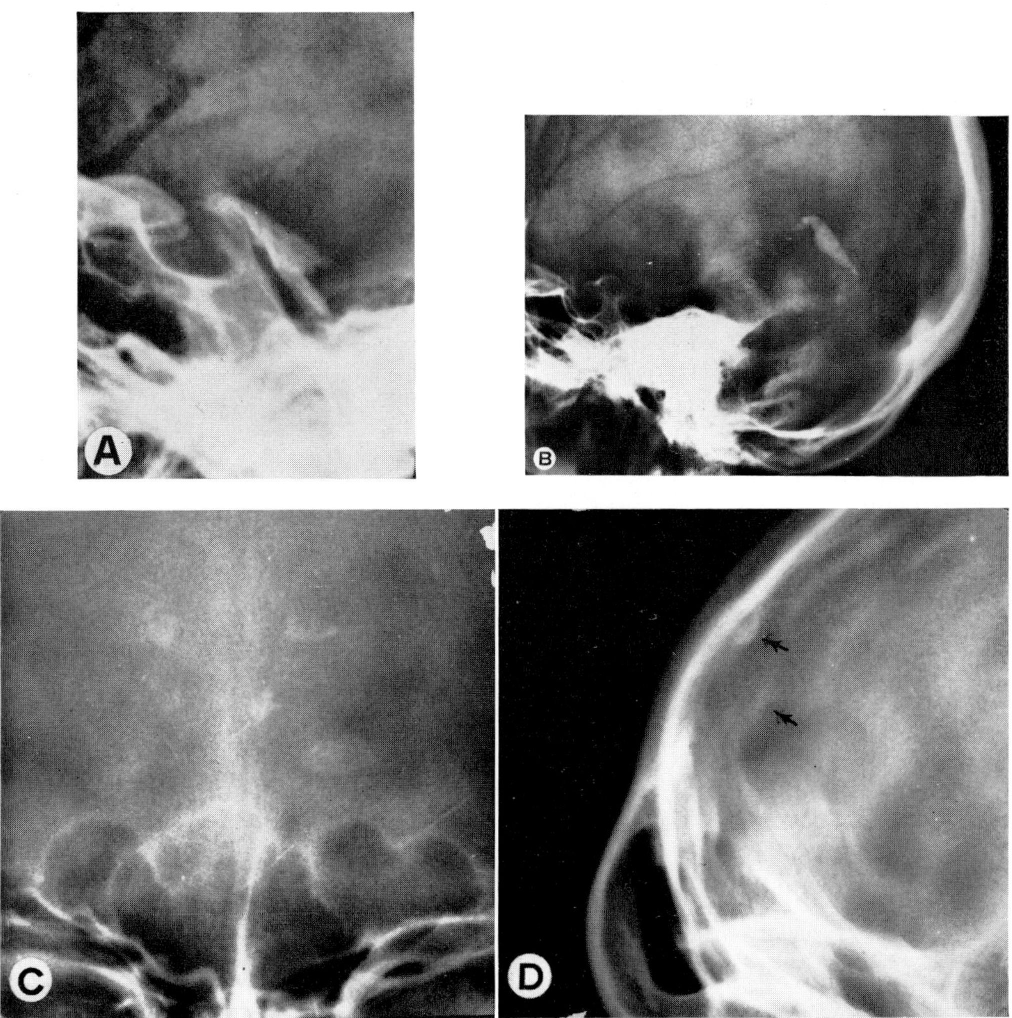

FIG. 156.—BENIGN MEMBRANOUS CALCIFICATION

Physiologic calcification frequently occurs in the portion of the tentorium extending from the sella turcica to the petrous tip, usually called the petroclinoid ligament (A). Ossification as well as extensive calcification often is seen. Calcification in the tentorium and falx cerebelli (B) is not as common as in the falx cerebri. When found, the calcification frequently is near the apex of the tentorium or along its lateral attachments. Calcification in arachnoid granulations may be seen as scattered, well defined calcified nodules. They occur most frequently in the parasagittal areas (C). The lateral film (D) shows them frequently to be smoothly rounded intracranially and based on the inner table of the skull (*upper arrow*).

taken for basilar artery or other pathologic calcification. Calcification in the apex of the tentorium may be mistaken for a displaced calcified pineal gland (fig. 156).

The *diaphragma sellae* is said to be calcified in approximately 3 per cent of individuals, most often in its lateral attachments, and occasionally bony bridging between the anterior and posterior clinoid processes is found. The deposits appear as transverse linear shadows extending from the anterior to the posterior clinoid processes. Often the calcification is bilateral. The changes should not be mistaken for arteriosclerosis of the

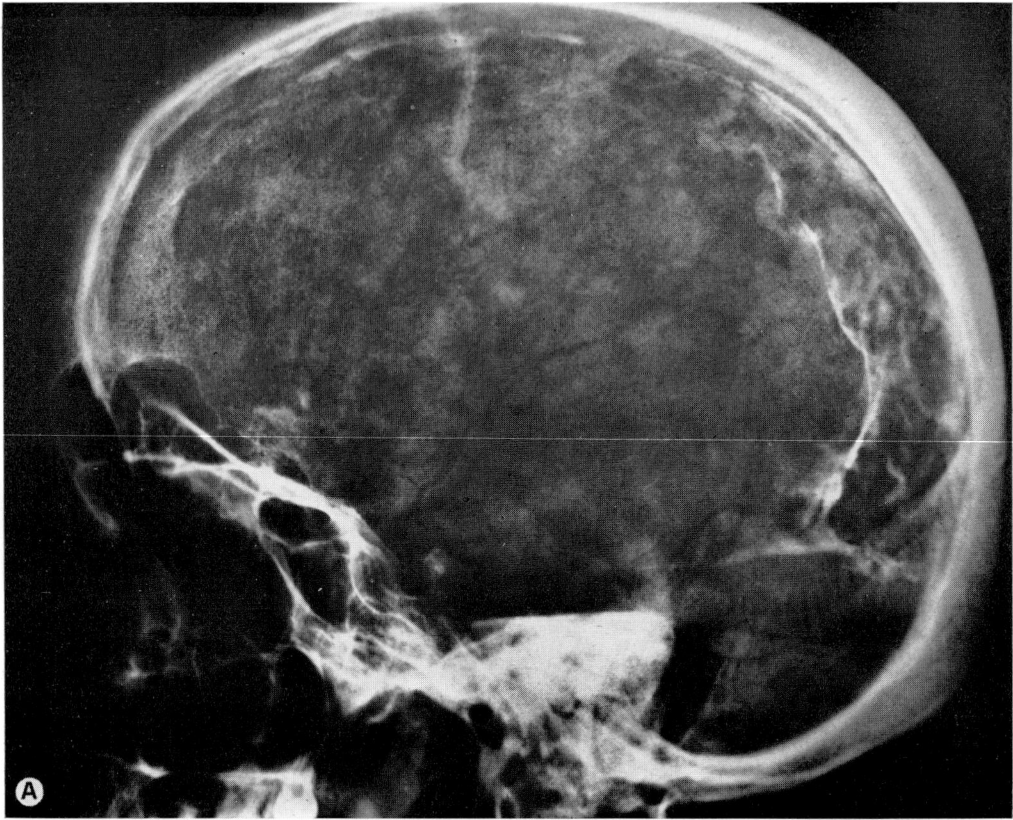

Fig. 157.—Calcified Subdural and Epidural Hematomas

Subdural hematomas of long standing may exhibit calcification, predominantly in the membranous capsule of a lesion. In some areas, irregular calcification may be present throughout the organized hematoma, as shown posteriorly (A). Epidural hematomas also may be found to contain calcium. In the case shown (B), the calcification was discovered two years after a ventriculogram. The ventricles were very large at the time of the initial examination, and the frontal portion of the brain apparently collapsed after removal of a large amount of fluid, causing epidural hemorrhage.

internal carotid arteries (fig. 161), since the cavernous portion of the carotid artery is below the level of the clinoids.

Membranous calcifications often causing difficulty in diagnosis are the solitary or multiple scattered *dural plaques*, and the calcified *arachnoid granulations*. The dural plaques are thin, flat, dense calcifications, and were observed by Dyke (1941) to be present in 5 per cent of adult patients. The calcified arachnoid granulations are rounded and usually 3 to 4 mm. in diameter. They most frequently are found parasagittally along the superior longitudinal sinus. Any of the arachnoid granulations within the cranium may exhibit calcification. When they are removed from the midline and isolated, however, they may be difficult to distinguish from small tumors.

Subdural hematoma. A subdural hematoma of very long standing, at least several years, may exhibit calcification and even ossification. As time passes, a hematoma may undergo organization and calcium may become visible in the degenerating connective tissue. Curvilinear calcium deposits that parallel the contour of the cranial vault may be seen in both the inner and outer mem-

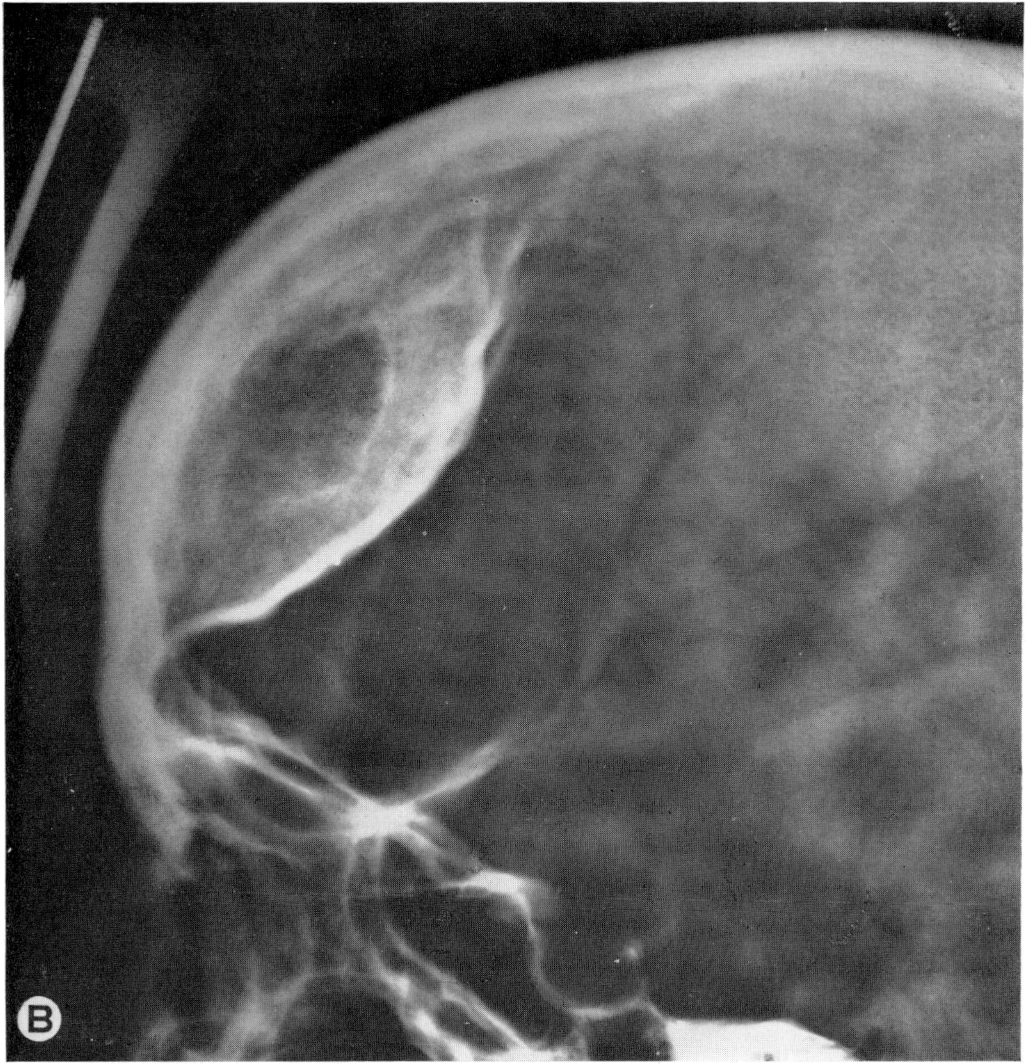

Fig. 157

branes of the hematoma (fig. 157). Between the smooth calcium lines representing the membranes, irregular plaques of calcium may be deposited. Very large hematomas may dissect along the superior surface of the tentorium where similar calcification may be visible. Calcified hematomas may be bilateral as well as unilateral.

It is expected that calcified subdural hematomas will be seen rarely in the future. The more prompt and thorough attention given head injuries under modern management should greatly reduce the number of overlooked and neglected cases. In the past, these patients usually were seen because of post-traumatic degenerative cerebral changes. Occasionally, radiologic evidence of cerebral atrophy accompanying calcified subdural hematoma that resulted from injury early in life is seen as hemicranial hypertrophy of the bones of the vault and of the paranasal and mastoid sinuses (fig. 616).

Subdural or extradural hemorrhage may result from sudden decompression of greatly dilated ventricles during ventriculography. Delicate meningeal vessels may be torn by collapse of ventricles and cerebral tissue that previously had been under the pressure of internal hydrocephalus. Such a hematoma may go unrecognized because of pre-existing neurologic abnormalities. The hematoma may become organized and calcified in the same way as a hematoma resulting from external trauma (figs. 604 and 606).

Meningiomas. Because of the calcareous deposits present in many meningiomas, Virchow assigned to them the name "psammomas." Meningiomas are of several types, and it is the fibrous tumor that has a very heavy connective tissue stroma in which psammoma bodies are found to a marked extent. Meningiomas constitute up to one-fifth of all intracranial tumors, and in a very high percentage of cases they may be diagnosed from plain roentgenograms. Meningiomas indicate their presence by hyperostosis, increased vascularity, and other effects on the bony skull, and frequently, sufficient calcium is present in a tumor to make it visible in plain skull films. In some instances, a psammomatous meningioma may be outlined in its entirety by calcium (fig. 146). The calcium is laid down in fine flecks in the whorls of the tumor and the many thousands of small deposits of calcium may produce a cloudlike shadow of increased density in the roentgenogram.

Meningiomas have several sites of predisposition (fig. 135), but fibrous tumors in any location may be psammomatous. Generally, the tumors are global and they may be centrally calcified, peripherally calcified, or exhibit diffuse homogeneous calcific density. Occasionally, the center is dense while the peripheral portion gradually becomes reduced in density, and radiating calcified spicules may be present at the margins.

The visible calcification in a psammomatous meningioma usually gives an indication of the size of the tumor. The pathologic specimen may be identical in size and form to the shadow of pathologic calcification visible in the roentgenogram (figs. 146 and 148). The size of a tumor manifesting itself by hyperostosis, on the other hand, is impossible to predict, unless secondary changes of an intracranial mass are present.

Tuberculous meningitis. In children who recover from tuberculous meningitis there is a very high incidence of intracranial calcification, approaching 50 per cent, according to Lorber (1958). The incidence has increased greatly since the introduction of effective antituberculous drugs. The calcification is more common in the basal meninges than in the cerebral substance, although occasionally it occurs in both places. The lime salts are deposited in the meningeal exudate covering the base of the brain, most often above the sella turcica.

In a sizable group of patients studied by Lorber, the calcification became visible in roentgenograms between 15 months and 3 years after recovery from the disease. The calcification may consist of a single small granule, but in the majority of patients clusters of calcium shadows are present. The deposits may appear ringlike or as a conglomerate mass. The location of the calcification in the interpeduncular and chiasmatic cisterns is characteristic, but when extensive, a calcific collar may be found encircling the midbrain. Without adequate clinical information, the finding of suprasellar calcification in a blind child may at first suggest a craniopharyngioma. A normal-appearing sella turcica and the absence of increased intracranial pressure at this stage of the disease process are helpful in arriving at the correct diagnosis.

Calcification of the Hypophysial Region

The differentiation of the various calcifications occurring in and about the sella turcica is a frequent problem of radiologic diagnosis, as just noted in connection with the deposits of healed tuberculous meningitis. The nature and extent of symptoms and signs produced by a variety of lesions in this area may be very similar, predominantly visual, endocrine, and hypothalamic. Radiologic examintion often is the most definitive preopera-

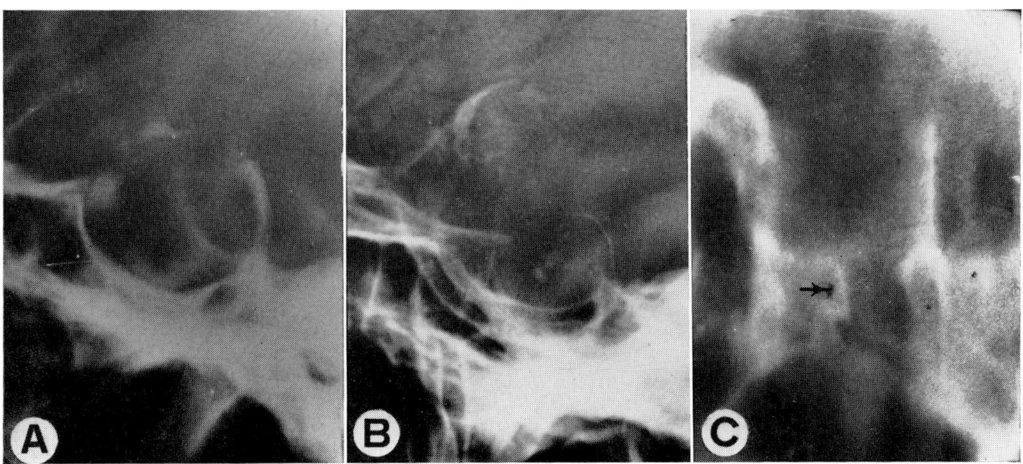

FIG. 158.—CRANIOPHARYNGIOMA

Craniopharyngiomas of the solid type may be contained largely within the sella turcica, which usually is very large. Calcification may be found within the substance of the craniopharyngioma, inside of the pituitary fossa, or in the tumor capsule (A). With cystic craniopharyngioma, calcification is very common and may be found at a considerable distance above the sella turcica (B). The position of the calcium does not indicate the upward extent of a cystic craniopharyngioma and frequently the calcareous deposits are confined to the sella or immediately suprasellar regions. When the sella turcica is large, a persistent craniopharyngeal canal (*arrow*) should lead to the diagnosis of craniopharyngioma, even in the absence of calcification (C).

tive method of differentiating between the more common lesions of the hypophysial region. Even plain films often serve to identify parasellar tumors through recognizable differences in the nature of gross calcification and associated bony changes.

While the calcifications in and about the hypophysial area form a heterogeneous group, justification for considering them together and at this juncture may be found in the difficulty in identification experienced by many students of neuroradiology. The appearance of meningiomas and the calcification following basilar arachnoiditis have been described. Calcified aneurysms of the circle of Willis and calcified gliomas of the hypothalamic area will be described later in more detail but are to be considered in the differential diagnosis of calcified lesions of the hypophysial region. The true hypophysial calcifications occur owing to developmental abnormalities and neoplastic lesions of the pituitary gland itself. In addition, certain tumors of the basisphenoid which sometimes involve the hypophysis in their growth must be included among the diagnostic considerations.

Craniopharyngioma. The most common tumor to produce recognizable suprasellar calcification is the craniopharyngioma. While the tumor is most commonly encountered in childhood, the occurrence of craniopharyngioma later in life has been described more frequently in recent years and the authors have observed a typical example in a 67-year-old woman.

The craniopharyngioma arises in epithelial rests of the hypophysial duct, which takes its origin from the buccal epithelium of the embryo. A canal, the craniopharyngeal canal, is sometimes found normally extending from the hypophysial fossa to the under surface of the sphenoid bone and with craniopharyngioma, it may be large (fig. 158). The tumors of clinical significance are of two structural types. One is the small, usually walnut-sized solid tumor composed of simple squamous epithelium. These tumors almost always are

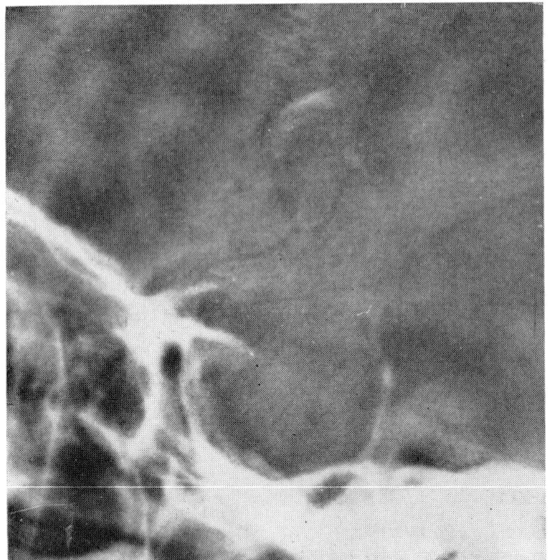

FIG. 159.—CALCIFIED PITUITARY ADENOMA

There is marked enlargement of the sella turcica in all directions, including depression of the floor into the sphenoid sinus and undercutting of the anterior clinoid processes. Calcification in the periphery of the adenoma is shown posteriorly and in its superior margin, 5 cm. above the sella turcica. There are no visible calcific deposits in the central portion of the tumor.

calcified (fig. 158). The second is the cystic type which may become very large and frequently involves the third ventricle in its upward extension (fig. 333). The latter cystic tumors are composed of columnar epithelium and because the cellular architectural arrangement comprises stellate forms that suggest the development of the enamel organ, they are called adamantinomas by some writers. The cyst walls are thick, being formed of dense connective tissue in which calcium usually is deposited in plaques.

Curvilinear calcium deposits are usually demonstrable along the superior extent of the mass and are said to occur in 70 to 80 per cent of patients. Any wall of the cyst may be calcified and calcium flecks may be visible in the central portion of the lesion. The solid lesions cause ballooning of the sella turcica and at the same time an increase in density of its walls. The *increased density* is in contrast to the sella enlargement of pituitary adenoma where thinning of the sellar boundaries occurs. In the cystic type of lesion there is often an elongated and shallow sella turcica with the clinoid processes and dorsum sellae most affected. Very small posterior clinoids and thin anterior clinoids with a well defined sella floor (except for the craniopharyngeal cleft) are findings favoring the diagnosis.

Pituitary adenoma. Gross degenerative changes in chromophobic pituitary adenomas are said to be unusual in any but very large tumors. The nutrition of these tumors is well maintained until they are massive, and the connective tissue is not abundant, usually being present only in thin strands. When calcification does occur in chromophobic adenomas, it may be found either in the central portion or in the wall of a cyst (fig. 159). In a study of 285 of Cushing's verified adenomas (1912 and 1932), Deery (1929) found calcium shadows within or just above the sella turcica in 7 per cent. No constant factors were found which might influence the development of calcium, such as the type of adenoma, the duration of disease, or the age of the patient.

Calcium in the capsule of the tumor may

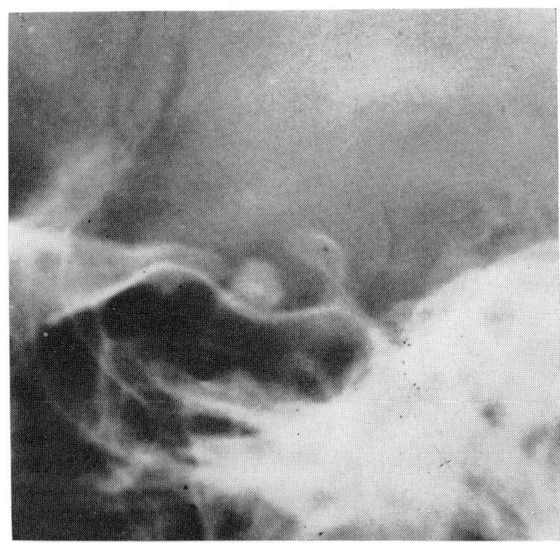

FIG. 160.—PITUITARY CALCULUS

Calcific deposits of sufficient size to be seen on radiographs may be found in the pituitary fossa in patients who have had a small pituitary adenoma which has become clinically inactive. The majority of such tumors are microscopic in size, and the calcification is not seen. Occasionally, small calcifications within the sella turcica may be demonstrated only by tomography.

(Revised 1963)

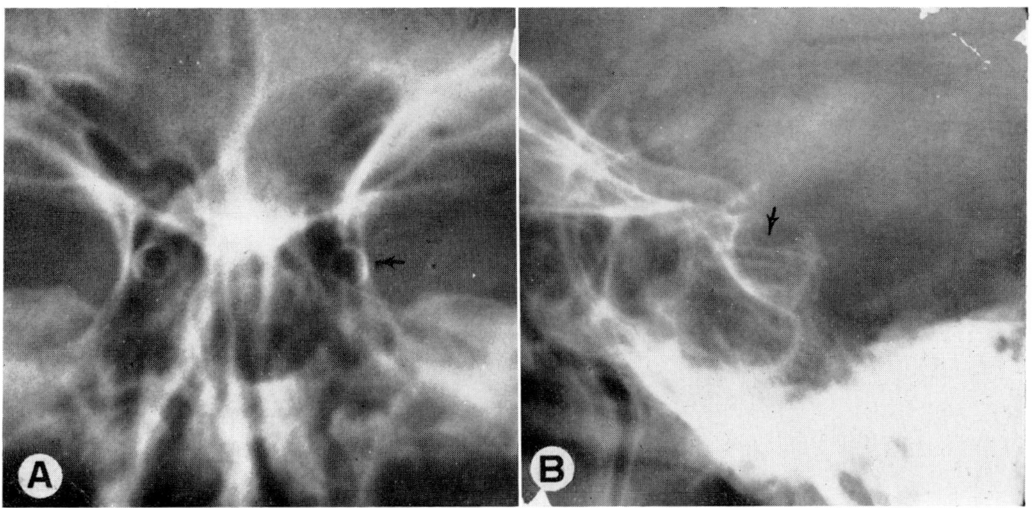

Fig. 161.—Carotid Artery Atherosclerosis

Calcification may be seen in the walls of the carotid artery when heavy deposits are present. In the frontal film (A), the shadows appear ringlike, as seen on end, in the cavernous segment of the artery (*arrow*). In the lateral film (B), the calcifications appear linear and parallel (*arrow*). Linear calcifications of simple degenerative vascular disease, not in aneurysms, usually are not projected above the level of the sella turcica. In some instances, extensive calcification may be seen spreading into the siphon and even into vascular branches.

extend well above the sella turcica in a conical form. The configuration is similar to the rather characteristic appearance of upward and forward extension of pituitary tumors found at pneumoencephalography (fig. 327). In the authors' experience, the incidence of calcification in pituitary adenoma is even less than that found by Deery. The presence of calcification may be misleading since it occurs so much more frequently in other lesions. The appearance of the sella turcica probably is the most helpful indication of the correct diagnosis.

Some investigators believe calcification is seen more commonly in the eosinophilic variety of adenoma, possibly because it grows more slowly (Courville, 1950). Spontaneous recession of small eosinophilic adenomas occurs frequently, and regressive changes occasionally are evident radiographically as calcareous deposits or bone formation within the sella turcica (fig. 160). The deposits have been called pituitary calculi.

Cranial tumor. Tumors arising from the base of the skull in the hypophysial region may produce bone or undergo calcification. Sizable *osteochondromas* may arise from the floor of the middle fossa. While more typically they destroy the skull base of the middle and posterior fossae and grow extracranially, a partially calcified intracranial mass may develop. The appearance resembles that of osteochondromas elsewhere with small islands of radiolucent cartilage remaining in a global or irregularly shaped mass. The margins may appear well defined but irregular. Other mesodermal tumors, such as *osteomas* and *fibromas*, may produce parasellar calcification. The sella turcica usually is intact and differentiation from sphenoid or middle fossa meningioma usually is more of a problem than confusion with hypophysial tumors.

Cranial chordomas characteristically arise in the clivus from the remnants of the rostral end of the fetal notochord. Clivus chordomas may extend into the sella turcica or a chordoma may arise within or anterior to the sella. Extensive sellar destruction may occur and calcium in varying amounts is found in the tumor in many instances (fig. 330). Some

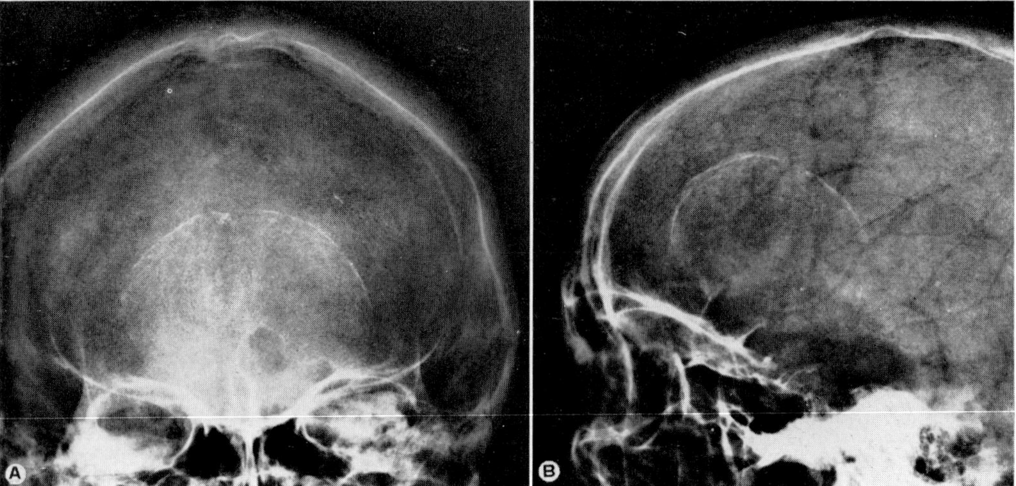

Fig. 162.—Calcified Subfrontal Aneurysm

A huge curvilinear calcium shadow is present which, in the frontal view (A), is seen to be centered in the midline above the olfactory groove. In the lateral view (B), the forward extent of the lesion in the inferior frontal area is well shown. The patient died suddenly several months after the films were made, presumably of rupture of the aneurysm.

of the visible calcium densities are the result of the inclusion of invaded sequestrated bone within the mass, while others result from true calcific degeneration in the tumor. Large numbers of tiny calcium shadows may be present in some chordomas, giving an indication of the size of the tumor from plain films. Bone destruction rather than new bone formation or calcification, however, is the most characteristic feature of chordoma and serves to differentiate it from sphenoid meningioma and other benign calcifying lesions of the hypophysial area.

Vascular Calcification

Arteriosclerosis or, more strictly speaking, *atherosclerosis*, is the cause of visible vascular calcification in many aging patients; it may be seen early in life secondary to other disease or even as a primary process. Lime salts readily accumulate in the fatty material deposited in the intima. The cerebral vessels are among those most commonly affected by atherosclerosis. Of the several major vessels usually involved, the calcium deposits are most easily seen in the cavernous portion of the carotid arteries where these vessels are projected through thin bone and air sinuses. In frontal view, the carotid artery appears ringlike as seen end on through the ethmoid areas (fig. 161). The lateral projection reveals the calcified vessels as transverse linear streaks superimposed upon the sella turcica or sphenoid sinus. Transverse linear or vertically convex calcium shadows extending above the level of the clinoid processes usually indicate aneurysmal dilatation of the artery. Vertically linear calcium deposits may extend upward above the anterior clinoid processes in cases of extensive arteriosclerosis and even may be observed to arborize into the usual anterior and middle cerebral arterial patterns. Basilar artery changes, while very common, are not readily seen because of the overlying dense petrous portions of the temporal bones.

Arterial aneurysms. The majority of arterial aneurysms result from a congenital weakness of the vessel wall, usually a deficiency of muscular tissue in the media. The elastic membrane of the intimal coat may be present or absent. As compared with vessels in other parts of the body, the cerebral arteries have extremely thin walls in proportion to their size, the difference depending on thinness of the external and middle vas-

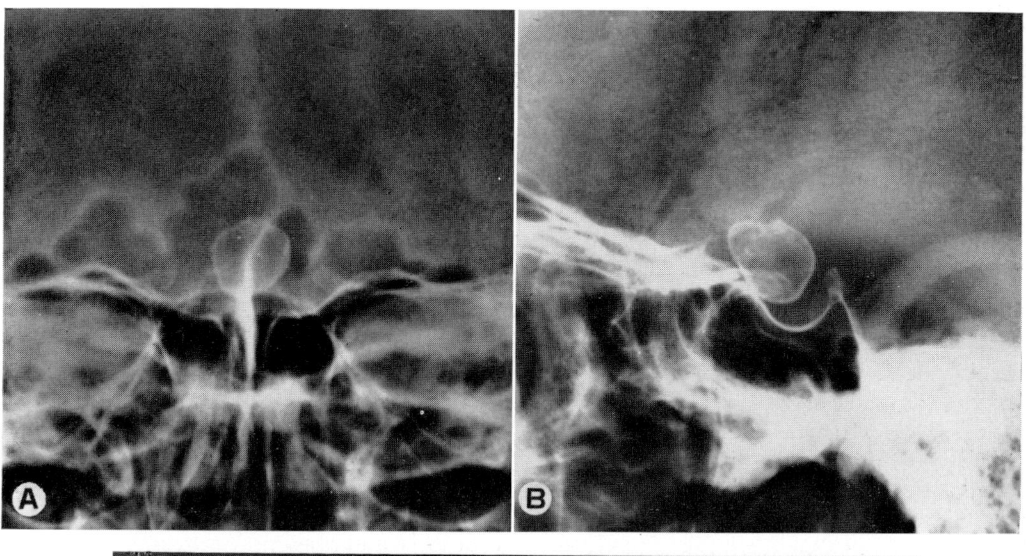

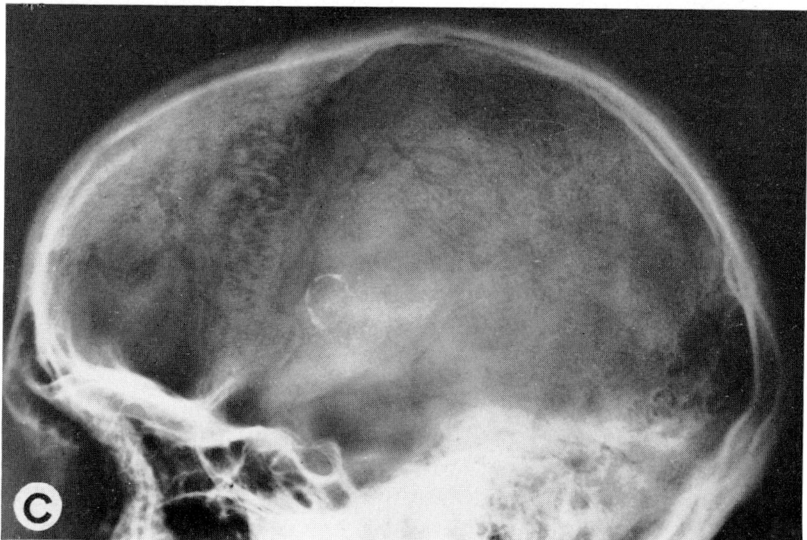

FIG. 163.—CALCIFIED SUPRASELLAR ANEURYSM

The ringlike calcified wall of an aneurysm resting on the dorsum sellae is present, and the lateral view (B) shows that the posterior-inferior margin of the lesion projects into the pituitary fossa. The frontal film (A) shows the precise midline location of the aneurysm. In another case (C), the incompletely calcified wall of an aneurysm of the middle cerebral artery is shown.

cular coats (Courville, 1950). This may play an important part in the high incidence of cerebral aneurysms. Most often the muscular coat deficiencies are at the bifurcation of larger vessels. In the majority of cases, only one aneurysm is found, although it is not unusual for them to be multiple.

The congenital arterial aneurysms usually undergo progressive development. In time, the force of the blood pressure on the point of weakness results in distention and the formation of a sac, the walls of which are made up of intima and adventitia, with little or no media. The wall of the aneurysm may become tissue paper thin, and this may lead to rupture. The sizes of aneurysms vary

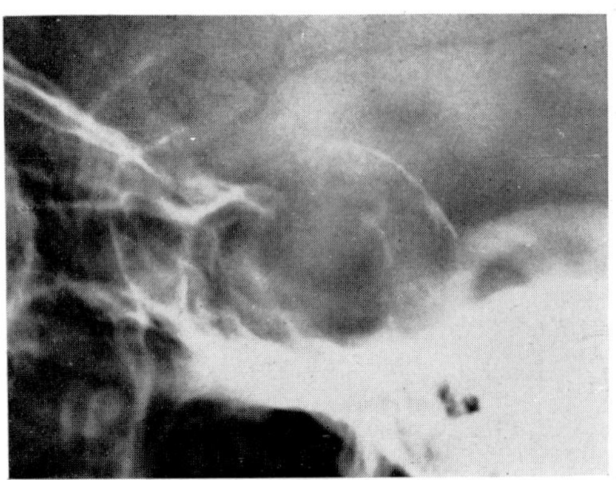

FIG. 164.—ANEURYSM OF THE INTERNAL CAROTID ARTERY

Calcification has occurred in the wall of a partially thrombosed aneurysm of the cavernous portion of an internal carotid artery. The curvilinear calcific line, located in the dome of the aneurysm wall, extends well above the level of the sella turcica. In addition, there is extensive erosion of the sella, including its clinoid processes, more marked on the side of the lesion.

considerably from those that are very small to those that occupy appreciable space and behave like tumors (fig. 162).

Atherosclerosis develops frequently in the intima of the aneurysmal sac, and it is through this process that the curvilinear calcification visible in radiographs develops (fig. 164). The calcium lines occurring in aneurysms are smoother and thinner than are found in tumors, and their ringlike or shell-like configuration affords ready identification (fig. 163). In the majority of cases, when calcification is present the aneurysm is partially thrombosed and sometimes completely so (fig. 164).

Aneurysms of the cerebral arteries also may be of the mycotic (inflammatory) type, fusiform (atherosclerotic) or dissecting (owing to arterial trauma). By far the most common type of aneurysm encountered is the saccular or congenital arterial aneurysm with the fusiform aneurysm of atherosclerosis next most common. The basilar artery is particularly inclined to the development of a fusiform type of pathologic change.

Calcified arterial aneurysms most often are found along the course of the internal carotid artery and on the circle of Willis. They may, however, be found arising from any cerebral vessel and are not unusual along the course of the middle cerebral artery (fig. 163). An aneurysm of the carotid artery, particularly of the cavernous portion, often produces erosion of the sella turcica which frequently is unilateral (Sosman and Vogt, 1926). Either the posterior or anterior clinoids or the sellar floor may be more affected, depending upon the location and size of the lesion (fig. 164). Other basal structures including the basal foramina may exhibit erosion. Whenever an aneurysm is considered a possible explanation for an intracranial curvilinear, partial or complete ringlike or shell-like calcium deposit, an angiogram should be carried out before any major procedure is undertaken. With unilateral sella turcica erosion, even without curvilinear parasellar calcification, angiography would be the first step toward establishing a definitive diagnosis.

The soft tissue calcification designated *metastatic calcification* by Virchow occurs not only in severe hyperparathyroidism but in any condition in which the serum contains excessive amounts of calcium and phosphorus, particularly chronic renal insufficiency, vitamin D poisoning and metastatic diseases of the bones (Albright and Reifenstein, 1948). The precipitation of calcium is apt to occur wherever there is localized alkalosis, especially in organs excreting acid, such as the lungs, the stomach, and the kidneys. Calcium salts also may be deposited in the internal elastic membrane of the intimal layer of the arteries. Predisposing intimal disease is not necessary for the deposition of lime salts in hyperparathyroidism. It is of interest that the arteries are prone to develop calcification on the basis of high blood calcium levels while calcification within the cerebral substance is facilitated by elevation of the interstitial rather than the serum calcium (figs. 165 and 178).

Cerebral vascular malformations. Vascular malformations of the face and scalp are common, and occasionally such a change may be associated with a cerebral malformation, as in the Sturge-Weber syndrome

(Revised 1963)

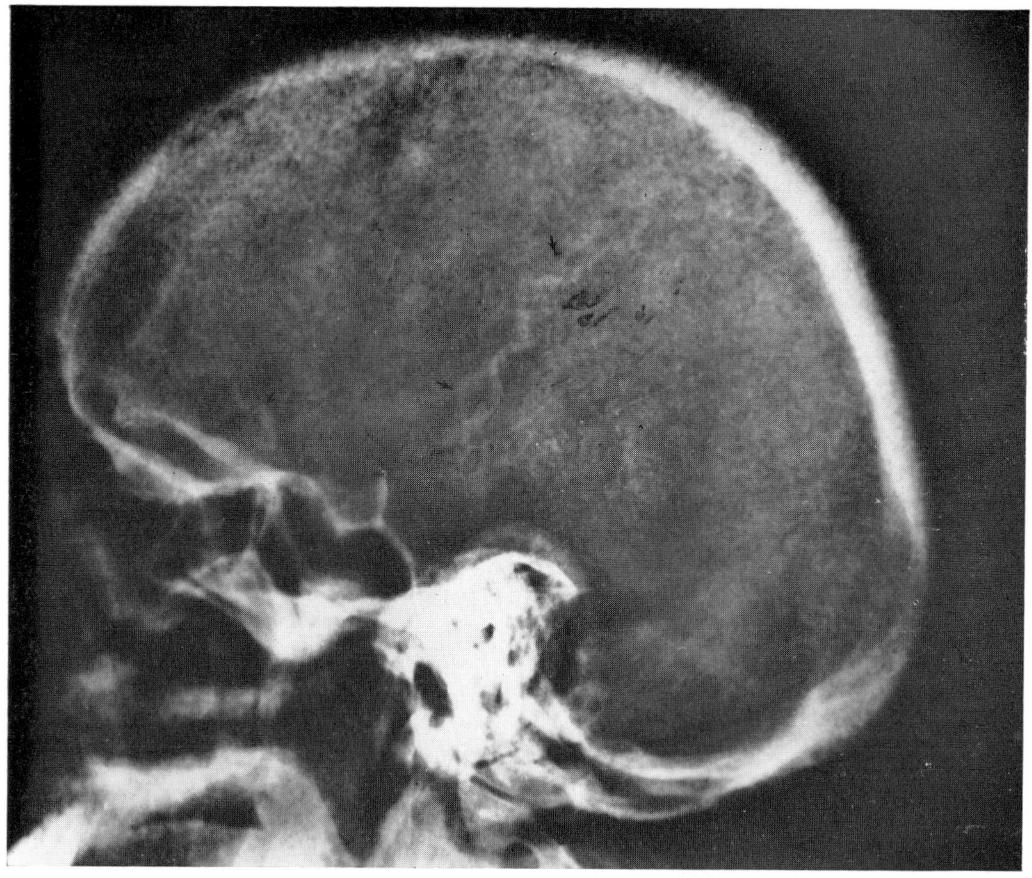

FIG. 165.—METASTATIC VASCULAR CALCIFICATION

In a case of hyperparathyroidism, rather extensive calcification has occurred in the vessels of the head, including smaller branches of both the internal and external carotid systems. The course of many vessels can be traced (*arrows*) owing to the deposition of calcium in normal vessels and also because of decalcification of the superimposed osseous structures. In the parietotemporal region, a broad area of slightly increased density is present, suggesting early plaque-like deposition of calcium which sometimes is seen in the early healing stage of the disease, following treatment.

(encephalotrigeminal angiomatosis). The clinical features of this syndrome are variable but include a convulsive state, a dermal nevus, mental retardation, glaucoma, and hemiplegia. The fundamental cerebral lesion is a *venous angioma* of the leptomeninges which is thought to result in faulty cerebral circulation. Numerous venous rather than arterial or capillary channels comprise the angiomatous malformations of the pia. The abnormal veins do not extend into the cerebral substance. Numerous intracerebral capillaries, however, appear to be a part of the pathologic process. Vascular changes of fibrosis, hyaline degeneration, and calcification occur. Concomitantly, there is a loss of underlying brain cells, gliosis, and the deposition of calcium in the parenchyma of the cortex (Yakovlev and Guthrie, 1931).

The underlying cortex usually exhibits several concentric layers of calcification in both the gray and white matter. The outer zones contain coarse, closely packed calcium granules which obliterate cortical architecture while in the deeper zones, finer deposits are loosely distributed among areas of relatively normal brain. The parenchymatous degeneration and gliosis providing the foun-

(Revised 1963)

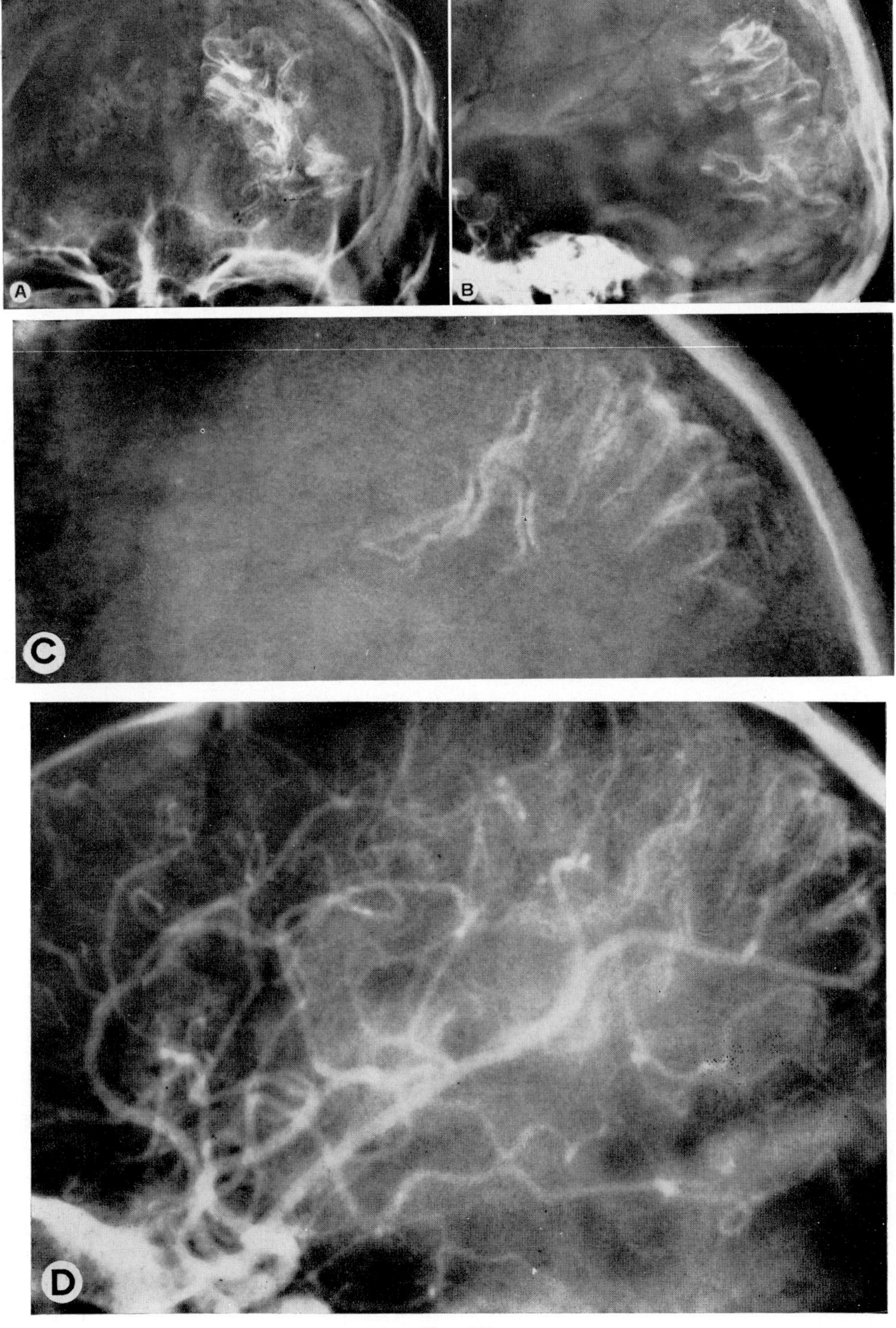

Fig. 166

(*Revised 1963*)

dation for the calcification is thought to result from capillary stagnation caused by the pial angiomatosis (Peterman *et al.*, 1958). Radiologic evidence of very large areas of calcification may be found in approximately two-thirds of patients. Usually the calcium deposits are situated at the occipital pole of the brain, although frontal pole lesions do occur. The calcification characteristically is disposed in parallel linear, serpentine, or convoluted configurations. Usually, the outline of contracted convolutions and narrow sulci are easily recognized (fig. 166). Extensive localized or generalized cerebral hypoplasia or atrophy often is present. The cortical calcification may be observed well away from the inner table of the skull, and large overlying subarachnoid fluid spaces may be outlined by gas at pneumography. The calcification along the medial surface of the cortex often will show that the superior longitudinal sulcus is not in the midline, but displaced in the direction of the lesion. Compensatory hemicranial hyperplasia may be present on the ipsilateral side and convolutional markings may be reduced or absent.

Angiography has been found to reveal vascular lesions in approximately one-half of the patients examined (Taveras and Poser, 1959). In addition to the venous angiomas, thrombotic lesions, anomalies of the dural sinuses, and arteriovenous malformations were found. Angiography will demonstrate the angiomas before calcification occurs and should be carried out in suspected cases of encephalotrigeminal angiomatosis, especially if surgical excision is contemplated.

Venous angiomas also may take the form of a simple varix or single dilated vein; of a serpentine angioma, consisting of a dilatation and tortuosity of one or more large veins; or of a complex racemose angioma. Single linear calcium deposits may be visible radiologically in some of these lesions, and this radiologic finding may be the only clue to the cause of the patient's symptoms, which is often epilepsy.

Arteriovenous malformations or angiomas may exhibit somewhat similar linear calcium shadows, sometimes parallel, or a large number of small punctate calcifications having a lacelike appearance. The former type of calcification may be in blood vessels while the latter usually is in adjacent atrophic brain. Differentiation from calcification occurring with venous angioma can be made in some cases by the presence of deep channels in the bone caused by associated dilatation of meningeal vessels. These wide, elongated, tortuous bony vascular channels result from an arteriovenous shunt, producing increased venous pressure and increased blood flow. Other arteriovenous malformations may contain sacculations with curvilinear or ringlike mural calcification (fig. 316). Associated with the shell-like calcification, and extending some distance from it, stippled deposits also may be present, suggesting the true nature of the vascular lesion. The amount of calcium discernible radiologically in no way suggests the size of the vascular malformation, but angiography readily will demonstrate its extent.

Localized Intracerebral Calcification

Physiologic calcifications. The *pineal gland* is the most common intracranial structure to calcify sufficiently to be visible in roentgenograms. The calcified pineal is visible in the skull films of more than 50 per cent

Fig. 166.—Meningeal Angiomatosis

As a result of vascular malformations in the meninges and superficial portions of the cortex, such as the Sturge-Weber syndrome, degeneration of neural tissue with calcification may occur in the cortical layers beneath the cerebral surface. The calcification frequently has a convoluted configuration. Evidence of more deep-seated atrophy also is shown, with the medial margin of the convoluted calcification situated well to the left of the midline of the cranial cavity (A). In the lateral view (B), the calcification shows that the cerebral surface has fallen away from the inner table of the skull in the posterior parietal region, a distance of 2 cm. In another case (C), the extent of calcific degeneration is shown. In spite of the large appearance of the artery (D), an angioma did not fill. The straightening of the vessel conceivably could be the result of ventricular enlargement due to atrophy with porencephaly.

(Revised 1963)

of patients of all ages. Regressive changes in the pineal body begin early in life and calcification occurs in its connective tissue stroma. The changes, which are evident in the form of calcareous deposits, occur not only with increasing frequency but in increased amount after the age of 20 years.

The calcifications seen in the pineal may be small punctate shadows or the entire gland may be replaced by hyalinized and calcified connective tissue. Usually, the calcification is ovoid with the long axis in the sagittal plane of the skull, measuring up to 1 cm. in length and 0.5 cm. in width. Occasionally, the regressive changes may take the form of cyst formation, and the capsule of the pineal may encompass a body of clear fluid. Calcification in the capsule of such cysts explains the occasional spherical or ringlike form of calcification of the pineal.

The calcified pineal body is a structure of great utility since normally it is situated in the midline, and lateral dislocation results frequently when brain tumors are present. Displacement of the pineal gland in radiographs as a finding of lateralizing significance in the presence of brain tumor was first described by Schüller (1912). Several methods for determining pineal displacement in the sagittal plane have been described. It must be appreciated also that a normally placed pineal may be a very useful negative finding in neurologic diagnosis. See page 1.27.

Habenular calcification was described by Stauffer, Snow, and Adams (1953) as an entity distinct from calcification of the pineal body. The calcification does not occur in the habenular commissure itself, but in the hindmost portion of the tela chorioidea of the third ventricle, which is attached at its posterior limit to the habenular commissure. The shadow is produced by the aggregation of myriads of psammoma bodies as occurs with chorioid calcification elsewhere. When seen in lateral radiographs, habenular calcification takes the shape of the letter C and can be seen to be distinctly separate from the pineal shadow. The attachment of the chorioid to the habenular commissure and its position as a cap over the anterior surface of this structure explains the characteristic configuration. The term habenular calcification is recommended for convenience, even though the calcium is not in, but anterior to, the habenular commissure.

Habenular calcification occurs almost as frequently as calcification in the pineal body. In 20 per cent of patients, visible habenular calcification is present without the pineal being discernible in lateral radiographs. The clinical importance of habenular calcification is that isolated deposits may lie at or forward of the anterior limits of the normal pineal position in the sagittal plane according to localizing charts and devices and be mistaken for a displaced pineal.

Slightly more than 10 per cent of patients of all ages exhibit calcification in the *chorioid plexus*, and the percentage is greatly increased if patients below the age of 20 years are excluded. The calcification occurs through a process of proliferation of cells of the pia arachnoid, followed by the formation of dense collagenous and fibrous reticular networks in which calcium salts are deposited. In radiographs, the calcium deposits usually appear as a collection of punctate calcific shadows, which may vary from a small visible fleck to an aggregate over 1 cm. in diameter. In other instances, the calcification may appear linear, crescentic, or ringlike, or it may be an irregular amorphous solid mass of calcium. The large calcific aggregates have been described as resembling a popped kernel of corn. The shell-like calcifications are associated with chorioid cysts, which are common.

Some degree of asymmetry of chorioid calcification is common, and it may be unilateral. Malbin (1948) and others have described mobile chorioid plexus calcification which changes position with a change of posture, and therefore even chorioid glomus calcium deposits may not be symmetrical. Psammomatous calcification may occur in the chorioid plexus at points other than in the glomus and the habenular area, and occasionally these deposits may gain sufficient size to be visible as solitary intracerebral calcifications (Wood, 1944). These aberrant calcium shadows may be seen anywhere along the course of the chorioid plexus in the

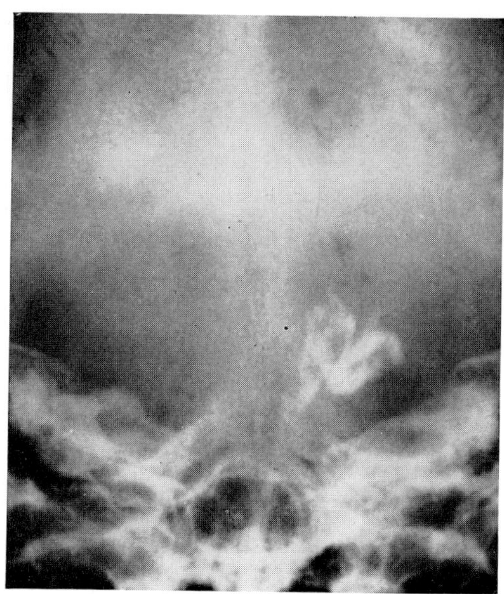

Fig. 167.—Calcified Brain Abscess

A well defined but irregular calcium shadow is present, which presumably is the inert residue of an abscess of mastoid origin that had occurred many years prior to the radiographic examination. The exact type of infection responsible for such lesions usually cannot be determined even histologically because of the extensive calcification and nonspecific nature of the inert residue.

lateral ventricles, but they are most common near the foramen of Monro. Calcification may occur in the tela chorioidea of the 3d ventricle or in the chorioid plexus in the roof of the 4th ventricle.

Inflammatory calcifications. Intracranial calcification produced by *brain abscess* occurs much less frequently today than in the past. The calcification is the end result of the disease process and does not occur during the active stage. Approximately one-half of all brain abscesses are the result of metastatic septic emboli from a distant focus, usually either the lungs or the heart, and, under these circumstances, they often are multiple. More than one-third of brain abscesses result from mastoiditis and sinusitis. Otogenous brain abscesses usually are of the adjacent type and occur with approximately equal frequency in the temporal lobe and the cerebellum. Calcific deposits found unexpectedly in these areas often are residues of abscesses that have been well handled. The abscesses develop capsules consisting of layers of connective tissue of varying thickness and density which are formed from the adventitia of regional blood vessels (Courville, 1950). If the abscess is evacuated or heals spontaneously, the focus is reduced to a contractile scar which in time becomes hyalinized and calcified.

A calcified brain abscess has no characteristic form. Often the calcium is quite dense, and the margins of the lesions well defined (fig. 167). Irregular central radiolucent areas may be present. Usually, the lesions do not exceed 1 to 2 cm. in diameter. Their temporal or cerebellar location adjacent to an abnormal mastoid and the absence of increased intracranial pressure to suggest tumor are good clues to the correct diagnosis.

The most common *granulomatous infection* to result in intracranial calcification is tuberculosis. Over 60 per cent of tuberculomas are multiple, and these often are associated with tuberculous meningitis. The single tuberculoma may be large and act like a tumor. They occur most frequently in children and in adolescents, and in these younger age groups are seen more often in the cerebellum. Tuberculomas are common in Indians and in other persons of low racial resistance to tuberculosis.

Tuberculomas of the brain exhibit a typical reaction at their margins consisting of epithelioid cells, lymphocytes, plasma cells, and tuberculosis giant cells. In the center of the lesion there is usually a structureless area, not caseated as in lymph nodes but instead a dense fibrotic reaction with hyalinization occurs. The majority of tuberculomas do not develop calcification visible in radiographs. In some cases, however, a well developed capsule may form, limiting the lesion. Calcium first is laid down in the central hyalinized area and in the capsule, and eventually the lesion may become calcified in its entirety (fig. 168). As with pyogenic abscess, the calcified tuberculoma has no characteristic form. The calcium deposits often are heavy, and at the time calcification of the tuberculoma becomes visible, there is no evidence of an expanding intracranial

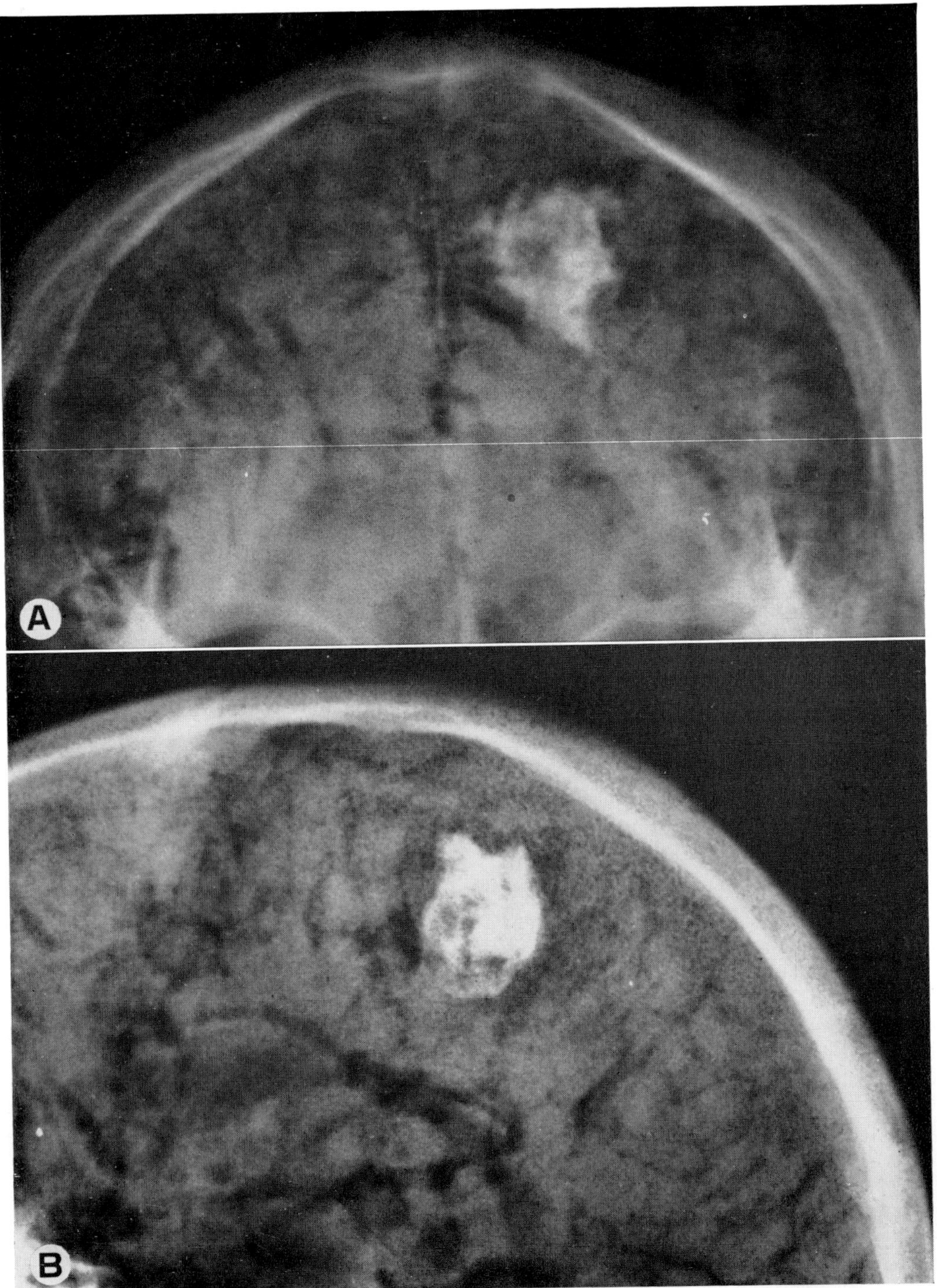

FIG. 168.—CALCIFIED TUBERCULOMA

A well defined calcium deposit measuring 2 cm. in diameter was found in the parasagittal portion of the anterior parietal lobe. The frontal pneumogram (A) shows subarachnoid gas outlining a number of wide, deep sulci in the neighborhood of the lesion, and there is no evidence that the mass occupies a greater volume than is denoted by the calcified portion. Several prominent sulci are shown in the lateral view (B) anterior to the calcified lesion. The lesion occurred in a Hopi Indian who had convulsions. (Courtesy of Dr. Walter Hileman, Tucson, Arizona.)

(Revised 1963)

process. Figure 168 illustrates localized cerebral atrophy around the calcified contracted residue of a solitary tuberculoma.

A number of other lesions may result in the formation of granulomatous masses within the cerebral substance, but their incidence is lower than the occurrence of tuberculomas. *Sarcoidosis* involving the central nervous system is being reported with increasing frequency. The *gumma* is one of the least common intracranial tumors found today. It is a focal periarterial granulomatous formation which develops into a local growth and may be of any size. The structure of the gumma includes a heavy overgrowth of connective tissue. Usually, it is not possible definitely to differentiate gumma from tuberculoma by pathologic methods. Among rare granulomas are included also the cerebral lesions of actinomycosis, coccidioidomycosis, torulosis, and other fungus diseases.

Hemorrhagic calcification. Unidentified solitary intracerebral calcifications often are labeled as being the end result of *intracerebral hemorrhage*. The exact nature of some lime deposits can never be determined, even at the time of microscopic examination, since they are amorphous masses that have no distinguishing features. A study of the pathologic processes occurring with intracerebral bleeding suggests that calcification should not occur frequently. Gross intracerebral hemorrhage, which the patient survives, ultimately undergoes resolution, and with its disappearance the cavity becomes smaller through the restoration of marginal brain architecture, the disappearance of edema, and ventricular enlargement. A capsule usually does not develop about an intracerebral hematoma, and for this reason a gross connective tissue scar is not the common end result of the lesion, as is the case with abscess. Nevertheless, it is quite possible that intracerebral calcification may, in some instances, be the result of old hemorrhage. A well established instance was reported by Grantham and Smolik (1942) in which a sizable rounded homogeneously calcified mass developed in one cerebral hemisphere in connection with a hemorrhagic event. The authors have encountered several cases in which prior intracerebral hemorrhage was the only logical explanation for the presence of a calcific lesion. The calcifications are most often amorphous deposits with irregular but well defined margins. Their size varies from very small to several centimeters; the usual size that we have encountered is 1 to 2 cm. When such a calcification occurs in the basal ganglia, it is not easily confused with the multiple symmetrical calcifications of hypoparathyroidism (Mascherpa and Valentino, 1959). The frequent occurrence of multiple small hemorrhages following needle puncture for ventriculography has been emphasized by Lindgren (1954).

Tumors of the brain. In discussing *gliomas* in this section, it is obvious that we consider the multiple calcific foci of tumors, whether fused or unfused, as a solitary aggregate or localized collection of calcification. Occasionally, a sizable tumor will exhibit only one small fleck of calcium, but, more often, multiple calcifications are clustered together in a mass.

Vascular occlusion and thrombosis are the causes of degenerative changes in the central portions of gliomas. Regressive and necrotic changes are due almost exclusively to progressive impairment of the tumor blood supply. Slow restriction of the blood supply produces central cystic and calcific changes. Rapidly growing tumors cause hemorrhage through invasion of blood vessels, and the more malignant tumors also attack larger blood vessels with resultant brain softening.

The glioma group, which comprises approximately 50 per cent of all brain tumors, exhibits significant amounts of calcification on microscopic examination in one-third of instances (Weed, 1914). Roentgenographic evidence of calcification can be found in approximately 10 per cent of patients with gliomas (Sosman, 1927), and even higher occurrences have been described. The careful study of stereoscopic roentgenograms unquestionably facilitates detection of tumor calcification and results in a higher accuracy of diagnosis of these lesions.

Of the glioma series, *oligodendroglioma* shows the highest incidence of gross calci-

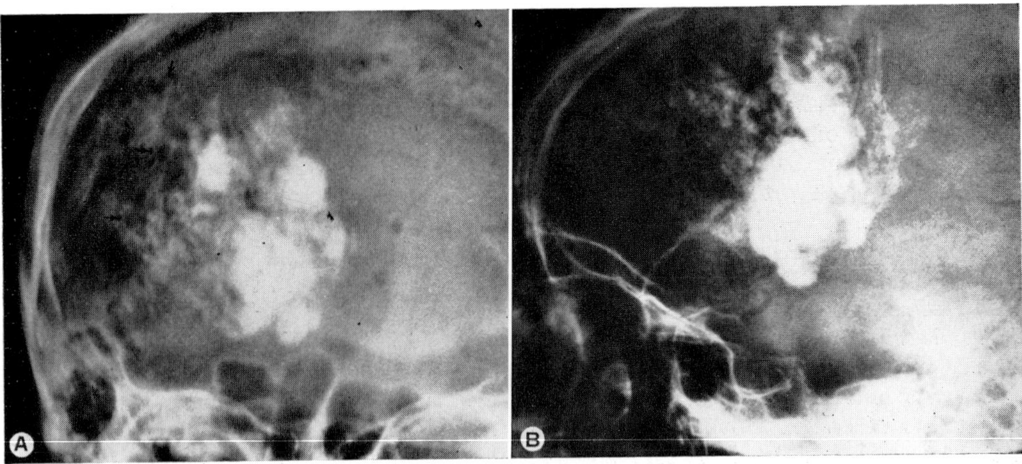

FIG. 169.—CALCIFIED OLIGODENDROGLIOMA

A very large calcified tumor is present in the right frontal lobe with some portions of the tumor exhibiting unusually dense masses. The lateral view (B) shows numerous strandlike anterior calcific extensions as far as the inner table of the skull. The frontal film (A) shows local pressure erosion of the inner table of the skull overlying the tumor. Numerous rounded osteolytic areas are present (*arrows*) which simulate those shown in Fig. 66, which resulted from thinning of the dura and herniation of brain into the bone.

fication (fig. 169). This is a tumor of the deep central white matter of the cerebrum of adults. The tumor is very cellular but relatively slowly growing. Its intercellular material is made up of strands of connective tissue and processes of tumor cells. The incidence of calcification may be more than 50 per cent.

Astrocytomas may contain radiologically visible calcification in 20 to 25 per cent of instances, since the tumor has a tendency to undergo calcific as well as cystic degeneration (fig. 170). In the central part of the tumor, calcareous deposits frequently are found in vessel walls as well as in fibrosed necrotic tumor substance. Although astrocytomas calcify less frequently than oligodendrogliomas, the astrocytoma is the leading cause of gliomatous calcification, since astrocytoma is by far the more common tumor. Mixtures of glial cells occur frequently in these slowly growing tumors, and preoperative differentiation of predominant cell type in calcified gliomas usually cannot be made.

Ependymomas exhibit calcification much less frequently than astrocytomas and oligodendrogliomas. Ependymomas arising in the lateral ventricles or cerebral white matter apparently have a great tendency toward cystic and calcareous change. Evidence has been collected that in young persons, large tumors of the frontal areas containing small

FIG. 170.—CALCIFIED GLIOMA

Irregular linear calcific shadows are present, projected through the parietotemporal portion of the skull in the first examination (A). The scattered linear deposits, varying in width, length, density, and direction, but grouped, are those usually associated with the calcification occurring in astrocytoma. Because of other disease, intracranial surgery could not be carried out, but a tumor dose of 3000 roentgens was delivered to the tumor by means of orthovoltage equipment. Examination one year later revealed the over-all area of the calcification to be smaller. Closer grouping of the calcifications is evident; the two prominent oblique deposits projected through the midparietal region were separated by 5 cm. at the first examination and by 3 cm. at the second examination. In addition, some of the inferior deposits appeared to be situated at a higher level. Some increase in the number and extent of the calcium deposits has occurred, indicating further tumor degeneration under therapy. The patient's clinical response paralleled the improvement indicated by the films.

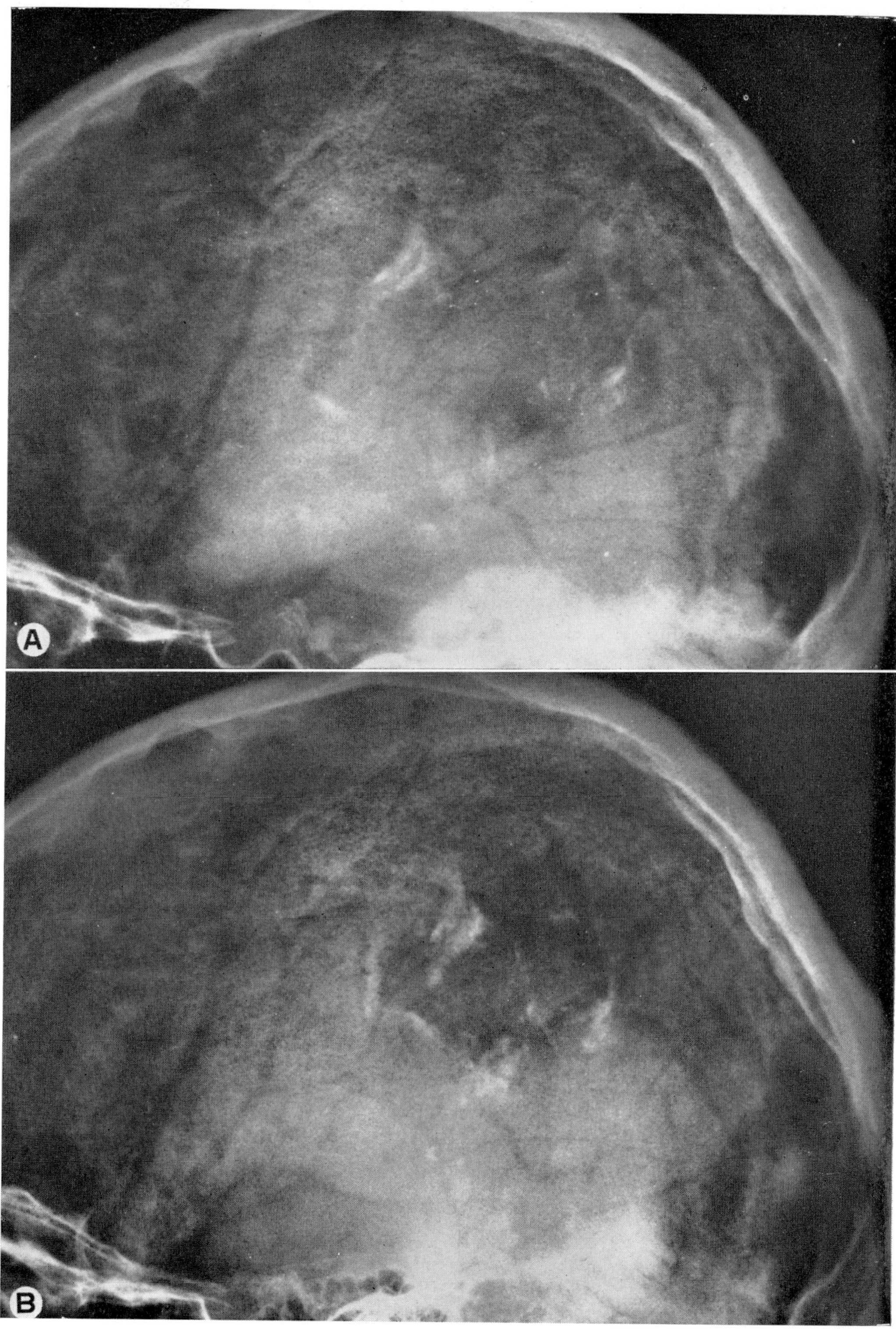

Fig. 170

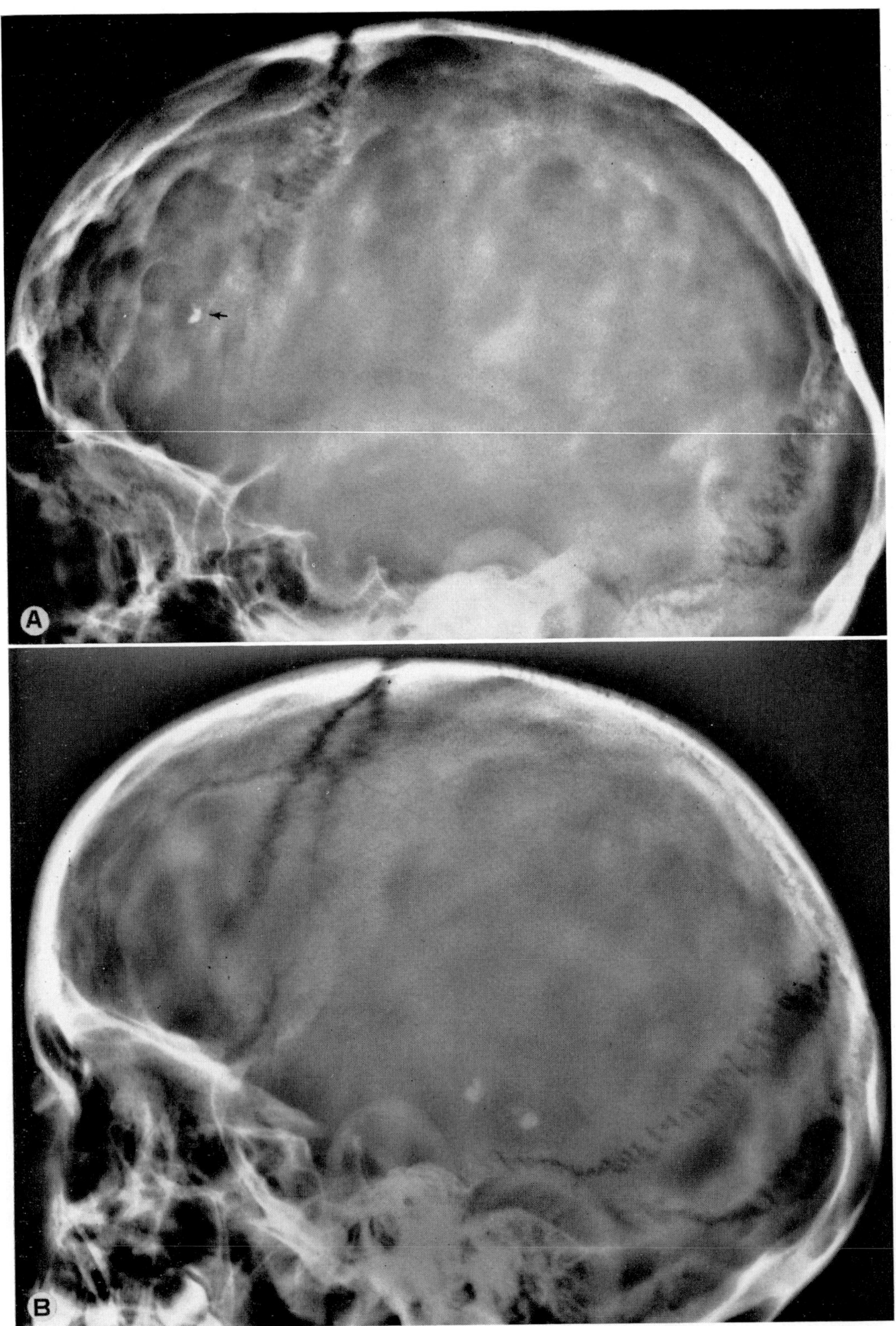

Fig. 171

(*Revised 1963*)

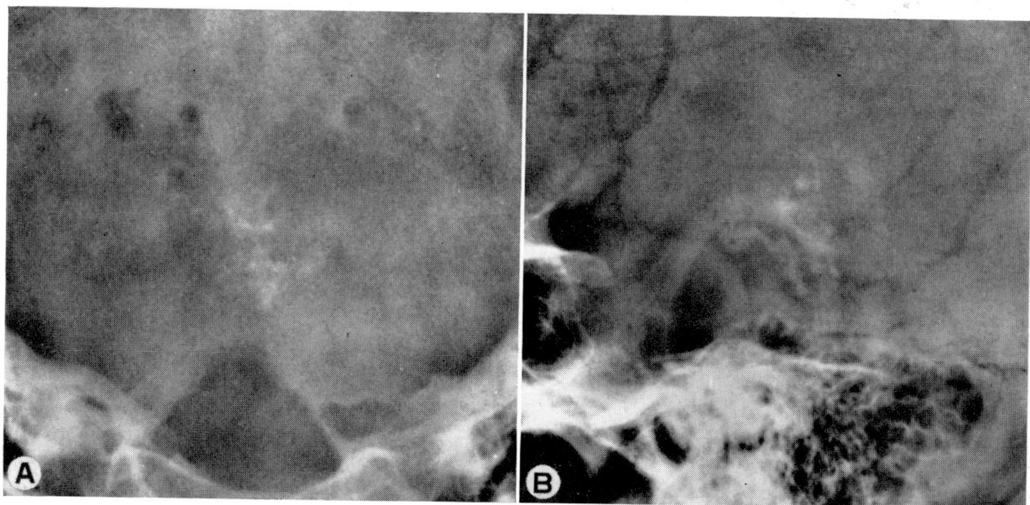

FIG. 172.—PINEALOMA

The frontal film (A) shows irregular conglomerate shadows of calcific density in the midline, covering an area of 2 cm. The lateral film (B) shows the calcific collection, irregular in outline, to be situated above and behind the sella turcica, which is atrophic. Any large calcification in the pineal region suggests the possibility of pinealoma, even though the calcified mass is not irregular and infiltrating, as in this case. (Courtesy of Dr. Colin Holman, The Mayo Clinic.)

amounts of calcium usually are ependymomas. Such an example is shown in Figure 171, which illustrates marked changes of increased intracranial pressure with a small solitary calcium deposit in the anterior fossa.

The *ganglioglioma* is a benign granular tumor composed of adult ganglion cells and astrocytes. The tumor has an abundant connective tissue stroma and calcific deposits are found often in the central portions.

Glial tumors arising in the *pineal body* often exhibit lime salt deposits. Evidence of pineal calcification is unusual under 10 years of age, and its presence should suggest the possibility of pinealoma. Large amounts of calcification in the pineal region, which extend beyond the usual limits of the normal pineal body, also should suggest neoplasm (fig. 172).

The calcifications found in radiographs produced by all gliomas may be punctate, amorphous, trabecular, or arborizing in appearance (fig. 170). Trabecular calcification is most characteristic of glial tumors. Even when the central part of the tumor exhibits an extensive conglomerate calcium collection, the marginal areas usually continue to display the typical linear tapering calcification, suggesting infiltration of normal brain substance by neoplastic tissue (fig. 169). Sizable areas of neoplastic calcification may be present and in rare instances may extend across the midline. Lengthy sweeping streaked arcuate deposits may occasionally be seen. In other instances, the shadows may resemble a cumulus cloud and occasionally, in such cases, differentiation from meningioma may be difficult. This is particularly

FIG. 171.—EPENDYMOMA

A solitary calcium deposit is present in the frontal region (*arrow*) in the case of a child who had a massive ependymoma of the frontal lobe (A). Local bone erosion is shown along the vertical portion of the frontal bone adjacent to the tumor, in addition to changes of generalized increased intracranial pressure. In another case (B), a solitary calcium deposit was found in the temporal lobe and projected in this view anterior to the pineal gland, which is displaced downward and backward. Small areas of calcification occurring in large tumors of the cerebral hemispheres in young patients frequently denote ependymoma.

true if the calcified glioma is near the cerebral surface. In general, however, a tumor with cloudlike calcification which has an arc of its periphery interrupted by the calvaria may be diagnosed as a meningioma with reasonable certainty.

More difficulty is experienced in identifying tumors in which irregular and atypical calcification occurs. Punctate or amorphous deposits and ill defined aggregates are most difficult to diagnose. Such calcifications occur in the brain substance in a variety of nonexpanding lesions, such as old inflammatory processes. Differentiation of atypical glioma calcification from calcified scars in plain films often depends on the presence or absence of increased intracranial pressure. Pressure changes may be assumed to indicate that the calcification is associated with an expanding intracranial lesion and the calcium deposit then is of localizing value. The absence of abnormal pressure does not always mean the opposite. Many authorities believe that unexplained calcification in the cerebral substance is an indication for an immediate definitive examination such as pneumography, angiography, or intracranial exploration. Certainly the minimum attention such a finding deserves is careful clinical follow-up study for an extended period of time, and serial skull roentgenograms for evidence of a change in the appearance of the calcification. In general, calcification in a glioma is an indication of a slowly growing tumor; survival is usually more prolonged and it is not uncommon to see patients with calcified gliomas live for 10 or 15 years or longer controlled by surgery or radiotherapy or both.

Teratomas, dermoids, and cholesteatomas frequently exhibit calcification. Teratomas of the cerebrum may be seen in the newborn and may become massive, with calcium of various forms scattered throughout the neoplasm. Teratomas and dermoids occur also in the region of the pineal body and in the cerebellum. In some instances, such tumors of the pineal may exhibit not only calcification but fat, the fatty portion surrounding the calcium as a zone of diminished density (Camp, 1950). Bone and dental elements may be found in dermoids and teratomas. Cholesteatomas occasionally exhibit deposits of calcium, which may appear as multiple curvilinear shadows of varying arcs grouped together in one portion of the brain. This distribution results from the deposition of calcium in the walls of the cystic tumor. Intraventricular cholesteatomas may develop in relation to the chorioid plexus and may become very large. Calcification in true *angiomas*, encountered most commonly in the cerebellum, is rare. When retinal angiomas are associated, these often exhibit calcification.

Multiple Intracerebral Calcifications

Tuberous sclerosis. *Bourneville's disease* is one of the neurocutaneous syndromes which includes such conditions as von Recklinghausen's disease (neurofibromatosis), von Hippel-Lindau's disease (neuro-occular angiomatosis) and Sturge-Weber-Dimitri's disease (encephalotrigeminal angiomatosis). Tuberous sclerosis is manifest clinically by mental retardation, convulsions, sebaceous adenomata of a butterfly distribution on the face, skeletal abnormalities, and developmental urologic disorders. Most patients present only one or two of the clinical manifestations and for this reason radiologic findings assume greater importance.

The neuropathologic changes of importance are the presence of abnormal areas of gray matter scattered throughout otherwise normal-appearing cerebral and cerebellar cortex. The cortical malformations consist of isolated masses of gray matter made up of abnormally developed nerve cells and neuroglia, which apparently pursue a course of development independent from that of the remaining cortex. Nodules of glial tissue are found protruding into the ventricular cavities. The cortical and ventricular masses frequently undergo degenerative change and calcification and their disposition in the cortex and ventricular wall is a clue to the nature of the lesion. The calcification of the intraventricular masses is more common in our experience.

Skull films usually exhibit multiple scattered calcium deposits that vary in size from

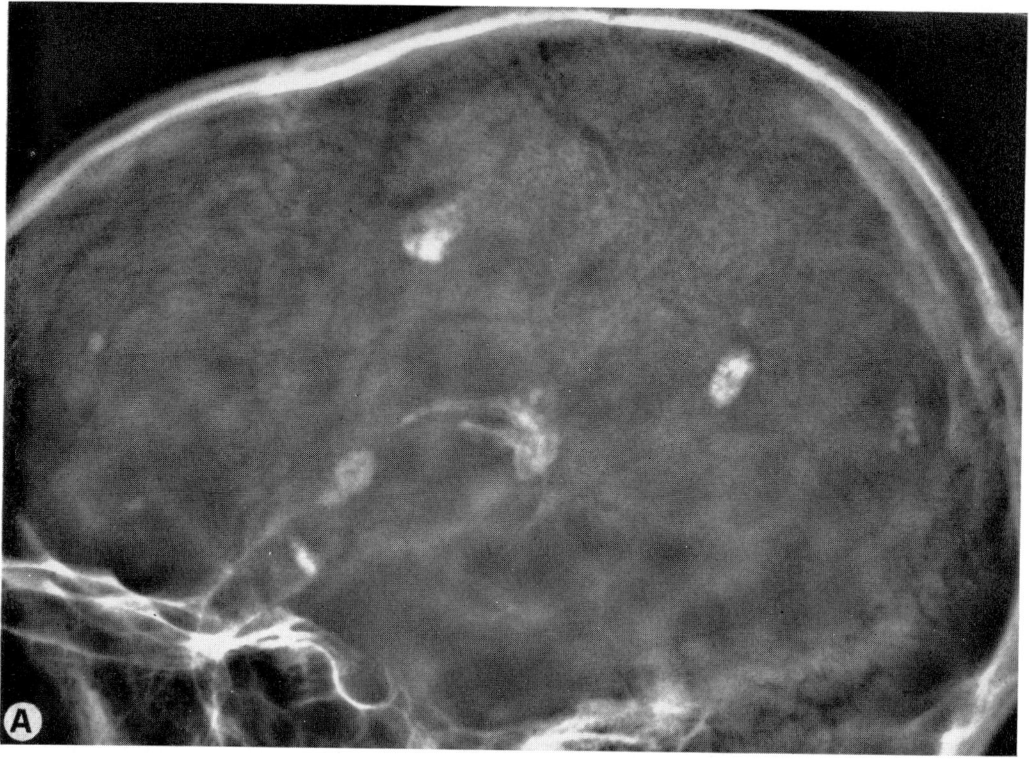

FIG. 173.—TUBEROUS SCLEROSIS

The nodular lesions of tuberous sclerosis frequently undergo calcification. Often the deposits are found along the ventricular walls and most often are rounded in configuration (see fig. 232). In other instances (A), curvilinear calcifications may be found in the region of the basal ganglia resembling postinflammatory changes. In another case (B), an unusually large oval calcification was found in the lateral portion of the frontal lobe.

very small to approximately 1 cm. Some calcifications may be several centimeters in diameter (fig. 173). The calcification often is rounded or oval, but through coalescence of nodular calcifications, irregular forms may develop. The calcifications usually are in close relationship to the wall of the lateral ventricle and sometimes the wall of the third ventricle. Calcification at a distance from the ventricular wall also is observed in the cerebral cortex, in the white matter, in the basal ganglia, or in the dentate nuclei (Holt and Dickerson, 1952). At pneumography, the ventricles are frequently large, and characteristic nodular masses of variable size are found encroaching upon the gas outline of the lateral ventricles. The cortical malformations, so conspicuous at necropsy, usually are not well visualized in pneumograms.

(Revised 1963)

In addition to the intracranial calcification, other radiologic findings of diagnostic importance may be encountered. These include localized areas of increased or decreased density of the skull which were found in a sizable percentage of the cases studied by Holt and Dickerson. Cystic changes and periosteal thickening of the bones of the hands and feet may be present. Urography may disclose renal malformations.

The nonsuppurative *encephalitides* comprise a host of neural disorders which are difficult to classify. Radiologic methods are not useful in the diagnosis of the majority of the lesions of this group. In a few isolated instances, however, radiologic findings may be helpful. *Toxic disorders* may occur as a result of systemic infections and inflamma-

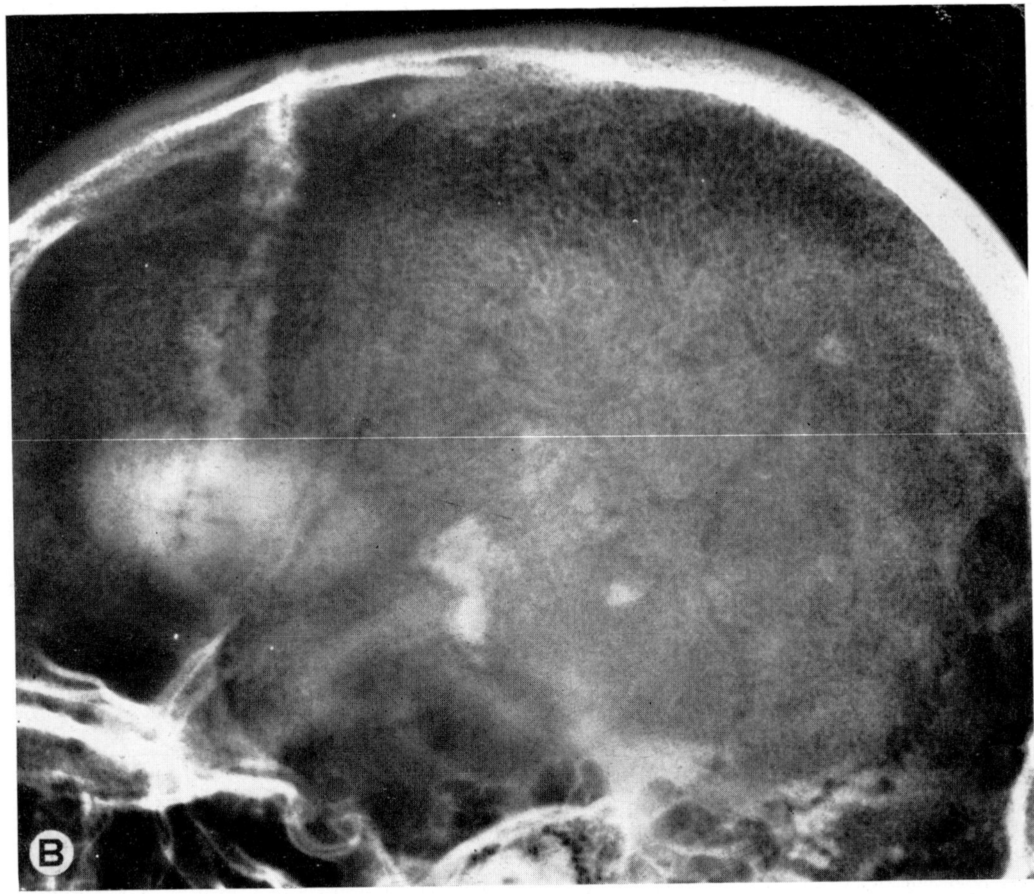

FIG. 173

tory diseases of the meninges. The toxic effects of carbon monoxide inhalation, of tetanus, and of botulism are said to result in cerebral calcifications in patients who survive such exposures.

Cytomegalic inclusion disease. Of the numerous neurologic disturbances produced by filtrable viruses, only one is known consistently to result in intracranial calcification. The causative agent is the salivary gland virus that probably infects a large proportion of the population at an early age. Generalized cytomegalic inclusion disease is an intrauterine infection that in its most serious form causes stillbirth or fatal neonatal illness. Death commonly occurs as a result of hemolytic processes caused by abnormal antibodies. No significant illness has been recognized in the mothers of infected infants, and the occurrence of the abnormality in the child is usually a surprise. The diagnosis is often suggested by the finding of intracranial calcification and may be established by the presence of characteristic cells in the urinary sediment.

The intracranial calcifications found in cytomegalic inclusion disease are multiple scattered deposits which are stippled, nodular, or curvilinear in appearance. The calcification characteristically is periventricular (fig. 174). As a result of the viral infection, extensive cerebral damage with marked dilatation of the ventricles takes place. Deposits may, however, occur in any portion of the brain substance, and calcification in the basal ganglia is common. This distribution is similar to that often seen in toxoplasmosis from which differentiation can be impossi-

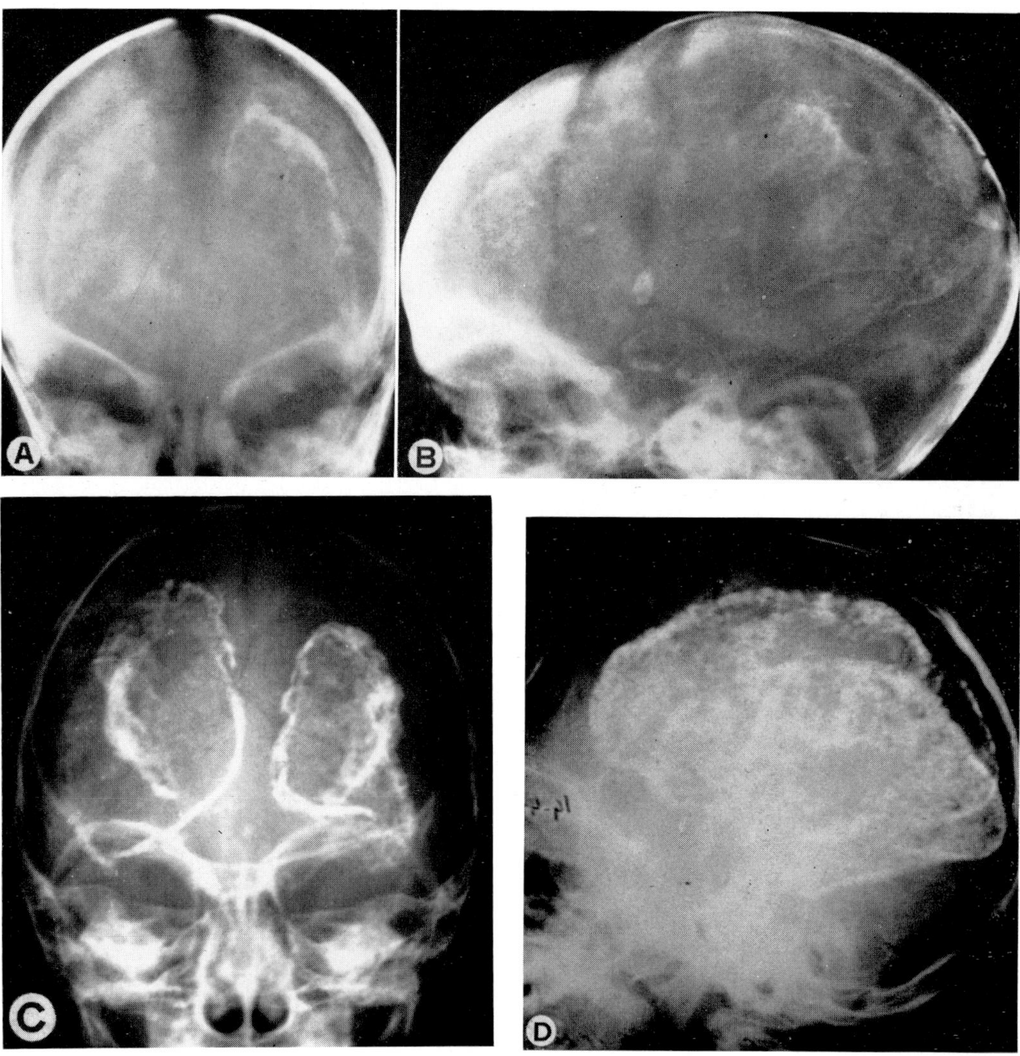

FIG. 174.—CYTOMEGALIC INCLUSION DISEASE

A newborn infant exhibits periventricular calcification (A). In addition, nodular calcifications are present in other portions of the thin brain overlying the dilated lateral ventricles (B). In another case, extensive periventricular calcification is shown in an infant with microcephalus (C and D). The films in the latter case were sent to Dr. John Caffey from Poland for consultation, and the referring physician is unidentified.

ble. At one time it was thought that the neonatal occurrence of calcification in cytomegalic inclusion disease distinguished it from the calcification of toxoplasmosis, which usually is seen after the first year of life. More recently, however, the calcification of toxoplasmosis has been described as occurring in the neonatal period.

Parasitic diseases. Numerous animal parasites act as causative agents of nervous system disease. In the protozoan infestations of malaria, trypanosomiasis, and toxoplasmosis, encephalitis is a prominent manifestation of the disease process. Scattered parasites of the metazoan group may affect the central nervous system. Radiologic examination may be of value in diagnosis when calcification results or when characteristic

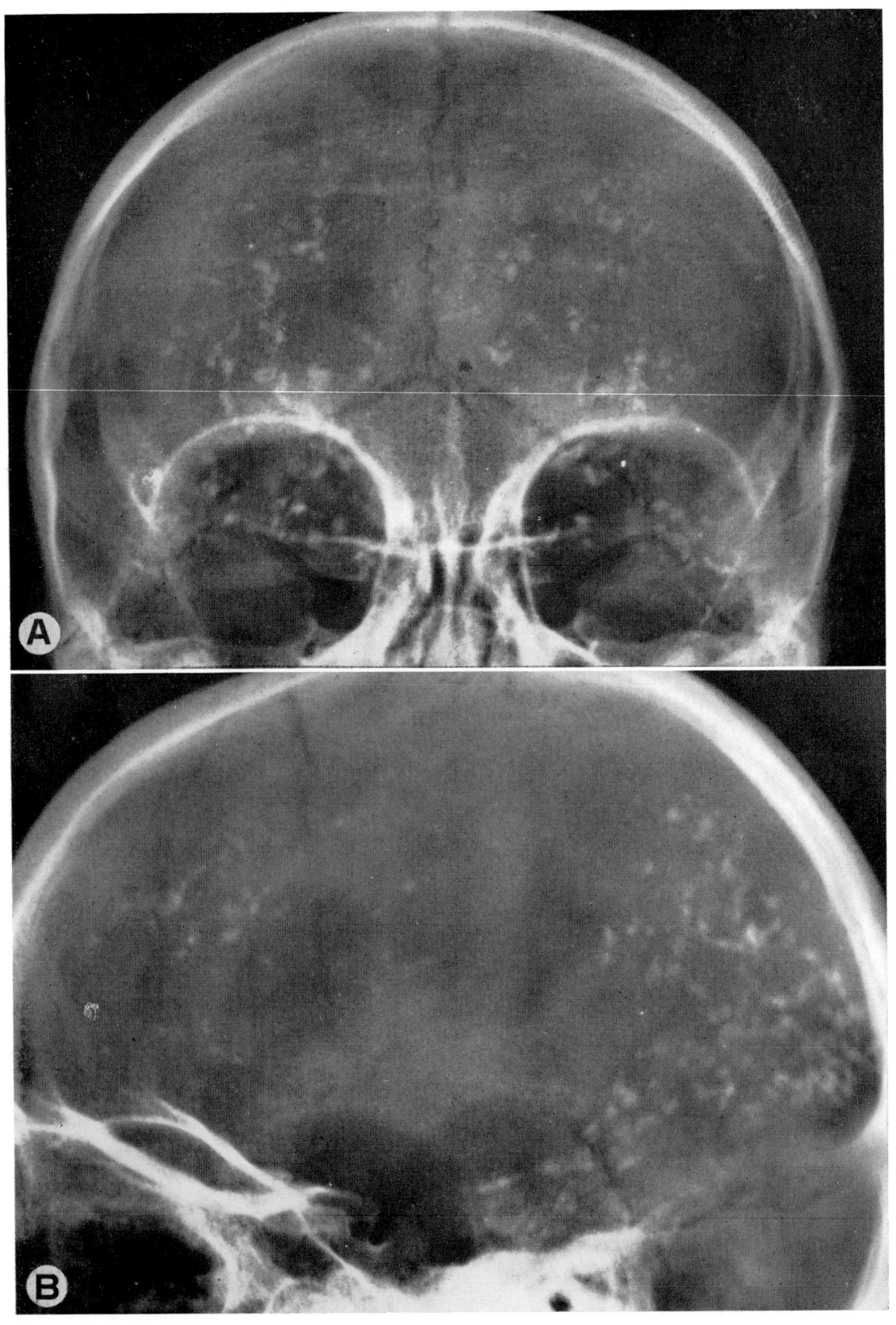

FIG. 175

(*Revised 1963*)

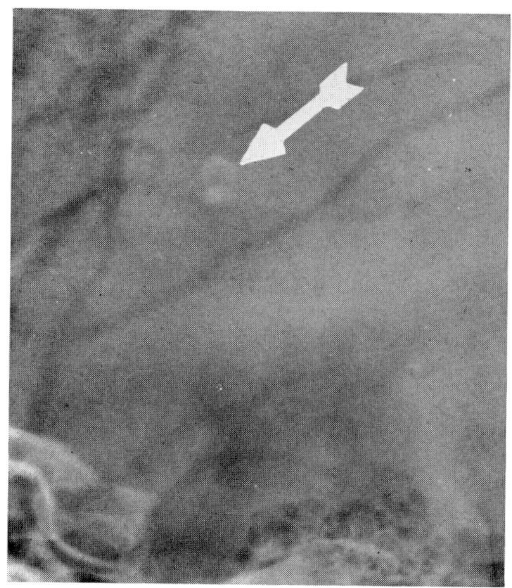

FIG. 176.—CYSTICERCOSIS
The lesions of cysticercosis often undergo calcification and vary considerably in size (see text). In some instances, the calcification may be ringlike (*arrow*). It is sometimes possible to identify a nodular shadow in relation to the ring which may be the residue of the parasite.

changes are produced in air studies or myelograms. Calcification may occur in the inert parasite or in the inflammatory and hemorrhagic residues of tissue reactions.

Of the protozoan diseases, *toxoplasmosis* most often produces radiologically visible calcification. The majority of patients are infected in utero. The fundamental lesions are widely disseminated miliary granulomas. Profound cerebral damage occurs characterized by necrosis and resultant calcification (fig. 175). The syndrome of convulsions, chorioretinitis, hydrocephalus, and calcareous deposits in the brain is characteristic. The calcifications are both nodular and curvilinear, the former usually scattered through the brain and the latter most commonly seen in the basal ganglia.

Tissue encystment (*Cysticercus cellulosae*) in the nervous system is a serious complication of infestation of man by *Taenia solium* (pork tapeworm). In the brain, the embryos most often are inclined to establish themselves in the basilar meninges or in the fourth ventricle, but in the encephalitic form, they are situated in nervous tissue (7 per cent of cases). Convulsions are among the most frequent neurologic disturbances. Small cysts may be found throughout the brain in which dead and sometimes calcified immature parasites are present. The cystic calcifications appear curvilinear or spherical and at times the location of the calcified embryo may be seen in profile attached to its ringlike calcified shell (fig. 176). The parasite may appear scaphoid but more often it has a round nodular appearance. The embryos usually are evenly calcified and of about the same size (1 to 2 mm.). The ringlike shadows of the calcified cysts are more variable in size but the majority average 0.5 cm. in diameter. In the past, the disease was seen frequently in British troops returning from military service in India. Until recently, the disease has been prevalent in Latin America, and its occurrence has been reported in Northern Mexico. Isolated cases are encountered in the United States from time to time.

The occurrence of calcification in *metastatic tumors* of the brain has been described from pathologic studies. In several instances, the size of the calcium deposit present in the pathologic specimen has indicated that it might be visible in radiographs. As yet, no radiologic correlation with these pathologic observations has been made.

In 1929, Geyelin and Penfield described an *endarteritis* producing multiple subcortical calcifications of the brain which was associated with epilepsy and mental deterioration. Examination of pathologic specimens revealed that the calcification occurred at the

---

FIG. 175.—TOXOPLASMOSIS
A multitude of nodular calcifications are present scattered throughout the brain of a young child (A). The frequently occurring curvilinear deposits in the basal ganglia are not present in this case. The disposition of the calcification posteriorly and inferiorly in the lateral view (B) suggests deposition in cerebral tissue overlying large ventricles. The child had microcephalus, and the films show thickening of the skull and premature narrowing of the sutures.

(*Revised 1963*)

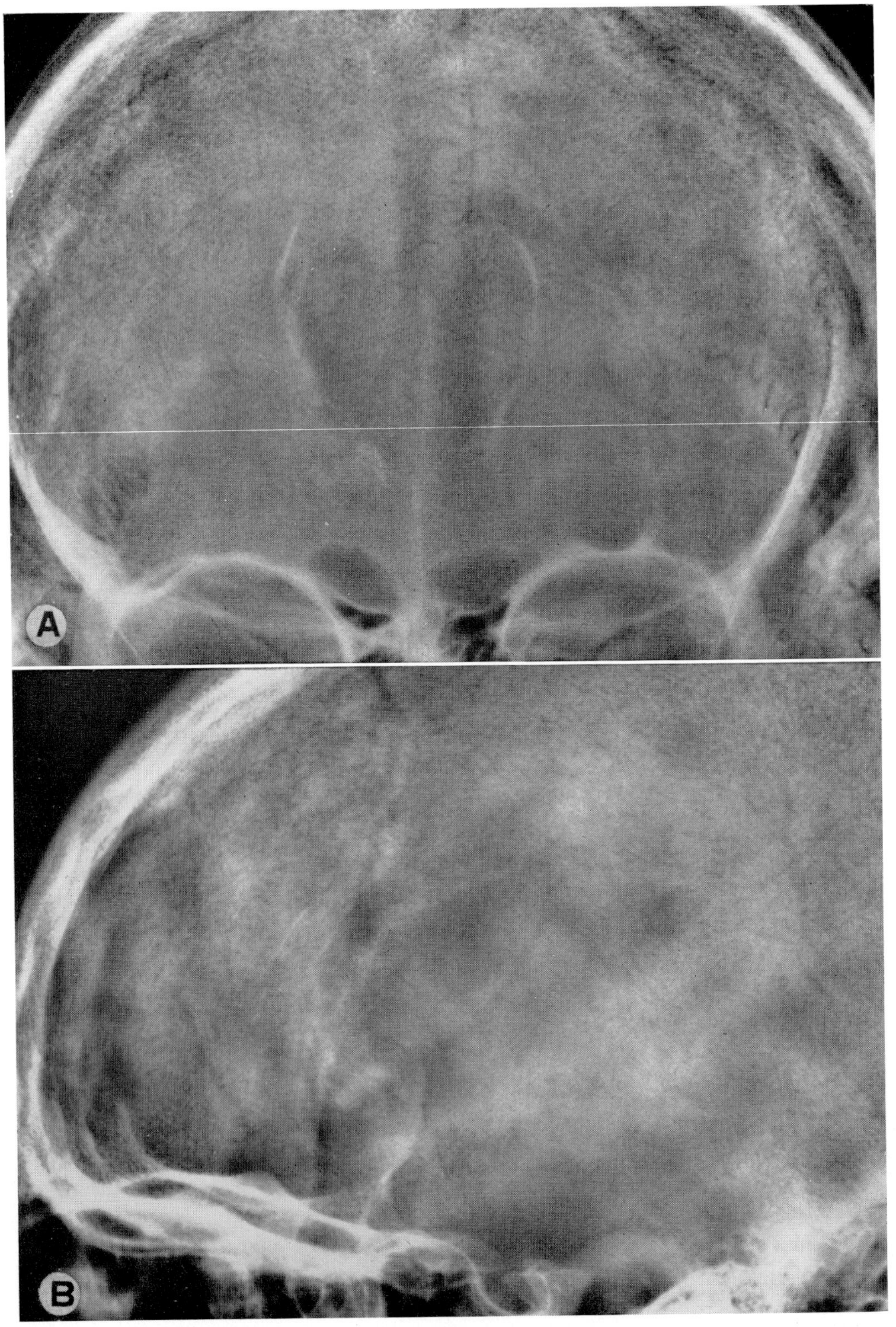

Fig. 177

(Revised 1963)

junction of the gray and the white matter in areas where there was a circumscribed alteration of cerebral tissue resulting from vascular insufficiency. Patchy gliosis was found about blood vessels, both arteries and veins. Calcification was present in the nodular glial scars as well as in the blood vessels themselves. There was no disturbance of calcium metabolism in these patients. The authors entitled the condition endarteritis calcificans cerebri.

Symmetrical calcifications. The most common form of symmetrical intracranial calcification is that which occurs in the *chorioid plexus*. Schüller (1912), who also described pineal calcification, was the first to mention the roentgenographic demonstration of calcification in the chorioid. The greatest clinical significance of chorioid calcification is the displacement that may occur with expanding intracranial lesions. Since chorioid plexus calcium deposits often are unilateral and are related to habenular calcification and other physiologic processes, they have been discussed earlier in this section.

A *lipoma* occurring in the corpus callosum often is directly visible as an area of diminished density because of the adult fat that it contains. In frontal view, the margins of the lesion are usually outlined by symmetrical linear calcium shadows which assume a V shape (fig. 177). The calcification takes place in the capsule of the lipoma. The theory of Klotz that tissue calcification occurs through fatty degeneration and the formation of a calcium soap is recalled.

The description of symmetrical cerebral calcification, particularly of the *basal ganglia* and often of the *dentate nuclei*, associated with hypoparathyroidism as related by Eaton, Camp, and Love (1939), was a significant development in the field of calcification (fig. 178). The groundwork for these depositions of calcium is not a pathologic process. The occurrence of colloid material is so common in the anterior half of the globus pallidus and in the dentate nucleus of the cerebellum that its presence is considered essentially normal (Ostertag, 1930, and others). The colloid deposits develop in and about the finer cerebral blood vessels and subsequent calcification takes place, apparently the result of some abnormality of the interstitial fluids which nourish them. Albright and Reifenstein (1948) have thrown some light on the mechanism by explaining that in hypoparathyroidism there is an excess of ionic calcium in the interstitial tissues, while the circulating calcium values are low.

Parathyroid insufficiency apparently is only one of several diseases that produce a disturbance of cerebral metabolism resulting in the deposition of calcium in colloidal material. Approximately two-thirds of patients with basal ganglia calcification do not have hypoparathyroidism. King and Gould (1952) described symmetric dense nodules of subtentorial calcification in the dentate nuclei in two patients who did not have hypoparathyroidism.

In *lipoid proteinosis*, bilateral calcification may be found deeply seated in the temporal regions. Frontal films may show the deposits through the orbits, while in lateral projections the calcification may be superimposed upon the sella turcica.

Several years ago, Kahn, Lion, and Zimmerman (1939) described a single case of symmetrical calcification in the *cerebral cortex* in a patient whose clinical picture simulated Pick's disease. Radiographs disclosed extensive calcification overlying both cerebral hemispheres, which was disposed in a linear and convoluted pattern, suggesting the configuration of the gyri. Neuropathologic examination of brain tissue revealed

---

Fig. 177.—Lipoma

Fatty tumors rarely may be found in the region of the corpus callosum and septum pellucidum. When there is a large proportion of adult fat and the lesion itself is large (A), the lesion may be identified because of its radiolucency. In such cases, there is frequently marginal calcification about the lateral aspects of the midline tumor, as in this case. The lateral film (B) reveals a comma-shaped shadow of decreased density occupying the usual region of the septum pellucidum, and there are curvilinear calcific densities anteriorly, probably in the rostrum of the corpus callosum. (Courtesy of Dr. Colin Holman, The Mayo Clinic.)

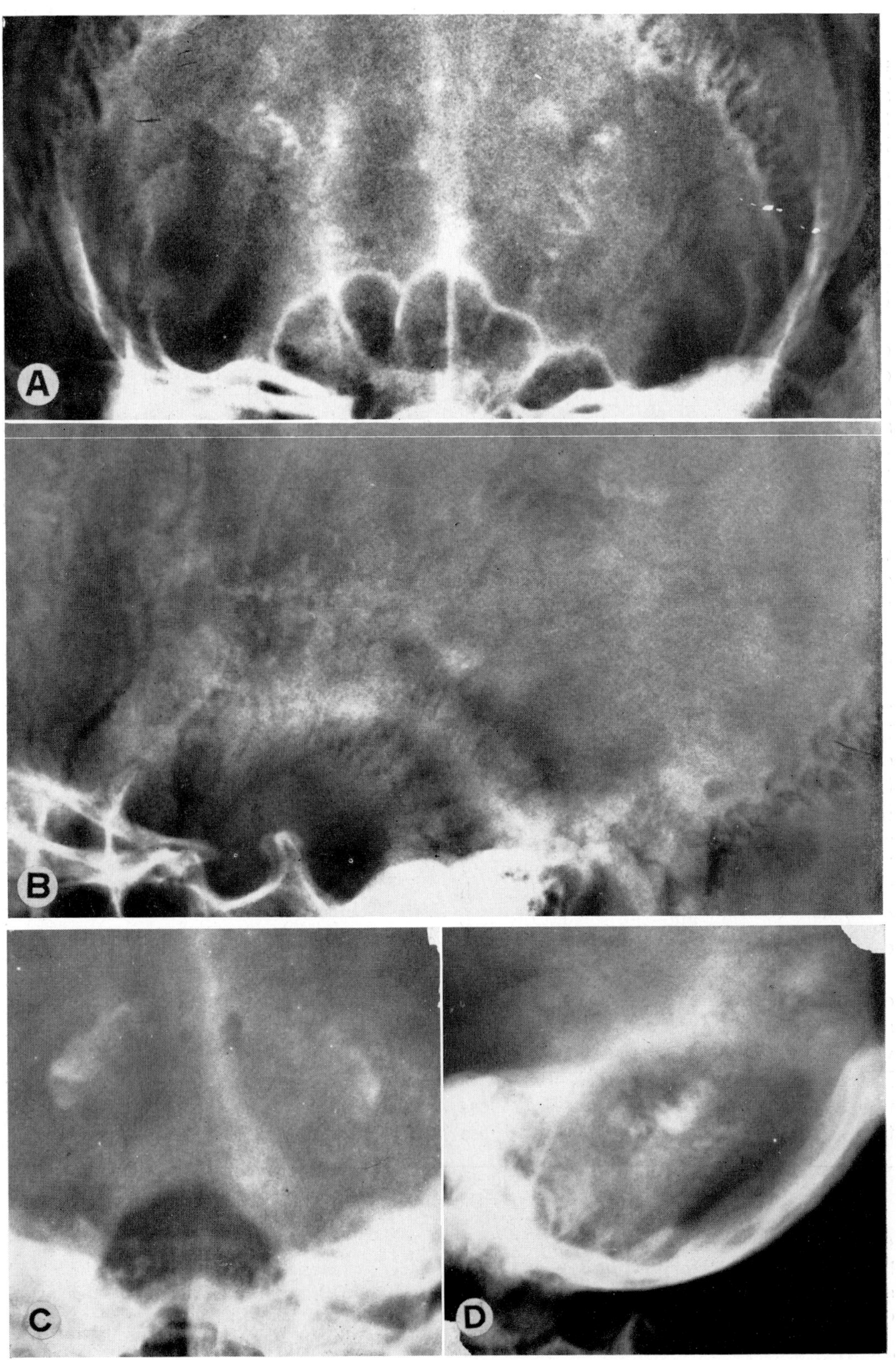

Fig. 178

(*Revised 1963*)

calcification in and about cortical capillaries similar to that found by Eaton, Camp, and Love (1939), and others in the region of the basal ganglia and dentate nuclei. The patient had clinical and chemical hypoparathyroidism as a result of previous thyroid surgery. As yet, no similar observations have been described.

INTRACRANIAL PNEUMOGRAPHY

Intracranial pneumography may be defined as the use of a gas for the radiographic depiction of the brain and its surrounding structures. The term is considered to include the procedures described originally by Dandy as ventriculography and pneumoencephalography as well as the numerous later technical modifications of gas injection techniques. For the sake of completeness, the intentional or inadvertent filling of cystic cavities with gas should be included under pneumography and the use of substances of increased density to demonstrate the ventricular system and abscess cavities will be discussed in this section.

The discovery of cerebral pneumography was the result of an accident. In 1912, a patient presented himself to Dr. W. H. Luckett of New York City because of headache which persisted for approximately 10 days following a head injury. Recently acquired apparatus was used by Dr. W. H. Stewart to obtain radiographs of the patient's head which revealed an intracranial pneumatocele of the frontal region which communicated with the ventricles of the brain. It was not until 1918, however, that Dandy intentionally replaced ventricular fluid by gas for the purpose of obtaining radiographs of the cerebral ventricles. The following year, Dandy conceived the idea of introducing air into the subarachnoid space by spinal puncture and allowing it to seek its own course into the ventricular system.

The choice of a special procedure for radiologic examination of the brain is the subject of a separate discussion. Once an "air study" has been decided upon, it remains for the radiologist, together with his technical assistants, to carry out the procedure according to a predetermined routine but subject to individual modification. The technique should not be rigid to the extent of posing an obstacle to special maneuvers to demonstrate certain specific areas of the brain. Nevertheless, there is considerable merit in having a basic routine. Each examination should be tailored to the individual problem, but it is advisable not to eliminate those routine films whose value has been amply demonstrated by experience. Pneumography now may be considered as a group of procedures comprising ventriculography, cisternal pneumoencephalography and lumbar pneumoencephalography, the latter being subdivided into global, selective, and controlled. Each type of gas injection is designed to meet specific clinical problems, as will be described subsequently.

Fig. 178.—Hypoparathyroidism

Calcification may be found in the basal ganglia in some cases of hypoparathyroidism, and it may also occur without the specific endocrine disturbance. The symmetrical deposition is best shown in frontal films (A). In lateral view (B), the multiple calcifications usually are projected in an arc (see also fig. 209). Calcification may be found also in the dentate nuclei of the cerebellum (D). In many instances, the calcification is symmetrical (C).

(*Revised 1963*)

Technique

PNEUMOENCEPHALOGRAPHY

Filling of the cerebral ventricles with gas is usually associated with headache and restlessness of varying degrees of severity and some type of premedication ordinarily is prescribed. Patients with degenerative cerebral disease suffer less acutely than those with normal brains and brain tumors. Narcotics, including Demerol, generally are to be avoided because of their depressant effect on vital centers whose function may be jeopardized by the disease process being investigated and particularly the tendency to cause hypotension with the patient in upright position. Paraldehyde and Avertin have been in use for many years for their hypnotic and anodyne effects and apparently are safe in spite of the pallor, perspiration, and shallow respiration that are produced. Ether should not be used since it causes swelling of the brain which results frequently in failure of the ventricles to fill with gas.

Barbiturates probably are the most widely used type of preparatory drug for pneumoencephalography at the present time. Atropine or scopolamine are advised, usually in addition to the basic barbiturate premedication. Whenever possible, medications should be of sufficiently small doses to allow the patient to cooperate with physicians and technicians during the procedure; relatively large doses of atropine are beneficial in reducing morbidity. Patient cooperation is essential to obtain good upright films and films with special positioning of the head. If heavy sedation is necessary, the valuable usage of upright films may be lost unless a special chair in which the patient is strapped in position is available. The patient should fast prior to the examination because of the frequent occurrence of vomiting.

Equipment and Preparation

The technique for a pneumoencephalogram should be as simple as possible. It should be executed in an orderly manner according to a standard routine or according to a prearranged plan designed by the radiologist to solve a particular diagnostic problem. The surgical instruments, preparatory solutions, and drapes required are few, and the most basic x-ray apparatus need consist only of an upright Bucky device and a horizontal x-ray table. It is possible to use a tilting fluoroscopic table for both purposes. If available, however, a specially constructed radiographic head stand will greatly facilitate the procedure (fig. 179). Such devices will allow easier positioning of the head and more accurate angulation of the x-ray tube than more rigid general purpose apparatus.

A number of different encephalographic chairs have been devised, and for the upright portion of the procedure some suitable type of seat for the patient is essential. The patient should be firmly supported and made as comfortable as possible. A chair that the patient can straddle, which gives support to the chest in leaning forward and which provides an arm rest or grasp, is desirable. An ordinary fluoroscopic chair serves the

Fig. 179.—Equipment Used for Pneumoencephalography

A freely flexible radiographic head stand, with adapted chair and table, greatly facilitates pneumography (A). The Bucky device and tube arm may be raised or lowered as a unit. The cassette holder may be rotated on its own axis. The counterbalanced radiographic tube arm may be swung about the Bucky device in an arc in two directions. The tube may be turned in its trunnions for precise angulation and alignment. A well-padded chair with a chin rest of adjustable height is fixed to the base of the head stand to place the patient in proper relationship to the film holder. The patient can be seated comfortably straddling the pneumographic chair and is supported by broad straps (B). A lumbar puncture is performed in the usual manner, using the Bucky device to support the head in the desired position (C).

(*Revised 1963*)

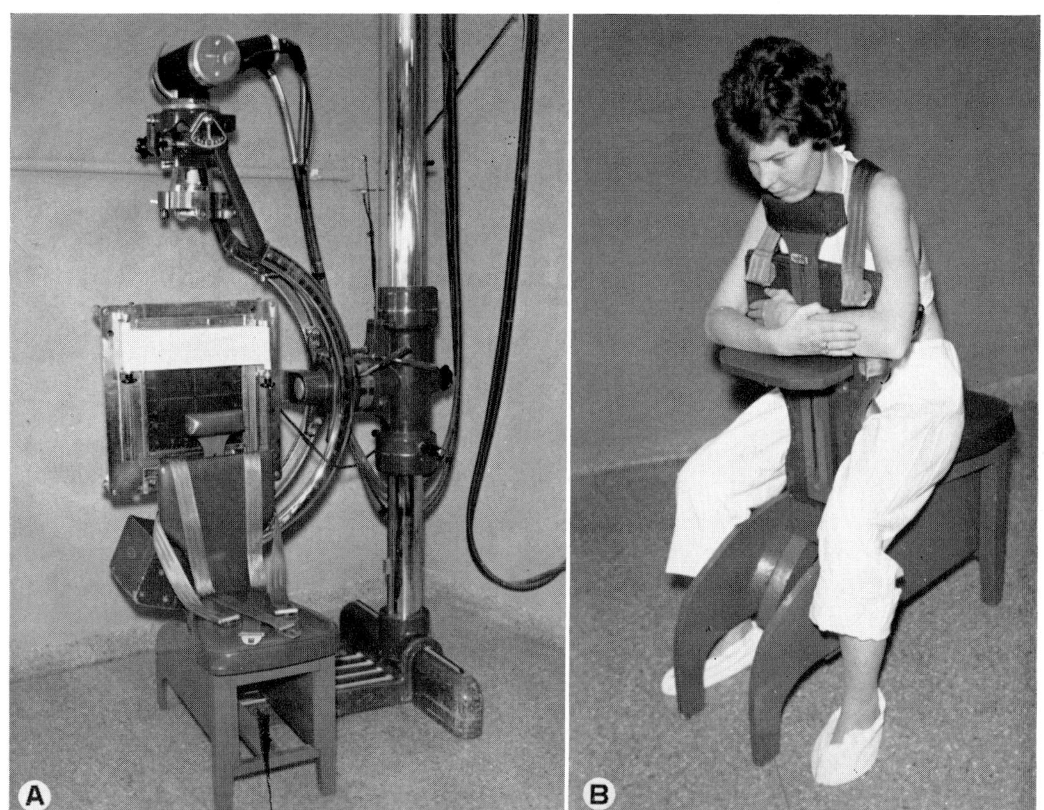

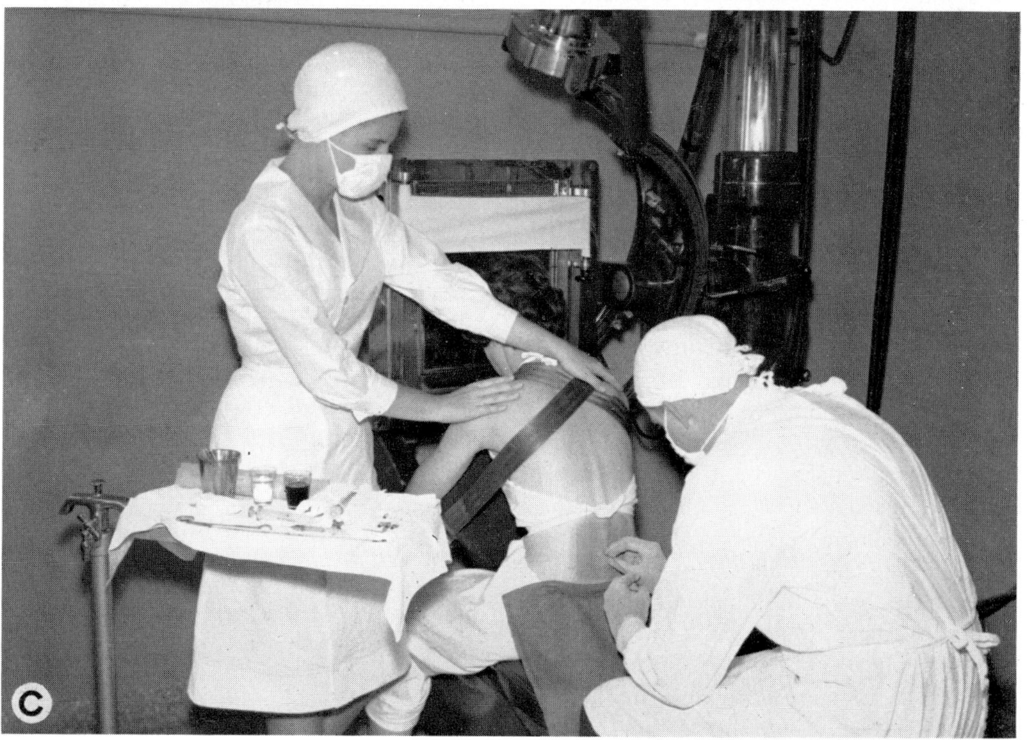

Fig. 179

(Revised 1963)

purpose very well in the absence of more elaborate special seats. Such a standard chair may be modified easily to provide an arm rest and a movable chin rest that can be used in extending or flexing the head for special positions. The face of the Bucky device will provide the best and most unencumbered support for the head (fig. 179). Pressure points should be padded and a safety belt may be used to protect the patient from falling and to assist him in maintaining a straight sitting posture. A swivel stool, placed at a slightly lower level than the patient, will provide a convenient seat for the operator.

In addition to the relatively simple seat just described, which can be used for the majority of patients, it is desirable to have a specially constructed somersaulting chair which may be used in selected cases. This chair must be rigid in its construction and well padded. The chair encloses a patient more fully than the usual seat, since the back must be supported. An aperture in the back of the chair is provided for performing the lumbar puncture. Wide belts are used to prevent the patient from moving appreciably, even when inverted. Rotation of the patient on his own axis as well as somersaulting should be possible. Movement of the chair should be smooth and even, through a well geared mechanism or motor drive. Degrees of angulation of the chair in both vertical and horizontal planes should be well marked. While many designs for such chairs have been created, one that has been found satisfactory for use of the somersaulting technique is illustrated in Figure 180.

A number of gases have been used to visualize the cerebrospinal fluid pathways. Air was the first substance to be used and is still the most widely used. Oxygen has been thought by some to be advantageous since it is absorbed more quickly and a lower incidence of headache has been reported. Carbon dioxide is absorbed too quickly to be useful. Helium, nitrogen, hydrogen, and neon have been employed by some workers. When room air is used, some simple method of purification is advocated.

Fluid and Gas Exchange

After preparation of the skin of the back with iodine and alcohol and the placing of protective drapes, the lumbar puncture is made with the patient in the sitting position (fig. 179). From this point on the procedure may take one of several courses, as previously mentioned. Once a puncture has been made, however, the operator is committed to whatever consequences may develop as a result of interference with the cerebrospinal fluid pressure. A false sense of security may be gained by withdrawing only a small amount of cerebrospinal fluid or abandoning the procedure at this point in the face of a high cerebrospinal fluid pressure, inasmuch as leakage of cerebrospinal fluid through the needle hole into the epidural space may occur. This has the same effect as the removal of a sizable quantity of fluid. Nevertheless, the manometric pressure should be determined at this point, and if grossly elevated for the sitting posture (more than 50 mm. above the level of the foramen magnum or more than 500 mm. of water), special precautions should be taken. Under normal circumstances, samples of cerebrospinal fluid should be obtained for cytologic and chemical studies, if these have not been carried out previously. If a cell count is to be done, 3 cc. of fluid are removed prior to the injection of any air since the count may be altered rapidly by the presence of foreign material.

Three generally different basic techniques of fractional pneumoencephalography are in wide use today and there are, of course, many modifications. All are descendents of the technique described by Dandy in 1919. Each is particularly useful for different types of patients and for different clinical problems. The three will be described in turn.

The first, or classical technique, may be referred to as *global pneumography*. Relatively large quantities of gas are used in connection with this type of study for visualization of the cerebral sulci as well as the subarachnoid cisterns and the ventricles. The second technique, *selective pneumography*, employs less gas, instilled as small

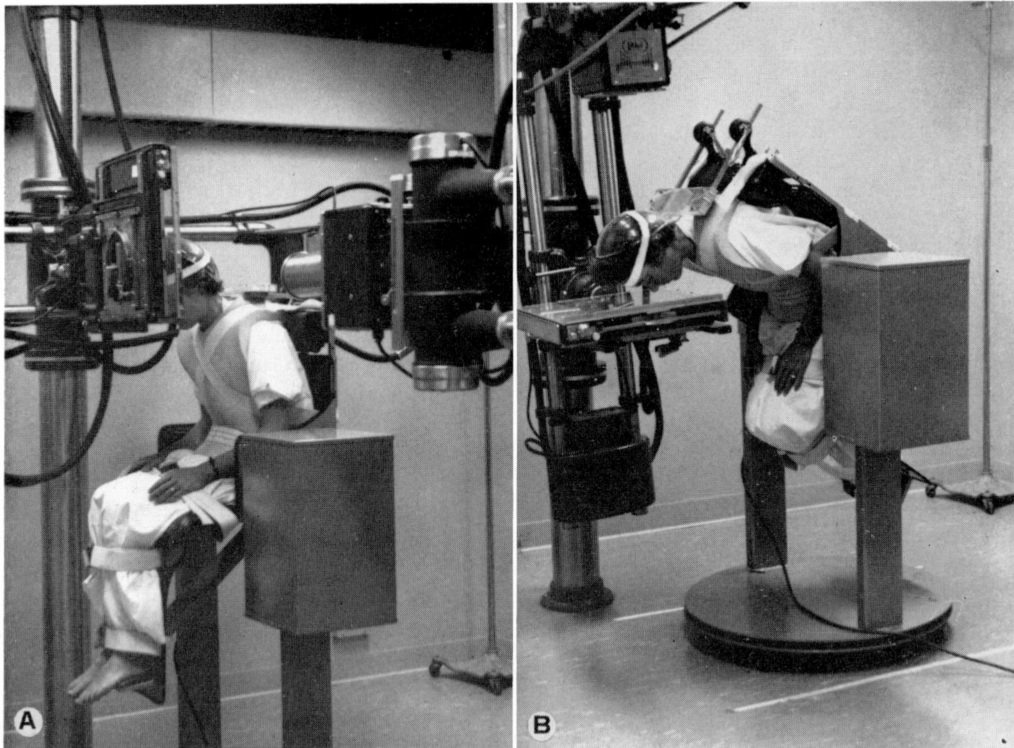

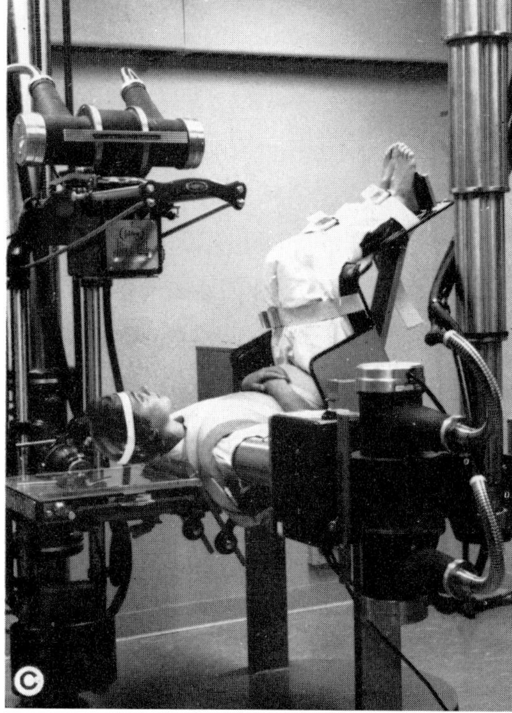

(Revised 1963)

Fig. 180.—Use of the Somersaulting Chair for Pneumoencephalography

In the initial phase of the examination (A), the patient is placed in the usual position for pneumoencephalography. Minor variations in the position of the head may be effected by flexion and extension of the head or by tilting the chair. After the desired amount of air has been injected, the patient may be placed in the prone position first (B) and films made with the vertical and horizontal beam. The patient then is made to complete the forward somersault, and the supine films are made (C). This maneuver will trap air in both temporal horns. In other cases, the order in which the films are made can be altered to suit the particular problem.

portions of the total amount used. In this procedure, repeated small injections and tailored positioning of the head in upright position are combined to visualize advantageously the subarachnoid cisterns. At the same time, the cerebral ventricles are satisfactorily seen and there is a minimum of laterally disposed subarachnoid gas to interfere with visualization of the central structures. *Controlled pneumography* involves the use of a *somersaulting chair*. With this technique, a relatively small quantity of gas is directed into the ventricular system following which it may be moved about at will by rotating the patient in the chair (fig. 180). Any patent portion of the ventricular system may be outlined by this method with a minimum of distraction by superimposed shadows.

The first, or global, technique will be presented at some length, since in connection with this discussion the various radiographic positions of pneumography will be described. This does not imply that this technique is the most widely applicable, although it may be for the clientele of a certain medical practice, while in another institution one of the other methods is most often employed. The procedure selected should be based first on clinical indications and, second, the method of procedure must be modified by the radiologist, depending on his findings as the examination progresses.

Global pneumography. Without attempting to describe in detail the factors that affect the choice of procedure under various clinical circumstances, it may be said that this technique is most applicable to those cases in which full visualization of the ventricular system and subarachnoid space is desired. Such examinations should be reserved for uncomplicated situations, that is, for patients who have no clinical, radiologic, or other evidence of an intracranial mass. The examination may be carried out to exclude brain tumor, but only when such a pathologic process is not strongly suspected. For example, a patient who has the onset of epilepsy late in life may have for the basis of his seizures a small tumor, although there is no other manifestation of such a neoplasm. In an attempt to find a surgically remediable irritative focus, intracranial pneumography may well be indicated. The examination should serve to differentiate a tumor or other space-occupying process from a nonexpanding lesion of the brain. Similarly, atypical mental changes may be an indication for global pneumography when cerebral atrophy is suspected clinically and when it is desirable to confirm the diagnosis or evaluate the extent of organic change.

According to classical techniques, the amount of air injected is always less than the quantity of fluid withdrawn. Some expansion of the gas is anticipated with a change from room to body temperature. Absorption, however, probably begins as soon as the gas is injected, and in many patients it proceeds rapidly. Lindgren (1949) has advocated the use of gas under slight pressure. Following lumbar puncture, no fluid is removed but a small volume (7 to 10 cc.) of gas is injected into the subarachnoid space. Under these circumstances, the gas may move more freely and there may be less disturbance of cerebrospinal fluid dynamics. Regardless of which method is adopted, the subsequent exchange of cerebrospinal fluid and gas is fractional and small exchanges in volumes of 10 cc. or less appear to be least disturbing to the patient. Davidoff and Dyke (1951) recommended that in the average case a total of 60 to 80 cc. of cerebrospinal fluid be withdrawn and that a correspondingly smaller total amount of gas (usually 50 to 70 cc.) be injected. In a normal patient, this represents a replacement of approximately 50 per cent of the total cerebrospinal fluid volume. Since the capacity of the normal ventricles may be less than 15 cc., it is obvious that to visualize the subarachnoid cisterns and sulci requires much more air than filling of the ventricles only. Ultimate determination of the quantity of gas to be used is dependent on film findings after the first gas injection, as described subsequently.

The total amount of gas used by current workers varies, but ordinarily it is much less than under the plan just described.

After the first injection under pressure, 5 to 10 cc. of cerebrospinal fluid and gas are exchanged until the total desired quantity is introduced. The head is positioned to direct the gas first into the posterior fossa cisterns and the ventricles and then into the general subarachnoid space. The course of the initially injected gas is determined by radiographs which are viewed by the radiologist before further injection is made. In some clinics, a Polaroid cassette is employed to make certain that the gas is in the subarachnoid and not the subdural space and that the ventricular system is patent. Such a survey study is not, however, a substitute for the taking of regular films at this time since the photographic paper does not afford sufficient detail for definitive interpretation.

Many variations of any basic technique can be introduced. Most important, however, is a clear idea of the movement of the air in the head depending on various factors, chiefly gravitational with change in the head position but, also, abnormal local conditions causing modification of the intracranial anatomy. Once this is well understood, it is possible to modify a technique to meet any special situation which may arise in the course of the examination. The primary goal of all radiologic examinations is optimum visualization of the structure being investigated. Whatever needs to be done to fulfill this goal will be required, but there are several ways of achieving the same result. The method of choice is that one which offers the highest percentage of success with, at the same time, the greatest amount of safety for the patient.

The *radiographic projections* used in pneumoencephalography are similar to those described in connection with examination of the skull and are described in accordance with the recommendations of the World Federation of Neurology, Problem Commission of Neuroradiology. Greater use is made of the horizontal x-ray beam in connection with pneumography since demonstration of the effects of gravity on movement of gas and fluid in the ventricles and in the subarachnoid space is all-important. In addition, it is frequently essential in the interpretation of vertical beam films to visualize in a right angle view the disposition of fluid and gas in the closed system, and stereoscopic films are not always a satisfactory substitute for horizontal beam examination. Positioning of the patient and alignment of the x-ray apparatus is of utmost importance. After spinal puncture and before fluid-gas exchange, the head is flexed and immobilized (fig. 181). The technician should be prepared to take three films in quick succession, beginning with a lateral view made with a grid-front cassette placed beside the patient's head. As soon as the first 10 cc. of gas have been injected, the stilette is replaced, and the operator withdraws from the radiation area. By this time the cisterna magna and fourth ventricle should be filled with gas and the lateral exposure with the horizontal x-ray beam can be made (fig. 181). Robertson (1957) has shown that gas ascends very rapidly to the cisterna magna and is temporarily arrested in the cerebellomedullary area. After displacement of fluid in this cistern, gas enters the fourth ventricle through the foramen of Magendie, where it may appear as early as five seconds after lumbar injection (fig. 181). Shortly thereafter the aqueduct of Sylvius and posterior portion of the third ventricle fill with gas.

Gas filling of the ventricles takes place probably by way of the foramen of Magendie. Fluid may come out through the foramen of Magendie or, possibly simultaneously, fluid flows out through the foramina of Luschka while air enters mainly through the foramen of Magendie. To assure fourth ventricular filling, therefore, it is necessary to have the head in such a position that the air can pass through the foramen of Magendie as soon as it gets into the cisterna magna. With the head only slightly flexed, air will enter the fourth ventricle without necessarily filling the cisterna magna. On the other hand, if the head is fully flexed, it is necessary to lower the fluid-air level in the cisterna magna to the plane of the foramen of Magendie before air enters the ventricles. In a patient who has a large cisterna magna, such as the one illustrated in Figure 221, injection of a considerable amount of air

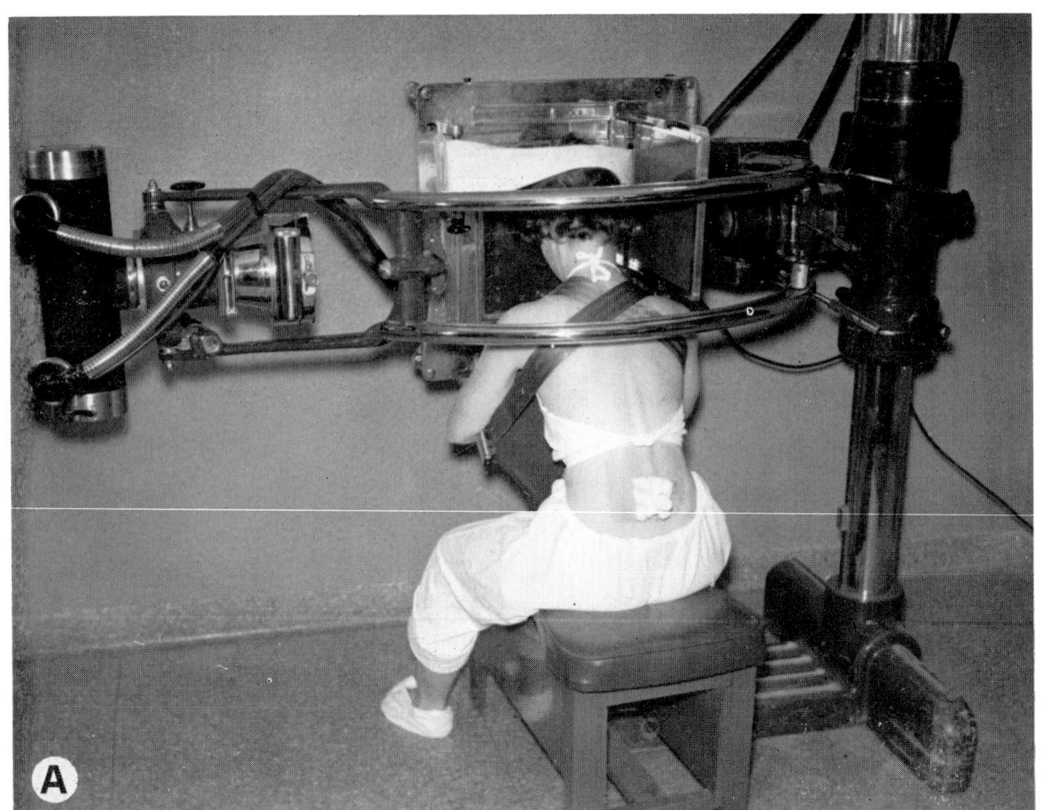

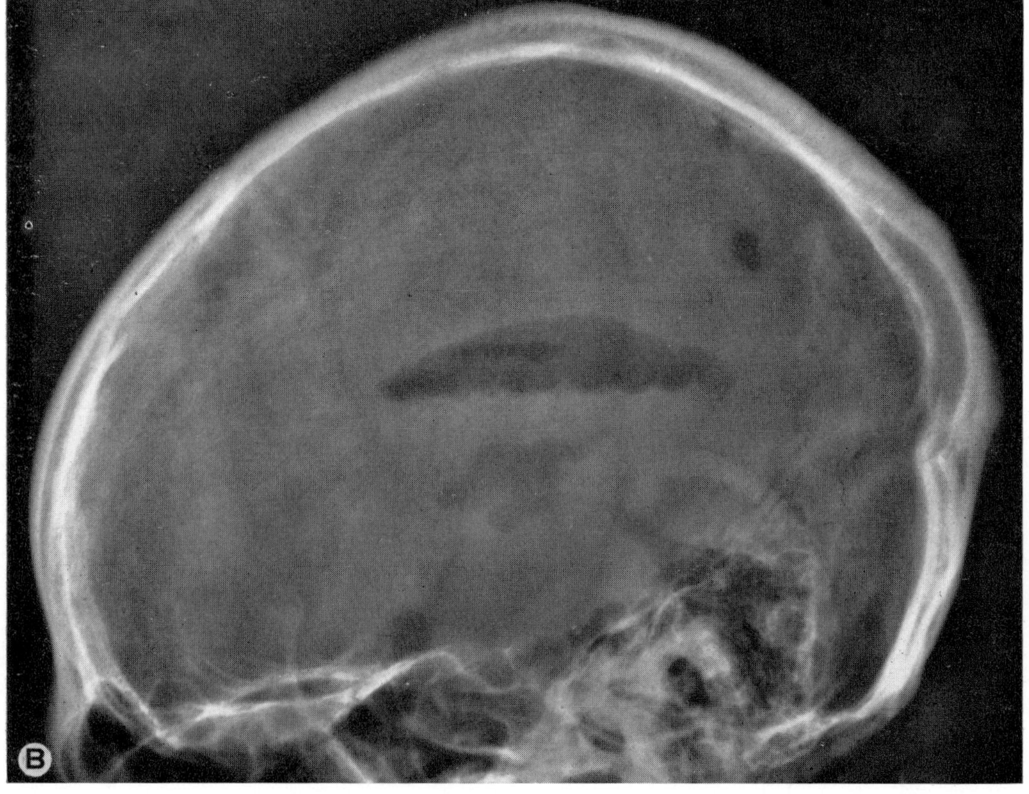

Fig. 181

(Revised 1963)

may be required if the head is held in flexion. However, in these cases, if the head is extended slowly, air will quickly enter the ventricles as the fluid level reaches that of the foramen of Magendie. On the other hand, if the cisterna magna is small, air will enter the ventricles even with the head fully flexed when approximately 15 cc. of gas have been injected. The average capacity of the cisterna magna is 7 to 10 cc., but large cisternae magna are relatively common.

Following exposure of the lateral film, the x ray tube is placed behind the patient and a film is made without moving the head. The latter film is made by a posteroanterior half axial (reverse Towne) projection of the x-ray beam. In the routine examination, this film is intended to provide a frontal view of the posterior portion of the cisterna cerebellomedullaris and other posterior fossa cisterns, the fourth ventricle, the iter, and the posterior third ventricle (fig. 182).

The initial injection of gas affords the best opportunity of the entire examination for visualization of the posterior fossa structures. Visualization of the fourth ventricle and aqueduct of Sylvius is essential for all complete examinations. With gas trapped in those structures by positioning as described, unencumbered depiction is possible. Later attempts at demonstration may be impaired by extensive distribution of subarachnoid and ventricular gas producing superimposed shadows. Even tomograms taken later in the examination, as advocated by some, are not as satisfactory as demonstration of the isolated gas-filled ventricular pathways.

Another important aspect of the initial gas injection is the estimation of ventricular position, configuration, and volume. Dyke and Davidoff championed this early evaluation of ventricular status and its use as a guide to subsequent procedure. Numerous examples of avoidable complications have been observed which resulted from the disregarding of ventricular status as demonstrable by such "scout" evaluation films.

The most helpful scout or survey film is one that demonstrates the lateral and third ventricles in frontal projection, the iter and fourth ventricle having been previously radiographed. After exposure of the posteroanterior half axial film, the head is slowly extended until the forehead and nose touch the film (fig. 183). This maneuver causes the first gas injected to enter the lateral and third ventricles. After fixation of the head in this position by a head clamp or restraining band, a straight posteroanterior exposure is made, using the Bucky device and a straight horizontal x-ray beam. Following exposure of this third film, the patient is allowed to relax in a position of semiflexion of the head and the three films are processed before the examination is allowed to proceed.

The three films are examined by the radiologist for evidence of posterior fossa subarachnoid or ventricular abnormality, and for higher ventricular filling, size, and displacement. The upper cervical region also should be included on the first lateral film. If gas has not entered the cranial cavity, the cause should be sought. Herniation of the cerebellar tonsils through the foramen magnum or a tumor of the high cervical or foraminal region may be demonstrated (fig. 197). Such a finding is an indication to terminate the procedure.

If gas has entered the cranium but not the ventricles, the cause may be faulty positioning or a large cisterna magna, as previously described, rather than disease. The size of the cisterna cerebellomedullaris is readily ascertained from the initial lateral

Fig. 181.—Lateral Examination during Ventricular Filling

The head is immobilized by means of a cloth band with the forehead resting on the face of the Bucky device (A). The orbitomeatal line is inclined 15 degrees below the horizontal. A cassette is placed beside the patient's head in a holder, which is part of the apparatus, and a lateral exposure is made utilizing the horizontal x-ray beam. The first radiograph obtained should allow good visualization of the upper cervical subarachnoid space, cisterna magna, fourth ventricle, aqueduct of Sylvius, and the posterior portion of the third ventricle (B). Varying amounts of gas may be found in the lateral ventricles at the time of the first exposure.

(Revised 1963)

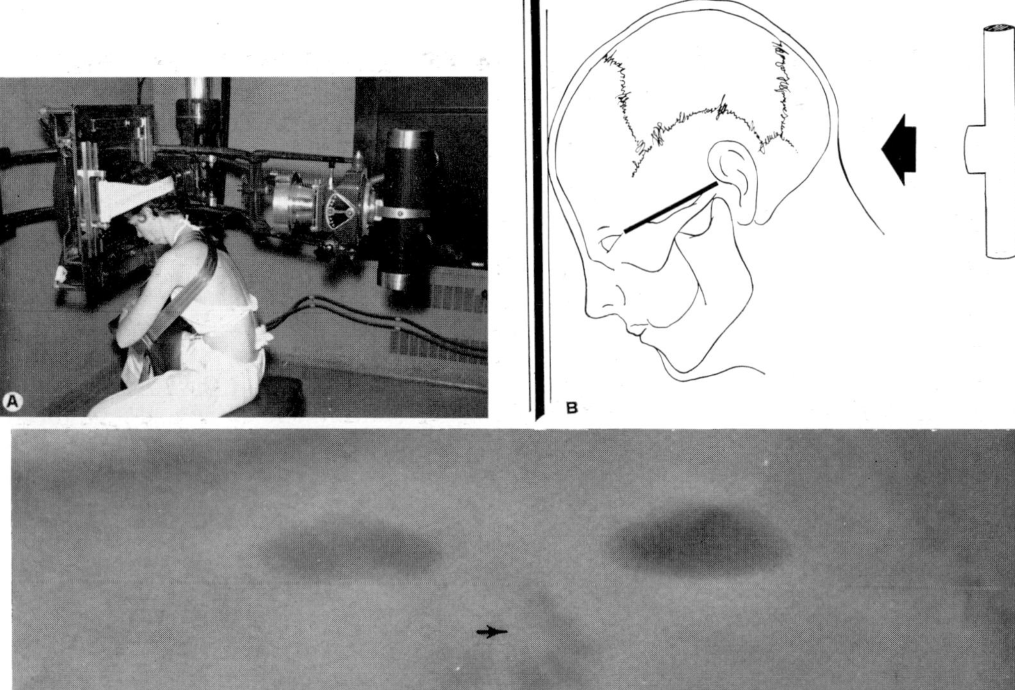

FIG. 182.—FRONTAL EXAMINATION DURING VENTRICULAR FILLING

Without moving the patient, the x-ray tube is swung 90 degrees in the horizontal plane (A). A frontal film is made in posteroanterior half axial projection as rapidly as possible after obtaining the first (lateral) radiograph. The horizontal central ray makes an angle of 15 degrees with the orbitomeatal line (B). If the neck is not flexible or if, for other reasons, the head cannot be easily positioned, the tube must be lowered and the central ray angled upward, more than is shown in A, and B, to obtain a true posteroanterior half axial view.

The frontal filling film (C) usually depicts well a number of important posterior fossa structures: the cisterna magna (*containing lower central vertical arrow*); the narrow shadow of the vallecula (*above lower central arrow*) leading to the fourth ventricle; the ventricle, which is round in this projection except for flattening of its superior margin (*upper vertical arrow*); the cerebellar tonsils, which are outlined medially and inferiorly by cisternal gas. Gas extending from the central portion of the cisterna magna laterally and upward fills the cerebellopontine recess on each side (*lateral arrows*). On one side, the petrosal vein is visualized. Gas in the quadrigeminal cistern outlines the pineal gland (*transverse arrow*). If the shadow of the posterior portion of the third ventricle is superimposed upon the fourth ventricle and the quadrigeminal cistern, a complex composite image results. Gas frequently is found in the aqueduct of Sylvius in this projection.

(Revised 1963)

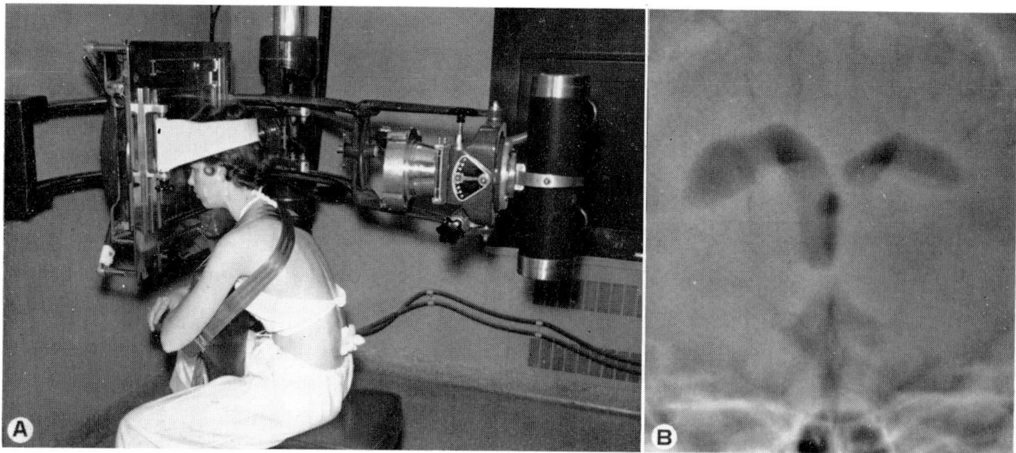

FIG. 183.—UPRIGHT STRAIGHT FRONTAL EXAMINATION

The patient's head is extended until the forehead and nose touch the face of the Bucky device (A). The orbitomeatal line is perpendicular to the film and the central ray is parallel to this line. The film obtained (B) shows filling of the lateral and third ventricles. At this time, there is often better filling of one lateral ventricle than the other. Asymmetrical filling may not be significant, but, if there is enlargement on one side, the larger ventricle often fills with greater facility. The fourth ventricle in this projection appears quadrilateral in shape, if the lateral recesses are well filled. The film is particularly useful to estimate ventricular volume and to decide how much additional gas should be injected.

film. Narrowing, if present without ventricular filling, may be particularly significant since this precedes foraminal herniation. If ventricular filling does occur, the presence or absence of displacement or deformity of the cerebellum or brain stem must be determined.

If the posterior fossa structures visualized in the first two films appear normal, the third film in straight posteroanterior projection then gives the best guide to further procedure. This film usually will reveal whether or not there is a shift of the lateral and third ventricles from their normal position which, if present, would contraindicate continuing the examination. If the ventricles are normally placed and of normal size, the operator resumes a fractional exchange of fluid and gas in 10 cc. quantities until a total of approximately 50 cc. (40 cc. additional) have been replaced. When the ventricles are enlarged, a proportionally large amount of gas must be used to visualize all portions of the ventricular system and subarachnoid space well. Even for global pneumography, it is advisable not to exceed an exchange of 100 cc., even in well marked examples of cerebral atrophy. Throughout the exchange subsequent to the taking of the first three films, the head is fixed in a position of slight flexion with the hairline against the Bucky device. This position should assure further filling of the ventricular system. Either concomitant with ventricular filling or subsequent to its completion, except for dependent fluid reservoirs, the gas will fill the cerebral subarachnoid space.

When ventricular filling does not occur following the initial injection and no abnormality is visible on the first series of three films, the replacement of 10 cc. of fluid by gas should be repeated, carrying out the same positioning and radiographic maneuvers as before. If the ventricles remain unfilled, usually it is useless to continue the exchange beyond 20 to 30 cc. In some clinics, the exchange of fluid and gas is continued up to 40 to 50 cc. if no obvious pathologic process is present on the scout films, in order to gain maximal information concerning the subarachnoid space. When the gas injection is concluded prematurely because of defective ventricular filling, the

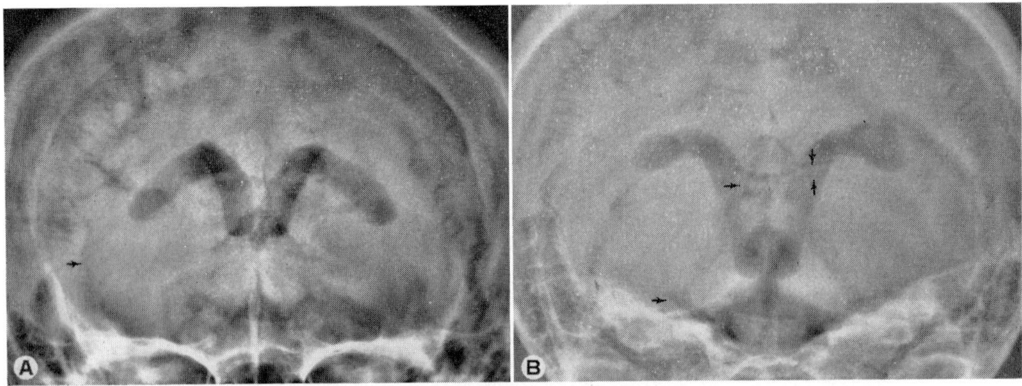

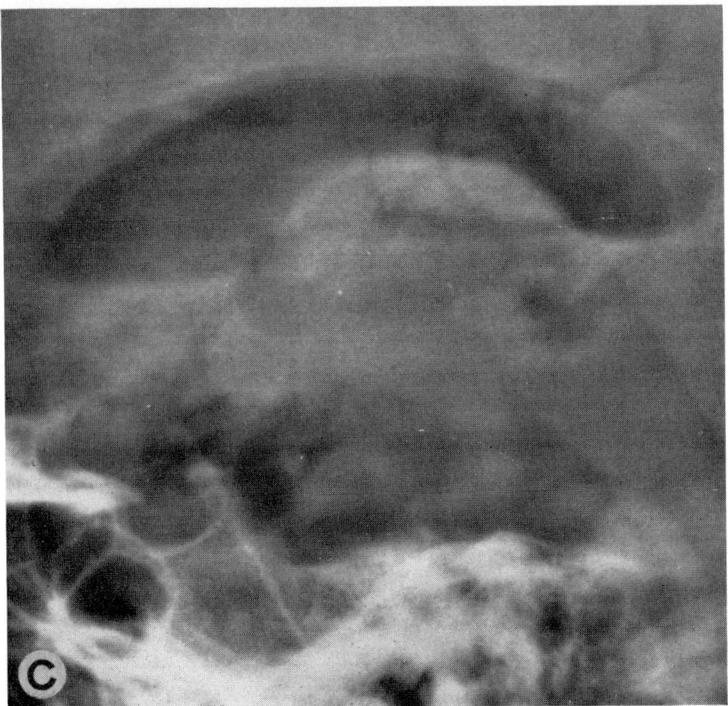

Fig. 184.—Upright Examination after Completion of Gas Injection

The posteroanterior straight frontal view (A) reveals the size, position, configuration, and degree of symmetry of the lateral ventricles. The roofs of the ventricles are particularly well shown, together with the distribution of gas in the subarachnoid space over the cerebral convexity. Gas also is present about the island of Reil (*arrow*).

A posteroanterior half axial projection (B) reveals the posterior fossa basal cisterns and the posterior communicating cisterns well distended. The lateral communicating channels extending dorsally around the brain stem often are well-shown. The channel from the cerebellopontine recess (*lower transverse arrow*) to the quadrigeminal cistern (*upper transverse arrow*) is outlined bilaterally. The retrothalamic space may be seen in frontal views in some cases, extending outward on each side from the quadrigeminal cistern. In this instance, a double shadow is cast (*vertical arrows*), thought to be the result of gas behind both the pulvinar and the upper posterior aspect of the thalamus.

The lateral upright film is most valuable to outline the lateral ventricular roofs (C). In some instances, gas beneath the base of the brain in the cisterns allows excellent visualization of these structures.

(*Revised 1963*)

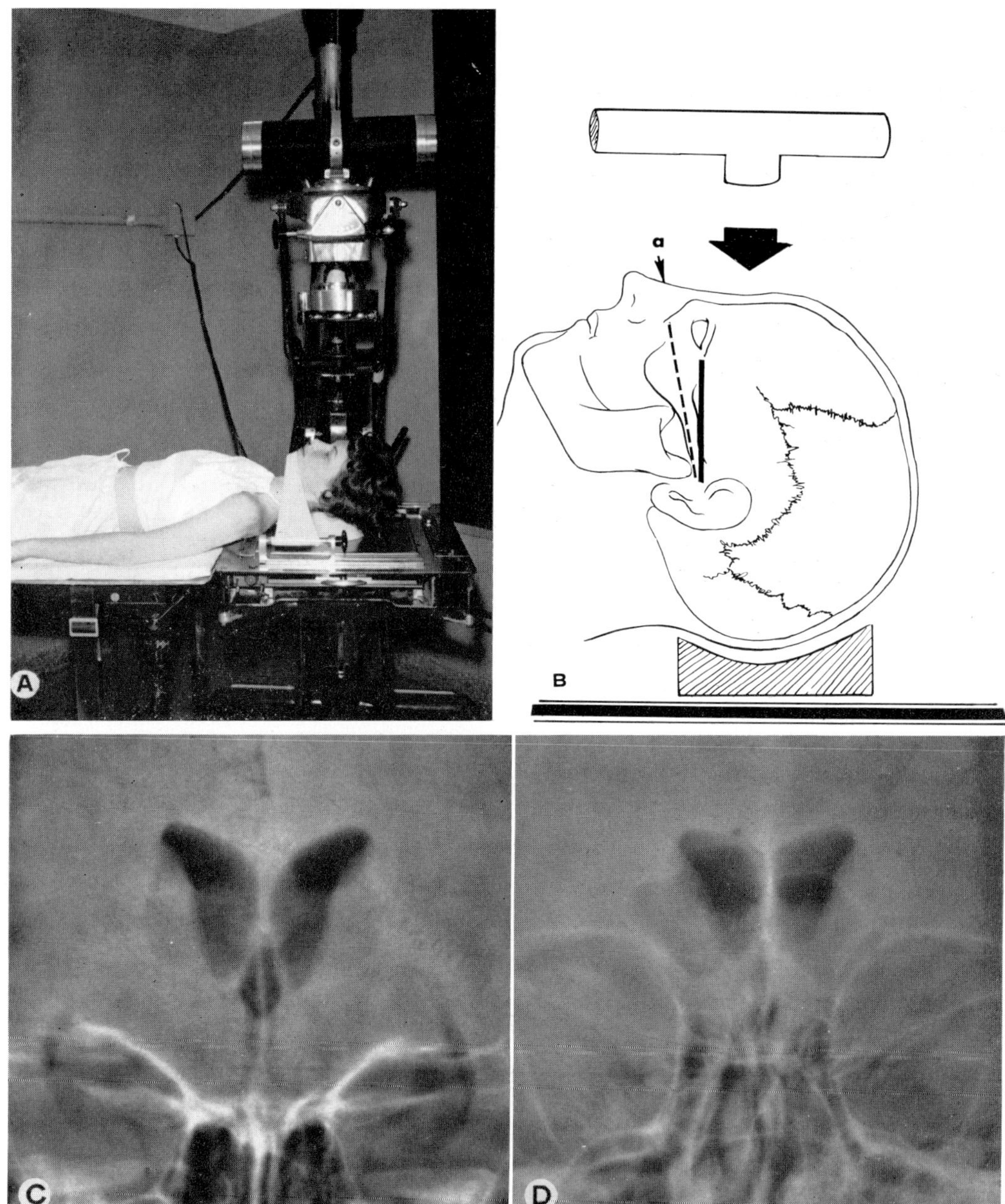

FIG. 185.—FRONTAL EXAMINATION IN SUPINE POSITION

The Bucky device is turned to horizontal position and placed at the head of the table upon which the patient reclines (A). A restraining band is used to fix the head in slight flexion with the orbitomeatal line perpendicular to the film in the Bucky tray. The vertical x-ray beam is directed through the nasion parallel to the orbitomeatal line (B).

The straight anteroposterior pneumogram (C) reveals the forward portions of the lateral and the third ventricles outlined by gas. In the normal frontal projection made in this position, the internal and external auditory canals will be shown projected through the central portion of the orbits. If the projection is made along Reid's base line—with the central ray directed through the point "a", as shown in (B)—a slightly different pneumogram is obtained. In the latter case, the petrous pyramids are projected along the lower orbital margins (D) and the facial structures usually obscure visualization of all but the lateral ventricles.

(Revised 1963)

entire series of films should be taken. Frequently considerable information may be gained from study of the gas filled subarachnoid spaces alone.

When the operator has concluded the gas injection, the needle is withdrawn and the final frontal and lateral views in upright position are obtained (fig. 184). In order to obtain a straight lateral view, it may be necessary to turn the patient almost sideways in relation to the Bucky device. Some workers believe that stereoscopic examination in these two projections is essential, and there is no question that stereoscopic study is most helpful in diagnosis in many instances.

The second half of the pneumographic procedure, or the horizontal radiographic examination, is begun by placing the patient supine on the examining table. In ventriculography, the examination is usually limited to the series of recumbent films. An ordinary flat radiographic or fluoroscopic table may be used. As with the upright examination, however, a flexible craniographic device used in conjunction with an examining stretcher or a separate 12 by 12-inch Bucky diaphragm placed on top of or at the head of the radiographic table will facilitate true projections (fig. 185). These devices are particularly useful if a patient has a rounded chest or a short stiff neck. The patient should be turned as infrequently as possible during the horizontal examination and the films exposed in as quick a succession as is feasible.

Frontal and then lateral pneumograms are taken with the patient remaining supine. For the supine films the head should be elevated slightly by a radiolucent pad or block under the occiput (fig. 185). This elevation will overcome natural extension of the neck and help prevent projection of the facial structures and paranasal sinuses over the ventricles in the frontal view. It will also allow complete inclusion of the occipital area in the following lateral view made with a cassette beside the head.

The head is tilted until the orbitomeatal line is perpendicular to the film. A straight anteroposterior view is taken with the central ray directed vertically through the center of the cranium and parallel to the orbitomeatal line. To insure sinus-free depiction of the ventricles, although with considerable distortion, an anteroposterior half axial projection also may be made at this point in the examination. The distortion which results affords even better visualization of the anterior horns than the straight frontal film (fig. 186). When the straight anteroposterior supine view is obtained stereoscopically, the shift of the x-ray tube should be along the long axis of the body and not in a transverse direction, although for the anteroposterior half axial projection, a transverse shift is allowable.

After exposure of the frontal films, the patient remains undisturbed in the supine position and the x-ray tube is swung 90 degrees to a point beside the head in order to obtain a lateral view with the horizontal beam (fig. 187). A grid-front cassette is again employed and ordinarily a single film is taken, although some workers advocate that all of the horizontal films be made stereoscopically (Childe, 1961). The right angle views made in this manner without moving the patient, and presumably without altering the disposition of gas in the ventricles and subarachnoid space, allow very satisfactory identification, lateralization, and comparison of anatomic structures.

The patient then is turned to the prone

Fig. 186.—Anteroposterior Half Axial Projection

The radiographic tube is shifted 20 to 25 degrees from the perpendicular (A) and the central ray is directed through the plane of the external auditory meatus (B). The radiograph thus obtained usually provides good visualization of the anterior half (tip) of each frontal horn and the forward portion of the third ventricle. There is distortion by the angled projection, particularly of the frontal horns, which appear elongated (C). Such distortion may be advantageous in visualizing the lateral, inferior, and medial aspects of the frontal tips, because superimposition of the more posterior ventricular segments is eliminated. The temporal horns also may be well-demonstrated in a modified superior-inferior view (see also Fig. 191).

(Revised 1963)

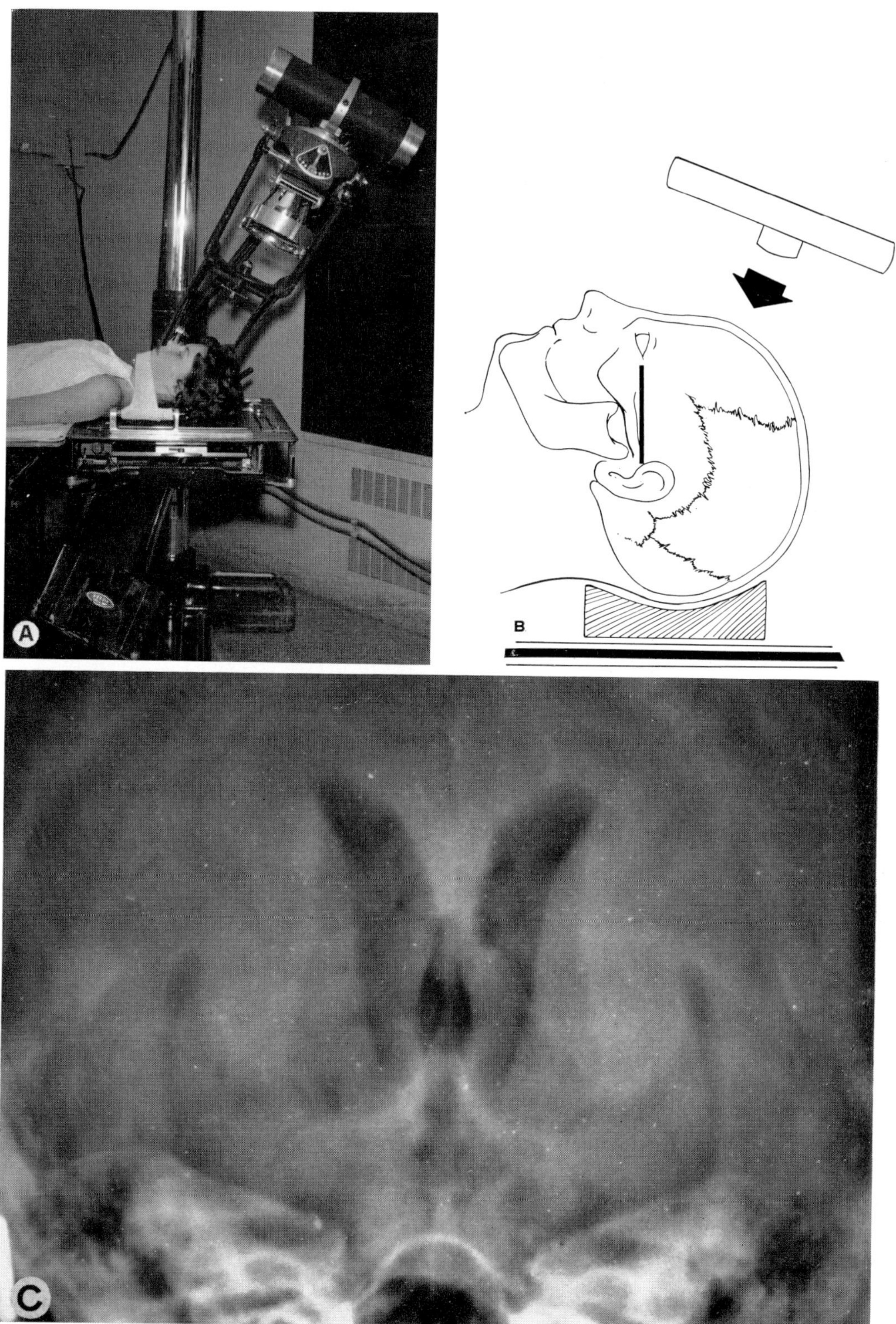

Fig. 186

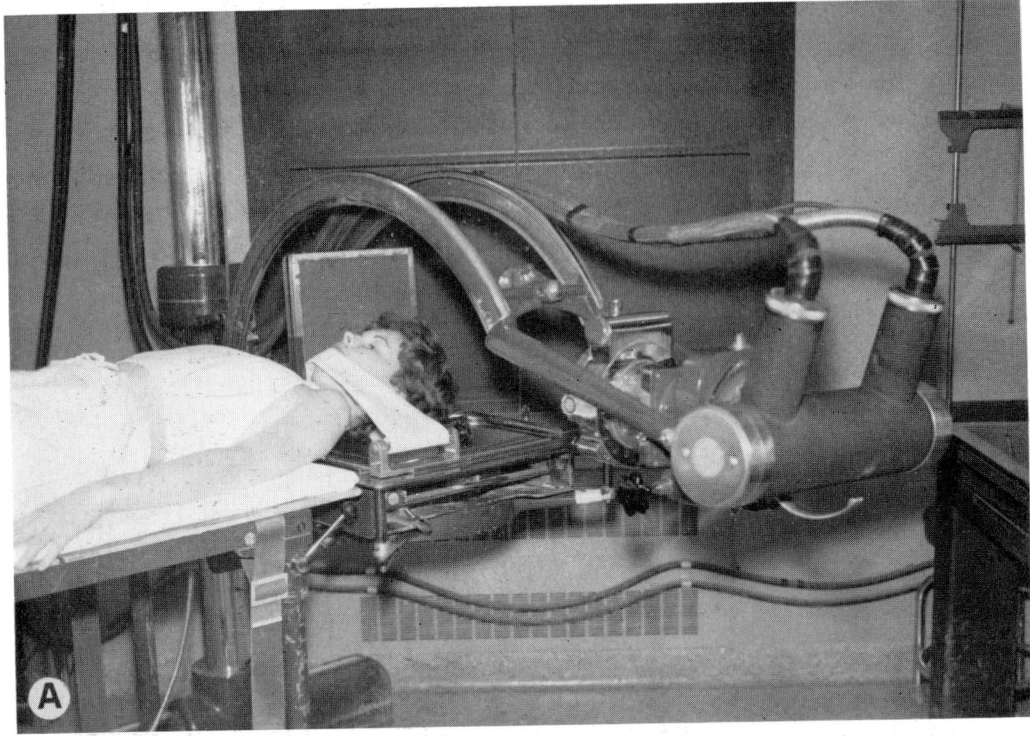

FIG. 187.—LATERAL EXAMINATION IN SUPINE POSITION

The patient remains undisturbed from the position shown in Figs. 185 and 186. A cassette is placed beside the patient's head and the radiographic tube is swung to an opposing position (A). The lateral supine pneumogram (brow-up lateral view) (C) is to be compared with the frontal film illustrated in Fig. 185. Varying degrees of fluid will be found in the dependent portions of the ventricles which prevents visualizaion of posterior segments, often to a greater extent than shown. A fluid-gas shadow is visible in each of the ventricles. Fluid remaining in the apical portion of the fourth ventricle should not be misinterpreted as a true reduction in height of this structure.

If a flexible headstand, which is separate from the radiographic table that supports the patient, is used, the surface of the Bucky device may be placed below (or above) the plane of the patient's body (B). With the patient supine, lateral examination in a position of hyperextension is accomplished with ease. In this position, gas enters the most anterior and inferior portions of the lateral ventricles and of the third ventricle, which are placed uppermost. The position is particularly effective for demonstrating abnormalities in the region of the foramen of Monro and in the hypothalamic portion of the third ventricle (see Fig. 260).

position while the x-ray tube remains beside the patient in position for a horizontal exposure. The side of the brain on which an abnormality is suspected should be uppermost as the patient is turned. The prone position usually is the most uncomfortable for the patient to maintain because of pressure on the face and the necessity of keeping the arms by the sides. It is also the most difficult for the technician since the roundness of the forehead induces rotation off axis. A support, such as a pillow or cushion, under the chest and a small pad under the chin will remove some pressure from the face and allow easier positioning and fixation of the head, or the Bucky device can be moved lower than the table top (fig. 188). After exposure of the lateral view, the x-ray tube is swung to the overhead position and, again, without disturbing the patient or gas distribution, a straight posteroanterior Bucky film is made employing a vertical

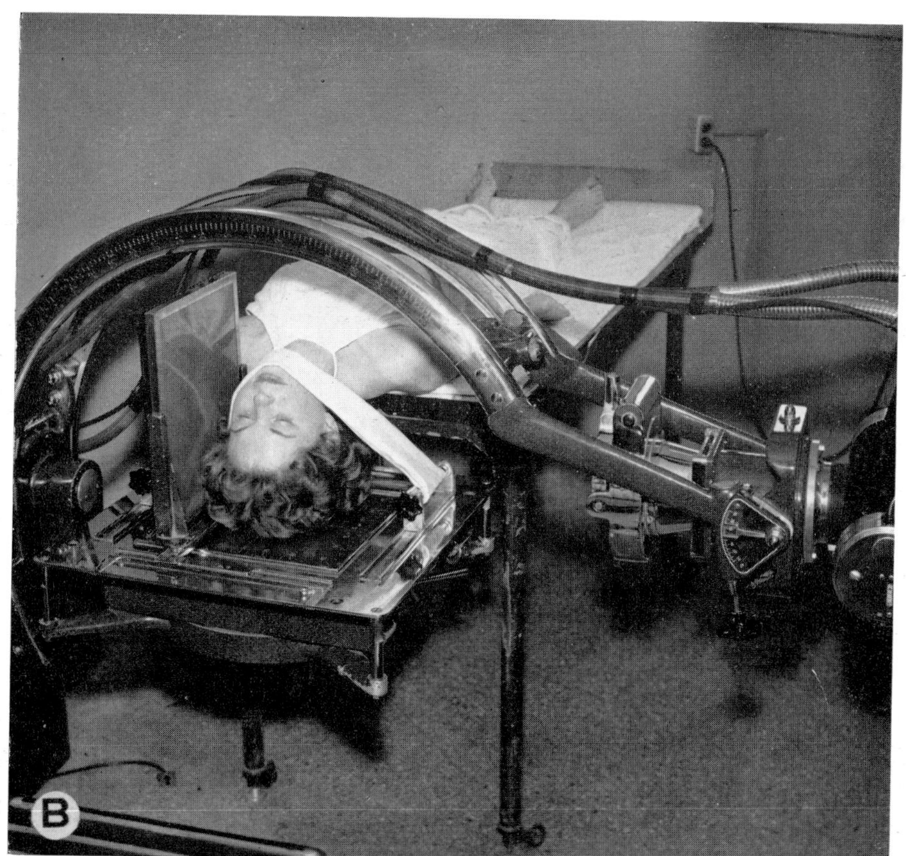

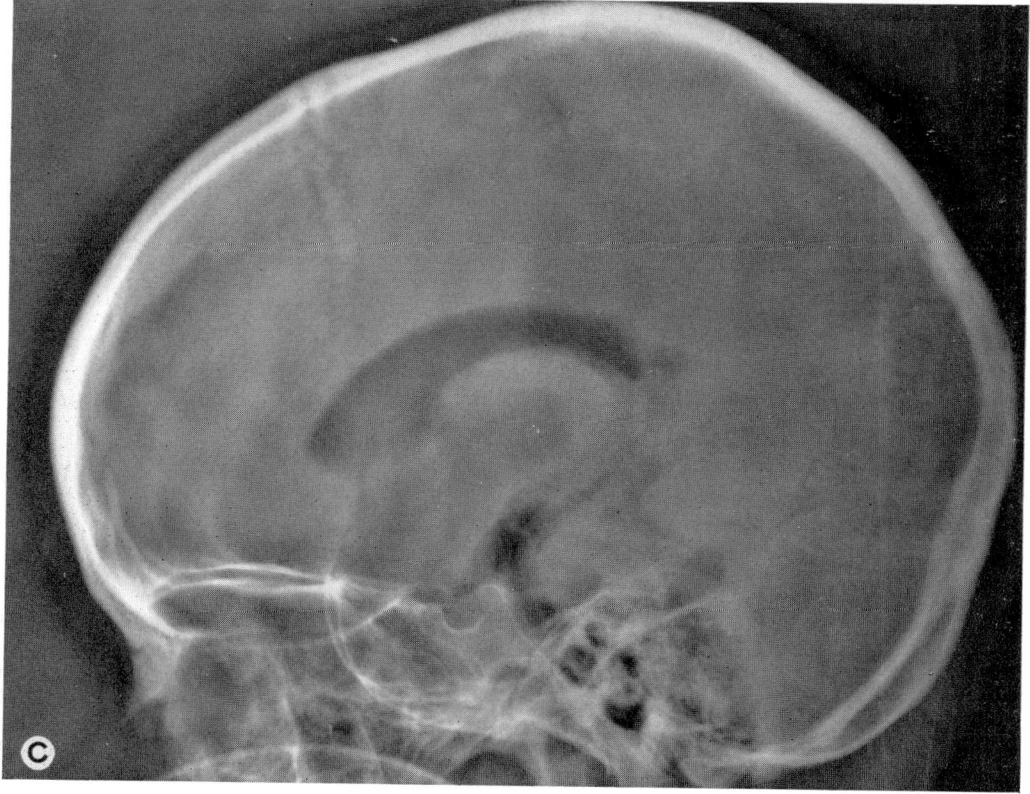

FIG. 187

(*Revised 1963*)

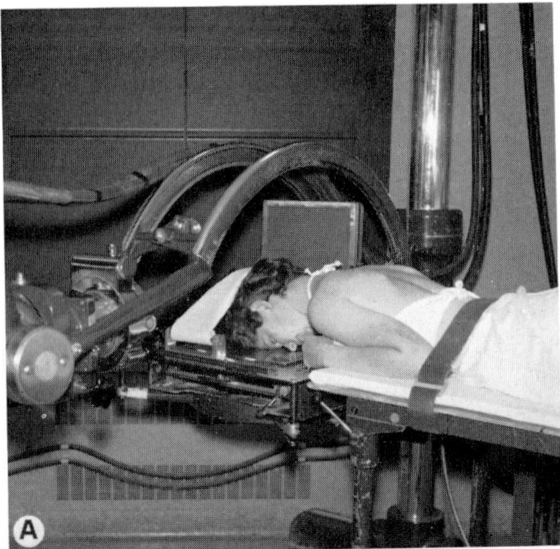

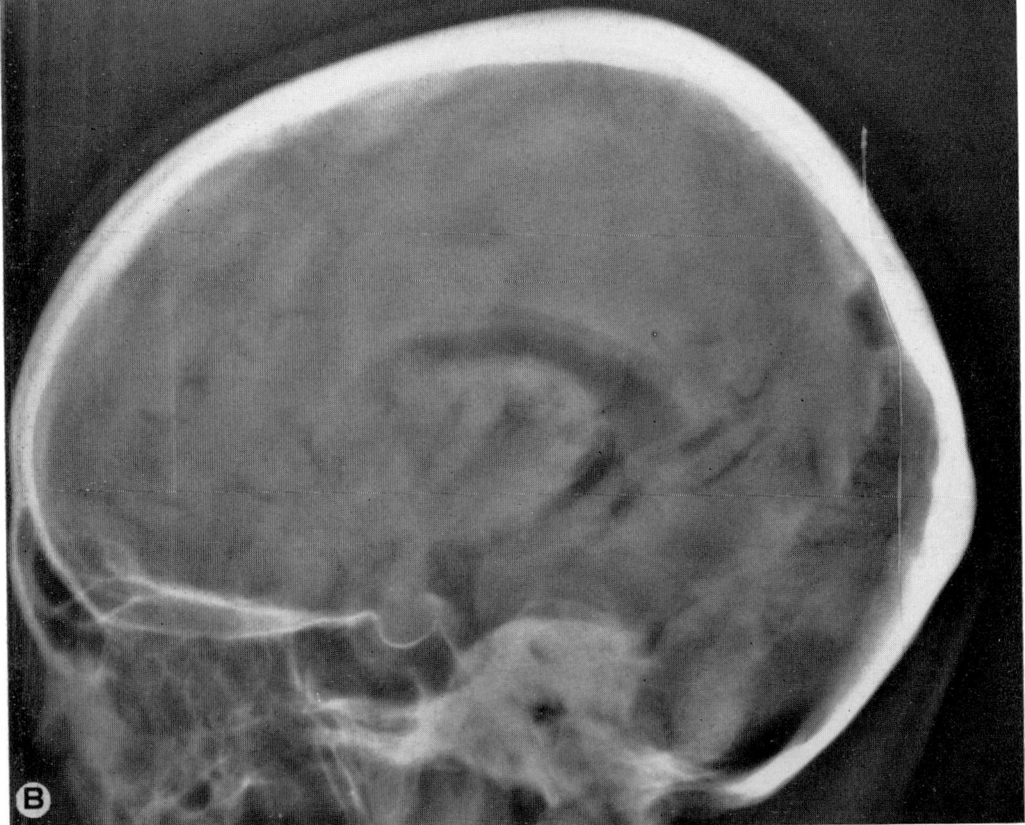

Fig. 188.—Lateral Examination in Prone Position

The position of the radiographic tube is not changed from that shown in Fig. 187. The patient is turned to prone position and a lateral view (brow-down lateral) is obtained using a grid-front cassette beside the patient's head (A). The horizontal beam film demonstrates the posterior (superior) portions of the ventricular system outlined by gas, while the anterior (dependent) portions are filled with fluid and are not visualized (B). The posterior part of the third ventricle, the cerebral aqueduct, and the fourth ventricle may be well-demonstrated in this view, in addition to the lateral ventricular atria and occipital horns.

(Revised 1963)

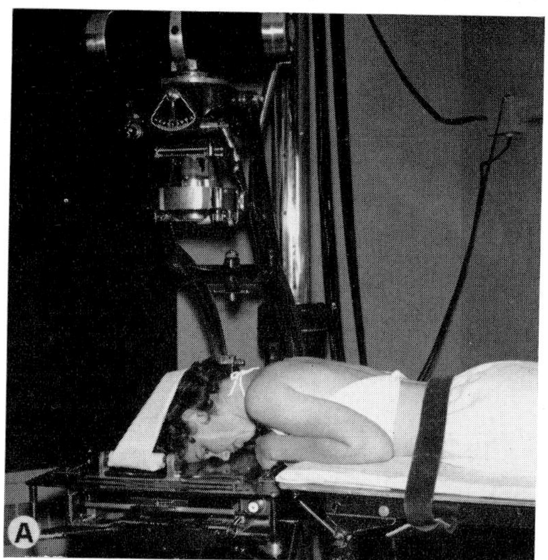

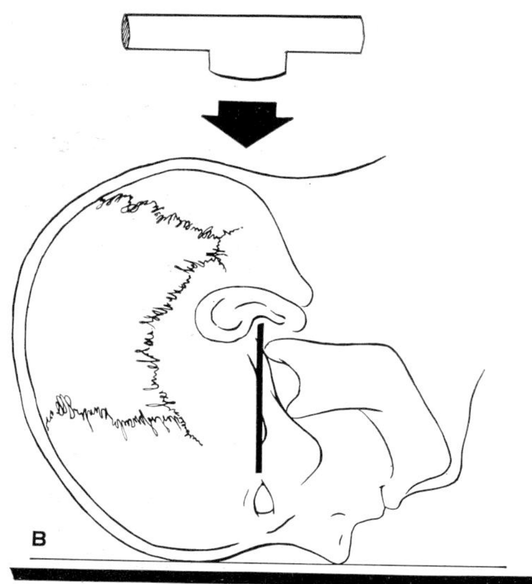

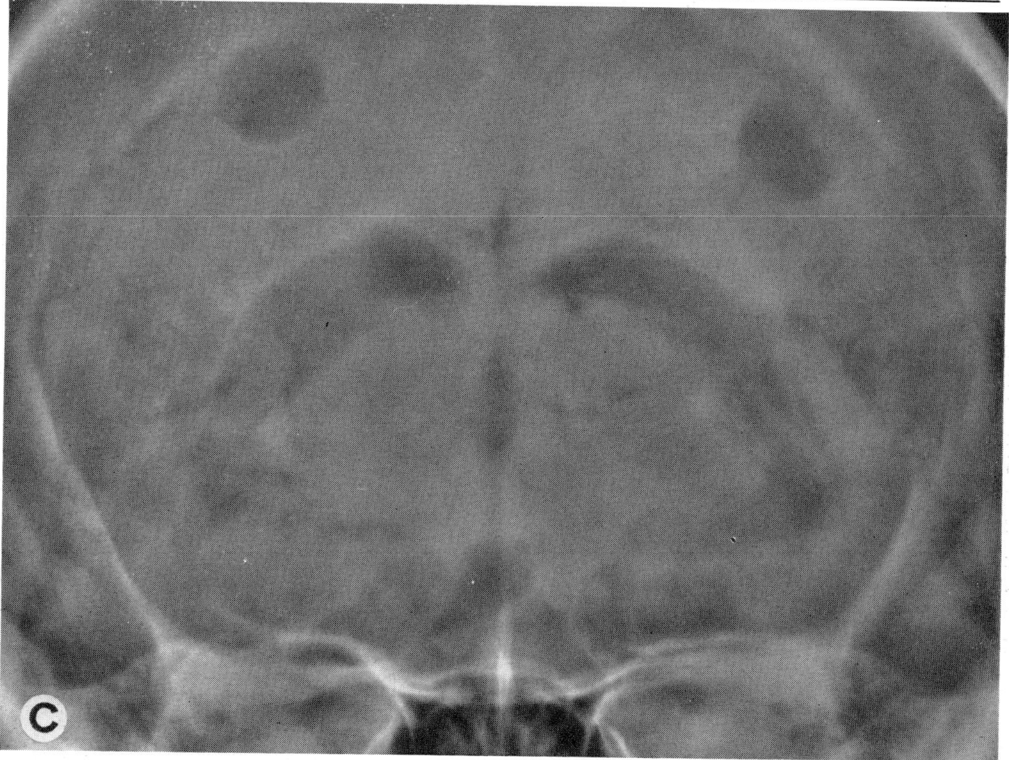

Fig. 189.—Frontal Examination in Prone Position

The patient remains prone, with the forehead against the center of the Bucky device and the nose resting lightly on the table (A). The orbitomeatal line again is perpendicular to the film. The central beam is directed vertically downward from the overhead radiographic tube through the inion and parallel to the orbitomeatal line (B).

The straight posteroanterior radiograph reveals gas distributed in the posterior portions of the lateral and third ventricles (C), the disposition being the same as that shown in Fig. 188. The temporal horns are filled to a varying extent, depending upon the quantity of fluid that remains trapped in these extensions. Sufficient gas frequently passes caudad from the third ventricle to outline the sylviduct and the fourth ventricle.

(Revised 1963)

x-ray beam (fig. 189). Stereoscopic views in this projection are easily obtained. Another view may be made in reverse half axial projection, but this is not done routinely.

The patient remains essentially prone, but the shoulders are turned to an oblique position and the neck is turned until the midsagittal plane of the head is perfectly horizontal. Either side may be examined first, but if one cerebral hemisphere is suspected clinically of being the site of disease, this side should be placed uppermost first. The corresponding arm may be brought forward and the fist used as a support for the chin. A pillow, or triangular block, is useful to support the upper chest in oblique position. The head is fixed in as nearly perfect horizontal plane as possible without rotation or twisting or depression of the vertex on its own axis (fig. 190). To accomplish this, the special head device or separate Bucky device at the head of the examining table is a great advantage since it may be raised or lowered to help bring the head into horizontal plane. The head should be firmly fixed by a restraining band or, preferably, a head clamp. The x-ray tube, which has remained overhead, is adjusted for a stereoscopic examination, and the pair of lateral exposures is made. Stereoscopic lateral films are always made in this position since ordinarily a right angle frontal view is not included in the routine. Sometimes, however, the frontal view taken with the horizontal x-ray beam is indicated (fig. 194).

The final routine set of films is made in exactly the same manner as just described, with the opposite side of the head uppermost.

While our routine calls for precise positioning of the head for the lateral horizontal views, it is of interest that some workers advocate slight tilting of the head by lowering of the vertex and elevating the face in an attempt to visualize better the temporal horns. Since the anterior tip of the temporal horn turns medially, it may contain a small fluid residue in true horizontal position and it is reasoned that the tilting will drain the temporal tip and allow gas to pass to its anterior extremity. Our experience teaches that in such off-plane projections, more important portions of the ventricular system often are inadequately visualized and facial and mastoid structures may be thrown into undue prominence. It is felt that a standard reproducible projection is more reliable than one which is geometrically untrue and which invites inaccurate, if not careless, positioning. On the other hand, there may be considerable value in carrying out several maneuvers routinely in connection with examination in lateral position. When the head is turned from frontal to lateral position, or from one side to the other, gentle rotation of the head on the neck forward, backward, and from side to side will cause gas in the dependent ventricle to ascend to the higher cavity through the interventricular foramen. During the maneuver, the vertex should be held high in relation to the base and downward rotation minimized in order to prevent excessive escape of gas from the third to the fourth ventricle and subarachnoid space. In this way, the anterior tip of the temporal horn can be emptied of fluid and a greater volume of the entire upper ventricle filled with gas. Even a deformed temporal horn often may be visualized in this way and since demonstration of the temporal area is

Fig. 190.—Lateral Examination in Recumbent Position

The head and shoulders are turned until the midsagittal plane of the skull is parallel to the Bucky device (A). From the overhead radiographic tube a vertical beam is directed at a point ¾″ above the external auditory meatus (B). The lateral aspects of the uppermost lateral ventricle are visualized to best advantage in this position (C). Since the temporal horn is the highest portion of the ventricular system, the structure should be well distended with gas unless an abnormality exists. The extreme anterior temporal tip, which turns medially, may contain some fluid and not be shown in its entirety. If a small quantity of gas remains in the dependent lateral ventricle, it usually is situated in the anterior portion of the ventricular body and posterior part of the anterior horn. Portions of the ventricular system caudad to the interventricular foramen may be outlined in varying degree. The sulci on both the medial and the lateral aspects of the brain often are well visualized.

(Revised 1963)

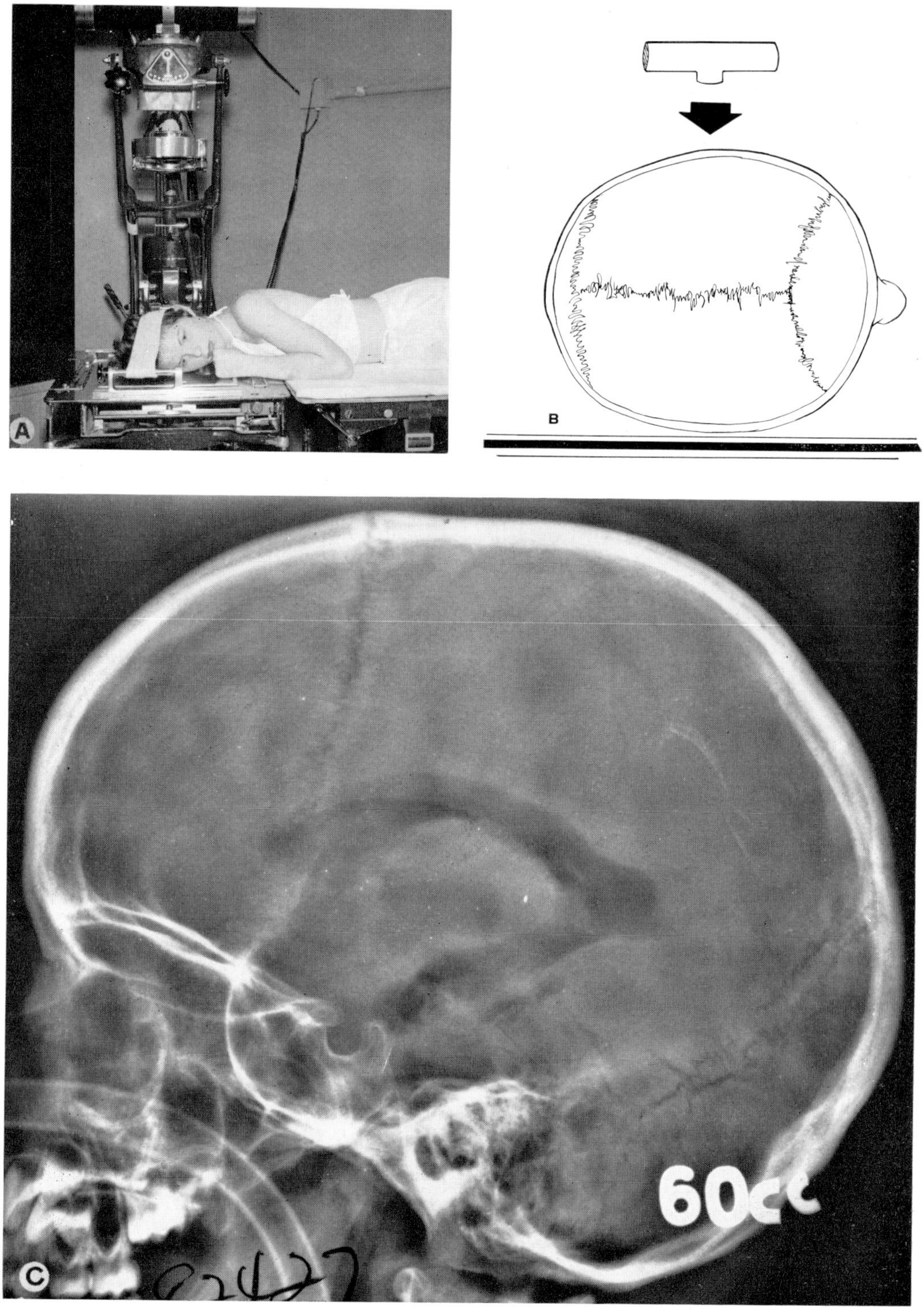

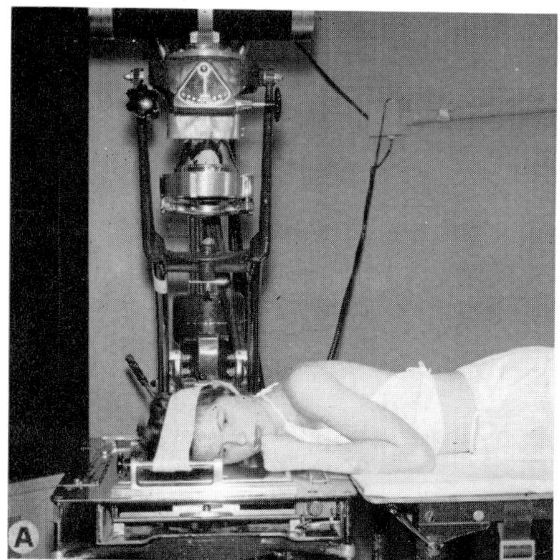

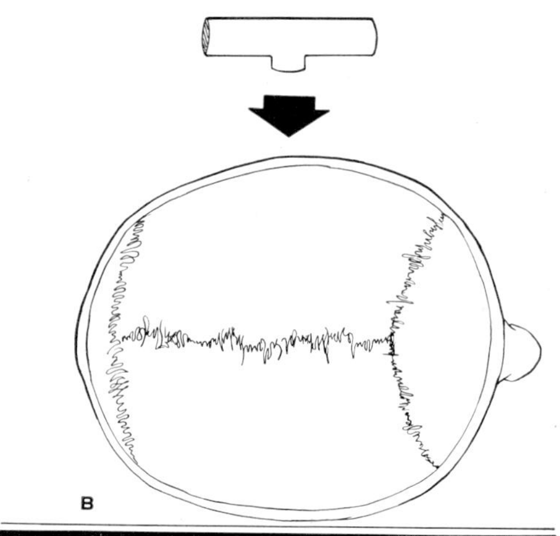

Fig. 190

the principal purpose of the recumbent lateral views, it is worthwhile to insure as full filling as the anatomic status allows. (See also under "Ventriculography.")

Selective or differential pneumography. In recent years, advocates of the use of smaller quantities of air for pneumoencephalography have become more numerous, and a considerable amount of writing on this subject has appeared in the literature. The term "selective (or differential) pneumogram" refers to the use of relatively small amounts of gas injected in little quantities with the flow of gas directed into channels of special interest by positioning of the head. Ventricular and subarachnoid pathways thus filled may be visualized without the superimposition of excessive collections of overlying gas. The examination is most suitable for the diagnosis of extracerebellar tumors of the posterior fossa, including both axial and extra-axial lesions. In the latter group particularly, and in the diagnosis of acoustic neurinoma specifically, the procedure is one of great utility. Patients with lesions of the suprasellar region or other tumors extending into the cisterns rostral to the posterior fossa also are suitable candidates for this type of air study.

Advantages of using small quantities of gas are lessened discomfort to the patient and apparent reduction in the complication rate. In some instances the diagnostic quality of pneumograms is actually improved by use of smaller amounts of gas for reasons just described. The concept that the use of the smallest amount of gas possible is best for the patient, provided the diagnostic quality of the examination is not impaired, appears to have considerable merit.

One of the obvious causes for increasing popularity of selective pneumography is the mounting statistical evidence that pneumoencephalography is less hazardous in the presence of subtentorial tumors than in the presence of supratentorial lesions. At one time the reverse was thought to be the case. To visualize well the posterior fossa structures, considerably less gas is needed than when visualization of the entire ventricular system is attempted. Furthermore, the greater use of cerebral angiography in recent times as the first procedure in cases of suspected supratentorial tumor has markedly decreased the incidence of complications which result from subfalcial and incisural herniation following pneumography. In the great majority of cases, differentiation can be made clinically between supratentorial and infratentorial lesions, and angiography or pneumography chosen as the first procedure for evaluation accordingly.

Various authors recommend different amounts of gas for the first injection, but the exact amount does not appear to be critical. Greater in importance than the quantity of gas used appears to be the taking in rapid sequence of the three radiographs recommended previously. Because visualization of the fourth ventricle and aqueduct are essential, the first (lateral) exposure should be made within 10 seconds after completion of the injection.

Ordinarily, 15 cc. of gas are injected in fractions of 5 cc. each. The first 5 cc. are injected with the hairline of the patient touching the Bucky device (about 25 degree angulation of the canthomeatal line with the plane of the film). Five cubic centimeters of cerebrospinal fluid are removed. This is followed by the injection of 5 cc. of air with the head extended slightly in order to fill the pontine cistern. The head is held in that position for about 10 to 15 seconds and then returned to its initial position. By flexing the head, the air in the pontine cistern will fill the lateral recesses of this cistern (also called cerebellopontine cisterns). Five cubic centimeters of cerebrospinal fluid are now removed, followed immediately by the injection of the third 5 cc. of air. To obtain greatest visualization of structures with the least amount of gas, the position of moderate flexion of the head recommended above appears to be optimum because it allows filling of the fourth ventricle without prior full distention of the cisterna magna.

In the cases where a tumor is suspected clinically, the above technique is modified at the beginning. *No cerebrospinal fluid is removed* and only 10 cc. of gas are injected. The fractions of gas used in such cases are

3 cc., 3 cc., and 4 cc. before exposing the three films recommended above.

The lateral exposure made with a grid-front cassette beside the head is followed as rapidly as is feasible by a frontal Bucky film. Without moving the head, an exposure in a posteroanterior half axial projection is made to obtain a semiaxial view of the posterior fossa structures. Again without delay, the head is extended until the forehead and the nose are against the Bucky device and a straight posteroanterior projection is obtained. The head is returned to a position of moderate flexion where it is maintained while the three initial films are rapidly processed.

After these films are viewed, a decision is made about how the examination is to continue. This decision will be guided by what is seen on the films, and no general rules can be given, although the following comments in regard to negative findings can be made. If the initial films reveal no contraindication, and the ventricles appear to be normal in size, the injection of additional gas for a total of 25 to 30 cc. may be elected. If unobstructed ventricles of large size are outlined, the procedure of limiting the study to small amounts of gas may be discarded and additional quantities that are proportionate to the estimated size of the ventricles may be used. At the completion of the air injection, the needle is withdrawn, and after an upright straight posteroanterior view and a lateral view are obtained, the patient is placed horizontal where pairs of right angle roentgenograms in supine, prone, right, and left lateral positions are obtained. The latter films are similar to those described first in conjunction with global pneumography and will give best visualization of the supratentorial areas. In general, the outlining of the posterior fossa structures is best controlled with the patient in upright position, while visualization of supratentorial structures is best accomplished with the patient horizontal.

Controlled pneumography. There are advantages in performing pneumoencephalography in specially constructed chairs that permit the patient to rotate 360 degrees along a horizontal axis (fig. 180). When using such a device, the technique of pneumoencephalography has to be varied accordingly. These devices permit the performance of the entire examination with relatively small amounts of gas (20 cc.) and without removing the needle, which may be advantageous in case it becomes necessary to add more air later on in the examination. Likewise, some air may be removed at the end, if desired. One of its biggest advantages is the ability to perform pneumoencephalography in unconscious or anesthetized patients because they are securely strapped to the chair, thus avoiding the usual difficulties encountered in these cases. The examination is expedited and valuable time in instituting treatment of the patient may be saved through satisfactory radiologic diagnosis of problem cases. For the most part, cooperative patients are examined by another method, although if a temporal or a hypothalamic tumor is suspected clinically, the controlled placing of gas in the ventricles may facilitate diagnosis in these instances. The somersaulting chair may be very useful also at ventriculography in the diagnosis of tumors obstructing or deforming any portion of the ventricular system.

For the portion of the examination usually performed in the sitting position, the head may be placed against the Bucky device and films made in straight posteroanterior projection and in lateral view, made with greater or lesser degrees of flexion as in any other method. When these films have been obtained, the patient is then rotated to a supine position, and brow-up lateral and anteroposterior views with two different angulations of the tube are made. After this, the patient is again tilted head-up and rotated into the prone position, followed by the taking of straight posteroanterior and lateral prone views. The frontal films may be made using two different angulations of the tube, if desired.

Up to this time, the anterior portions of the temporal horns have not been visualized. To accomplish this, from the prone position, the patient is somersaulted. As the patient's head passes inferiorly, the temporal horns

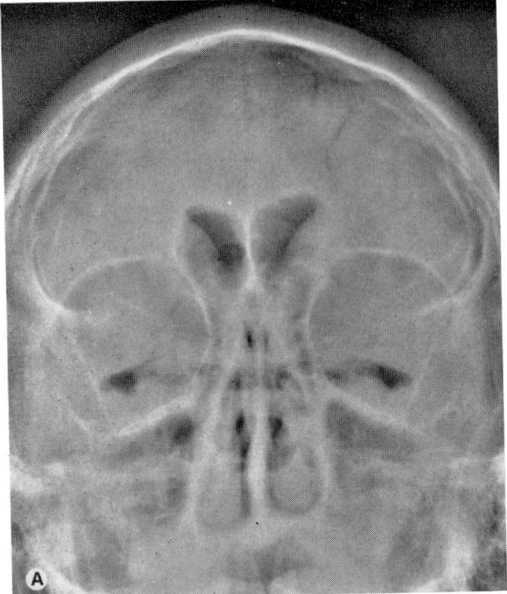

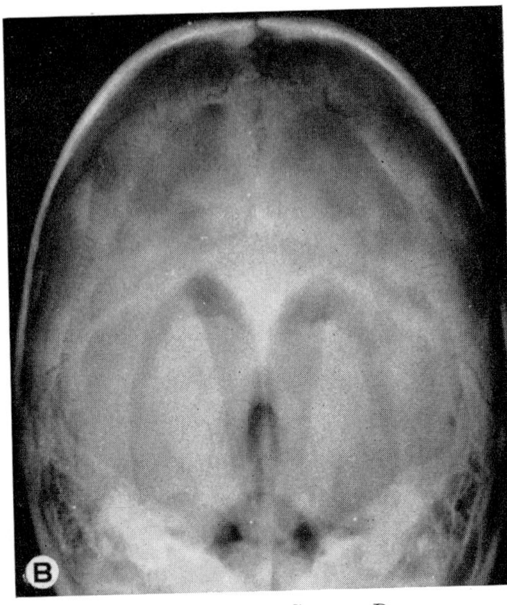

FIG. 191.—FRONTAL AND SUPERIOR VIEWS OF THE TEMPORAL HORNS IN SUPINE POSITION

After trapping gas in the temporal horns (see text), the horns may be radiographed through the orbits using the alternate projection shown in Fig. 185. With the patient supine, the x-ray beam is directed along Reid's base line. The anterior temporal tip and the forward portion of the body of the temporal horn are viewed axially (A).

In the anteroposterior half axial view, a modified superior-inferior depiction of the temporal horns is provided (B). The medial curvature of the temporal horn at its anterior end gives this portion of the horn a configuration which has been likened to the bowl of a spoon (see also Fig. 186).

are completely filled, and as his head is brought over to a supine position, both temporal horns will remain distended. At this time, (1) stereoscopic lateral views are made using the horizontal x-ray beam, followed by (2) frontal films of the temporal horns made through the orbits, and also (3) films made in the half axial projection (figs. 191 and 186).

When the somersaulting chair is used, there is never any difficulty in visualizing the anterior portion of the third ventricle if there is only a very small amount of gas present. Likewise, there usually is no difficulty in refilling the posterior portion of the third ventricle or the aqueduct and fourth ventricle. In order to fill the latter structures, a backward somersault is used, starting from the supine position and letting the patient's head go under him.

It is only rarely that the vertical beam lateral views are required. Vertical beam lateral views, which have been used by many workers for years, are intended principally to outline the temporal horns. Visualization of the temporal horns, however, is more easily accomplished as explained above and better distention is obtained since in lateral recumbent position the medial portion of the temporal horn is still filled with fluid. Nevertheless, if vertical beam lateral views are desired, the patient is placed in the supine position, the straps are loosened, and the head is turned to either side. An additional advantage of the somersaulting chair, shown in Figure 180, is that in order to correct slight rotation in frontal alignment it is not necessary to move the patient's head, which may produce rotation in other planes, but it is possible to rotate the entire patient in the chair the desired number of degrees when a head clamp attached to the chair is used. If a head clamp on the Bucky device is used, the correction of the rotation must be made in the usual manner.

Unless there is a special reason to remove the patient from the department as soon as possible, he remains on the radiographic table or in the somersaulting chair until all of the films are processed and viewed by the radiologist. Any unsatisfactory films may be repeated immediately while sufficient gas remains in the ventricles. If certain portions of the ventricles or subarachnoid space are not visualized adequately for diagnosis, appropriate films may be repeated or special maneuvers may be carried out and supplemental films made to help clarify the problem.

VENTRICULOGRAPHY

It is not within the province of this section or the qualifications of its authors to discuss the techniques of ventricular puncture, their relative merits, and the methods of exchange of ventricular fluid and gas. Suffice it to say that this is a procedure for the neurosurgeon which is usually carried out in the operating room but which sometimes, in emergency, is performed in the radiology department by means of the twist drill.

Routine Procedure

Following the injection of gas, the patient is taken to the pneumographic room, usually in a light plane of anesthesia, and attended by an anesthetist as well as the neurosurgeon or his assistants. The presence of an endotracheal tube may make the radiographic procedure more difficult. In the positions requiring flexion of the head and neck, particular care must be taken to avoid obstruction of the airway through bending or buckling of such a tube in the pharynx.

The examination should be carried out as expeditiously as possible and without interference with maintenance of desired anesthesia, since intracranial surgical procedures will be required immediately following ventriculography for a high percentage of patients. It is our custom to assign two technicians to carry out ventriculography. Only the horizontal series of pneumograms is prescribed as a routine. The procedure, therefore, may consist of as few as 10 films. As soon as each set of films is exposed, it is taken to the dark room and processed immediately with the result that by the time the final film is taken, the first films are available for viewing. Unless unusual difficulties are encountered, the entire procedure should not require more than 15 to 20 minutes. In the authors' departments, it is customary for the radiologist and neurosurgeon to view the films together as soon as they are fixed. Any repeat films required are taken immediately and if supplemental procedures are deemed desirable, they are executed at once.

Supplemental Procedures

Upright films are not a part of the ventriculographic routine but, on occasion, they may be considered essential to visualize better the ventricular roofs if not shown in horizontal films. If gas has escaped into the subarachnoid space, upright films may afford good demonstration of the superior and inferior surfaces of the brain. Considerable manual effort may be required in anesthetized patients to obtain the optimum position before the upright Bucky device, but we do not hesitate to carry out upright ventriculography if it is thought that helpful diagnostic information will be gained. If a somersaulting chair is available, the patient may be transferred to this device for the taking of upright or other additional films. Such a piece of equipment is most useful for examining anesthetized patients, as previously described. Various ingenious carriages and flexible radiographic table tops have been designed for free rotation of the patient in horizontal position, which also may be useful adjuncts in carrying out the horizontal portion of the examination.

When the ventricles are not well dilated or, if for some other reason, only a small amount of gas has been instilled at ventriculography, a common problem is visualization of the aqueduct of Sylvius and the fourth ventricle. Nonobstructing posterior fossa lesions occur with sufficient frequency to make visualization of the lower ventricular pathways imperative for a complete examination. In some instances, manipulation of the head suffices to complete the study with the gas already present in the ventricles. On other occasions, additional gas may be required which may be instilled by a repeated ventricular puncture or by an injection into the lumbar subarachnoid space, as for pneumoencephalography. If the latter is to be carried out, some neurosurgeons will prefer to have a catheter in a lateral ventricle and others tap the ventricles to allow air to escape in the sitting position, but this is a matter of surgical judgment in the individual case.

Combined ventriculography - pneumoencephalography. The ventriculogram-pneumoencephalogram combination is a reliable procedure and although time consuming and exhausting for the patient, it probably is the most satisfactory solution for incomplete ventricular visualization in the majority of instances. For this purpose, the patient is placed in the pneumoencephalographic chair and the head flexed to facilitate ventricular filling. A total of 10 cc. generally are all that will be required to outline the posterior fossa structures well with few exceptions, and after this amount has been introduced, the lateral and posteroanterior half axial views (or the first two films of the pneumoencephalogram series) are exposed. The films are processed immediately and in the majority of instances, the status of the fourth ventricle and iter will be clarified sufficiently to terminate the examination.

Central ventriculography. A procedure to visualize selectively the third ventricle, aqueduct of Sylvius, and fourth ventricle was described by Azambuja *et al.* (1956) and consists in the introduction of a flexible rubber catheter through the foramen of Monro after the placing of frontal burr holes. The examination is most suitable for patients who have extremely dilated venticles in whom an obstructive lesion in the region of the posterior third ventricle, the iter, or fourth ventricle is present. Once the catheter is placed within the third ventricle, the patient is taken to the pneumographic room and, after placing him in the prone position, 5 cc. of gas are injected through the catheter. Immediately thereafter a lateral film is made with the horizontal x-ray beam and a stereoscopic pair of vertical beam straight posteroanterior views also are taken. These radiographs usually are sufficient in the majority of instances to demonstrate the posterior third ventricle, the aqueduct of Sylvius and the fourth ventricle if the obstruction is not complete. The advantages of central ventriculography are that it is not necessary to remove any cerebrospinal fluid, and there are no confusing overlying shadows within the lateral ventricles covering the area of greatest interest in the posterior third ventricle and posterior fossa. The presence of long-standing obstructive lesions can be suspected by the length of the clinical history and by the appearance of the plain film radiographic examination of the skull in most instances.

Positive contrast examination. Although the use of substances of metallic density to visualize cerebral structures has been carried out for over a quarter century, more extensive notice has been given to the method in recent times. Thorotrast (thorium dioxide) was one of the first substances used, and because of its miscibility with water, it produces very satisfactory visualization of the cerebrospinal fluid spaces. Introduction of thorium dioxide produces no immediate reaction, but because it is a colloidal suspension, eventually the contrast material will behave like particulate matter and produce a leptomeningeal inflammation. Irritation of the ependyma with production of ependymitis and obstruction of the aqueduct of Sylvius and resultant hydrocephalus may occur (Dyke, 1941). In addition, the concern that has developed regarding the latent effects of the radioactivity of Thorotrast makes it unacceptable in many instances.

The use of Lipiodol in the ventricular system was described by Balado and Carillo in 1935. More recently, Pantopaque has been used for the same purpose. The third ventricle, aqueduct of Sylvius, and fourth ventricle can be demonstrated very satisfactorily by this means (fig. 192). The small amount of contrast material used allows only a minor portion of the ventricular system to be outlined, especially if the ventricles are enlarged, but direction of its flow by fluoroscopy through the foramen of Monro will allow positioning of the material strategically at the location of a posterior obstruction. A chief objection to the use of Lipiodol and Pantopaque is their persistence in the ventricular cavities in the presence of obstruction, or in the subarachnoid spaces for an indefinite period of time. Lipiodol, like Thorotrast, may induce an ependymitis and adhesive arachnoiditis, and it is doubtful that Pantopaque can be regarded as innocent of the production of latent inflammatory reactions.

Radiopaque contrast media are seldom used by the authors because gas has proven satisfactory in almost all instances. Occasionally, however, difficult problems arise in the differentiation of obstructive and communicating hydrocephalus, and in the diagnosis of posterior fossa tumors, and in these cases Pantopaque may be a useful material (fig. 298). Under these circumstances, it is undesirable to inject a large amount of gas into markedly dilated ventricles because of the danger of collapse of the brain and hematoma formation (fig. 196). However, with somersault techniques it is possible to fill any portion of the ventricular system with a very small amount of gas. Other methods of determining ventricular patency exist, such as the use of organic dyes and radioactive materials. Generally speaking, the injection of radiopaque materials into the ventricles or the passage of such media into the basal cisterns and ventricles following lumbar injection, as described by Malis (1958), are rarely superior to the proper use of gas and are reserved for judicious use in highly selected cases.

In infants, Pantopaque ventriculography is easily performed by fontanelle puncture and the injection of 1 to 2 cc. of contrast material into a lateral ventricle. The injection should be made, if feasible, with the face dependent in order to allow collection of the Pantopaque in the anterior horn. Following this, the head is extended, and the body usually slightly elevated, to allow the contrast material to pass through the foramen of Monro. When the material is collected in the third ventricle, the child is turned quickly to a supine position. Some workers prefer to place the patient upright at this point with the head slightly extended. In either event, filming should be carried out quickly since, if there is an incomplete obstruction, the contrast material may pass out of the ventricles very rapidly into the subarachnoid space.

It is our practice to place the occiput, when the patient is turned supine, on a small radiolucent pad to elevate the head from the radiographic table and depress the chin. A lateral view is made immediately, employing the horizontal x-ray beam and a grid-front cassette placed beside the patient's head. This is followed as rapidly as possible by a half axial projection, using an angled vertical x-ray beam, the film ordinarily being made with the Bucky device. The two films described usually are adequate to demonstrate a point of obstruction and deformity of the posterior third ventricle, iter, or fourth ventricle, if present. In children, the use of fluoroscopy is not as essential as in the case of adults, since the manipulation may be repeated if not successful on the first try. Avoiding fluoroscopic exposure, however, would appear to be a minor consideration under such circumstances, and better results are assured if it is used. Repuncture and a second Pantopaque injection, if required, certainly are more hazardous.

In adults, fluoroscopy is employed routinely because of the relative immobility of the patient, as compared with an infant, and the need for delicate manipulation and rapid filming when the contrast material has reached the desired location. The examination is begun with the patient sitting sideways in front of an upright tilting fluoroscopic-radiographic machine with spot film attachment. For these examinations, the footboard of the table is raised to a height

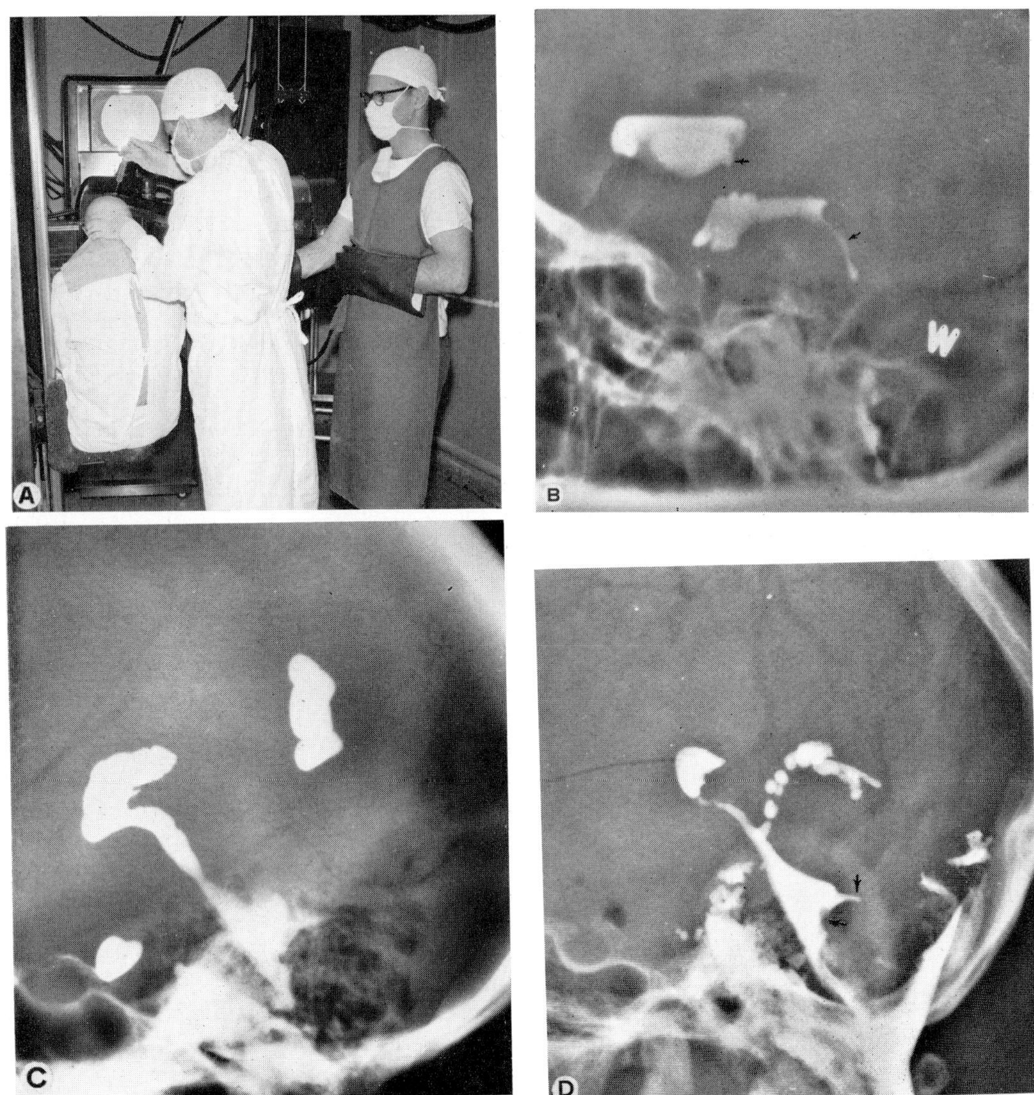

FIG. 192.—PANTOPAQUE VENTRICULOGRAPHY

In adults, positive contrast ventriculography is carried out under fluoroscopic control, with the patient upright. The foot rest of the fluoroscopic table is used as a seat for the patient. One to 2 cc. of contrast material are injected into the atrium of one lateral ventricle (A). The head is well flexed to cause the contrast material to descend into the anterior horn, following which its course is guided under fluoroscopy.

Spot films (B) are made as the contrast material passes through the foramen of Monro (*upper arrow*) to fill the dependent portion of the third ventricle and spill over into the aqueduct of Sylvius (*inferior arrow*). When a sufficient quantity (0.5 to 1 cc.) of contrast material has entered the third ventricle, the fluoroscopic table is tilted to horizontal with the patient in supine position (see text). The contrast material in the third ventricle (B) thus is trapped in the posterior portion of the third ventricle, the cerebral aqueduct, and the fourth ventricle, if there is no obstruction (C). The examination should include frontal views made with the spot film device when the patient is upright, an anteroposterior Bucky film made with the patient supine, and horizontal beam lateral views in both positions. The contrast material also passes readily into the subarachnoid space through the foramen of Magendie and the suitable to make a comfortable seat for the patient. With conventional apparatus, the patient faces to the fluoroscopist's right. The neurosurgeon is to the left, behind the patient, at the open portion of the fluoroscopic arm. Through a previously placed posterior burr hole, a needle is inserted into a lateral ventricle. The needle, however, could be inserted in the operating room and the patient brought to the Radiology Department with the needle in place. The patient's head is flexed sharply, and 1 to 2 cc. of Pantopaque are injected (fig. 192). Under these conditions, the material should pass promptly into the anterior horn of the lateral ventricle. Following the injection, the ventricular needle is removed. Under fluoroscopic guidance, the head is extended slowly and the contrast material flows posteriorly until it passes by gravity through the foramen of Monro.

After the contrast material has been collected in the third ventricle, the head is extended even further to cause the Pantopaque to enter the posterior portion of the third ventricle. It may be necessary to move the patient forward and arch the back slightly. Under fluoroscopically guided hyperextension, the contrast material fills the posterior third ventricle and, if patent, the aqueduct and fourth ventricle are visualized. At this time, lateral radiographs are made employing the spot film device. If the contrast material passes into the fourth ventricle, the degree of extension of the head may be reduced slightly for the patient's comfort. Such lateral spot films usually involve some magnification but, because of the good contrast afforded by the radiopaque material, satisfactory ventricular outline ordinarily is obtained. After satisfactory spot filming in lateral projection, either to demonstrate a point of obstruction or to demonstrate patency of the ventricular pathways, the patient is turned 90 degrees to face the radiologist. Frontal spot films then are made. The need for spot filming is attested by the fact that instances have been encountered in which sizable posterior fossa tumors were present, displacing the fourth ventricle, but in which the positive contrast material passed fairly rapidly out of the ventricular system and into the spinal subarachnoid space. Apparently the strong force of gravity on Pantopaque accounts for this occurrence under circumstances in which gas could not be made to traverse the narrowed lumen. For the same reason, cinefluorography has been found a valuable adjunct and is now frequently used rather than spot films. The upright frontal spot films or the frontal cinefluorographic record usually provide a rather distorted image but are satisfactory to show a lateral deformity or displacement of the fourth ventricle or aqueduct.

Following the obtaining of this film record, and with the patient's back against the fluoroscopic table, the table is tilted downward to the horizontal position. As horizontal is approached, the footboard of the table which had acted as a seat is removed. With the patient supine, the occiput is slightly elevated on a radiolucent block and lateral and frontal views are obtained as described in connection with the examination of infants. The latter films usually are of excellent quality if the contrast material has not disappeared from the ventricular system by the strong force of gravity and provide the greatest assistance in precise radiologic diagnosis.

One other technique employing Pantopaque may be best mentioned at this point. Following the method of Malis (1958), which has been called rhombencephalography, Pantopaque injected into the lumbar subarachnoid space may be passed into the

---

foramina of Luschka. Positive contrast myelography serves to outline narrow spaces that cannot be satisfactorily demonstrated by gas.

Another method of positive contrast examination involves the cephalic passage, with the patient supine, of a large amount of Pantopaque which has been injected into the lumbar subarachnoid space (D). The technique, which has been termed rhombencephalography, provides excellent radiographic detail of anatomic structures, such as the dorsal recesses of Retzius (*upper arrow*) and the chorioid plexus (*lower arrow*), but is generally considered unnecessary for clinical diagnosis (see text).

(*Revised 1963*)

fourth ventricle and occasionally into more rostral portions of the ventricular system (figs. 192 and 219). Relatively large quantities of contrast material must be employed, however, and this is considered undesirable. Furthermore, the uncertainty of results has tended to make the authors prefer other methods involving chiefly the use of air.

Tomography. This procedure is a valuable adjunct for the demonstration of midline structures or lesions at pneumography and, in the past, has found extensive use. The procedure was more popular when great reliance was placed on vertical beam radiography before the advent of high speed-high definition grid-front cassettes and flexible tubestands which allow wide application of the horizontal beam examination. In addition, global pneumography and large volume ventriculography were the universal procedures at the time and it was frequently necessary to utilize tomography to visualize central areas now readily seen through differential or selective techniques. Current infrequent use notwithstanding, it is desirable to have available in the room where pneumographic procedures are carried out an attachment for body section radiography. Any of the various movements carried out by commercially available tomographic devices are satisfactory for the clinical purposes of pneumographic diagnosis. The use of a multilayer film holder will reduce radiation to the patient, although only two or three sections are needed in the majority of instances and conventional methods are regarded as entirely safe.

Conventional tomography is more helpful at ventriculography than in pneumoencephalography. In the latter, the use of upright films made during the filling phase of the examination usually allows unencumbered visualization of the cisterna magna, the fourth ventricle, the iter, and even the third ventricle. At ventriculography, however, it is important to determine with certainty the caudal extent of gas movement in order to diagnose a supratentorial or infratentorial deep seated obstructing lesion, and some of the areas in question may be obscured by dilated lateral ventricles. It must be said, however, that vertical beam tomography, which, for the most part, requires that the head be placed in lateral recumbent position, is practically useless in modern pneumography where smaller amounts of gas are used. Under these conditions, there is usually an insufficient quantity of gas present to fill the lateral ventricles and also outline the third ventricle, aqueduct of Sylvius, and fourth ventricle.

Autotomography. This is a method of utilizing the horizontal x-ray beam in body section techniques and is applicable to differential pneumography and other upright examinations. It is a good substitute for the more elaborate apparatus and maneuvers required for horizontal beam tomography employing Bucky devices and other specially designed commercial equipment. The method first was described by Vallebona (1930) and again, apparently independently, by Ziedses des Plantes (1950). The modern application of autotomography has been summarized by Schechter and Jing (1960) and Schechter and de Gutiérrez-Mahoney (1962). Suffice it to say that the method is now chiefly used in connection with selective pneumography to visualize the fourth ventricle in frontal and lateral projection. Rather than having the radiographic tube and film move synchronously, they remain stationary and the patient provides the required motion. By gently and evenly oscillating the head in a smooth side-to-side motion, either voluntarily or passively, the objects about the craniovertebral axis are clearly visualized while those at a distance are obscured (fig. 193). Thus, the configuration of the fourth ventricle may be demonstrated more clearly than in conventional projections and deformity or displacement can be more readily recognized.

Other maneuvers. The *temporal horns* may be very difficult portions of the ventricular system to visualize and evaluate and the problem has been the subject of extensive study by several workers. Lindgren (1948) has stressed the importance of study in both lateral and frontal projections made with the patient supine. The variation in visualization and appearance with angula-

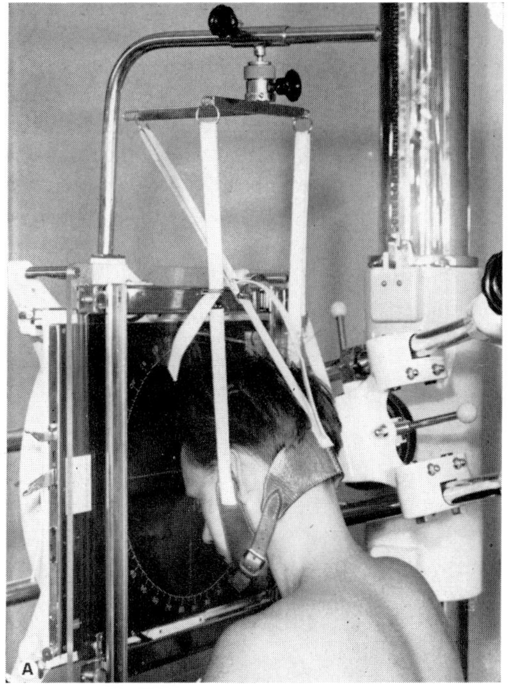

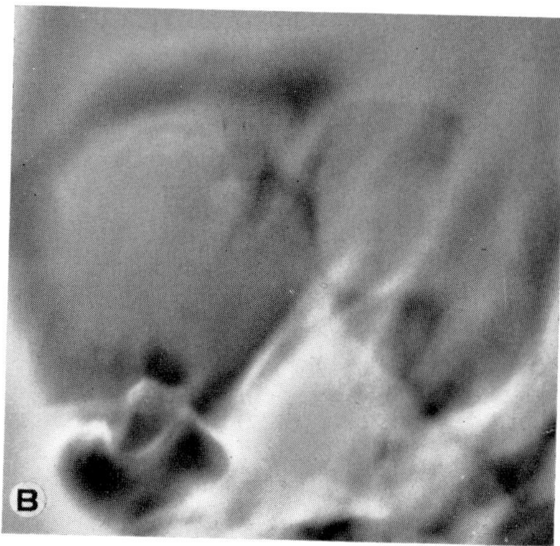

FIG. 193.—AUTOTOMOGRAPHY

In order to avoid use of the elaborate apparatus required to obtain tomograms with the horizontal x-ray beam, it is possible to move the patient's head about its axis to provide the required motion. Ordinarily, the patient can voluntarily rotate the head on the neck in a smooth oscillating motion, while a lateral film made with the horizontal x-ray beam is exposed. In less cooperative patients, a head halter may be required (A). Reins may be attached to the supporting straps at the level of the patient's ears and the head moved rhythmically by pulling one rein and then the other. Thus, the operator can remain behind the patient in a position which is remote from the x-ray beam.

The films obtained provide clinically satisfactory depiction of structures about the craniovertebral axis, while those more laterally placed are obscured (B). The radiograph may be compared with Fig. 181 for its relative freedom from superimposed mastoid air cell shadows in the region of the fourth ventricle.

tion of the tube or of the head in supine position is well recognized and several anatomic variations are described. In the technique advocated by Lindgren, one horn is filled at the time. Horizontal beam supine lateral views and vertical beam frontal films are required. The latter are obtained by projecting the temporal horn through the orbit, using a 20-degree cephalad angulation from the orbitomeatal line. Another frontal view in anteroposterior half axial projection is taken.

A preferable way of examination is to fill both temporal horns simultaneously, using a forward somersault maneuver with the patient in a rotating chair and to take stereoscopic lateral supine views and the two anteroposterior views described above (figs. 185, 186, and 187). The stereoscopic lateral views permit visualization of both temporal horns and obviate the need for repeated maneuvers.

The simplest maneuver to fill one temporal horn consists in placing the patient in the lateral position on the side opposite that being filled for several minutes to allow as much air as possible to enter the uppermost ventricle. Then the patient is placed in the supine position. The views described are made. The maneuver is repeated for the opposite side. The technique of filling only one temporal horn becomes necessary when there is insufficient air remaining in the lateral ventricles for simultaneous visualization of both sides.

While the films described will give adequate information about the temporal areas in most instances, the temporal relationship to the third ventricle, to the lateral aspect of the skull and the symmetry of the two sides may require special frontal views. The anteroposterior half axial projection may allow satisfactory visualization when the horns are well filled and a good comparison of the two sides is possible. A frontal view with the head in lateral position, employing the horizontal x-ray beam, may allow better visualization of the lateral aspect of the temporal horn in its entirety, but will not show the medial portion which remains filled with fluid (fig. 194). The head position is similar to the conventional lateral recumbent examination, except that the head is elevated above the table by a block or pad. The patient may be more comfortable lying straight on his side with the head supported in line with the spine. Using a grid-front cassette, the x-ray beam is directed either posteroanteriorly or anteroposteriorly, as the case may be. After the side of suspected abnormality is examined, a film of the opposite side usually is made for comparison. Strictly comparable films are not obtained if one film is anteroposterior and the other posteroanterior. By swinging the patient on his stretcher around to the opposite end of the headstand, similar projections can be obtained. The resulting film should show the uppermost ventricle almost completely filled with gas, except for some cerebrospinal fluid usually remaining in the anterior horn and body of the ventricle against the midline. Some gas usually is trapped in the anterior portion of the dependent ventricle.

The region of the *atrium*, the *posterior part of the temporal horn* and the *occipital horn*, if present, may be visualized well in a prone position favored by Robertson (1946) in which the head and neck are extended beyond the examining stretcher or table and flexed until the vertex becomes the most dependent portion of the patient. The atria and posterior part of each temporal horn may be well visualized in such a projection. Lindgren (1948) accomplishes somewhat similar visualization by placing the patient in ordinary prone position and having the tube angled approximately 35 degrees in a caudocephalad direction. The position of more extreme flexion, recommended by Robertson, may provide visualization of the inferior wall of the posterior part of the temporal horn and of the atrium in lateral view made with the horizontal beam. The position is used by Childe (1961) in connection with ventriculography to visualize the third ventricle and posterior fossa structures. The dependent head is agitated to induce filling of the posterior part of the third ventricle, the aqueduct of Sylvius, and the fourth ventricle. With the patient prone, three frontal views are made. The first is taken with the tube angled caudocephalad 5 degrees below the posteroanterior half axial plane. A second is made with the tube moved cephalad 5 degrees for a stereoscopic shift, and a third film is made after moving the tube a similar distance further cephalad. In this way, two stereoscopic pairs of films are produced, the first and second films being mates as are the second and third. Childe recommends such duplication of stereos as often helpful in visualizing the aqueduct of Sylvius, the fourth ventricle, and cisterna magna.

The region of the *foramen of Monro* and *anterior third ventricle* may be visualized well by use of a position of hyperextension, essentially the reverse of that just described. With the patient supine, the head and neck are extended over the end of the examining table until the region of the vertex again is most dependent (fig. 187). Examination only in lateral projection in this position is feasible, employing the horizontal x-ray beam and grid-front cassette, since the facial and basal areas overlie the cranium in superior view. Examination in the hyperextension position is easy to execute and ideal for demonstrating the effects of suprasellar or hypothalamic masses on the third ventricle (fig. 260). At ventriculography, the position may be useful

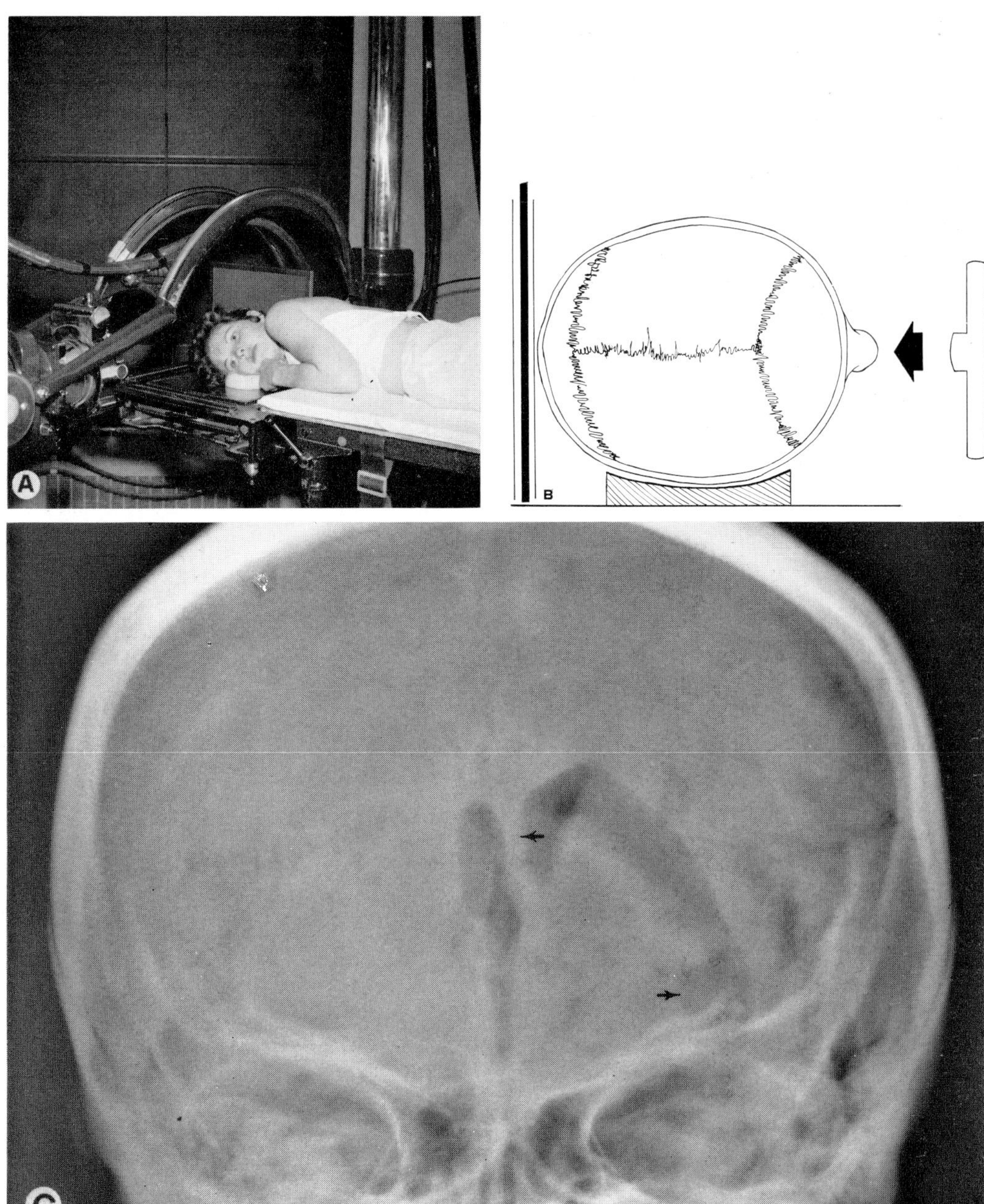

Fig. 194.—Frontal Examination of a Temporal Horn in Lateral Recumbent Position

The patient occupies the same position used to obtain the classical lateral view (see Fig. 190). The horizontal x-ray beam and a grid-front cassette placed behind the patient's head are employed (A and B). In the frontal radiograph (C) the superior portions of the uppermost lateral ventricle are outlined by gas. The lateral margin of the temporal horn thus is well depicted. Visualization of the anterior temporal tip, which turns medially, will vary, depending upon the amount of fluid that remains trapped in this portion of the horn (*lower arrow*). The medial wall of the ventricular body and anterior horn may be obscured by fluid remaining in these segments (*upper arrow*). Some gas often is trapped in the medial portion of the dependent ventricle (compare with Fig. 190). Filling of the third and fourth ventricles may occur in varying degree. Very frequently the sulci of the lateral aspect of the uppermost hemisphere are well outlined.

(Revised 1963)

to visualize obstructing lesions of the foramen of Monro, such as colloid cysts.

The use of *television-monitored fluoroscopy* and *cinefluorography* are in the stage of development at the present time. Both appear promising and the usefulness of the latter has been described in connection with Pantopaque ventriculography. The techniques are of significant clinical value in myelography. For the most part, cinefluorography in neuroradiology has been utilized in the study of human physiology and evaluation of its clinical usefulness has begun only recently.

Methods of visualization on television and cine filming of the flow of gas in the subarachnoid pathways and ventricles in conjunction with injections in upright position are under study. Such techniques may have particular application in the area of selective pneumography. Limited experience has disclosed that a fleeting visualization of the subarachnoid pathways frequently is obtained on only a few frames of the cinefluorographic record, similar to opacification of cardiac segments. Thus, one cerebellopontine cistern may be seen filled for only a fraction of a second, following which the gas passes on to another area. Tumors of the eighth cranial nerve may be demonstrated or excluded by cinefluorography, employing very small quantities of gas, in cases in which conventional methods require repeated gas injections and the exposure of multiple films. Although the full potential of television controlled air injection and cinefluorographic recording of intracranial pneumography are not known, the prospect of a valuable contribution to neuroradiology by these media is good.

Morbidity and Complications

A certain degree of morbidity usually accompanies any gross disturbance of a physiological system, such as the cerebrospinal fluid circulation. In the case of pneumoencephalography, morbidity is a significant consideration, but also small, when compared with the information that usually is gained, provided the indication for the examination is sound. In addition, there is a calculated risk of complications, but again, the incidence should be low if some avoidable complications, such as certain herniations, can be reduced to a minimum through the proper selection of patients (see "Selection of Diagnostic Procedure"). As will be described below, the nature of the patient's fundamental intracranial disease is more often related to the development of complications and even the severity of morbidity than other factors, which often play a minor role.

MORBIDITY

Headache is by far the most common symptom associated with pneumoencephalography, and in many instances it may be severe and prolonged. The great majority of patients experience some degree of headache, and its absence may be of significance since many patients who do not complain of this symptom are found to have cerebral atrophy of degenerative, inflammatory, or other origin. In some instances, the head pain begins as a subjective sensation related to the cephalad flow of gas. Some patients will describe vividly paresthesias, occasionally formication, as the gas passes through the neck and into the cranial cavity, the sensations often being suboccipital and temporal in location. A painful pressure in the head often is described, frequently related to the frontal region.

Headache may lead to apprehension, dizziness, and faintness, without objective evidence of a significant circulatory disturbance. As a result, an occasional patient may become uncooperative and difficulty may be experienced in maintaining the upright posture. As stated earlier, proper pre-

(Revised 1963)

medication is important in preventing excessive morbidity of this type. Adequate barbiturate sedation is the most reliable method in the experience of most workers. Morphine and its substitutes do not appear to be superior in avoiding these symptoms, and it is generally conceded that the degree of patient cooperation is much less when they are used, particularly with regard to reasonableness and maintenance of the upright posture.

Other symptoms are largely related to the *vegetative* nervous system. Exactly why such symptoms are produced is not entirely clear, but it has been suggested that the presence of foreign material, such as gas, produces an irritation of these centers, many of which are along the ventricular walls. Following headache, nausea and vomiting are the most frequent disorders encountered, usually preceded by the customary salivation, respiratory tract mucous secretion, and cold perspiration. For this reason, fasting prior to the examination is recommended as part of the routine preparation, and the support of barbiturate sedation by atropine or scopolamine is advised. In the great majority of patients, nausea and vomiting are not related to brain stem compression. Instead, and in line with the concept just mentioned, it would appear more likely that salivation, perspiration, nausea, and vomiting are related to gas entering the fourth ventricle and affecting the adjacent medullary centers.

Usually next in frequency of occurrence are pallor, coldness of the skin, and chilliness of the patient. These changes often are associated with slowing of the pulse and a reduction of body temperature. Although slow, the pulse usually is of good quality. A slow pulse of poor quality may be found and, rarely, a rapid weak pulse may develop. When an increased pulse rate occurs, there is usually also an increase in the respiratory rate and an elevation of body temperature. In the majority of patients, as is mentioned later, some elevation of blood pressure occurs. In the minority of patients, lowering of the blood pressure is found.

Depression, muscular weakness, and drowsiness may be only the aftermath of vomiting. Severe restlessness may have more serious implications and may be followed by syncope and collapse in severe cases. A prompt response to stimulants, the administration of oxygen, and supportive treatment as described below can be expected unless a complication develops. Cyanosis has been observed to be a frequent occurrence by some investigators.

Although numerous attempts have been made to relate morbidity to certain disease processes, particularly tumors, such direct relationship rarely can be found. The symptoms appear to be related more to the individual than to disease, and normal persons frequently suffer the most severe morbidity. Lack of morbidity, however, has been related fairly well to the presence of cerebral atrophy. It is not unusual for such patients to complain of no headache, to experience no untoward symptoms during the examination, and to be normally active soon after the procedure. Therapeutically beneficial effects have been ascribed to pneumoencephalography (Penfield, 1927, and Gardner, 1929).

On the other hand, there is very convincing evidence that the morbidity that accompanies pneumoencephalography is directly related to the volume of gas which is used for the examination. The quantity of fluid removed may play a complementary role (Slosberg and Bornstein, 1955). The smaller the quantity of gas employed for the examination, the less significant the morbidity. In recent years, much less gas has been used for pneumography than in the past, and a reduction of morbidity and also of complications has resulted. Morbidity is most severe when complete replacement of cerebrospinal fluid by gas is carried out, as was once the practice in many clinics.

Not only the severity of morbidity but its duration is affected by the quantity of gas employed. Headache and other symptoms may not reach their height immediately but may be greatest 3 to 6 hours after completion of the examination. While the symptoms usually are markedly alleviated by the following day, it is not uncommon to have significant morbidity for two to three days. In some instances, symptoms may persist for a week. With the use of smaller quantities of gas, the duration of morbidity is reduced proportionately.

Changes in the cerebrospinal fluid may be found by laboratory examination following pneumoencephalography. There is an almost immediate pleocytosis following the first injection of gas. Polymorphonuclear leukocytes are the main element of the cellular increase. The reaction occurs with such rapidity that it is desirable to obtain samples of cerebrospinal fluid for cell count as soon after the puncture is made as feasible, consistent with the technique of study in use.

Chemical as well as physical changes in the cerebrospinal fluid composition take place, and often an elevation of sugar and albumin can be demonstrated. The greatest change in cerebrospinal fluid composition usually occurs within 12 hours after completion of the examination, and under normal circumstances, the cellular and chemical components have returned to their original level by 36 to 48 hours. No clear-cut relationship between cerebrospinal fluid changes and clinical findings can be satisfactorily defined. Again, the volume of gas used appears to be all-important, the extent of cerebrospinal fluid change corresponding most closely to the quantity of gas injected.

Inflammatory meningeal reactions following pneumoencephalography also are encountered, and it is difficult to say whether the milder reactions are part of the morbidity of the procedure or whether they constitute an infection which is well handled by the patient. In some individuals, the irritative effect of replacement of fluid by gas can conceivably produce a stiff neck and elevation of temperature. In these cases, there is usually persistent headache and often vomiting. On laboratory examination, inflammatory changes in the cerebrospinal fluid are found. A latent period of 24 to 48 hours usually is connected with this type of inflammatory meningeal process, which appears to support the thesis that the process is the result of infection.

All of the symptoms, signs, and laboratory findings connected with pneumoencephalography which have been described usually will disappear spontaneously within 24 to 72 hours after the examination. In some instances, specific as well as supportive treatment will be required. For the most part, however, treatment is purely symptomatic. Bed rest is advised for the first day, and forcing of fluids may reduce the duration of morbidity. Some workers advocate the administration of caffeine sodiobenzoate intramuscularly immediately after the examination, followed by the oral administration of caffeine-phenacetin-aspirin combination as required.

The inhalation of oxygen both as a preventive and therapeutic measure has been advocated. The breathing of 95 per cent oxygen for one hour before the examination is considered by some to reduce the severity of symptoms. There is considerable evidence in the literature that the breathing of oxygen after encephalography accelerates absorption of the gas which is injected and the inhalation of oxygen before pneumography may prevent excessive nitrogen from diffusing into the cerebrospinal fluid. Some workers place the patient in an oxygen tent routinely, following completion of the procedure (Robertson, 1957). In the average case, the patient is fairly comfortable after the first 24 hours, although headache may occur in the upright posture, and, when feasible, it is desirable to have the patient remain inactive for two to three days.

The morbidity of ventriculography is more difficult to assess than that of pneumoencephalography. Many common symptoms pertain. When heavy medication or general anesthesia is used for either ventriculography or pneumoencephalography, some symptoms, such as nausea and vomiting, may be more properly ascribed to the anesthetic agent than to the injection of gas. When subsequent intracranial surgery is required after ventriculography, the effects of the surgical procedure and its morbidity supervene. Generally speaking, the morbidity of ventriculography should be less than that of pneumoencephalography, subtracting anesthetic effect, but there are certain complications in connection with ventriculography that do not pertain to pneumoencephalography and vice versa.

COMPLICATIONS

As in all radiologic procedures involving instrumentation, complications occasionally occur in conjunction with pneumoencephalography. In general, the complications may be divided into two groups, which may be termed for convenience medical and technical. It will be seen subsequently that the technical complications very frequently are of medical import, since they very frequently occur in the presence of organic disease of the brain.

Medical Complications

Transient *meningeal inflammation* occurring 24 to 48 hours after intracranial pneumography is mentioned above. While in the majority of these instances clear-cut evidence of inflammatory changes (indicated both by clinical findings and alteration of the cerebrospinal fluid composition) is found, it is usually not possible to identify causative microorganisms. While this type of nonspecific inflammatory reaction is not uncommon, true *meningitis* is seldom seen. With reasonable care, the incidence of infection should be very low, certainly much less than one per thousand. While the *Bacillus pyocyaneus* was indicted by Kerman *et al.* (1943) as a significant offender, the authors have never encountered a meningeal infection of this type.

Blood pressure changes. Some alteration in the blood pressure, usually an elevation, occurs in connection with pneumoencephalography in most patients. While in some patients there may be no appreciable alteration in blood pressure during or after the procedure, Meyer (1932) found that an elevation of as much as 100 mm. Hg occurred in some patients. A rise or fall in the blood pressure, even of considerable magnitude, is not necessarily a harbinger of complication. In the majority of instances, the blood pressure will return to its basic level in 1 to 2 hours. Elevations drop to normal, usually without incident. Even when there is lowering of the blood pressure resulting in syncope, recovery usually is prompt with stimulation.

Lowering of the blood pressure may, on occasion, be the cause of more serious incidents. *Hemiplegia* may occur in the case of patients with unilateral carotid vascular disease who are subjected to pneumoencephalography. It is frequently not possible to segregate patients with neurologic disturbances, the basis of which is vascular insufficiency, from patients who have degenerative neurologic disturbances of other origins. If the proper diagnosis could always be anticipated clinically, angiography rather than pneumography would be selected to confirm the diagnosis in these instances. However, it is inevitable that many patients with unilateral vascular insufficiency will be subjected to pneumoencephalography and, if there is a substantial drop in blood pressure in this particular group of patients, hemiplegia may be encountered. The majority of the patients who developed hemiplegia during examination by the authors had only a transient paresis with complete or subtotal recovery within a few weeks.

Subarachnoid *bleeding* from aneurysms or vascular malformations may occur as a result of elevation of the blood pressure during pneumoencephalography. Further mention of such occurrences is made below in discussing hemorrhage. Whenever such leakage is encountered, the examination should be terminated promptly, since additional manipulation may incite further hemorrhage. Other complications which may be encountered in connection with blood pressure changes include *pulmonary edema,* which may be immediate but which may be seen also after a latent period. *Coronary occlusion* may be precipitated by pneumoencephalography, presumably either by abrupt lowering or elevation of blood pressure. Fortunately, such complications are not encountered often, and it is doubtful that a direct correlation

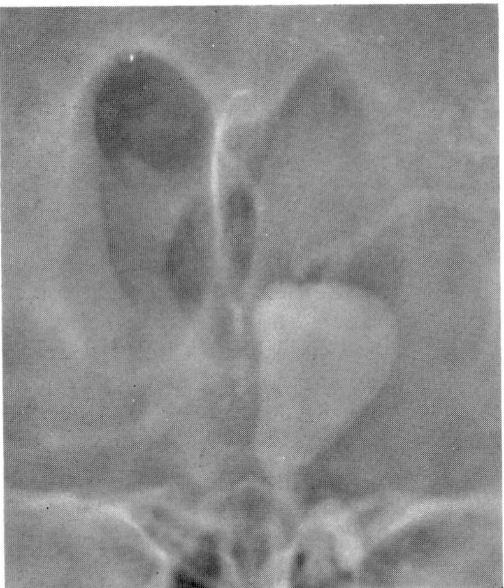

Fig. 195.—Hemorrhage during Pneumoencephalography

While a pneumoencephalogram was being performed, the cerebrospinal fluid—which at first was clear—became sanguinous. An angiogram, performed subsequently, revealed a large saccular aneurysm of the carotid bifurcation. The aneurysm later was proven to be the source of the subarachnoid hemorrhage.

with pneumoencephalography can be made in the majority of instances.

Hemorrhage. Intracranial bleeding may be encountered as a direct or indirect complication of pneumography. Hemorrhage may occur at a number of different sites and under a variety of circumstances. By and large, hemorrhage as a complication of pneumography is seen more frequently with ventriculography than as a result of pneumoencephalography.

At pneumoencephalography, *subarachnoid hemorrhage* may occur from vascular malformations, including arterial aneurysms. In some instances, this is thought to be an indirect complication, caused by the elevation of blood pressure that frequently occurs during the examination, as mentioned above. While it is preferable to examine all patients suspected of having such vascular disease by angiography, it is not rare for such lesions to give rise to bizarre symptoms and signs or to epileptic seizures which cause the decision for a pneumographic examination to be made. It appears unlikely that pneumography incites the primary episode of bleeding from such malformations very often, but more probable that the examination produces a recurrence or an aggravation of bleeding from a previously established site. Instances have been encountered in which the cerebrospinal fluid was clear at the outset of the pneumoencephalogram, but on later withdrawal the fluid was found to be sanguinous as a result of leakage from a congenital aneurysm, later confirmed by other methods (fig. 195). The appearance of blood in the cerebrospinal fluid at any time should suggest the possibility of leakage from a pathologic intracranial source. Unless the operator is convinced that the presence of blood can be accounted for by the needle puncture, or previous needling in the recent past as evidenced by clearing of the fluid as the examination progresses, the procedure should be terminated.

The incidence of *subdural hemorrhage* resulting from pneumoencephalography is not known, since the collection of a small quantity of blood in the subdural space may go unrecognized. It is not uncommon, however, as is described below, for gas to enter the subdural space for technical, anatomic, or pathologic reasons. If careful monitoring of pneumoencephalography is not practiced, large quantities of gas may be injected into the subdural space. Under these circumstances, there may be tearing of small cerebral veins passing through the dura-arachnoid membranes on their way to the dural sinuses. It has been suggested that a pre-existing subdural hematoma favors the entrance of gas into the subdural space or that the two occur together sufficiently frequently to justify a strong suspicion of subdural hematoma when subdural gas is demonstrated (Crosby and Dennis, 1956). As is mentioned below, the subdural collection of gas indeed raises a strong suspicion of intracranial disease, since pathologic processes often are present. Brain tumor is the lesion most often associated with a subdural gas collection and degenerative diseases are

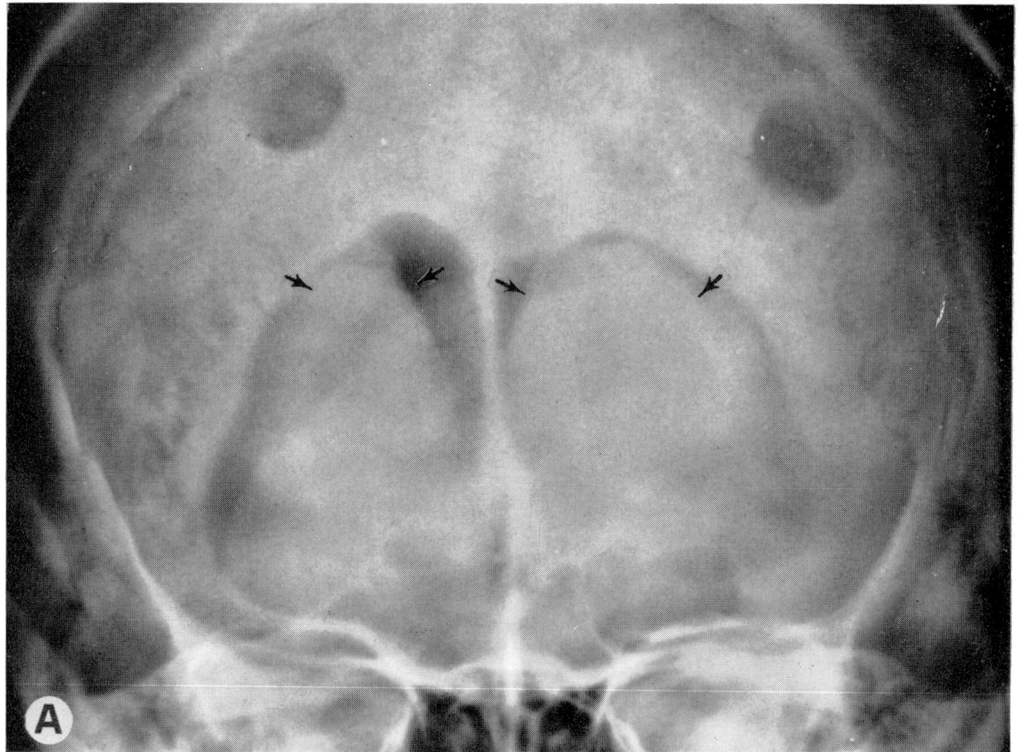

FIG. 196.—HEMORRHAGE OCCURRING AS A RESULT OF VENTRICULOGRAPHY

Enlargement of the shadow of the thalamus may be caused by the trauma of a ventricular needle. Ventriculography (A) performed with difficulty because of the small ventricles, reveals enlargement of the shadow of the thalamus on each side (*arrows*) with narrowing of the lumen of the ventricular atrium. A pneumoencephalogram, performed six weeks after the ventriculogram, reveals that the thalamus has reverted to a normal appearance bilaterally, and the atrial lumen restored (see Fig. 189, same patient). Similar findings were shown on lateral views made at each of the examinations. Presumably, edema and hemorrhage, following multiple needle penetrations in an attempt to puncture a small or misplaced ventricle, are the basis for the enlargement of such normal structures.

Ventriculography performed in the presence of greatly dilated ventricles, with the replacement of a large quantity of cerebrospinal fluid by gas, can result in a collapse of the brain on one side. A large epidural hematoma has developed in the frontal region with flattening of the entire anterior aspect of the ventricle (B). The patient had hypertensive hydrocephalus owing to obstruction of the aqueduct of Sylvius (*lower arrow*) by a cerebellar tumor. A pressure diverticulum of the medial wall of the lateral ventricle is shown near the junction of the atrium and ventricular body (*upper arrow*).

second in frequency. In a group of patients studied by Scheinberg and Yahr (1955), subdural hematoma was not one of the common conditions with which the subdural collection of gas occurred. It would appear that subdural gas dissection is more often the cause of subdural hemorrhage than the effect.

At ventriculography, some type of intracranial hemorrhage is not uncommon, although in the majority of instances it does not affect the fate of the patient. On the other hand, the authors have knowledge of one instance in which fatal hemorrhage occurred during ventriculography. In this patient, a child with congenital anomalies, a misplaced dural sinus was opened at the time of ventriculography and exsanguination occurred. Bleeding from the bone and from the meninges, rather stubborn to control, is encountered frequently.

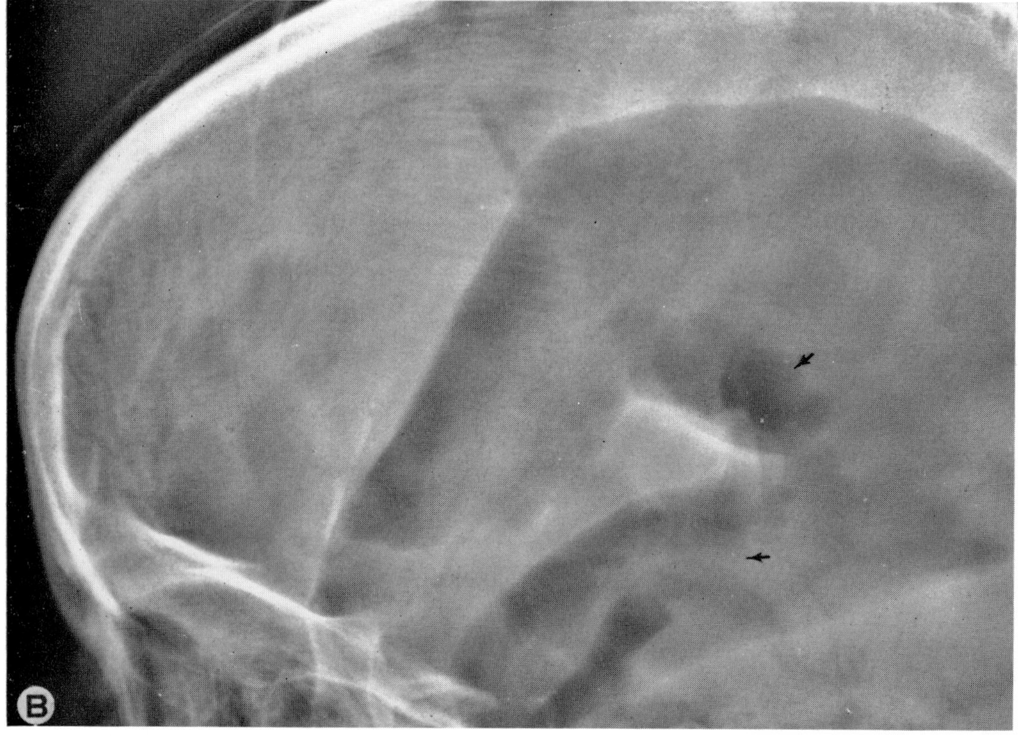

Fig. 196

Intracerebral hemorrhage occurs at ventriculography more often than other types of intracranial bleeding. The frequent finding of multiple small hemorrhages along the tract of the needle inserted for ventricular puncture has been emphasized by Lindgren (1954). The authors have been impressed with the occurrence of swelling in the parietal area, presumably edema and hemorrhage, following multiple needle penetrations in an attempt to puncture an elusive lateral ventricle. In cases in which air insufficient for diagnosis is instilled into the ventricular system or when rapid absorption of gas has occurred prior to filming, second injections occasionally are made to better visualize the ventricles. In a number of such cases, evidence of ventricular deformity has been found on the second set of films which was not present on the first, and this can be explained by needle trauma. An incorrect diagnosis of parietal tumor can easily be made under such circumstances.

Intraventricular hemorrhage may result from trauma by the needle to a vessel of the ventricular wall or to the chorioid plexus. A mistaken diagnosis of intraventricular tumor is quite possible if the circumstances of development of such hematomas are not understood, since, in some cases, they may be very large (Dyke, Elsberg, and Davidoff, 1935).

Epidural hematoma and *subdural hematoma* may occur as a result of ventriculography, but usually not owing to direct trauma. More often, they occur in patients who have hydrocephalus, especially children, in whom large quantities of ventricular fluid are removed and replaced by gas. The removal of fluid and absorption of gas results in ventricular and cerebral collapse with tearing of veins at fixation points, often extradurally or subdurally. In the experience of the authors, such hematomas have been found most often at a frontal pole of the brain, although occasionally they may be found elsewhere (fig. 196). Such a hematoma may even undergo calcification and be visible in a plain skull roentgenogram (fig. 157).

Herniations. Downward herniations of the supratentorial contents through the tentorial incisura and of the posterior fossa contents through the foramen magnum constitute important sources of potential complication in pneumoencephalography. By lowering pressure in the spinal canal, such as may be produced by removal of cerebrospinal fluid, it is possible to increase pre-existing herniations of the intracranial contents or to provoke a herniation which was not previously present. Even when no cerebrospinal fluid is removed during pneumoencephalography, it is still possible to have a relative lowering of the intraspinal cerebrospinal fluid pressure due to leakage of the fluid through the needle hole into the epidural space. Leakage into the subdural space is less significant because the pressure gradient is preserved, inasmuch as the fluid is still within the dura.

If the fluid pressures are taken in the spinal canal during pneumoencephalography, it is found that injection of air without the removal of cerebrospinal fluid causes a temporary elevation of cerebrospinal fluid pressure which lasts several minutes and then the pressure returns to normal. On the other hand, when a quantity of 10 to 20 cc. of cerebrospinal fluid is removed, the intraspinal cerebrospinal fluid pressure goes down and remains low for a considerable time, as long as 30 minutes or even longer, even though some air may be injected. The slow rise to normal following the removal of a significant amount of cerebrospinal fluid is even more prolonged in patients who have a brain tumor than in normal individuals. It is probable that patients who have an intracranial tumor have a reduced volume of cerebrospinal fluid in the subarachnoid space and the removal of an amount of 20 cc. may represent a fairly high percentage of the available fluid under these circumstances. For this reason, it is highly advisable to inject air without removing fluid in any patient in whom a strong suspicion of the presence of an intracranial mass exists

clinically. The initial amount injected should be possibly no more than 10 cc., and thereafter increments of 5 cc. are added if further information is needed following the inspection of the initial films (see "Technique").

In our experience, *tonsillar herniations* (herniations of the cerebellum through the foramen magnum) are the most frequent form of hernia seen by pneumoencephalography. They do not affect the fate of the patient in the majority of instances. Downward displacement of the cerebellar tonsils is associated with a fairly high percentage of tumors of the cerebellum and a much smaller percentage of tumors of the brain stem or extra-axial structures. Any bulky tumor, however, either posterior fossa or supratentorial, can be associated with downward displacement of the cerebellar tonsils. It is for this reason that attention should be given first to the air triangle at the junction of the cervical spine and skull in the initial lateral film taken during pneumoencephalography. Any tonsillar shadow that projects below the level of the foramen magnum should be regarded with suspicion as regards abnormality, although an occasional normal patient will have a tonsil that extends beyond the foramen magnum. It is common to find that the dark air shadow in this region will obscure the tonsillar herniation, and it is almost always necessary to hold the film against a bright light. This step should never be neglected.

A low position of the cerebellar tonsils is not necessarily a contraindication to the addition of more air. More care should be exercised, however, if additional gas is injected and, particularly, no fluid should be removed. Sometimes the cerebellar tonsils will be at a level halfway between the foramen magnum and the atlas, but air still is seen posterior and anterior to the tonsil. This slight degree of tonsillar herniation is usually indicative of a posterior fossa mass lesion and it is rarely a sign of great danger. On the other hand, if the cerebellar tonsillar shadow is seen to reach below the posterior arch of the atlas, this should be considered as severe tonsillar herniation and extreme care should be taken.

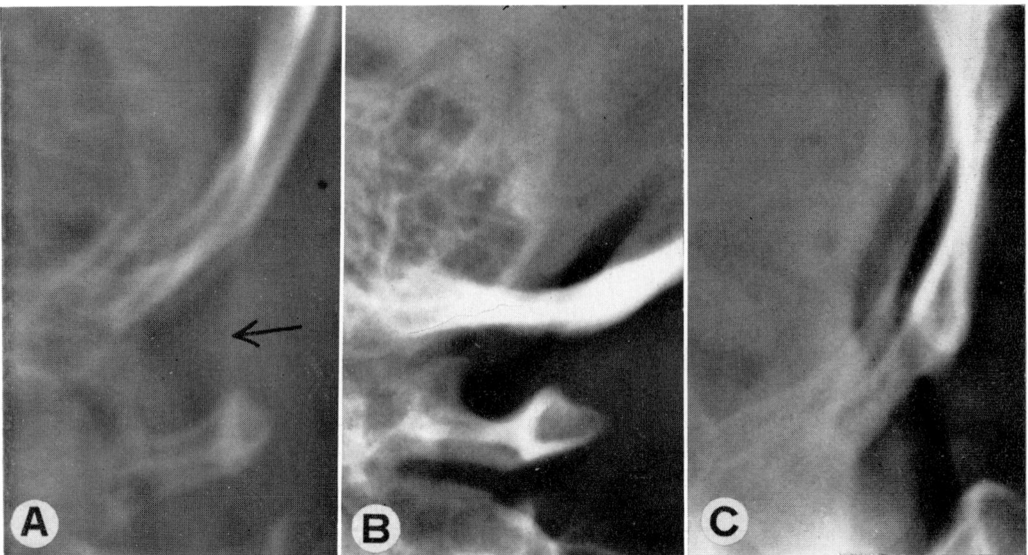

FIG. 197.—HERNIATION OF THE CEREBELLAR TONSILS

The first filling film of the pneumoencephalogram should disclose, under normal circumstances, a sizable gas collection posterior to the upper cervical spinal cord (A). The space is generally triangular (*arrow*), expanding upward to fuse with the posterior extension of the cisterna magna behind the cerebellum. The cerebellar tonsils are just above the rim of the foramen magnum and behind the gas shadow of the vallecula. The over-all appearance of the gas collection is that of a large check mark. The first film of the pneumogram should be examined carefully, with a strong light if necessary, for the possibility of narrowing or obliteration of the spaces, denoting tonsillar herniation.

Acute tonsillar herniation (B) produces obliteration of the air triangle behind the cervicomedullary junction (see also Fig. 295). In the presence of chronic tonsillar herniation (C), some space behind the dislocated tonsils ordinarily is preserved (see also Fig. 242). Ventricular filling ordinarily does not occur in the presence of either type of herniation.

On the basis of pneumographic findings, *acute* and *chronic tonsillar herniations* may be recognized. In acute severe herniation the tonsils occupy the entire width of the air triangle behind the upper cervicomedullary junction (fig. 197). In these cases, no significant air space is seen behind or in front of the herniated cerebellar tonsil. Sometimes it is difficult to be sure of this because of the normal relative radiolucency of this area as compared with the skull. This is particularly true because the lower margin of the herniated tonsil may overlie the arch of the atlas or the axis and may thus be inconspicuous. Any difference in the relative radiolucency of the air column behind the cervical cord when the cervical area in the neighborhood of C2 or C3 is compared with that of C1 should raise the question of tonsillar herniation. In doubtful cases, tomography may be necessary. Autotomography usually demonstrates the tonsillar herniation adequately.

Chronic tonsillar herniation is seen in slowly growing tumors of the posterior fossa; it is part of the Arnold-Chiari malformation. Characteristically, a sizable air space is seen posteriorly between the herniated tonsils and the dorsal margin of the spinal canal and foramen magnum. In some cases it is impossible to separate the tonsillar shadow from that of the upper spinal cord and medulla (figs. 197 and 242). In these cases, if there is no filling of the fourth ventricle, it is not possible to differentiate by pneumography herniation caused by a tumor from an Arnold-Chiari malformation. Liliequist (1960) has indicated that in cases of Arnold-Chiari malformation a strip of air can be seen along the anterior aspect of the herniated

(*Revised 1963*)

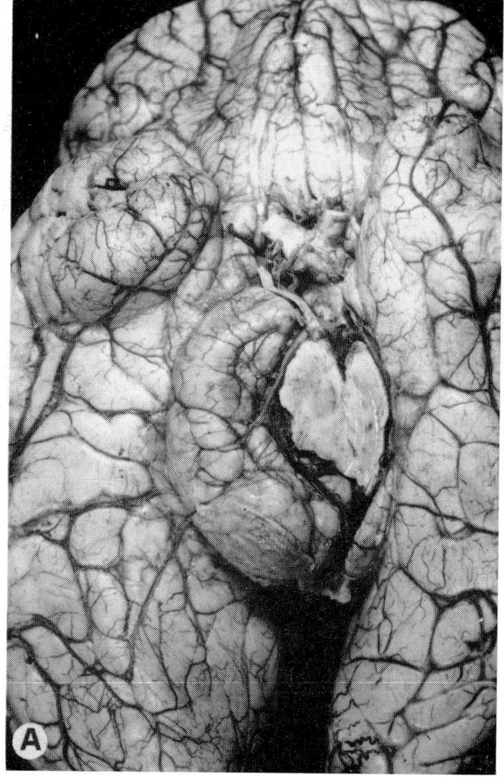

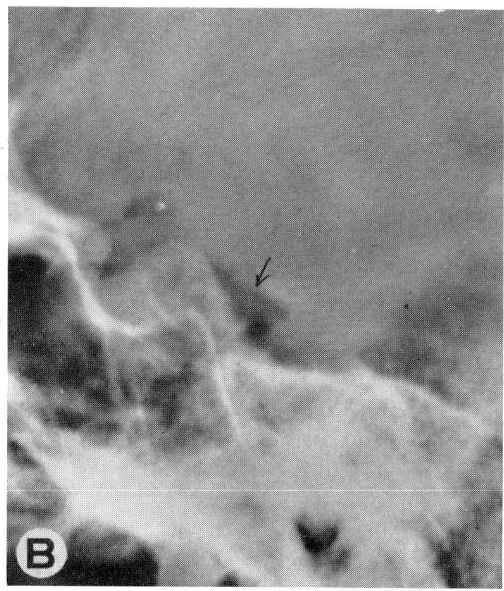

FIG. 198.—DOWNWARD TRANSTENTORIAL HERNIATION

The base of the brain exhibits swelling of the hippocampus on the right (A), owing to almost complete downward transtentorial herniation of this structure. The midbrain is deformed by displacement to the opposite side; the ipsilateral half is compressed by the hippocampus, and the contralateral portion is indented by the resistant tentorial edge. Mesencephalic edema and petechial hemorrhages are present owing to venous stasis and rupture.

Severe herniation of the hippocampus through the tentorial incisura is present, producing obstruction of the cisterna interpeduncularis (B). The head of the air column in the cistern outlines an oblique line (*arrow*), sloping downward and backward from the top of the dorsum sellae, which represents the margin of the markedly dislocated hippocampus.

In less severe herniations, gas may extend higher in the cisterna interpeduncularis; the margin of the dislocated hippocampus then extends straight backward from the sella turcica (C). In some instances a dilated third ventricle, or a suprasellar mass, may simulate a hippocampal herniation (D). Ventricular obstruction has resulted from aqueduct gliosis; the third ventricle bulges far downward to erode the sella turcica and to obstruct the cisterna interpeduncularis (*arrow*).

tonsil which represents an elongated vestibule of the foramen of Magendie. If no air is seen in front of the herniated tonsil, it is difficult to differentiate this herniation from an intramedullary tumor unless an elongated and downwardly displaced fourth ventricle also is seen.

Only one tonsil may herniate while the one on the opposite side remains in normal position. This may be demonstrated in some cases in the frontal projection.

(Revised 1963)

Ventricular filling frequently does not occur in the presence of tonsillar herniation and, because the demonstration of this abnormality is an indication for increased caution often necessitating termination of the procedure, ventriculography must be carried out to arrive at a diagnosis in these cases.

Downward transtentorial herniation of supratentorial contents through the incisura is a frequent finding at pneumoencepha-

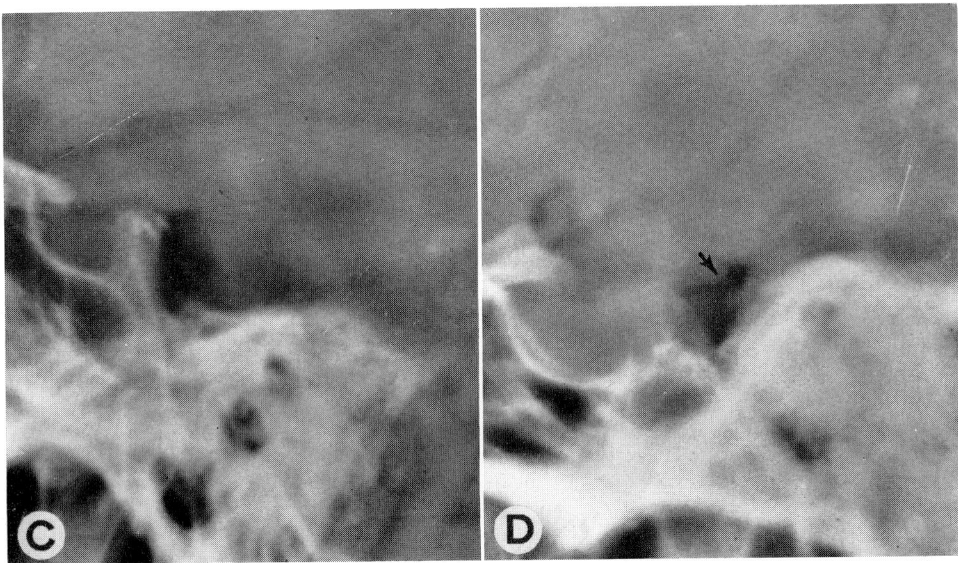

Fig. 198

lography in cases ill-suited for this type of examination and is often associated with the patient's demise. In recent times, due to the prevalence of cerebral angiography in the diagnosis of lesions of the supratentorial space it is infrequent, in our experience, to demonstrate transtentorial herniations by pneumoencephalography.

Anterior hippocampal herniations produce a posterior displacement and flattening of the corresponding peduncle. The pressure causes elevation of the corresponding side of the quadrigeminal plate which can be demonstrated by pneumoencephalography. Middle and posterior herniations of the hippocampus produce a flattening of the midbrain which is displaced toward the opposite side of the incisura and downward. The contralateral side of the midbrain is thus compressed against the edge of the tentorium, which may lead to the production of pyramidal tract signs homolateral to the herniation. Bilateral herniations are not uncommon, particularly in patients with bilateral subdural hematoma and large frontal tumors; they lead to a pear-shaped deformity of the upper brain stem.

Various dislocations and deformities of the cisterns as well as obstruction of the cisterns may be demonstrated when herniation occurs. The aqueduct of Sylvius is often compressed and deformed and this leads to a lack of filling of the ventricular system by pneumoencephalography which is observed commonly in the presence of supratentorial tumors and also in the case of cerebellar tumors. Middle and anterior hippocampal herniations produce a deformity or an obstruction of the cisterna interpeduncularis, particularly if the herniation is bilateral. The lower the defective filling of this cistern, the more severe the herniation (fig. 198). Obstruction of the cisterna interpeduncularis is not always due to herniation and may be produced by suprasellar tumors. In the case of herniation, however, the defect tends to be generally horizontal with either a straight or finely irregular margin. Contrariwise, with suprasellar tumors the gas margin is rounded or lobulated and is not horizontal in position (figs. 326 and 328). A markedly enlarged, bulging third ventricle may also produce such a deformity (fig. 198). Sometimes the entire lower margin of the herniated hippocampus can be outlined by air. In frontal projections, a deformity of the quadrigeminal cistern may be seen. The quadrigeminal tubercle is elevated on the corresponding side with anterior herniations or it may be depressed with posterior or

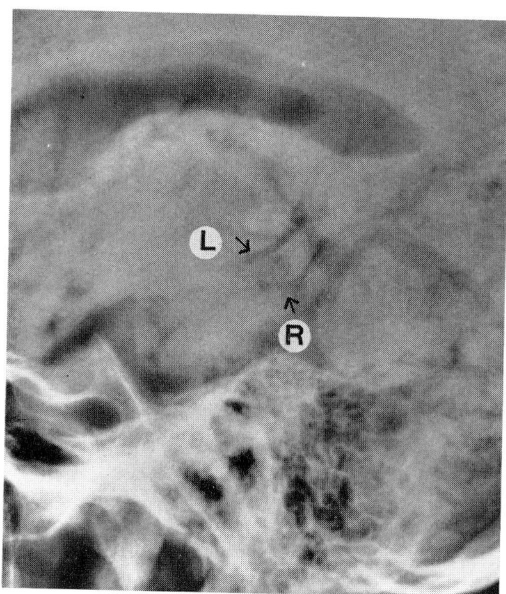

Fig. 199.—Unilateral Downward Displacement of Retrothalamic Cistern

Displacement of one retrothalamic extension of the quadrigeminal cistern downward and backward is present (*arrow with letter "R"*), as compared with the opposite retrothalamic space. The displacement, occurring in this case as a result of a temporal lobe tumor, suggests impending posterior transtentorial herniation of the hippocampus.

complete herniations. Likewise, the retrothalamic cistern may show downward displacement on one side in comparison with the opposite side (fig. 199). Such displacement is not necessarily a sign of herniation and may be produced by a neoplasm which enlarges the thalamus or which displaces the thalamus backward. The shadow of the quadrigeminal plate or of the aqueduct may be tilted backward, and this is an indication either of an anterior herniation or of an anteriorly placed supratentorial tumor that is low in position which is causing backward tilting of the brain stem.

Upward transtentorial herniation is common in tumors of the posterior fossa. Upward herniation has received less attention than downward extension. Ventriculography may cause an exaggeration of a pre-existing upward tentorial herniation which may, in some cases, result in the patient's demise. The most common manifestation of upward transtentorial herniation is elevation of the floor of the third ventricle (fig. 200). Unilateral upward herniation may produce an indentation of the posteroinferior aspect of the third ventricle which can mimic the deformity produced by incisural space-occupying tumors. Upward herniation of the cerebellum posteriorly may encroach on the quadrigeminal cistern and even may produce displacement of the cistern behind the splenium of the corpus callosum. The latter cistern may, in some instances, become concave downward instead of convex, as is normally the case.

In addition to transtentorial herniations, other supratentorial herniations that are fairly common should be considered. These include (1) herniation of the base of the

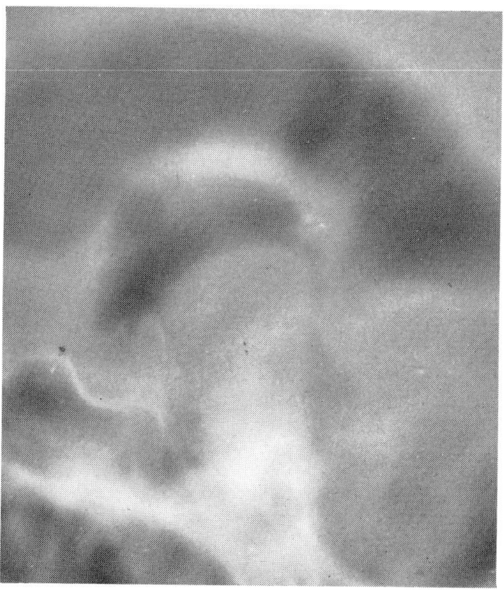

Fig. 200.—Upward Herniation at the Tentorial Incisura

The tomogram of a patient with a large cerebellar tumor reveals marked forward displacement of the fourth ventricle. The fourth ventricle also is elevated by the caudally situated tumor, and its height is reduced by compression. Pressure exerted on the brain stem produces upward displacement of the floor of the third ventricle and a reduction in height of the third ventricular lumen posteriorly (see also Figs. 297 and 323).

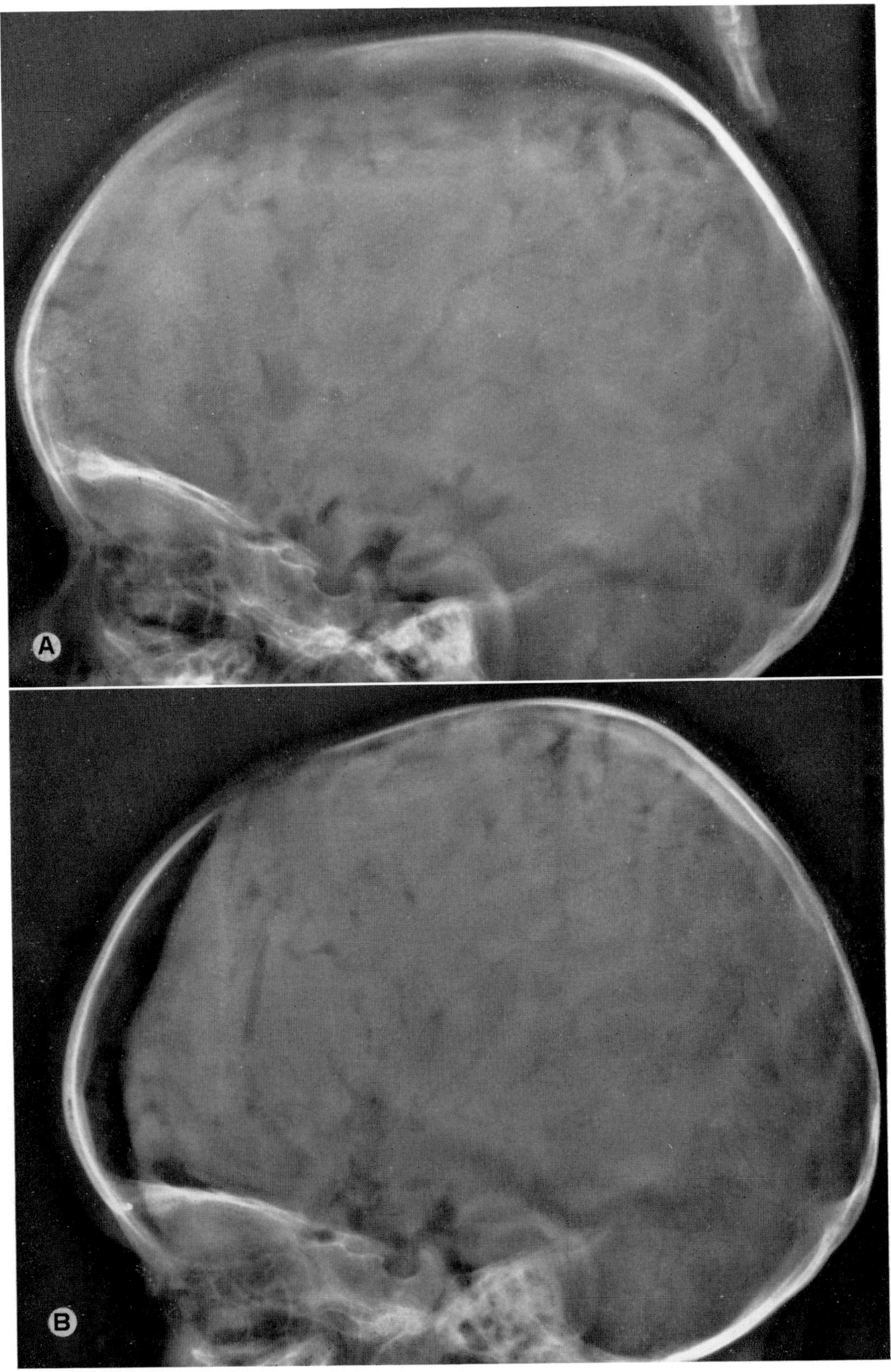

Fig 201

frontal lobe behind the sphenoid ridge, (2) herniation of the gyrus rectus behind the tuberculum sellae, (3) subfalcial herniations or midline shifts which are discussed in detail under hemispheric tumors (see "Supratentorial Extraventricular Masses").

Retrosphenoidal herniations are common in the case of anterior frontal tumors and particularly with frontopolar tumors. The herniations are responsible for backward displacement and flattening of the tip of the temporal lobe which occurs. It is not uncommon to find that air studies are erroneously interpreted as indicating an extension of a frontal tumor into the temporal lobe. Angiographic findings may be connected with this type of herniation and are discussed briefly under "Angiography."

The *gyrus rectus herniation* also may be found in frontal lobe tumors and was seen in one case of pseudotumor cerebri. Gyrus rectus herniation can cause compression of the optic chiasm and bitemporal hemianopia may result. In the case of pseudotumor cerebri mentioned, there was no filling of the ventricles by pneumoencephalography but air in the suprasellar cisterns presented a curved configuration which corresponded exactly with the pathological appearance found later at autopsy.

Further details on herniations are given in the pneumographic section on "Intracranial Tumors" and the angiographic section "Diagnosis of Brain Tumors."

Mortality. It is difficult to ascertain a valid figure for the incidence of death directly related to pneumoencephalography. The importance of pneumoencephalography as a causative or contributory factor in death is evaluated differently by various writers. The temporal profile of events leading to death may involve not only pneumoencephalography but possibly subsequent angiography or ventriculography and intracranial surgical exploration. It appears quite probable that in many instances pneumoencephalography may be the first link in a chain of events leading to death, but in most instances it is not possible to single out any one of the events as the sole cause of the patient's demise, as described in connection with herniations.

In addition to the complications that have been described, any of which may, too frequently, lead to the patient's death, *air embolism* is a fatal event occasionally encountered. Two such cases were reported by King and Otenasek (1948), one in an adult and the other in a young infant. The authors have encountered one such case, also occurring in a young child. Sudden death occurred during the procedure in all instances. The authors' case resembled those of King and Otenasek in that the exact portal of entry of gas into the vascular system could not be determined precisely at necropsy although sizable quantities of gas were found in the vascular system, including the heart chambers. King and Otenasek suggested that the mechanism involved the tearing of a small vein entering one of the dural sinuses, which allowed ingress of air into the venous system. This thesis is borne out by the case of our experience mentioned, inasmuch as the major portion of the gas entered the subdural space, separating widely the surface of the brain from the inner table of the skull (fig. 201).

The over-all death rate in conjunction with pneumoencephalography appears to be in the neighborhood of 0.25 per cent. In a group reviewed, five deaths occurred in a series exceeding 3,000 cases. This compares well with the 0.22 per cent described by

Fig. 201.—Large Subdural Gas Collection Producing Fatal Air Embolism

Films were made immediately after death in the case of a patient who suffered fatal air embolism during pneumoencephalography. The upright film shows that almost all of the gas is in the subdural space between the vertex and the superior cerebral surface, with essentially no subarachnoid gas present (A). The supine lateral film reveals a similar very wide separation of the frontal poles of the brain from the frontal bone (B). Wide separation of the surface of the brain from the inner table of the skull apparently produced tearing of a vein at its junction with a dural sinus, allowing gas to enter the venous system. Necropsy in the case illustrated revealed sizable quantities of gas in the vascular system, including the heart chambers.

Davidoff and Dyke (1951). Three of the authors' cases had supratentorial tumors that resulted in herniations following pneumoencephalography. There were no posterior fossa tumors in the series. A fourth patient died as a result of subarachnoid hemorrhage from an aneurysm, while the fifth was the child mentioned above who had fatal air embolism. The incidence of one death in 600 pneumoencephalograms compares favorably with the complication rate for most anesthetic agents. Inasmuch as three of our five cases, and two of the cases described by Davidoff and Dyke, would under normal circumstances now be examined by angiography rather than pneumoencephalography, it is to be anticipated that a further reduction in the mortality rate can be expected in the future.

Technical Complications

Defective filling of the ventricular system and subarachnoid space at pneumoencephalography may result from (1) incomplete filling of the ventricles despite the presence of patency, (2) nonfilling of the ventricular system despite the presence of gas in the subarachnoid space, and (3) entrance of gas into the subdural space rather than the subarachnoid space.

1. Incomplete or inadequate filling of the ventricular system for diagnosis despite the injection of a sufficient quantity of gas into the spinal canal occurs fairly frequently. Whenever defective filling of any portion of the ventricles is observed, it first must be assumed that it is the result of disease unless proven otherwise. Proof to the contrary consists in absence of deformity of any portion of the ventricles outlined, lack of displacement of midline or other ventricular structures, absence of dilatation, or other changes.

Failure of filling of one lateral ventricle occurs not infrequently as a result of physiologic disturbances, which are temporary, or owing to faulty technique. Frequently, improper positioning of the head can be the cause of nonfilling of one lateral ventricle. Re-examination in positions designed to visualize the unfilled areas with gas should be carried out. It is often desirable to allow the patient to remain in one position for a period of time, since in some instances too rapid filming accounts for insufficient gas having entered a lateral ventricle. If, for example, the right lateral ventricle is not filled and all other portions of the ventricular system appear normal, the patient should be placed in the left prone position with the midsagittal plane of the head horizontal, and he should be allowed to remain in this position for from 3 to 5 minutes. During this time, gentle rocking of the head backward and forward or raising and lowering of the head in relation to the horizontal plane may be carried out. Some workers use manual tapping of the cranium as an adjunct since this is thought to facilitate the bubbling of gas through the fluid system, particularly through narrow pathways such as the foramen of Monro. In addition, rotary maneuvers may be carried out. Special projections may be obtained with the head variously disposed, to establish that maximum opportunity for gas to pass through a narrow ventricular segment has been provided.

In children examined under ether anesthesia, one portion of the ventricular system may not fill. In these cases, edema of the brain probably accounts for the nonfilling. Undoubtedly, similar transient swellings occur in other patients which are not on the basis of disease. In such instances, we have found it helpful to administer urea in intravenous drip in one-half the dose employed for intracranial surgery. Urea causes prompt removal of fluid from the brain in most instances, and frequently incomplete ventricular filling then becomes complete.

At ventriculography, also, the use of urea may be an invaluable adjunct, even in pathologic states. It is not infrequent that only one lateral ventricle can be punctured at the time of ventriculography. While this may be fortuitous, more often it is caused by deformity, displacement, or collapse of the ventricle that cannot be entered. If good filling of the ventricle on the contralateral side is obtained, then the administration of urea may allow gas to enter the abnormal ventricle and better define the pathologic process which is present. In this way, it may be possible to avoid other procedures, such as further attempts to tap the ventricle on the abnormal side or cerebral angiography, to confirm the presence of disease, and to localize it for surgical treatment.

Inadequate ventricular filling for diagnosis may occur at pneumoencephalography as a result of failure of sufficient gas to enter the head, even though an adequate quantity has been injected into the lumbar area. In these instances some technical problem, such as displacement of the needle partially into the subdural or extradural space, probably is the most common cause. In other instances, malformations of the meninges may account for loss of gas injected.

Most often, perhaps, the cause of inadequate ventricular filling for diagnosis is not failure of the gas to enter the cranial cavity but its retention in the cranial subarachnoid space and nonentrance into the ventricular system. In these cases, faulty positioning of the head or an incompetent cisterna magna (see p. 1.305) may be the basis for the difficulty.

Partial or inadequate ventricular filling does not have as serious a connotation as absence of filling of an entire segment of the ventricular system. In a group of more than 2,000 patients reviewed by Scheinberg and Yahr (1955), partial but nonocclusive ventricular filling inadequate for diagnosis was found in 83 patients. Only four of the patients subsequently were found to have brain tumors, an incidence of 5 per cent. Such an incidence of occurrence of brain tumor is to be expected in patients undergoing pneumoencephalography; therefore, partial general filling by itself probably should be given little weight. As indicated, it probably is (1) a transient physiologic change interfering with normal mechanisms rather than an organic process or (2) on a technical basis, often faulty positioning during the injection of gas or during subsequent filming.

2. Complete failure of ventricular filling, on the other hand, very frequently is of great pathologic significance. In this group are considered patients in whom a satisfactory fluid-gas exchange is accomplished following lumbar puncture and in whom films show the gas to be in the cranial subarachnoid space but not in the ventricular system (fig. 202). While the same factors just considered under partial filling may conceivably be at play in some instances, this usually is not the case. For the most part, correlation is not clear between nonventricular filling and (1) the performance of a previous lumbar puncture with gas passing extra-arachnoidally, (2) the type of gas used, or (3) the type of anesthetic agent. Ether, however, is well known as an agent causing cerebral edema and is now seldom employed. Accurate statistics, therefore, on the effect of ether are not readily available.

The true significance of nonfilling is shown by the high incidence of pathologic processes that are encountered by diagnostic study subsequent to pneumoencephalography. In the group examined by Scheinberg and Yahr, successful subarachnoid filling and failure of the ventricles to fill was the most common type of unsatisfactory pneumoencephalogram analyzed. Gas entering the subdural space was second in frequency. In some instances, both subarachnoid and subdural gas were present without evidence of gas entering the ventricles. *Approximately one-half of such patients were found to harbor a brain tumor.*

Some patients who had nonfilling at pneumoencephalography, in the series just cited, had second pneumoencephalograms attempted. When the pneumoencephalogram was repeated because gas had entered the subdural space at the first sitting, and such patients were found to have ventricular nonfilling after a satisfactory subarachnoid injection on a second sitting, 70 per cent had a brain tumor.

Thus, it is seen that complete failure of ventricular filling at pneumoencephalography has a serious connotation, inasmuch as the majority of the patients in whom such defective filling is observed have a brain tumor. The authors' experience corresponds very closely to the various reports separately

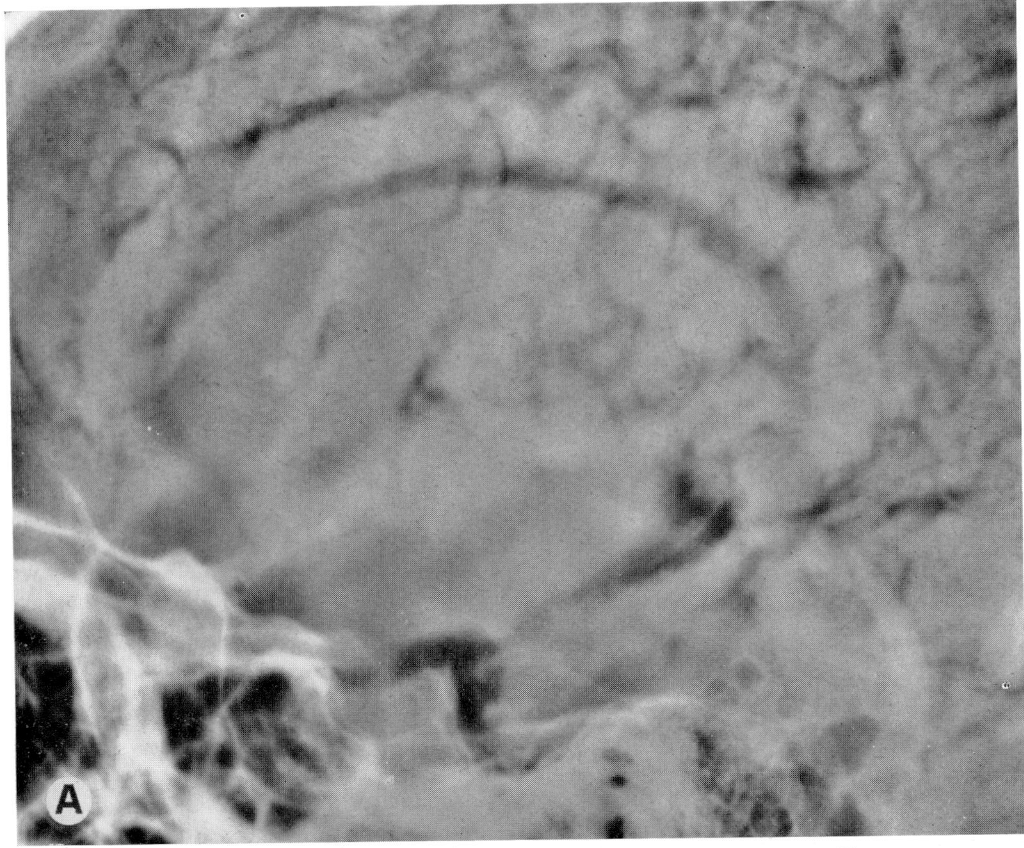

FIG. 202.—INTRACRANIAL SUBARACHNOID GAS WITHOUT VENTRICULAR FILLING

A large quantity of gas is present in the cranial subarachnoid space but no filling of the ventricular system is shown (A). Approximately one-half of patients exhibiting nonfilling of the ventricular system—despite the presence of gas in the cranial subarachnoid space—have a brain tumor (see text). In this instance, the subarachnoid space appears dilated, particularly with respect to the posterior communicating channels, because the anterior pathways are obstructed by a hypothalamic tumor. Dilatation of the callosal sulcus and cingulate sulcus also is shown; the anterior portion of the callosal sulcus is narrowed and the sulcus elevated as a result of ventricular dilatation.

In a second case (B), the subarachnoid gas outlines the tumor itself, a large pituitary adenoma with suprasellar extension. Such abbreviated examinations frequently are diagnostic, and resorting to ventriculography or angiography may not be necessary. A full series of films should be made, even though the ventricles do not fill.

published regarding such findings. In some instances, urea may be used in an attempt to salvage a satisfactory diagnostic examination and, indeed, it may have a therapeutically beneficial effect as regards prevention of herniation. Again it may be pointed out that considerable information may be gained from films made in various projections where no ventricular filling occurred (fig. 202).

3. Subdural gas has been thought in the past to be largely a technical complication, or one related to malformation of the meninges, as previously noted. By others, it has been considered to have significance as regards the presence of subdural hematoma (see "Head Injuries and Their Complications"). It appears more likely that subdural gas, or combined subdural and subarachnoid gas, with nonfilling of the ventricles has a similar implication to that just discussed. The

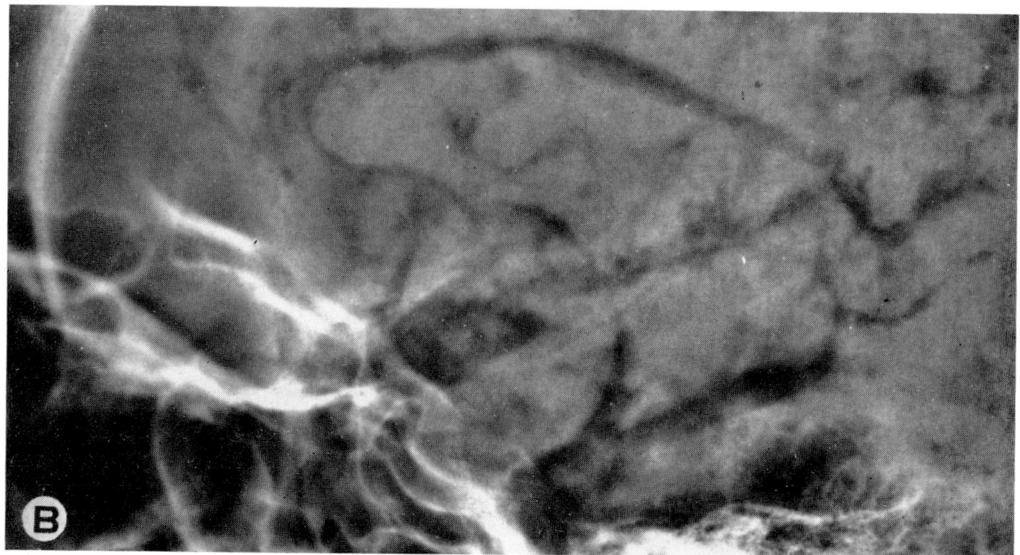

FIG. 202

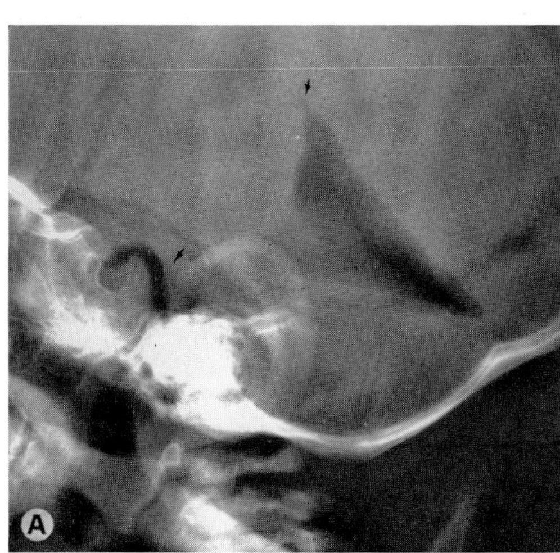

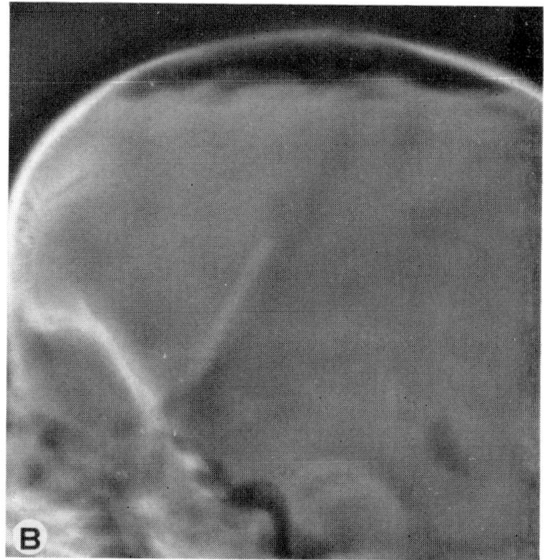

FIG. 203.—GAS IN THE SUBDURAL SPACE AFTER INITIAL INJECTION

Gas has collected entirely in the subdural space (A), both around the sella turcica (*lower arrow*) and beneath the tentorium (*upper arrow*). In another case (B), subdural gas is present also between the inner table of the skull and the cerebral surface. The beaked or hooklike collection of gas above and behind the sella turcica is often a valuable indication of a subdural injection and should not be mistaken for gas in the subarachnoid cisterns. After such a finding is encountered on the preliminary film, and when ventricular filling does not occur with a second injection of gas following adjustment of the spinal needle, the procedure should be abandoned.

incidence of brain tumor is almost as high when subdural gas collections occur as is the case when subarachnoid extraventricular collections are found. We have come to view nonfilling of the ventricles (the main body of injected gas either in the subarachnoid or subdural space) with ominous implication as regards the probability of brain tumor.

Whenever nonfilling of the ventricles is encountered in the preliminary films, or when ventricular filling does not occur promptly after a second injection of gas following adjustment of the needle, the procedure should be abandoned (fig. 203). The patient then should be examined by ventriculography if a posterior fossa tumor is suspected or by angiography if a supratentorial lesion is considered more likely.

ANATOMY

For the purposes of this discussion, pneumographic anatomy may be divided into several major sections, although basically there are two prime areas of consideration (1) the cerebral ventricles, (2) the subarachnoid space. In radiologic diagnosis, however, the lateral ventricles must be related to the cerebral sulci, the third ventricle to the suprasellar subarachnoid space, and the fourth ventricle to the basal and the communicating cisterns, as well as numerous other interrelations. One of the more important relationships is that of pneumographic anatomy to angiographic anatomy, which the authors will attempt to integrate. While we will rely on classic concepts as much as practicable, some clinically helpful departures will be described in connection with both normal and pathologic conditions.

Attention has been given previously to maneuvers designed to fill predominantly either one or the other of the principal fluid spaces with gas, since it is unusual in modern practice to carry out extensive cerebrospinal fluid drainage and outline completely both the ventricular and subarachnoid areas. Nevertheless, some degree of subarachnoid filling occurs frequently at ventriculography and varying degrees of mixed filling almost always occur at pneumoencephalography. It should be possible to localize and identify all of the gas shadows visualized in pneumograms and to say with a high degree of certainty whether their appearance is normal or abnormal, taking into consideration the extent of filling which is present.

The cerebral ventricles normally consist of four ependymal lined cavities which communicate with each other and with the subarachnoid space. Paired lateral ventricles are contained in the central portions of the cerebral hemispheres, the third ventricle is located largely within the supratentorial portion of the brain stem, and the fourth ventricle lies on the dorsal aspect of the brain stem of the posterior fossa. The foramina and channels which connect the ventricles to each other are narrow, and frequently are the site of obstructing lesions. The interventricular foramina connect the two lateral ventricles and the foramen of Monro connects the lateral ventricles with the third ventricle, forming the stem of a Y-shaped passage. In his original article in 1783, Monro described and illustrated well the ostia connecting the three ventricles, and it is not considered improper to refer to the confluence as well as the individual connections as the foramen of Monro. The third and fourth ventricles are joined by a narrow midline canal running through the midbrain, the aqueduct of Sylvius or iter. The fourth ventricle communicates with the cisterna magna through its central foramen, the foramen of Magendie, and through the paired foramina of Luschka at the extremities of its lateral recesses. The intracranial subarachnoid space may be divided into (1) the basal cisterns, which are large fluid pools beneath the inferior surface of the brain, (2) the peripheral subarachnoid space, overlying the cerebral convexities, and (3) the communicating cisterns, which connect the basal reservoirs with the general fluid space of the convexities.

LATERAL VENTRICLES

The lateral ventricles are the largest and most readily distinguishable structures at pneumography. Anatomists subdivide each lateral ventricle into five segments, usually designated the anterior (or frontal) horn, the ventricular body, the atrium, the posterior (or occipital) horn, and the temporal (or inferior) horn. Further subdivision has been made, such as the classical designations of Retzius in which the lateral ventricular body is divided again into anterior third, middle third, and posterior third. In some institutions ventricular components are numbered for surgical guidance and medical record convenience. The authors prefer to relate lateral ventricular anatomy to three structures, almost always well visualized at pneumography. In addition, the points are standards of reference in cerebral angiography. More detailed discussion of pneumographic-angiographic relationships are given in connection with the pneumographic classification of brain tumors to be presented subsequently.

The *first* reference point is the *foramen of Monro* which, in the lateral view, is projected through the center of the angiographic Sylvian triangle (figs. 204 and 205). Portions of the brain forward of the plane of the foramen of Monro may be termed "preforaminal." Similarly, cerebral hemispheric segments above this point may be designated "supraforaminal" and segments behind may be called "postforaminal" (fig. 206). The *second* reference point, the *atrium* or trigone, is of larger proportions, but since gas tends to pool in this ventricular confluence, it is almost always outlined, even in pneumograms of poor quality. In lateral view, the atrium is projected just behind the posterior extremity of the Sylvian triangle of the angiogram, and thus, the "retro-Sylvian" area of angiography corresponds to the "periatrial" area of pneumography. The *third* point of reference is the *temporal horn*. The temporal ventricular segment is clearly related to vessels of the Sylvian fissure, which lies above the horn, and the substance of the temporal lobe. Almost all morphologic alterations of the temporal region are reflected both in the pneumogram and in the angiogram.

The frontal, or anterior, horn is that portion of the lateral ventricle that lies forward of, or anterior to, the foramen of Monro. The frontal horn extends first forward, thence laterally (at approximately a 45-degree angle) and ventrally to end in a rounded termination in the substance of the frontal pole. The body of the lateral ventricle extends backward from the interventricular foramen to a less well-defined point in the region of the splenium of the corpus callosum. The ventricular body is an arched cavity, becoming more narrow as its extends backward, before widening into the ventricular atrium. The anterior and middle thirds of the ventricular bodies are closely applied, but the posterior third diverges from its mate and, at the same time, turns downward to enter the largest part of the ventricle, the atrium. The atrium comprises that portion of the lateral ventricle in relation to the splenium of the corpus callosum, which represents a confluence of the posterior extremity of the ventricular body and the posterior segment of the temporal horn, together with their junction with the occipital horn, or its vestige. The atrium is generally crescent-shaped, concave anteriorly, and often wide in its central portion, toward which both the ventricular body and temporal horn expand. The central portion of the atrium and the center of the third ventricle, including the massa intermedia, and the pineal gland inclusion are in the same general transverse body plane. From the atrium, the temporal horn extends downward and forward obliquely, at an angle varying in degree, depending to a considerable extent upon the shape of the cranium. The temporal horn in its posterior portion continues the divergence begun by the posterior ventricular body and bows laterally. Anteriorly the temporal horn turns rather sharply medialward and downward, to end approximately 3 cm. from the anterior temporal lobe tip.

(*Revised 1963*)

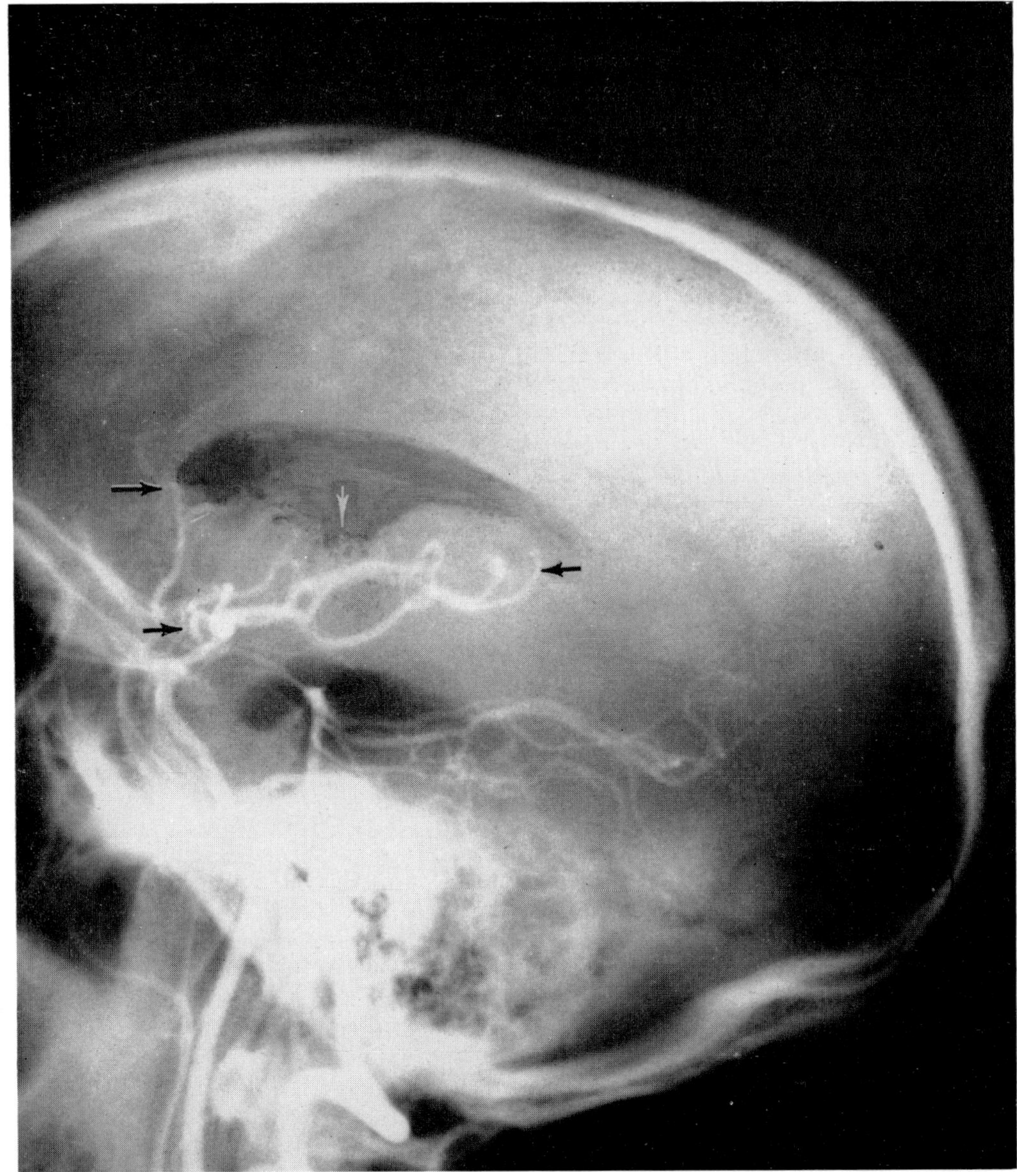

FIG. 204.—COMBINED PNEUMOGRAM AND BRACHIAL ANGIOGRAM (EARLY ARTERIAL PHASE) IN PATIENT WITH CHROMOPHOBE PITUITARY ADENOMA

An angiogram was performed shortly after completion of a pneumoencephalogram; it serves to demonstrate the pneumographic-angiographic relationship of the foramen of Monro (*white arrow*) to the angiographic Sylvian triangle (*black arrows*). The film was made with the patient supine and shows residual gas in the anterior horns, anterior portions of the ventricular bodies, and in the temporal horns. Arborization of the middle cerebral artery in the insular region is triangular in disposition; the foramen of Monro is projected through the central portion of the triangular collection of vessels. The relationship may be used as a point of cross reference for the localization of angiographic and pneumographic findings in lateral views (see text).

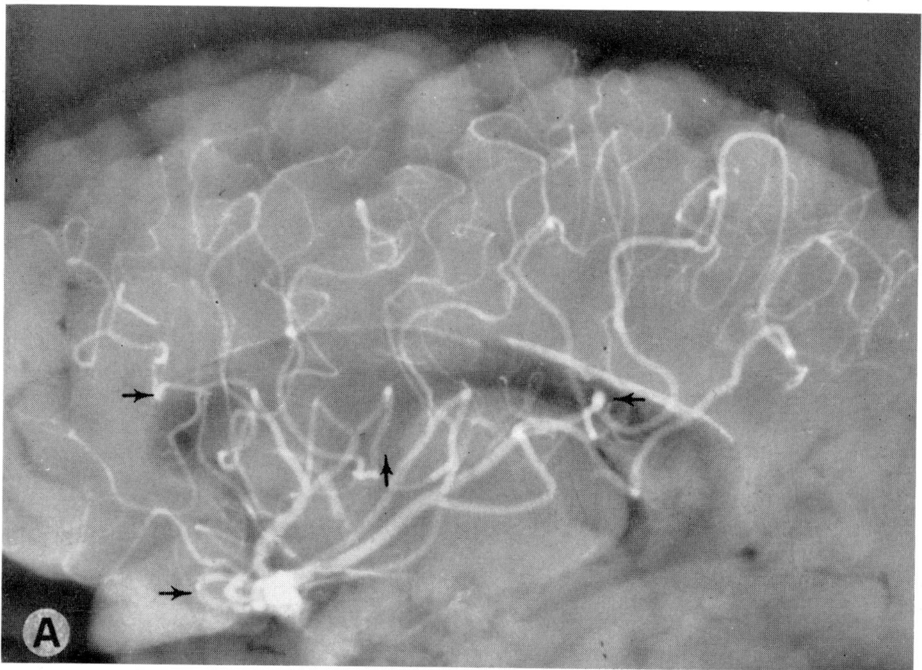

Fig. 205.—Sagittal Relationships between the Lateral Ventricle, the Middle Cerebral Artery and the Internal Cerebral Vein

A lateral radiograph of an isolated cerebral hemisphere is shown, in which the lateral ventricle is filled with air and a middle cerebral artery has been injected with opaque material (A). The corners of the angiographic Sylvian triangle are indicated (*transverse arrows*) and the location of the foramen of Monro (*vertical arrow*) in the center of the triangle is evident (see Fig. 204). In addition, the relationship of the atrium of the lateral ventricle to the Sylvian triangle is demonstrated. The periatrial portion of the cerebral hemisphere in pneumograms corresponds to the retro-Sylvian portion of the brain in angiograms. The temporal region of the pneumogram, with its gas-filled temporal horn, corresponds to the infra-Sylvian area of the angiogram.

The venous phase of a cerebral angiogram, made following a pneumoencephalogram, demonstrates additional ventriculovascular relationships (B). The confluence of the chorioidal vein and terminal vein (thalamostriate vein) to form the internal cerebral vein on each side constitutes the venous angle of the angiogram (*transverse arrow*). The union occurs at the foramen of Monro (*vertical arrow*). The foramen of Monro seen at pneumography and the venous angle seen in the late phases of angiography provide for further cross reference between lateral pneumograms and angiograms. (Courtesy of Dr. Giovanni Di Chiro, National Institutes of Health, Bethesda, Maryland.)

The occipital horn is the only portion of the ventricular system exhibiting a high degree of variability in appearance. The occipital horn is absent or rudimentary in a large percentage of patients. A well developed occipital horn is present only in approximately 10 per cent of individuals, and in these instances it extends backward and medialward from the atrium toward the occipital pole. There is also a slight upward slope from its origin in the atrium. Most often the occipital horn has the appearance of a small finger-like projection of fairly uniform width, with a rounded tip. It is not infrequent for the occipital horn to be tapered almost to a point, while at other times it may be somewhat bulbous and even flared. Development on the two sides may be totally different to the extent that one occipital horn may be absent while the other is well developed.

(*Revised 1963*)

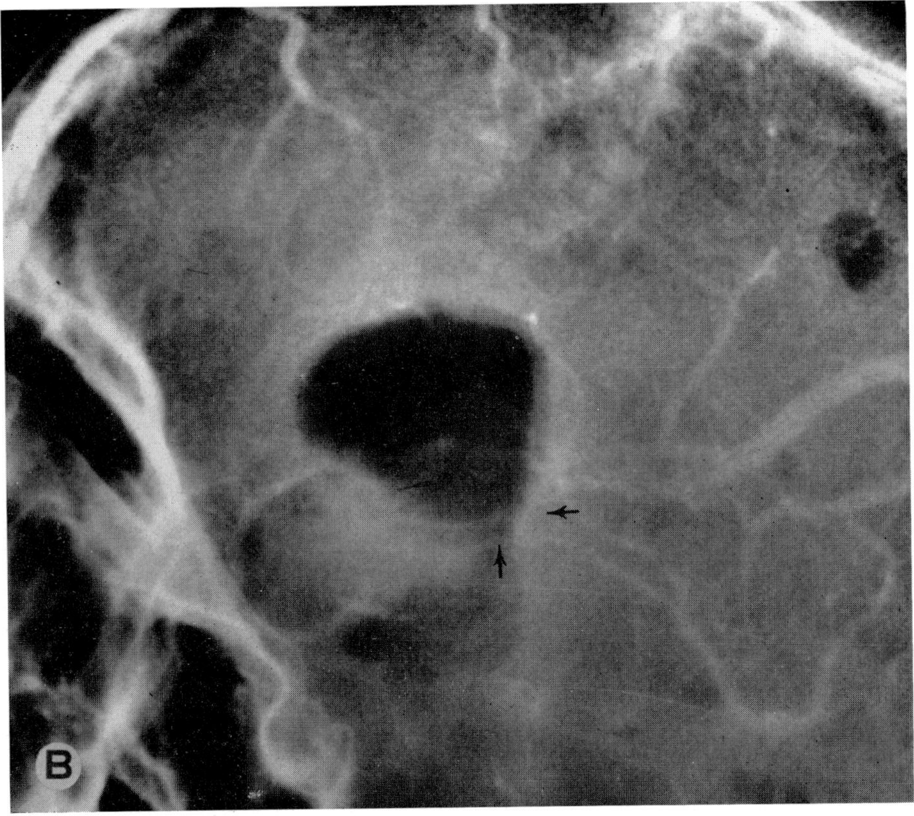

Fig. 205

Surface Projection

The lateral pneumogram accomplishes by its very nature a projection of the lateral ventricles onto the bony skull, since the air density of the ventricles and the bone density of the skull are both visible and are superimposed. Except for subarachnoid gas over the convexities, which outlines various gyri and sulci, the soft tissues of the brain between the ventricles and cranium are not visualized. The sulci are inconstantly visualized, however, particularly when small quantities of gas are used for pneumoencephalography, and at ventriculography, the cerebral surface is seldom seen. It is desirable, therefore, to have a good concept of cranio-cerebro-ventricular relationships and to be able to associate cranial landmarks and ventricular deformities with cerebral surface structures, even though the latter are not seen (fig. 207). Similarly, in comparing angiograms and pneumograms it is necessary to have cross reference points, as previously mentioned, and to project mentally both vascular and ventricular structures onto the cerebral surface, through which surgical approaches are made.

The classical anatomic approach is to establish a lobar relationship of the ventricular system to the brain. For this purpose, the Taylor-Haughton lines provide a satisfactory guide (fig. 208). These lines, which were developed primarily as surgical topographic landmarks in 1900, interestingly enough employed radiologic methods, then in their infancy, to establish their validity. Taylor and Haughton (1900) placed malleable wire in the major fissures and sulci of the brain of anatomic specimens and also marked principal cranial landmarks with tin wire. The fixed brain with the metallic markers was replaced in the skull and radio-

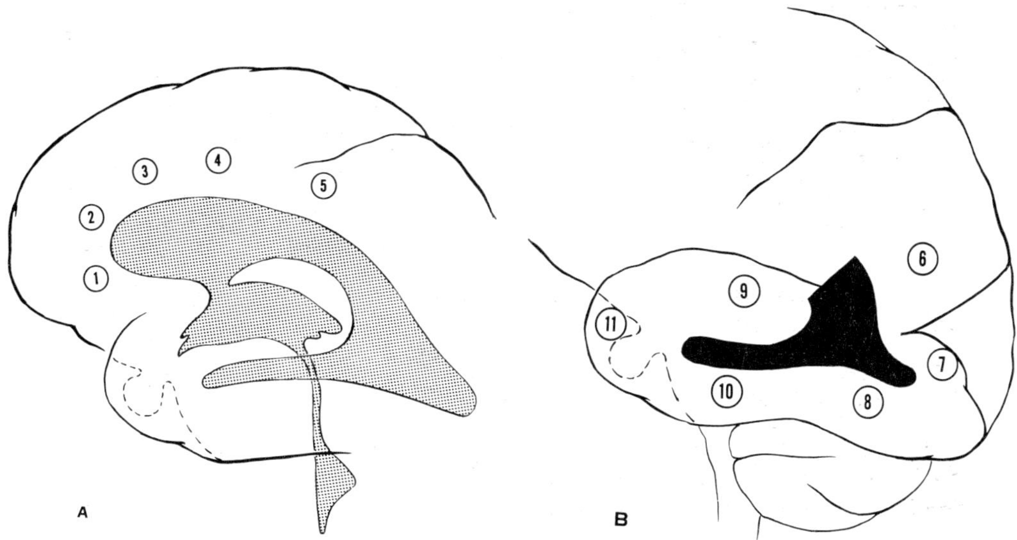

Fig. 206.—A Scheme of Hemispheric Division from the Lateral Pneumogram

Anatomic reference in the pneumogram may be integrated with angiographic localization (see Fig. 422). The anterior and superior portions of the hemisphere may be divided into segments which may be related to the foramen of Monro and, therefore, to the angiographic Sylvian triangle (A). The portions of the frontal lobe forward of the foramen of Monro may be divided into inferior preforaminal (1), anterior preforaminal (2), and superior preforaminal (3). Areas 1, 2, and 3 correspond to the frontal localizations at angiography. Area 4 may be denoted as supraforaminal and area 5 as postforaminal. The areas correspond generally to the angiographic anterior supra-Sylvian area and the posterior supra-Sylvian area, respectively.

Posterior and inferior hemispheric localization may be related to the ventricular atrium and temporal horn (B). The segment above the atrium may be referred to as superior periatrial (6), the segment which is predominantly occipital may be called posterior periatrial (7), and the area below and behind the trigone—generally related to the posterior portion of the temporal lobe or the superior surface of the tentorium—may be designated inferior periatrial (8). These areas, 6, 7, and 8, correspond to the angiographic localizations of superior retro-Sylvian, posterior retro-Sylvian, and inferior retro-Sylvian. The main portion of the temporal lobe may be subdivided into superior (9), anterior (11), and inferior temporal (10), in relation to the temporal horn. These divisions correspond to the infra-Sylvian area of the lateral angiogram.

graphic exposures made to relate these principal cerebral divisions to plain skull and topographic anatomy.

The radiologist may quickly draw out the position of the Rolandic and Sylvian fissures of the brain on one film of a pneumoencephalogram with the aid of only a flexible rule. The first step is to identify in the lateral pneumogram the inion, or the external occipital protuberance, and the nasion, or the midpoint of the frontonasal suture at the root of the nose. The tip of the flexible rule is placed at the nasion and the rule is bent to conform as closely as possible to the outer table of the skull. The semicircumferential distance to the inion is noted, and the one-half, one-quarter, and three-quarter points are marked on the x-ray film with a wax pencil. A string or wire may substitute for the rule, and sometimes more accurate points may be obtained in this way, although they are generally not necessary for clinical purposes. Following the marking of the five points on the film (the nasion, the quarter circumferential point, the midpoint, the three-quarter point, and the position of the inion), several lines are then drawn which relate the radiographic depiction of the lateral ventricle to the external surface of the brain. A line is drawn from the lower

(Revised 1963)

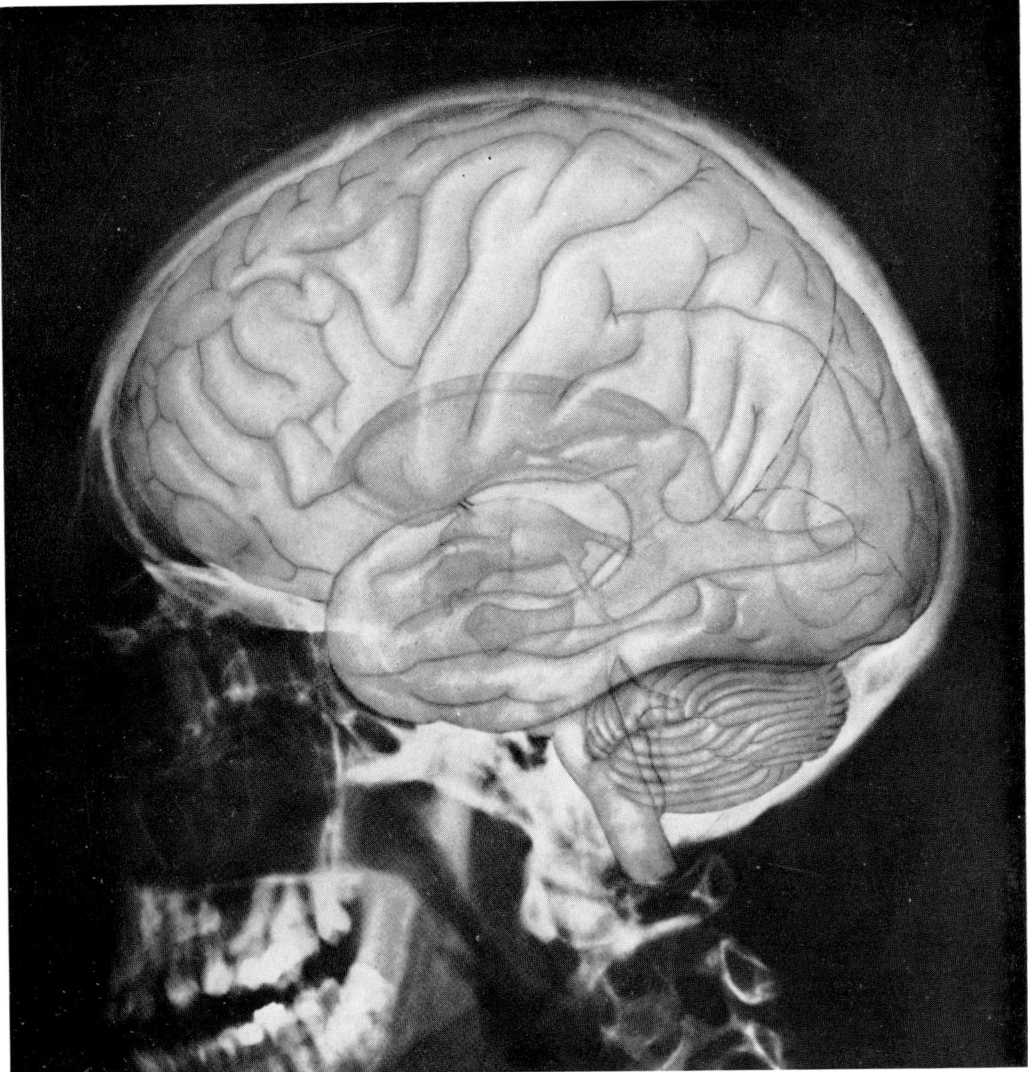

Fig. 207.—Composite Radiograph of the Skull and Artist's Drawing of the Brain, Showing the Cerebral Ventricles

Within the intracranial area of a lateral radiograph, a drawing of the lateral cerebral surface has been made. The parieto-occipital and calcarine fissures, on the medial aspect of the brain, have been added as dotted lines. The projected relationship of the ventricular system to the surface structures of the brain, and to cranial topographic points (see Fig. 8), is demonstrated. (Courtesy of Mr. William S. Cornwell, Rochester, New York.)

margin of the orbit through the center of the external auditory meatus (Reid's base line). A dotted line is then drawn from the external auditory canal to the anterior 25 per cent point on the arch of the cranial vault. The nasion and the 75 per cent circumferential point to the inion are aligned and the point of intersection with the dotted line previously drawn is marked. This intersection identifies the Sylvian point of the brain. A solid line is drawn from the Sylvian point backward and upward 7 cm. on the axis from the nasion to the 75 per cent distance point and this represents the extent of the Sylvian fissure on the cerebral surface.

The posterior margin of the head of the

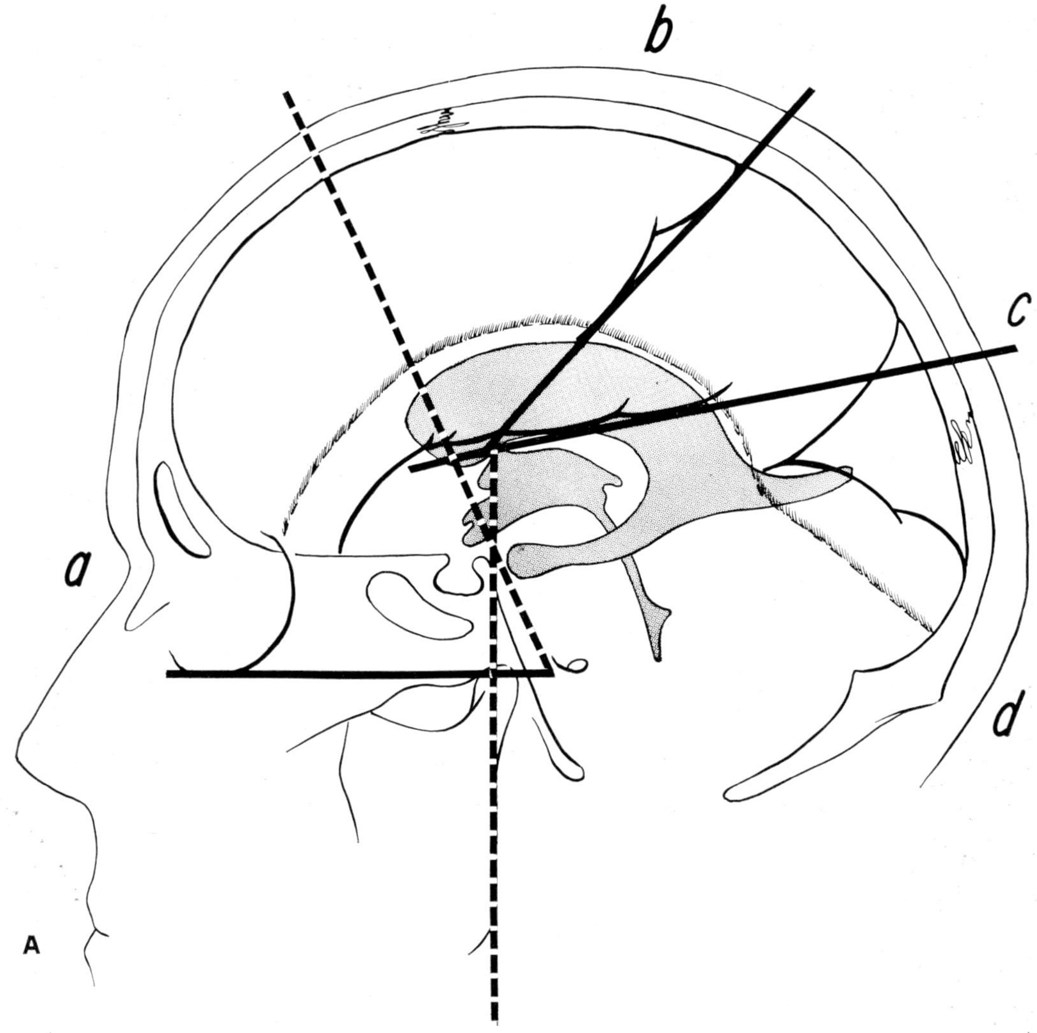

FIG. 208.—CLASSICAL DEPICTION OF CRANIO-CEREBRO-VENTRICULAR RELATIONSHIPS ACCORDING TO THE METHOD OF TAYLOR AND HAUGHTON

Using points that can be located clinically and in radiographs, a series of lines is constructed to determine the location of the Rolandic and Sylvian fissures on lateral films, or on the surface of the patient's head (see text). Ventricular deformities thus may be related to lobar divisions of the brain by means of the lines. In the sketch (A), the location of the parieto-occipital fissure and the position of the falx and tentorium also have been drawn. Only a flexible rule is required to locate the Taylor-Haughton lines on the lateral pneumogram (B).

mandible then is identified and a dotted line is drawn through it vertically and perpendicular to Reid's base line to intersect with the line of the Sylvian fissure. A mark is made one inch posterior to the midway point from the nasion to the inion along the arch of the vault. A solid line is drawn from this point to intersect on the Sylvian fissure with the vertical dotted line just described. This latter solid line conforms generally to the position of the Rolandic fissure. In this way, a clinically workable definition of the posterior boundary of the frontal lobe and the superior boundary of the temporal lobe may be determined on radiographs. The occipital lobe is small and comprises that portion of the cerebral substance directly posterior to the atrium, or that portion of a

(Revised 1963)

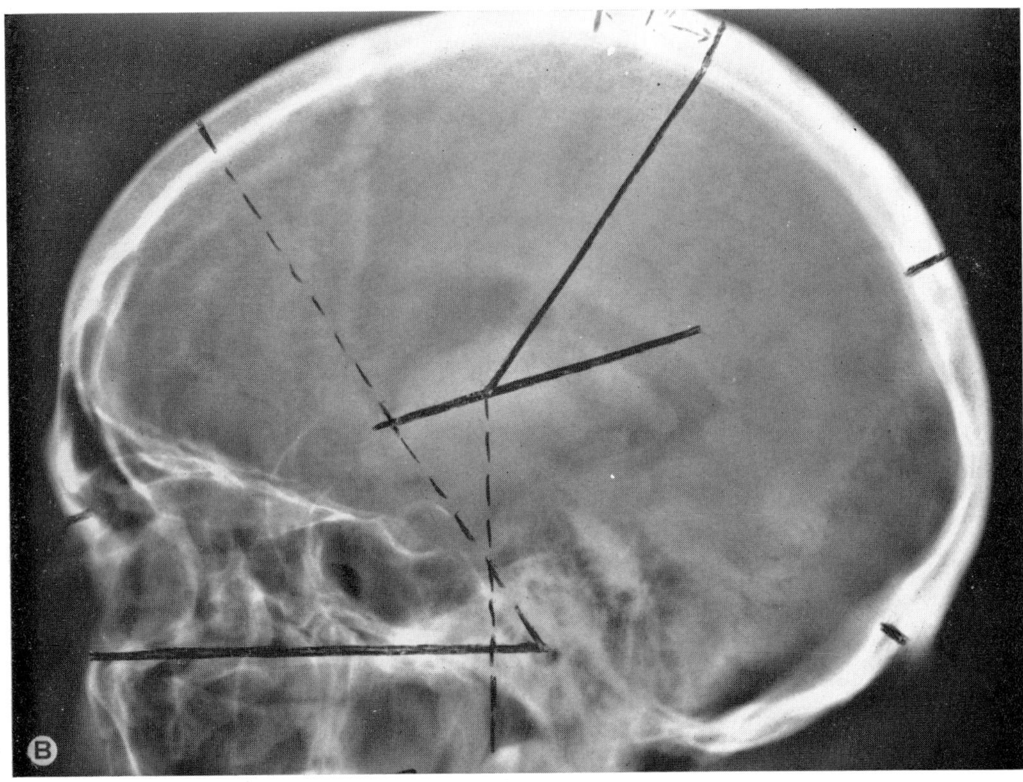

FIG. 208

cerebral hemisphere into which an occipital horn extends, if it is developed.

The relating of pneumographic structures and abnormalities to the lobes of the brain is more accurate than associating them with the overlying cranial bones. Even so, difficulty may be encountered in determining whether a certain variation from normal is in the frontal or parietal lobe, because of the obliquity of the dividing fissure. For this reason, and because of lobar deformities and boundary displacement which may develop with disease, the Taylor-Haughton lines are not as useful in clinical work as they otherwise might be.

Frontal Horn

The frontal lobes, which contain the frontal horns and anterior portions of the ventricular bodies, are the most highly evolved parts of the brain and constitute approximately one-half the mass of the cerebrum. From the lateral aspect the frontal lobe is demarcated by the lateral fissure (Sylvian fissure), from the temporal lobe, and by the central sulcus (Rolandic fissure), from the parietal lobe, the radiographic topographic depiction of which has been described. The Rolandic fissure, although one of the chief landmarks of the brain, probably can be more correctly considered as a sulcus, since in man it usually does not extend downward to intersect with the lateral or Sylvian fissure. The precentral sulcus often is more conspicuous in pneumograms and often does extend into the lateral fissure. The convolutional pattern of the brain in man exhibits considerable variation both anatomically and radiologically, but by drawing the Rolandic fissure on the lateral pneumogram and constructing a line parallel to and approximately 1.5 cm. forward of the Rolandic fissure, the motor area of the frontal lobe may be defined satisfactorily for clinical purposes.

(Revised 1963)

The motor area is one of the major divisions of the frontal lobe. Its functions are perhaps the best understood of any portion of the brain and, because of the significant implications for surgical procedures in this region, localization of pneumographic changes in relation to the motor strip is highly important.

The large lateral aspect of the frontal lobe, forward of the precentral sulcus, is divided into three sections by fissures extending transversely. These fissures, or more properly sulci, are the superior and inferior, and they divide the premotor portion of the brain into the superior, middle, and inferior frontal gyri (fig. 215). These sulci form convoluted curves, paralleling the arched superior cerebral surface. The inferior frontal sulcus often is the more prominent of the two main frontal sulci on the lateral aspect of the brain. The inferior margin of the lateral ventricle generally follows the course of this sulcus. The portion of the brain forward of the anterior horn is irregularly convoluted and this area may be referred to generally as the anterior pole of the brain, or the frontal pole. Lesions arising in this area will be shown later to have a different effect upon the appearance of the ventricle than those which arise in the ventricular coronal planes.

The *anterior horn*, extending forward, laterally and inferiorly from the foramen of Monro, is bounded medially by the septum pellucidum in its posterior portion and further forward by the pillars of the fornix and partially by the corpus callosum. The anterior extremity terminates in a blind pouch in the substance of the frontal pole, and is surrounded by radiating fibers of the corpus callosum. Inferiorly, the anterior horn outlines the rostrum of the corpus callosum and fornix. Laterally, gas in the posterior one-half of the anterior horn bounds the head of the caudate nucleus while further forward the lateral margin is formed by the central white matter of the frontal lobe.

Varying degrees of filling of the anterior horn will result in different pneumographic appearances. In the anteroposterior half axial projection, or when only a small amount of gas is present in the lateral ventricles, the divergence appears exaggerated in frontal view. In the same projection, the variation in filling on the two sides may be so conspicuous that depression of one ventricular roof is suggested. When only a very small amount of gas is present, sufficient only to fill the forward portion of the anterior horn, the obliquely placed "shield-like" configuration is all that is seen in frontal films. When only the anterior horns are filled, there is no reason to take antero-posterior half axial views, but, if there is more complete ventricular filling, the projection may serve to throw the anterior horns clear of other air shadows, thus allowing independent depiction.

When there is gas filling of the anterior horn as far back as the foramen of Monro, the typical "butterfly" configuration of the ventricular system in frontal projection is the usual finding superimposed on the "shield." The lateral margin of each posterior segment, as previously mentioned, is formed by the head of the caudate nucleus. In this coronal plane the ventricles are separated by the septum pellucidum and their roofs formed by the corpus callosum (fig. 209).

In lateral projection the anterior horns usually have a smoothly convex superior surface, formed by the radiating fibers of the anterior portion of the corpus callosum. The inferior surface often is slightly concave downward, resulting from superior projection of the head of the caudate nucleus. The anterior extremity of the frontal horn forms an arc between the corpus callosum and caudate nucleus. The width of the arc varies to some extent on the two sides, and from one individual to another. A prominent anterior horn may result in a "bulbous" configuration (fig. 225), a moderate degree of which may be a normal variation, but marked prominence of such a form may indicate atrophy. In some individuals an indentation of the ventricular roof at the level of the junction of the anterior horn and the body may be present and contribute to the bulbous appearance of

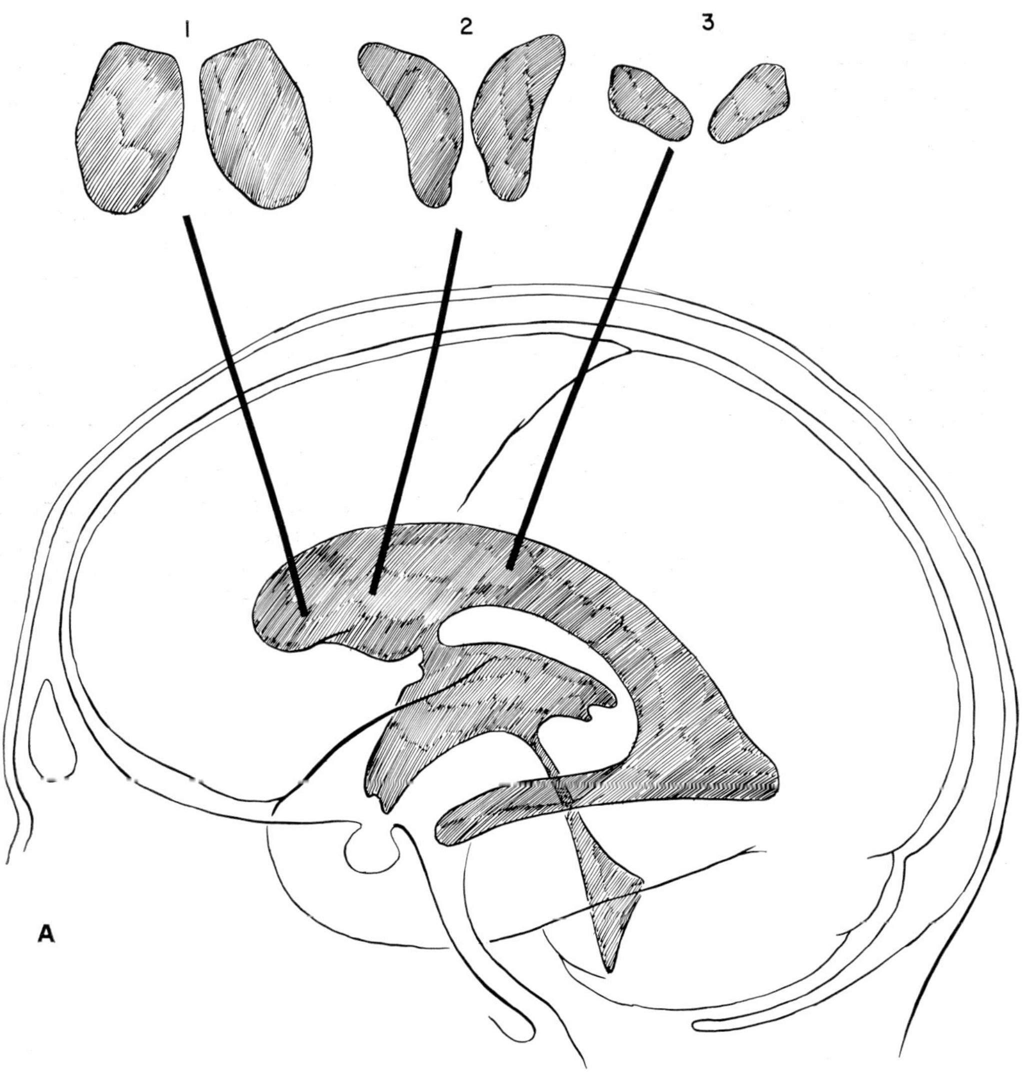

Fig. 209.—Segmental Origin of Shadows Contributing to the Outline of the Lateral Ventricle in the Frontal Pneumogram

Analysis of the composite shadow of the lateral ventricle, as seen in anteroposterior projection with the patient supine, reveals that it is formed by three major components (A). If there is isolated filling of the forward portion of the anterior horn, the configuration is that of a shield (1). The posterior half of the anterior horn is indented on the lateral side by the head of the caudate nucleus, resulting in a triangular ventricular configuration. The two ventricular segments in this plane resemble a "butterfly" (2). The ventricular body is roughly quadrilateral in cross section (3). The segments usually are superimposed, forming a composite shadow which is partially resolved by films made in anteroposterior, half axial projection (see Fig. 186).

Calcification in the basal ganglia, seen in some cases of hypoparathyroidism, enhances the shadow of the caudate nucleus in pneumograms. The relationship of this anatomic structure to the lateral ventricular wall (B) and its position in the posterior portion of the anterior horn (C) are brought out by the "double contrast" of calcification and gas.

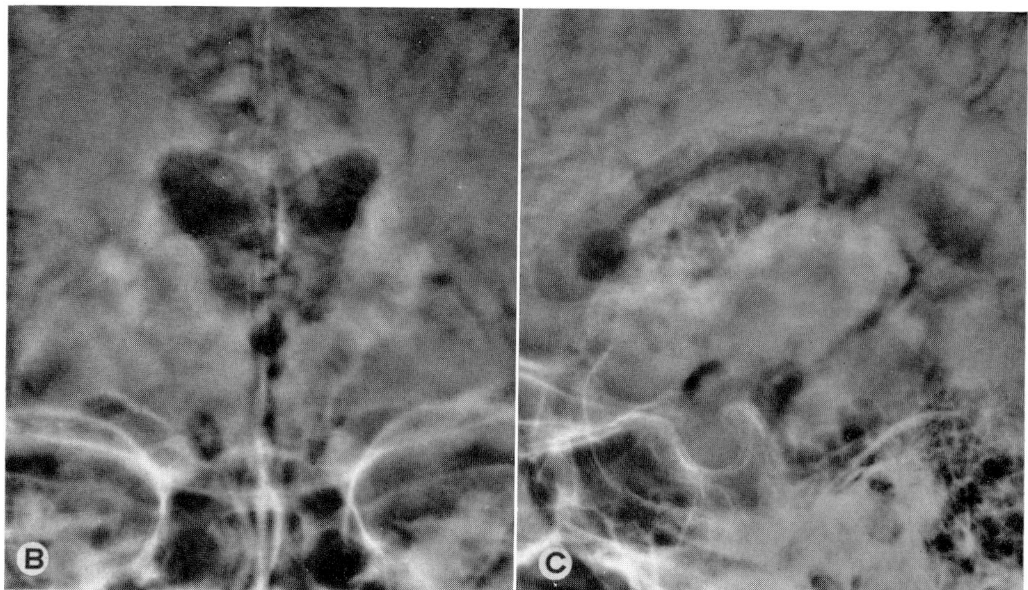

Fig. 209

the anterior horn. This indentation or "nick" was thought by Lindgren (1941) to be the result of a condensation of fibers of the corpus callosum extending across the ventricle. Davidoff and Dyke (1951) considered it more likely to be an irregular development of brain.

Body

The *ventricular body* extends from the interventricular foramen of Monro to the coronal plane of the splenium of the corpus callosum, where it joins the atrium. The body is arched superiorly along a curved line, usually continuous with the anterior horn as seen laterally. In frontal projection the ventricular body is generally quadrilateral in shape, having a medial wall (the septum pellucidum), a roof (the corpus callosum), and a lateral and inferior boundary formed by the basal ganglia laterally and by a group of structures, including a margin of the thalamus, along the ventricular floor. The lateral wall slopes approximately at a 45-degree angle, sometimes straight, but more often exhibiting varying degrees of medial convexity, corresponding to the lateral margin of the posterior half of the anterior horn (fig. 209). There is some variation between the anterior, middle, and posterior thirds of the bodies as seen in frontal pneumograms, but generally the relationships are similar. In the anterior portions the ventricles are more angular laterally. This lateral and dorsal angulation usually is well defined, and the angle is sharp. Any apparent alteration of the lateral ventricular angle should be examined with a high degree of suspicion. Narrowing of the lateral angle always suggests an expanding lesion, especially if it results from some degree of flattening of the ventricular roof. Widening or rounding of the angle most commonly is the result of degenerative or atrophic processes. Some degree of blunting, however, is quite consistent with a normal ventricular appearance, particularly in older individuals.

In the frontal projection, the structures forming the inferior and lateral walls of the ventricle are, beginning medially, (1) the body of the fornix, (2) the chorioid plexus, (3) the thalamus, (4) the terminal vein, and (5) the caudate nucleus, which extends lateralward and upward to form the lateral angle with the corpus callosum. The boundaries thus comprise alternating neural and vascular structures. A visible projection of

(*Revised 1963*)

the chorioid plexus into the ventricular lumen may serve to separate the thalamus from the medially placed fornix.

In the lateral film the ventricular floor is formed by the caudate nucleus anteriorly and posteriorly by the dorsal surface of the thalamus. Other structures such as the terminal vein and chorioid plexus also form portions of the ventricular floor, but they usually are not distinguishable in the lateral view of the ventricular body even on stereoscopic study. Irregularities along the floor, of minor extent, often are the result of variations in the appearance of the chorioid plexus. Usually, however, the floor of the lateral ventricle in lateral projection appears smooth and continuous in outline.

The *posterior portion of the ventricular body* and the superior portion of the atrium may be related topographically to the parietal lobe of the brain. The anterior boundary of the parietal lobe is formed by the central sulcus (Rolandic fissure), but there is not sharp demarcation on the lateral cerebral surface between the parietal and the occipital and temporal lobes. The parietal lobe, however, may be divided into three parts. The first is the forward portion or postcentral gyrus, situated between the Rolandic fissure and the postcentral sulcus, the sensory counterpart of the precentral gyrus or motor area (fig. 215). A transverse line, the intraparietal sulcus, divides the larger, more posterior part of the parietal lobe into superior and inferior lobules. The superior is occupied principally by the superior parietal gyrus. The inferior parietal lobule may, if desired, be further subdivided into the supramarginal gyrus and the angular and the posterior parietal gyri. The Sylvian fissure at its posterior end has a prominent ascending ramus, and the supramarginal gyrus is situated about both banks of this sulcal extension. The superior temporal sulcus, at the posterior extremity, has a backward extension about parts of which the angular gyrus is situated.

The posterior third of the ventricular body diverges laterally and inferiorly into the splenium of the corpus callosum and the appearance in frontal projection becomes more rectangular. The medial wall is formed by the splenium of the corpus callosum, while the fornix is inferior. Fibers of the corpus callosum extend laterally over the roof of the posterior body, while the white matter of the depths of the parietal lobe form the lateral boundary. The floor of the posterior third of the ventricular body is formed by the thalamus medially, lateral to which are the chorioid plexus, the fornix, and the hippocampus. The posterior ventricular body enlarges gradually into the atrium, which exhibits a similar but expanded quadrilateral configuration.

Atrium

The *atrium* or trigone connects the posterior portion of the ventricular body with the temporal horn, and, if present, with the occipital horn. The points of demarcation between the ventricular body and the atrium, and between the atrium and the temporal horn, are less well defined than most other ventricular landmarks. The anterior wall of the atrium is formed by the fornix and posterior aspect of the thalamus or pulvinar. If a line is drawn from the most posterior point of the convexity of the anterior atrial wall to the center of the occipital horn or its vestige, then a line drawn perpendicular to the first, at its anterior extremity, will roughly demarcate the points of junction with the ventricular body and temporal horn. The portion thus designated in the lateral roentgenogram will have a semilunar configuration with varying degrees of fullness in different individuals. The atrium is normally the most expanded portion of the ventricle and is often the first place where abnormal enlargement may be noticed as a result of degenerative changes.

The posterosuperior and posteroinferior aspects of the atrium are gently curved, and generally are smooth in outline. The extreme posterior aspect will vary in appearance, depending upon whether an occipital horn is present or not. In some instances, with absence of the occipital horn, the smooth curve of the posterior wall from above and below will be continuous. Frequently, however, along the posterosuperior margin and just above the base of the occipital horn, there is an indentation of the ventricular curve as a result of prominence of the calcar avis and forceps major. This often affects the occipital horn more than the atrium.

Within the atrial lumen, on the anterior aspect, the glomus of the chorioid plexus is visible as a rounded shadow producing a filling defect in the atrial gas outline at pneumography. In the majority of instances this shadow is broad based but in some instances may be more pedunculated and mobile. The shadow is usually found in the anterior central portion of the atrium, but frequently is more prominent superiorly and expansion of the chorioid plexus may extend into the ventricular body. The shadow is 1 cm. in diameter on the average and often is larger. The surface may be smoothly rounded or multilobulated. Calcific degeneration of varying extent frequently is found in the glomus and moderate asymmetry of size and appearance of the glomus on the two sides is commonplace.

In frontal views the atrium appears as a diverging, elongated quadrilateral gas shadow slightly wider superiorly than ininferiorly. From the ventricular body the atrium extends laterally at an angle of approximately 35 to 40 degrees and downward to reach the temporal horn. The marginal angles of the atrium are not as sharp as those observed in the main portion of the ventricular body and some degree of blunting in this region frequently is found under normal circumstances. Superiorly, the atrial shadow fuses with that of the similarly diverging oblique posterior segment of the ventricular body. Inferiorly, it connects with the curving shadow of the posterior aspect of the temporal horn, and just above this the darker rounded or disc-shaped shadow of the occipital horn may be superimposed.

Temporal Horn

The *temporal horn* or inferior horn may be divided into two parts, the body and the tip. The body of the temporal horn is a tubelike or finger-like forward and downward extension from the atrium, 4 cm. in length and generally of uniform caliber, although frequently it may taper slightly from backward forward. The horn ends approximately 3 cm. behind the temporal lobe tip and this extremity is projected in lateral pneumograms just behind the dorsum sellae. The superior aspect of the roof of the temporal horn is formed chiefly by the tapetum of the corpus callosum, and to a slight extent by the tail of the caudate nucleus. The floor is formed by the hippocampus and throughout most of the length of the temporal body the hippocampus indents the medial as well as the inferior wall to a significant degree. Therefore, on cross section the temporal horn has a crescentic shape. The main portion lateral to the hippocampus may be called the lateral cleft and that portion above the hippocampus the supracornual cleft. The former occupies an essentially vertical plane and the latter a generally horizontal plane (fig. 210). Thus, the axis of the x-ray beam will have a considerable effect on the appearance of the gas collections in these two right-angled compartments (Childe and Penfield, 1937). Anteriorly, the hippocampus becomes flatter (*pes hippocampi*) and over this flattened portion of the hippocampus the anterior extremity of the ventricle turns downward and medially to form the temporal tip. At the tip the lateral portion of the floor is formed by the collateral eminence, the degree of prominence depending upon the depth of the collateral fissure over which the cerebral substance of the eminence extends (figs. 191 and 210). The chorioid plexus extends along the superior and medial aspect of the temporal horn in the supracornual cleft throughout its length.

The appearance of the temporal horn in the frontal pneumogram depends on the projection used to make the radiograph. In anteroposterior halfaxial projection the anterior aspect projects downward and as it reaches the tip, it expands "spoonlike" (figs. 186 and 191). In the anteroposterior projection taken with the vertical x-ray beam parallel to Reid's base line, the patient supine, the anterior aspect is partly

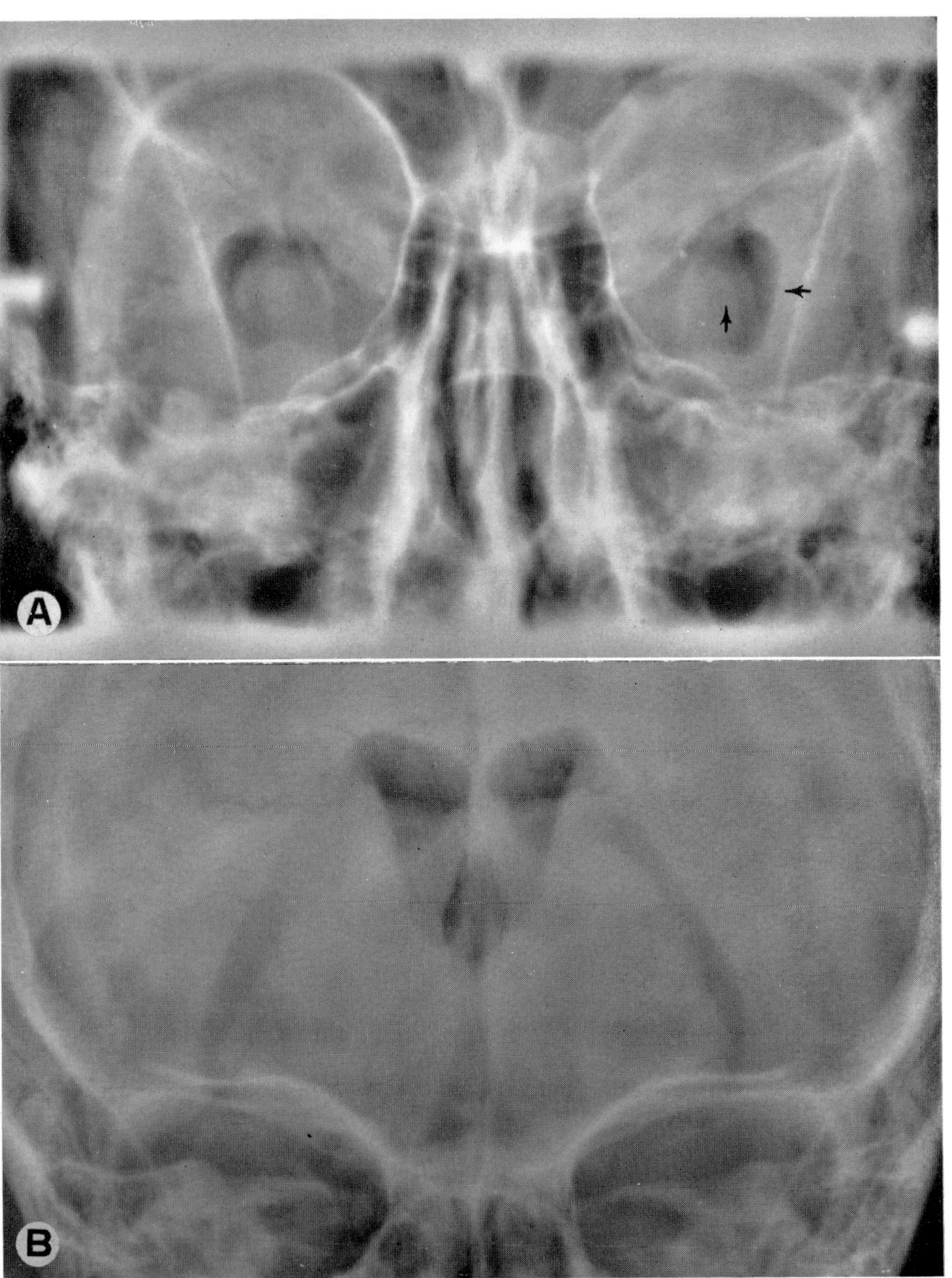

Fig. 210.—Frontal Demonstration of the Temporal Horns

A film made through the orbits (along Reid's base line) provides an axial view of the temporal horns (A). The superior transverse portion of the horn (supracornual cleft) is at right angles to the lateral cleft (*transverse arrow*). The hippocampal shadow along the medial wall of the horn is prominent (*vertical arrow*). More anteriorly, the hippocampus is reduced in height, and the flatter portion (pes hippocampi) allows medial and downward turning of the horn to form the anterior temporal tip. In some cases, the collateral eminence is more prominent (see Fig. 191). In other instances, special films are not required. Frequently, routine frontal views (B) will show the anterior portion of the temporal horn well, and be adequate for clinical diagnosis.

(*Revised 1963*)

superimposed on the posterior portion and its appearance is similar to that of a true coronal section through this region of the temporal lobe.

With the head in lateral recumbent position, the uppermost temporal horn is the highest point of the ventricular system, and if gas is present in the lateral ventricles, filling of the temporal horn should occur in all instances. *Failure to visualize the uppermost temporal horn under these circumstances should always be regarded as a finding of pathologic significance.*

In topographic projection on the lateral aspect of the brain the temporal horn is visualized through the middle temporal gyrus. Mass lesions arising in this plane commonly affect the temporal horn directly, with compression and occlusion (fig. 282). Lesions arising higher in the superior temporal gyrus area may deform the ventricle without occlusion while those arising in the inferior temporal gyrus frequently elevate the temporal horn, sometimes with striking displacement, but commonly without occlusion.

The portion of the temporal lobe best understood functionally is the invaginated portion of the Sylvian fissure. This is the portion of the temporal lobe opposing the island of Reil and upon which transverse temporal convolutions are located. The most anterior portion of these convolutions is the transverse temporal gyrus, or the gyrus of Heschl. This area receives the impulses of audition, and in right-handed individuals the transverse temporal gyri on the left side exhibit a greater degree of complexity than those on the contralateral side.

The true temporal medial surface, facing toward the midsagittal plane, is the oldest part of the lobe. Inferiorly, the inferior temporal gyrus has an extension on the medial side which is continuous posteriorly with an enlarged segment often termed the fusiform gyrus. Above this is situated the hippocampal gyrus, with its medial protrusion, the uncus. These portions of the brain are concerned traditionally with olfaction. The type of cortex present suggests, on histologic study, a more primitive form of neural tissue than that exhibited elsewhere by the neocortex.

(Revised 1963)

Occipital Horn

The *occipital horn*, or posterior horn as previously stated, is the most variable portion of the ventricular system. The marked variability of the occipital horn, and even its absence in normal brains, was pointed out by Curran as early as 1909. The occipital horn varies from a small teatlike structure projecting backward from the atrium to a well developed fingerlike projection extending posteriorly and slightly ventrally from its atrial origin; the posterior extremity may project to a point within 1 to 2 cm. of the occipital bone. In some instances the tip of the occipital horn is well rounded while at other times it may be bulbous or even flared, simulating a fishtail. Frequently, the occipital horn will be straight and taper almost to a point.

Variations to be recognized are the indentations at the base of the occipital horn, frequently affecting also the posterior superior margin of the atrium, as previously described. They result from the varying degrees of development of the calcar avis and posterior forceps of the corpus callosum. Full development of the calcar avis and forceps major apparently is the basis for the obliteration of the occipital horn on one or both sides. The characteristic findings are the presence of a shallow or deep notch at the rostral extremity of the horn on the medial side (calcar avis) above which is another prominence, the bulb (posterior forceps).

In frontal projection, the occipital horns are not well demonstrated unless they are reasonably well developed. In posteroanterior prone pneumograms, when the occipital horns have the best opportunity to fill, they appear as rounded or disclike areas of air density, superimposed upon the atrial portion. When long, the occipital horns are found to turn medially toward their termination. The horns are perhaps best seen when small but equal amounts of gas are present on the two sides outlining only these posterior extensions (fig. 211).

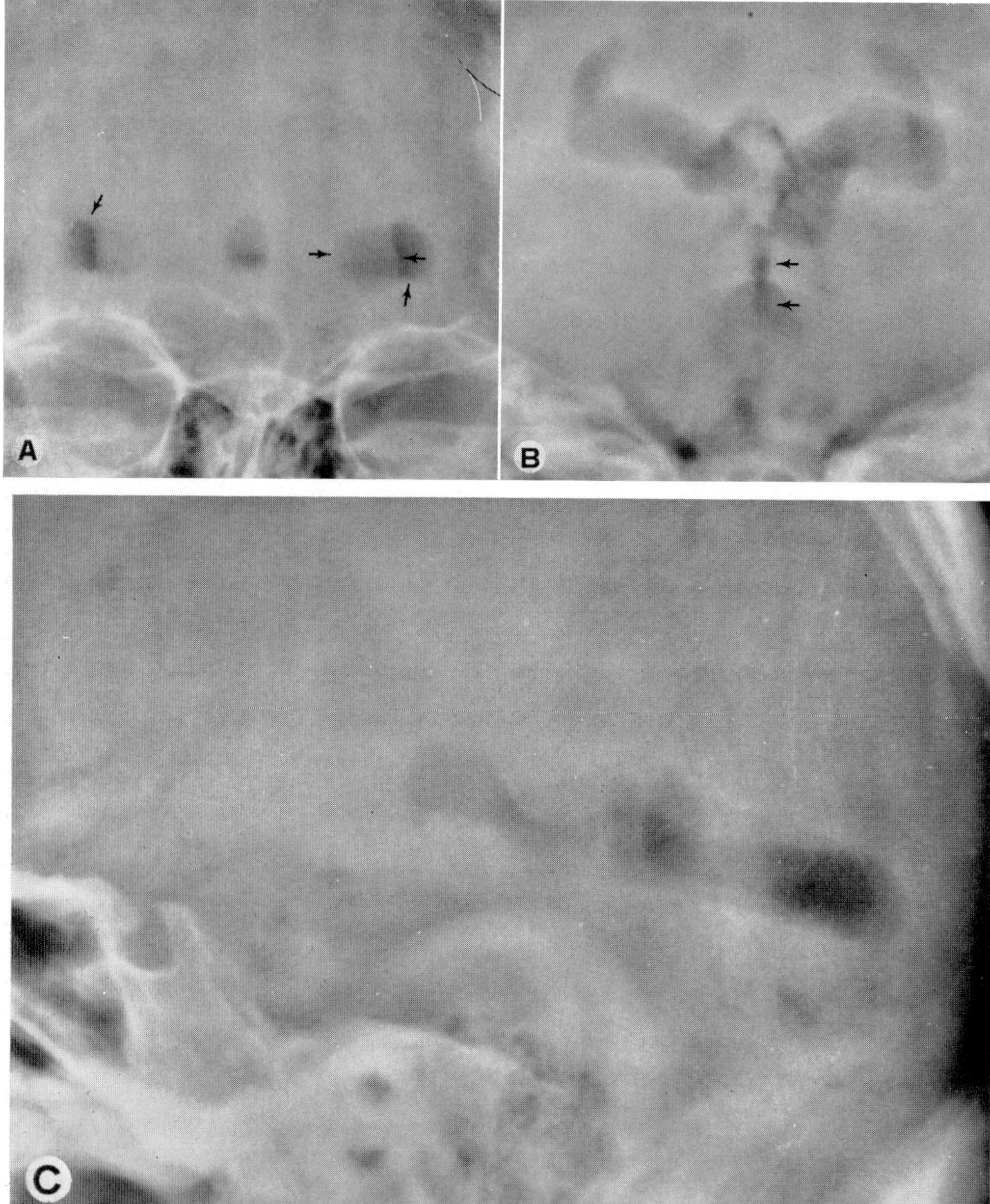

FIG. 211.—OCCIPITAL HORNS AND POSTERIOR PORTION OF THE THIRD VENTRICLE

Films made 24 hours after pneumoencephalography show isolated collections of residual gas in the posterior portions of the lateral and third ventricles. When poorly developed, the occipital horns appear disclike, superimposed upon the shadow of the atrium in the frontal projection. When more fully developed, the occipital horns exhibit double contours in frontal view (A). The anterior portion of the occipital horn is the darker portion of the shadow, and it is lenticular, owing to the calcar avis (*lateral transverse arrow*); the collateral eminence (trigone) often produces a flattening of the inferior portion of the horn (*lower vertical arrow*); the lumen of the occipital horn may be narrowed superiorly and medially by the bulb, formed by the posterior forceps of the corpus callosum (*arrow on reader's left*). The

(Revised 1963)

The *occipital lobe* is demarcated on the medial aspect of each cerebral hemisphere. The parieto-occipital fissure is a prominent landmark extending downward and forward at an angle of approximately 45 degrees from the region of the lambda, or the junction of the parietal or occipital bones. The calcarine fissure runs almost perpendicular to the parieto-occipital fissure, resulting in a Y-shaped configuration, the stem directed forward. On both banks of the calcarine fissure and extending into the depths of it is situated the primary visual area of the brain, the fibers originating in the superior part of the retina terminating upon the superior bank of the calcarine fissure and those from the inferior half of the retina terminating on the lower bank. The main portion of the occipital area above the calcarine fissure is called the cuneus, while that below is the lingual gyrus. The occipital lobe has only a small circumferential extension upon the lateral aspect of the brain at the extreme posterior pole of the hemisphere. Forward of this, but projected through the occipital lobe on the medial side, is the posterior parietal gyrus. It is possible, therefore, for expanding lesions arising in the true parietal lobe to affect the occipital horn on its lateral aspect, while those arising medially are true occipital lobe lesions. This serves to recall a similar unusual lobar-ventricular relationship, that of the Rolandic fissure to the ventricular body. In this region, expanding lesions in the posterior portion of the frontal lobe and anterior portion of the parietal lobe can produce identical deformities of the ventricle. For these and other reasons to be discussed later, precise lobar localization of lesions producing ventricular deformities is not always feasible and other schema of classification may be preferable. Thus, the area behind the ventricular atrium, as seen in lateral pneumograms, may be referred to as posterior periatrial, regardless of whether the cerebral substance under consideration is strictly in the parietal or in the occipital lobe anatomically (fig. 206).

Measurements

The *volume* of the ventricular system has been determined by various investigators. One of the more reliable evaluations is the result of the work of Bull (1961). The ventricular system was found to contain no more than 15 to 20 cc. of fluid in the average case. Last and Tompsett (1953) considered 20 to 25 cc. to be the usual range of ventricular volume from their study of casts. Ventricles of more than 25 cc. capacity apparently are abnormally large, in the majority of instances. By and large, the lower portion of the ranges described (15 to 20 cc.) is the more normal situation. The lower limit, however, is less important than the upper, since in a number of normal patients studied by Bull, a ventricular volume of less than 10 cc. was found.

Linear *measurements* of various aspects of the ventricular system are approximations, based on averages, taken from examination of a large number of pneumograms. Generally they serve to confirm the presence of ventricular deformities, since a considerable range exists between the minimum and maximum normal measurements in different individuals which may be related to differences in the shape of the head. A number of useful measurements of reference exist, however, as the result of the observations of Dyke, Davidoff, and others. Those related to the lateral ventricles are more numerous in consideration of the frontal pneumogram, while in the lateral view the various measurements are more significant in relation to the

---

posterior portion of the occipital horn extends medially, as it passes backward in the central white substance of the occipital lobe, casting a lighter shadow when gas filled (*medial transverse arrow*).

The medial curving of the posterior horn is shown in the posteroanterior half axial projection of another case (B). The aqueduct of Sylvius is demonstrated, joining the third and fourth ventricles; the superior and inferior ostia appear rounded (*arrows*), and the main portion of the iter foreshortened, resulting in an appearance resembling a small dumbbell. The lateral view (C) reveals well-developed finger-like projections of the occipital horns, extending downward and backward from the region of the atria, in this case measuring 4 cm. in length. A large suprapineal recess also is gas filled.

(*Revised 1963*)

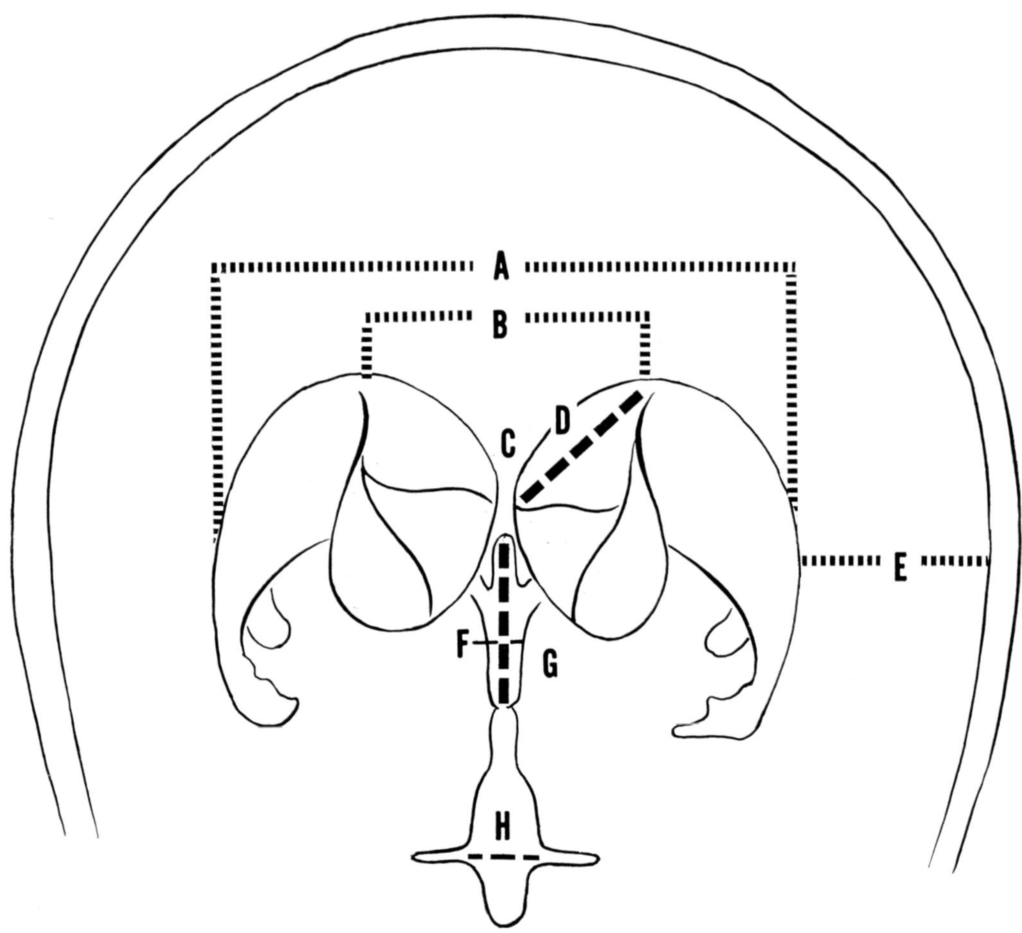

Fig. 212.—Normal Ventricular Measurements of the Frontal Pneumogram

Measurement	Minimum	Maximum	Average
	cm.	*cm.*	*cm.*
A. Spread of lateral ventricles	6.5	9.0	7.5
B. Width of bodies, lateral ventricles	2.0	4.0	3.5
C. Width of septum pellucidum	0.1	0.3	0.2
D. Oblique width of ventricular body	1.5	2.4	2.0
E. Temporal horn to skull	3.5	4.5	4.0
F. Width of third ventricle	0.3	0.7	0.4
G. Height of third ventricle	2.2	3.0	2.5
H. Width, floor of fourth ventricle	1.5	2.0	1.7

midline third and fourth ventricular structures (figs. 212 and 213).

In frontal pneumograms, the maximum distance between the lateral angles of the ventricular bodies should not exceed 4 cm. More recent experience suggests that even this measurement is generous and if a transverse distance greater than 3.5 cm. is found, the films should be scrutinized for other evidence of ventricular enlargement.

Often rounding and blunting of the lateral ventricular angles is present. A method of

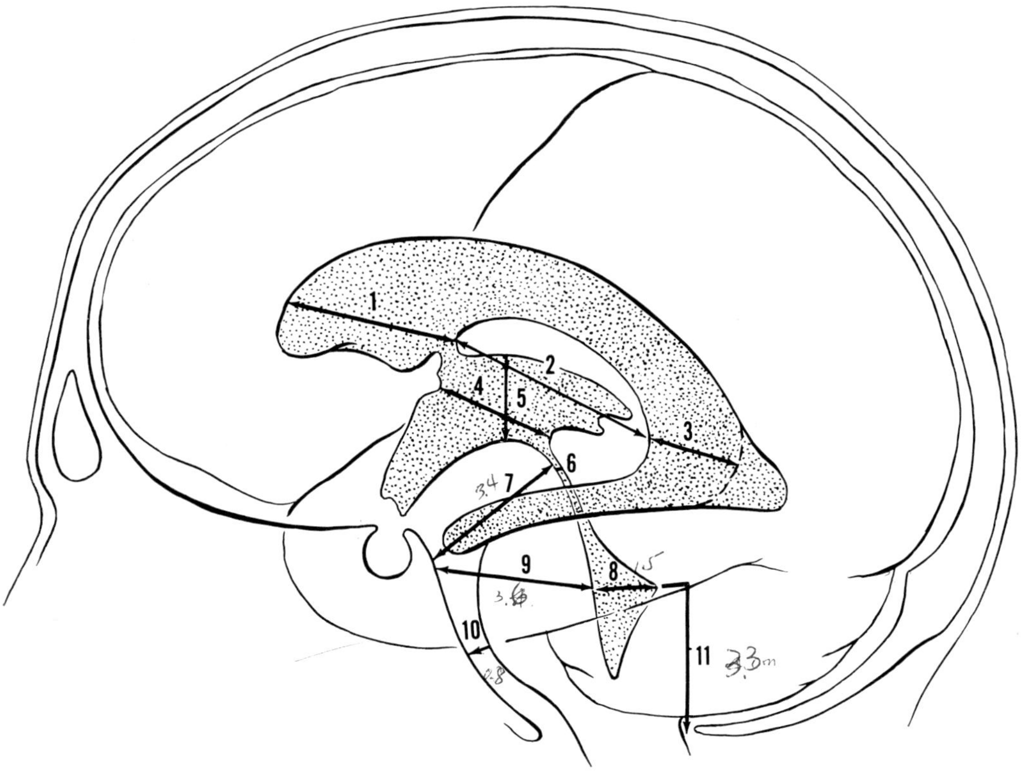

FIG. 213.—NORMAL VENTRICULAR MEASUREMENTS OF THE LATERAL PNEUMOGRAM

Measurement	Minimum	Maximum	Average
	cm.	*cm.*	*cm.*
1. Length of anterior horn	2.5	4.0	3.5
2. Length of ventricular body	3.5	5.0	4.5
3. Width of atrium	1.5	3.0	2.3
4. Foramen of Monro to aqueduct	2.3	2.8	2.5
5. Central height of third ventricle	1.2	1.6	1.5
6. Caliber	0.1	0.2	0.15
7. Aqueduct to dorsum sellae	3.0	3.9	3.4
8. Height of fourth ventricle	1.0	2.0	1.5
9. Fourth ventricle to sella	3.3	4.0	3.6
10. Width pontine cistern	0.5	1.2	0.8
11. Fourth ventricle to foramen magnum	3.0	4.0	3.3

ventricular measurement is advocated by the authors, not dissimilar to that of Jirout (1948). Because the lateral angle is the earliest area to show changes when ventricular enlargement occurs, it appears that a method based on measurement of this portion of the ventricle is capable of showing minimum ventricular enlargement.

A measurement is taken on a line perpendicular to the oblique diameter of the *body* of the ventricle (not the frontal horn), as indicated in Figure 214, 0.5 cm. from the lateral ventricular extremity. In adults over 30 years of age, a measurement of 9 mm. is the upper limit of normal. A measurement of 10 to 12 mm. is considered as 1 plus enlargement, 13 to 15 mm. as 2 plus, 16 to 19 mm. as 3 plus, and 20 mm. or over as 4 plus

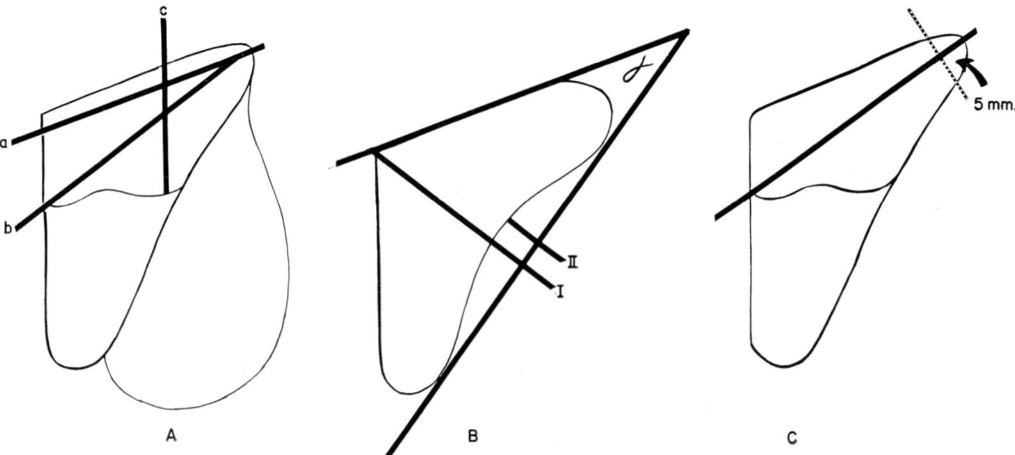

FIG. 214.—MEASUREMENT OF THE LATERAL VENTRICLES

A method of measuring the ventricular body is shown, as advocated by Robertson (A). From a point near the top of the lateral angle, a line is drawn below and parallel to the ventricular roof (a); another line is drawn obliquely from the lateral angle to the junction of the floor with the septum pellucidum (b). The normal measurement of ventricular width along the first line (a) was found by Robertson to be less than 2 cm.; the oblique width of the ventricular body (b) was found by Last and Tompsett to range between 1.5 and 2.4 cm. (an average of 2.0 cm.). The thickness of the ventricular body (c) was found by Last and Tompsett to average 0.6 cm.; the maximum measurement rarely exceeded 1.0 cm. in their series.

Jirout devised indices that relate to the posterior portion of the anterior horn (B). The normal lateral angle in this plane is between 20 and 35 degrees. Measurement along a line constructed from the superior medial angle of the ventricle perpendicular to the lower arm of the lateral angle normally is less than 1.5 cm. (I). A parallel line, marking the greatest indentation of the ventricular side wall (II), is related inversely to the length of Line I and the degree of the angle (when the angle and measurement I increase, there usually is flattening of the side wall).

A simple method of clinical value for determining ventricular enlargement is shown in (C). The measurement is taken along a line perpendicular to the longest oblique diameter, 5 mm. from the ventricular edge, in the body of the lateral ventricle (not the frontal horn). A measurement of 10 to 12 mm. is considered as 1 plus dilatation; 13 to 15 mm. is considered as 2 plus dilatation; 16 to 19, as 3 plus; 20 mm. or more is "4 plus" enlargement. In younger individuals (under 30 years of age), a measurement of 7 mm. is considered as the upper limit of normal, and 8 to 12 mm. would be considered as "1 plus" ventricular dilatation; otherwise, the same measurements pertain at all ages after childhood.

enlargement. In adults under 30 years of age, 7 mm. is considered as the upper limit of normal and 8 to 12 mm. is considered as 1 plus enlargement.

The lateral ventricles are separated by the septum pellucidum which normally measures no more than 2 mm. width. When there is considerable enlargement of this structure in frontal view, an anomaly or pathologic process is to be suspected. Also, in frontal views, the occipital horns generally are separated approximately 6 cm. at their bases and the maximum divergence of the temporal horns is 8 to 9 cm., rarely more than 8.5 cm. Cranial shape has some effect. The distance from the temporal horn to the inner table of the skull is, on the average, 4 cm. Any gross variations in these latter measurements should alert one to the possibility of a mass lesion, either central or lateral to the temporal horn.

In the lateral projection, the roofs of the anterior ventricular bodies usually are situated 5 to 6 cm. from the vertex of the skull. Other measurements of value in connection with the lateral ventricles are the distance from the anterior extremity of the ventricle to the frontal pole (4 to 5 cm.) and a similar distance from the middle of the atrium to the occipital pole (5 to 6 cm.). Other measurements of ventricular structures may be useful. Various measurements are shown diagrammatically in Figures 212 and 213, and cross reference is made to these numbers in connection with anatomic and pathologic considerations of various areas of the brain.

Vast amounts of cerebral tissue exist peripheral to the ventricular system. Because of the distances, tumors arising in only slightly different places may reflect somewhat similarly upon the gas outline of the ventricles. Unfortunately, most abnormal measurements reflect gross changes and careful attention must be given to minor alterations of ventricular appearance which may, or may not, be supported by measurable variations from the normal in pneumograms.

CEREBRAL SULCI

In their monograph, *The Normal Encephalogram*, Davidoff and Dyke illustrate extensively the depiction of the various sulci and convolutions on the lateral aspect of the brain in pneumograms. The sulci of the convexity are the most inconstant structures visualized in pneumoencephalograms and with the smaller amounts of gas used for modern encephalography, they are less frequently visible and identifiable today than in the past. The anatomic relationship of the ventricular system to the lateral topographic surface is more practically made by the drawing of the imaginary lines described than by the recognition of occasional lateral sulcal shadows demonstrated. On the other hand, the fissures and sulci on the medial aspect of the brain are much more commonly outlined together with specific cerebral structures, even when small quantities of gas are used, since there is a more natural flow of gas through the larger central subarachnoid pathways than through the narrow lateral channels. The relationship of the lateral ventricles to gas-outlined structures on the medial aspect of the brain is possible in a high percentage of lateral pneumograms and also very often in frontal pneumograms.

Medial

Gas usually is present in some part of the superior longitudinal fissure (longitudinal cerebral fissure or interhemispheric fissure), which is the major cleft between the cerebral hemispheres and in which the falx cerebri is located. The superior longitudinal fissure extends from just above the ventricular roof at the corpus callosum to the vertex and can be seen in frontal films made either upright or horizontal in which it appears as a dark, linear, gas shadow. Occasionally, a white line, representing the falx, is visible in the gas shadow.

There are four major sulci on the medial aspect of each hemisphere which extend laterally and perpendicular to the superior longitudinal fissure and which may be visible in either lateral or frontal view. These are the callosal, cingulate, parieto-occipital, and calcarine sulci. The *callosal sulcus* is one of the most conspicuous surface markings shown in pneumograms, often measuring as much as 2 to 3 mm. in width. It appears in the lateral film as a dorsally arched, curvilinear shadow, extending longitudinally through the central part of the cranial cavity, and if the entire extent of the corpus callosum is outlined, it may appear as an elongated letter C lying on its side with the open side down (fig. 202). Anteriorly, the callosal sulcus is projected well above the ventricular roof, while posteriorly it is essentially on the same level as a result of the divergence of the ventricles and the extension of the posterior portion of the corpus callosum between them.

In some instances, a superior angulation may be found in the curve of the callosal sulcus in the postforaminal region. Posterior to this point, the callosal sulcus may be quite straight and slope downward and backward as an oblique line rather than a curvilinear shadow. Anteriorly, gas extending over the genu of the corpus callosum may

(Revised 1963)

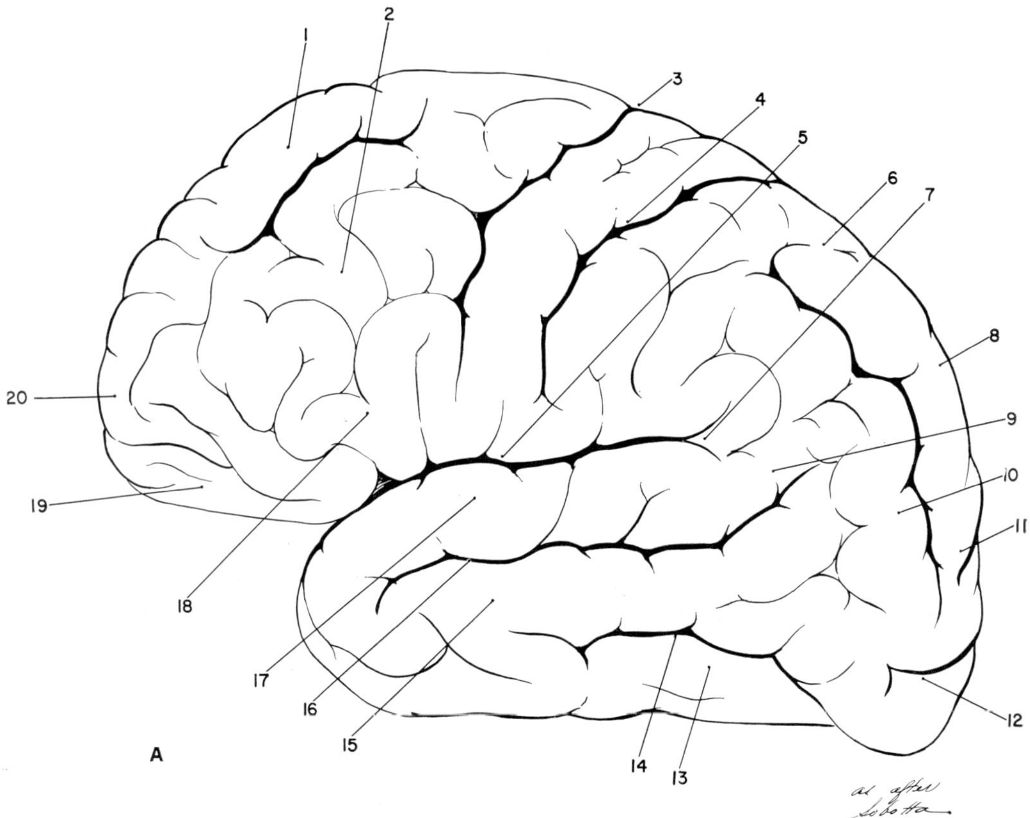

FIG. 215-A.—LATERAL CEREBRAL SURFACE

(1) Superior frontal (supramarginal) gyrus. (2) middle frontal gyrus. (3) precentral sulcus. (4) central cerebral (Rolandic) fissure. (5) lateral cerebral (Sylvian) fissure. (6) postcentral sulcus. (7) supramarginal gyrus. (8) superior parietal lobule. (9) angular gyrus. (10) inferior parietal lobule. (11) parieto-occipital fissure. (12) transverse occipital sulcus. (13) inferior temporal gyrus. (14) middle temporal sulcus. (15) middle temporal gyrus. (16) superior temporal sulcus. (17) superior temporal gyrus. (18) inferior frontal gyrus. (19) orbital gyri. (20) frontal pole.

be as much as 1.5 cm. forward of the anterior horn. The callosal sulcus over the genu bends sharply downward and then backward, and gas may occasionally be seen extending over the rostrum into the region of the cisterna lamina terminalis. At its posterior end, the callosal sulcus extends over the enlarged callosal commissure, or the splenium of the corpus callosum. Gas extending over the splenium is continuous with the shadow of the quadrigeminal cistern to be described subsequently.

Immediately above the corpus callosum on each side is the *cingulate gyrus*, which generally parallels the direction and configuration of the corpus callosum in its anterior three-fourths. Posteriorly, it bends around the splenium and through a narrow isthmus connects with the hippocampal gyrus on the medial aspect of the temporal lobe. In lateral pneumograms, the sulcus is visible approximately 1 cm. forward of the genu of the corpus callosum, and from this point it passes upward and backward in a smooth curve to terminate in wavy undulations in the superior periatrial region. Thus, the cingulate gyrus is outlined by gas in the callosal sulcus below and the cingulate sulcus above. The width of the band of soft

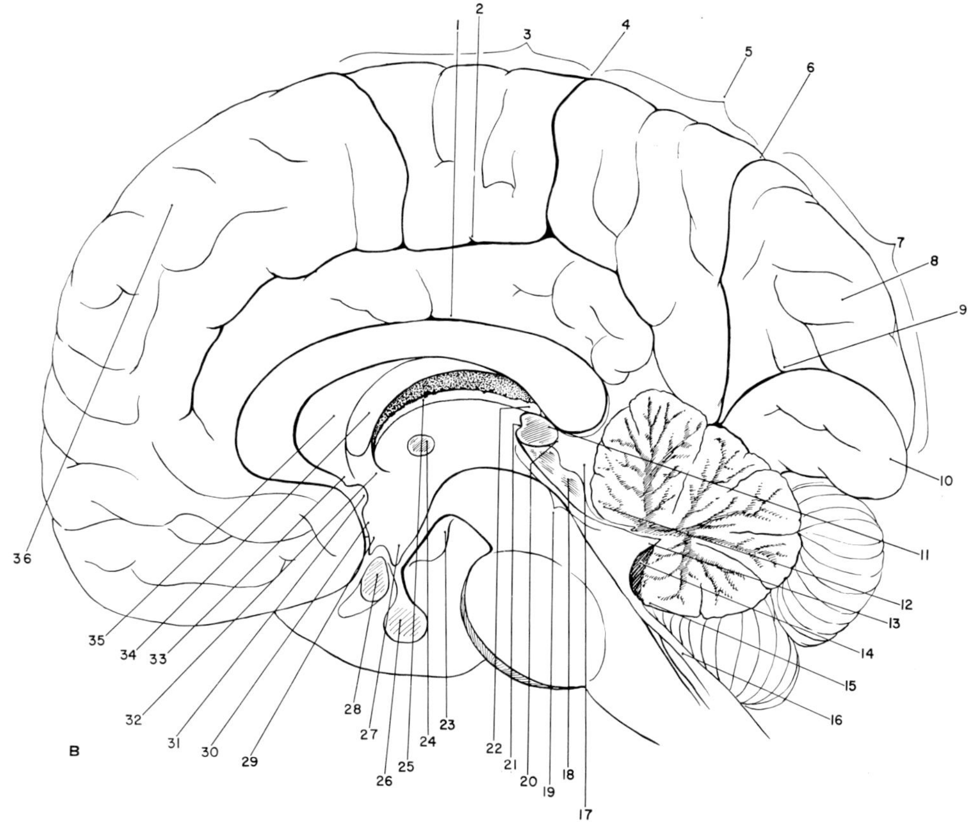

Fig. 215-B.—Medial Cerebral Surface

(1) Callosal sulcus. (2) cingulate sulcus. (3) paracentral lobule. (4) posterior limb of cingulate sulcus. (5) precuneus. (6) parieto-occipital fissure. (7) cuneus. (8) superior parietal lobule. (9) calcarine fissure. (10) occipital pole. (11) pineal gland (epiphysis). (12) cerebellomedullary recess of quadrigeminal cistern. (13) fourth ventricle. (14) chorioid plexus. (15) foramen of Magendie. (16) caudal extension of fourth ventricle under the obex. (17) quadrigeminal cistern. (18) quadrigeminal plate. (19) aqueduct of Sylvius (cerebral aqueduct or iter). (20) infrapineal recess of quadrigeminal cistern. (21) pineal recess. (22) suprapineal recess. (23) tuber cinereum and mammillary body. (24) massa intermedia (middle commissure). (25) tela chorioidea of third ventricle. (26) pituitary gland (hypophysis). (27) infundibular recess. (28) optic chiasm. (29) optic recess. (30) lamina terminalis. (31) anterior commissure. (32) foramen of Monro. (33) rostrum of corpus callosum. (34) fornix. (35) septum pellucidum. (36) superior frontal (supramarginal) gyrus.

tissue density representing the cingulate gyrus is approximately 1 cm.

The *parieto-occipital fissure* is not ordinarily seen in pneumograms. The fissure arises dorsolaterally on the convexity of the hemisphere and extends upward to the superior edge of the hemisphere from which it extends downward and forward on the medial surface. The termination of the fissure is projected approximately 1 cm. ventral to the splenium of the corpus callosum. Between the parieto-occipital fissure posteriorly and the upward extension of the cingulate sulcus anteriorly, the quadrate lobe or precuneus is located. The *calcarine fissure* extends from the parieto-occipital fissure sharply downward and backward toward the tip of the occipital pole. The portion of brain between the calcarine and parieto-occipital fissures is the cuneus (fig. 215).

Other structures of significance situated

(*Revised 1963*)

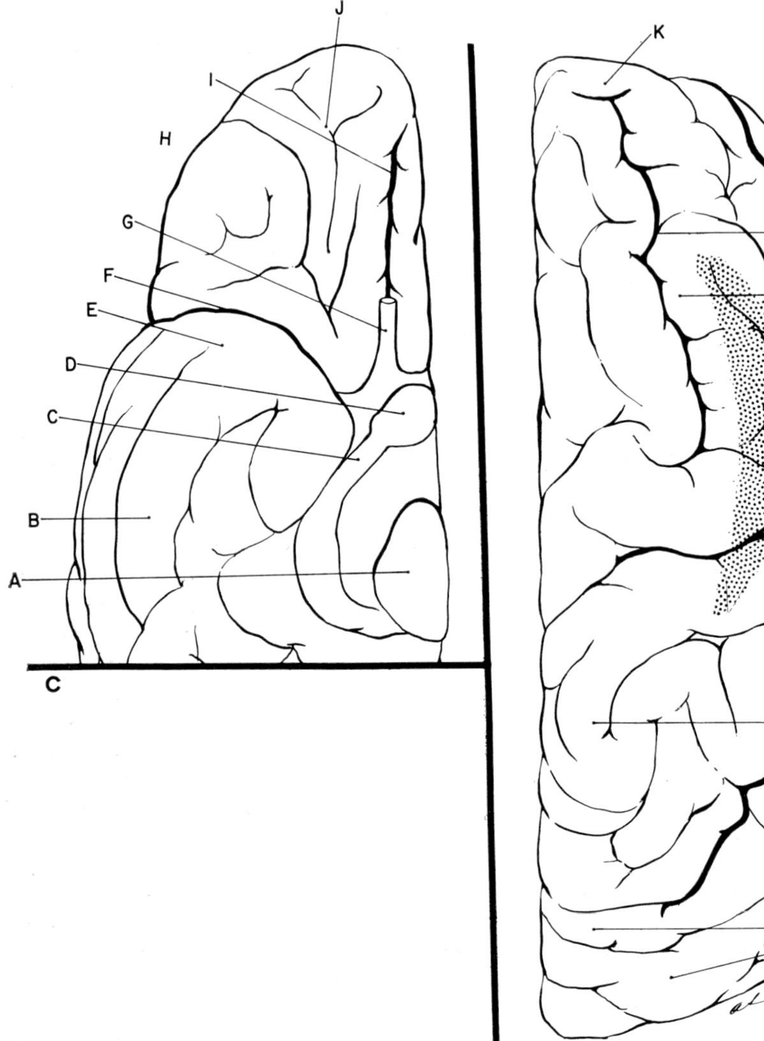

Fig. 215-C.—Inferior Cerebral Surface

(A) Midbrain. (B) inferior temporal gyrus. (C) hippocampal gyrus. (D) uncus of hippocampal gyrus. (E) inferior surface of temporal pole. (F) lateral cerebral (Sylvian) fissure. (G) olfactory nerve. (H) lateral orbital gyrus. (I) olfactory sulcus. (J) anterior orbital gyrus.

Fig. 215-D.—Superior Cerebral Surface

(K) Frontal pole. (L) inferior frontal sulcus. (M) superior frontal sulcus. (N) middle frontal gyrus. (O) Island of Reil (insula). (P) central cerebral (Rolandic) fissure. (Q) postcentral sulcus. (R) interparietal sulcus. (S) superior parietal lobule. (T) inferior parietal lobule. (U) superior occipital gyri.

on the medial aspect of the brain may occasionally be seen in lateral pneumograms. The medial hemispheric extensions of the precentral and postcentral gyri, or the motor and sensory strips, form the *paracentral lobule*. The central sulcus itself, or Rolandic fissure, may or may not extend over the hemispheric edge and indent the dorsomedial aspect of the brain. In either case, the division of motor and sensory areas is not gross medially, contributing further to the difficulty of differentiating precisely between frontal and parietal lesions at pneumography, as previously pointed out. Only the anterior half of the paracentral lobule belongs with the frontal lobe. When there is a strongly developed cingulate sulcus, the paracentral lobule may be visualized, limited inferiorly by the cingulate sulcus, and posteriorly by a dorsal extension of this sulcus. Anteriorly, the paracentral lobule is bounded by the medial extension of the superior frontal gyrus, preferably called the marginal gyrus. Between the paracentral lobule and the cuneus of the occipital region is the precuneus or quadrate lobule of the parietal lobe. Anteriorly, this subdivision is bounded by the upwardly directed limb of the cingulate sulcus and behind by the parieto-occipital fissure. Inferiorly, the subdivision is bounded by the subparietal sulcus which is not seen very frequently in pneumograms.

In frontal pneumograms, in addition to the superior longitudinal fissure containing the falx, the callosal and cingulate sulci frequently are visible. The callosal sulci on the two sides usually are visualized as narrow, undivided linear gas shadows extending outward essentially perpendicular to the superior longitudinal fissure for a distance often of 5 mm. Medially, the sulci of the two sides open into the superior longitudinal fissure, occasionally flaring superiorly, which results in a small, triangular space. Some consider the space of sufficient prominence to call this area the cistern of the corpus callosum. The inferior margin or free edge of the falx is at the superior angle of the space or cistern. As seen in frontal films, the corpus callosum is limited above by the callosal sulci and the gas in the lateral ventricles below. Its thickness is variable and may be as much as 12 mm. in frontal projection.

Also visible in the frontal pneumogram is the cingulate sulcus which usually appears as a narrow transverse shadow parallel to the callosal sulcus and approximately 1 cm. superior to it on each side. This sulcus is often deep and may project as much as 1.5 cm. from the midline. The soft tissue shadow on each side between the cingulate sulcus and the callosal sulcus is the cingulate gyrus. Occasionally, some of the other sulci described above on the medial aspect of the brain may be visible in frontal pneumograms but superimposition on the ventricular system and on the bones of the facial area renders them difficult to recognize. Identification in lateral projection usually is more satisfactory.

In the frontal lobe area a few other sulci may be worthy of mention since they may, from time to time, be seen in pneumograms, usually a lateral view. The anterior limb of the cingulate sulcus separates the cingulate gyrus from the marginal gyrus, and visualization of this portion of the sulcus is common. Ordinarily, however, the cingulate sulcus is not visible forward of the point where the callosal sulcus takes its sharp downward turn. A few sulci of the supraorbital portion of the frontal lobe are seen frequently. On the medial aspect posteriorly is the paraolfactory area bounded behind and above by the posterior paraolfactory sulcus. In lateral pneumograms the sulcus appears as a curvilinear shadow projected vertically above the planum sphenoidale and then forward beneath the anterior inferior extremity of the corpus collosum. The sulcus is continuous with the ventral extension of the anterior portion of the callosal sulcus and provides a communication between the latter and the cisterna lamina terminalis. An important clinical consideration of the posterior paraolfactory sulcus is that it may be displaced as a result of certain tumors arising in the region of the sella turcica and along the olfactory groove.

In frontal pneumograms, the olfactory sulci, which extend upward lateral to the gyrus rectus of each side, should not be confused with the crural cisterns. The former usually are seen only in anteroposterior views made with the patient supine. The sulcal shadows originate close together near the midline and extend upward at an angle of 60 degrees from the horizontal, diverging in a V-shaped manner. The cisternal shadows are further apart at their origins and diverge at angles of 45 degrees from horizontal. Further anterior on the mesial surface of the ventral portion of the frontal lobe, is the main rostral sulcus extending transversely forward from the central plane of the paraolfactory area. Other minor rostral sulci

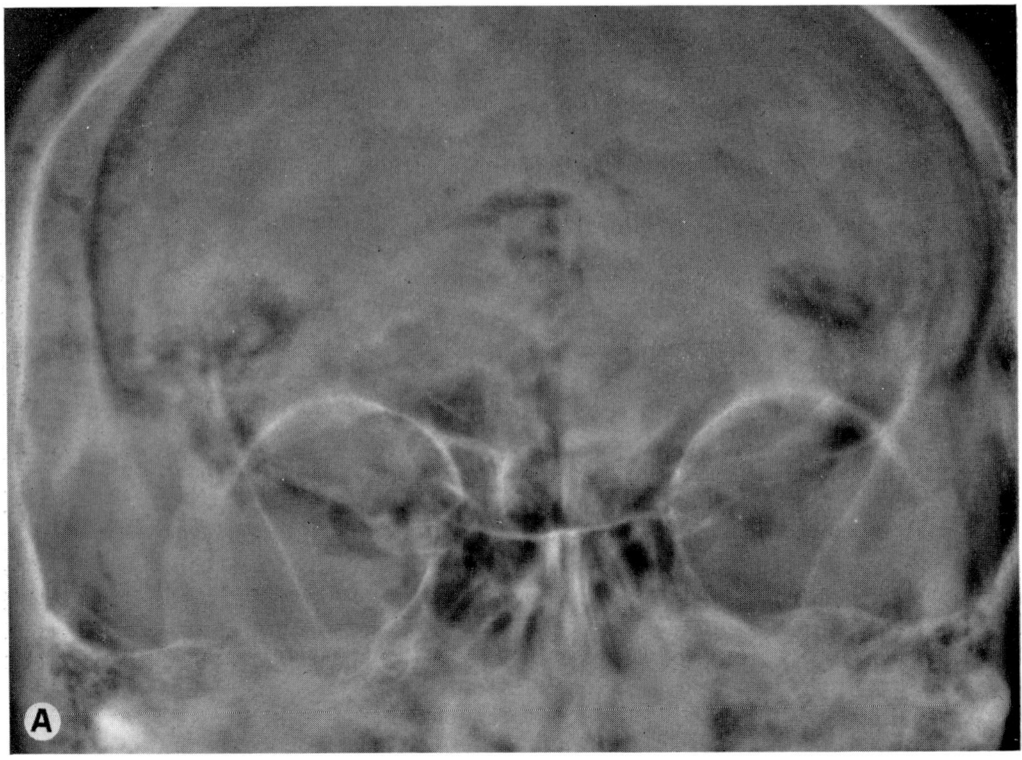

Fig. 216.—Sulci of the Island of Reil

The circular sulcus of Reil separates the insula from the opercula; it appears as a curved saucerlike collection of gas extending upward and medially above the superior wall of the orbit, as seen in frontal view (A). Gas in the Sylvian fissure extends outward from the circular sulcus to the lateral surface of the brain. In lateral view, the sulci of the island of Reil are projected through the third ventricle and the anterior inferior portion of the lateral ventricle (B); their location corresponds to the arborization of the middle cerebral artery, forming the angiographic Sylvian triangle (see Figs. 204 and 367). The foramen of Monro is projected through the central portion of this area. The short sulci of the island of Reil are visible anteriorly, following generally the plane of the base of the triangle (*anterior arrow*); the long sulci are directed upward and backward toward the apex of the triangle, just forward of the plane of the ventricular atrium (*posterior arrow*). In the case illustrated, all of the sulci are more prominent than usual because of atrophy.

are present which further subdivide this portion of the medial frontal cortex into a number of small gyri.

Island of Reil

In addition to the standard frontal, parietal, temporal, and occipital lobes of the brain, some anatomists group certain structures which are in proximity and which serve certain basic functions, calling them the fifth and sixth lobes. These are the island of Reil (also called the central lobe) and the *limbic lobe* on the medial aspect of the cerebral hemisphere. The limbic lobe includes the cingulate gyrus, its posterior extension known as the isthmus, and its continuation into the hippocampal gyrus. There is considerable resemblance between the cingulate gyrus, the isthmus, and the hippocampal gyrus, both histologically and physiologically. The classical responses produced by stimulation of various parts of the limbic system are visceral, including alterations of blood pressure, respiratory rate, gastrointestinal motility, and other similar effects. There is no particular radiologic advantage

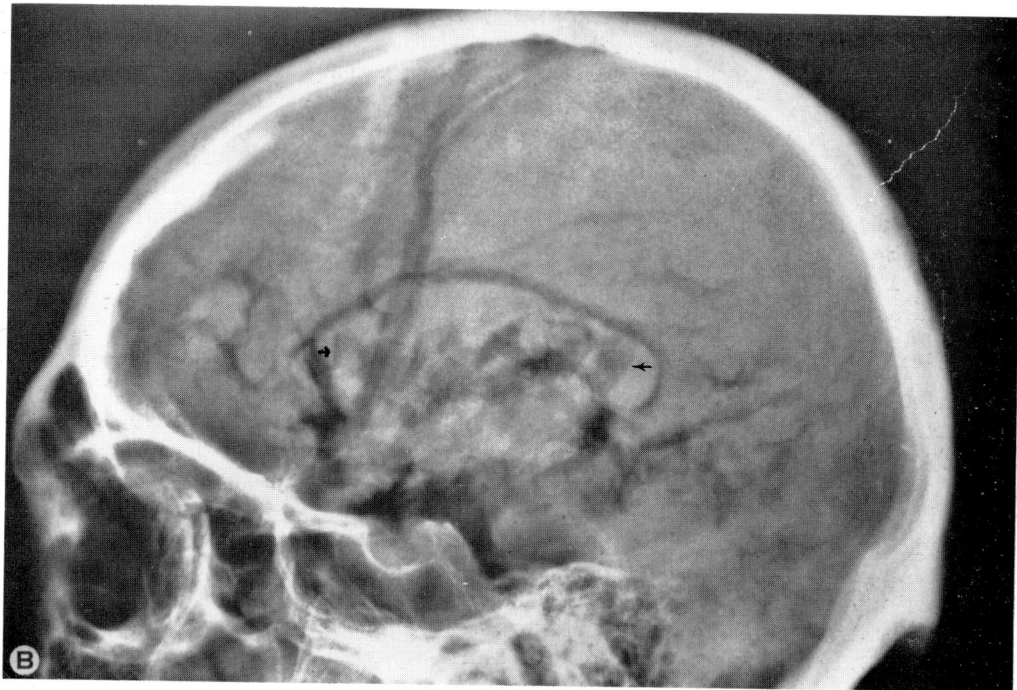

Fig. 216B

in considering the limbic system as a separate lobe of the brain.

On the other hand, the *insula (island of Reil)* frequently is visualized in pneumograms and is an excellent pneumographic-angiographic point of cross reference. The island of Reil, insula, fifth lobe, or central lobe is in the depths of the Sylvian fissure and is visible grossly only by separating the frontal and temporal lobes. Part of the invaginated tissue in this region belongs to the frontal lobe, while other portions of the cerebrum covering the insula are derived from the frontal, temporal, and parietal lobes. This central lobe is actually a triangular island of cortical tissue, as the name implies.

The portions of the temporal, frontal, and parietal lobes covering the insula are known as the opercula. The insula is separated from the opercula by the infolding of the brain sometimes referred to as the circular sulcus of Reil. In frontal pneumograms air frequently outlines this circular sulcus which appears as a curved disclike collection of gas above and lateral to the temporal horn. The circular sulcus may be as much as 3 cm. in length and several millimeters in width as seen in frontal films. In straight anteroposterior views, it is often projected upward and slightly medially at an angle of approximately 20 degrees from the lateral end of the superior wall of the orbit. Air in the Sylvian fissure is often seen to extend from this shadow to the lateral surface of the brain (fig. 216). Gas collections in these areas become very prominent in the presence of relatively mild degrees of cerebral atrophy. In lateral projection, some of the sulci and gyri of the island of Reil may be visualized. Their projection is at the level of the third ventricle and the inferior portion of the lateral ventricular body. The long sulci extend as far backward as the plane of the atrium. The foramen of Monro is projected through the central portion of this triangular area. The island of Reil is of importance in angiography also, since the middle cerebral artery divides into several branches on the surface of the insula forming the angiographic "Sylvian triangle" (see "Anatomy" under "Angiography"). *The area is of great radiologic importance since it provides a foundation for the integration of pneumographic and angiographic anatomy* (figs. 204 and 205).

Lateral

The sulci on the lateral aspect of the brain have been discussed earlier in connection with the surface projection of the ventricular system. The lateral sulci are not as often visualized as the medial, particularly when relatively small amounts of gas are used for pneumoencephalography, in accordance with modern methods. Furthermore, the lateral view must be depended upon almost exclusively for visualization of these sulci. The frontal film is not of great value in visualizing the lateral sulci; at least, the lateral sulci are not seen well in comparison with the medial fissures, which can be identified frequently and with a high degree of accuracy. The Sylvian fissure often is visible in frontal view. In addition, some of the sulci of the frontal and occipital poles can be identified occasionally in anteroposterior or posteroanterior pneumograms. A good method of appreciating the sulcal anatomy of the cerebral convexity, however, is by the study of stereoscopic lateral recumbent pneumoencephalograms. A nearly ideal method of studying the pneumographic anatomy of the sulci is the use of multiple sagittal tomograms, as advocated by di Chiro (1961). Some degree of sulcal filling on the lateral surface should be seen in normal cases, even when small fluid-gas exchanges are performed. Filling of the sulci on one side and not on the other is highly suggestive of disease, either subarachnoid adhesions or obliteration of sulcal spaces by pressure.

The lateral or Sylvian fissure is perhaps the most readily recognized of the lateral cortical markings. The lateral extension of the fissure begins at a point projected above the sella turcica and extends backward and upward for a distance of approximately 7 cm. prior to turning upward to a short terminal extension in the superior periatrial region (figs. 207 and 215). It usually is not necessary to draw the Taylor-Haughton lines to identify the Sylvian fissure, since the marking is strong. Occasionally, however, a parallel cleft, such as the superior temporal sulcus, may be prominent and may be indistinguishable from the lateral fissure unless guide lines are constructed.

The central or Rolandic fissure, on the other hand, often is not a strong surface marking. Frequently, the precentral sulcus is more prominent. Even at the time of surgical exposure, it may be difficult to identify the motor area with certainty unless electrical stimulation is carried out. Construction of the Taylor-Haughton lines, therefore, may be of considerable assistance in anatomic study of the frontoparietal convexity by pneumography. When seen, the Rolandic fissure appears slightly S-shaped, with the curves reversed; superiorly, the concavity is forward and inferiorly it is concave dorsally. It generally divides the superior aspect of the convexity into an anterior and posterior half as it extends obliquely upward and backward from just above the forward portion of the Sylvian fissure. When prominent, the transverse superior and inferior frontal sulci may be visualized. Similarly, other sulci of the hemispheric convexity occasionally may be identified.

THIRD VENTRICLE

The third ventricle is a narrow midline cavity essentially contained within the supratentorial portion of the brain stem (diencephalon). The third ventricle has been described as having a trapezoid shape in sagittal section (fig. 213). In coronal section, the anterior portion appears as a narrow cleft, while the posterior portion has a more fusiform or rounded configuration. Anteriorly, the third ventricle communicates with the lateral ventricles at the foramen of Monro and caudally it empties into the aqueduct of Sylvius.

The third ventricle can be divided into two major sections by a line drawn perpendicular to the roof through the massa intermedia.

The portion of the third ventricle forward of this line usually is referred to as the anterior or hypothalamic portion of the third ventricle, while the part posterior to the line is the posterior portion of the third ventricle or the prepineal portion. The anterior portion viewed laterally is somewhat cone-shaped, bending forward and downward to a point just above the sella turcica. The posterior portion, as viewed from the side, is smooth and rather square, except for indentations and outpouchings along its posterior wall. The ventricular roof is smoothly curved and superiorly convex. The floor of the third ventricle parallels the roof and is continuous with the anterior wall of the aqueduct of Sylvius and the floor of the fourth ventricle in a smoothly arched line.

Topographically, the third ventricle is projected in lateral view between the ventricular body and the temporal horn and generally its shadow overlies the superior temporal gyrus and the squamous portion of the temporal bone (fig. 207). From the suprasellar region, the third ventricle extends upward and backward at an angle of approximately 90 degrees from the plane of the dorsum sellae and clivus.

Bridging the third ventricle and forming portions of its boundaries are several commissures. The largest and most conspicuous of these at pneumography is the middle or gray commissure, usually referred to as the *massa intermedia.* In some instances, where there is poor filling of the third ventricle by gas, the shadow of the massa intermedia blends with the outline of the lateral walls and roof of the ventricle. Under these circumstances, the size and configuration of the commissure cannot be determined and a false impression of a filling defect in the superior portion of the third ventricle may be gained. In the average case, however, the massa intermedia is well defined in lateral view as a round or oval shadow measuring up to 1 cm. in anteroposterior diameter. Although the massa intermedia extends across the lumen of the third ventricle to join the thalami of the two sides, it usually is not seen in frontal projection. Occasionally, the massa intermedia may be absent.

The *anterior wall* of the third ventricle, and the rostral boundary of the hypothalamic portion, is limited above by the foramen of Monro. Just inferior to this, the anterior columns of the fornix bound the third ventricle, below which is a rounded structure, the *anterior commissure* (fig. 215). Extending downward for some distance to the termination of the third ventricle inferiorly is the thin lamina terminalis. This also forms the anterior boundary of the *optic recess* of the third ventricle, the anterior of the two inferior recesses between which the optic chiasm is seated. Caudal to the optic chiasm, the anterior inferior third ventricle extends downward into a funnel-shaped ventral extension, the infundibular recess. Between the two recesses is the chiasmatic notch formed by the optic chiasm (fig. 226).

The floor of the third ventricle is formed anteriorly by the thin tuber cinereum which extends backward from the infundibulum in a curved manner to the mammillary bodies. The latter structures are generally in the coronal plane of the massa intermedia, or slightly anterior to it. The floor of the posterior portion of the third ventricle is formed by the cerebral peduncles.

The *third ventricular roof* is lined by a thin epithelial membrane, the velum interpositum, and covered by important vascular structures, most conspicuous of which are the chorioid plexus and internal cerebral veins (fig. 401). The chorioid plexus of the third ventricle is continuous with that of the lateral ventricles and extends as parasagittal strips of venous plexus running throughout the entire length of the third ventricular roof. Posteriorly, the plexus curves downward and the two portions terminate in the suprapineal region.

The posterior wall of the third ventricle derives its greatest clinical importance from the presence of the pineal gland in this area. The suprapineal recess forms the posterior superior boundary of the ventricular cavity, and this is situated above the pineal body and the habenular commissure. The pineal

(Revised 1963)

recess extends into the gland usually as a notch, although it may penetrate as deeply as 4 mm.

In frontal pneumograms, the appearance of the third ventricle is dependent upon the amount of gas which is available to fill the different portions of the ventricular cavity which, in turn, often depends upon the position of the head. In the supine position, the anterior half of the third ventricle normally appears as a midline narrow radiolucent band projected just above the bony structures of the cranial floor. In the prone posteroanterior view, when only the posterior half is filled, the shadow usually is wider resulting in a rounded or oval configuration. Often the outlet of the third ventricle into the aqueduct of Sylvius is visualized as a superimposed small darker rounded shadow. Occasionally, a large massa intermedia may be visualized in frontal projection extending across a wide third ventricle, and if the suprapineal recess is well developed, this may be visualized in the posteroanterior view as an exaggeration of the posterior superior margin of the third ventricular shadow.

The appearance of the third ventricle in lateral projection of the pneumogram varies considerably with the position of the head. Under ordinary circumstances, some fluid remains in the dependent portion of the ventricle with the result that only the uppermost segment of the third ventricular lumen and its walls are outlined. Through combined viewing of upright, prone, and supine lateral pneumograms, essentially all of the anatomic structures bounding the third ventricle which have been described above can be visualized. In some instances, however, the quantity of ventricular gas may be so small that a "hanging head" lateral view with the patient supine may be required to distend the hypothalamic portion (fig. 187). In other cases, in which the somersaulting chair is used, the position of ventricular gas may be readily controlled and the anterior third ventricle visualized when only very small quantities of gas have been introduced. When other cerebral and cranial structures interfere with good visualization of the third ventricle and when there is full filling of the ventricular system with gas, tomographic examination in the midsagittal plane may be the best answer for visualization of the third ventricle and its anatomic components. Visualization of the third ventricle also may be accomplished by autotomograms in lateral projection with the head hanging (fig. 187) if an abnormality of the area is anticipated. In the average case, when detailed visualization of the third ventricle is necessary, the required radiographic procedures are carried out during a later phase of the examination and films are usually made with the patient in supine or prone position. Ordinary lateral recumbent tomograms made with the vertical x-ray beam may occasionally give additional information in cases of posterior third ventricular obstruction by pinealoma.

In addition to the technical factors affecting the appearance of the anterior third ventricle in lateral pneumograms, anatomic variants of the superior surface of the sphenoid bone and of the optic pathways are responsible for different configurations and relationships. The hypothalamic recesses may be almost on, or well above, a line drawn from the nasion to the tuberculum sellae (fig. 226). The striking normal variations of this region were the subject of an important report by Bull in 1956.

Third ventricular *measurements* have been established and a normal range determined by a number of workers. The practicability of applying such measurements to the third ventricle in pneumograms is somewhat less than the value of measuring lateral ventricular structures, the iter, and fourth ventricle. The most constant measurement apparently is from the inferior margin of the foramen of Monro to the aditus of the aqueduct of Sylvius, which is essentially the distance from the anterior to the posterior commissure. Enlargement of the third ventricle, when it occurs, usually is most conspicuous in the hypothalamic portion and in the recesses, not only the optic and infundibular recesses but that of the suprapineal area. The suprapineal recess varies greatly in size, particularly in length, and it is normally commonplace to find an extension of 1 to 1.5 cm. behind the midpoint of the pineal gland. Its termination may be somewhat bulbous in configuration (see "Anatomic Variants"). When there is increased ventricular pressure of some duration, the suprapineal recess may become extremely dilatated and this has been referred to as a pressure diverticulum of the third ventricle (fig. 240).

In some cases, the measurements of greatest clinical value are those defining the height of the third ventricle in lateral view and the width in frontal view. On the average, the width of the third ventricle is only 0.5 cm. and enlargement often is noticeable first as an increase in width. Later there may be gross widening with bulging of the side walls to the point of rounding. In lateral view, the height of the third ventricle usually is not more than 1.5 cm. in its midportion (fig. 213). Increased height usually occurs by means of upward bulging of the roof. Of perhaps more clinical value is reduction in height of the third ventricle as a result of elevation of the floor, which may be seen in tumors which infiltrate or displace upward the midbrain and peduncles. In general, measurements applied to the third ventricle are not particularly useful in detecting the presence and location of expanding lesions, since the limits of variation are not exceeded until it is quite apparent from inspection that some enlargement or localized reduction in caliber has occurred. Measurements may be useful in quantitating the degree of involvement, particularly before and after various types of treatment.

The *pineal gland*, pineal body or epiphysis is situated at the posterior extremity of the third ventricle and projects into the ventricular lumen by virtue of its partial envelopment by the suprapineal recess and the aditus of the iter. For this reason, the pineal is most conveniently considered in connection with the third ventricle, particularly as regards tumors of the diencephalon. Mention has been made earlier of the relationship between the pineal and the habenular commissure in connection with the calcific degenerations that occur in these structures.

The pineal body is cone shaped with its base directed anteriorly and embedded in the posterior wall of the third ventricle. The posteriorly directed apex lies essentially free in the quadrigeminal cistern. Above the pineal is the splenium of the corpus callosum while inferior to it is the quadrigeminal plate, which often is affected early by the development of pineal tumors which exert pressure upon it with characteristic occular disturbances. Normally, however, the pineal body is separated from the quadrigeminal plate by the infrapineal recess, an anterior extension of the quadrigeminal cistern. The posterior portion of the third ventricle extends backward over the superior aspect of the pineal as a suprapineal recess, as previously noted, and separates the pineal body from the corpus callosum. The suprapineal recess is usually narrowed or obliterated in the presence of pineal tumor corresponding to the encroachment downward upon the quadrigeminal plate. The pineal recess of the third ventricle actually extends into the substance of the pineal body as a narrow projection. The recess is bounded by the diverging superior and inferior laminae which connect the pineal body with other parts of the brain through the habenular commissure and posterior commissure, respectively.

Because the pineal body is almost surrounded by gas of the third ventricle and its recesses and by gas in the communicating cisterns, the body is usually quite conspicuous in pneumograms, particularly in lateral projection. In the frontal pneumogram, made with the patient prone, the pineal body appears as a midline rounded shadow of soft tissue density approximately 5 mm. in diameter demarcated by the third ventricular and cisternal gas collections. In lateral pneumograms, and particularly in midsagittal laminagraphic sections, the pineal and its associated recesses are readily visible. The length of the pineal gland varies from 7 to 10 mm., on the average. The length of the suprapineal recess, in the average case, is about 5 mm., although it may be very long as noted elsewhere (see "Anatomic Variants"). The measurable height of the suprapineal recess from the top of the pineal to the tela chorioidea varies with the degree of gas filling of the third ventricle. At its origin from the third ventricle, the height may be 3 to 5 mm. The pineal recess is not visible in many normal encephalograms; but in some instances it may appear as a thin gas line extending as much as 4 mm. backward into the pineal substance. All of the findings relating to the pineal gland are intensified when the pineal contains calcium, and visualization also is improved by the use of sagittal tomograms.

AQUEDUCT OF SYLVIUS

The aqueduct of Sylvius, or iter, extends as a narrow canal through the midbrain and connects the third ventricle with the fourth ventricle. According to most anatomists, the aqueduct extends from the caudal margin of the posterior commissure, where it is continuous with the third ventricle, to the lower end of the quadrigeminal plate at the margin of the inferior colliculus, beyond which it opens into the fourth ventricle. The length of the aqueduct of Sylvius varies between 1.5 and 2.0 cm., and in some instances it may be slightly more; its diameter is 1 to 2 mm. (fig. 213). It has been pointed out that the caliber is not even throughout, being greatest in the central portion of the midbrain, and in earlier periods this was sometimes referred to as the mesencephalic ventricle. At the third ventricular end, slight narrowing of the aqueduct occurs as a result of its passage beneath the posterior commissure, and similarly slight narrowing occurs caudally beneath the inferior colliculus.

The slope of the iter varies somewhat with the shape of the head. Generally, however, the structure is dorsally arched and although there is almost a 90-degree change in direction of the cerebrospinal fluid pathway from the third to the fourth ventricles, the degree of arc described may vary slightly in different individuals. From the outlet of the third ventricle the aqueduct extends almost straight backward but soon turns into a gentle bend which continues until the direction approaches vertical. The floor of the aqueduct in its posterior portion is continuous in a straight line with the floor of the fourth ventricle.

Because of its small size, the gas-filled aqueduct does not outline anatomic structures per se but indicates more the position, slope, and course of the mesencephalon in which it is contained. Secondary changes resulting from tumors and disease processes, near and remote, are common because the aqueduct serves as one of the several bottlenecks of the ventricular pathway by virtue of its strategic location and small size. The relationships of the midbrain and its aqueduct to the rigid tentorium and its incisura form the basis not only for cerebrospinal fluid circulatory disturbances within the ventricular system but also in the communicating cisterns. Nearby tumors and herniations may displace, compress, and occlude the iter. Inflammatory processes frequently produce symptoms as a result of aqueduct involvement, and this structure is the site of many congenital malformations, the latter being a principal cause of hydrocephalus in infancy.

In the frontal pneumogram made with the patient prone, the upper portion of the aqueduct is visualized as a small, rounded shadow of diminished density superimposed upon the posterior third ventricle. The mid and distal portions appear as a midline linear shadow extending downward to terminate in the upper fourth ventricular outline. Here, also, the lowest segment may be seen on end and appear rounded in some projections. After the ventricles are filled, the best position for distention of the posterior portion of the third ventricle affords the best visualization of the aqueduct. Thus, prone, inverted and forward "hanging head" positions all may be useful to demonstrate the iter at ventriculography or during the later maneuvers of pneumoencephalography. No

(Revised 1963)

special positions are needed, however, to demonstrate the aqueduct in filling films made in the upright posture (fig. 181). Advantage always should be taken of the high degree of contrast provided by exposures made when gas first passes through the aqueduct. Failure to visualize the iter, at least in lateral projection, constitutes an incomplete examination and requires additional special procedures to rule in or out disease.

The slope, curvature, caliber and relationships of the shadow of the iter in pneumograms conform essentially to the anatomic features of the midbrain canal that have been described. Because of the great importance of the secondary changes which occur in the aqueduct associated with various intracranial lesions, its patency, size and direction must be very carefully examined. Since the tentorium is rigid, it is the lower part of the aqueduct that is displaced most readily with posterior fossa tumors. This is particularly true of cerebellar tumors, which are ideally situated to exert the greatest effect of displacement upon the lower midbrain. Numerous other lesions to be described exert equally important effects upon higher portions of the iter.

Because of the frequency of displacement of the aqueduct, reflected particularly in lateral pneumograms, numerous measurements have been made along its course. Measurements of the position of the aqueduct are among the more reliable standards recommended as clinically useful at pneumography. The most commonly applied measurement is that from the midaqueduct to the dorsum sellae which various investigators have found to be approximately 3.5 cm. in the average case (fig. 213). It should be stated that the actual measurements are dependent on the degree of magnification of the structures in the radiograph. When a short anode film distance is used (less than 36 inches), the above measurement cannot be applied.

Ascertainment that an aqueduct exceeds 2 mm. caliber usually is a pneumographic finding of limited value since dilatation can be recognized readily by inspection when this measurement is approached. Measurements less than the average are not ordinarily significant. Such a measurement must be interpreted in relation to the total degree of ventricular filling and the transient nature of aqueductal distention as recognized more recently from cinepneumographic studies. A localized segment of constant narrowing, however, with dilatation cephalad may be more informative and indicative of the presence of a localized stenosis (fig. 241).

Without resort to measurement, displacement of the iter often can be appreciated by drawing a line along the ventral aspect of the shadow of the aqueduct and extending it caudally. Since the lower aqueduct is almost straight, the line should follow along the floor of the fourth ventricle and, if extrapolated further, it should extend into the central part of the cervical vertebral canal. Other methods for estimating the normal position of the aqueduct are given in connection with the discussion of "Intra-axial Posterior Fossa Tumors."

FOURTH VENTRICLE

The fourth ventricle is a caudal continuation of the ventricular system from the lower end of the aqueduct of Sylvius. Anatomically, the fourth ventricle extends from the caudal margin of the inferior colliculus to the obex, which is a band of tissue on the dorsal aspect of the inferior portion of the medulla oblongata and which connects the fasciculi gracilis as they diverge rostrally after ascending from the spinal cord. From its cephalic end, the fourth ventricle expands in three directions (each lateral and posteriorly) until it reaches its greatest size at the level of the fastigium or the summit of its furthest posterior extension. The summit (or apex) and greatest lateral extensions are angular and essentially in the same plane. Caudad to the summit and lateral angles,

(Revised 1963)

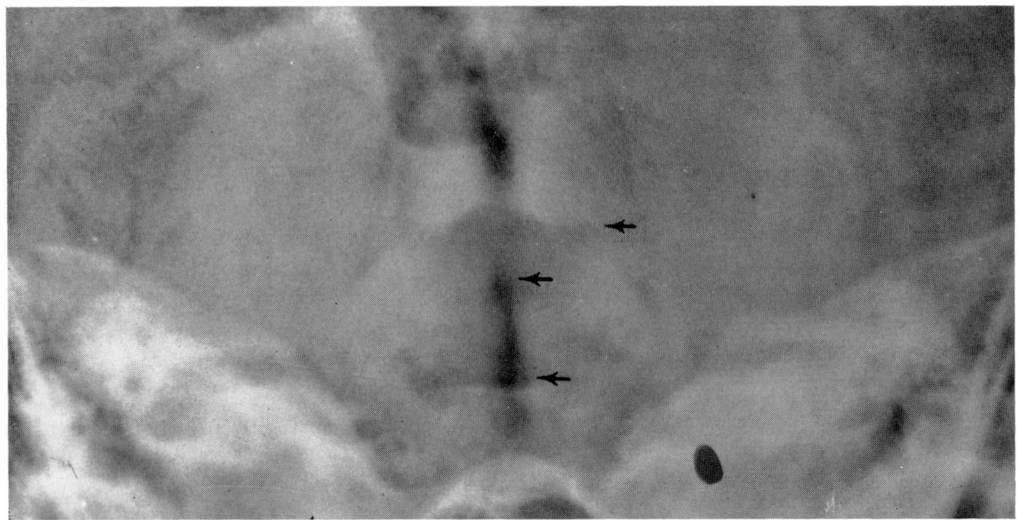

FIG. 217.—POSTEROANTERIOR HALF AXIAL DEPICTION OF POSTERIOR FOSSA STRUCTURES

A radiograph made during the filling stage of pneumography, shows the lateral recesses of a slightly dilated fourth ventricle. The recesses appear roughly as triangular lateral extensions from the lateral angles of the fourth ventricle, extending symmetrically outward from the main ventricular shadow (*upper arrow*). At the caudal end of the fourth ventricle, the foramen of Magendie is visualized (*middle arrow*) at the top of the vallecular cleft (*lower arrow*).

the fourth ventricle narrows sharply to a point beneath the obex, just described; it is potentially continuous with the central canal of the spinal cord. Because the portion of the fourth ventricle cephalad to the summit changes size more gradually than the caudal portion, the cephalic segment is longer. For this reason, the shape in frontal view is not truly rhomboid; it is described by Robertson as resembling an inverted kite when viewed from behind. In three dimensions, the configuration somewhat resembles an umbrella tent stretched unevenly. The average length of the floor of the fourth ventricle has been established as 3.2 cm. from the casts of Last and Tompsett (1953). Approximately three-fifths is rostral to the summit and two-fifths caudal. The summit usually lies just below the plane of greatest ventral expansion of the pons.

The fourth ventricle lies between the anterior surface of the cerebellum and the posterior surface of the pons varolii and superior portion of the medulla oblongata. Anatomically, the fourth ventricle is considered a part of the latter structures. The immediate roof of the fourth ventricle is formed superiorly by the anterior medullary velum, a caudal extension of the quadrigeminal plate. The cephalic portion of the fourth ventricular roof may have a slightly curved configuration in lateral view due to indentation of the superior (anterior) medullary velum by the lingula of the cerebellar vermis. At the fastigium or apex of the fourth ventricle, the anterior medullary velum is continuous with the (posterior) inferior medullary velum which forms the roof of the caudal portion of the fourth ventricle. The caudal roof very often has a ventrally convex configuration rather than being straight because of the posterior application of the nodulus of the cerebellum. In addition, there is intralumenal protrusion of the chorioid plexus of the fourth ventricle which is attached to the inferior surface of the ventricular roof (fig. 192). Retzius (1892) described two small dorsal extensions (recesses) of the fourth ventricle on each side of the fastigium and these occasionally may be visualized (figs. 192 and 219). Just caudad to the chorioid plexus, along the midsagittal plane of the ventricular roof, is a small orifice, the foramen of Magendie, which is a principal connection between the ventricular system and the subarachnoid space. Through this opening, the fourth ventricle is continuous with the vallecular cleft of the cisterna magna (fig. 217). Caudal to the foramen of Magendie, the fourth ventricular roof extends briefly to the obex.

The lateral aspects of the fourth ventricle are formed principally by the cerebellar peduncles and medullary eminences. The floor is formed by the pons varolii and the upper half of the medulla oblongata. As it extends outward beneath the brachium pontis, it tapers toward the lateral angle of the irregular rhomboid or diamond configuration of the fourth ventricle. The lateral angles are essentially in the plane of the apex and somewhat below the ventricular center. Projecting further outward and forward as well as slightly caudad are the lateral recesses of the fourth ventricle (figs. 183 and 217). These extensions empty into the lateral recesses of the medullopontine cisterns through the foramina of Luschka. The lateral recess is long and narrow, sometimes finger-like, while at other times, especially when dilated, it is tortuous and resembles somewhat the appearance of the fallopian tube. The chorioid plexus extends into the lateral recesses and occasionally may protrude through the foramina of Luschka. It is not rare for the foramina of Luschka to be closed. There is good evidence that under ordinary circumstances at pneumoencephalography the air injected into the lumbar subarachnoid space enters the ventricular system through the foramen of Magendie while ventricular fluid passes out principally through the foramina of Luschka (Davidoff and Dyke, 1951).

Lateral View

In pneumograms, *visualization of the fourth ventricle is all important.* Numerous techniques and special projections have been described previously. In the lateral projection, the fourth ventricle has one of the most constant appearances of any ventricular structure. The shadow is roughly triangular in shape and conforms to the anatomic configuration previously described, including the indentations of the lumen produced by the chorioid plexus and segments of the cerebellar vermis. In films made during the filling phase, the paucity of interfering gas shadows may make it possible to locate the point of the foramen of Magendie. Gas in the lower end of the fourth ventricle may maintain continuity dorsally with the subarachnoid gas extending into the vallecula. The slope of the fourth ventricle is at an angle of approximately 75 degrees in relation to Reid's base line, but the direction may vary slightly with the shape of the head. The floor of the fourth ventricle diverges cephalad from the plane of the clivus, while the two are closer together caudad; the line of the fourth ventricular floor, when extended, should pass through the central portion of the foramen magnum.

Frontal Views

In contrast with the lateral view, the frontal appearance of the fourth ventricle is variable, depending chiefly on projection. In most instances, a moderate degree of flexion of the head (at least 15 degrees) is required to fill and visualize the ventricle satisfactorily. Even during the early filling phase, there may be superimposition of the fourth ventricle on other structures. With the head flexed and the patient upright, the cisterna magna is superimposed on the fourth ventricle; the upper portion of the latter may be superimposed upon the aqueduct and part of the third ventricle. With extension, gas passes forward into the anterior cisterns and the fourth ventricular outline (if still filled) is then seen in combination with anterior subarachnoid gas shadows.

In the earlier stages of filling, and sometimes even when fully filled in upright posture, the fourth ventricle appears generally rounded in the usual frontal projection with moderate flexion (fig. 218). It may be readily recognized and differentiated from

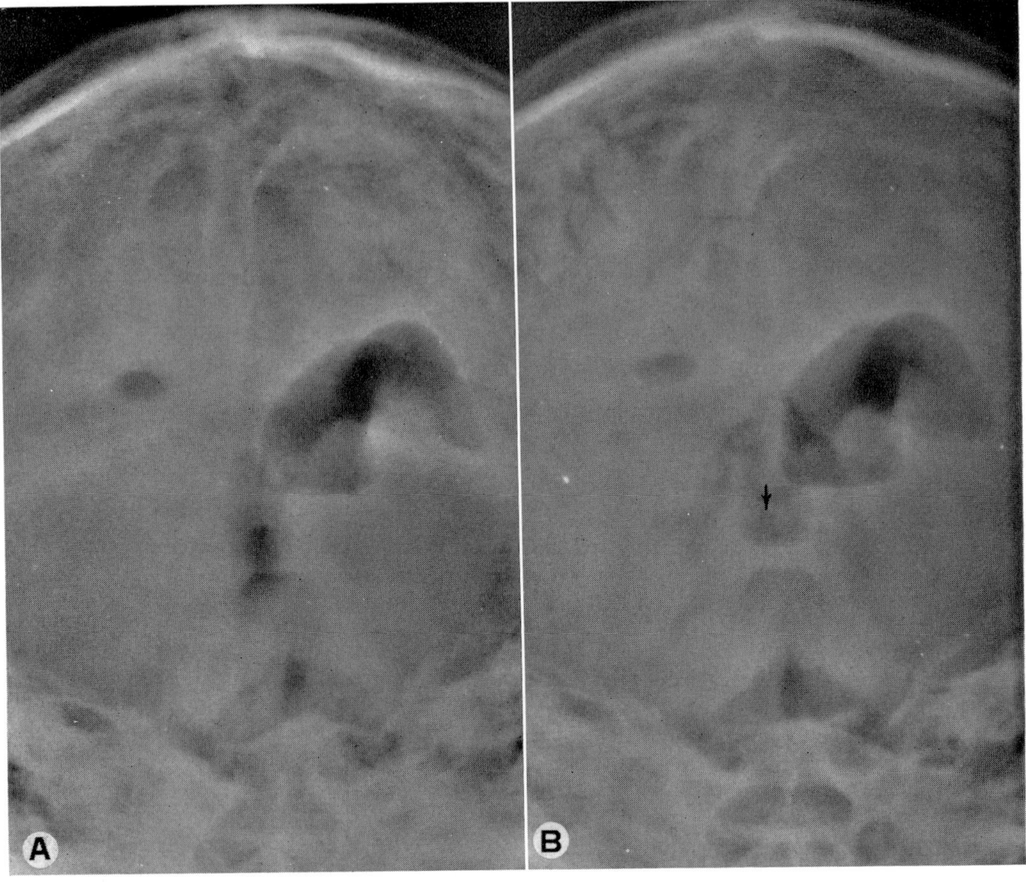

Fig. 218.—Effect of Positioning on Posterior Fossa Structures

The first filling film was made with slight rotation of the head present (A). The vallecula, fourth ventricle, aqueduct, and third ventricle are malaligned, and the possibility of displacement cannot be excluded under these circumstances.

A second film was made after repositioning of the head (B). The fourth ventricle is midline in position and regular in outline, demonstrating the normal slight flattening of the shadow of the fourth ventricular roof usually seen in this projection (*arrow*). The symmetry of the posterior communicating cisterns is well shown.

the various structures upon which it is superimposed by the fact that the top of the rounded shadow is flat. It appears as though a segment has been removed from the circular outline of the structure. The point of communication through the foramen of Magendie with the subarachnoid space between the tonsils (vallecula) is often well shown. The linear shadow of the aqueduct is foreshortened and superimposed on the gas outline of the third ventricle, the degree of superimposition depending on the quantity of gas that has entered the third ventricle. The asymmetrical diamond shape of the ventricular floor is not seen, but when the head is positioned for the straight postero-anterior projection, the upper half is demonstrated and appears roughly triangular in outline (fig. 183).

Ordinarily, the recesses are not seen. The superior posterior recesses of Retzius may occasionally be seen in lateral projection, especially when positive contrast examination is performed (fig. 192). In the usual filling frontal views, the lateral recesses may be visualized if the fourth ventricle is dilated. Under these circumstances, there is also some enlargement of the lateral recesses which may appear as tortuous tubular extensions extending outward and cephalad. Also in the presence of ventricular dilatation the fourth ventricular outline may become irregular and later deformed. Again in lateral view, with enlargement of the posterior fossa subarachnoid spaces as well as the fourth ventricle, a very wide communication between the fourth ventricle and the vallecula may be demonstrated and in some instances there may be apparent absence of a segment of the posterior medullary velum.

In the posteroanterior projections, the effect of rotation on the appearance of the fourth ventricle is quite significant. Every attempt should be made to align the head precisely so that the midline structures of the third ventricle, aqueduct, midportion of the fourth ventricle, and the vallecula are in a straight line. Even mild degrees of rotation of the head will result in an apparent lateral deviation of the fourth ventricle, which may be mistaken for displacement by a mass. Recognition of the presence of rotation by visualization of bony landmarks and measurements as described elsewhere will help to avoid errors of this nature (fig. 218).

Measurements

Along with the aqueduct of Sylvius, the fourth ventricle provides an important landmark for the application of measurements. Numerous authors have laid down pneumographic measurements including Sahlstedt (1935), Dyke and Davidoff (1940), Robertson (1941), Sutton (1950) and Last and Tompsett (1953). As noted earlier, the length of the fourth ventricle from the posterior end of the inferior colliculus to the obex varies from 3 to 3.5 cm. Trisecting this line, the junction of the middle and posterior thirds should be approximately beneath the fastigium of the fourth ventricle. A line drawn from the apex perpendicular to the floor reveals the fourth ventricular height to be on the average 1.5 cm. The maximum measurement is 2.0 cm. A line drawn from the same point along the ventricular floor to the junction of the posterior clinoids and dorsum sellae averages approximately 3.5 cm. The minimum distance along this line is 3.3 cm., while the maximum measurement obtained by most authors is 4.0 cm. (fig. 213). These measurements are important since the height of the fourth ventricle and its distance to the dorsum are reduced with cerebellar tumors and increased with pontine and other lesions anterior to the fourth ventricle. Another measurement obtained in the lateral view is from the apex of the fourth ventricle to the base of the posterior fossa, and this varies between 3 and 4 cm. The wide variation is caused in large part by the great differences in shape of the occipital bone.

In frontal projection, the width of the fourth ventricle is 1.5 to 2 cm., the measurements being taken from the lateral angles but not including the recesses, when visualized. The width and height of the fourth ventricle are generally about the same, the width being very slightly greater in most instances. However, one may be checked against the other. When fourth ventricular dilatation occurs as a result of atrophy or hydrocephalus, the fourth ventricle usually enlarges in both coronal and sagittal planes. Numerous tumors of the posterior fossa, particularly those of the pons, cause flattening of the fourth ventricle with reduction in height and increase in width.

Relative measurements frequently are as informative as absolute ones and may be applied without reference to published tables. One of the most widely used measurements of the fourth ventricle is Twining's line. A line extending from the tuberculum sellae to the torcular Herophilii, when divided in two, should have its midpoint fall within the fourth ventricle, usually along the ventricular floor or just posterior to it. Twining's line is often referred to as the "TTT line." Another similar relative measurement of value is that suggested by Sahlstedt. This line is drawn from the dorsum sellae through the junction of aqueduct and fourth ventricle to the inner table of the skull. When the line is trisected, the ventriculosylviductal union should be at the meeting of the anterior and middle thirds of the line. As valuable as measurements may be, both absolute and relative, to confirm a suspicion of abnormality, the possibility of abnormality first must be appreciated. This is best achieved through a good understanding of ventricular anatomy and normal pneumographic morphology and topography. As previously noted, a vertical line drawn along the floor of the fourth ventricle and under the obex normally extends into the spinal cord just behind the center, since the fourth ventricle is potentially continuous, after a ventral jog, with the central canal of the spinal cord. The line along the fourth ventricle also should point to the central portion of the foramen magnum. Any significant shift of the fourth ventricle from its normal position in the sagittal plane results in malalignment of the fourth ventricular floor which should be readily recognizable.

SUBARACHNOID CISTERNS

The subarachnoid cisterns are the large cerebrospinal fluid pools that are situated principally about the base of the brain but which extend about various infolded portions, sometimes as relatively narrow channels separating anatomic structures. The cerebral cisterns are part of the general cranial subarachnoid space, the total fluid content of which is appreciably greater than that of the ventricular system. Visualization of the subarachnoid cisterns may be equally as important as visualization of the ventricular system itself, particularly in the diagnosis of tumors of the posterior fossa. In instances in which the ventricles do not fill, examination of the subarachnoid space may be all important and frequently is sufficient for diagnosis.

The cisternal fluid spaces generally take their names from anatomic structures that they surround or with which they are variously in contact. The cisterns may be divided into two general groups: (1) those of the basal regions between the inferior brain surface and the floor of the skull, and (2) those which provide communicating pathways between the basal cisterns and the general subarachnoid space over the cerebral convexities. The latter also serve to separate several infolded major portions of the brain. It may be advantageous to consider the cisterns according to the following classification. In the listing, synonyms of the preferred terms are given in parenthesis.

A. Basal Cisterns
- I. Posterior fossa
  - 1. Cisterna magna (cisterna cerebellomedullaris)
    - Cerebellar portion
    - Vallecula
    - Medullary portion
  - 2. Cisterna pontis
    - Central portion (medial reservoir)
    - Lateral portions (lateral pontine cisterns)
    - Cerebellopontine recesses (lateral recesses)
  - 3. Cisterna interpeduncularis and its extensions
    - Intercrural cistern (dorsal section cisterna interpeduncularis)
    - Crural cisterns (peripeduncular extensions cisterna interpeduncularis)
- II. Middle fossa
  - 1. Suprasellar cistern
    - Prechiasmatic portion
    - Postchiasmatic portion
  - 2. Parasellar cisterns

B. Communicating Cisterns
- I. Anterior channels
  - 1. Cisterna lamina terminalis
  - 2. Sylvian cisterns
- II. Posterior channels
  - 1. Lateral—left and right around brain stem (circummesencephalic cistern, cisterna ambiens)

(Revised 1963)

2. Dorsal—quadrigeminal cistern and its extensions
   - Superior cerebellar space (posterior extension)
   - Cerebellomedullary recess (inferior extension)
   - Retrothalamic spaces (lateral extensions, wings of cisterna ambiens)
   - Cisterna velum interpositum (anterior extension)
   - Pericallosal space (superior extension)

Basal Cisterns

Posterior fossa. The *cisterna magna* is the most capacious of the subarachnoid cisterns, and from this feature it derives its name. The main portion of the cisterna magna is situated posterior to the medulla oblongata and inferior to the cerebellum. It extends downward to join the subarachnoid space of the spinal canal, and therefore in the midsagittal plane it is triangular in shape bounded by the occipital bone inferiorly and posteriorly, by the cerebellum superiorly, and by the medulla anteriorly (figs. 219 and 221). The apex points into the *vallecula*, a small valley between the cerebellar tonsils, and toward the foramen of Magendie. Ordinarily, the cistern contains between 5 and 10 cc. of cerebrospinal fluid, but it may be considerably larger without denoting cerebellar atrophy or hypoplasia. Because of the relationship of the cistern to the cerebellum and the medulla oblongata, it is formally known as the *cisterna cerebellomedullaris* (Key and Retzius, 1875). Its anatomic extent is not limited to the posterior areas but it encircles the brain stem and extends laterally as well (fig. 220). The anterior portion of the cisterna cerebellomedullaris is termed by Robertson the *medullary cistern*, while the posterior extension behind the cerebellum may be called the cerebellar portion.

The cisterna magna is a relatively free space with wide separation of the pia and arachnoid but a cavity within which varying numbers of arachnoid trabeculae are present. The lateral and posterior superior extent of the cistern is limited by a reapproximation and partial fusion of the arachnoid and pia as the cerebellar expansion approaches the bony skull. Beyond this superiorly and laterally, the pericerebellar subarachnoid spaces are narrow. The pia-arachnoid limiting membrane accounts for the relatively sharp termination of the cistern behind the inferior portion of the cerebellum and the presence of an acute angle at the termination. The membrane also prevents free egress of gas over the posterior and lateral aspects of the cerebellar hemispheres to the superior surface, under normal circumstances. When air continues upward behind the cerebellum to fill the superior cerebellar space, we speak of an "incompetent" cisterna magna. The position of the limiting membrane, or location of the fusion between arachnoid and pia, accounts for the great variation in size of the cisterna magna (fig. 221). In some cases, the cistern may reach the undersurface of the tentorium, whereas at other times it is very small. Occasionally, the cisterna magna extends supratentorially through a defect in the tentorium at the posterior attachment of the latter. In one case, this supratentorial extension (which does not communicate with the supratentorial subarachnoid space) caused an area of thinning of the inner table of the occipital bone. Lesser degrees of thinning are observed in other cases where an extremely large cisterna magna is present.

The anatomic structures bordering the cisterna magna and extending into it are generally segments of the medulla oblongata and cerebellum. The anterior wall is formed by the medulla oblongata and inferior roof portion of the fourth ventricle. The *vallecula* is a midline upward extension of the cisterna magna between the tonsils of the cerebellum. Superiorly and posteriorly, the vallecula is limited by the cerebellar vermis proper. The vallecula should be in midsagittal plane in normally positioned frontal pneumograms. It has the configuration of a high isosceles triangle with the apex directed superiorly. Gas usually outlines the cerebellar tonsils fairly well since they project into the lumen of the cisterna magna. The tonsils may be

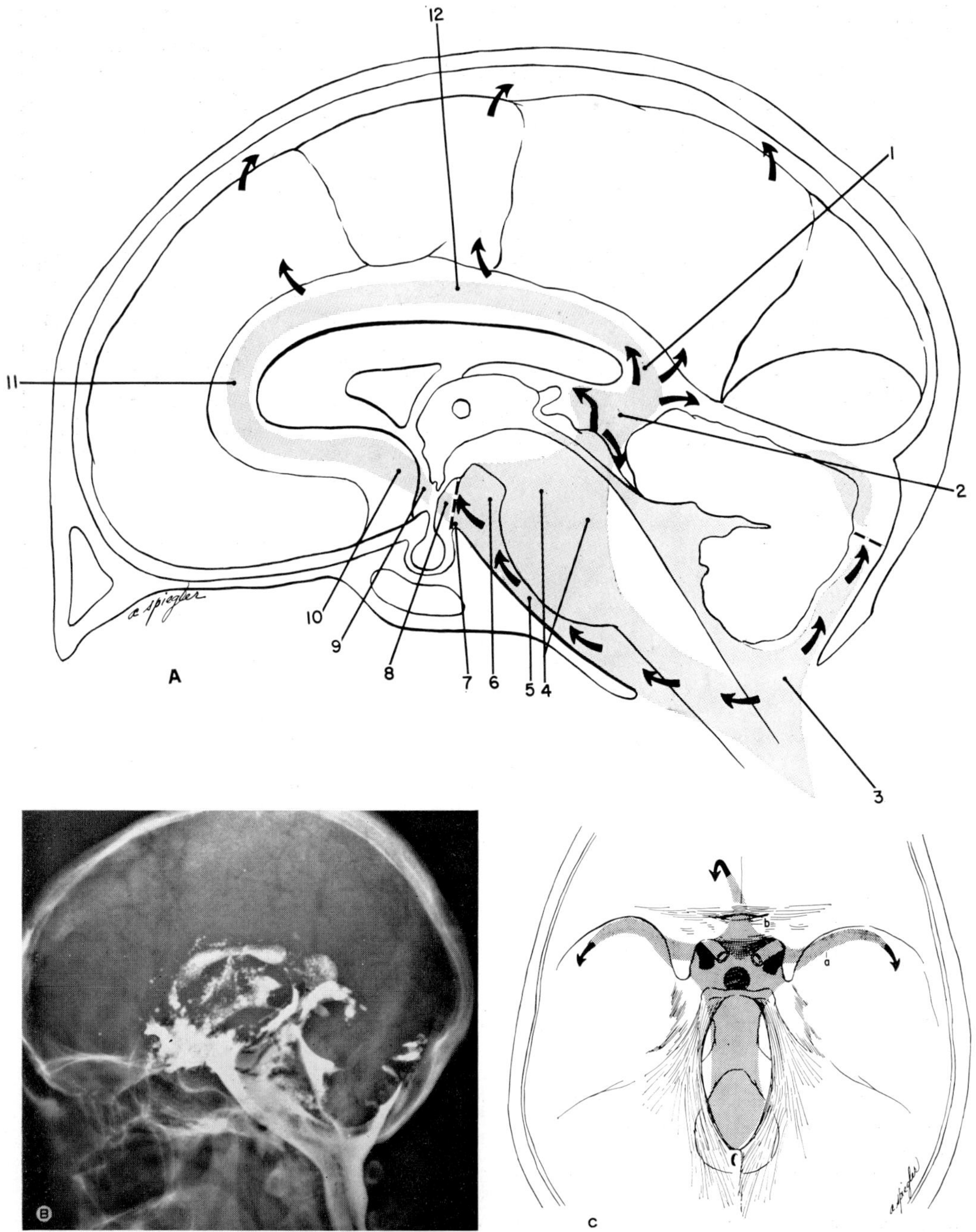

Fig. 219.—Anatomic Division of the Basal and Communicating Cisterns

The majority of the major cisterns are visible in the lateral pneumogram. In the sketch (A), the main cerebrospinal fluid pathways are shaded. From the cisterna magna (cerebellomedullaris) (3), the main course is rostral and upward through the pontine (5) and interpeduncular (6) cisterns. Fluid then flows in one of two main directions: it may continue forward, or be funneled in a broad thin band from the lateral extensions of the basal cisterns through the lateral communicating channels around the brain stem (4) into the quadrigeminal cistern (2). The forward passage of gas at pneumography may be im-

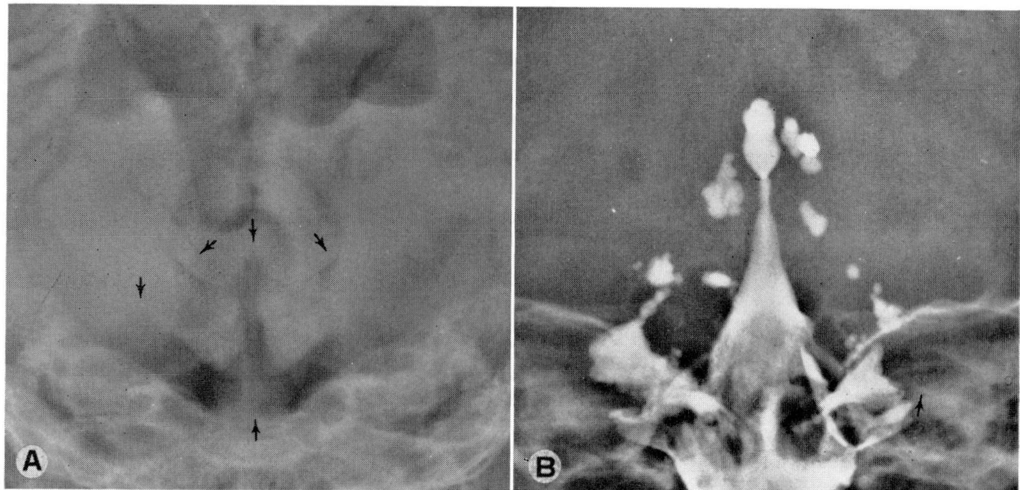

FIG. 220.—FRONTAL PROJECTION OF THE POSTERIOR SUBARACHNOID CISTERNS

A posteroanterior half axial view (A) shows gas in the cisterna magna (*lower central vertical arrow*), continuous above with the shadow of the vallecula (isosceles triangle) between the cerebellar tonsils. The cerebellopontine recesses are large in this case, allowing good depiction of their form (*lateral vertical arrow*). Gas is shown in the intercrural cistern (dorsal portion of cisterna interpeduncularis), superimposed upon the shadow of the vallecula and the fourth ventricle in this projection (*upper vertical arrow*). The central intercrural shadow is continuous with gas extending laterally around the cerebral peduncles into the crural cisterns (*oblique arrows*). The film also shows gas in the right and left lateral channels around the midbrain, communicating with the quadrigeminal cistern above.

Cisternal anatomy may be demonstrated well by filling the subarachnoid channels with radiopaque fluid (B). In the case shown, Pantopaque is present in the cisterna magna and cerebellopontine extensions, one of which is deformed by a small acoustic neurinoma (*arrow*). The interrupted contour of the lateral communicating channels and the quadrigeminal cistern are outlined; (compare with (A)). The iter and fourth ventricle are opacified in the center of the figure; the triangular extensions of the lateral recess of the fourth ventricle are illustrated. (Courtesy, Dr. B. Wolff, New York.)

slightly asymmetrical normally and thus occasionally produce some midline distortion of the vallecula; however, such asymmetry is usually minimum in normal persons, since the tonsils are essentially paired paramedian structures. The anterior and inferior margins of the cerebellar hemispheres proper bound the lateral expanse of the cisterna magna

---

peded by the membrane of Liliequist (7); normally, the delay is only temporary, and the postchiasmatic (8) and prechiasmatic (9) portions of the suprasellar cistern then fill. The thin cisterna lamina terminalis (10) is shown diagrammatically as the main forward channel providing communication to the callosal sulcus (12) through the subarachnoid space around the rostrum (11). A corresponding communication is through the subarachnoid space around the splenium (1). A number of important subarachnoid extensions visible in lateral view are not indicated in the diagram; additional lateral channels and cisternal recesses are not visible in the lateral projection (see text and Fig. 220).

In pneumograms performed the modern way, it is unusual to see all of the cisternal and communicating spaces filled with gas on one film. For anatomic purposes, a radiopaque cast of portions of the cerebrospinal fluid pathways may be created by filling the subarachnoid cisterns with Pantopaque (B). (Courtesy, Dr. Bernard Wolff, New York.)

A full axial view of the middle fossa cisterns by pneumography is difficult to obtain. In the sketch (C), the course of the central and lateral cisterns is shown diagrammatically. The largest lateral communicating channel, the Sylvian cistern (a), extends outward behind the sphenoid ridge, having a configuration resembling the long horn of a steer. The main forward pathway through the cisterna lamina terminalis and the pericallosal communicating channel is indicated (b).

(Revised 1963)

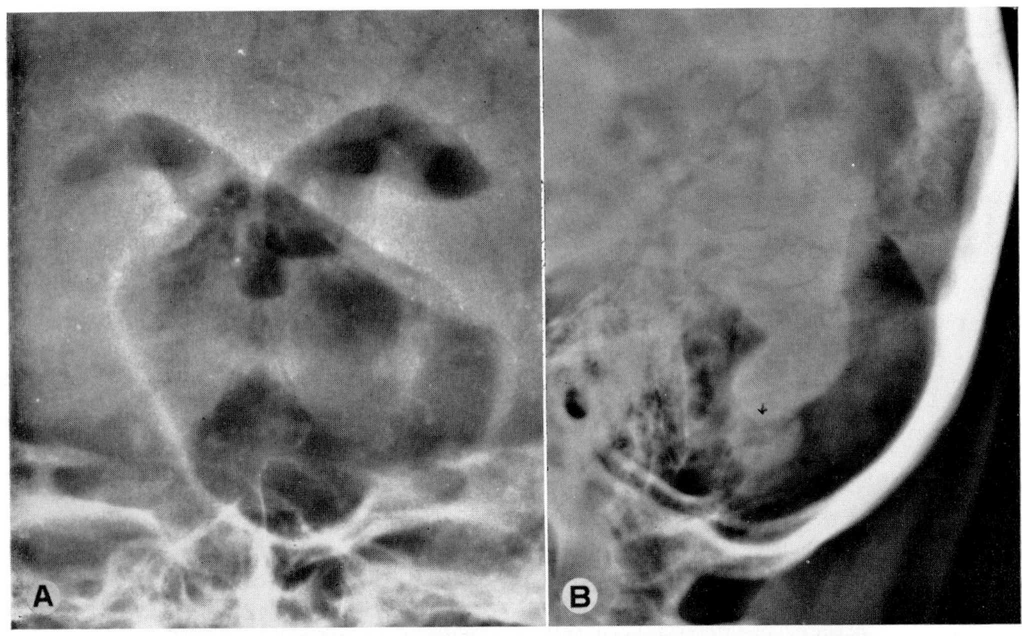

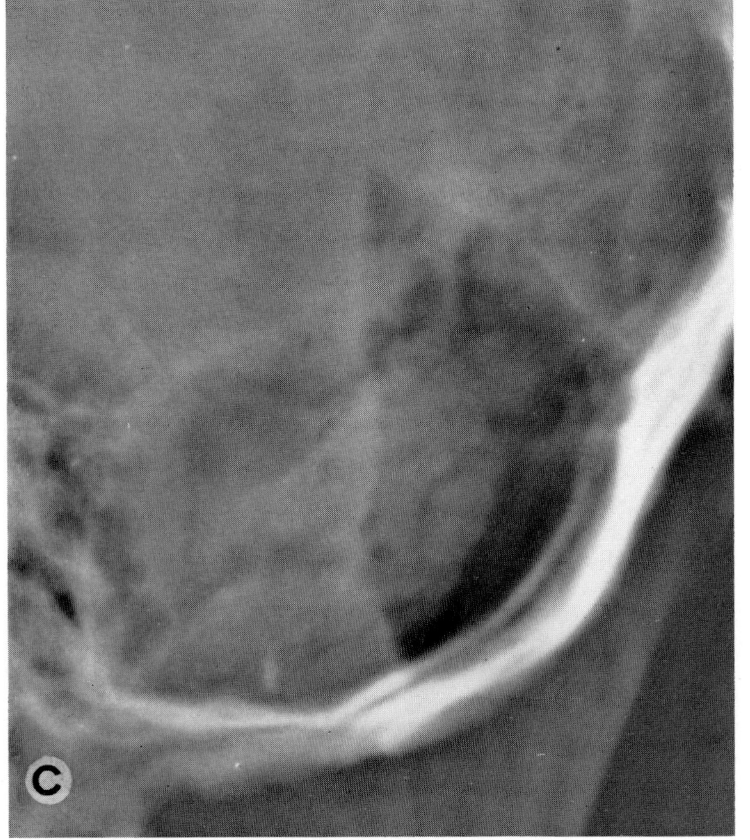

Fig. 221

(Revised 1963)

and the degree of their presentation into the cistern is dependent upon the location of the lateral limiting membrane previously described.

Anteriorly, the cisterna cerebellomedullaris is continuous around the brain stem through its medullary portion with the *cisterna pontis*. The cisterna pontis is divided into a medial single midline segment and the two lateral portions. Leading outward from the lateral portions are the cerebellopontine recesses. The central portion of the cisterna pontis is a sizable cavity which separates the anterior aspect of the pons varolii from the clivus of the sphenoid and basiocciput. The lower section is projected through the petrous and mastoid portions of the temporal bones and often is not well seen except in laminagrams and other films made with special techniques. The anterior boundary of the cisterna pontis is the sloping or gently curved clivus. The posterior boundary is the ventral convexity, or belly, of the pons which is usually clearly outlined in normal lateral pneumograms. Inferiorly, the pontomedullary notch indicates the point of fusion of the pons and medulla. Superiorly, another constriction of the brain stem is outlined as the ventral convexity of the pons curves more sharply backward toward the cerebral peduncles. Gas in the upper part of the central portion of the cisterna pontis clearly demarcates this surface configuration as the pontine cistern fuses above with the cisterna interpeduncularis.

The medial reservoir of the pontine cistern is bounded incompletely by two lateral membranes situated parallel to the basilar artery, with the result that they form a cerebrospinal fluid canal in which the basilar artery is contained. The basilar artery usually can be seen in pneumograms as a linear shadow several millimeters in diameter running parallel to the anterior boundary of the pons, to which it is usually closely applied and attached by subarachnoid trabeculae. Frequently it can be followed upward, diverging from the brain stem as it enters the cisterna interpeduncularis, as far cephalad as its entrance into the circle of Willis.

The degree of filling, the size, and the shape of the medial portion of the cisterna pontis are very important in pneumographic diagnosis of lesions arising in various sections of the posterior fossa. The lateral portions also are extremely important, since visualization of these areas and their recesses has a specific application in the diagnosis of cerebellopontine angle tumors. Each lateral (cerebellopontine) recess extends to and along the posterior surface of the petrous bone, which forms one of its principal boundaries and which it outlines quite discretely in frontal films designed for this purpose (fig. 220). Above, each lateral extension of the cistern is limited by the tentorial attachment to the petrous bones. The cerebellum and its peduncles form the posterior boundary. The inferior boundary is an arachnoid membrane which arises along the medullopontine notch but which allows free communication with the cisternal spaces below. Posteriorly, the lateral divisions of the cisterna pontis also communicate with the cisterna magna.

The *cisterna interpeduncularis* is the rather

Fig. 221.—Variation in Size of the Cisterna Magna

A large cisterna magna is present which is "competent" but which extends high behind the cerebellum as a result of high position of the limiting membrane (A). The exceptionally dark gas shadow may obscure cerebellar structures and give a false impression of smallness of the cerebellum (B). The upper margin of the vallecula is shown in the lateral view (*vertical arrow*); the vallecula usually cannot be seen in this projection with the usual quantities of gas present. The cerebellar tonsils are shown extending downward into the large cistern (*transverse arrow*). Just above the *arrow* is the tonsillar notch.

A very large cisterna magna is present with gas extending over the superior surface of the cerebellum (C). The lateral film, made with the horizontal x-ray beam and with the head well flexed, shows how large quantities of gas can be trapped in a capacious cisterna magna before filling of the other cisterns and the ventricles can begin. When a cistern of this order of size is encountered, the head should be extended in order to accomplish ventricular filling (see text).

(Revised 1963)

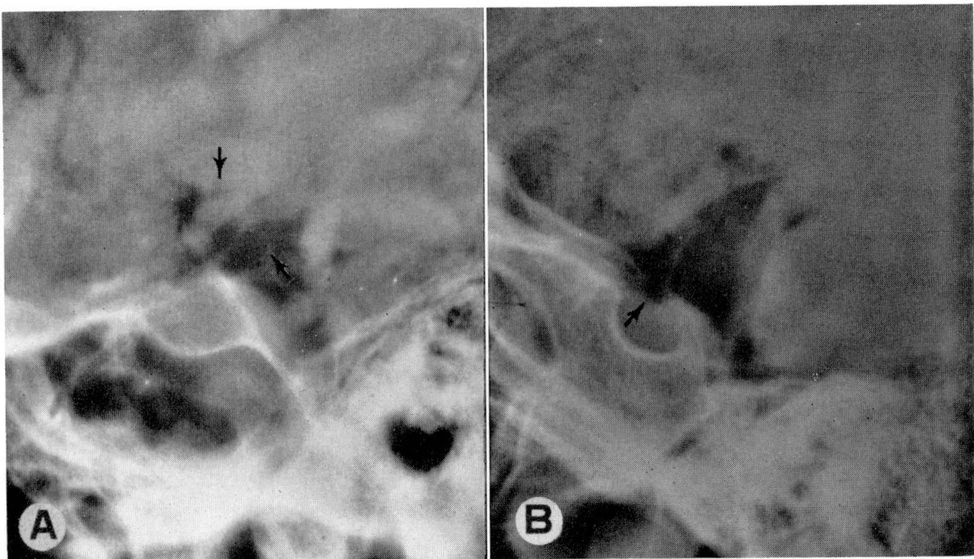

FIG. 222.—MEMBRANE OF LILIEQUIST

The cisterna interpeduncularis is bounded anteriorly by the membrane of Liliequist, above and behind the sella turcica (A). The membrane separates incompletely the upper portion of the cisterna interpeduncularis from the suprasellar cistern; it often is seen in the lateral pneumogram extending from the posterior clinoid processes to the hypothalamus, at the anterior margin of the mammillary bodies (*posterior arrow*).

The subarachnoid space above the sella turcica (suprasellar cistern) may be divided into two compartments that are separated by the optic nerves and chiasm (*anterior arrow*). The portion of the suprasellar cistern forward of the optic pathways is designated the prechiasmatic portion of the suprasellar cistern (termed by others the cisterna chiasmatis); the space between the optic pathways and the membrane of Liliequist, the main body of the cistern, may be called the postchiasmatic portion.

In another case, the membrane of Liliequist is unusually well shown, curving upward and backward from the posterior clinoid processes to the hypothalamus (B). The diaphragma sellae is sharply outlined (*arrow*).

wide space, appearing roughly triangular in sagittal plane, situated anterior to and extending between the cerebral peduncles. The name is considered to be a poor choice of terms which has resulted in confusion regarding the anatomy of the area. The cistern is bounded anteriorly by the dorsal surface of the sella turcica at the level of the *membrane of Liliequist*, which extends from the posterior clinoid processes to the hypothalamus, just anterior to the mammillary bodies (fig. 222). The membrane is slightly concave posteriorly and its thickness and density vary. While ordinarily it produces only a transient delay in passage of gas from the cisterna interpeduncularis forward into the suprasellar area, the membrane may cause significant interference with communication between the cisterns posterior to the sella turcica and those above this structure. Superiorly, the cisterna interpeduncularis is in contact with the structures along the posterior portion of the floor of the third ventricle. Posteriorly, it extends into the space between the cerebral peduncles and faces the superior margin of the pons varolii. Some authors consider the cisterna interpeduncularis to extend forward above the sella turcica to the region of the optic nerves and to have a correspondingly wide lateral extension. It would appear preferable, however, to consider the suprasellar cisterns separately for better clinical orientation.

Numerous anatomic structures often can be identified in the interpeduncular area in lateral pneumograms, including cranial nerves and important vessels along the base of the brain. Such identification is of academic interest but rarely of clinical importance unless, for example, an abnormal shadow can be related to a vascular outline. Even then, the connection is better made by angiography.

The cisterns of the crura cerebri (peduncles of the cerebrum) are only dorsal and anterior extensions of the cisterna interpeduncularis. In speaking of the cisterna interpeduncularis, reference generally is made to the triangular space just described as seen in the lateral view. The frontal projection demonstrates the crura (legs or pillars) and their adjacent cisterns to best advantage. The midline dorsal extension of the cisterna interpeduncularis is the *intercrural cistern*; it is triangular in frontal view, projecting upward into the interpeduncular space (fig. 220). In films made with exaggerated flexion of the head, the intercrural cistern may be superimposed on the vallecula. The intercrural cistern may be identified in the composite shadow by the well rounded configuration of the cerebral peduncles on each side of the cistern.

The peripeduncular extensions, or *crural cisterns*, are forward, lateral, and upward projections which separate the peduncle from the hippocampus of the medial aspect of the temporal lobe on the two sides. The crural cisterns may be 2 cm. or more in length. Together, the appearance of the intercrural and crural cisterns has been likened to a three-pointed crown, as viewed from behind (figs. 220 and 236). Identification of the crural cisterns by their divergence at an angle of 45 degrees from the horizontal and their differentiation from the olfactory sulci, which have a greater degree of angulation, has been mentioned earlier.

Middle fossa. The *suprasellar* cistern is the principal space above the sella turcica and is intimately related to the optic pathways. It is wide from side to side and, except for the membrane of Liliequist, it is in free communication with the cisterna interpeduncularis. Many authors still consider the major portion of the suprasellar cistern to be a segment of the cisterna interpeduncularis, although clinically they are quite apart.

(Revised 1963)

Lindgren (1957) has suggested that the entire midline space anterior to the membrane of Liliequist be called the *cisterna chiasmatis.*

The suprasellar cistern consists of two main portions: (1) the larger midline space above the sella turcica, previously referred to as the anterior part of the interpeduncular cistern, and (2) the smaller cisterna chiasmatis. The authors prefer to regard the space anterior to and above the optic chiasm and nerves (the cisterna chiasmatis) as the prechiasmatic portion of the suprasellar cistern. The area behind and below the optic chiasm is termed the postchiasmatic portion of the suprasellar cistern. The latter varies considerably in size from patient to patient. The width corresponds to that of the sella turcica. The height and anteroposterior measurements are quite variable and in some patients, the space is very large. The post chiasmatic portion of the suprasellar cistern is bounded posteriorly by the band of Liliequist, superiorly by the structures which form the anterior portion of the floor of the third ventricle (chiefly the tuber cinereum), anteriorly by the optic chiasm and nerves, and inferiorly by the diaphragma sellae. A very large number of anatomic structures border or pass through this cistern, both vascular and neural (fig. 222). There is extensive literature dealing with the ability to visualize specific structures in the basal cisterns of this region but, aside from the main vascular trunks and the optic pathways, it is difficult to be certain that one is dealing with a specific anatomic entity in any given case.

Along the floor of the cistern, a transverse line of demarcation between the gas shadow of the pneumogram and the soft tissue contents of the sella turcica usually is visible. The outlet of the sella turcica is bounded superiorly by the dura mater and its arachnoid reflection which together are known as the diaphragma sellae. This shadow usually extends from just below the anterior and middle clinoid processes along the tuberculum to a point just beneath the posterior clinoid processes at the junction of the clinoids and dorsum (fig. 222). In some instances, the level of the diaphragm is appreciably lower, even in the presence of a pituitary gland of normal size. Projection of the diaphragm above the clinoid level, however, is not normal. Superior arching or suprasellar extension in a dome or conelike manner usually indicates an intrasellar mass lesion.

The suprasellar cistern inferiorly extends into the hypophyseal subarachnoid space around the stalk of the pituitary gland. The arachnoid membrane continues through the diaphragma sellae where it spreads out over the surface of the pituitary gland. Just beneath the diaphragma sellae, where the arachnoid diverges to be applied closer to the pituitary surface, a small subarachnoid space exists but this does not ordinarily fill with gas in pneumograms. In the presence of increased intracranial pressure, the hypophyseal subarachnoid space may enlarge or, with ventricular obstruction, the infundibular recess of the third ventricle may protrude into the sella turcica, depressing or excavating the normal soft tissue shadow to a remarkable degree.

The *parasellar cisterns* communicate freely with the midline suprasellar cistern, from which they extend outward and forward. Each space follows the internal carotid artery and is partially bounded by arachnoid reflected from the artery to the Sylvian fissure. From its location above and forward of the cavernous sinus, each cistern soon empties into a Sylvian cistern between the inferior surface of the frontal lobe and the anterior tip of the temporal lobe, a transverse opening with which the parasellar space is continuous.

Communicating Cisterns

Anterior channels. In the midline above the prechiasmatic portion of the suprasellar cistern, there is a very thin extension of the cisterna chiasmatis along the anterior wall of the hypothalamic portion of the third ventricle. This is named for the anatomic structure it bounds, the *cisterna lamina terminalis*. There is no firm anterior boundary of either the cisterna chiasmatis or the cisterna lamina terminalis. Forward to these areas, fluid and gas fill the general frontal subarachnoid space and sulci.

The cisterna lamina terminalis serves as a principal communicating pathway by joining the inferior end of the callosal sulcus located beneath the rostrum of the corpus callosum. The callosal sulcus bends around the rostrum, extending superiorly and then posteriorly. Through this large sulcus there is communication with the superior longitudinal fissure on the medial surface of the brain. In addition, the cisterna lamina terminalis joins laterally the Sylvian cisterns. The proximal portions of the anterior cerebral arteries and the anterior communicating artery are contained in the cisterna lamina terminalis. Posteriorly, the cistern is separated from the lumen of the third ventricle only by the thin lamina terminalis; this anatomic feature has been utilized in connection with an operation to relieve hydrocephalus in which an artificial opening is made between the ventricle and cistern.

The other anterior communicating channels are the *Sylvian cisterns*. The spaces are paired, extending laterally on each side from a parasellar cistern as mentioned above. The Sylvian cistern is a transverse space between the inferior surface of the frontal lobe and the anterior tip of the temporal lobe. Each extends slightly upward as it progresses from its medial to its lateral end. The cistern parallels the sphenoid ridge behind which it is located. Anteriorly and medially, the Sylvian cistern is in communication with the cisterna lamina terminalis. Laterally, the cistern is continuous with the general subarachnoid space over the surface of the brain with which it communicates by means of the subarachnoid space of the Sylvian fissure. The depth of the cistern is approximately 1.5 cm., and its transverse length approximately 3 cm., depending on the length of the transverse portion of the middle cerebral artery which it follows before turning to enter the Sylvian fissure (fig. 223).

Posterior channels. In order to reach the spaces behind the brain stem, cerebrospinal fluid or gas must pass around the brain stem by lateral and posterior extension from the basal cisterns. This communication is accomplished through left and right lateral channels extending around the brain stem in a jacket-like manner. The lateral

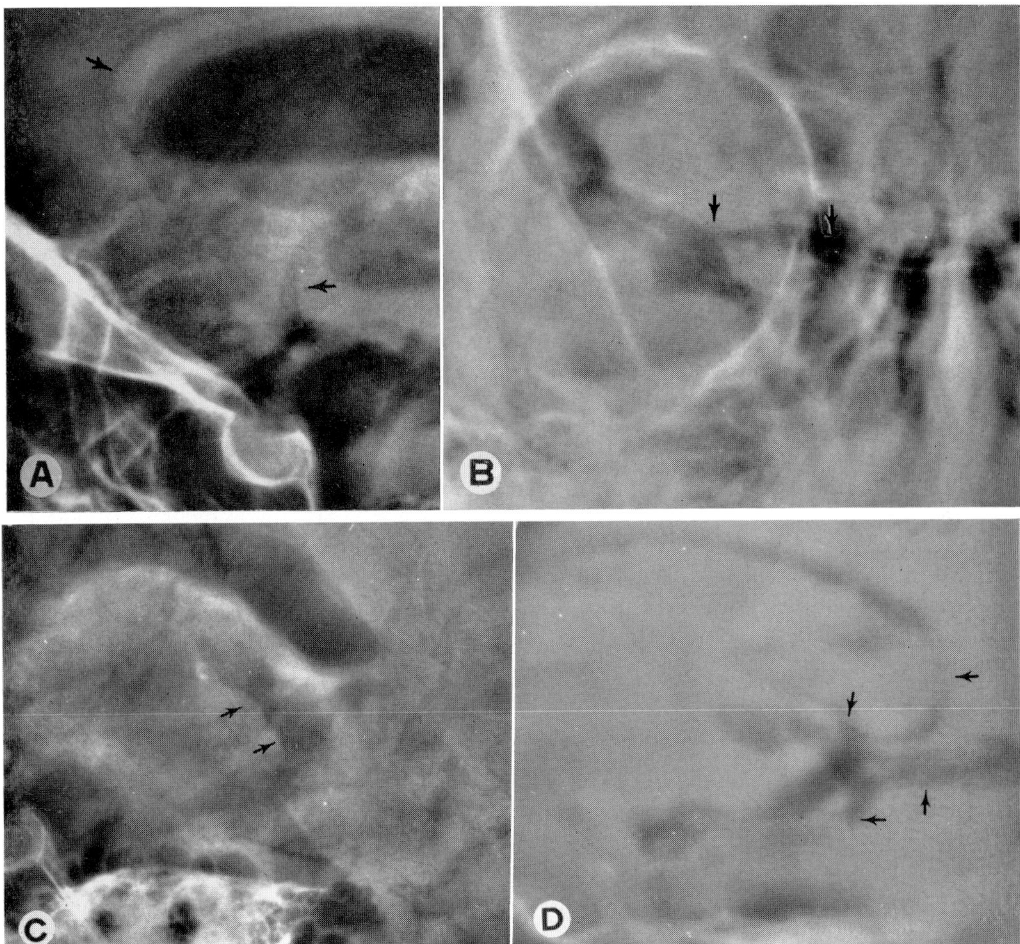

FIG. 223.—ANTERIOR AND POSTERIOR COMMUNICATING CISTERNS

The anterior communicating pathways are best seen in lateral projection (A). The cisterna lamina terminalis, anterior to the third ventricle, extends upward from the region of the prechiasmatic portion of the suprasellar system (*lower arrow*); the cistern communicates forward and around the rostrum of the corpus callosum through the anterior extension of the callosal sulcus (*upper arrow*). Beside the sella turcica anteriorly, and behind the medial end of the sphenoid wing on each side, is the parasellar cistern, poorly visualized because of the superimposed air sinus shadows; its lateral and forward extension is the Sylvian cistern (see also Fig. 219).

The Sylvian cistern and its communication with the Sylvian fissure are better visualized in frontal view (B). The cistern extends laterally, parallel to and behind the sphenoid ridge (*arrows*); it is wide based on the parasellar cistern medially, and tapers laterally, the configuration resembling a steer horn (see Fig. 219). The lateral extension of this communicating channel is to the subarachnoid space of the cerebral convexity and the Sylvian fissure.

The dorsal subarachnoid communication from the base of the brain to its cortical surface is through the quadrigeminal cistern. The cistern is best visualized, together with the quadrigeminal plate (*arrows*), when the retrothalamic extensions are not superimposed (C). Midsagittal tomograms often show the posterior communicating channels to advantage (D). The quadrigeminal cistern is mainly behind the collicular plate; a posterior extension is into the superior cerebellar space (*lower vertical arrow*); an inferior extension is into the cerebellomedullary recess (*lower transverse arrow*); a superior extension is through the pericallosal space (*upper transverse arrow*), from the superior quadrigeminal confluence (*upper vertical arrow*) to the callosal sulcus (cistern) on the medial hemispheric surface.

(Revised 1963)

communicating spaces serve to transport cerebrospinal fluid from the basal cisterns to the large dorsal space, the quadrigeminal cistern. At some levels, when viewed in cross section, the subarachnoid space around the midbrain appears as a cylindrical sleeve, while at other brain stem levels it approaches more a triangular configuration.

The ambient nature of the cerebrospinal fluid pathways encompassing the brain stem has led to use of the terms cisterna ambiens and circummesencephalic cistern. The communicating channels around the brain stem, however, do not constitute a separate cistern; in order to encompass the brain stem, segments of multiple cisterns must be listed. Thus, the ventral subarachnoid cisterns and their recesses communicate through left and right lateral channels posteriorly to the dorsal (quadrigeminal) cistern and its recesses. The quadrigeminal cistern, in turn, is a communicating cistern, superiorly to the cerebral subarachnoid space and posteriorly to the cerebellar subarachnoid space. For these reasons, it appears advisable to limit use of the term "cisterna ambiens" in an all-inclusive connotation and consider the cisternal segments facing various aspects of the brain stem according to divisions which ordinarily can be recognized in pneumograms.

The *quadrigeminal cistern* is so named because among the most important structures that it embraces are the quadrigeminal plate and the quadrigeminal bodies. Earlier, this space was referred to as the cisterna venae magnae cerebri, because the great cerebral vein is situated in the superior portion of the quadrigeminal cistern. The quadrigeminal cistern is a rather large space which forms something resembling a distribution point for cerebrospinal fluid or gas upward into the major medial sulci, posteriorly over the cerebellar surface and anteriorly and inferiorly into several ramifications between various infolded and deeply situated cerebral structures (fig. 223). As just noted, inflow of fluid is from the lateral communicating cisterns under ordinary circumstances. Fluid or gas also may pass posteriorly and upward from the cisterna magna over the posterior surface of the cerebellum to reach the quadrigeminal cistern in subjects having an "incompetent" cisterna magna.

Anteriorly, the quadrigeminal cistern faces the quadrigeminal bodies and the pineal body with its associated third ventricular recesses. Superiorly, the splenium of the corpus callosum generally bounds the cistern, and the great cerebral vein (vein of Galen) is located here. Posteriorly, the cistern straddles the free edge of the tentorium and faces the tentorial attachment of the falx cerebri and its related structures. Inferiorly, the quadrigeminal cistern is bounded by the upper promontory of the cerebellar vermis.

A posterior extension of the quadrigeminal cistern is the subarachnoid space over the superior surface of the cerebellum (cisterna cerebelli superior). At the junction of the quadrigeminal cistern and the supracerebellar space, the communication is wide and posteriorly it extends in a funnel-shaped manner into a fairly constant and relatively narrow space extending over the dorsal surface of the cerebellum. Inferiorly, extension of the quadrigeminal cistern is into the space between the anterior surface of the cerebellum and the upper portion of the fourth ventricle. The anterior medullary velum is a very thin structure which bounds this cisternal extension anteriorly. Because of the thinness of the velum it may appear, on occasion, that subarachnoid gas is continuous with gas in the fourth ventricle. This is never the case normally, although it is one of the weak points of the ventricular system where a pressure diverticulum may develop (figs. 244 and 324).

One of the structures along the anterolateral aspect of the quadrigeminal cistern on each side is the pulvinar of the thalamus. An extension of the cistern facing the thalamus is present on each side which courses 2 to 3 cm. lateralward, forward and downward. At pneumography, gas extending around the thalamus into this cleavage space has a winglike configuration when viewed posteroinferiorly. For this reason, Lindgren (1950 and 1957) called the space the lateral *wing of the cisterna ambiens*. The same cleft is called by others the *retrothalamic space, retrothalamic extension, retrothalamic portion,* or *retropulvinarian portion* of the quadrigeminal cistern. In the past, the retrothalamic space was often mistaken for the outline of the posterior part of the cisterna ambiens in lateral pneumograms; however, this space is actually perpendicular to the cisterna ambiens, which is only seen in reverse half axial views. With few exceptions, the retrothalamic cistern is represented by a thin curvilinear shadow which crosses the center of the quadrigeminal plate between the upper and lower quadrigeminal tubercles (fig. 223). Ordinarily, the retrothalamic cistern is not visible in frontal views because it is too thin to cast a shadow unless this cisternal space is enlarged on a congenital basis or secondary to atrophy. In infants, it is often shown well. In occasional cases, the upper portion of the retrothalamic cistern can be seen in frontal projection as a linear shadow extending upward and laterally; rarely a double shadow is seen produced by the upper margin of the thalamus above and the superior aspect of the pulvinar just below (fig. 184).

An anterior extension from the quadrigeminal cistern is the *cisterna velum interpositum.* This space is more often outlined in children than in adults and its visualization may be considered an anatomic variant, similar to the cavum (fig. 227). In children, the space often is quite wide, whereas in adults it is small and represented as a thin air shadow on the radiograph. Occasionally, it will be found as a large space in adults. The space is formed by two foldings of the arachnoid over the roof of the third ventricle. It is situated between the fornix above and the chorioid plexus and the epithelial roof of the third ventricle below. Anteriorly, the cisterna velum interpositum stops just behind the foramen of Monro. The cistern is generally triangular, having a long, trumpet-like configuration with its base posteriorly. Filling also may occur through the lateral wings or retrothalamic spaces which are continuous with and terminate in the cisterna velum interpositum.

(Revised 1963)

By a superior and posterior extension (pericallosal space), the quadrigeminal cistern also communicates with the callosal sulcus. The channel curves backward and up over the splenium and then extends forward over the body of the corpus callosum to become the callosal or supracallosal sulcus or cistern. By this route, a large portion of the cerebrospinal fluid reaches the superior longitudinal fissure along the medial aspect of the brain in a good percentage of cases. It is evident, therefore, that fluid may pass freely in the subarachnoid space anteriorly around the rostrum of the corpus callosum from the cisterna lamina terminalis to reach the superior longitudinal fissure. Fluid passes posteriorly around the splenium of the corpus callosum from the quadrigeminal cistern to the same fissure. Fluid also passes laterally around the temporal lobes to reach the lateral cerebral fissures. Thus, there are two principal channels communicating with the general subarachnoid space on the medial aspect of the brain and two channels supplying the convexities. In addition, numerous minor sulcal ramifications are present.

Radiologic Features

The majority of the major cisterns described can be seen in both frontal and lateral pneumograms. Some of the ramifications, however, can be seen only in certain views, or are best seen in special views such as the reverse half axial projection or tomograms. Furthermore, the technique employed in the injection of gas and positioning of the head during the injection materially affect the cisterns that fill.

Lateral view. While the structures visualized will vary with the quantity of gas used and the selectivity of the injection, all of the cisternal fluid spaces aforementioned can be seen in lateral view with the following exceptions: (1) the lateral portions of the cisterna pontis and the cerebellopontine recesses, (2) the intercrural and crural cisterns, (3) the lateral communicating channels around the midbrain (unless dilated), and (4) the vallecula of the cisterna magna (inconstant). All other major subarachnoid cisternal enlargements may be seen in lateral projection if there is optimal subarachnoid filling by gas.

Pneumograms made with the head in flexion result in full filling of the cisterna magna followed principally by ventricular filling, as described elsewhere. The general configuration of the cisterna magna in pneumograms conforms to that of the anatomy described and is quite familiar to radiologists. The outline of the inferior cerebellar margin in the early lateral pneumogram may be of importance to diagnose cerebellar expansion by an intrinsic mass. Herniation or impending herniation of the cerebellar tonsils may be seen. The superioinferior length of the cisterna magna from the top of the vallecula to the foramen magnum may measure 2 cm. Similarly, an anteroposterior measurement from the medulla oblongata to the posterior angle of the cisterna magna beneath the limiting membrane is usually 2 cm. In some instances, apparently normal variations, the cisterna magna may be considerably larger without denoting cerebellar hypoplasia or degeneration (fig. 221).

The anterior extension of the cisterna magna and its junction with the cisterna pontis usually is not clearly seen in the ordinary lateral pneumogram because of the density of the overlying temporal bones. When deformity and distortion are suspected, tomograms may be used to visualize the anterior medullary surface. This may be necessary with tumors of the clivus, tumors of the margin of the foramen magnum, and in basilar impression. The inferior margin of the pons and its junction with the medulla together with the membranes that bound the medial and inferior aspects of the lateral compartments of the cisterna pontis cannot be seen. In the average case, the upper two-thirds of the pons is clearly visible between the midline pontine gas shadow and the fourth ventricle; the lower third usually is obscured by the petrous areas. In some instances, it may be difficult to visualize ideally even the upper two-thirds of the pontine region and its associated cisterns without tomography, when the mastoid sinuses are unusually well developed.

Measurements concerning the distance from the fourth ventricle to the dorsum sellae and other measurements related to the fourth ventricle and iter have been given and their significance mentioned. A supplementary measurement is the distance from the ventral aspect of the pons to the clivus at the narrowest point of the cistern; the median width for normal patients is 0.5 cm. (fig. 213). A maximum normal measurement of 1.2 cm. and an average of 0.8 cm. are recognized; a normal minimum is difficult to establish because of variations in filling of the cisterna pontis at pneumography.

Passing upward along the anterior pontine margin in the encephalogram, the shadow arches backward, sometimes fairly sharply, and the interpeduncular cistern is then visualized. The basilar artery does not follow the sharp superior convexity of the pons but diverges from it to extend in a smoother arc up into the lumen of the cisterna interpeduncularis. Occasionally, the basilar artery may be followed to the highest point of the cistern, and it may even indent the floor of the third ventricle.

There are no measurements applicable to cisterns other than the ones above that are of clinical importance. Incomplete filling of the communicating subarachnoid pathways and the blending of shadows in the suprasellar cisterns are so common that it is impractical to apply measurements to these regions. It is more satisfactory to rely on deviations from anatomic appearances and asymmetry, particularly in the frontal view, for clues to the presence of disease. In the suprasellar region, the midline postchiasmatic portion is seen with a high degree of consistency in the lateral pneumogram. Failure of filling of this region must be regarded with strong suspicion as regards the possibility of a tumor. In lateral films made in the supine position, or in tomograms, the cisterns further forward frequently can be visualized, particularly the narrow cistern in front of the optic chiasm. The Sylvian cisterns often can be seen in such brow-up films end on just behind the sphenoid wings.

Two of the most prominent structures visualized in the lateral pneumogram are the comma-shaped retrothalamic cisterns, which usually are demonstrable extending from the midpeduncular area backward and upward to cross the midportion of the quadrigeminal plate. The two extensions usually are completely or partially superimposed. The shadows may appear quite wide, measuring 2 to 3 mm. in diameter. Anteriorly and inferiorly, each retrothalamic space ends against the uncus and has a flared configuration which occasionally may be evident in the lateral pneumogram.

Frontal views. Cisterns meriting extra study in the frontal pneumogram are (1) the lateral extensions of the cisterna pontis (cerebellopontine recesses), (2) the lateral aspect of the cisterna magna (cerebellomedullaris), (3) the left and right lateral communicating channels over the dorsolateral aspect of the brain stem, best seen in reverse half axial views, (4) the crural cisternal projections from the cisterna interpeduncularis, which also are seen best in reverse half axial projections. In addition, the olfactory sulci usually are seen only in frontal projections with the patient supine.

Gas extending outward from the lateral portion of the cisterna pontis forms a somewhat triangular and laterally elongated shadow along the posterior surface of the petrous bone and below the tentorium; it is angled upward approximately 30 degrees from the horizontal. The angle varies somewhat with the degree of flexion of the head used to make the radiograph and also varies with the slope of the petrous pyramids. The recess serves to outline the petrous margin and is clinically important since it is obliterated by tumors, usually neurinomas of the eighth nerve. If the recess is visible in the presence of tumor, it usually is elevated.

When the cerebellopontine recesses are completely filled, they have the configuration shown in Figures 184 and 220. They are normally symmetrical, but asymmetries are seen, often due to incomplete filling. It is common to encounter one side better filled than the other, or one cistern may not be filled at all. This is usually due to slight tilting of the head to one side when the head was extended and then flexed again to fill the cisterns (see "Technique"). In order to correct this situation, 5 cc. of gas should be injected with the head moderately extended, followed within 15 seconds by flexion of the head, this time slightly tilted toward the side showing greater filling. If after repeating this maneuver two or three times there is still no filling of a cerebellopontine recess, an abnormal situation such as a cerebellopontine angle tumor, or sometimes adhesions, must be considered.

A small round dense shadow is often seen in the cerebellopontine recess, laterally, produced by a tentorial vein. The shadow of the fifth nerve is often visible in the medial portion of the extension.

The crural cisterns are at a slightly greater angle than the cerebellopontine recesses from the transverse plane. Inferiorly, their bases are separated approximately 2 cm. and their length is approximately the same. The cisterns visualized at pneumography usually are quite thin shadows, corresponding to the narrow space between the peduncle and hippocampus on each side.

In the absence of ventricular filling, total reliance must be placed on evaluation of the subarachnoid space at pneumography. Frequently, the information that can be gained from careful examination of the subarachnoid spaces and the appearance of adjoining neural structures is sufficient for accurate diagnosis without resorting to other special radiologic procedures.

ANATOMIC VARIANTS

In this section, brief consideration will be given to a number of anatomic variants commonly encountered, almost all of which are incidental findings and have no known pathologic significance. Certain writers consider several of these variants to be developmental abnormalities. In some cases, they are associated with true congenital malformations, usually cerebral hypoplasia. Hypoplasia is discussed in the section on hydrocephalus. The variants may be related either to the ventricular system or the subarachnoid space.

Lateral Ventricles

The ventricular contours are relatively constant, except for the occipital horns, where variation is the rule. Nevertheless, some minor variations of configuration of the lateral ventricles may be encountered in the region of the frontal horns and in the ventricular body. Portions of the ventricular walls may be absent, such as the interventricular septum. The chorioid plexus contained within the ventricles may vary considerably.

Septum pellucidum. Agenesis of the septum pellucidum is relatively rare but partial absence of the septum is found occasionally at pneumography. Perforations of the septum pellucidum may occur secondary to internal hydrocephalus which may produce small or extensive defects. In the typical case of agenesis of the septum pellucidum, a simple single ventricular cavity is present without other anomalies. The ventricles are not usually enlarged but when dilatation occurs, it usually is mild. Secondary perforations of the septum, on the other hand, are associated with very large ventricles.

The recognition of agenesis of the septum pellucidum is usually easy when the frontal pneumogram is viewed. The thin white line separating the two lateral ventricles is absent, no vestige ordinarily being seen in this projection. In some instances, a small midsagittal projection is present into the confluent ventricular cavity from the roof. Films made in upright posture will demonstrate a common gas-fluid level across the midline (fig. 224).

In lateral view, a comma-shaped area of intensified radiability is present extending from the anterior horn to the posterior half of the ventricular body. The head of the comma shadow is in the preforaminal portion of the anterior horn with rapid tapering of the intensified radiolucent shadow in the postforaminal region. The rather sharp, dorsoventral tapering found with absence of the septum pellucidum differentiates it from the smoothly rounded configuration of a gas-filled cavum septum pellucidum along its posterior aspect. While the diagnosis is obvious from the frontal projection, there is also no difficulty in recognizing this defect from the lateral view alone on films made with the horizontal x-ray beam. In this position there again will be a common gas-fluid level in the two ventricles.

While absence of the septum pellucidum is of no importance by itself, many of the patients are examined by pneumography because they have convulsive seizures. The presence of slight rounding of the lateral angles and a first degree enlargement by measurement found in some cases suggests the possibility of structural deficiency of cerebral tissue.

Cysts of the septum pellucidum are of two varieties, those which communicate freely with the ventricular system and those which do not. The former are much more frequently encountered than the latter. In the case of noncommunicating cysts, it may be difficult to differentiate these benign variants from primary tumors of the septum pellucidum or tumors which involve this structure secondarily (see "Intraventricular Tumors"). Cysts which are noncommunicating at the time of the initial filming at pneumography may be found to contain gas at a later time if delayed films are made several hours after completion of the formal examination. Since such cysts are more frequently found in children, both by pneumography and necropsy, it has been suggested by Davidoff and Epstein (1950) that the condition is one which must often correct itself as an individual grows older.

The septum pellucidum is a double membrane covered by ependyma, the leaves of which are separated by a slitlike space or potential space. Through developmental variation, the space between the membranes may be wide, occasionally more than a centimeter. The cyst which results is often associated with a smaller but similar cavity further posteriorly, the *cavum Vergae*, and the two together are often referred to as the fifth and sixth ventricles of the brain.

The cavum septum pellucidum is bounded

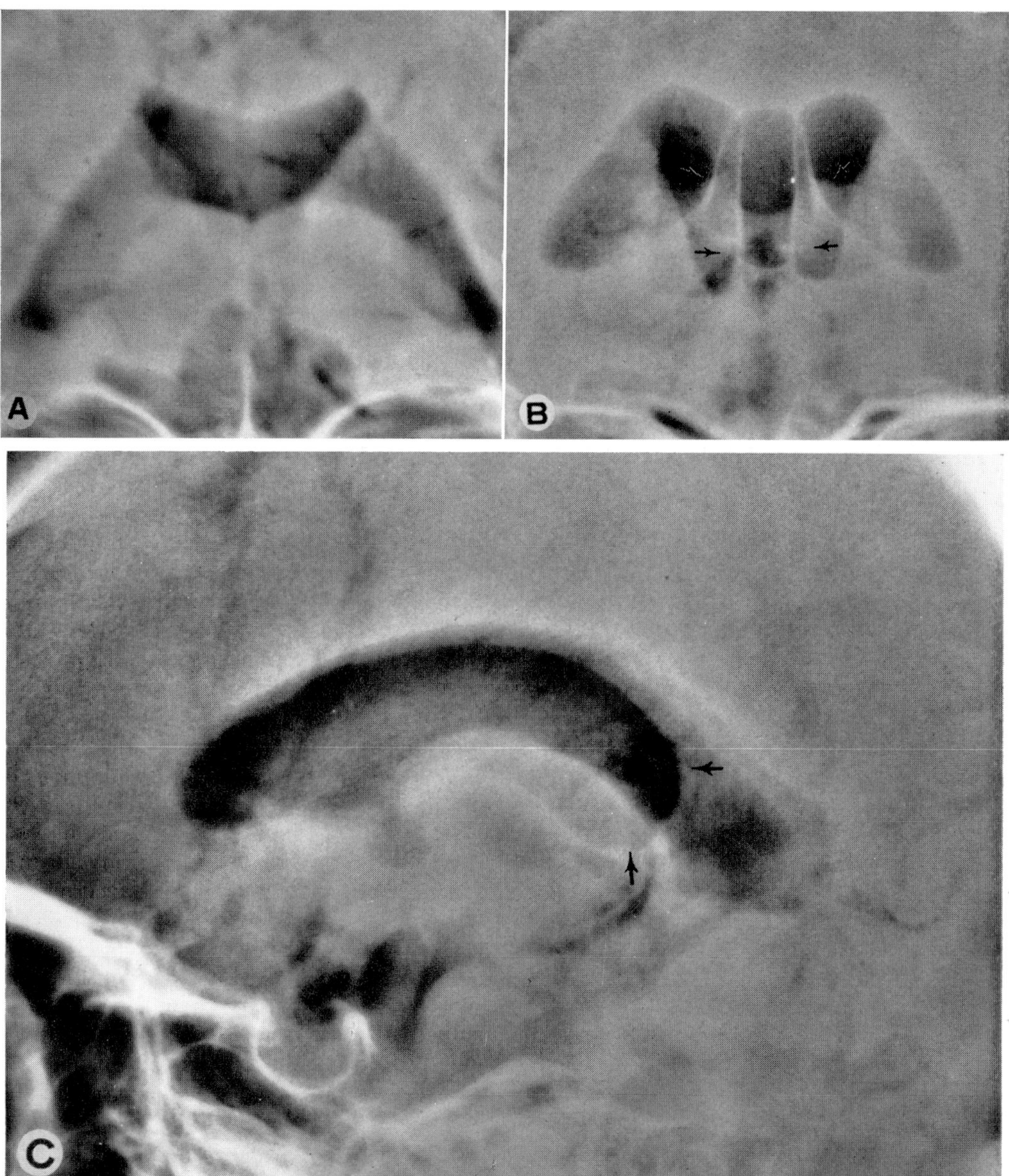

Fig. 224.—Anomalies of the Septum Pellucidum

Absence of the septum pellucidum ordinarily is easily recognized in the frontal projection (A). The central white line of the septum may be partially or completely absent; a common fluid level in the two lateral ventricles will be shown in films made with the horizontal x-ray beam.

The combined shadows of a cavum septum pellucidum and cavum Vergae are shown in frontal view (B). A ribbonlike shadow of air density is present in the midline anteriorly between the lateral ventricles, bounded by the parallel white lines of the leaves of the septum pellucidum (*arrows*). Further posteriorly, in the region of the cavum Vergae, the midline cavity is wider because the walls of the posterior ventricular bodies diverge. In lateral view, the dark shadow projected through the anterior horns and ventricular bodies represents the confluent shadows of the two cava, the anterior and posterior extremities being marked by *transverse arrows* (C). While the cavum Vergae is projected predominantly above the ventricular floor, it may extend below, as in this case (*vertical arrow*), and differentiation from a cavum vellum interpositum must be made (see Fig. 227).

(Revised 1963)

superiorly and anteriorly by the corpus callosum, the genu forming the anterior boundary. The anterior floor is formed by the rostrum of the corpus callosum and the anterior commissure. The posterior and inferior margins are formed by the anterior pillars of the fornix. Communication, if present, is with the third or lateral ventricles, sometimes both.

The cavum may be readily recognized in the frontal pneumogram where it appears as a third gas-filled space between the shadows of the lateral ventricles. The cavum is in the midline and is separated from the lateral ventricles by the two leaves of the septum pellucidum which appear as very thin, parallel white lines on either side of the central cavity (fig. 224). In lateral view, the cavum septum pellucidum is an elongated radiolucent shadow, concave downward along both its superior and inferior borders. The anterior and posterior extremities are smoothly rounded with the result that the over-all configuration is sausage-shaped. The top of the cavity is usually slightly below the ventricular roof, because the lateral ventricular angles are projected above it. The floor is essentially on the same level as the corresponding portion of the lateral ventricles. The anteroposterior extent is slightly less than that of the septum pellucidum itself. For the most part, the cavum septum pellucidum is of anatomic interest only. As with absence of the septum pellucidum, however, associated neural deformities may be present which account for the clinical disturbances leading to pneumography, usually epileptic seizures. Recognition of the true nature of a cavum septum pellucidum is important, however, when there is defective filling of a lateral ventricle as a result of intracranial tumor. If a gas-filled cavum septum pellucidum is mistaken for one lateral ventricle under these circumstances, false localization may result.

The *cavum Vergae* is not truly a cavity of the septum pellucidum but is closely related to it and may communicate with the latter. Rarely, a *cavum Vergae* may be found as an isolated accessory cavity. The superior boundary is formed by the body of the corpus callosum and the posterior margin by the splenium of this structure. Anteriorly, the cavity is bounded by the body of the fornix and the lateral walls are the posterior pillars of this structure. The floor is formed by the transverse fornix (psalterium). Thus, the *cavum Vergae* is a shallow, horizontal cleft between the inferior aspect of the corpus callosum and the posterior central portion of the body of the fornix. The *cavum Vergae*, like the cavum septum pellucidum, may exist as a cavity communicating with the ventricular system or as a noncommunicating fluid-containing compartment; the two cava may intercommunicate.

In frontal pneumograms, the communicating *cavum Vergae* appears as a midline cavity projected between the lateral ventricles. In lateral view, when both cava are present, the posterior end of the cavum septum pellucidum is not roundly blunted but an hourglass configuration develops with a second rounded compartment present behind the construction. Such a form suggests intercommunication or that the two compartments are in contact, if not communicating. When isolated, a communicating *cavum Vergae* may resemble a large olive and appear as an area of increased radiolucency projected through the junction of the ventricular body and atrium. The superior margin of the cavum is below the level of the ventricular roof, while the floor is on the same level as the floor of the lateral ventricles. Care should be taken not to confuse a *cavum Vergae*, which is above the fornix, with the cavum velum interpositum, which is beneath this structure. The latter is seen much more frequently than the *cavum Vergae*, as described below. Whenever it is desired to visualize any of these midline cavities to better advantage at pneumography, midsagittal tomography is recommended.

Ventricular configuration. Variations in ventricular configuration may be cornual or corporal. Among the latter, variations in ventricular size are to be considered as well as mural irregularities which may locally alter ventricular configuration, particularly in the region of the ventricular roof.

In earlier discussion, the variation in normal ventricular size has been described. Ventricular volume was studied by Bull (1961), who found between 7 and 20 cc. as the normal range of total ventricular capacity, with an average of 15 to 16 cc. Last and Tompsett (1953) considered 20 to 25 cc. more usual from their study of casts. The upper limit of normal is variable, but a volume in excess of 25 cc. probably is out of normal range. Various measurements to determine abnormality of ventricular size have been given earlier in this section.

As seen in frontal view, the lateral ventricles are remarkably symmetrical at pneumoencephalography in the average case, considering the many technical and physiological influences upon ventricular filling. Some degree of ventricular asymmetry, however, frequently is seen and may be considered within normal limits. Differences in the maximum width of the ventricular bodies up to 2 mm. are not of pathologic significance in the majority of instances. When a lateral ventricle is at the borderline between normality and enlargement, it is usually difficult to say whether this is a developmental variation or an acquired, usually degenerative, change. In younger individuals, a difference in size is more often on the basis of the former, and frequently a larger frontal or ethmoid sinus will be noted on the side of the larger ventricle. In older individuals, ventricles only slightly larger than average are not necessarily abnormal since there is a slowly progressive reduction in size of the brain after middle life. Often the frontal horns exhibit changes of atrophy earlier and to a greater degree than the ventricular body. The greatest degree of normal variation occurs in the region of the atria. One atrium frequently is found to be much more fully rounded than the other on postero-anterior pneumograms. In this region, a difference in width of the ventricles of as much as 5 mm. may be present without any apparent pathologic significance.

The most important consideration in connection with ventricular asymmetry is the difference in appearance which develops as a result of a small tumor. Narrowing of the lateral angle of a lateral ventricle may be the most significant clue in the early diagnosis of a supratentorial extraventricular mass and should lead the observer to seek confirmatory evidence of such a lesion elsewhere in the pneumogram. One of the most common mistakes in interpretation of pneumograms occurs owing to the larger, normal ventricle being considered slightly enlarged while the smaller, abnormally narrow ventricle is considered to be the normal structure. This error may be avoided by giving careful attention to the appearance of the lateral angle. The lateral corner, if truly angular, may be narrowed by pressure since a slightly rounded contour is the normal configuration.

A troublesome condition in pneumographic diagnosis is *coarctation* of the walls at the lateral angle of one ventricle, which was described by Davidoff in 1946. This variation occurs in an otherwise normal ventricular system. In the frontal pneumogram, the outer edge of the roof of the involved lateral ventricle is lower, the angle sharper, and the ventricular width less than on the opposite side. In these instances, as contrasted with the deformity of parasagittal tumor, no corroborating evidence of a mass is found on the other views made at pneumography. There is no dislocation of midline structures and no other ventricular deformity with coarctation (fig. 225).

Occasionally, an extra gas shadow may be visible in frontal films superimposed upon the inferior portion of the anterior horn. In lateral view, this is seen to be a blunt forward extension of the horn which may project as much as 1 cm. beyond the usual plane of the ventricular limit. This projection is sometimes referred to as a diverticulum of the frontal horn. Apparently it is caused by a defect in the anterior forceps of the corpus callosum. The variant may be unilateral or bilateral.

It is common to find, in lateral view, one or several sessile projections downward along the supraforaminal or superior preforaminal portion of the ventricular roof (fig. 225). The deformity is caused by radiations of the corpus callosum, which may be unilateral or bilateral. Lindgren (1941) referred to the indentations as condensed fibers of

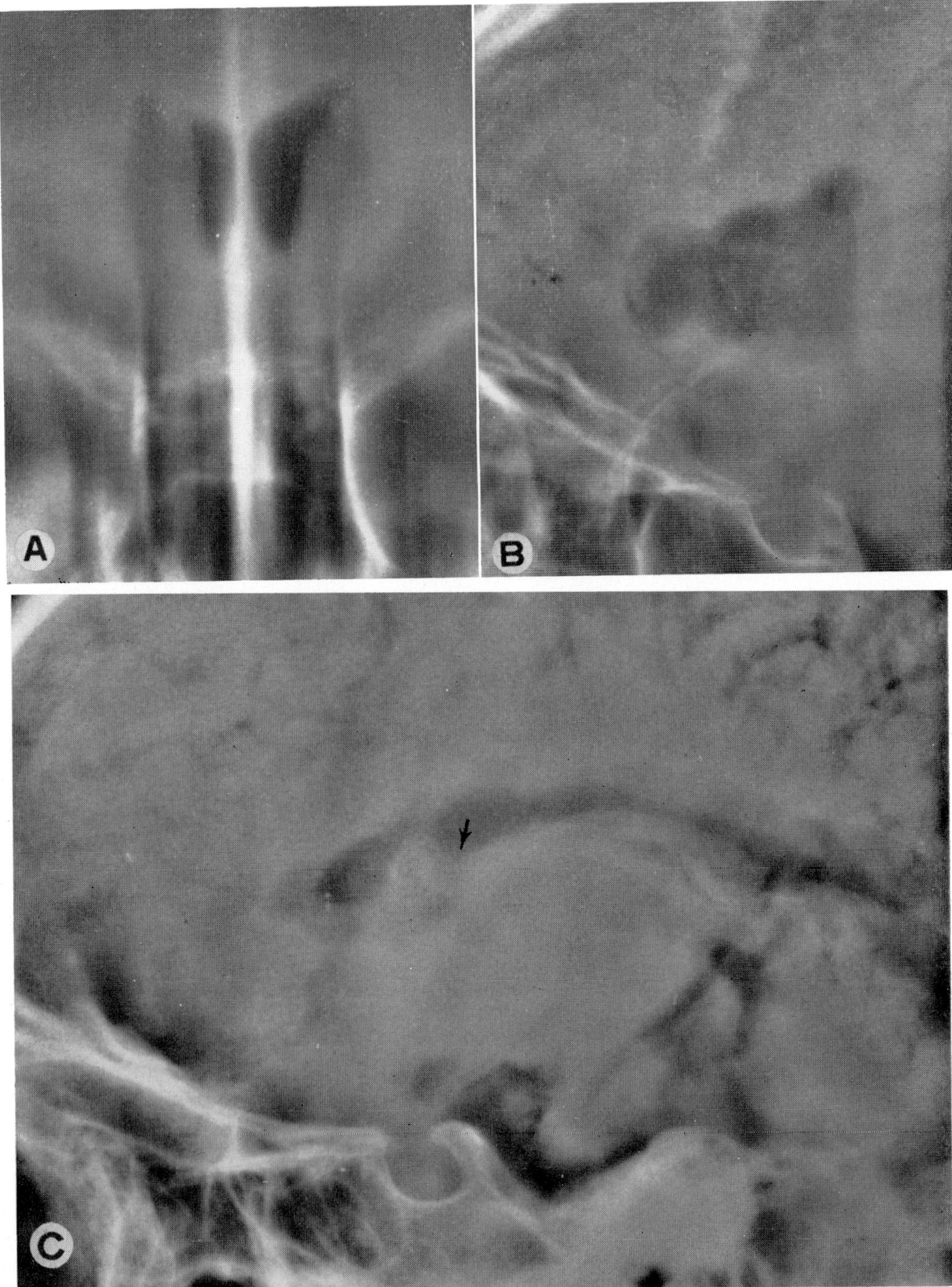

Fig. 225.—Variations of Ventricular Contour

Coarctation of the walls of the right lateral ventricle at the lateral angle is shown in an otherwise normal appearing ventricular system (A). The outer edge of the ventricular roof on the right is lower than on the left, and the lateral angle of the ventricular body is sharper. The width of the ventricular body is less than on the opposite side.

(Revised 1963)

the corpus callosum extending across the ventricle. Similar shallow indentations may be observed further posteriorly along the roof of the body, in some instances. There is usually no problem in differentiating the defects from tumor. The possibility of tuberous sclerosis may be suggested but the clinical and other radiologic manifestations of this condition, particularly calcification, are missing.

In the region of the atrial roof, the forceps major of the corpus callosum may exhibit varying degrees of prominence along the superior boundary of the trigone. At the junction of the superior wall of the atrium and the occipital horn, if present, the calcar avis (hippocampus minor) often produces an indentation of the ventricular lumen. The defect results from a deep lateral projection of the calcarine fissure which causes an invagination of the ventricular wall. The resulting notch in the ventricular outline may be of considerable size and depth. The defect is best seen in the lateral view, but the calcar avis also affects the medial wall of the atrium and occipital horn (fig. 211). Just above the calcar avis, the posterior forceps of the corpus callosum produces another medial indentation, the bulb of the occipital horn.

Variations along the ventricular floor are seen occasionally, and for the most part these are irregular defects owing to differences in development of the chorioid plexus. Different degrees of prominence of the caudate nucleus, fornix, and thalamus may cause minor changes in curvature and slope of the ventricular floor and side walls. Further posteriorly, prominence of the thalamus and fornix may encroach upon the base of the trigone or anterior wall of the atrium. In such cases, if the choroid glomus is prominent, the anteroposterior measurement of the atrium may be quite small.

The work of Last and Tompsett (1953), who made accurate measurements from ventricular casts, substantiates the belief that asymmetry of the occipital horns is the rule. It was found that the length of the occipital horn from the posterior portion of the atrium to the occipital tip varied between 0 and 3.4 cm. When a developed occipital horn is present, the average length is 2.0 cm.

The notch of the calcar avis may be of such prominence that in some positions, gas in the atrium may be separated from the gas shadow of the occipital horn. Under these circumstances, the occipital horn may appear as a separate cavity but should not be mistaken for an area of porencephaly. More important, when the occipital horn is absent, the shadow of the calcar avis combined with the posterior forceps of the corpus callosum may produce a sizable indentation which should not be mistaken for a periatrial tumor.

Chorioid plexus. Variations in the chorioid plexus of the lateral and third ventricles are common. Radiologic evidence of variants of the chorioid plexus of the fourth ventricle is not encountered frequently.

The chorioid plexus of the lateral ventricle is a horseshoe-shaped structure extending from the anterior portion of the temporal horn to the foramen of Monro. In the temporal horn, the plexus passes along the medial aspect of the ventricular roof in the supracornual cleft to the atrium. In the atrial region, there is normally an abundant amount of plexus tissue along the anterior wall, the glomus of the chorioid plexus. The chorioid plexus extends forward from the atrium to the foramen of Monro as one of the structures forming the floor of the body of the lateral ventricle. At the foramen of

---

A defect in the anterior forceps of the corpus callosum may result in a bilateral forward extension of the anterior horn (B). The wavy configuration of the ventricular roof is caused by irregular radiations of the corpus callosum extending across the ventricle.

An accessory glomus of the chorioid plexus is shown along the floor of a lateral ventricle just above the foramen of Monro (C). The mass of chorioid tissue appears attached to the floor of the ventricular body at its anterior extremity, just before the plexus passes through the foramen (*arrow*). Occurrence of accessory glomera most commonly is at this site; they frequently contain calcium, as in the case illustrated.

(Revised 1963)

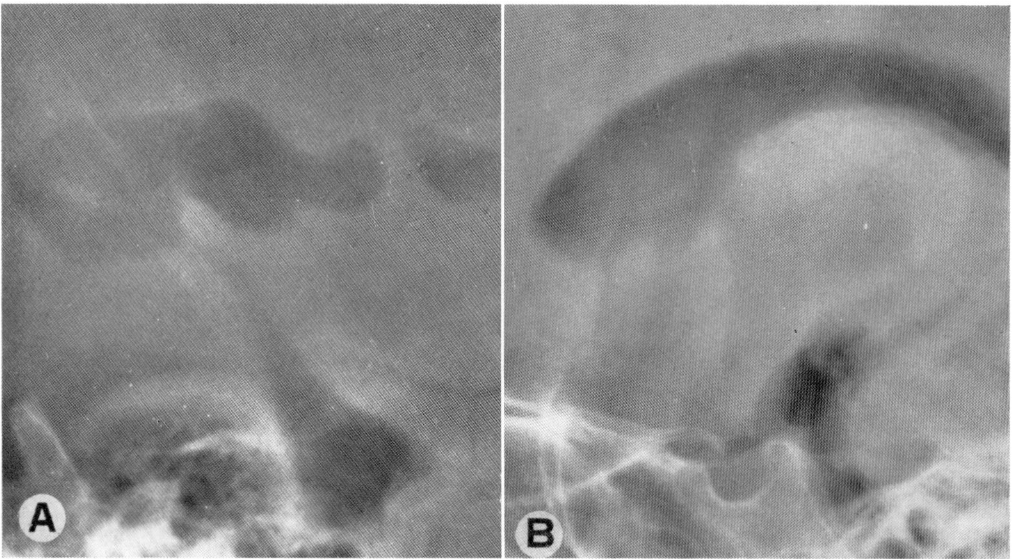

FIG. 226.—VARIATIONS OF THE THIRD VENTRICULAR RECESSES

A very large suprapineal recess may be found in an otherwise normal-appearing ventricular system (A). The most frequent variation is an elongation of the recess (see Fig. 211). In some instances, as in the case illustrated, there also is an increase in height and width of the recess.

Downward extension of the hypothalamic portion of the third ventricle is quite variable (B). In some normal cases, the optic and infundibular recesses are situated as much as 1 cm. above the sella turcica, and frequently more (see also Fig. 192). The distance from the tuberculum sellae to the chiasmatic notch between the optic and infundibular recesses may vary from one to more than two centimeters.

Monro, the plexus joins its mate from the opposite side and after passing through the foramen of Monro continues along the third ventricular roof posteriorly as the tela chorioidea. There is no chorioid tissue in the frontal horn or occipital horn.

Variations in the region of the chorioid glomus of the atrium are abundant. Asymmetry is quite common. In some instances, one chorioid glomus may be only 0.5 cm. in diameter, while the other may be very large, producing a conspicuous filling defect in the atrial outline. The glomus may be oval as well as globular, and in such instances the major diameter of the ovoid may measure 2 cm. or more. In many instances, the atrial enlargement of the chorioid plexus is more elongated or spindle-shaped.

A difference in position of the glomus on the two sides is common. In some atria, the glomus will be found directly behind the thalamus. In other instances it will be near the junction of the atrium and ventricular body or it may be found near the posterior portion of the temporal horn. The glomus may be pedunculated and move about within the cavity of the ventricle with change in posture of the head.

The chorioid plexus of the ventricular body also is variable in appearance. Mainly, it is quite low and flat and blends with the other structures of the ventricular floor. In other patients, however, it is quite prominent and clearly visible in the frontal pneumogram where it appears as an irregular elevation 2 or even 3 mm. in width. In some instances, accessory glomera may be found in the ventricular body (Wood, 1944). These enlargements may have a diameter of 5 mm. or slightly more. The common site of occurrence is near the foramen of Monro but small enlargements may be found anywhere along the course of the plexus in the ventricular body (fig. 225).

(Revised 1963)

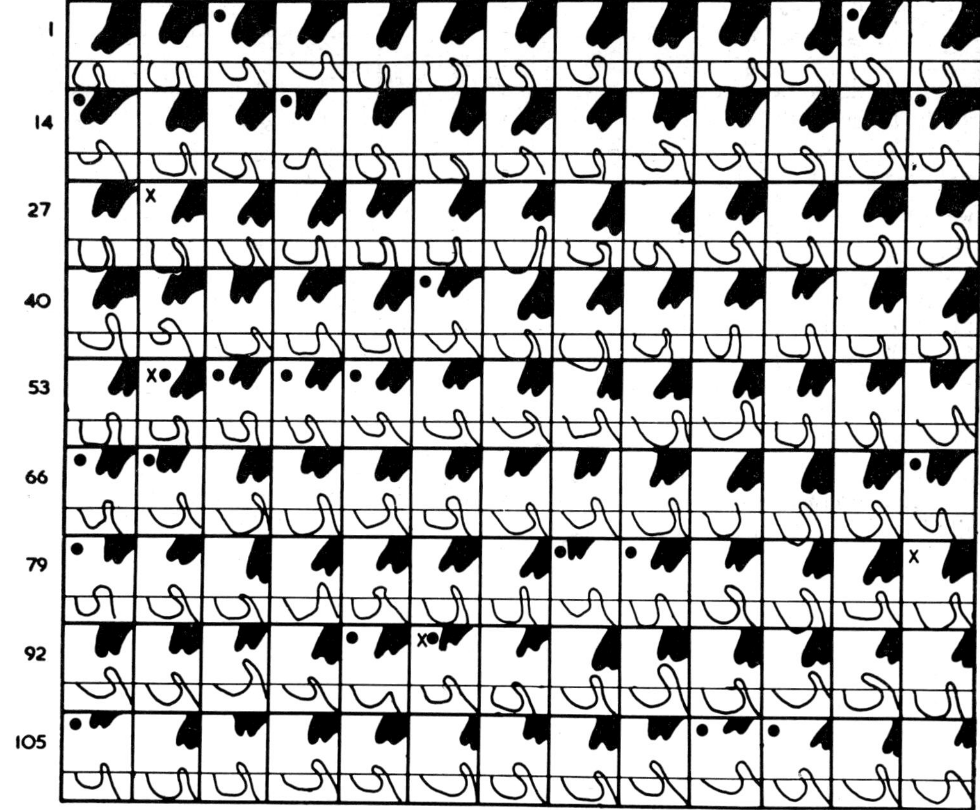

Fig. 226-C.—Tracings of 117 Normal Third Ventricles

Considerable normal variation in configuration of the anterior recesses, as well as in their position (C), is encountered (see text). (Courtesy of James Bull, M.D., F.R.C.P., F.F.R., London.)

Calcification is common in the localized enlargements of the chorioid plexus or glomera (see "Intracranial Calcification"). In some instances, only small punctate deposits are visible radiologically, while in other instances extensive conglomerate masses of calcium are evident. Calcium deposits of small size may be seen in the accessory glomera of the ventricular body, particularly near the foramen of Monro. Small deposits rarely can be identified in the region of the tela chorioidea of the third ventricle and in the chorioid plexus of the fourth ventricle.

At ventriculography, the chorioid shadow may be found to be enlarged as a result of trauma from the needle tip when an atrial puncture has been carried out (Dyke, Elsberg, and Davidoff, 1935). On these occasions, the traumatized glomus may be markedly enlarged as a result of hemorrhage within the chorioid tissue and may fill more than half of the atrial lumen. The large size or unilateral presence of such a mass should not lead to an erroneous diagnosis of intraventricular neoplasm (fig. 196).

Third Ventricle

The third ventricle is relatively constant in its general configuration. There is, however, some variation in the height and width of the third ventricular cavity, the variation being much greater in frontal projection than in lateral view. Differences in height probably are related more to projection and degree of ventricular distention by gas than to normal variation in size.

Recesses. Variation is more common in

the region of the hypothalamic recesses and the peripineal recesses than in the main portion of the third ventricle. Bull (1956) found remarkable differences in the relation of the hypothalamic cavity to the sella turcica in normal subjects. Variations in position of the optic recess of the third ventricle may be gross (fig. 226).

Enlargement of the suprapineal recess is one of the most common variants of the third ventricle. Robertson (1957) reported its occurrence in 2 per cent of patients. In some instances, the suprapineal recess is large in height and width, and it is frequently very long. In one of the cases examined by Robertson, the recess measured 4 cm. in length. The same author, performing pneumoencephalography on conjoined twins united at the vertex, found a huge curved outpouching from the posterior portion of the third ventricle extending to a point that ordinarily would be located near the midpoint of the sagittal suture. Mirror images of the ventricular system were found in the twins, and the fundi of the pouches were separated by a distance of only 2 mm. In the former case with the 4-cm. length suprapineal recess, a large parieto-occipital bone defect was present.

It is postulated that a large suprapineal recess develops owing to varying degrees of interference with the downward migration of the third ventricle which accompanies growth of the cerebral hemispheres. It has been suggested that the suprapineal recess is a vestige of the pineal eye. The hypothesis is that the pineal organ was once a complex structure composed of a median eye, situated in the midsagittal plane, and a related glandular structure connected with the third ventricle. In some reptiles, a median eye is thought to represent the upper portion. In mammals, only the glandular portion together with some commissures and other neural elements are found (Robertson, 1957, and Keith, 1954).

Ordinarily, the suprapineal recess is a small cavity at the posterior superior extremity of the third ventricle, above the pineal body and habenular commissure. It extends backward beneath the corpus callosum into the quadrigeminal cistern for varying distances. It is not unusual in a normal individual to find a posterior extension of 1 to 1.5 cm. behind the midpoint of the pineal body. The height of the recess also varies, but in the average case it does not exceed 2 to 3 mm. When the length exceeds 1 cm., the terminal portion frequently points upward toward the parietal region, a miniature of the very large recess found in connection with the developmental abnormalities mentioned above (figs. 226 and 238).

Usually, a conspicuous suprapineal recess is not of pathologic or clinical significance. In the case of hypertensive hydrocephalus, there may be marked dilatation of the recess which then may be called a pressure diverticulum of the third ventricle. The wall may become so thin in some instances that it ruptures. A communication then is established between the third ventricle and quadrigeminal cistern, providing a rare spontaneous decompression of the internal hydrocephalus.

The pineal recess is extremely variable in size and development. In the majority of pneumograms it is not sufficiently filled with gas to be visible. In some instances, however, there is an invagination of the pineal body by the posterior portion of the third ventricle to a depth of 4 to 5 mm. The infrapineal recess is not an extension of the third ventricle but is a fluid space extending forward from the quadrigeminal cistern between the inferior surface of the pineal body and the superior portion of the quadrigeminal plate.

Pineal gland. The great variations in the appearance of the pineal gland as regards both size and shape are well recognized and have been mentioned elsewhere (see "Intracranial Calcification"). One variant, the cystic pineal gland, may be worthy of reemphasis at this juncture. Such cysts are thought to develop within the pineal body owing to distention of an obliterated portion of the embryologic pineal diverticulum. In plain films, a ringlike calcium shadow often is present about the periphery, resulting from calcific degeneration in the parenchymal portion. Cases have been encountered in which a cystic pineal body more than 1 cm. in diameter was present. In the pneumogram, a large rounded indentation of the third ventricle is found, resulting from a mass which corresponds to the calcified wall of the cyst visible in plain films. Associated narrowing of the aqueduct of Sylvius has been reported in some instances of cystic pineal body. While the authors have observed an apparent narrowing just behind the aditus in one instance, there was no interference with ventricular filling and no correlation with clinical findings could be made. Cases which have been followed by plain films have shown no change in the size of the calcific ring with the passage of time.

Subarachnoid Space

Variations in the subarachnoid space are too numerous to discuss as a separate entity. Instead, their consideration is integrated with discussion of pathologic conditions as they affect the cisterns and general subarachnoid pathways. Only two variants will be mentioned here.

Cisterna magna. The cisterna magna is extremely variable in size, as has been mentioned earlier. It may communicate freely with the subarachnoid space over the superior surface of the cerebellum and may even extend above the usual plane of the tentorium. The main significance of the variation in size of the cisterna magna is its technical effect on ventricular filling. The presence of unusually large cisternal reservoirs may require the use of undesirable quantities of gas, unless proper positioning of the head is carried out to compensate for the trapping of gas (see under "Technique"). The occurrence of such a large cisternal cavity does not denote cerebellar atrophy in the majority of instances (fig. 221).

Cavum velum interpositum. The *interventricular cavum* (cavum velum interpositum) is a space that passes forward from the quadrigeminal cistern above the roof of the third ventricle. The cavity develops owing to an unusual separation of the crura of the fornix. Because the crura diverge more widely than normally, there also is an increased separation of the ventricular atria.

(Revised 1963)

The quadrigeminal cistern, situated medial to the crura, is unusually wide and deep. The thalami are widely separated. The narrow space extending between the spread thalami is the cavum velum interpositum. Above, the cavity is bounded by the fornix anteriorly and hippocampal commissure posteriorly. The floor is bounded by the roof of the third ventricle anteriorly, and the suprapineal recess or pineal body posteriorly.

A cavum velum interpositum is found fairly frequently at intracranial pneumography. As is the case with the cavum septum pellucidum and *cavum Vergae*, the variation is found more commonly in children, and the same question may be raised as to whether spontaneous obliteration of the cavity may not occur with the passage of time. As far as is known, no pathologic state is associated with the presence of the interventricular cavum. In a group of children studied by Zellweger (1951), mental retardation was a prominent part of the clinical picture and significant anomalies, such as defects of the corpus callosum, were found in several cases.

In pneumograms, the interventricular cavum may be seen in frontal as well as in lateral projection. In lateral view, the roof of the interventricular cavum is projected just beneath the floor of the posterior portion of the lateral ventricular body. The floor of the cavity is projected above the posterior portion of the third ventricular roof. It will be recalled that the floor of the *cavum Vergae* parallels the floor of the lateral ventricle. Therefore, there should be no difficulty in differentiating the two cavities. The interventricular cavum may be wide and lentil-shaped or narrow and curvilinear. When narrow, it often is crescent-shaped, paralleling the curve of the floor of the body of the lateral ventricle and the anterior wall of the atrium (fig. 227). The curved gas shadow may pass forward almost to the foramen of Monro. Posteriorly, there may be either a wide or an inconspicuous communication with the quadrigeminal cistern.

In frontal projection, the interventricular cavum is rounded or oval in shape. The midline cavity and the shadow of the septum pellucidum are superimposed in anteropos-

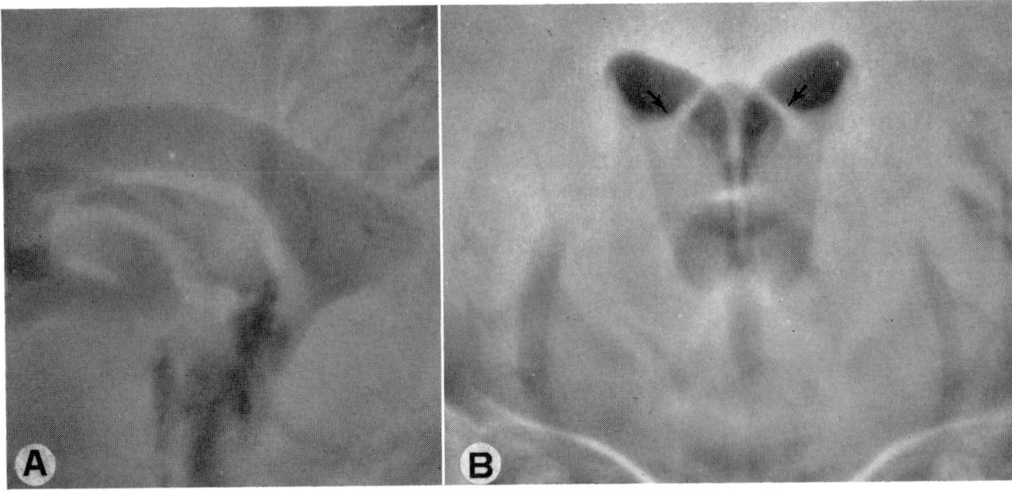

Fig. 227.—Cavum Velum Interpositum (Interventricular Cistern)

The interventricular cistern is an enlargement of the anterior extension of the quadrigeminal cistern to form a cavum above the roof of the third ventricle (A). In this case the third ventricle is deformed by a suprasellar tumor. The cistern may extend as far forward as the foramen of Monro. The cavity is wide posteriorly and tapered anteriorly; both the superior and inferior walls are ventrally concave. The result is a comma-shaped shadow, projected between the outline of the lateral ventricles and the roof of the third ventricle. In lateral view, the top of the interventricular cistern usually is not projected above the level of the lateral ventricular floor, and should not be mistaken for a cavum Vergae (see Fig. 224).

In frontal view (B), the interventricular cistern appears as a midline cavity upon which the shadow of the septum pellucidum is superimposed. The cavity is situated between the wide space caused by a developmental separation of the thalami. The medial walls of the posterior portions of the lateral ventricles also are widely separated (*arrows*), with narrowing of the ventricular lumina.

terior views. The shadow of the interventricular cavum also is superimposed upon the enlarged triangular shadow of the quadrigeminal cistern, the apex of the triangle directed superiorly. The base is wide, for reasons explained above. The thalamic shadows are more widely separated than usual in the frontal projections, and there is often a corresponding increase in width of the ventricular bodies themselves.

Development of the subarachnoid space is thought to occur owing to the outflow of cerebrospinal fluid from the fourth ventricle. Factors effecting cerebrospinal fluid circulation during embryonic life, therefore, may exert considerable influence on the size of the cisterna magna and, indeed, the development of all of the cisterns. The natural process of fusing of adjacent membranes opposes the development of cisternal cavities in prenatal life. The height of cerebrospinal fluid pressure may have a significant effect at this stage on the cleavage of cellular layers. How much influence a high prenatal pressure may have in the development of some of the variants described is not known.

Hydrocephalus

Because satisfactory pneumography includes visualization of the ventricular system a change in size should be one of the most readily appreciated alterations when the ventricles are abnormal. The common change in size is enlargement, although a few disease processes are associated with small ventricles. The precise upper limit of normal ventricular size is difficult to define; an average adult range has been given under "Anatomy" (figs. 212 and 214). In early life, the ventricles usually are small, with sharply defined anatomic boundaries and angles as previously described. With advancing years, there is usually some gradual enlargement of the lateral ventricles and the corners may be less angular. Lateral ventricles which measure more than 4 cm. across the roofs of the two ventricular bodies are, with few exceptions, abnormally large. In some instances, ventricles which measure less than 4 cm. in transverse diameter may suggest, to the experienced eye, evidence of enlargement when minor changes in form are present. Rounding of the lateral or of the inferior angle, a reduced prominence of the side wall or other alteration in slope of a ventricular boundary may accompany mild enlargement. A method of measurement which has been found satisfactory for daily use to confirm enlargement of the ventricular body is shown in Figure 214. Evidence of enlargement often may develop first in the region of the anterior horn and in the atrium of the lateral ventricles; although some normal asymmetry may occur, the earliest changes of ventricular dilatation or hydrocephalus may be detected in these segments. Enlargement of the third ventricle is more often a late rather than an early manifestation of hydrocephalus, while fourth ventricular enlargement may be a predominant or even isolated finding in the presence of certain cerebellar hypoplastic or degenerative disease processes.

Hydrocephalus as used here is a widely encompassing term and not limited merely to the extreme examples of ventricular dilatation commonly seen in connection with the infantile developmental abnormalities. Ventricular enlargement may be conveniently divided into two general types: (1) hydrocephalus *ex vacuo* and (2) obstructive hydrocephalus. The first type also may be referred to as *hypotensive*, while the second may be called *hypertensive* hydrocephalus. The former results chiefly from supratentorial lesions of various types; since this variety is ordinarily not accompanied by clinical or radiologic evidence of increased intracranial pressure, pneumoencephalography, rather than ventriculography, ordinarily is the procedure of choice. Unfortunately, in the majority of instances the changes of hydrocephalus *ex vacuo* are not reversible and in only a few instances can satisfactory treatment be instituted.

(*Revised 1963*)

Hypertensive or obstructive hydrocephalus, on the other hand, usually requires treatment to relieve the obstruction and the increased pressure. The majority of obstructions result from neoplasm, although numerous nontumorous conditions produce obstruction, particularly in younger individuals. (Tumors will be dealt with in a later section.) The majority of non-neoplastic obstructing lesions are infratentorial in location; and, because there is frequently clinical and radiologic evidence of increased intracranial pressure, ventriculography is usually required to demonstrate the obstructed site.

HYPOTENSIVE HYDROCEPHALUS

This type of hydrocephalus, also called *hydrocephalus ex vacuo* (by virtue of a vacuum), may be caused by either congenital or acquired disease. The majority of congenital lesions are the result of maldevelopment of neural tissue. They may vary from the severe form of cerebral agenesis to a relatively well localized area of cerebral hypoplasia. In other instances, the neural changes may be secondary to vascular disease, to infection, and to numerous other acquired pathologic conditions.

Cerebral Hypoplasia

Hypoplasia may be generalized or focal and, as previously mentioned, may vary tremendously in the extent of failure of brain development. In addition, various specific maldevelopments may occur which may overshadow the generalized hypoplasia because of their striking pneumographic appearance. An example is agenesis of the corpus callosum, which is often described as an entity but which is never isolated and constitutes only the most obvious and conspicuous change in the midst of various less dramatic malformations.

An enormous number of maldevelopments of the brain have been described pathologically, and the pneumographic appearances associated with these maldevelopments have

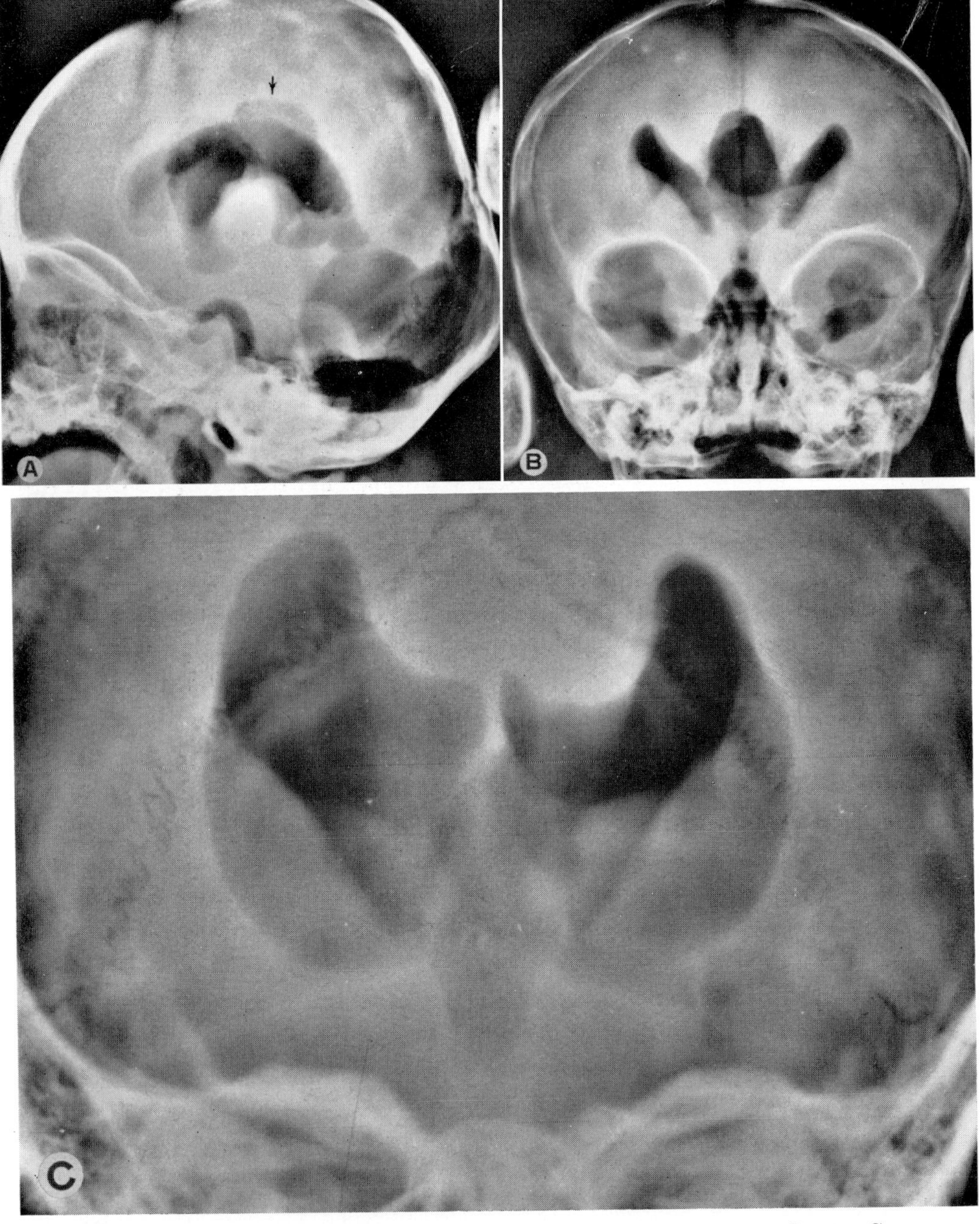

Fig. 228.—Cerebral and Cerebellar Hypoplasia with Agenesis of the Corpus Callosum

The lateral view reveals a cranium which is small by absolute measurement, and in relation to the facial structures, indicating microcephalus (A). The anterior fontanelle is narrow for the patient's age. There is enlargement of the ventricles and of the subarachnoid space, both above and below the tentorium. The findings indicate generalized hypoplasia of cerebral and cerebellar structures, and intracranial hypotension. Upward extension of the third ventricle above the level of the lateral ventricular roofs can be seen (*arrow*).

(Revised 1963)

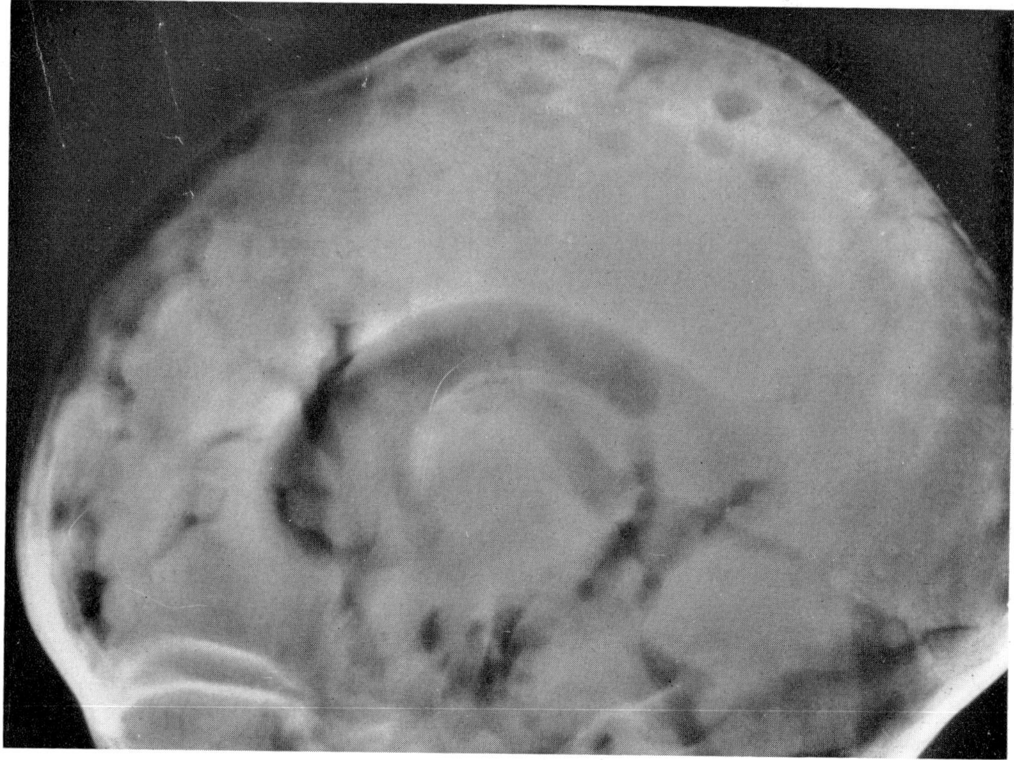

FIG. 229.—CORTICAL HYPOPLASIA

In some instances, widening of the subarachnoid space over the cerebral convexity may denote cerebral hypoplasia or degeneration, even in the absence of ventricular enlargement. The cerebral sulci exceed 3 mm. in width and extend deeply between the gyri; the latter often are flat and have beveled margins. In infants, caution must be exercised in diagnosing cortical hypoplasia without other changes. The frontal gyri often appear small early in life, but when pneumoencephalography is performed in later years, an essentially normal appearing cortical surface may be found (see Fig. 230). In the case illustrated, a pneumogram performed two years later revealed further enlargement of the subarachnoid space and a mild degree of ventricular enlargement had supervened. An interventricular cistern is present.

been described in the living by many authors. No attempt will be made to describe the pneumographic changes associated with all of the pathologic maldevelopments that can occur. In the majority of instances, the skull is small and this may be unilateral if the hypoplasia is predominantly or entirely on one side. In a fair number of instances, however, a relatively normal skull size is maintained. In these cases, the smallness of the intracranial soft tissue shadows and the very large fluid spaces, either ventricular or subarachnoid, may be very striking (fig. 228). Sometimes it appears that there is only a thin membrane overlying certain portions of one lateral ventricle, while in other areas

---

The frontal projection also shows upward extension of the enlarged third ventricle between the separated (developmentally unapproximated) lateral ventricles, resulting from a specific maldevelopment of the corpus callosum, in addition to the general hypoplasia (B). In other instances, in which the corpus callosum is not as greatly malformed centrally, the third ventricle does not extend as high; however, the lateral ventricular roofs are defective, and the latter structures extend upward and laterally in a hornlike manner (C).

(Revised 1963)

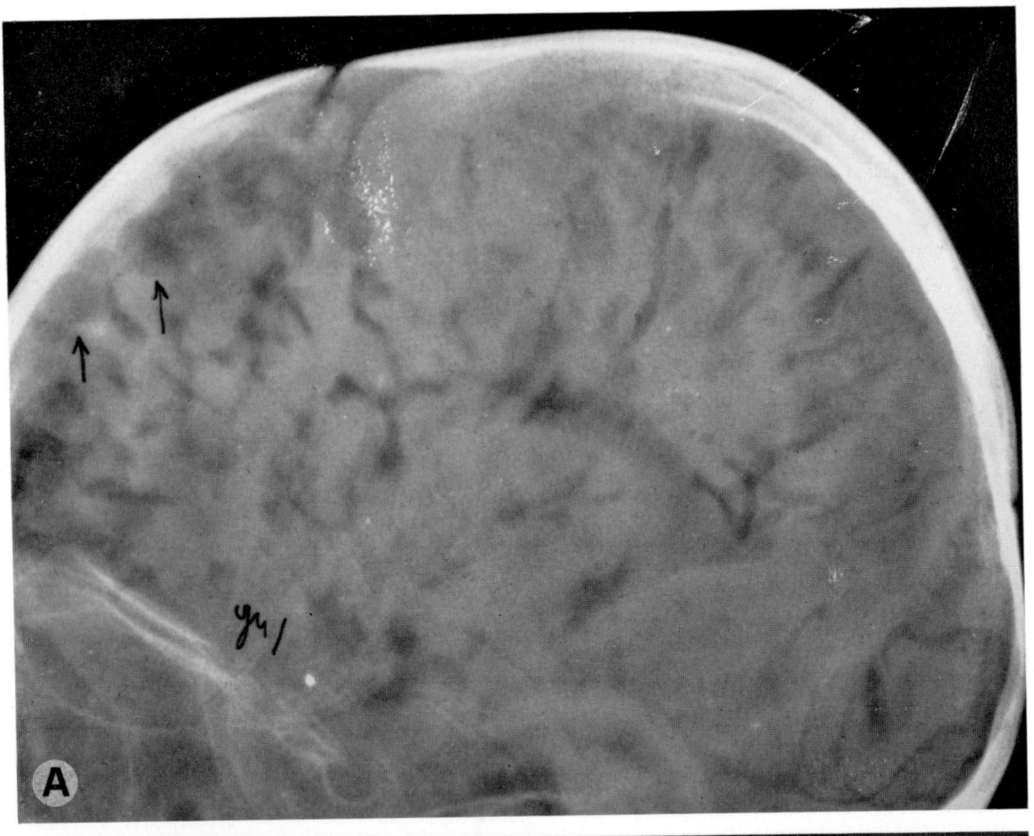

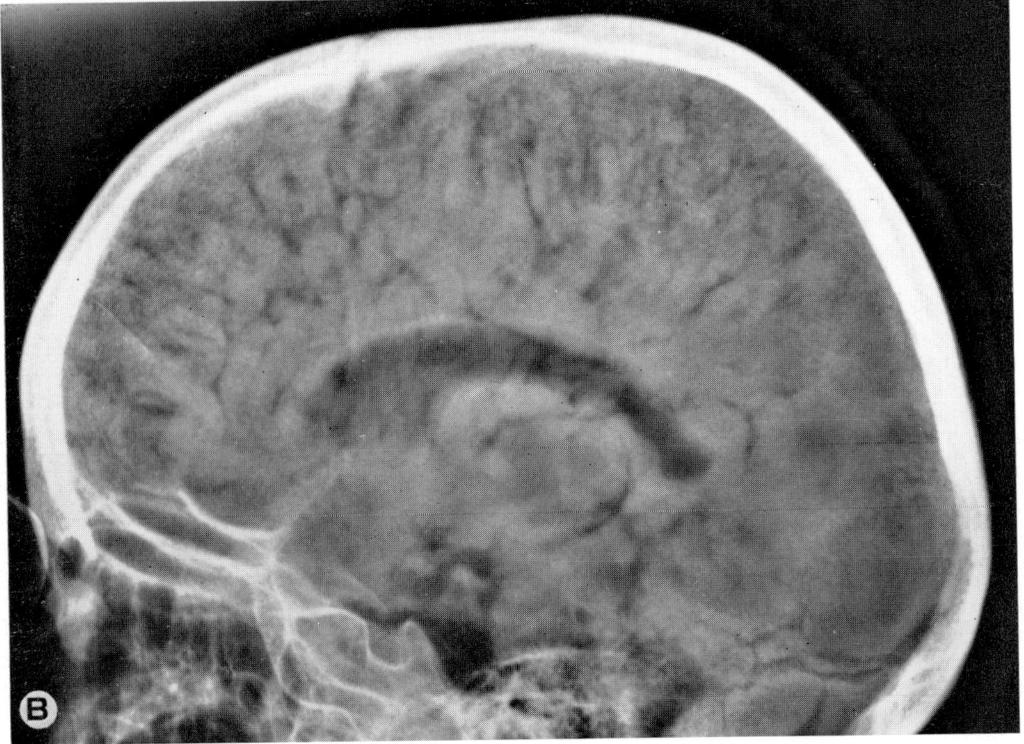

Fig. 230

(Revised 1963)

cerebral tissue measuring 1 to 2 cm. in thickness may be present. The enlarged ventricle may exhibit "ribbing," thought to be the result of crossing veins and other resistant structures, but this is more common in the hypertensive type of hydrocephalus. In other instances, the enlarged ventricle may appear compartmented and the sections may fill inconstantly. It is now considered unwise, in the presence of markedly enlarged ventricles, to substitute large quantities of gas for fluid (see "Morbidity and Complications"). For this reason there may be difficulty in obtaining a clear pneumographic picture of anatomic details when there is marked hypoplasia.

At the other end of the spectrum is found unilateral atrial enlargement or the unilateral presence of an occipital horn, both of which are considered normal variations. Between these two extremes, there are varying degrees of ventricular enlargement and cisternal and sulcal enlargement (figs. 229 and 230). Widening of the subarachnoid space over the cerebral convexity, and deeply extending wide cerebral sulci between rather flat beveled gyri, may be indicative of cerebral malformation or degeneration, even in the absence of ventricular enlargement. Sulci measuring 2 mm. in width in pneumograms are prominent and those measuring 3 mm. are abnormally wide (fig. 237). Similarly, cerebellar folia which appear small and which are separated by large gas collections indicate cerebellar hypoplasia or atrophy (fig. 231). Simple enlargement of the cisterna magna does not denote disease.

A few of the specific anomalies which have received widespread attention in the pneumographic literature may be worthy of brief description; for instance, agenesis of the septum pellucidum, agenesis of the corpus callosum, and the hemicranial and hemicerebral changes described by Dyke, Davidoff and Masson (1933). Failure of development of the septum pellucidum has been described under "Anatomic Variants."

Agenesis of the corpus callosum is a convenient term to denote a group of changes associated with defective formation of this structure. The term agenesis may be incorrect in many instances since the roof structure may be only partially malformed or partially absent. Frequently, there is rather generalized hypoplasia of one or both cerebral hemispheres associated with the corpus callosum abnormality. Failure of this large commissure to bridge the hemispheres causes the ventricles to remain separated from one another. With the lateral ventricles separated and the corpus callosum absent, the third ventricle can enlarge and extend upward along the midline, and often this occurs to a remarkable degree (fig. 228). When the vertical extension of the third ventricle is not so great, subarachnoid gas outlining the superior longitudinal fissure may extend downward further than usual.

In the frontal projection of the pneumogram, a rather characteristic appearance is presented. The lateral ventricles are concave medially, and their superior aspects often are pointed and hornlike in configuration. Frequently, however, there is rounding of the ventricular outlines associated with enlargement from generalized hypoplasia. The falx cerebri may extend down normally and produce an indentation of the enlarged third ventricle. The frontal horns often are malformed. While there is no specific clinical picture associated directly with agenesis of the corpus callosum, mental changes are commonly found. The pneumographic changes associated with this specific malformation were described by Davidoff and Dyke in 1934; in most of their patients the pneumogram was performed because of convulsive disorders.

Fig. 230.—Normal Infantile Cortex Simulating Hypoplasia

The pneumogram of a one-year-old infant, who developed convulsive seizures, exhibits wide deep sulci, and apparently small gyri (*arrows*), over the frontal portion of the brain (A). A second pneumogram, made at the age of four years, reveals a normal cortical and ventricular appearance (B). In infancy, allowance must be made for gyri which are normally small at this stage of brain development (compare with Fig. 229).

(Revised 1963)

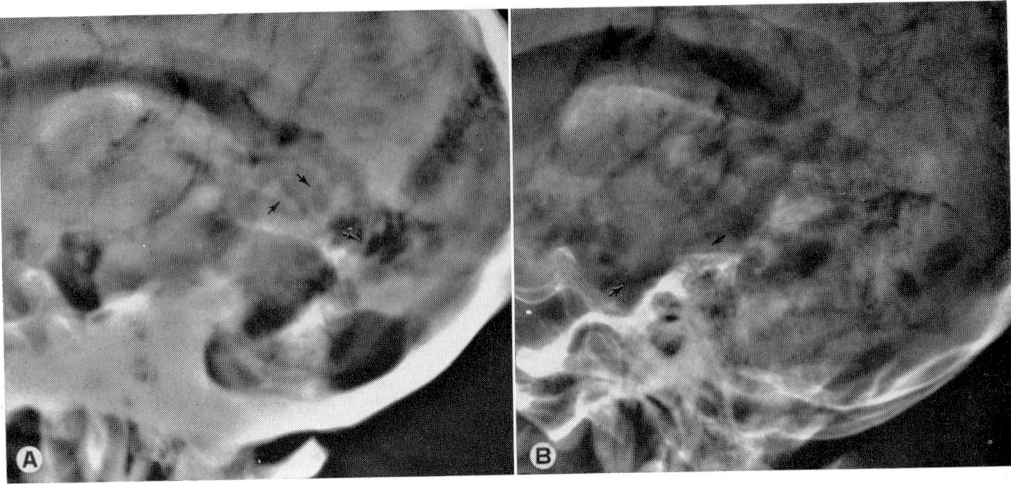

FIG. 231.—CEREBELLAR HYPOPLASIA AND ATROPHY

Hypoplasia of the cerebellum occurs in connection with generalized maldevelopment of the brain (see Fig. 228), but occasionally it may be seen as an isolated entity (A). The fourth ventricle is moderately enlarged; the cisterna magna is much larger than usual, although not incompetent; gas in the subarachnoid space over the cerebellar hemispheres outlines numerous small maldeveloped cerebellar folia (*arrows*). Atrophy of the cerebellum is not rare as an independent finding (B). In the case illustrated, the clinical entity of olivopontocerebellar atrophy was diagnosed. Except for a small brain stem shadow—between the floor of the fourth ventricle and the dorsal margin of an enlarged cisterna pontis (*arrows*)—the appearance cannot be differentiated radiologically from other types of cerebellar atrophy, or from cerebellar hypoplasia.

Cerebellar Hypoplasia

Cerebellar changes may be found as a fragment of general hypoplasia of the brain or, more rarely, as an independent entity. The diagnosis must be based on demonstration of actual smallness of the cerebellum, and it is helpful to find absolute enlargement of the fourth ventricle. Because the size of the cisterna magna varies tremendously, the diagnosis of cerebellar hypoplasia or atrophy cannot be made on the basis of large size of the cisterna magna as an isolated finding. The combination of (1) a wide cisterna magna, not sealed off in the usual way but communicating widely with the subarachnoid space over the cerebellum, (2) a wide foramen of Magendie joining the cistern with a large fourth ventricle, and (3) actual smallness of the cerebellum, constitutes good evidence of cerebellar hypoplasia. Frequently, there is enlargement of the anterior cisterns owing to smallness of the brain stem. In some instances of hypoplasia the cerebellar convexity is irregular and nodular, but the cerebellar folia are not prominent. The folia are quite conspicuous in atrophy, although shrunken, with deep, wide fluid spaces separating them (fig. 231).

In both frontal and lateral pneumograms, enlargement of the fourth ventricle should be evident. The abnormal cerebellar surface and wide circumferential subarachnoid space may be clearly shown in both views, as well as the large cisterna magna. Enlargement of the communication between the fourth ventricle and cisterna magna at the foramen of Magendie may be seen in the routine lateral pneumogram, but often it is best brought out in a midsagittal tomogram.

The size of the cisterna magna varies with the occipital cranial shape and, more importantly, with irregularities of meningeal development and attachment. Failure of development of the limiting membrane results in an "incompetent" cistern, with a wide communication between the cisterna magna and the subarachnoid spaces over the cerebellar surfaces. When the tentorial attachment is defective posteriorly, it is possible for the cisterna magna to extend upward for a considerable distance. Several cases have been seen in which the cistern extended as far upward as the lambda. The cerebellum in these cases was normal.

Meningoceles or meningoencephaloceles usually can be diagnosed clinically, but occasionally pneumography is useful to determine whether or not, and to what extent, cerebral herniation is involved in the anomaly. Similar protrusions may occur in the midline frontal region and elsewhere. They are most common in connection with the spine, and reference is made again to these lesions in the section dealing with myelography.

Specific Diseases

Tuberous sclerosis. This condition has been discussed earlier with regard to its pathologic background, in the section dealing with "Intracranial Calcification." The nodules of multiple cerebral sclerosis are scattered throughout the hemispheres and are quite commonly found in the subependymal regions of the ventricles. The resultant changes in pneumograms were described in 1935 by Berkwitz and Rigler. In some instances, no ventricular abnormalities are found. More often, however, there is moderate enlargement of the ventricular system; the ventricular walls, particularly the roofs, exhibit irregular nodular indentations varying in size up to 2 cm. and occasionally larger (fig. 232). The diagnosis may be suspected by the radiologist from plain film examination. The pneumographic finding of ventricular marginal irregularities with calcium deposits contained in the nodular masses is usually indicative of tuberous sclerosis. In other cases, the subependymal glial masses are seen in the pneumoencephalogram in the absence of calcification; the descriptive term "candle drippings" has been used to describe them. Partial obstruction in the region of the foramen of Monro is frequently found in these cases, and true tumors (usually mixed gliomas or ganglio-gliomas) may be associated.

Toxoplasmosis. The parasitic infestation has been mentioned in the section on "Intracranial Calcification," at which time some of its clinical and pathologic features were described. The calcifications are scattered and often asymmetrical. The deposits vary in size from 1 to 2 mm., and conglomerate shadows are common. One of the most characteristic findings is the presence of curvilinear deposits of calcium in the region of the basal ganglia (fig. 175).

Cerebral damage from toxoplasmosis is most severe when infection occurs during the prenatal period. Adult encephalomyelitis resulting from toxoplasmosis does occur, but the chronic changes of cerebral degeneration and calcification so prominently associated with infantile and congenital toxoplasmosis apparently do not occur. In children, the condition may be a varied combination of internal hydrocephalus and communicating hydrocephalus. In the majority of patients, the head is small and normal in shape, with the bony thickness occasionally increased. Mixed findings are accounted for by the combined effect of destruction of cerebral substance by the parasitic disease and occasional obstruction of the aqueduct of Sylvius as a result of ependymitis.

While in almost every instance an air study will show ventricular enlargement, the enlargement usually is in connection with microcephalus and hydrocephalus with hypotension, rather than elargement of the head from ventricular hypertension. Very frequently the ventricular dilatation is asymmetrical, indicating the random effect of the protozoan destructive process. If there is a small head with calcification, a pneumogram frequently is not done; when this procedure is carried out, it usually will reveal irregular and asymmetrical ventricular dilatation. Ventricular enlargement of a marked degree frequently is found in the region of the lateral ventricles, with moderate dilatation of the third ventricle and less marked involvement of the fourth ventricle. In patients who have enlargement of the head and hypertension, pneumography frequently will show an obstruction of the aqueduct of Sylvius. The basal cisterns usually are unobstructed and of normal size. When gas is disposed over

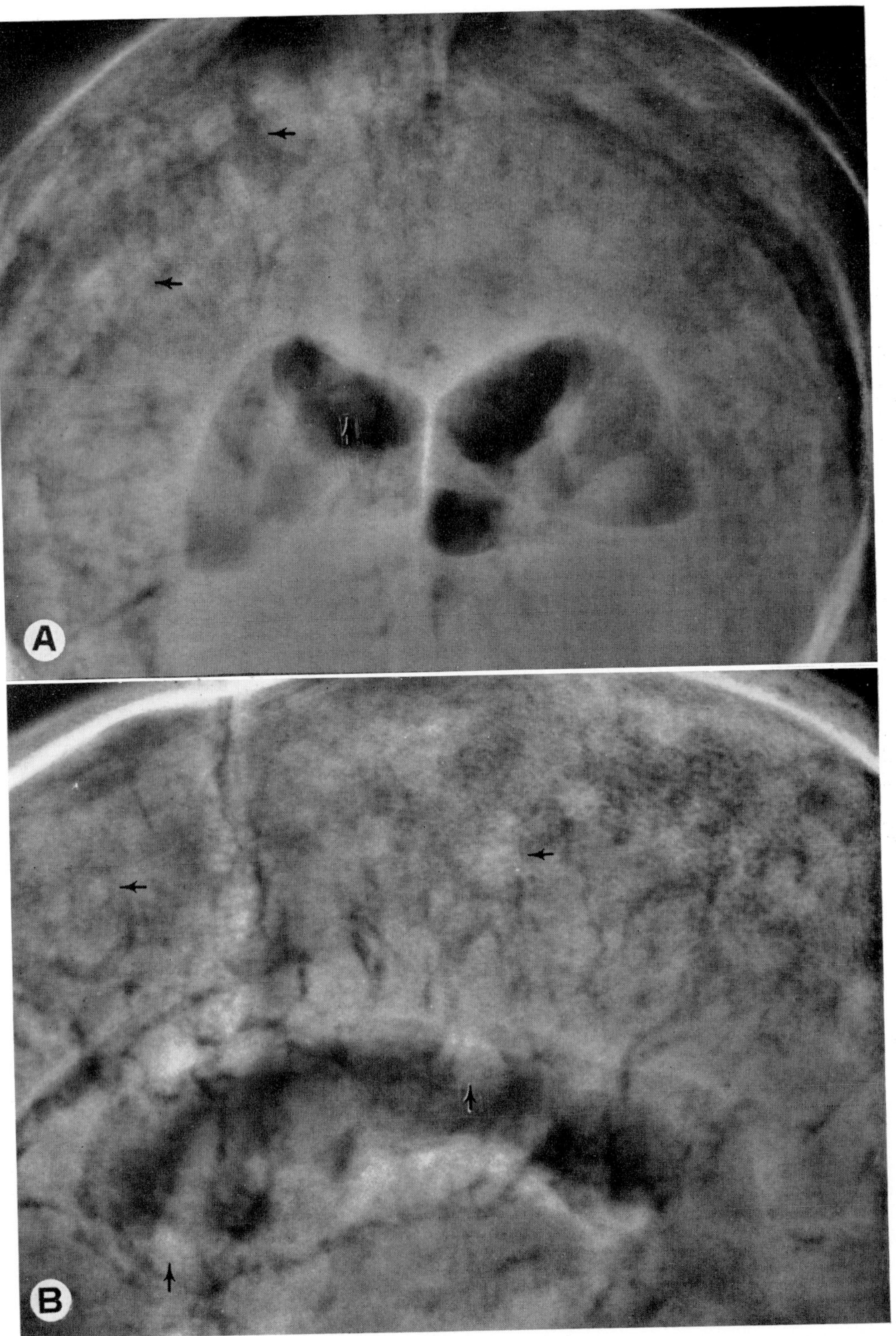

Fig. 232

(*Revised 1963*)

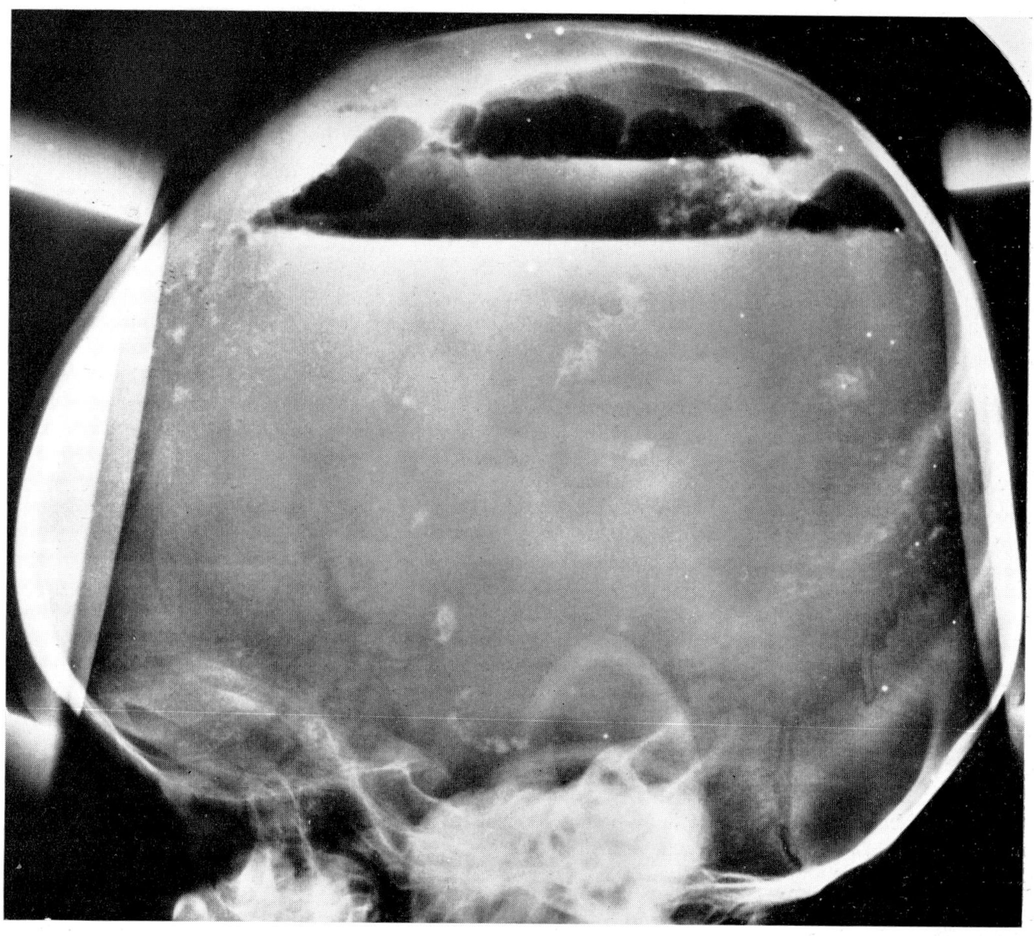

Fig. 233.—Cytomegalic Inclusion Disease

The lateral pneumogram reveals markedly dilated ventricles, only a small amount of fluid having been replaced by gas. The upright film reveals very thin cerebral cortex remaining on both sides; the thickness is less than 5 mm. at several points. Numerous calcified postinflammatory residues are scattered throughout the brain.

the convexities, wide, deep cerebral sulci usually are visualized. To establish the diagnosis clinically, the finding of a bilateral chorioretinitis in the region of the macula is most important.

Cytomegalic inclusion disease. Viral encephalitis is another of the prenatal inflammatory processes associated with marked cerebral destruction. The disease process appears to be increasing in incidence. The salivary gland virus is the chief offending agent, usually occurring among mothers who have developed no immunity, and is particularly prevalent in mothers of rural

---

Fig. 232.—Tuberous Sclerosis

Ventricular enlargement is shown, both in the frontal view (A) and the lateral projection (B). Multiple nodular irregularities are present, extending into the lumina of the ventricles from the roofs, the side walls, and the ventricular floors (*vertical arrows*). In addition, there are nodules of abnormally developed cerebral tissues scattered throughout the hemispheres (*transverse arrows*). A number of the nodules of multiple cerebral sclerosis contain visible calcium deposits.

(*Revised 1963*)

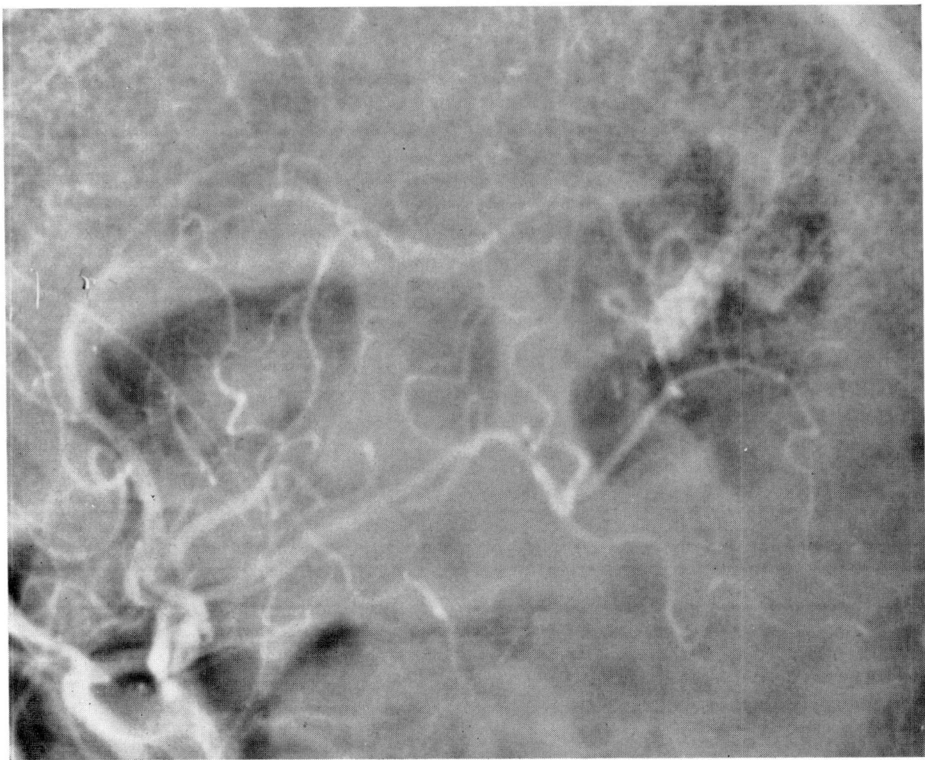

FIG. 234.—ARTERIOVENOUS MALFORMATION WITH FOCAL CEREBRAL ATROPHY
The combined pneumogram-angiogram shows a moderate-sized gas collection, outlining a well demarcated area of loss of cerebral substance that immediately surrounds an arteriovenous malformation. Mild enlargement of the ipsilateral ventricle was present.

origin. As with toxoplasmosis, the pneumographic changes are those of marked ventricular dilatation, usually with a small head, but enlargement of the head is more common than in toxoplasmosis. Here, the meninges are found to be involved by a meningoencephalitis more often than an ependymitis is seen. Therefore, the obstruction occurs most often at the outlet of the fourth ventricle as a result of the arachnoiditis. In the majority, however, there is such extreme cerebral damage that difficulty may be encountered in determining how much dilatation is due to loss of substance and how much is present owing to surgically correctible obstruction.

Any systemic inflammatory disease occurring in women during pregnancy may affect the fetus, either generally or as regards one organ or system, if it is of sufficient severity. The specific processes of toxoplasmosis and cytomegalic inclusion disease, however, selectively affect the nervous system and usually result in malformations of the brain. A number of other inflammatory processes result primarily in obstructive phenomena and will be described in the section dealing with hypertensive hydrocephalus.

If pneumoencephalography is attempted, the ventricles may not fill because of basal adhesive arachnoiditis. At ventriculography, large ventricles usually are found. The overlying cortex may be very thin in some areas (fig. 233). The diagnosis may be suspected by the radiologist even before an air study is done because of the calcification demonstrated on plain films. A periventricular distribution of pathologic calcification is most characteristic of the condition (fig. 174). The calcium deposit of cytomegalic inclusion disease may be present at birth.

Vascular Lesions

Another common cause of hydrocephalus *ex vacuo* is congenital vascular disease. *Arteriovenous malformations* may cause focal or, less often, generalized ventricular enlargement. The size and extent of the arteriovenous malformation is the most important factor relating to the ventricular change.

While these angiomatous malformations may be purely arterial or purely venous, the majority are arteriovenous, with chronic shunting of blood from the arterial to the venous system. In any event, there is not a normal capillary circulation in the region of the lesion. The lesions may occur in any portion of the brain, although they are most commonly hemispheric and in the distribution of the middle cerebral artery. More than one main arterial trunk may feed into the shunt, and there may be blood supply from the opposite hemisphere. Meningeal vascular abnormalities of the Sturge-Weber type also invoke cerebral degeneration. Serial radiologic observation often will reveal progressive calcification developing in the brain substance in the region of the lesion. More extensive description will be found in the sections dealing with angiography and calcification. In occasional cases, hypoplasia of a large part of one hemisphere occurs; the medial aspects of the hemispheres may be dislocated from the midline toward the side of the lesion.

If a pneumogram is done early in life, there may be no ventricular abnormality in the average case of arteriovenous malformation. In severe cases, however, generalized ventricular dilatation may be found even in infancy. There is often a disproportionate focal enlargement near the lesion. In unusual instances, there is, instead, a focal ventricular deformity suggesting a mass in the region of the lesion. This may be due to the sheer overabundance of vessels. In other cases, intracerebral hemorrhage, which is frequent, may produce evidence of a mass.

McRae and Valentino (1958) found changes in the pneumogram in 33 out of 35 cases of angiomatous malformation. In the patients with superficial angiomas, cortical atrophy as well as local or generalized ventricular enlargement was found. In the central angiomas the picture may be that of ventricular obstruction. Even in the absence of hemorrhage, either type of lesion is capable of producing findings suggestive of a mass lesion (fig. 234).

The consideration of angiomatous malformations leads into an area where it is often difficult to separate congenital and acquired defects. While the basic angiomatous lesion is a congenital malformation, it enlarges with growth of the patient. As noted above, pneumographic evidence of loss of substance may be absent early in life and found in later years. A history of birth injury or trauma soon afterward is often not available, even though such an event has occurred. Changes resulting from such trauma are, of course, acquired and may lead to generalized atrophy, hemiatrophy, or focal atrophy. Perinatal sepsis also may result in impaired brain growth, and it may not be clear at a later period whether the end result is a congenital hypoplasia or atrophy secondary to an acquired disease process. The brain may be affected directly, as previously noted, or the primary damage may be meningeal with secondary cerebral changes. In addition, such infections may affect vessels with the development of mycotic arterial changes or, more often, thrombosis on the venous side, with extensive loss of cerebral substance. Congenital syphilis may result in pneumographic changes similar to that found in the acquired form. In some instances, the changes may be reversible, as illustrated by the report of Wyatt and Carey (1939).

Hemihypoplasia and Hemiatrophy

When cerebral hemihypoplasia occurs, or when cerebral hemiatrophy develops early in life—especially during the first two years—certain pneumographic and cranial changes may be found which are rather characteristic. The resultant combination of findings was described in 1933 by Dyke,

Davidoff and Masson and subsequently was given the imposing title of *cerebral hemiatrophy or hemihypoplasia with homolateral hypertrophy of the skull and sinuses.* This means essentially that, when hemihypoplasia is present or when hemiatrophy occurs early in life, stimulation for skull growth by brain expansion is reduced. Other compensatory cranial changes occur to take up the relative vacuum. This is a natural phenomenon and is seen in normal patients with asymmetry of the ventricles; the side of the larger ventricle often can be suspected by the cranial changes of hemihypertrophy observed in plain films. With clinically significant hemihypoplasia the degree of ventricular enlargement and the extent of cranial changes may be striking (fig. 616). Similar changes, developing from acquired atrophy in infancy, may be based on trauma, inflammation, or vascular malformations and occlusions.

In pneumograms, the more significant changes are seen in frontal projection. There is an asymmetry of the lateral ventricles, the maldeveloped or damaged side containing a dilated rounded ventricle, with the other ventricle frequently normal in appearance. Because the change is hemispheric and congenital (or acquired early in life), there is usually a shift of the midline structures toward the side of disease. In some instances, the degree of shift may be marked (fig. 616). This is in distinct contrast to unilateral cerebral atrophic changes acquired later in life, with which dislocation of midline structures is an unusual finding (fig. 288). Dyke cautioned against the pneumographic diagnosis of tumor, which is usually the cause of dislocation of midline structures later in life. The appreciation of bony changes, Dyke advised, may be used for radiologic differentiation between hypoplasia and tumor.

Filling of the subarachnoid space is inconstant over the diseased hemisphere. In hypoplasia, and particularly in the case of inflammation and trauma, there may be such a degree of arachnoiditis that there is poor filling of the subarachnoid space on the ipsilateral side. If filling does occur, there is usually enlargement of the subarachnoid space, and gas may outline coarse sulci, or there may be other large abnormal collections over the hemispheric surface.

The *cranial changes* that occur are not always equally developed. In some patients certain changes may predominate while others are relatively inconspicuous. Any combination of these cranial alterations can provide the basis for the correct diagnosis. The majority of changes are again best recognized in frontal projection. Usually, the slope of the skull on the involved side is greater and less well rounded than on the opposite normal or relatively normal side. Frequently, there is considerable thickening of the cranial vault, which may be either an increase in width of the diploic space, thickening of the inner and outer tables, or both. Convolutional markings are frequently reduced or absent on the side of the hemihypoplasia. From the plain films it is often possible to determine the location of structures ordinarily midline in relation to the skull, since development on the normal side may produce an eccentric location of the falx.

Along the floor of the skull the sinuses and basal bony structures may enter into the hypertrophy. The crista galli deviates toward the side of the diseased hemisphere. The air sinuses of the paranasal and mastoid regions enlarge to take up the available intracranial space, and there is often some exaggeration of the slope of the sphenoid ridge. The ridge may exhibit some thickening. The frontal and sphenoid sinuses are enlarged on the side of the disease process, and often the frontals are asymmetrical to a marked extent. The ethmoid sinuses also participate in the enlargement to a marked degree, and supraorbital ethmoids frequently are found. The mastoid sinuses on the abnormal side are ordinarily enlarged, and the petrous ridge may exhibit considerable elevation. This elevation is caused by increased aeration of the petrous portions of the temporal bone and by compensatory elevation, particularly when the predominant portion of the cerebral change is posterior.

(*Revised 1963*)

Atrophy

The use of the terms hypoplasia and atrophy perhaps should not be regarded too critically. Atrophy suggests a loss of substance, while hypoplasia, used strictly, implies that substance has not developed. Pneumographically, there is no essential difference between hypoplasia and atrophy; with either there may be ventricular enlargement, sulcal enlargement, cisternal enlargement, or combinations of the three. Differentiation between hypoplasia and atrophy is more readily made on a clinical basis than radiologically. A radiologic clue, however, is the size of the head. If the head is small, and occasionally thicker than usual, the probability is that there has not been the usual degree of stimulation of cranial growth by a normally growing brain. If, on the other hand, the head is normal in size and there is no obstructive element, this indicates that the brain has grown normally but, as a result of disease, one or several portions has degenerated, and the shrunken portion has been replaced by cerebrospinal fluid.

Microcephaly is the purest form of cerebral hypoplasia which is likely to be encountered in pneumographic work, since the more severe forms of agenesis, such as anencephaly, usually are not compatible with life. A radiologic attempt to differentiate atrophy and hypoplasia is of very doubtful value; the radiologic findings constitute only one facet of a very complex clinical problem. Maldevelopment *in utero*, arrested development at various stages of postnatal life, some element of interference with the cycle of cerebrospinal fluid production, circulation, and absorption, all are possible bases for hypoplasia, and upon these acquired pathologic processes may be superimposed.

Acquired hydrocephalus ex vacuo finds one of its purest causes in trauma, since the chain of events causing degeneration can be related to an insult with a definite point in time. Head injuries and their complications will be taken up in a separate section. The degenerative changes following injury may be general or focal. Localized changes of porencephaly occurring beneath a head injury or skull fracture often can be clearly related to the traumatic episode. On the other hand, the development of porencephalic cysts may follow cerebral damage of varied origin.

(Revised 1963)

One specific type of traumatic episode, not commonly considered under the heading of head injuries, is that associated with intracranial surgical procedures. This may well be considered here. Whenever the brain is manipulated surgically, some degree of degenerative change often follows. Simple retraction of the brain in the treatment of purely extracerebral lesions, such as aneurysms and pituitary adenomas, may cause frontal or temporal atrophy with localized enlargement of one or more portions of a ventricle. A local degenerative change almost always occurs if the surgical procedure involves incision of the brain substance. Changes are more marked if there is removal of normal or diseased tissue. Amputation of a portion of a hemisphere will, of course, be associated with the replacement of this area by a large fluid space, since the brain itself has no regenerative power. Such findings become important in the case of pneumograms performed postoperatively. Recurrence of an intracranial tumor may be masked by the loss of cerebral substance and its replacement by fluid. This condition may occur owing to growth of the recurrent tumor into the free space produced by the loss of substance, or the displacement of normal structures into the free space without characteristic deformity.

Vascular insufficiency is a common cause of cerebral atrophy. In patients with generalized atherosclerosis, atrophy of the cortex and deeper white matter is evidenced at pneumography by widening of sulci and enlargement of cerebral ventricles. Enlargement of the lateral ventricles is usually disproportionate to enlargement of the third and fourth ventricles. Nevertheless, varying degrees of third ventricular enlargement are often found. Fourth ventricular enlargement with atrophy of cerebellar folia may occur independently as previously described.

With the more frequent use of angiography, in addition to pneumography, for

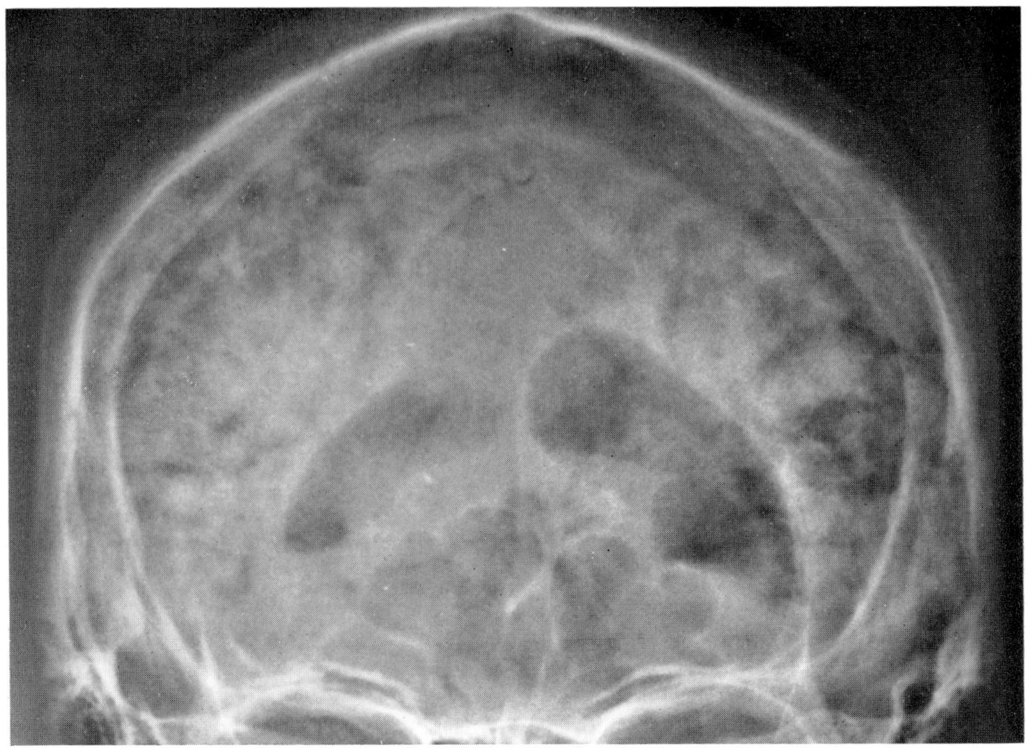

Fig. 235.—Hemicerebral Atrophy Following Middle Cerebral Artery Thrombosis
A frontal pneumogram reveals moderately severe unilateral ventricular dilatation, and ipsilateral enlargement of cortical sulci, denoting hemicerebral atrophy. The patient had suffered a stroke five years before the pneumogram, and for several months prior to the examination there had been mental deterioration (same case as illustrated in Fig. 562).

diagnosis, the vascular basis of clinically atypical degenerative changes often is established. In many patients occlusion of a portion of the internal carotid or vertebral system may cause a progressive neurologic deficit, simulating brain tumor. When pneumography is performed in these cases, a degenerative rather than an expanding lesion is, of course, demonstrated. In the past, reconciliation of the clinical picture with pneumographic changes often has been difficult. Angiography has provided a means of confirming major vessel insufficiency and explaining a progressive clinical picture in the presence of atrophy (fig. 235).

After cerebral embolism, atrophic changes similar to those resulting from carotid thrombosis are observed, although it is unusual to have occasion to investigate such patients by pneumography. Ecker (1945) and Robertson (1957) have emphasized the occurrence of hemiatrophy owing to cerebral ischemia which follows injury to the internal carotid artery in the neck—either severe direct damage to the vessel, resultant thrombosis, or perivascular constrictive changes. The frequent occurrence of vascular narrowing following carotid puncture for cerebral angiography, particularly when there is extraluminal injection with resultant transient clinical symptoms, is well known. While transient clinical symptoms are common, permanent changes secondary to ischemia, such as atrophy, are not encountered often, according to Crawford (1956).

What relationship *arterial aneurysms* may have to cerebral atrophy is not nearly as clear as the role of other vascular lesions just described. Yet, it has been observed in numerous instances that unilateral atrophy is not an unusual finding on the side of an arterial aneurysm, particularly some of the larger aneurysms of the circle of Willis. Whether the aneurysm itself in some way produces a relative ischemia of a homolateral portion of the brain, or whether other anomalies of the circle of Willis are the basis for relative insufficiency, usually is not evident. The ipsilateral atrophy usually is of mild degree. Bilateral ventricular enlargement, sometimes marked, is often found in patients who have had one or more episodes of subarachnoid hemorrhage from aneurysm.

In addition to the conditions that have been described, in which atrophy is demonstrable at pneumography, there are many others in which the atrophy is not often found during life, because pneumography is not required for diagnosis. These include the degenerative changes associated with chronic toxic states, chronic neurologic disorders, and certain psychiatric conditions, such as the psychoses. There is also a group of atrophies of unknown origin, such as simple idiopathic cerebral atrophy and Pick's disease, in which pneumography is more important for diagnosis.

Lead poisoning frequently results in an encephalopathy. The severity of exposure is more important than chronicity, according to Williams *et al.* (1933). In the later stages of disease there may be considerable generalized ventricular enlargement and cortical shrinkage (Dyke, 1941, and McKhann, 1932). In the case described by McKhann, the cerebral damage was predominantly unilateral. The ventricle on one side was considerably enlarged and there was a shift of the ventricular system toward the ipsilateral side. In the more acute cases, usually young children with cerebral edema, the plain films show widening of the major sutures (fig. 71). Pneumography is not ordinarily employed in acute lead intoxication, and when performed, it usually is unrevealing. *Other chronic toxic states*, such as uremia and habitual overindulgence in the use of alcohol, barbiturates, and certain narcotics, may be associated with atrophy (Robertson, 1957).

Encephalitis of viral origin, or encephalopathy following the exanthemata, may cause permanent cerebral damage. Davidoff and Epstein (1950) describe the pneumographic findings in eight patients with chronic neurologic disturbances following epidemic encephalitis. For the most part, the changes consisted of generalized atrophy, both central and cortical. In a number of cases there was unusual enlargement of the basal cisterns. No disproportionate focal changes were found in the region of the basal ganglia. In children who had encephalopathy associated with the exanthemata, the same investigators found varying degrees of ventricular enlargement, but cortical atrophy was very striking (fig. 236).

General paresis is usually associated with a disproportionate enlargement of the cerebral subarachnoid space, as compared with the ventricular size. The latent changes affect primarily the gray matter of the cortex and pneumograms demonstrate enlarged sulci, sometimes 4 to 5 mm. wide. The convolutions appear shrunken and atrophic. Whenever there is marked cortical atrophy with relatively normal ventricles, the possibility of general paresis should be considered (fig. 237).

Numerous primary neurologic disorders, including Huntington's chorea, Wilson's disease, idiopathic dystonia, Little's disease, athetosis, and Friedreich's ataxia have been investigated by pneumography. No pathognomonic pneumographic patterns have been found. In some patients, the ventricular system is normal; more frequently, there is ventricular dilatation, diffuse cortical degeneration and, in some, irregular porencephaly.

In Schilder's disease, there is progressive degeneration and sclerosis of the white matter. Cases have been encountered in which pneumography was an important procedure to differentiate Schilder's disease from brain tumor. In a few young children examined by the authors a progressive clinical picture suggested brain tumor. This impression was strengthened by absolute enlargement of

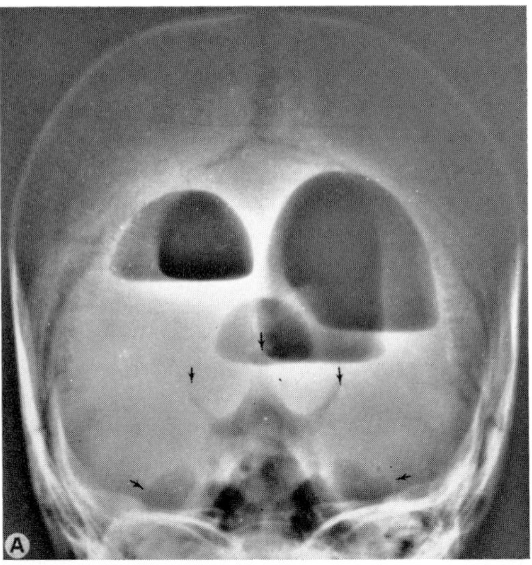

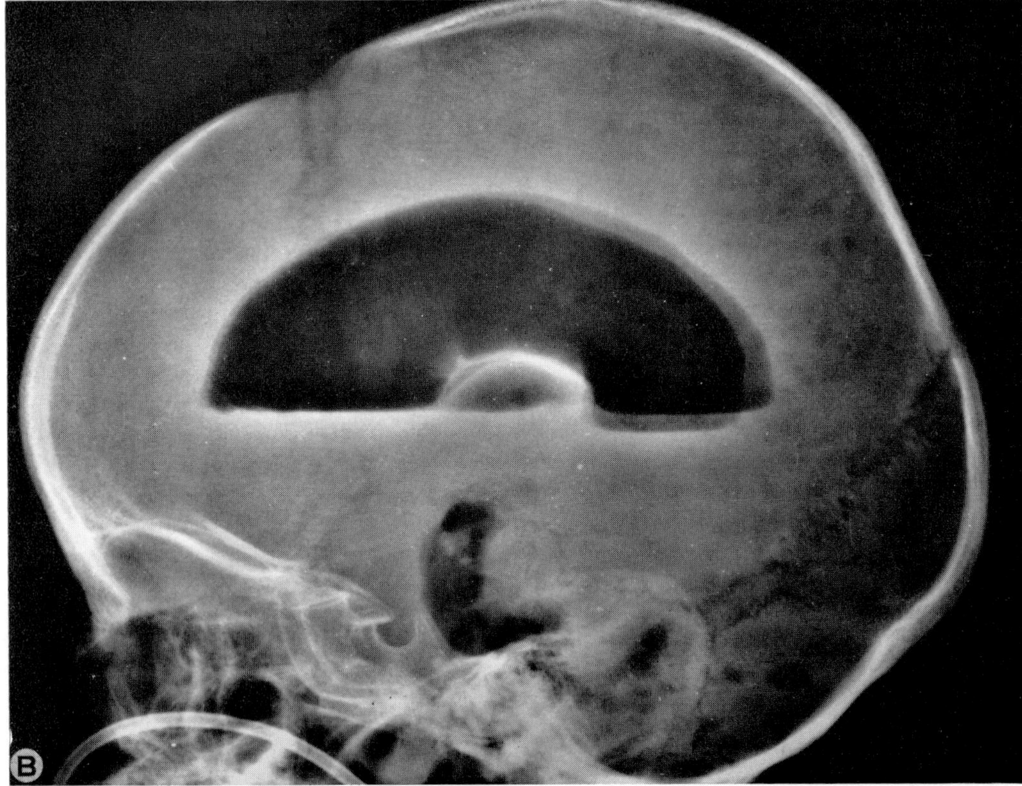

Fig. 236.—Generalized Cerebral Atrophy Following Infection

A child (18 months) had a severe attack of meningoencephalitis one month prior to the pneumogram, during which he had a high fever for one week. The infection slowly subsided under antibiotic therapy, but convulsions and a profound neurologic deficit developed. The frontal pneumogram (A) shows marked, and fairly symmetrical, dilatation of the lateral ventricles, and gross enlargement of the third ventricle. Gas in the enlarged intercrural and crural cisterns (*upper arrows*), demonstrates well the head during a period of observation. At pneumography, however, the ventricular system was normal in these cases. In later stages of the disease, however, ventricular dilatation develops owing to profound atrophy. A similar clinical problem may arise in connection with atypical cases of multiple sclerosis. In this condition, the ventricular enlargement usually is more often mild to moderate, and the cortical and cisternal enlargement may be most prominent.

Two specific types of dementia, usually referred to as *presenile dementia*, are Alzheimer's disease and Pick's disease. Many reports have appeared concerning the pneumographic findings in these conditions since they were reported by Flugel in 1932. The value of pneumography stems from the fact that the diseases may be insidious in onset and progressive in nature, with mental impairment, motor and speech disturbances, and convulsions. Pneumography, therefore, frequently serves to differentiate the presenile dementias from tumor.

In the typical case, there is rather marked ventricular enlargement which is usually symmetrical. A prominent feature often is disproportionate enlargement of the anterior and temporal horns. In other instances, cortical atrophy with dilatation of the subarachnoid space may be prominent. Pathologically, the findings in the two diseases are quite similar. It is not feasible, therefore, to try to differentiate, on the basis of pneumograms, the two conditions from each other, or even from other causes of cerebral atrophy.

A specific clinical entity of pneumographic interest is *olivopontocerebellar atrophy*. Because the clinical picture is usually diagnostic, pneumography is not required; under some circumstances, however, an air study is carried out. The pneumogram usually reveals (1) small cerebellar folia and wide, deep hemispheric sulci, (2) enlargement of the subtentorial subarachnoid space, (3) disproportionate smallness of the pons, although the whole brain stem may be of less than average size, (4) enlargement of the gas shadows of the cisterna pontis and cisterna interpeduncularis, (5) varying degrees of enlargement of the fourth ventricle (fig. 231). Apart from the syndrome of olivopontocerebellar atrophy, simple cerebellar atrophy may occur as previously noted. Here, as with cerebellar hypoplasia, the diagnosis rests not on the presence of a large cisterna magna, but on definite evidence of loss of cerebellar substance by surface changes and fourth ventricular enlargement.

One of the most outstanding pneumographic enigmas is *simple cerebral atrophy*. The clinical diagnosis is often difficult to establish; in some instances, increased intracranial pressure is observed, as evidenced by papilledema. Epilepsy, even that beginning later in life and sometimes focal in origin, is more often associated with degenerative disease than brain tumor. The cerebrospinal fluid may exhibit pathologic changes, similar to those found with tumor. A rapidly progressive clinical course occurs in some patients. Pneumography often is the only definitive way of establishing a diagnosis during life and of avoiding unnecessary surgical procedures.

The basis for simple atrophy is varied and may be a summation effect of several fundamental processes. Hereditary and congenital alterations of growth and development may be factors which, by themselves, are insufficient to produce clinical changes. The cumulative effects of trauma, infections, and vascular insufficiency may be superimposed on a congenital deficiency, to result in such cerebral degeneration.

Pneumography, while extremely valuable in the diagnosis of cerebral atrophy, also may be of some prognostic value by defining the extent of changes present. It is particularly important in the evaluation of epilepsy,

---

the configuration referred to as a "three-pointed crown" (see text). There is enlargement also of the cerebellopontine recesses (*lower arrows*). In the lateral view (B), the pontine and interpeduncular cisterns are dilated; the absence of gas in the communicating cisterns and over the cerebral surface raises the question of a postmeningitic obstruction of these channels, in addition to the postinflammatory cerebral degeneration. The cerebrospinal fluid pressure, however, was low.

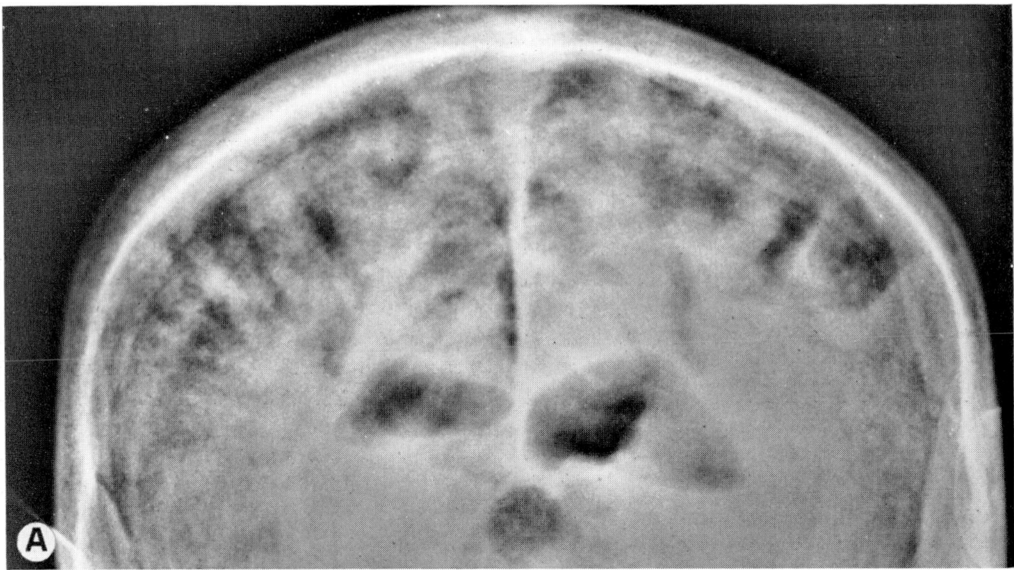

FIG. 237.—ATROPHY OF THE CEREBRAL CORTEX

If a luetic infection results in general paresis, it frequently produces a disproportionate enlargement of the cerebral subarachnoid space as compared with ventricular size, through cortical atrophy. Both frontal (A) and lateral (B) views in the case illustrated show gross sulcal enlargement; a few of the sulci measure slightly over 1 cm. in width; the shrunken convolutions are reduced not only in width but in height. The ventricles exhibit mild generalized enlargement.

In another case, an elderly patient with advanced cerebral arteriosclerosis exhibits marked cortical atrophy, which is disproportionate to ventricular size (C). In occasional instances, such as the cases illustrated, a definite etiology may be ascribed to cerebral atrophy, either cortical or deeply seated; in the majority of patients, however, the exact cause usually is obscure.

especially if the surgical treatment of epilepsy is under consideration (Penfield and Erickson, 1941, and Childe and Penfield, 1944). In the majority of patients with epilepsy, the pneumogram will show generalized ventricular and subarachnoid enlargement. In some cases, a focal area of cortical atrophy may be found; in others, an area of poor subarachnoid filling may be demonstrated, due to adhesions. Either suggests a focal lesion responsible for the convulsions.

In the average case of cerebral atrophy, there is generalized ventricular enlargement. Usually, the lateral ventricles are affected to the greatest extent. The third ventricle exhibits mild to moderate enlargement in most instances. The fourth ventricle may or may not be enlarged, depending on the presence or absence of infratentorial changes. Measurements to quantitate ventricular enlargement are given under "Anatomy."

Ordinarily, with simple atrophy, the ventricular enlargement is bilateral, but it may be prodominantly on one side. The subarachnoid space also is enlarged, in a typical case. A pneumographic diagnosis of atrophy, predominantly cortical, may be made when there are enlarged sulci, without ventricular changes. General paresis has been mentioned as the prototype. Contrariwise, a pneumographic diagnosis of atrophy, predominantly central, is permissible when the ventricles are dilated, but the subarachnoid space is not enlarged. It must be remembered, however, that long standing, partially obstructing lesions of the posterior fossa may simulate cerebral atrophy. For this reason it is essential to demonstrate clearly all of the posterior fossa structures both in lateral

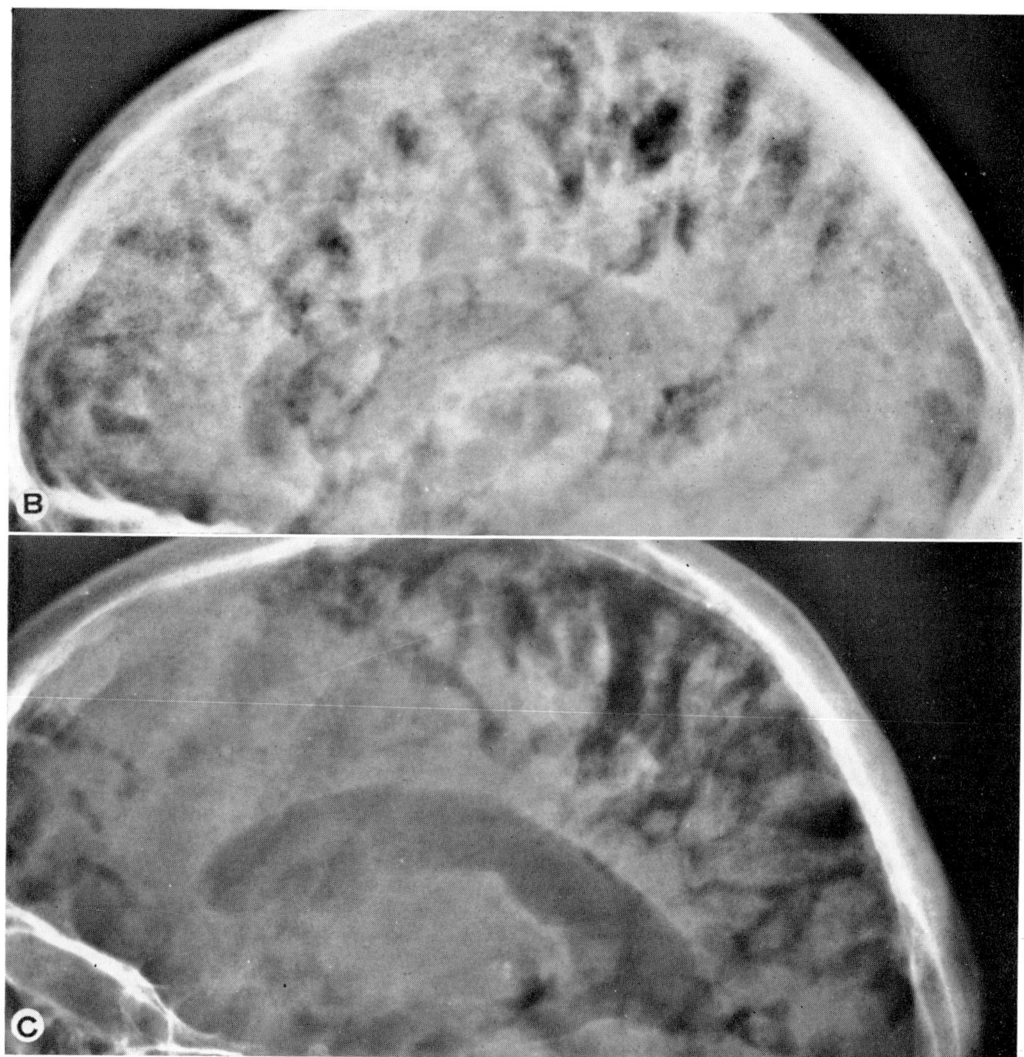

FIG. 237

and frontal projections before reaching a conclusion.

As noted earlier, it is not always easy to judge between mild unilateral enlargement of a lateral ventricle and the changes produced by a small hemispheric tumor. When a lateral ventricle is only slightly narrowed at its angle by the pressure of an adjacent tumor, it may not be recognized as abnormal. Instead, it may be thought that the contralateral normal ventricle exhibits mild atrophy, by comparison. The point is re-emphasized because of the importance of diagnosing tumors early in their development. The width of the lateral angle and the slope of the ventricular roof may be the best clues for differentiation of the two processes.

(Revised 1963)

Difficulty may be encountered, also, in deciding when cerebral sulci are abnormally large. Before an evaluation is made, it is essential to have all of the details concerning the technical aspects of the examination. The use of substances which shrink the brain, such as urea, must be known, and judgment must be made concerning the appearance of the cortical markings in relation to the quantity of gas used for the examination. A cortical cerebral sulcus is considered enlarged when it measures over 3.0 mm. in width. When large quantities of gas are used, the subarachnoid gas over the surface of the brain may give the impression of cortical atrophy. If no actual enlargement of sulci—indicating shrinkage of two adjacent gyri—is present, cortical atrophy can not be diagnosed. Localized areas of cortical atrophy in the neighborhood of Pacchionian granulations are common.

The correlation of pneumographic and pathologic findings associated with cerebral atrophy is not altogether satisfactory. Indeed, examination of the autopsy specimen usually fails to reveal not only the cause but also the presence of premortem loss of cerebral mass, except in severe cases, or in certain specific conditions. The most commonly observed instances of slight, nonobstructive, ventricular dilatation are nonspecific and the pathologist is unable to detect them after fixation of the brain.

HYPERTENSIVE HYDROCEPHALUS

The second main category of hydrocephalus is obstructive or hypertensive hydrocephalus. (In this section, discussion of neoplastic causes will be excluded.) In the majority of instances, the changes are of congenital origin; some result from inflammatory conditions, traumatic episodes, and a few other causes.

The non-neoplastic conditions which result in obstructive hydrocephalus occur in one of three places: (1) in the aqueduct of Sylvius, (2) at the outlets of the fourth ventricle, or (3) along the extraventricular cerebrospinal fluid pathways. In a high percentage of patients, some type of surgical treatment is instituted, either a direct approach to the site of obstruction or some type of bypass procedure. In some instances, particularly in early infancy, the degree of obstruction and irreparable brain damage may be so great at the time the patient is first seen that surgical intervention is not advisable.

Aqueductal Obstructions

Congenital. The classical, and the most common, example of hydrocephalus in this category is infantile obstructive hydrocephalus resulting from congenital malformation of the aqueduct of Sylvius. The malformation usually is an atresia, resembling atresias occurring in the gastrointestinal tract and elsewhere in the body. The columns of ependymal cells which ordinarily are well aligned to form the wall of the lumen of the aqueduct do not proliferate properly or join in the usual manner. Often multiple blind pockets, or isolated microscopic cavities, are present along the usual course of the iter rather than a point of true focal narrowing of an otherwise normal lumen. The grade of the obstruction in the iter depends on the extent of the blind ending of the malformed channels, and the number which join, even though abnormally, to allow the transmission of cerebrospinal fluid. Complete obstruction rarely exists; even though radiologically gas and other substances may fail to pass through the narrow channels, some fluid frequently can get through. For this reason, discrepancies often exist between dye tests (in which an organic dye is injected into the ventricular system and recovered after lumbar puncture, if any patency exists) and the use of gas which, when injected into a fluid medium, does not pass as readily through narrow channels because of surface tension.

Clinically, the head usually is enlarged at birth, or begins to enlarge soon thereafter. Lateral and third ventricular dilatation is the basis for the cranial enlargement, owing to the inadequacy of cerebrospinal fluid passage through the aqueduct of Sylvius. Ventriculography is readily performed in these patients by puncture of a lateral ventricle through the anterior fontanelle, although a burr hole may be used. Robert-

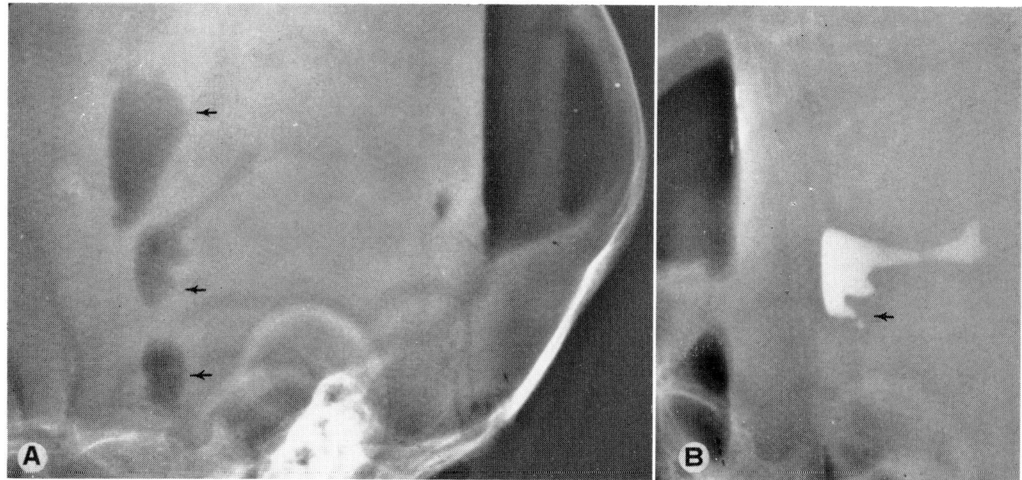

FIG. 238.—CONGENITAL OBSTRUCTION OF THE AQUEDUCT OF SYLVIUS

A lateral pneumogram made with the patient prone (A) shows marked dilatation of the lateral ventricles with only 0.5 cm. thickness of cerebral cortex posteriorly. The central of the three anterior gas shadows depicts the posterior portion of the dilated third ventricle at its outlet (*middle arrow*). The two third ventricular gas projections above are the pineal recess and suprapineal recess, respectively. The shadow above the third ventricle represents lateral ventricular gas trapped in a compartmented portion of the ventricular body (*upper arrow*). The shadow below the third ventricle is a similar gas collection in a temporal horn (*lower arrow*). A supine lateral film was made following the installation of Pantopaque into a lateral ventricle and passage of the opaque substance into the third ventricle (B). The obstruction of the aqueduct of Sylvius (*arrow*) shown by the conventional ventriculogram is confirmed.

son (1957) has had considerable success in demonstrating the caudal limit of the obstructive process by the injection of 10 cc. of gas by the lumbar route. In some instances, a combined ventriculogram-pneumoencephalogram is required; in selected patients, as previously described, small amounts of radiopaque material may be used to define the site of obstruction (fig. 238).

Contrary to the practice of a number of years ago, it is now the consensus that the smallest quantity of gas consistent with diagnostic accuracy should be injected into the ventricles by fontanelle puncture. The large quantities of gas formerly used frequently resulted in ventricular collapse, with tearing of meningeal vessels and hemorrhagic complications (fig. 196). Ten cubic centimeters of gas injected into even markedly dilated lateral ventricles may be adequate to give all the information that is required, and we recommend that not more than 50 cc. be used, to avoid complications.

(Revised 1963)

In infancy, somersaulting of the patient may be executed manually to control the position of gas in the ventricles. In older patients, a specially constructed somersaulting chair provides equal control of the ventricular disposition of gas (see "Technique"). If, for some reason, the point of obstruction cannot be determined with a small quantity of gas, then use of a positive contrast material probably is less hazardous than the injection of additional gas.

The radiographic examination in hydrocephalus may well begin with upright frontal and lateral films made at a six-foot distance. Examination under such teleroentgenographic conditions is not absolutely necessary, but it does have the advantage of providing a nearly accurate measurement of cortical thickness without application of correction factors. It also allows ready comparison of measurements from one case to another.

The use of a six-foot distance to estimate cortical thickness was suggested by Scarff

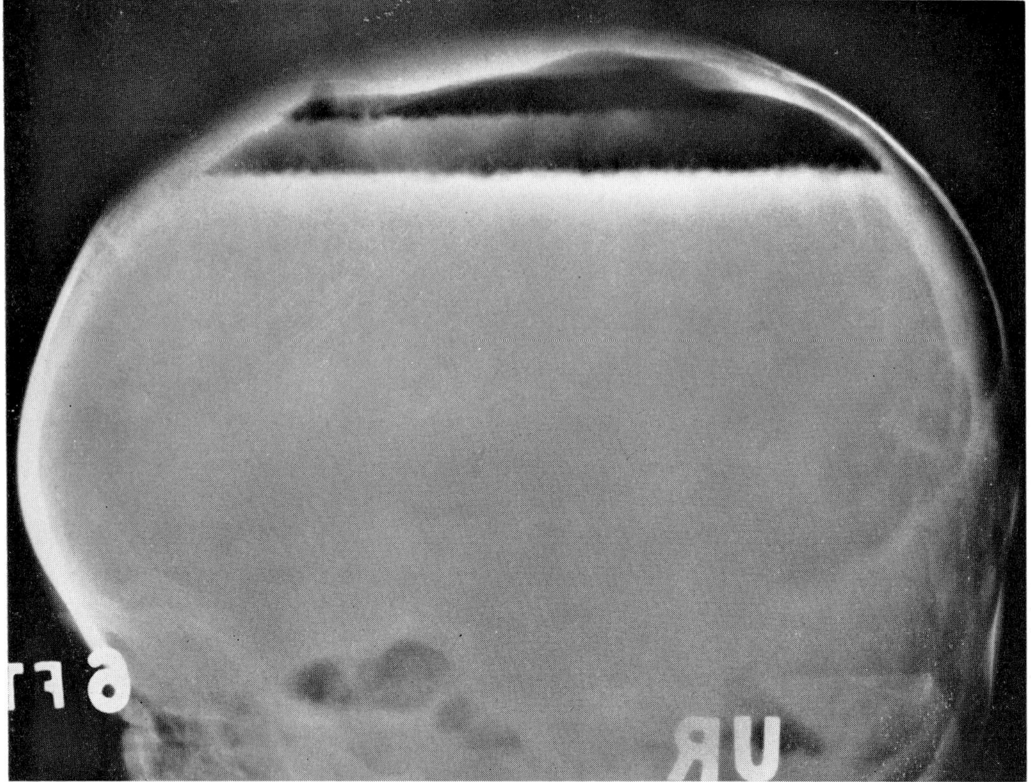

Fig. 239.—Method of Determining Cerebral Thickness in Hydrocephalus

Upright films made at a 6-foot distance provide a means of measuring the thickness of remaining cerebral tissue under standard conditions. Lateral films are made also in supine and prone position, and a frontal upright examination is included. Measurement of the thickness of cerebral substance between the dilated ventricle and inner table of the skull has been suggested as a reliable index for the selection of patients for corrective surgical procedures. A uniform cortical thickness of 2 cm. will usually assure an average intellectual developement, whereas a thickness of less than 1 cm. will preclude an acceptable result.

(1952), who used measurements obtained as a guide to the selection of patients for operative procedures (fig. 239). If the cortical thickness was found to be 1 cm. or greater at its thinnest point, then these patients were given the benefit of a corrective procedure. If the cortex was found to be less than 1 cm., then the patients were considered inoperable, because excessive cerebral damage was considered to be present for a satisfactory clinical result, particularly from the standpoint of patient intellect. A recent long-term follow-up of the patients operated upon, largely on the basis of this radiologic criterion, has proved that this is a satisfactory method of determining operability.

Some patients who have sufficient thickness of cortex to be operable (from this standpoint alone) may have associated congenital abnormalities which contraindicate surgical treatment. Such changes can be appreciated by pneumography, but would be missed if a simple fontanel puncture for study of the subdural space, and for estimation of cortical thickness is carried out.

Following the upright films, the ordinary horizontal views are made in order to exclude tumor. Since small quantities of gas are used, stereoscopic views often are omitted because this type of study gives little additional information. For infants, inverted films are taken after lifting the child by the feet, starting from the supine position. Such views may be invaluable to visualize the foramen of Monro, the third ventricle, the iter, and other areas, when small amounts of gas are employed.

In the congenital type of aqueductal obstruction, the atresia usually begins high, just caudal to the outlet of the third ventricle. Often a short, tapering gas projection is shown bending backward and downward from the region of the aditus, the length of which usually does not exceed 3 to 4 mm. In some instances, essentially no projection beyond the posterior end of the third ventricle may be demonstrated by air, although a short projection may be shown with opaque material. In the average case of congenital hydrocephalus caused by aqueduct atresia, no gas or positive contrast material will pass caudal to the proximal aqueduct. The tapering gas shadow which is seen does not deviate from the normal course of the aqueduct. Rare congenital tumors, such as hemangiomas and occasionally other types of midbrain neoplasms, may result in a slight displacement.

The lateral and third ventricles rostral to the aqueduct exhibit varying degrees of dilatation without evidence of a filling defect or deformity by tumor. The lateral ventricular dilatation is not always symmetrical; one ventricle sometimes is considerably larger than the other. The overlying cerebral tissue may be extremely thin and occasionally not demonstrable in pneumograms. Compartment-like areas may be found which have almost the appearance of thin-walled cysts, sometimes with incomplete septa or with "ribbing" due to crossing blood vessels. These rather localized outpocketings are referred to by some as *diverticula.* In addition to the rather local changes, general differences in cortical thickness may be seen. It is not infrequent to find an extremely thin frontal or occipital cortex, particularly the latter, with paper thin cerebral tissue overlying these areas and fairly good presentation of brain tissue elsewhere. In these instances, there is no abrupt point of thinning but a gradual transition.

Because of the large amount of fluid, the solid brain remaining may exhibit unusual mobility, particularly when moderate to sizable quantities of ventricular fluid are replaced by gas. Mobility often is evident in infants when the patients are inverted to show the point of arrest of the passage of gas. In some instances, such a change in posture may show the obstructed aqueduct dislocated as far forward as the suprasellar region (fig. 238). Care should be taken not to interpret this dislocation resulting from mobility as being displacement by a tumor. This type of difficulty may be largely avoided if a small amount of Pantopaque, usually 1 to 2 cc., is injected into the ventricle without the removal of any fluid. There is not as much movement of the brain with change in posture when the intraventricular pressure is maintained. It is not difficult in infants, with or without fluoroscopic control, to direct the contrast material through the enlarged foramen of Monro into the third ventricle; thence, into the obstructed aqueduct. We prefer to attempt diagnosis with gas initially; if this is not satisfactory, Pantopaque is instilled and its course controlled by fluoroscopy, to expedite the examination.

Acquired. Benign acquired obstruction of the aqueduct of Sylvius, or stenosis, results from a gliosis which may narrow the aqueduct at any point or throughout its entire length. There may be thickening of the ependymal lining, but the most prominent microscopic change is subependymal, where scarring caused by proliferation of astrocytes and other glial elements is found. The reaction is inflammatory, although frequently not postinfectious; at least historical or objective evidence of infection often is lacking. Occasionally, a true cause and effect relationship between meningitis or meningoencephalitis and the development of aqueduct stenosis can be established.

It is usually possible to diagnose correctly benign aqueductal stenosis, chiefly because of the funnel-like even tapering of the undisplaced aqueduct but also because of the marked internal hydrocephalus which results. There are very few acquired lesions that result in such a severe degree of hydro-

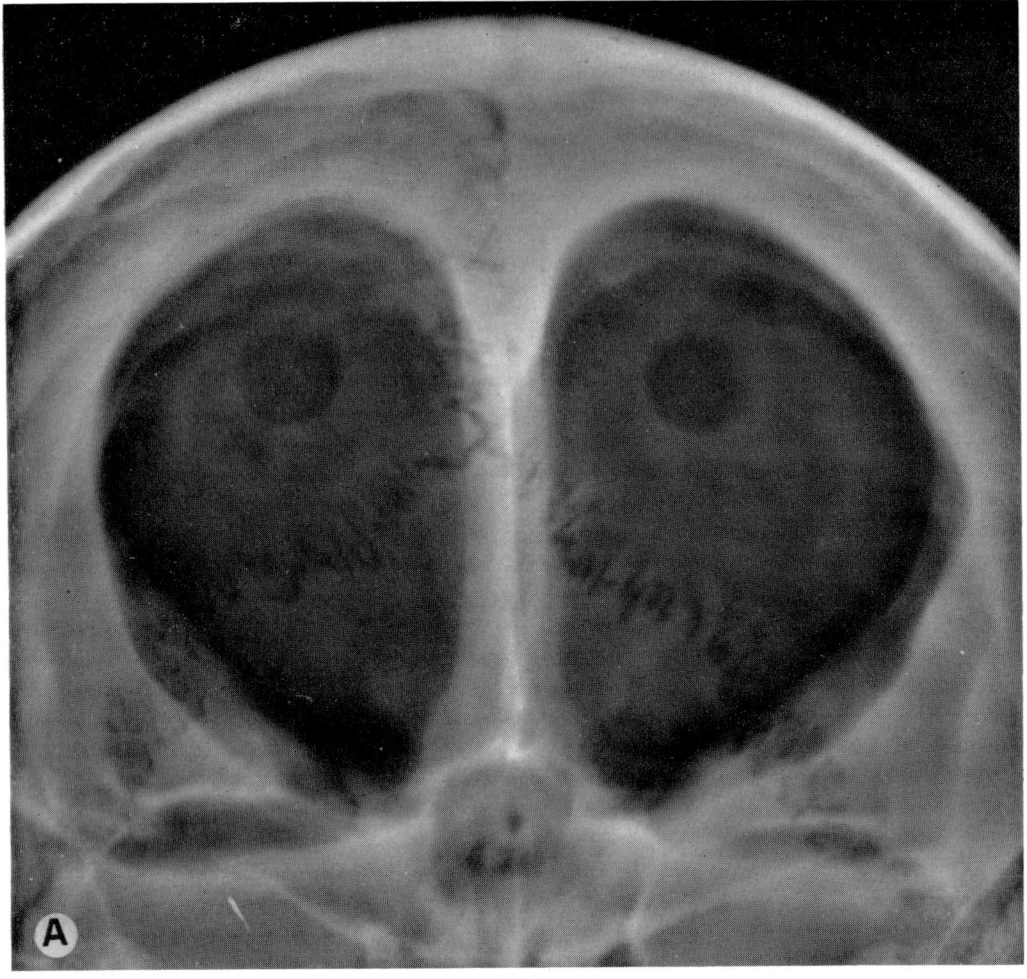

Fig. 240.—Aqueduct Stenosis

A severe degree of symmetrical ventricular dilatation occurs with benign acquired obstruction of the aqueduct of Sylvius (A). In lateral view (another case), the roofs of the ventricles are shown to be uneven in their upward extension (B). Small downward projections from the roofs of the dilated ventricles often are seen (*upper arrows*) due to crossing blood vessels which apparently provide more resistance to stretching than the cerebral substance. The hypothalamic portion of the third ventricle is markedly dilated with erosion of the sella turcica. In this view, the shadow of the enlarged temporal horn is superimposed upon the downward extension of the third ventricle (*lower arrows*). When a large amount of gas is used in the examination, as in this case, the exact point of obstruction at the outlet of the third ventricle, or lower in the aqueduct, may not be clearly seen without the use of tomograms (see Fig. 241).

cephalus as does aqueduct gliosis. Occasionally, a well differentiated glioma of the midbrain may produce clinical and pneumographic changes which are indistinguishable from benign gliosis of the aqueduct. The cause of the extreme hydrocephalus associated with aqueduct gliosis is thought to be the slow development of narrowing of the iter with repeated compensatory increases in ventricular pressure that keep the channel patent. Eventually, a high degree of obstruction occurs, which may exist over a long period of time, because there is no specific neurologic deficit to bring the patient to definitive diagnostic studies.

Patients with aqueduct gliosis usually re-

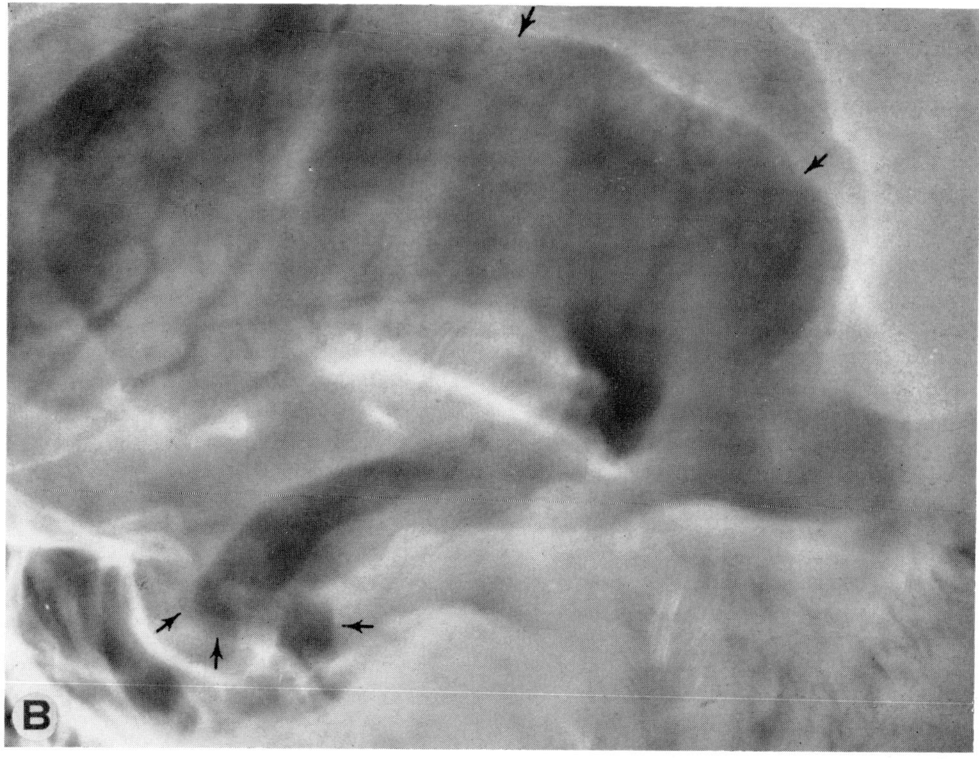

FIG. 240

quire ventriculography, or a combined ventriculogram-encephalogram, for definitive diagnosis. The remarkable degree of ventricular dilatation, which is found in many cases, should immediately alert the radiologist to the probability of a benign rather than a neoplastic process. A colloid cyst, or occasionally other tumors of the third ventricle, may produce a pronounced degree of lateral ventricular dilatation, but these are excluded when the large third ventricle fills promptly. If only a small amount of gas has been injected, which is desirable, a somersault or some other maneuver will be required to direct the gas to the point of obstruction in the aqueduct. The aditus and the proximal aqueduct are dilated, exhibiting the characteristic funnel-shaped deformity without displacement (fig. 241). In adults, tomograms may be useful after trapping the gas in the third ventricle but lateral tomograms with the patient prone cannot be obtained without special apparatus. However, autotomography is often satisfactory in these cases. Tomograms taken with the patient prone and with the head turned to the side require larger quantities of gas.

The benign lesions causing obstruction at the foramen of Monro, of the iter, and of the outlet of the fourth ventricle produce, as a result of long standing pressure of high grade, disproportionate local enlargements of the ventricles that have been called *acquired pressure diverticula* (Dyke, 1942). The lateral ventricles exhibit such localized pressure diverticula along the medial aspect of the atrium. Dyke described a case in which the diverticulum extended outward and beneath the tentorium. Occasionally, such diverticula may rupture, with spontaneous relief of the markedly elevated intraventricular pressure.

Another weak point mentioned earlier is the suprapineal area of the third ventricle. This recess is often enlarged in the presence

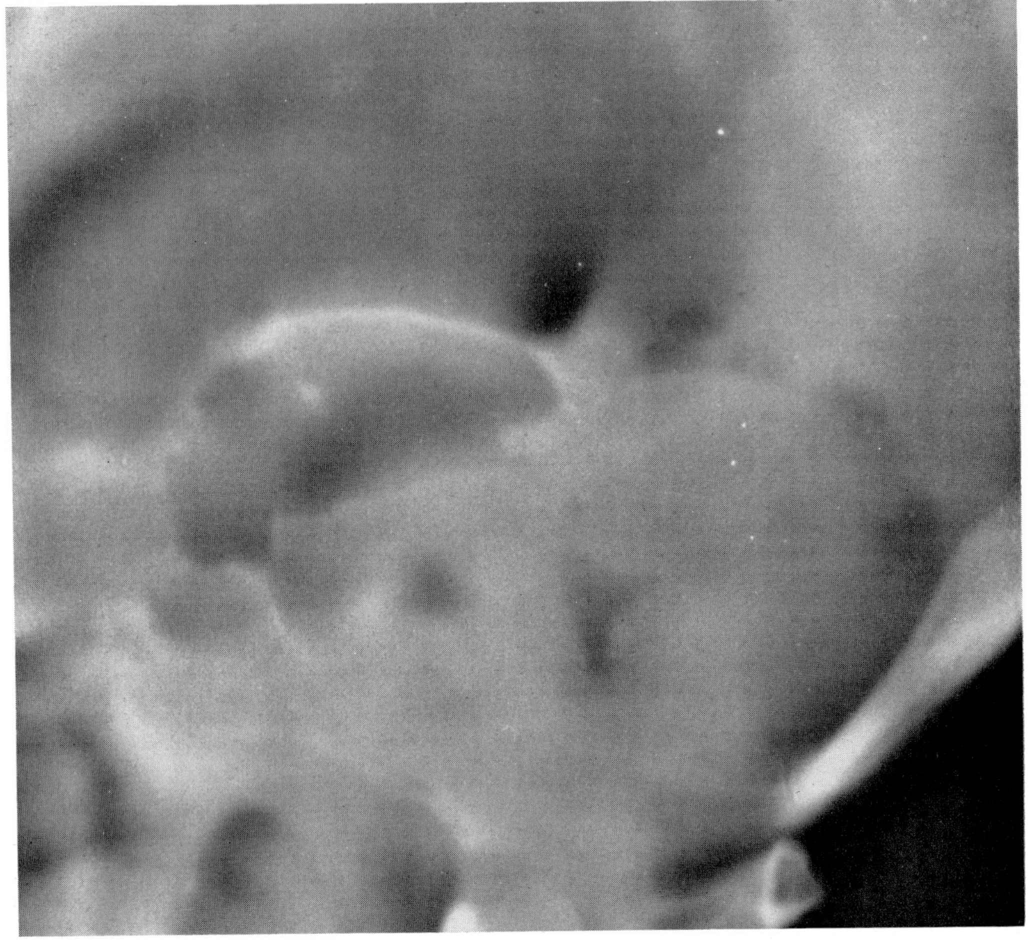

Fig. 241.—Aqueduct Stenosis

A midsagittal tomogram was made following combined ventriculography-pneumoencephalography. The ventricular system is markedly dilated as far caudad as the outlet of the third ventricle. The 10 cc. of gas injected into the lumbar subarachnoid space outline a small fourth ventricle. Between the third and fourth ventricles, an intermittent hairline shadow of the iter can be made out. Obstruction of the aqueduct in this case was postinflammatory, developing after recovery from meningitis, which must have produced also an ependymitis. The suprapineal recess is dilated as a result of high intraventricular pressure.

of high intraventricular pressure, even to the extent of becoming a pressure diverticulum, which extends backward into the upper part of the quadrigeminal cistern (figs. 240 and 241). Lesions producing chronic obstruction of the aqueduct of Sylvius most often are the cause of third ventricular diverticula; similar suprapineal distentions are found less frequently owing to fourth ventricular obstructions. Spontaneous rupture also may occur in this area, thereby establishing a communication between the third ventricle and the subarachnoid space.

Anteriorly, the gross enlargements of the optic and infundibular recesses, which may occur owing to obstructing lesions of the posterior part of the third ventricle, may be considered as diverticula. The sella turcica may be eroded to a remarkable degree by the enlarged pulsating recesses of a markedly dilated anterior third ventricle (figs. 64 and 244). The recess actually may project into

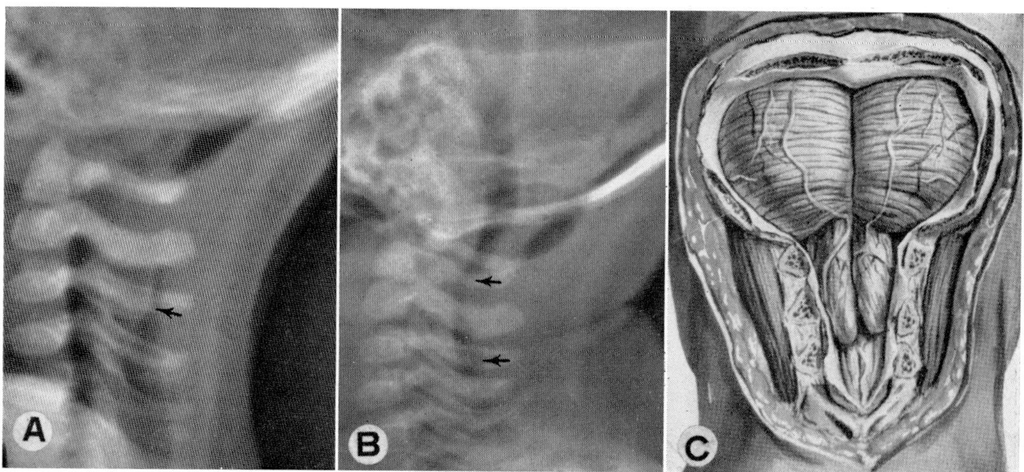

FIG. 242.—ARNOLD-CHIARI MALFORMATION

A lateral film, made after attempted pneumoencephalography (A), reveals a narrowing of the upper cervical subarachnoid space. At the level of C1 and C2, the spinal cord shadow is continuous with the caudally displaced medulla oblongata, and dorsal to it are the smoothly rounded inferior margins of the dislocated cerebellar tonsils (*arrow*). A small amount of gas passes behind the tonsils into the cisterna magna, a finding characteristic of chronic tonsillar herniation.

The lateral ventriculogram (B) revealed ventricular enlargement owing to the obstruction at the outlet of the fourth ventricle. The fourth ventricle is deformed, and a fingerlike caudal projection of the fourth ventricle (*arrows*) extends into the upper cervical region.

An artist's sketch (C) illustrates the anatomic relationships of the dislocated and elongated cerebellar tonsils through the foramen magnum and into the upper vertebral canal. (Courtesy of Dr. F. H. Netter and Ciba, New York.)

the pituitary fossa. Pituitary insufficiency may develop, and this, combined with the marked degree of sellar destruction shown on plain films, may lead to an erroneous diagnosis of pituitary tumor. At ventriculography, the distention of the hypothalamic portion of the third ventricle is usually clearly evident from supine lateral films (fig. 240). Midsagittal tomograms will demonstrate the actual impression of the third ventricle on the sella turcica to best advantage.

There may be some hesitancy to use opaque contrast material in patients with aqueduct gliosis because it has been reported that inflammation is invoked. While an arachnoidal reaction may be seen from time to time, evidence that ependymitis occurs is less convincing. If a diagnosis is not clear, however, the slight risk involved in using Pantopaque appears justified. If the obstruction is of the high degree found in the average case of aqueduct stenosis, a short circuiting operation usually will be required; therefore, the aggravation of inflammatory changes, which could result from the introduction of Pantopaque, probably will be of no consequence.

Some workers recommend the injection of a small amount of gas into the lumbar subarachnoid space to exclude with certainty the presence of a posterior fossa tumor. In the usual case of aqueduct gliosis, 10 cc. of gas injected from below will fill the posterior fossa cisterns and outline a normal appearing fourth ventricle and, occasionally, a segment of distal aqueduct (fig. 241). The combined ventriculogram-pneumoencephalogram procedures certainly give the fullest evaluation in any particular case. As noted earlier in connection with congenital hydrocephalus, Robertson (1957) has very successfully used pneumoencephalography alone for the diagnosis of aqueductal lesions. Unless followed by ventriculography, however, there would appear to be a strong possibility of overlooking a supratentorial tumor, particularly

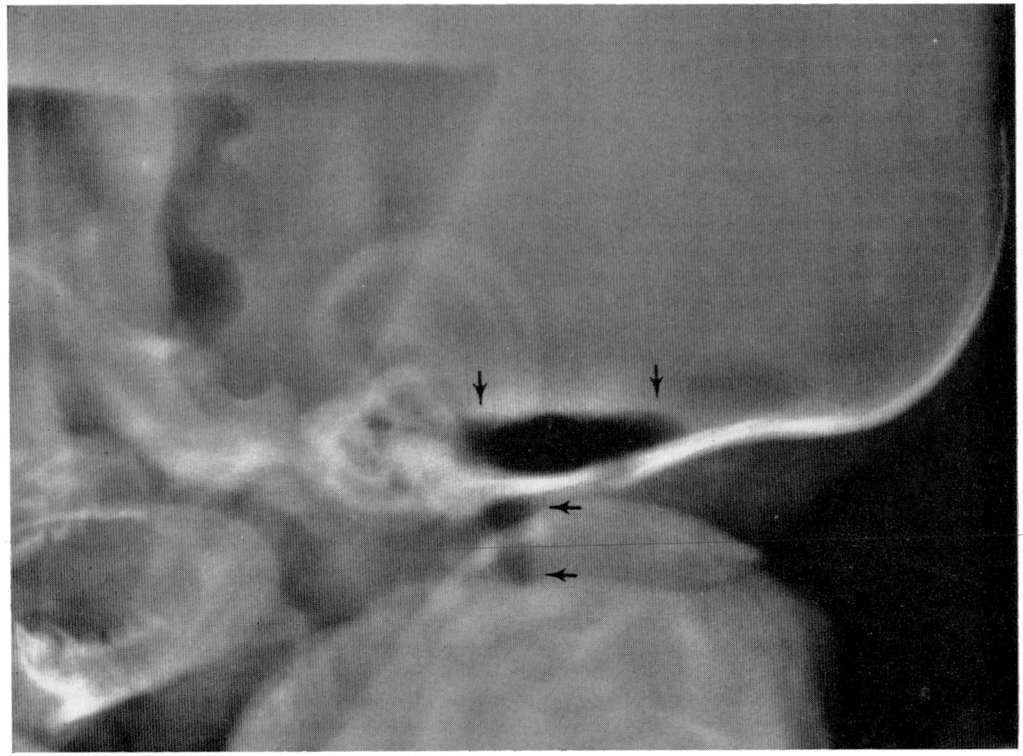

FIG. 243.—ATRESIA OF THE FORAMINA OF LUSCHKA AND MAGENDIE

The lateral ventriculogram, made with the infant inverted, reveals a markedly enlarged fourth ventricle which is only partially outlined by gas collected in the caudad portion (*vertical arrows*). The dilated ventricle is closely applied to the occipital bone. There is bulging of the caudal end of the fourth ventricle into the cervical canal to the level of C2 (*transverse arrows*). Failure of gas to escape from the dilated fourth ventricle into the spinal subarachnoid space, with the patient inverted, denotes lack of patency of the cerebrospinal fluid pathways.

one in the pineal region. In one of our cases, the combined procedures of ventriculography and pneumoencephalography allowed us to visualize the aqueduct throughout its length in a patient with stenosis following meningo-encephalitis. The aqueduct was of extremely small caliber throughout its length and only by filling it from both directions could the full length be demonstrated. Tomograms were helpful in visualizing the hairline shadow of the aqueduct.

Aqueduct stenosis in teen-aged children and adults is often produced by periaqueductal gliomas, which are slowly growing, infiltrating tumors. The tumors frequently do not produce enlargement of the brain stem; therefore, the correct diagnosis seldom is made except at necropsy.

Fourth Ventricle Obstructions

The *second major group* of conditions causing non-neoplastic hydrocephalus of the hypertensive type obstructs the outlet of the fourth ventricle at the foramina of Luschka and Magendie. Causes of obstruction at this point are various and include the Arnold-Chiari malformation, meningoceles, congenital cysts of the arachnoid, simple atresia of the fourth ventricular foramina, and basilar arachnoiditis. In some instances, platybasia, fusion deformities of the cervical spine, and other bony abnormalities may contribute to the fourth ventricular obstruction.

Arnold-Chiari malformation is a caudal displacement of the brain stem and cerebellum through the foramen magnum into the upper cervical area. It is often associated with other congenital defects, but it may exist alone. Because of the relative smallness of the cervical vertebral canal, the dislocated cerebellum may be tightly applied to the fourth ventricular roof and obstruct its outlets.

In the uncomplicated case, attempted pneumoencephalography will reveal an interference with cephalic passage of gas in the middle and upper cervical areas. A small amount of gas may pass through narrow pathways into the occipital region. Gas does not enter the ventricular system but, instead, outlines a large shadow (medulla oblongata) continuous with the cervical spinal cord and a smoothly rounded shadow dorsal to it, representing the dislocated cerebellum (fig. 242). The latter might be mistaken for an extramedullary tumor on the dorsal aspect of the spinal cord.

When ventriculography is performed, dilatation of the entire ventricular system is found. The fourth ventricle is deformed and elongated caudally, and its inferior extent may be visualized in the upper cervical region (fig. 242). The long finger-like projection of the fourth ventricle relates well to the downward extension of the brain stem and cerebellum, which is outlined by cervical subarachnoid gas at pneumoencephalography. As with examination of any midline area, tomography facilitates visualization.

Atresia of the foramina of Luschka and Magendie appears to be a more common cause of obstructive hydrocephalus in early life than has been appreciated in the past. The condition was described by Dandy in 1921, and its importance was re-emphasized by Walker (1944). Because of increased intracranial pressure, examination usually is by ventriculography; marked dilatation of the entire ventricular system without other deformity is the usual finding. The most important point in these cases, as well as in basilar arachnoiditis to be described subsequently, is to exclude a tumor blocking the outlet of the fourth ventricle. Frequently, the diagnosis of foraminal atresia or basilar arachnoiditis is one of exclusion; therefore, it must be made only after exhaustive attempts to demonstrate a neoplasm. Particular care must be taken not to overlook a tumor along the fourth ventricular floor at its lower end, such as a sessile ependymoma (fig. 245). The area often is difficult to visualize because of the overlying mastoid air cells and basal bony structures. It is recommended that sagittal tomograms be made routinely in the study of these patients, since diagnosis is so heavily dependent on the elimination of tumor as a diagnostic possibility. Inverted films also are very helpful in diagnosis.

In the typical case of atresia of the foramina of Luschka and Magendie, the lateral and third ventricular dilatation may be marked, as with aqueduct gliosis. In addition, however, a large aqueduct and large fourth ventricle with smooth walls will be shown. In the case of low fourth ventricular obstructions, the enlargement of the fourth ventricle usually is out of proportion to the enlargement of the third and lateral ventricles. Frequently, the lower end of the fourth ventricle will extend to the bony rim of the foramen magnum. The imperforate membranes may bulge into the vertebral canal. Inverted films, however, disclose no communication; gas fails to enter the spinal subarachnoid space from the fourth ventricle, and the ventricle ends caudally with a smoothly rounded margin (fig. 243). In some cases, almost the entire posterior fossa will be occupied by an enormously dilated fourth ventricle. Such a change has led to the erroneous conclusion that the fourth ventricle is a cerebellar cyst, even at the time of surgical exploration.

An occasional finding which causes alteration of the usual contour of the fourth ventricle is a pressure diverticulum of the roof, in the region of the thin anterior medullary velum. The ballooned ventricle projects into the quadrigeminal cistern at the cerebellomedullary recess (fig. 244).

Fourth ventricular obstructions of congenital origin may not manifest themselves clinically until the second or, occasionally, the third decade of life. Dilatation of very long standing may produce changes in the skull, consisting of enlargement of the pos-

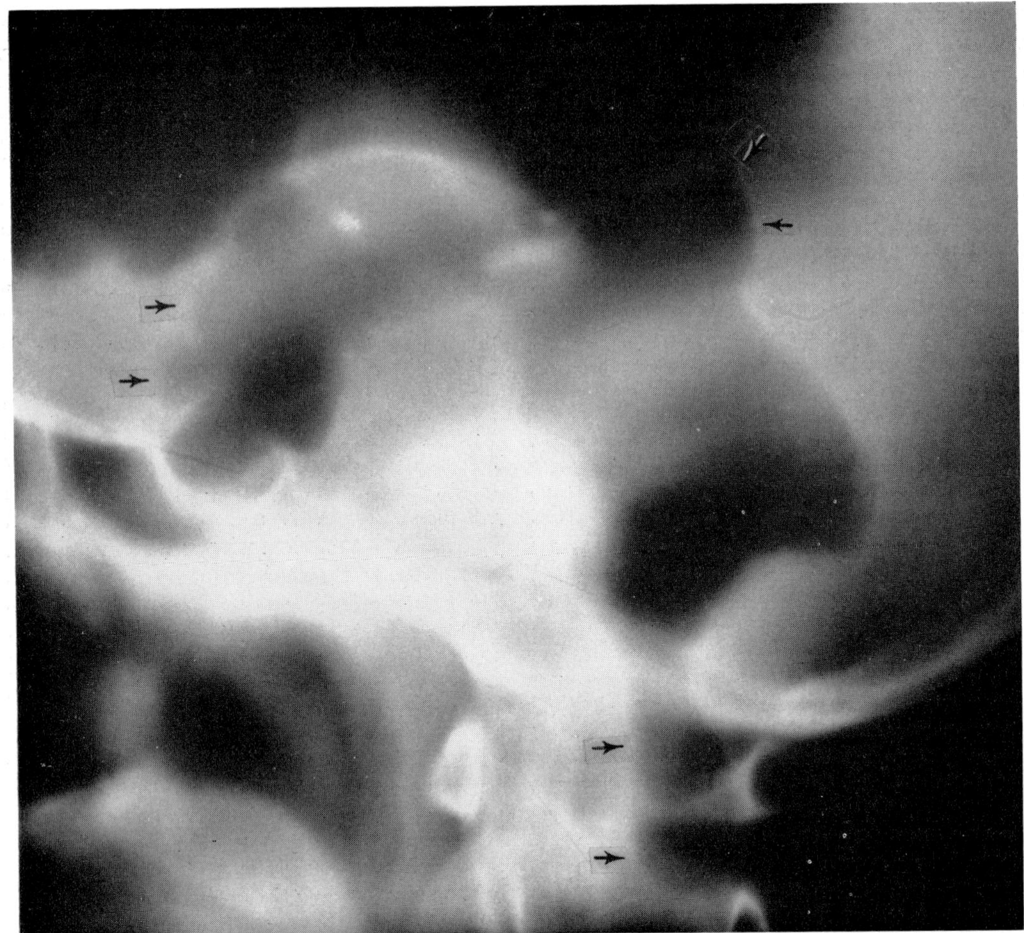

FIG. 244.—FORAMINAL ATRESIA AND PRESSURE DIVERTICULUM OF THE FOURTH VENTRICLE
A midline tomogram, made at ventriculography, shows a markedly enlarged fourth ventricle which is dilated out of proportion to other sections of the ventricular system. A projection of the fourth ventricle into the upper cervical region (*lower arrows*) is shown, similar to that illustrated in Fig. 243. The upper dorsal portion of the fourth ventricle has herniated at the thin anterior medullary velum into the area of the quadrigeminal cistern (*posterior arrows*), forming a pressure diverticulum. There is also bulging of the hypothalamic recesses of the third ventricle, and projections forward in the region of the lamina terminalis (*anterior arrows*), owing to high pressure in the third ventricle.

terior fossa and thinning of the bones (Bucy, 1939, and Taggart and Walker, 1942). The lateral sinus grooves may lie well above their ordinary position, and alterations in slope of the petrous ridges may be found. On the other hand, Davidoff and Epstein (1950) did not find evidence of enlargement of the posterior fossa in any of their cases, even though in some patients the fourth ventricle was extremely dilated.

Acquired basilar arachnoiditis cannot always be distinguished clinically or radiologically from congenital atresia. Many cases of basilar arachnoiditis can be related to a known inflammatory meningeal process or traumatic episode. At the time of surgical exploration, a milky, thickened arachnoid overlying the base of the brain, particularly over the outlets of the fourth ventricle, may be found. In other cases, there may be a thin membranous veil or band of tissue over the foramina; in still others, localized cystic

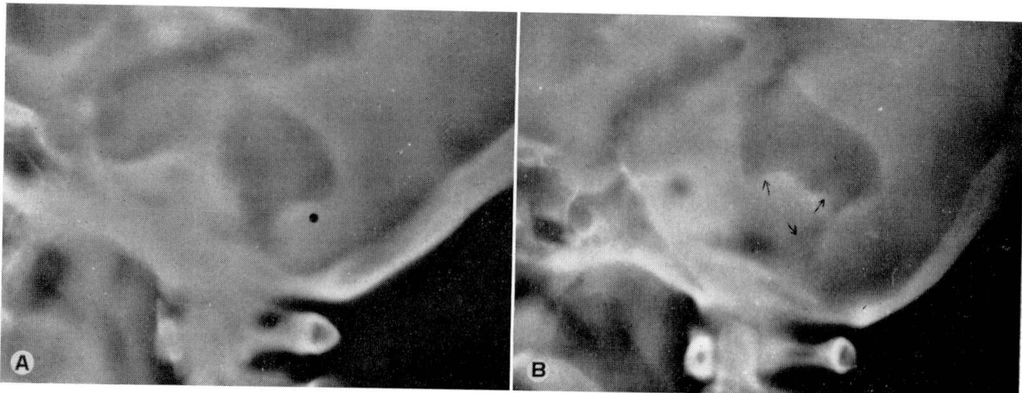

FIG. 245.—BASILAR ARACHNOIDITIS FOLLOWING MENINGITIS

A lateral tomogram, made at ventriculography, shows a moderately dilated fourth ventricle which is smooth in outline (A). The superior dorsal wall is straight, and there is slight bulging of the anterior wall. The caudal end of the fourth ventricle is dilated but does not extend lower than usual. No gas escaped into the subarachnoid space from the distended ventricular system. At the time of surgical exploration, an opalescent thickened arachnoid membrane overlay the base of the brain, obstructing the egress of fluid from the foramina of the fourth ventricle.

Benign fourth ventricular obstructions are to be differentiated from those caused by tumor. The midsagittal tomogram (B), made at ventriculography, demonstrates a mass in the caudal portion of the fourth ventricle blocking the lumen (*arrows*). Such low fourth ventricular tumors may be overlooked, particularly if they are sessile and along the anterior wall. The area may be obscured by superimposed mastoid air cells. In some cases, the dilatation of the fourth ventricle itself may allow the intraluminal mass to be surrounded by gas, thus obscuring the soft tissue shadow.

changes develop in the arachnoid, which may resemble a soft tumor.

The findings at ventriculography in posterior fossa arachnoiditis resemble those described under congenital atresia of the ventricular outlets, in the average case (fig. 245). The fourth ventricle may be larger in proportion to the lateral and third ventricles than in foraminal atresia; in other cases, for some unknown reason, the reverse is true. Again, the diagnosis is principally made by exclusion, employing the same criteria and techniques described in connection with congenital obstruction.

Metaventricular Obstructions

In the *third* type of hydrocephalus with increased pressure, there is no ventricular obstruction but free communication of the ventricles with the subarachnoid space. For this reason, this type of hydrocephalus is referred to radiologically as communicating hydrocephalus. There is always an obstruction of some type, but in communicating hydrocephalus it is outside of the ventricular pathways (fig. 246).

In a large number of patients, an obstruction to subarachnoid cerebrospinal fluid circulation is present at the tentorial incisura, obstructing the posterior communicating channels (fig. 236). In other cases, there is obstruction of the anterior communicating channels. There also may be an obstruction of the subarachnoid circulation over the cerebral convexities, preventing the fluid from reaching the arachnoid granulations, such as occurs with subdural hematoma. Failure of the absorptive mechanism itself is thought to be the cause of communicating hydrocephalus in many instances. This failure occurs owing either to a paucity of arachnoid villi, or some malfunction of those that are present. Certain abnormalities of sinus blood flow, such as thrombosis of the superior longitudinal sinus, may be the basis for a communicating hydrocephalus.

Generalized ventricular enlargement in

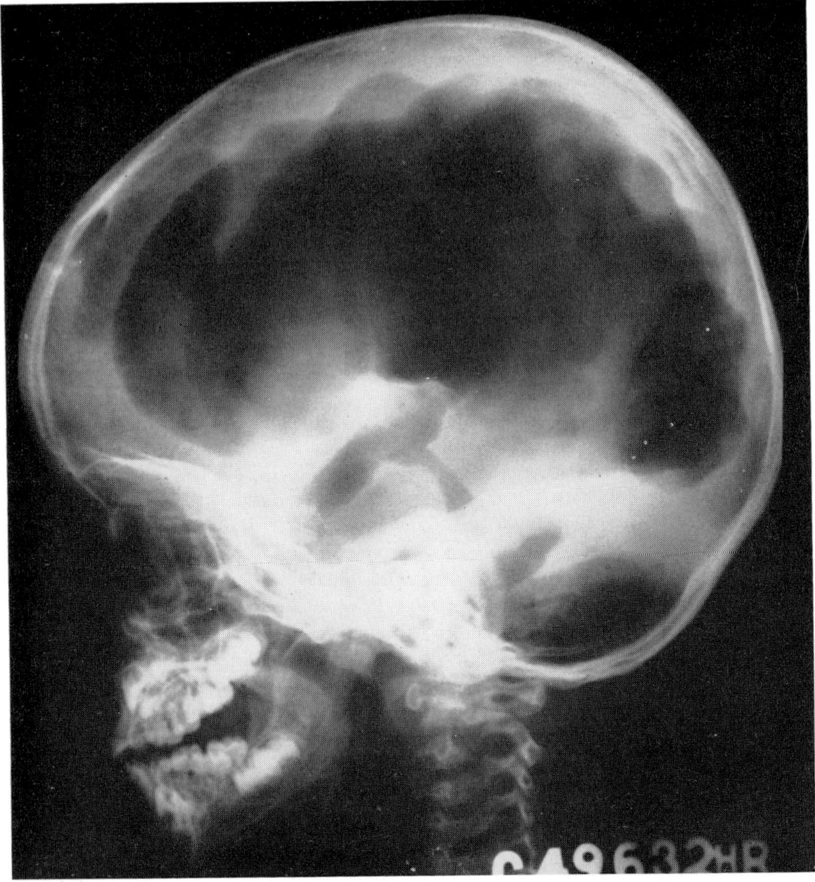

Fig. 246.—Communicating Hydrocephalus

There is marked enlargement of the entire ventricular system, and a free communication exists between the ventricles and the dilated subarachnoid pathways. In the case illustrated, there is widening of the subarachnoid space, even over the cerebral convexities; this indicates that cerebrospinal fluid absorption is ineffective for some reason, in this case presumably a congenital malformation of the Pacchionian mechanism. Communicating hydrocephalus may be caused by metaventricular obstructions in other portions of the subarachnoid space; the possibility of obstruction in the communicating cisterns was suggested by the findings illustrated in Fig. 236.

varying degrees is found at pneumography, depending upon the severity and duration of the circulatory interference. It should be possible to demonstrate a free communication of the fourth ventricle with the cisterna magna by ventriculography. Gas should be injected into the lumbar region only if it is necessary to study the subarachnoid space for the exact external site of obstruction in preparation for surgical treatment, such as division of the tentorium. In the majority of instances, proper choice between surgical procedures can be made if it is known with certainty whether the hydrocephalus is communicating or obstructive.

In the infant, pneumography also serves to exclude congenital tumors; it is particularly important to diagnose a chorioid papilloma, which produces communicating hydrocephalus through increased formation of cerebrospinal fluid. For this purpose, it may be necessary to add more gas than is used ordinarily, because these tumors are most frequently found in the atrium of the ventricle. The medial portion of the atrium cannot be visualized adequately with small amounts of gas, in the presence of extreme ventricular dilatation. Another lesion, subdural hematoma, should be considered in every case of cranial enlargement or communicating hydrocephalus; the high incidence of subdural hematoma in infancy, and its amenability to surgical treatment, make correct diagnosis imperative. Carefully performed pneumography is essential for a proper evaluation of any condition resulting in hypertensive hydrocephalus.

Intracranial Tumors

As used in this text, the term "tumor" refers to any type of space occupying lesion, whether it be a neoplasm, hematoma, abscess, cyst, or other type of mass. The tumor classification used is anatomic; discussion will be divided into five sections: (1) intraventricular tumors; (2) extraventricular supratentorial tumors; (3) intra-axial posterior fossa tumors; (4) extra-axial posterior fossa tumors; and (5) extra-axial suprasellar tumors. Certain lesions which are discussed in detail under other headings will be mentioned only in differential diagnosis.

INTRAVENTRICULAR TUMORS

General Considerations

Tumors occurring in the ventricles of the brain are among the most important studied by pneumography, usually ventriculography. Neoplasms presenting within the lumen of a ventricle constitute approximately 8 per cent of all brain tumors or 6 per cent of all tumors of the central nervous system (fig. 249). In spite of their relative infrequency, intraventricular masses are of great significance because: (1) they probably are the easiest of all tumors to detect by pneumography, (2) frequently they can be identified preoperatively, (3) many of the lesions are benign, and (4) operative removal often results in complete cure. With other, less favorable types of new growths, air study defines the extent of the lesion accurately and assists in more complete surgical or radiologic eradication.

The ease of diagnosis results from the direct contact of ventricular gas with the surface of the tumor. Thus, the presence, location, size, extent, point of origin, and the surface morphology of the lesion may be clearly evaluated. Since particular types of tumors arise in certain locations in the ventricles, the type of lesion present may be predicted with a fairly high degree of accuracy. Gas in contact with the tumor gives direct evidence of the neoplastic process, rather than indirect evidence, as is the case with tumors arising deep in the white matter. The direct demonstration of an intraventricular tumor at pneumography corresponds in accuracy to the tumor stain of angiography.

Intraventricular tumors have certain general features in common which tend to set them apart from other brain tumors. Clinically, many intraventricular tumors do not produce characteristic symptoms or neurologic signs which lead to a suspicion of their presence. The size of the tumor, for example, may have very little bearing on the symptoms related to it. The location of a tumor often is more important than size. Large tumors originating in the atrium may result in late symptoms; small tumors, which block the foramen of Monro or the iter, may produce obstructive symptoms while still quite small. Frequently there is no reliable neurologic localization. In many instances, the clinician does well to suspect a "midline" tumor and to recommend the procedure of choice, ventriculography, for confirmation. Since the majority of intraventricular tumors are associated with hydrocephalus, and through this phenomenon lead to neurologic consultation, the intraventricular tumors constitute a prime example of why causes of hydrocephalus should be defined, since many of the patients are potentially curable (see "Hydrocephalus").

Several intraventricular tumors have growth features in common, even though their tissue types differ. The tumors extend principally into the ventricular lumen, probably because it presents the least resistance to growth. Only some of the more basically

TABLE III

Type of Tumor	Cushing, 1932	Baker, 1943	Courville, 1950
	%	%	%
Glioma	43	50	34
Pituitary adenoma	18	4	5
Meningioma	13	16	12
Neurinoma	9	2	2
Congenital	6	3	2
Metastatic	4	15	26
Granuloma	2	4	14
Vascular	2	5	2
Miscellaneous	3	1	3

FIG. 247.—THE REPORTED PERCENTAGE INCIDENCE OF INTRACRANIAL TUMORS BY HISTOPATHOLOGIC TYPE (3627 CASES)

invasive types of tumors, chiefly gliomas, penetrate into neighboring neural structures to a significant extent. Ventricular dilatation occurs frequently, even when the lesions do not obstruct the ventricular pathways (the so-called *dilatation ahead of the tumor*).

In some instances, tumors are located strategically near a ventricular narrowing, such as the foramen of Monro or the outlet of the fourth ventricle. Such tumors may go through a repeated series of obstructive phenomena, first causing a block of the cerebrospinal fluid flow and then, through ventricular dilatation, the ostium may be stretched with relief of the obstruction. After a period of further growth, obstruction may occur again followed by ventricular dilatation and foraminal stretching. Consequently, it is not unusual for a ventriculogram to show a colloid cyst which does not completely obstruct the foramen of Monro, even though the lateral ventricles are markedly enlarged (fig. 259). In addition, it is well recognized that such tumors may block a foramen with the patient in one posture and not in another. The common clinical finding of headache with a change in posture is a clinical feature of colloid cyst that is often helpful for diagnosis.

Some tumors, particularly those of the chorioid plexus, incite an increased production of cerebrospinal fluid; by causing a production which keeps ahead of the subarachnoid absorptive system, a communicating type of hydrocephalus is established (fig. 252). In other instances, the effects of increased brain bulk and generalized increased intracranial pressure are thought to be the principal causes of ventricular dilatation. Not infrequently, tumors growing in the ventricular lumen will undergo fragmentation, with groups of cells metastasizing through the cerebrospinal fluid to seed to other parts of the ventricles and to the subarachnoid space. The occlusion of narrow ventricular channels, such as the aqueduct of Sylvius, may occur as a result of such tumor sequestration (fig. 253). It should be remembered that tumors may seed rostrally in the ventricular system as well as caudad.

Angiography occasionally is carried out as the first special procedure in an attempt to diagnose intraventricular tumors, since in many instances the central location of such lesions cannot be suspected clinically. In institutions where angiography is used as a "screening" procedure, the examination often is not diagnostic. Hydrocephalus is a common finding revealed by angiography in the case of intraventricular tumors. Vascular displacement may be demonstrated, either arterial or venous. An abnormal vascular supply of the tumor through chorioidal and other vessels may be found. Nevertheless, the various angiographic changes which may occur are not as specific as those seen at ventriculography. Because

TABLE IV

	%
Astrocytoma	40
Glioblastoma multiforme	22
Mixed glioma	9
Medulloblastoma	7
Ependymoma	7
Hemangioblastoma	7
Oligodendroglioma	5
Pinealoma	2
Chorioid papilloma	1
	100%

FIG. 248.—NEURAL TUMOR FREQUENCY BY HISTOPATHOLOGIC TYPE (NEUROLOGICAL INSTITUTE OF NEW YORK)

(Revised 1963)

TABLE V

	%
Frontal	24
Cerebellar	18
Temporal	15
Parietal	9
Brain stem	8
Spinal cord	7
Intraventricular	6
Thalamic	5
Pineal	3
Occipital	2
Hypothalamic	2
Corpus callosum	1

FIG. 249.—NEURAL TUMOR FREQUENCY BY ANATOMIC LOCATION (NEUROLOGICAL INSTITUTE OF NEW YORK)

increased intracranial pressure resulting from hydrocephalus is the rule with intraventricular tumors, ventriculography usually is carried out rather than pneumoencephalography. Ventriculography is the procedure of choice whenever a "midline" tumor is suggested by the clinical findings. Pneumoencephalography usually results in no filling or inadequate filling of the area of interest.

Intraventricular tumors may arise from any of the structures normally resident within the ventricular lumen, or from tissues occasionally occurring within the ventricle as a result of developmental abnormality. Tumors arising in the ventricular walls, either in the ependymal or subependymal layers, grow primarily into the ventricular lumen. Tumors arising more deeply—at some distance from the ventricular wall—may grow largely toward the ventricle, with the bulk of the mass contained within the lumen. Some lesions of the latter type, which undergo cystic changes, may rupture into the ventricle; a cavity within the tumor then is continuous with the ventricular lumen, and is itself outlined by gas injected at ventriculography. Ordinarily, however, deep tumors present only incidentally and occasionally into the ventricle. Such neoplasms which involve the ventricle by direct extension are not classed as true intraventricular tumors (fig. 271). In a similar manner, cerebellar tumors frequently involve the fourth ventricle by invasion, and vice versa. Many authors do not include primary fourth ventricular tumors in the intraventricular classification, but instead consider them with other tumors of the posterior fossa because the exact location of the primary site often cannot be established.

(Revised 1963)

Displacement is not a prominent feature of intraventricular neoplasms, even tumors of one lateral ventricle. Presumably this is because the tumor expands into the cerebrospinal fluid without soft tissue resistance. In some cases, however, a tumor of a lateral ventricle may attain such size that some lateral displacement must take place. More frequently, as has been described, there is symmetrical ventricular dilatation. Diagnosis ordinarily is dependent upon deformity, which results from general or segmental disproportionate dilatation, and the presence of a discrete filling defect in the ventricular lumen.

Lateral Ventricles

Lateral ventricular tumors may be divided into two groups: (1) non-neoplastic masses and (2) true neoplasms. The benign masses include intraventricular hematomas, foreign bodies, parasitic cysts, usually cysticercosis, and others.

Non-neoplastic. Intraventricular hemorrhage is commonly found at autopsy and is often a catastrophic event. Intraventricular hematomas, usually subependymal, are a very frequent finding in ventriculography owing to injury to the chorioid plexus and ventricular walls (fig. 196). More recently, Baker (1962) has described a number of cases of spontaneous intraventricular hemorrhage in which the pneumographic appearance resembles an intraventricular tumor (fig. 250). Apparently these masses result most often from subependymal hemorrhage which elevates the ependyma but which remains fairly well confined. In frontal view, the mass has a globular or a triangular configuration, even forming a cast of one lateral ventricle on occasions. Of diagnostic importance may be the length of the lesion along the ventricular floor in lateral view. The mass may extend from the foramen of

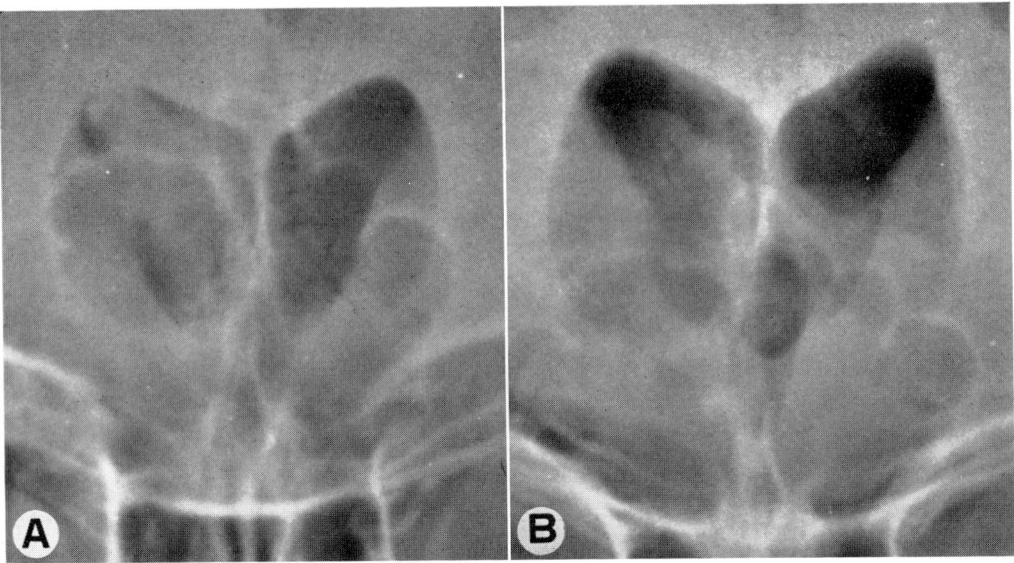

FIG. 250.—SPONTANEOUS INTRAVENTRICULAR HEMATOMA

A frontal pneumogram, made at the time of initial examination (A), reveals a soft tissue shadow obscuring the greater portion of the lumen of the right lateral ventricle. The soft tissue mass conforms generally to the shape of the ventricle. The frontal film of a pneumogram performed 10 days later (B) reveals an abnormal shadow remaining in the ventricular lumen, but it is much smaller. Confirmation of the diagnosis of an organizing hematoma was obtained.

Monro backward through the entire ventricular body to the region of the atrium. In one case observed (fig. 250), examination on two separate occasions showed a reduction in size of an intraventricular mass; this, together with clinical findings, would appear adequate to establish the presence of a contracting rather than an expanding process, and obviate unnecessary surgical intervention.

Normal cerebral structures and developmental variations may produce projections into the ventricular lumen, which should be recognized for their anatomic worth (fig. 225). Various congenital malformations, such as tuberous sclerosis, may be associated with nodular lesions of the ventricular wall, which may cause small filling defects within the lumen (fig. 232); it is unlikely that they are often mistaken for true intraventricular neoplasms. Parasitic cysts, while more common in the fourth ventricle, may occasionally occur as filling defects in the third ventricle, a lateral ventricle, or the subarachnoid space.

Since the *chorioid plexus* is an important anatomic component of the ventricles, lesions arising from this structure uniquely fall into the category of intraventricular masses. In the case of the lateral ventricles, a normal chorioid glomus may occasionally attain considerable size and be quite asymmetrical. In addition, such a mass may become pedunculated, and have appreciable mobility within the ventricular lumen by means of a stalklike attachment to the main body of the chorioid plexus. Large chorioid glomuses appearing first in a ventricular body and then in a temporal horn, with change in position of the head, have been described.

Enlargement of a chorioid glomus, as a result of hematoma formation at the time of ventriculography, was appreciated long ago by Dyke, Elsberg, and Davidoff (1935). Apparently, a hematoma results readily when a ventricular needle enters the extremely vascular structure of the chorioid glomus. Ordinarily, enlargement of the glomus shadow is seen unilaterally, although it may be bilateral. Rarely, when an oppor-

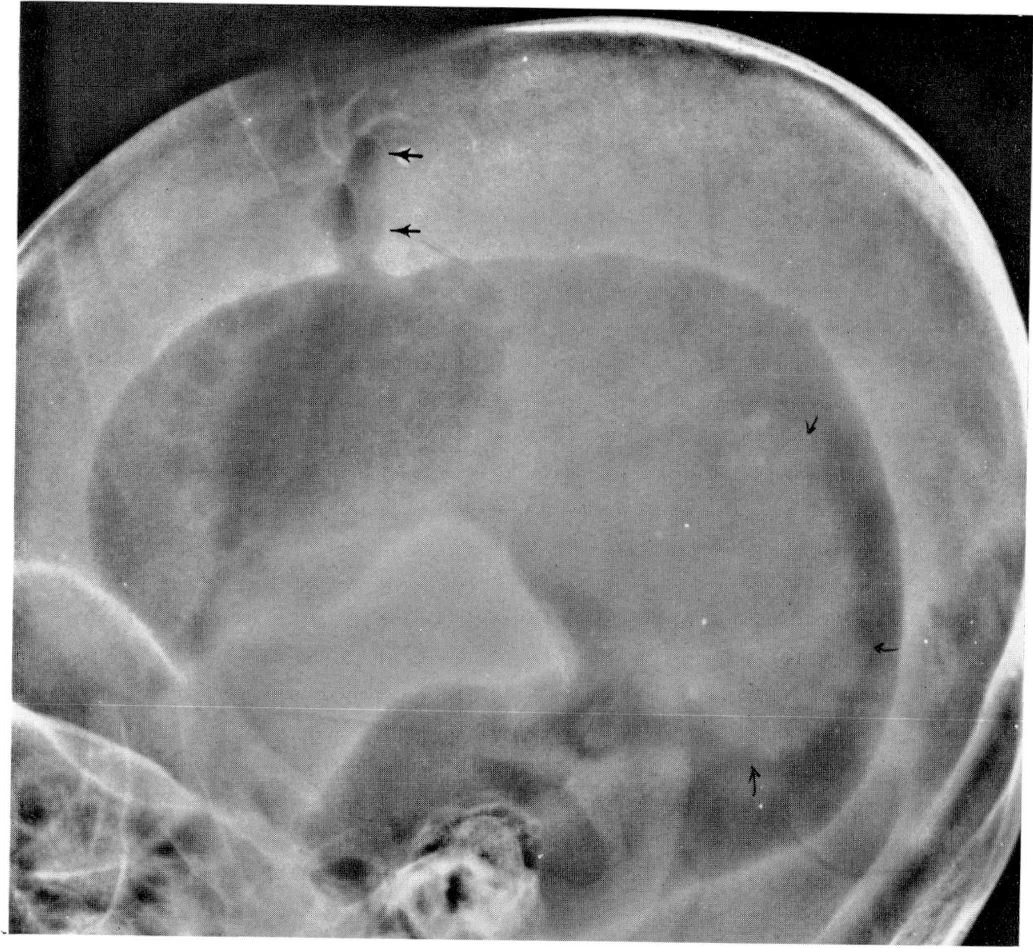

FIG. 251.—CHORIOID PLEXUS PAPILLOMA

The lateral ventriculogram reveals moderately severe hydrocephalus; a large tumor of the lateral ventricle is outlined by gas in the atrium and posterior portion of the ventricular body (*posterior arrows*). Gas covers all surfaces of the tumor, except the anterior aspect; the tumor appears to arise from the usual location of the glomus of the chorioid plexus. The surface of the tumor is finely irregular in contrast with epidermoidomas, and some glial tumors, which often have a grossly irregular surface. A sizable superior projection of gas into the cerebral substance of the supraforaminal region has occurred along the tract of the ventricular needle (*upper arrows*), and toward the anterior fontanelle, through which the puncture was made.

tunity is provided for subsequent visualization of the ventricles, the shadow of the enlarged chorioid glomus can be observed to become progressively smaller with the passage of time (one to two weeks).

Chorioid plexus papillomas. True tumors of the lateral ventricles of several varieties are encountered; the only neoplasm arising in a lateral ventricle which may not be seen outside of the ventricular system is the papilloma of the chorioid plexus. An important report on this subject was published by Matson and Crofton (1960), who reviewed the literature and described 16 additional cases of their own observed during a period of 17 years. The incidence, therefore, obviously is small, and it is generally agreed to be something less than 0.5 per cent of all intracranial tumors.

The tumor is seen most frequently during

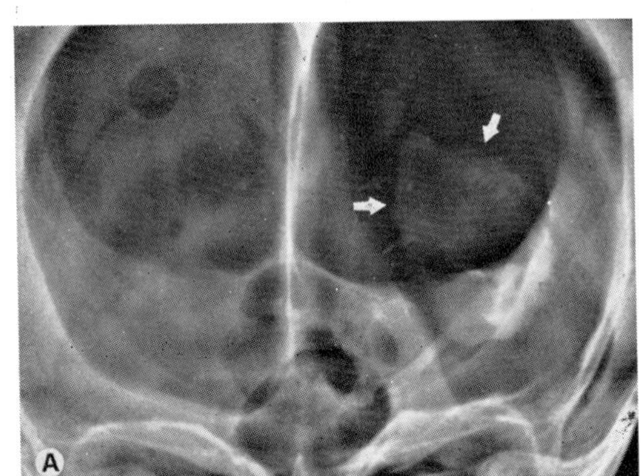

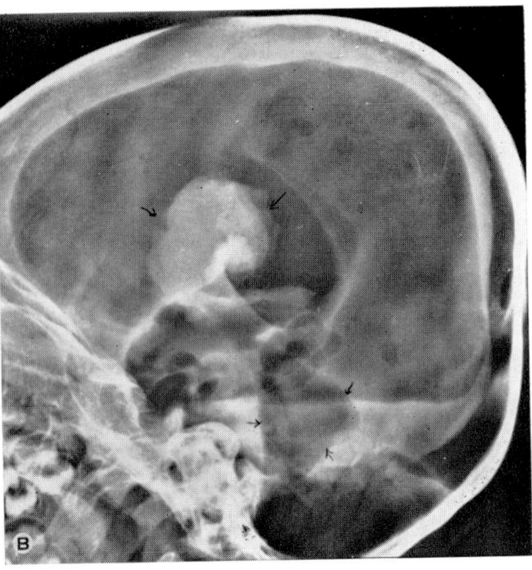

FIG. 252.—CHORIOID PLEXUS PAPILLOMA

Severe symmetrical ventricular dilatation is present. The frontal ventriculogram (A) reveals a 4 by 3 cm. mass in the ventricular lumen, surrounded by gas on four sides in this projection (*arrows*). The lateral ventriculogram (B) shows the tumor to be in the anterior portion of the ventricular body (*upper arrows*) and attached to the ventricular floor just behind the foramen of Monro. The third and fourth ventricles are markedly enlarged, and the latter structure (*lower arrows*) communicates widely with the cisterna magna. Gas is present posterior to the brain in the subdural space. The subdural collection may have occurred by leakage of ventricular gas through the puncture site of the thin overlying cortex (see Fig. 251), or it may have been injected inadvertently directly into the subdural space at the time of ventriculography.

the first decade of life, and very commonly during infancy. Matson and Crofton considered the tumor to be interesting because (1) occasionally it has a prenatal occurrence, (2) frequently there is associated communicating hydrocephalus, (3) commonly it has a benign noninvasive character with the possibility of total excision, (4) it has a histological relationship to normal ependyma and the normal chorioid plexus, and (5) some variants of the tumor closely resemble ependymomas.

The chorioid tumors are found most often in the lateral ventricles in children; the incidence is greater in the fourth ventricle in adults. Plain skull films frequently show changes resulting from increased intracranial pressure in children; megacephalus, resulting from hydrocephalus, with widening of sutures usually is found. Calcification, which is frequently seen in normal chorioid tissue, is not a feature of chorioid papilloma, particularly in children. In the majority of instances, the tumors have attained considerable size (3 to 6 cm. in diameter) by the time radiologic examination is carried out. The tumor surface is usually finely irregular, but may be lobulated. In the majority of cases, the finely irregular surface serves to distinguish the chorioid papilloma from the grossly irregular surface of the epidermoidoma (fig. 251). Occasionally, the surface is smooth, and in these cases differentiation from meningioma is not possible on the basis of the appearance of the tumor alone. Fragmentation with seeding to other portions of the ventricular system may occur. Histologic examination usually reveals a structure that resembles the normal chorioid plexus very closely. Malignant changes are rare, but may occur with invasion of adjacent neural structures.

At ventriculography, dilatation is almost always found, either on the basis of obstruction or as a result of overproduction of cerebrospinal fluid with a communicating hydrocephalus. The tumor mass itself often is very large, but still may incompletely fill the greatly dilated ventricle (fig. 252). The tumor origin usually is in the atrium; at other times it may arise near the foramen of Monro, or in other locations where large collections of chorioid tissue normally are found. Lateral ventricular dilatation usually is greater on the side of the tumor; in the majority of patients there is some displacement of midline structures away from the side of the mass. Dilatation often is greatest in the proximity of the tumor with less marked enlargement elsewhere. In a great many instances, however, there is generalized dilatation of the ventricular system and of the subarachnoid pathways. A number of instances in which porencephalic cavities were present near the tumor have been reported; in two of the patients described by Matson and Crofton the tumor was masked by the porencephalic cyst.

Liber and Lisa (1940) and McGuire, Greenwood, and Newton (1954) have reported angiomas of the chorioid plexus which are indistinguishable clinically or radiologically from true papillomas. Hemangiomas, however, are rare lesions. For all practical purposes, it may be said that intraventricular masses occurring in children are chorioid papillomas when they are (1) based along the lateral ventricular floor, particularly in the atrial region, (2) associated with pronounced communicating hydrocephalus, (3) finely irregular in outline and disproportionately large for the symptoms they produce.

The communicating hydrocephalus associated with chorioid papilloma is by far its most interesting feature. Quantitation of the excessive formation of cerebrospinal fluid is quite difficult. There is, however, a greatly increased epithelial surface present which is thought to account for the vast increase in cerebrospinal fluid production. Prompt and permanent relief of hydrocephalus usually occurs in all patients in whom a papilloma of the chorioid plexus is successfully removed; this would appear to be strong evidence in favor of the theory that the hydrocephalus is caused solely by overproduction of cerebrospinal fluid by the tumor, rather than some associated abnormality of the cerebrospinal fluid absorption.

Epidermoidomas. Epidermoid tumors constitute a general type of neoplasm frequently considered to be of "congenital" origin. The tumors were described by Cruveilhier (1829) who, because of the refractile and nodular surface, described the neoplasms as "pearly tumors." Mueller (1838) suggested the name cholesteatoma. Many epidermoidomas result from epithelial inclusions within the neural substance (Remak, 1854). While the epidermoids occurring in the bony skull all probably are of "inclusion" origin, those arising in the ventricles and even the subarachnoid space may begin as new growths from the epithelium of the chorioid plexus. The tumors grow very slowly and, when favorably situated, may be surgically extirpated.

In the tumor series described by Cushing (1932), epidermoidomas constituted less than 0.5 per cent of all intracranial tumors. Such lesions occurring in the bones of the skull, on the other hand, are very common. The intracranial tumors of importance are those which are found in the lateral ventricles, in the fourth ventricle, ventral to the pons, or in the cerebellopontine angle.

Grossly, the tumor surface has the appearance of mother-of-pearl. On histologic examination, the outer layers of the mass are composed of densely compact epithelial cells. The deeper portions of the lesion may exhibit a loose honeycomb-like arrangement of cells, resembling the structure of plants (Courville, 1950).

Hydrocephalus, particularly lateral ventricular enlargement, occurs as a result of obstruction or increased brain bulk, or both, produced by the tumor. The epidermoidomas occurring in a lateral ventricle are very irregular cauliflower-like masses. The atrium and body of a lateral ventricle are the most common sites of occurrence. Occasionally, they may be found in a temporal horn (fig. 253). Invasion of adjacent neural structures may occur, but extension usually is local and limited.

At ventriculography, the tumor, which

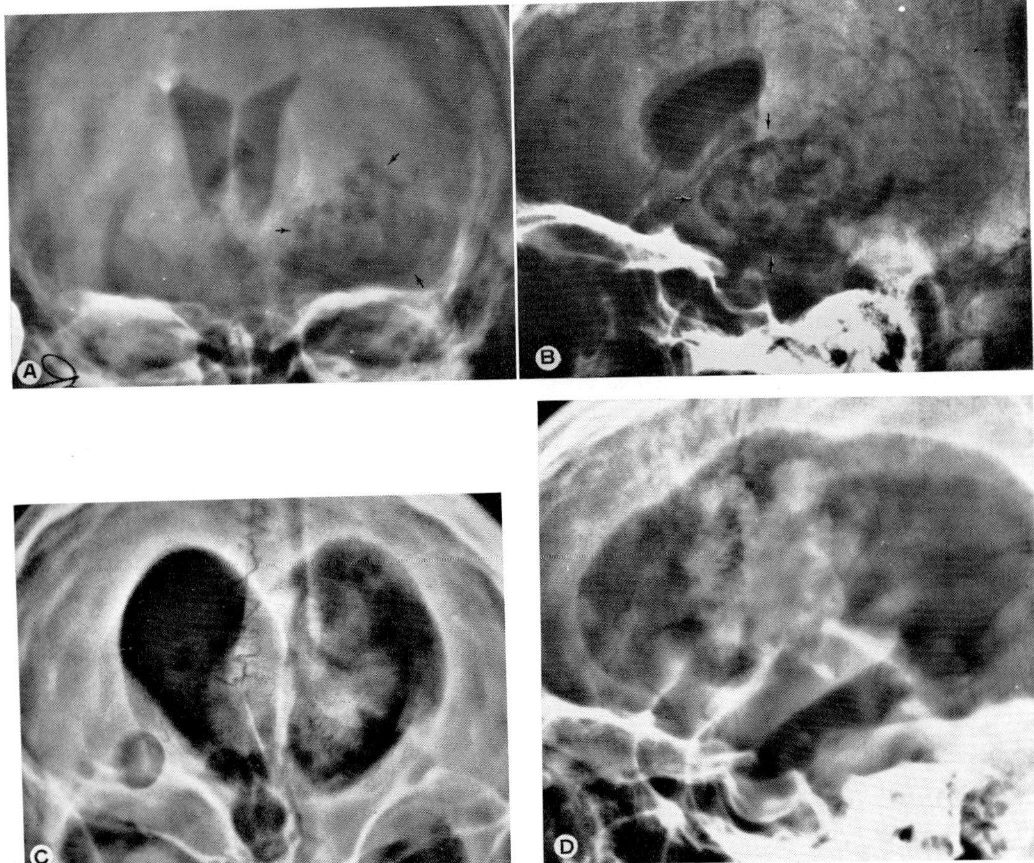

Fig. 253.—Epidermoid Tumor of the Lateral Ventricles

Films made with the patient supine show isolated dilatation of the left temporal horn and moderate ventricular displacement in the frontal pneumogram (A). A tumor with a very irregular surface occupies a large portion of the lumen of the temporal horn, resulting in a dappled appearance of the gas outline (*arrows*). In the lateral pneumogram (B), the dilated temporal horn is well demarcated (*arrows*); the lumen is almost completely filled by a mass with a grossly uneven surface, characteristic of epidermoidoma (see text).

In another case, the frontal ventriculogram (C) reveals a large tumor filling the medial portion of the left lateral ventricle and bulging across the midline. The tumor occupies the greater part of the ventricular lumen on the medial side. The lateral ventriculogram (D) shows the irregular cauliflower-like mass to be located in the supraforaminal portion of the lateral ventricle. The deep clefts, into which gas enters to give the tumor its rough, irregular appearance, are fairly characteristic of epidermoidomas. Several oligodendrogliomas, arising from the septum pellucidum, have been encountered which simulated the findings shown in this case. The large third ventricle is explained by fragmentation of the tumor surface and obstruction of the aqueduct of Sylvius by the separated particles of tumor.

may have grown slowly over a long period of time and attained considerable size, usually is sharply demarcated by gas with which it is in contact in an enlarged ventricle. The tumor itself may measure 4 to 5 cm. in diameter, and occasionally more. The mass is based on the ventricular floor—or roof of the temporal horn, third or fourth ventricle—apparently rooted in the chorioid plexus. The tumor may be outlined by gas over most of its surface, except where attached; in other instances, when the tumor arises in a temporal horn, only a portion of the surface may be in contact with the ventricular gas because the lumen is filled or blocked by the mass (fig. 253). Some tumors present in the lumen of both lateral ventricles, apparently having grown through the septum pellucidum, while still maintaining a predominantly intraluminal growth.

The degree of hydrocephalus varies and it may be localized or generalized, depending on the origin of the tumor. Epidermoidomas of the temporal horn, for example, may result almost exclusively in dilatation of that ventricular segment (fig. 253). In other instances, dilatation of the third and both lateral ventricles may occur acutely, as a result of tumor fragmentation with blockage of the cerebral aqueduct. More typically, there is a marked degree of dilatation of both lateral ventricles, which develops slowly over a long period of time, owing to the tumor's benign nature and slow growth.

The possibility of an epidermoid tumor should be suspected when a bulky mass is found in a lateral ventricle. Gas over the tumor surface reveals the rough, irregular form of the neoplasm. Characteristically, gas extends into the depths of the tumor through wide and deep clefts, producing the cauliflower appearance considered typical by Dyke (1941). The surface configuration is not as finely irregular as is seen with the typical chorioid papilloma; neither is the surface as coarse as ordinarily observed with ependymoma or oligodendroglioma. Occasionally oligodendrogliomas, which present within the ventricular lumen, appear as shaggy masses indistinguishable from epidermoidomas. The former type of tumor more often is based on the septum pellucidum, or arises in the third ventricle and extends to the lateral ventricles. Epidermoidomas usually arise from the ventricular walls when chorioid plexus tissue is present. Oligodendrogliomas frequently contain calcium.

Dermoid tumors also may be found in a lateral ventricle, on rare occasions. More commonly dermoids are encountered in the region of the pineal, in the cerebellum, or in the fourth ventricle. Usually the tumors are cystic; a large proportion contain calcific elements visible on plain films (see "Intracranial Calcifications"). The margins of dermoids may be smooth or lobulated, but the deep fissures found in the case of epidermoids do not usually occur with the cystic dermoids. True *teratomas* also may occur, but not as pure intraventricular tumors. These rare tumors have been described most often as occurring in the region of the epiphysis, the hypophysis or in anterior brain stem locations. The solid portions of the tumor contain tissues derived from the three germ layers and frequently there are sizable cysts and areas of hemorrhage. Large new growths occurring very early in life which contain calcific elements visible on plain skull films should suggest the possibility of teratoma, whether the lesion be in the sites previously listed or situated anywhere within the hemispheric cerebral substance.

Meningiomas. *Intraventricular meningiomas* usually do not manifest themselves clinically until they have grown for a long period of time and have attained considerable size. These lesions, like the chorioid papillomas and epidermoidomas, probably arise from the tissues of the chorioid plexus. They most often occur in the region of the trigone and take origin from the glomus. In some instances, the tumors may take the general configuration of the ventricular lumen and extend into the temporal horn (fig. 254). There often is moderate ventricular dilatation, frequently of the ipsilateral ventricle. The ventricular dilatation presumably is the result of pressure behind the bulk of tumor; dilatation of the opposite ventricle does not often occur except when obstruction takes place. Tumors originating near the foramen of Monro or in the third or fourth ventricle more readily produce obstruction and may produce symptoms early when the tumor is yet small (fig. 261).

This particular type of meningioma falls into the category that Cushing and Eisenhardt (1938) termed "meningiomas without dural attachment," which constitute only a small percentage of all meningiomas. Clinical diagnosis is difficult until late in the course of

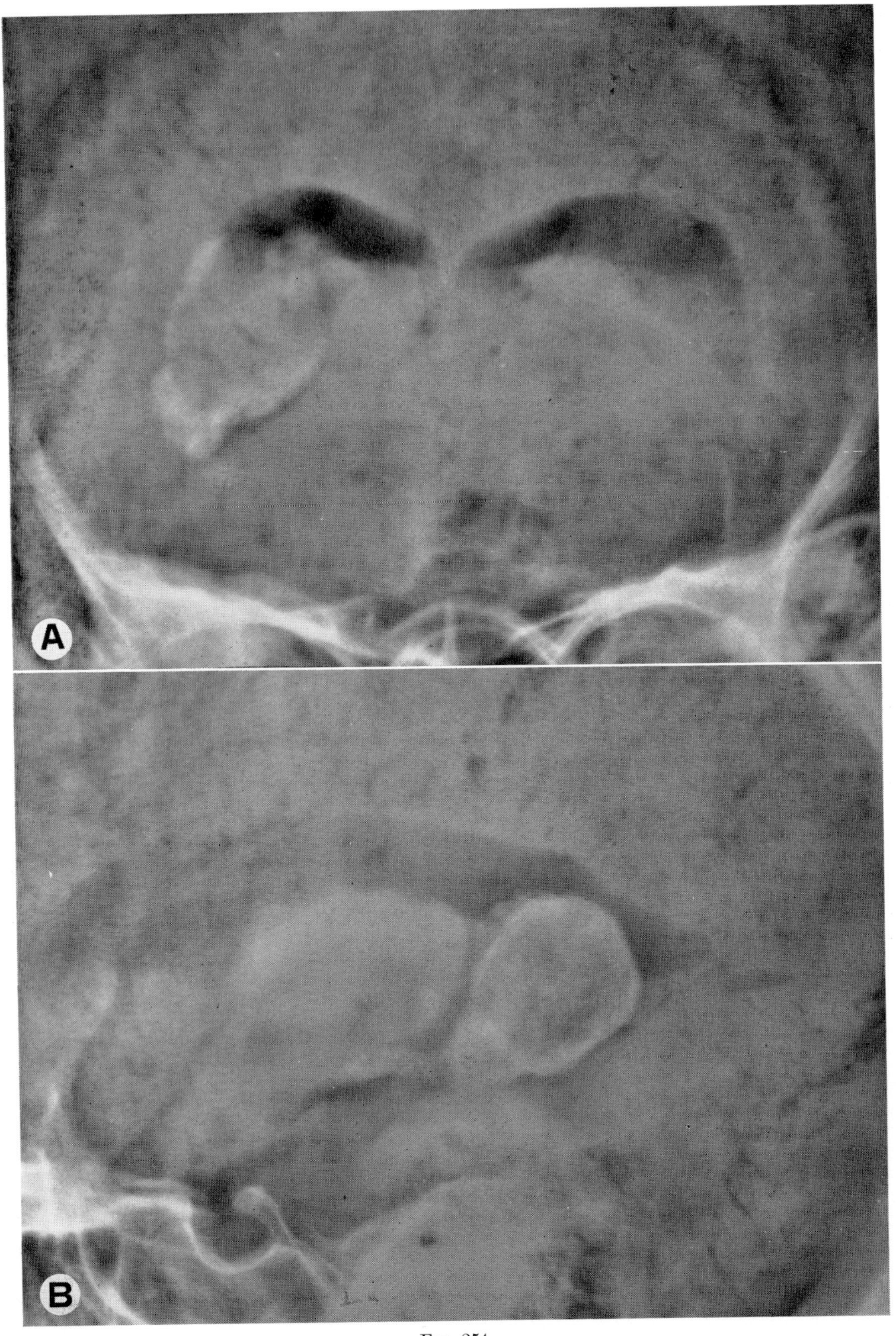

Fig. 254

(*Revised 1963*)

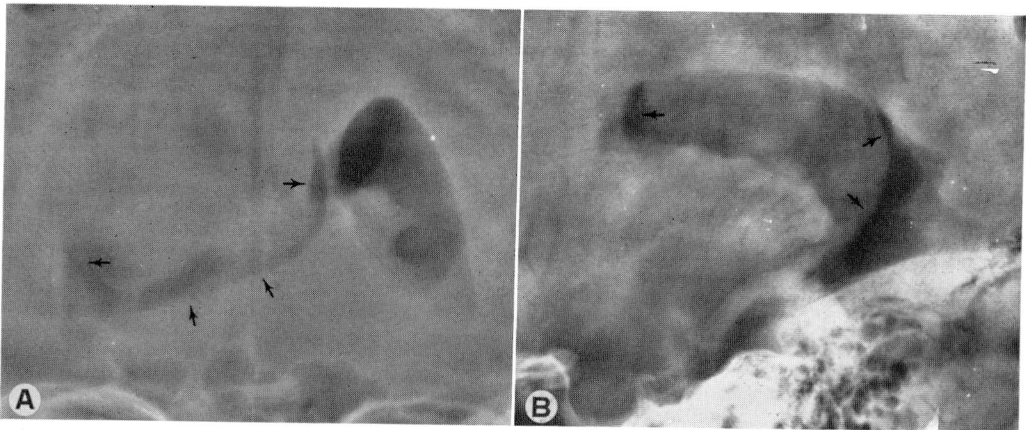

FIG. 255.—INTRAVENTRICULAR MENINGIOMA

A large, smooth mass is present in the posterior portion of the right lateral ventricle which largely obscures the lumen of the atrium in frontal view (A). Gas is shown extending medial and lateral to the tumor (*transverse arrows*) and also behind the lesion (*vertical arrows*): this gas does not clearly show the tumor outline. Because the tumor is of such size that it reaches the ventricular roof, no gas is shown over the superior surface of the tumor.

The lateral ventriculogram (B) shows that the tumor is based on the ventricular floor in the region of the atrium and posterior part of the ventricular body. This is the most common site of such tumors, which probably arise from the chorioid plexus. The smoothness of the tumor surface (*arrows*), and the location of the lesion are most helpful in making the correct diagnosis.

the disease. Calcification visible in plain films occurs in the minority of tumors that we have encountered; when present, the correct diagnosis may be strongly suspected from plain skull examination (fig. 254). At ventriculography, the tumor ordinarily is well demarcated by gas, the surface being smooth and even or exhibiting large lobulations. The presence of a large tumor in the atrium of an enlarged ventricle, with the smooth surface described, and occurring in a relatively young adult should suggest meningioma (fig. 255).

Displacement of the septum pellucidum and other midline structures is frequent but usually of moderate degree. The contralateral ventricle may be enlarged, the dilatation varying from mild to moderately severe. In the absence of obstruction, it is not as marked as is the case with chorioid papilloma. Frequently, however, tumors arising in the ventricular body or trigone will obstruct the ipsilateral temporal horn with striking disproportionate enlargement of this segment. Occasionally, a meningioma may extend into the lateral ventricle from the superior aspect and the point of origin then is not always clear. Some tumors of this type are so definitely intraventricular that aberrant chorioid origin is suggested, while others may arise from the inferior margin of the falx and grow predominantly downward. The latter are not true intraventricular tumors and do not have the sharply margin-

FIG. 254.—INTRAVENTRICULAR MENINGIOMA

A tumor with dense marginal calcification is present in the atrium of the right lateral ventricle, which extends downward into the temporal horn. The frontal film (A) shows a small amount of gas passing around the medial aspect of the tumor, which has widened the atrium. The lateral film (B) discloses the calcified mass to be comma-shaped, with a tapering extension forward into the superior cleft of the temporal horn, following the course of the chorioid plexus. The well defined mass contains dense marginal and conglomerate calcific nodules denoting the psammomatous nature of the lesion. (Courtesy of Drs. John Goree and Robert Reeves, Duke University School of Medicine.)

(Revised 1963)

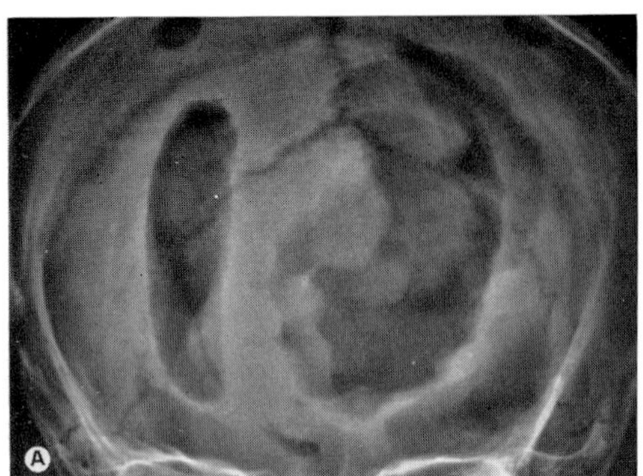
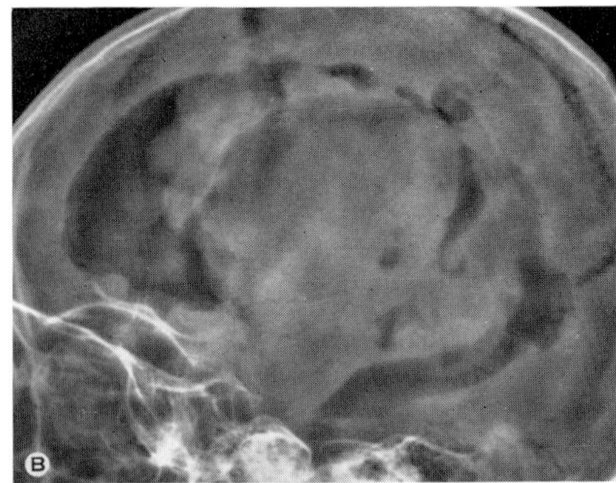

Fig. 256.—Ependymoma of the Lateral Ventricle

An enormous tumor is present, contained predominantly in the markedly dilated lumen of the left lateral ventricle. The frontal ventriculogram reveals the right lateral and third ventricles to be grossly displaced (A). A large multilobular mass, apparently based on the medial ventricular wall, extends in an irregular manner into the gas-filled ventricular lumen. The surface of the tumor is coarsely uneven, with ventricular gas extending into clefts between the large surface nodules. The lateral film reveals the tumor to extend from the anterior horn through the ventricular body and atrium into the temporal region (B).

ated outline characteristic of primary intraventricular tumors.

Gliomas. Tumors of the glioma group constitute by far the largest number of intraventricular tumors. The nodular glial masses occurring in tuberous sclerosis, which project into the lateral ventricles, have been described elsewhere. Usually, there is no difficulty in recognizing this process, since the intraventricular tumors are multiple and small and frequently contain calcium. Most often the nodules are located along the ventricular roof and are subependymal in location. Occasionally, such nodular glial collections may undergo neoplastic change.

Gangliogliomas are benign tumors which are relatively rare. The tumors are thought to be related to the polar spongioblastomas and are composed of adult ganglion cells and astrocytes (Courville, 1950). Connective tissue often is abundant and deposits of calcium frequently are found in the central portions of the tumors. The location of such tumors is said to be similar to that of the polar spongioblastomas, but the ones that the authors have encountered most frequently are those which arise along a ventricular boundary and project into the ventricular lumen. The masses are usually sharply demarcated and fairly smooth in outline. Such lesions may obstruct the foramen of Monro and result in hydrocephalus.

Ependymomas arise less frequently in the region of the lateral ventricles than in the fourth ventricle. We have, however, encountered such tumors presenting primarily as intraluminal masses and resembling somewhat an epidermoid tumor of a lateral ventricle (fig. 256). Such lateral ventricular lesions usually do not contain calcium.

The supratentorial ependymomas occurring in childhood and growing primarily as hemispheric lesions are described elsewhere. These tumors often attain considerable size. The presence of a bulky hemispheric tumor which contains a small amount of central calcific degeneration, occurring in a young individual, should always suggest the diagnosis of ependymoma (fig. 171).

While *oligodendrogliomas* are relatively uncommon glial tumors, constituting only about 1 per cent of some series (Davis, 1942), they are not infrequent lesions in the region of the ventricles and other deeply seated structures. It is frequently found that such tumors are not composed purely of oligodendroglial elements. Oligodendrogliomas may arise from the septum pellucidum. It is not infrequent for tumors arising in the septum to extend into both lateral ventricles, although the growth usually is asymmetrical and predominantly on one side.

Evidence of an oligodendroglioma may be found on plain film examination by the presence of deep-seated calcification in the brain (fig. 169). The calcification usually is irregular in outline with linear extensions from a central conglomerate collection of calcium. The calcium develops as a result of degenerative changes in the differentiated tumor by means of mechanisms previously described; this is related, in part, to the very slow growth characteristic of the neoplasm. Evidence of long-standing increased intracranial pressure is found in many instances on the plain skull films, manifested chiefly by extensive sella turcica damage. The increased pressure results either from the bulkiness of the tumor, ventricular obstruction, or a direct effect on the sella itself, in the case of third ventricular extension. Often a combination of factors is at work. In other instances, plain film changes of increased pressure may not be present even though the tumor may have attained remarkable size. In these instances, it appears probable that compensatory mechanisms may counteract the building up of high pressure. It is well known that such lesions, either oligodendrogliomas or astrocytomas or mixed lesions, may undergo malignant metaplasia at any time during their development. Often this is a late event in the case of the tumors under discussion. The radiologist should not be disturbed about his diagnostic impression, therefore, if examination of a surgical specimen reveals glioblastoma multiforme when the otherwise classical appearance of a long-standing oligodendroglioma has been observed. Under these circumstances, undoubtedly the surgeon has obtained only a marginal, unrepresentative portion of the entire lesion, although the prognostic implications of the finding of a high grade of malignancy in such a lesion are no less grave. In many instances, this metaplasia is the same reason that a patient who has harbored a benign lesion for many years finally presents himself for medical attention.

(Revised 1963)

At ventriculography, dilatation usually is present as a result of obstruction at the foramen of Monro or extension into the third ventricle. A large irregular filling defect usually is present in the dilated ventricles, often bilaterally, when the lesions have arisen from the septum pellucidum. A few smooth oligodendrogliomas have been encountered. The surface of the average tumor is grossly irregular with fissures into which gas may extend. If growth has occurred in this manner, the tumor may be indistinguishable from a cholesteatoma although the lobulations are not as numerous or the fissures as deep. Extension through the septum pellucidum, in the case of biventricular masses, favors oligodendroglioma; in one case, a bilateral cholesteatoma was observed. The presence of calcium is a finding in favor of a glial tumor; size is not a reliable criterion.

Astrocytomas, if pure tumors of this histologic type, do not provide as characteristic an appearance as do the massive, often shaggy oligodendrogliomas and the ependymal tumors. More often, the intraventricular presentation is incidental to the tumor's growth. In many instances, the tumor begins its growth in the basal ganglia, or some other neighboring structure, and tends to assume the character of a tumor of that location. No distinctive growth pattern can be ascribed to intraventricular astrocytomas.

The term *interventricular tumor* may be applied to cysts and neoplasms of the septum pellucidum, and to those tumors of the corpus callosum which grow downward into the septum without extending appreciably beyond this structure. The majority of cysts of the septum pellucidum communicate with the ventricular system and fill with gas at the time of pneumography. This is a developmental variation more properly called a cavum septum pellucidum, rather than a cyst, and the finding has been described elsewhere under "Anatomic Variants." Occasionally, however, a *noncommunicating cavum septum pellucidum* (septum pellucidum cyst) may occur. This cyst is, of itself, often innocuous, although other cerebral anomalies may be associated which do cause symptoms.

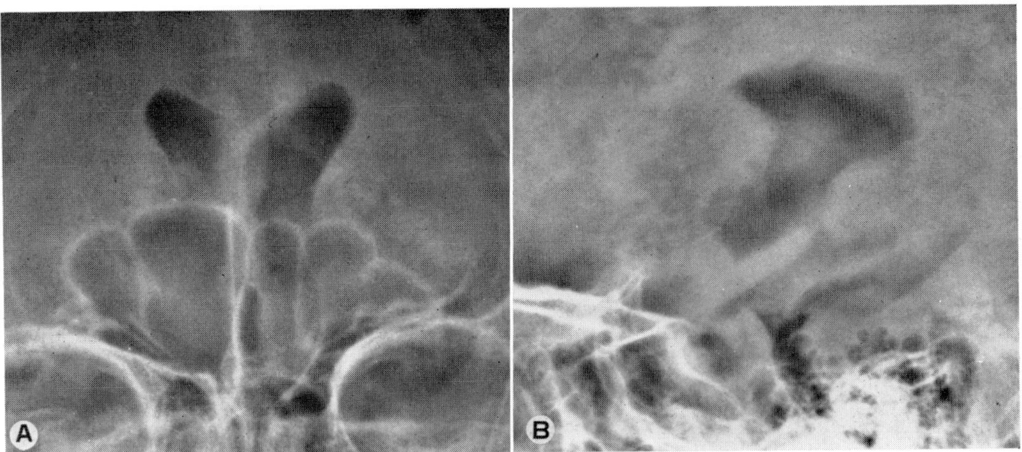

FIG. 257.—INTERVENTRICULAR ASTROCYTOMA

The frontal pneumogram (A) reveals a vertical midline mass superimposed upon the shadow of the septum pellucidum. The shadow is much wider than the normal thickness of the septum. The smoothness of the lesion in this view suggested the possibility of a septum pellucidum cyst, or noncommunicating cavum septum pellucidum. The frontal horn shadows, however, are not demonstrated. The lateral pneumogram (B) shows that the lesion is essentially preforaminal, growing backward along the septum pellucidum to the supraforaminal plane.

Ventricular obstruction develops in some cases. The pneumographic differentiation of cysts and solid tumors of the septum pellucidum is not always possible, if the former do not communicate with a lateral ventricle or with the third ventricle. Characteristically, the noncommunicating cavum septum pellucidum is smooth in appearance and has rounded, bilaterally convex margins. At other times, however, solid tumors may mimic this configuration, presenting a globular appearance in both frontal and lateral view. On the other hand, a noncommunicating fluid-filled cavum septum pellucidum may have straight parallel or asymmetrical borders and give no clue that the widened septum pellucidum shadow is the result of a fluid collection and not solid tissue. If immediate surgical intervention is not clinically indicated, then observation over a period of time, with a repeated pneumographic examination, gives the best radiologic indication concerning whether or not the process is a new growth (fig. 257).

The majority of interventricular tumors are gliomas, usually well differentiated astrocytomas or oligodendrogliomas, which have just been described. Other glial cellular elements may predominate in some neoplasms. Calcium deposits often are present in primary interventricular tumors, particularly those of the oligodendroglioma group. Tumors which arise in the *corpus callosum* and extend downward are more readily recognized as true tumors than those of the septum itself. Widening of the septum pellucidum occurs in the minority of patients with corpus callosum tumors but was considered sufficiently frequent to be included in the differential diagnosis of causes of widening of the septum pellucidum given by Lowman, Shapiro, and Collins (1948). In the authors' experience, extension of corpus callosum tumors into the septum is not a rare occurrence and two examples are shown in Figure 258. Roof deformities of the lateral ventricles with depression, ventricular spreading and narrowing of the lumen usually are sufficiently characteristic to cause no difficulty in establishing the primary site of such tumors as being in the corpus callosum.

Lipomas of the corpus callosum may extend downward into the septum; their frequent association with agenesis of the corpus callosum was described by List, Holt, and Everett (1946). In these instances, the

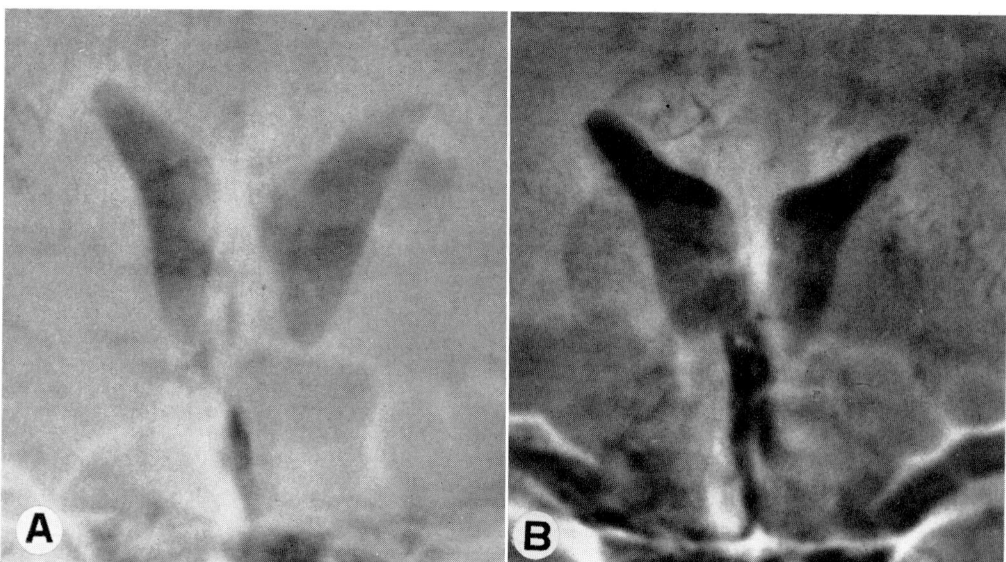

FIG. 258.—INTERVENTRICULAR EXTENSION OF GLIOMA OF THE CORPUS CALLOSUM

A frontal pneumogram reveals deformity of the roofs of the lateral ventricles with depression and spreading of the medial ventricular walls (A). Encroachment of the tumor upon the medial aspect of each lateral ventricle has resulted in an abnormally steep lateral and upward slope of the roofs; the width of the ventricular lumen on each side is reduced. The shadow of the interventricular septum is widened as a result of further downward extension of the tumor. In another case (B), the left lateral ventricle is affected more than the right side.

lateral ventricles are widely separated, but in others the degree of ventricular separation may be due only to the size of the interventricular extension of the fatty mass (fig. 177).

Occasionally, neural tumors metastasizing through the cerebrospinal fluid will result in implants on the septum pellucidum, as well as in other locations. The presence of septum pellucidum implants is only an incidental finding in most instances, and may be readily recognized by the multiplicity of the small nodular lesions and the presence of similar masses along other portions of the ventricular walls (fig. 265). Glioblastoma multiforme, pinealoma, and medulloblastoma are among the more frequent tumors to extend in this fashion.

While widening of the septum pellucidum has been described as an associated finding in a widely scattered variety of lesions, including tumors of the third ventricle and thalamus, the authors are inclined to agree with Lowman, Shapiro, and Collins (1948) that, in the average case with a technically satisfactory pneumogram, such lesions should not present difficulty in diagnosis. If one lateral ventricle is not filled because of obstruction, such as may result from the irregular growth of a corpus callosum tumor or a tumor of the septum itself, the width of the interventricular septum cannot be determined. Ordinarily, the septal shadow is very thin, measuring no more than 2 mm. on frontal pneumograms; any widening above 3 mm. requires explanation.

Third Ventricle

Included in this group of tumors, among others, are two lesions of great pneumographic importance, (1) the colloid cyst of the anterior portion of the third ventricle and (2) the pinealoma of the posterior half. The significance of the former lesion is its benign nature and amenability to complete surgical extirpation, without a tendency to recurrence. The pinealoma is one of the tumors of the brain which is most responsive to

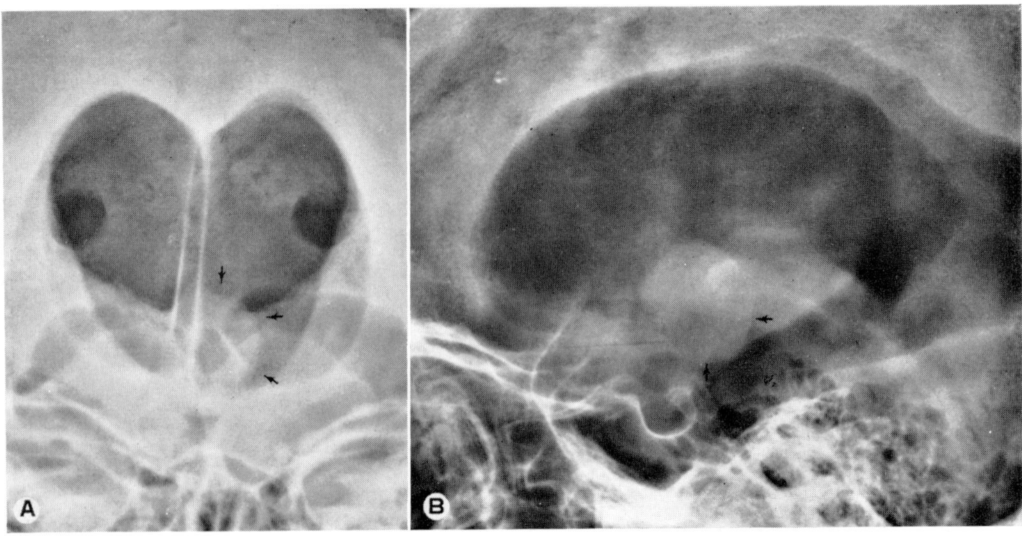

Fig. 259.—Colloid Cyst of the Third Ventricle

The frontal ventriculogram (A) shows a smoothly rounded tumor presenting in the inferior medial portion of the lumen of the left lateral ventricle (*arrows*). Both lateral ventricles are dilated symmetrically as a result of obstruction at the interventricular foramen. The lateral ventriculogram (B) shows that the tumor is also smooth in the right angle projection and slightly oval in configuration. Some gas has passed anterior to the mass into the third ventricle to outline the inferior and posterior aspects of the lesion (*arrows*). All sides of the tumor are sharply demarcated except for the posteromedial margin, where it is attached to the anterior extremity of the roof of the third ventricle. (C), Supine lateral view of same case.

radiation therapy; in many instances, its growth can be controlled for many years by this means. In addition, third ventricle tumors comprise a variety of glial lesions arising from the walls of this structure and those tumors of the suprasellar area which invade or involve the hypothalamic portion. Adamantinomas of the third ventricle proper have been described; in general, however, the hypothalamic effect of suprasellar lesions is secondary, and these processes are considered in more detail elsewhere.

Colloid cysts. These cysts are epithelial-lined masses containing a colloid material from which the lesion derives its name. Such cysts arise from residual epithelial cells of the paraphysis in the anterior portion of the roof of the third ventricle. The paraphysis is a thin-walled sac derived from the roof plate of the telencephalon; the foramen of Monro is the adult representation of the spot where the telencephalic vesicles originated from the third ventricle. Colloid cysts are loosely attached to the chorioid plexus of the roof of the third ventricle at the forward extremity of the plexus. The cyst wall is composed of a thin, fibrous capsule while the lining is of flattened epithelium, under pressure from the colloid material within.

If colloid cysts form at all, they ordinarily enlarge into lesions of clinical significance. This is thought to be true since small cysts are not often found incidentally at necropsy. Clinical importance results when these cysts grow to such size that they produce obstruction at the foramen of Monro. Often a high degree of dilatation of the lateral ventricles is found (fig. 259). The lesion may obstruct the communication of either lateral ventricle with the third ventricle or block the communication between the two lateral ventricles. Ventriculography is the procedure of choice, and the technique of ventriculography is of some importance. With ordinary radiographic equipment, it is usually necessary to tap both ventricles and inject an adequate amount of gas on both sides to outline at least one-fourth of the

(*Revised 1963*)

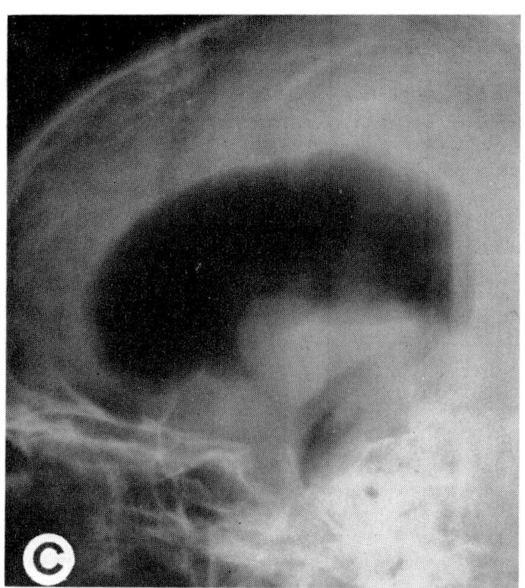

FIG. 259-(*Cont.*)—COLLOID CYST OF THE THIRD VENTRICLE

The supine lateral ventriculogram often shows the characteristic large olive-shaped mass completely outlined. When smaller amounts of gas are used for ventriculography, it may be necessary to use a hyperextended position or the somersaulting chair to control the position of the gas and to direct it to the region of the foramen of Monro. If the dome of a smooth convex mass presenting at the foramen cannot be partially outlined in this manner, it is not possible to differentiate a colloid cyst from a glioma of the third ventricle, or some other lesion obstructing the foramen of Monro.

ventricular lumen. Films with the patient supine then will demonstrate the anterior portion of the ventricles as far back as the foramen of Monro, and gas will be found in the region of the tumor, in the average case. If a supine hanging head lateral film is taken (fig. 187), less gas will be necessary to demonstrate the interventricular area. A significant reduction in the quantity of gas that must be injected is accomplished by use of the somersaulting chair; with this device the movement of small quantities of gas may be controlled, even if the ventricles are large, and the gas may be positioned at the ventricular confluence to outline a cyst, if present. Only the superior surface may be seen with the patient inverted, because the cyst may be forced further into the foramen. Lateral ventriculograms, particularly those made with the patient supine, often show that gas has passed anterior to the cyst into the third ventricle, thus allowing visualization of much of the circumference of the mass (fig. 259). The loose attachment of the cyst probably accounts for gas extending anterior to the lesion with the occiput dependent. The same mechanism undoubtedly explains the intermittent symptoms, and change of symptoms with posture, which may be a prominent part of the clinical picture.

The importance of making a firm diagnosis of a colloid cyst radiologically can hardly be overemphasized since the presence of such a lesion is a clear indication for surgical removal. Barring surgical complication, complete eradication of the disease process without danger of recurrence can be anticipated. A principal problem is the late presentation of the patient, or delayed ventriculography, with the result that ventricular dilatation has persisted for such a long time that pressure damage to neural tissue is not reversible. Any tumor presenting at the foramen of Monro should arouse a high degree of suspicion in the radiologist's mind regarding the possibility of colloid cyst; every attempt should be made to demonstrate a lesion in this region to its fullest extent in order to determine its morphologic characteristics.

In plain skull films there is usually no characteristic finding, since the cysts do not contain calcium. The presence of calcium in a tumor presenting at the foramen of Monro should lead one away from the diagnosis of colloid cyst. Ordinarily, only plain film evidence of increased intracranial pressure is found.

Although the cysts originate in the rostral extremity of the third ventricle, their presentation ordinarily is through the foramen of Monro into a lateral ventricle. The foramen is stretched to accommodate the tumor; often it is sufficiently dilated to allow the passage of cerebrospinal fluid in small amounts around the cyst, and also permit some gas to pass anteriorly at ventriculography in positions other than supine.

Only occasionally are colloid cysts found entirely within the third ventricle.

When there is a complete obstruction at the foramen of Monro, only the superior half of the cyst presenting into the lateral ventricle will be visualized. In such cases, the offending tumor will appear as a dome-like mass extending upward, slightly eccentrically, into the lateral ventricular lumen; it obliterates the inferior medial angle between the ventricular floor and the septum pellucidum. In many instances, the septum pellucidum will be bowed around the tumor with the result that the lesion will appear to present very nearly in the midline. The inferior angle of the ventricle contralateral to the side of presentation may be narrowed. The surface configuration of the colloid cyst always is very smooth along all aspects as seen in the various pneumographic views. When ideally visualized, there is a sharp angle between the tumor and the ventricular floor; there is no evidence of a broad-based attachment but rather seating directly into the foramen of Monro.

The shape of the tumor is usually oval but it may be round. The size is helpful in diagnosis since the greatest diameter rarely exceeds 2 cm.; more often it is closer to 1.5 cm. When there is failure of filling of the third ventricle at ventriculography, the tumor appears as a hemisphere with its base at the expected position of the foramen of Monro. If a small amount of gas does enter the third ventricle, not only the portion of tumor which has extended into the lateral ventricle is outlined, but also the anterior margin and often the inferior aspect is seen. Occasionally, a small amount of gas may even demonstrate the posterior inferior aspect of the cyst. In these instances, the complete configuration is most often oval, with the major axis extending through the foramen of Monro. The tumor has been described as resembling a "queen olive" in size, shape, and smoothness.

The degree of lateral ventricular dilatation can be quite marked; the extent of dilatation and its duration may be of considerable prognostic significance, as previously mentioned. It is not unusual to find that the lateral ventricles measure 8 cm. or more in their transverse diameter; in some instances, the dilatation may be asymmetrical. When asymmetry exists, the larger ventricle should be found on the side to which the cyst presents since the degree of foraminal obstruction is greater here. In some instances, however, the difference in size appears to be related to the degree of ventricular filling when gas is injected. Occasionally, it is found that the septum pellucidum has ruptured, owing to the presence of a high degree of increased intraventricular pressure with hydrocephalus. After rupture occurs, the pressure in the two ventricles is equalized, and a common air-fluid level is demonstrated in pneumograms made with the horizontal beam. Other pneumographic features of colloid cyst are inconstant and of little assistance in diagnosis. The cardinal features are, in summary: (1) marked ventricular dilatation, (2) an obstruction easily localized at the foramen of Monro, (3) a rounded or oval, smooth, slightly mobile mass in the foramen of approximately 1.5 cm. diameter, part or all of which can be demonstrated.

Hypothalamic. Other tumors of the anterior portion of the third ventricle are quite inconstant in their presentation. Frequently, they are indistinguishable from neoplasms originating in cerebral tissue and secondarily invading the third ventricle. In the *hypothalamic area*, the ventricular lumen frequently is obliterated and only the superior aspect of the neoplasm is outlined by gas (fig. 260). The tumor types encountered here are the astrocytoma, ependymoma, polar spongioblastoma, and an occasional epidermoid tumor. The hypothalamic recesses are common places for tumors metastasizing through the cerebrospinal fluid circulation to implant. When pineal tumors break out of their confinement in the posterior third ventricle, early seeding may be found in the hypothalamic region.

A mass demonstrated in the hypothalamic region usually carries a poor prognosis, as compared with other tumors of the third ventricle. Whether the tumor arises in the third ventricular lumen proper or whether it originates in subependymal layers or

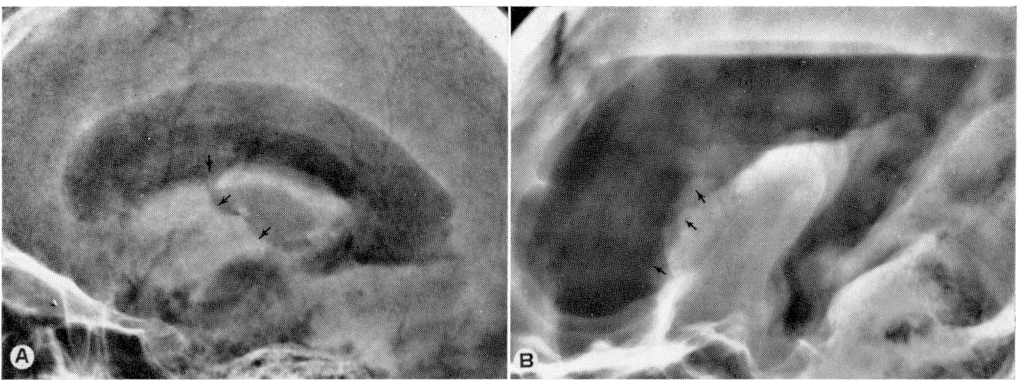

FIG. 260.—GLIOMA OF THE HYPOTHALAMUS

The anterior half of the third ventricle is obliterated by a soft tissue mass (A), the posterior extent of which is well demarcated by gas outlining its surface (*lower arrows*). The foramen of Monro (*upper arrow*), posterior to the lesion, is encroached upon and is slightly dilated, as are the lateral ventricles.

In another case (B), a hypothalamic fibrillary astrocytoma has occluded the lumen of the third ventricle, producing complete obstruction at the foramen of Monro. The lateral film, made in hyperextension (see Fig. 187), places gas against the tumor surface as it bulges into the lateral ventricles (*arrows*). The multilobular surface of the lesion presenting in the lateral ventricles does not suggest colloid cyst, but rather a solid tumor arising in the wall or lumen of the third ventricle.

neighboring tissues, extension into adjacent vital structures occurs relatively early. Because these tumors obliterate the inferior portion of the third ventricle, only the superior aspect of the tumor is outlined by gas. The demonstration of an irregular superior surface of tumor is almost always indicative of an infiltrating glioma (fig. 260). If the superior aspect of the mass is smooth, the pathologic process more often is of extraventricular suprasellar origin. Metastatic implants, however, may have a smooth superior configuration and may occlude only a small part of the anterior third ventricular lumen. In some instances, only the optic or infundibular recess may be obscured.

In spite of the fact that the tumors are situated above the sella turcica and obstruct the ventricular pathway, plain-film evidence of increased intracranial pressure frequently is absent, presumably because of the rapid growth of hypothalamic gliomas. Calcification also is uncommon in primary tumors of the hypothalamus. If the foramen of Monro is obstructed, there is usually lateral ventricular dilatation, but it is not as great as with more slowly growing lesions, such as colloid cysts. Under these circumstances, the tumor surface is usually not outlined with gas and it may be necessary to carry out a surgical procedure on an inoperable lesion in order to establish the diagnosis. Therefore, every effort should be made by the radiologist to visualize the surface of the tumor and to differentiate a true infiltrating hypothalamic glioma from a colloid cyst or other operable lesion obstructing the foramen of Monro. In the majority of institutions, it is considered desirable to attempt control of a primary hypothalamic glioma by radiation therapy. Hypothalamic granulomas, usually xanthomas, may occur alone or in association with generalized disease of the Hand-Schüller-Christian type. Tumors of other tissue types, similar to those found in the lateral ventricles, may rarely be encountered in the third ventricle. These include tumors of chorioid origin, meningiomas, and blood clots. Meningiomas of the third ventricle have a very smooth surface similar to those found in the lateral ventricle (fig. 261).

(*Revised 1963*)

Tumors arising along the third ventricular floor often originate in the cerebral peduncles or other parts of the brain stem. In these instances, there is a smooth elevation of the

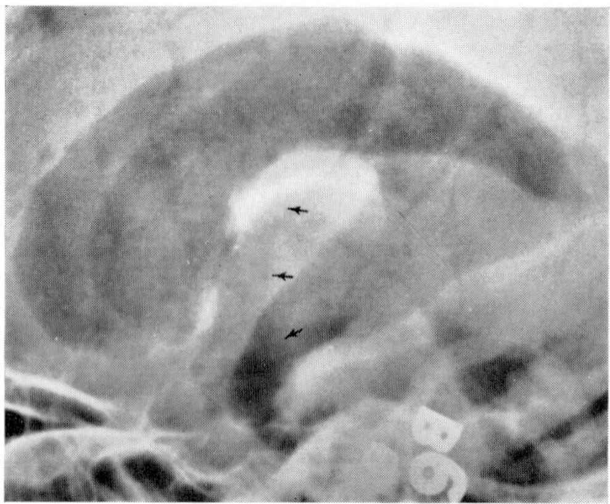

FIG. 261.—MENINGIOMA OF THE THIRD VENTRICLE

The lateral ventriculogram reveals an obstruction of the posterior portion of the third ventricle. The lumen of the posterior half of the ventricle is occluded by an interventricular tumor which has a very smooth convex anterior margin (*arrows*), extending from the roof to the anterior ventricular floor. A small amount of gas injected by the lumbar route shows the fourth ventricle to be normal in size and configuration.

ventricular floor posteriorly, with reduction in height of the third ventricle. With many cases of extraneural tumor, the third ventricle is displaced upward and forward. Tumors arising in the basal cisterns immediately inferior to the third ventricular floor affect the hypothalamus and result in deformities somewhat similar to those just described; the suprasellar tumors are discussed separately.

Pinealomas. The pinealoma is another principal tumor of the third ventricle. The tumors actually arise from the pineal body or epiphysis and some objection might be raised to classifying the tumors as intraventricular. However, the pinealoma usually extends forward and presents as a mass in the posterior portion of a dilated third ventricle, since the tumor often produces obstruction of the adit of the iter. On the other hand, there may be considerable posterior growth into the quadrigeminal cistern. Posterior extension and encroachment upon the colliculi result in the characteristic eye changes which allow clinical suspicion of the presence of a tumor of the pineal area. Growth even into the occipital region has been reported.

The most common type of pinealoma is a well circumscribed noninvading tumor composed of small, round cells; these chief cellular elements are situated among large cells with clear nuclei and abundant cytoplasm; both are imbedded in a fibrous tissue stroma. The tumors occur frequently in early life and may be associated with endocrine disturbances. Four out of five patients described by Davidoff and Epstein (1950) were below the age of twenty. More embryonic types of cells may be found in some pineal tumors simulating those of the primitive pineal body; these tumors are referred to as pinealoblastomas by some investigators. Dermoids and teratomas of pineal origin also have been reported.

Plain film changes associated with pinealoma are those usually related to increased intracranial pressure and unusual calcification in the pineal region. Since many of the tumors occur in young individuals, widening of the sutures frequently is observed. In older patients, pressure atrophy of the sella turcica occurs in the majority of instances. This atrophy is due usually to obstruction of the outlet of the third ventricle with pressure of a dilated anterior third ventricle upon the sella turcica. In some patients, plain film evidence of increased pressure may be questionable or absent. The presence of abnormal calcification or the displacement of normal calcification may occur with pinealoma. Degenerative calcification in a normal pineal body often is seen at the edge of a neoplastic area; under these circumstances, the normal appearing pineal shadow may be displaced, usually backward and lateralward, although it may be shifted in any direction. In young individuals, the presence of calcification covering a large area, even ringlike calcium deposits, should arouse a suspicion of pinealoma. Unusual, and often dense, calcifications may be found in the pineal region in the presence of dermoid tumors of the pineal.

Because of the usual presence of increased intracranial pressure clinically and radio-

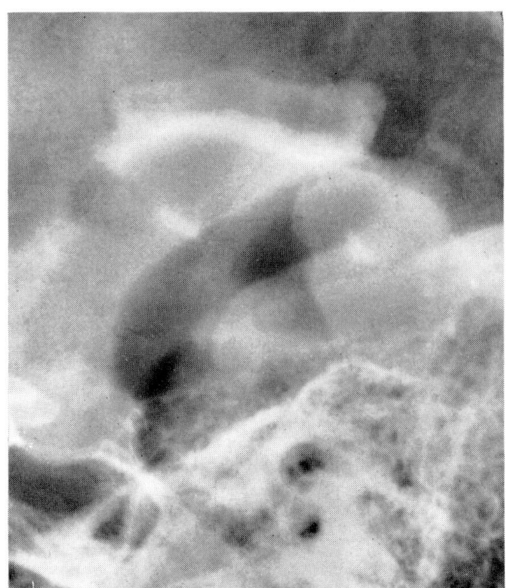

Fig. 262.—Pinealoma

A smooth, convex tumor shadow is present, extending forward into the prepineal portion of the third ventricle. The suprapineal recess is obliterated by upward growth of the mass. Downward growth has produced occlusion of the adit of the iter and obstructive hydrocephalus. A calcium shadow—in what appears to be the central portion of the tumor—is helpful in relating the neoplasm to its pineal origin.

logically, and the frequent presence of occular disturbances suggesting pinealoma clinically, ventriculography ordinarily is carried out rather than pneumoencephalography. Older reports cite marked lateral ventricular dilatation as characteristic of pinealoma. In the authors' experience, however, this is not always the case, probably because of earlier clinical diagnosis in recent years; one example of a nonobstructing pinealoma has been observed. Typically, however, there is moderate ventricular enlargement involving the lateral ventricles and the anterior portions of the third ventricle. There is no difficulty in filling the third ventricle at ventriculography. Gas trapped in this structure will demonstrate an obstruction of the outlet of the third ventricle in films made with the patient prone. Larger tumors with more prominent ventricular dilatation may be demonstrated readily with the head in lateral recumbent position provided there is sufficient gas to fill at least one ventricle completely. Midline tomograms are useful to better visualize the obstructing mass. In the great majority of patients no gas will be found in the aqueduct or fourth ventricle.

The tumor itself should be clearly visible because the anterior extremity is delineated by gas in contact with the mass. Small tumors appear smoothly rounded, rostrally convex, and occupy only the posterior part of the third ventricle (fig. 262). The adit of the iter is encroached upon early, in the average case, with obstruction of the ventricular pathways at this point. Small pineal tumors may be diagnosed before complete obstruction has occurred; characteristically, the suprapineal recess is narrowed or obliterated early in the growth of the tumor. Occlusion of the suprapineal compartment favors the diagnosis of pinealoma over other tumors which may invade the posterior portion of the third ventricle. The narrowed suprapineal space was thought characteristic of pinealoma also by Twining (1939); he used the term pseudorecess to denote this compromised third ventricular space.

When very large pineal tumors extend as far forward as the massa intermedia, they can obliterate the outline of this structure. With larger tumors, the anterior margin of the lesion may lose its smoothly rounded configuration and the advancing margin may have a straight or squared appearance (fig. 263).

In frontal view, moderate to marked lateral ventricular dilatation usually is found; the ventricles are of smooth contour unless tumor implants have occurred. The third ventricle usually is visible as a well rounded midline cavity into which the pineal mass projects. In the posteroanterior view, third ventricular gas may assume a crescentic configuration as a result of the gas being trapped posteriorly and over the superior aspect of the presenting mass. The crescent horns are pointed downward and frequently there is evidence of more tumor on one side than the other.

As has been mentioned earlier, pinealomas

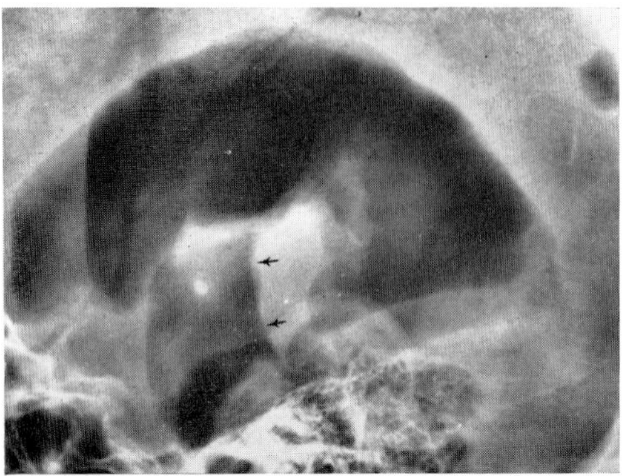

FIG. 263.—PINEALOMA

A large tumor of the posterior portion of the third ventricle is present, producing complete ventricular obstruction. The prone lateral ventriculogram reveals gas closely applied to the anterior margin of the tumor (*arrows*), which is fairly smooth in outline but straighter from the ventricular roof to the floor than the tumor shadow shown in Fig. 262. The suprapineal recess is obliterated, which is a common finding with pinealoma. Astrocytomas and ependymomas, arising in the prepineal portion of the third ventricle, may produce an indistinguishable ventriculographic appearance (see text).

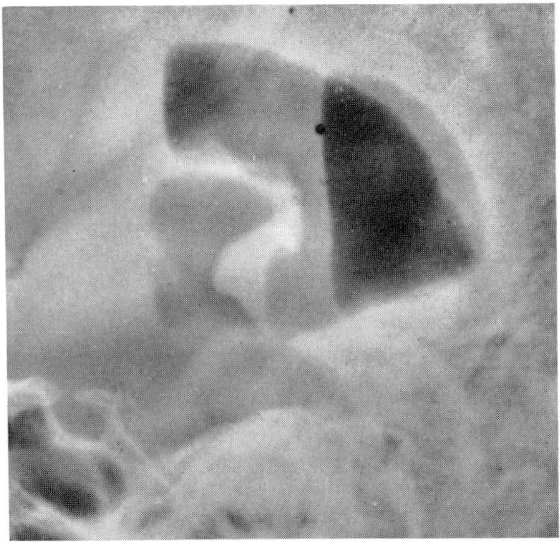

FIG. 264.—METASTATIC CARCINOMA OF THE PINEAL REGION

This is an unusual example of a metastasis from carcinoma of the lung presenting as a mass anterior and inferior to the calcified portion of the pineal gland. The tumor extends downward to obstruct the outlet of the third ventricle. The suprapineal recess is not obliterated; occlusion of the recess generally is considered to be an early growth characteristic of pinealoma (see text).

may grow beyond their well circumscribed station in the posterior third ventricle; direct extension occurs along the third ventricular floor in some cases; at other times, metastasis takes place through the cerebrospinal fluid, often to the anterior portion of the third ventricle where the optic or infundibular recess may become filled with tumor. Such extensions were at one time termed ectopic pinealomas (Horrax and Wyatt, 1947); Horrax (1947) emphasized pinealoma as a cause of diabetes insipidus. In the series of 79 tumors of the third ventricle reported by Cummins, Traveras, and Schlesinger (1960), there were 35 posterior third ventricle tumors. It is customary clinically and in literature to refer to almost all posterior third ventricle tumors as pinealomas, although only about three-quarters of these tumors are of pineal origin; the rest are astrocytomas or ependymomas. In the entire group, there were five distant pineal growths, two of which were on the spinal cord; the two in the suprasellar area, caused hemianopia as the first symptom.

While in the average case identification of a pinealoma can be made with reasonable certainty, occasionally other lesions may encroach upon the posterior aspect of the third ventricle and cause difficulty in diagnosis. Tumors of the quadrigeminal area, either gliomas, meningiomas of the tentorial margin or aneurysms of the great vessels in this region, may encroach upon the posterior aspect of the third ventricle. Metastatic carcinoma from the lung and from other organs may simulate pinealoma (fig. 264). A mass may be found not only at the usual pineal site, but there may be mural metastases in the lateral and third ventricles, including the hypothalamic area. Medulloblastoma and other tumors of the cerebellum growing upward may occasionally cause difficulty in diagnosis. Some cerebellar tumors also may be complicated by mural implants reaching the third and lateral ventricles through the cerebrospinal fluid (fig.

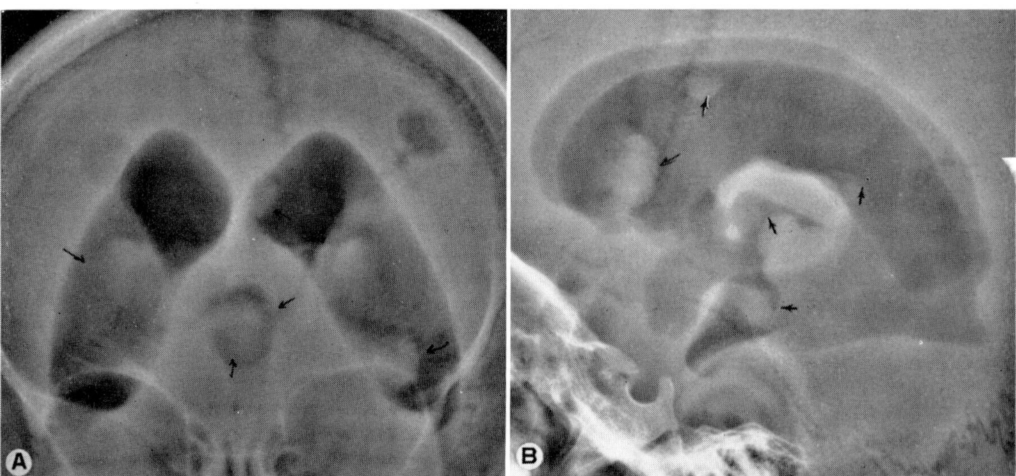

FIG. 265.—MULTIPLE INTRAVENTRICULAR METASTATIC DEPOSITS

A medulloblastoma of the upper cerebellar vermis has grown into or seeded to the pineal region. The lateral ventriculogram (B) shows the nodular configuration of the prepineal extension of the tumor which projects forward almost to the massa intermedia (*central arrow*). The ventricular obstruction is in the midaqueduct (*lower arrow*), characteristic of high cerebellar tumors or posterior tumors of the incisural region. Multiple metastatic deposits, varying in size, are shown also in the lateral ventricles (*upper arrows*). The frontal ventriculogram (A) shows symmetrical enlargement of the lateral and third ventricles which again are shown to contain multiple mural secondary deposits (*arrows*).

265). Tumors of the brain stem sometimes extend upward and gliomas spreading from neighboring structures may occlude the posterior third ventricle. In general, however, these lesions exhibit more displacement or compression than is usually associated with pinealoma; the characteristic appearance of the intraventricular presentation associated with pinealoma ordinarily is not mimicked.

Aqueductal tumors are rare and not considered as an entity, but as part of the midbrain glioma group. These tumors, together with aqueduct stenosis or gliosis, cause obstruction at or near the outlet of the third ventricle; in such cases, the configuration of the recesses and other normal structures along the posterior aspect of the third ventricle is preserved; often the shadows are more conspicuous than under normal circumstances, because of dilatation of the posterior third ventricle (fig. 306).

Fourth Ventricle

Tumors of the fourth ventricular cavity are considered here in the intraventricular group because they are distinct pathologically and because frequently they may be distinguished from other posterior fossa lesions pneumographically. The tumors which most satisfactorily fit into the category of intraventricular tumors of the fourth ventricle are those lesions which most obviously arise within it, and which remain almost completely intraluminal. Some slowly growing ependymomas, dermoid tumors, and chorioid papillomas are associated with the most classical pneumographic appearances.

Attempts to segregate intraventricular tumors of the fourth ventricle from other posterior fossa tumors, chiefly of the cerebellum and brain stem, are not as satisfactory as defining such tumors of the lateral ventricles. Frequently, ependymomas extend out between the cerebellar hemispheres, invade the medulla oblongata, and may extend through the foramina of Luschka into the basal cisterns. On the other hand, tumors such as medulloblastomas and astrocytomas, arising in the cerebellar vermis or other periventricular structures, very often in-

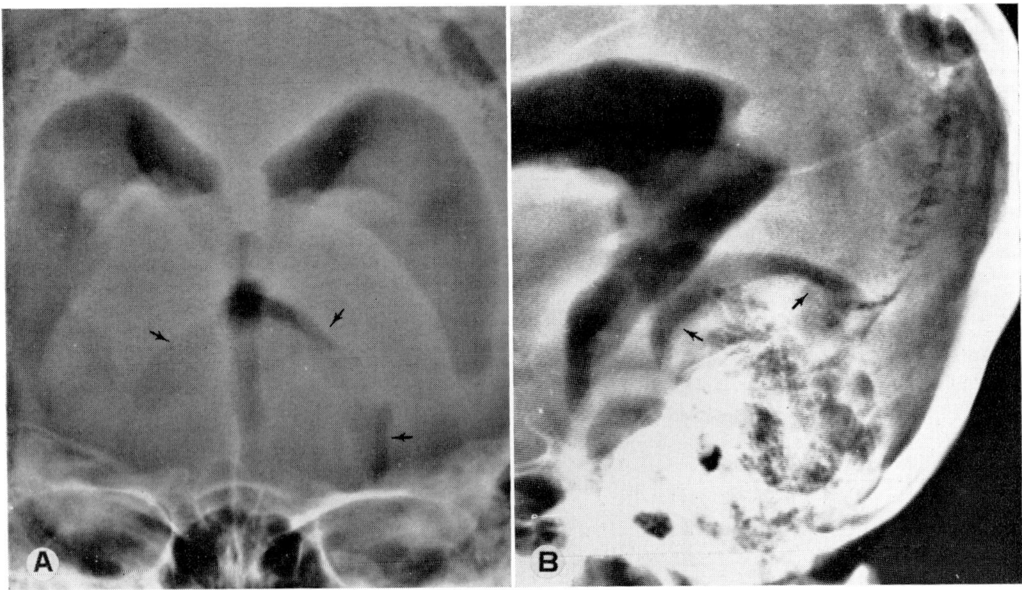

FIG. 266.—EPENDYMOMA OF THE FOURTH VENTRICLE

A large tumor is present in the lumen of the fourth ventricle, producing ventricular obstruction. The superior margin of the tumor appears well delineated in both the frontal (A) and lateral (B) ventriculograms. The remaining patent superior portion of the fourth ventricle proximal to the tumor is markedly dilated. The frontal ventriculogram (A) shows gas in the superior part of the fourth ventricle extending over the upper surface of the tumor and also outlining its left lateral aspect (*arrows*). The lateral film (B) also shows gas extending over the superior and posterior surfaces of the smooth, convex tumor (*arrows*). Apparently the tumor is wide-based in the caudal portion of the fourth ventricle and also along the right side of the ventricular wall.

vade the fourth ventricle during their growth. Other tissue types, including oligodendrogliomas and hemangioblastomas, also frequently involve the fourth ventricle. The tendency for medulloblastoma to invade the fourth ventricle is so common that in the series of fourth ventricle tumors described by Craig and Kernohan (1938) medulloblastoma outnumbered ependymoma by 50 per cent. Ependymomas of the supratentorial area, however, are by no means limited to the ventricular cavities and extensive hemispheric involvement may occur with such lesions.

Ependymoma is the prototype of fourth ventricular tumor, when it occurs completely enclosed within the ventricular lumen. Ependymal tissue is relatively abundant in the region of the fourth ventricle. The typical picture occurs in those instances in which a well circumscribed mass occurs in the caudal portion of the fourth ventricle. With slow intraluminal growth of the tumor, foraminal obstruction occurs with resulting dilatation of the fourth ventricle, sometimes disproportionate to dilatation of the third and lateral ventricles. It has been suggested that foraminal obstruction may alternate with foraminal patency, following ventricular dilatation, and this could well explain the unusual size of the fourth ventricle in some instances.

Dilatation of the fourth ventricle, up to a certain point, facilitates demonstration of discrete masses within its lumen at ventriculography. If the ventricle becomes too large, gas will encompass the tumor to such an extent that it may be more difficult to detect. Gas in contact with the tumor surface usually reveals it to have a multilobular convexity; a large portion of the tumor may be outlined in this manner by gas over

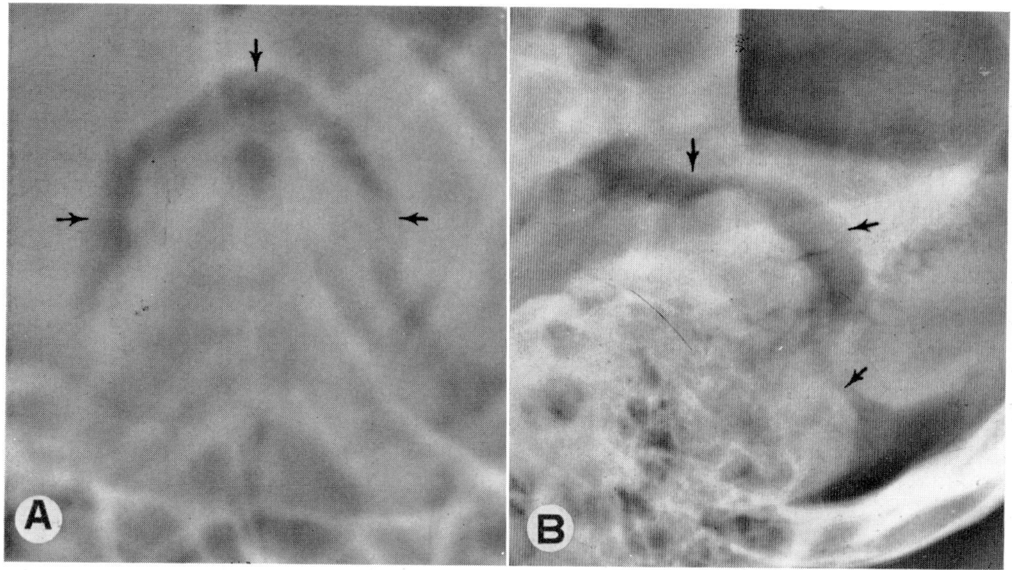

FIG. 267.—EPENDYMOMA OF THE FOURTH VENTRICLE

There is moderate ventricular dilatation even though the obstruction is incomplete. The frontal ventriculogram (A) reveals gas extending widely around a large mass in the central portion of the lumen of the fourth ventricle (*arrows*). The lateral ventriculogram, made with the patient prone (B), reveals a tumor with large surface lobulations extending backward into the dilated ventricular lumen (*upper arrows*) from the floor of the fourth ventricle; the residual lumen extends over the superior and posterior surfaces of the mass. A free communication between the fourth ventricle and cisterna magna is present (*lower arrow*). When the fourth ventricle is stretched to such an extent that it largely encompasses a lesion, the tumor outline may be obscured by the overlying ventricular gas unless tomograms are made (see Fig. 245).

several aspects of the lesion. Often it can be seen that the mass has a wide-based attachment along the ventricular floor or that it takes its origin from a lateral aspect of the ventricular cavity (fig. 266). Because of the overlying mastoids in some patients and the large amount of air actually present within the dilated fourth ventricle, as mentioned above, visualization of the intraventricular mass in lateral projection often is best accomplished by the use of tomograms (fig. 245). In other instances, lateral films made with the patient prone suffice very well to demonstrate the dilated, obstructed fourth ventricle and the tumor it contains. Frontal views, particularly posteroanterior films made with the patient prone, serve also to show the true intraluminal nature of the tumor (fig. 267).

Papillomas of the chorioid plexus of the fourth ventricle may present a pneumographic appearance somewhat resembling that described for the classical ependymoma, the location of papillomas being dorsal and caudal in their attachment. Papillomas have been described earlier in connection with tumors of the lateral ventricles; except in young children, however, they are most commonly found in the region of the fourth ventricle. Chorioid papillomas are capable of producing hydrocephalus by obstruction of the ventricular foramina, by overproduction of cerebrospinal fluid, or by both.

While at times it is possible for the radiologist to define tumors, such as circumscribed ependymomas, as being truly intraventricular, the fourth ventricular dilatation required frequently is not present. Instead, more often than not, the fourth ventricular lumen is occluded, either by a tumor growing within it or by collapse from adjacent invasion. This condition occurs frequently with ependymomas and is the rule in the case of other tumors which very often present in the fourth ventricle surgically and pathologically, such as the medulloblastoma and astrocytoma. With the latter, more invasive types of tumors, ventricular structures are not preserved and are not recognizable pneumographically. In other instances, displacement may be more prominent than ventricular obliteration, but in either instance the lesion itself is not clearly depicted. While a classical, circumscribed, intraventricular tumor, as described, should be readily recognized, the problem more often confronting the radiologist is to be certain of the presence of a posterior fossa tumor in the event of obliteration or displacement of the fourth ventricle. In these instances, therefore, the chief contribution of ventriculography is to establish with certainty the presence of a posterior fossa tumor and to determine the location of the bulk of its growth, whether in the cerebellum, in the brain stem, or in extra-axial areas. For this reason, many writers do not consider tumors of the fourth ventricle apart, but consider fourth ventricular involvement only a complication of the primary process through disturbance of cerebrospinal fluid circulation. It should be remembered, also, that extension of any tumor into the lumen of the fourth ventricle is favorable for seeding of the tumor to other portions of the central nervous system. The frequency of spinal cord and brain metastases from medulloblastoma growing into the fourth ventricle and into the subarachnoid space is well recognized. Similar distant seeding occurs with ependymoma and other glial tumors, with hemangioblastoma, and is said to occur with chorioid papilloma in numerous instances. The recognition of tumor extension into the fourth ventricle, either radiologically or surgically, may affect therapy, therefore, to the extent that postoperative radiation may be directed to wider areas than the site of origin of the tumor. Occasionally, when a classical intraluminal ependymoma is demonstrated arising from the ventricular floor, with obvious rooting in the brain stem, radiation alone may be used. Successful control of ependymoma of this type by radiation therapy over many years has been observed. McRae and Elliott (1958), in a review of posterior fossa tumors in children that was designed specifically to evaluate the radiologic signs that might lead to a radiologic differentiation, arrived at the conclusion that it is often not possible to differentiate between the two principal lesions, astrocytoma and medulloblastoma. Skull changes suggestive of long-standing increased pressure and calcification suggest astrocytoma, while normal skull roentgenograms favor medulloblastoma. Extreme ventricular dilatation suggests astrocytoma and demonstration of an intraventricular mass favors medulloblastoma.

EXTRAVENTRICULAR SUPRATENTORIAL TUMORS

The pneumographic diagnosis of mass lesions of the cereberal hemispheres has been overshadowed in recent years by the spectacular developments in vascular opacification techniques and a better understanding of angiography through experience in interpretation. Nevertheless, ventriculography and pneumoencephalography remain as dependable methods for visualization of cerebral structures. The untoward effects of pneumography, either pneumoencephalography or ventriculography, in the presence of actual or impending herniations are now well recognized, and must be weighed against the calculated risks involved in angiography.

The replacement of cerebrospinal fluid by less dense and less resistant gas often leads to an exaggeration of pre-existing dislocations of cerebral structures owing to tumor. Subfalcial herniation of midline structures, such as the septum pellucidum, frequently is seen following ventriculography when no evidence—or only minimum evidence—of midline vascular displacement is shown by prior angiography. Indeed, pneumography may facilitate the lateralization and localization of hemispheric tumors by exaggeration of anatomic dislocations; while this occasionally may be helpful it also may impair diagnosis and may force surgical intervention or jeopardize the patient's welfare.

It is significant that approximately 75 per cent of all brain tumors are hemispheric in location or originate in sites from which they affect the lateral and third ventricles. Even if spinal cord tumors are included, cerebral tumors constitute approximately two-thirds of all neoplasms of the central nervous system. The frontal lobes are the largest portions of the cerebrum and 50 per cent of cerebral lobar tumors or more than one-third of all supratentorial tumors are located in the frontal lobe areas (fig. 249). The temporal lobes form the next largest segment of cerebral tissue and one-fourth of all supratentorial tumors originate in the temporal areas. Parietal tumors form one-sixth of cerebral lesions; this means that three out of every four supratentorial tumors will be situated in the frontal, temporal, or parietal regions. This leaves one tumor in four to be found in the occipital lobes, the thalamic and hypothalamic (including suprasellar) regions, the ventricles and other special structures of the supratentorial portion of the brain.

With few exceptions, there are no truly reliable pneumographic changes which allow the absolute determination of etiology of cerebral mass lesions. Clues to identification are numerous and should be used to their fullest extent. Multiplicity of lesions, for example, does not always indicate metastatic neoplasms since multiple granulomas, abscesses, or hematomas may be encountered. Dumbbell-shaped gliomas also may give an impression of multiplicity. Deeply seated tumors near the ventricle most often are glial in origin but not necessarily so, since intraventricular meningiomas occur. Conversely, tumors near the cerebral surface may be gliomas rather than meningiomas, since such tumors may even present in the extracerebral spaces.

The accompanying list (fig. 247) shows the incidence of various types of brain tumors in the experience of three investigators with large series of cases. It is of interest to see the similarities and the differences in the incidence of various mass lesions in these three series; the three reports were made slightly more than a decade apart. Primary tumors, or gliomas, are by far the most common lesions encountered by all. Cushing's series is somewhat weighted by the large number of tumors of several types referred to him because of his expertness in management of these particular diseases. Of significance perhaps is the steady increase in the number of metastatic lesions and granulomatous processes found over the years; they now constitute a sizable proportion (40 per cent in some series) of cerebral masses, not including hematomas. It is important also to appreciate the shift in incidence of various types of brain tumors with advancing age. While the percentage of all gliomas in relation to other brain tumors may even be reduced beyond the age of 60 years, according to some reports, there is a distinct shift toward malignancy in older persons. Thus, while approximately 35 per cent of brain tumors beyond the sixth decade are gliomas, practically all are glioblastomas; the incidence of astrocytomas (1 to 2 per cent), oligodendrogliomas (1 per cent), and other well differentiated cell types are drastically reduced. The frequency of occurrence of meningiomas (28 per cent), acoustic neurinomas (12 per cent), and metastatic carcinomas (18 per cent) is high. More than 90 per cent of brain tumors in elderly patients fall into one of the four categories: glioblastoma, meningioma, metastatic carcinoma, and acoustic neurinoma. While attempts at identification of cerebral mass lesions is hazardous, radiologic impressions may affect treatment; every attempt must be made to identify disease processes as accurately as possible.

General Manifestations of Hemispheric Tumors

Although histologic identification is not always possible, localization by pneumography is feasible with a high degree of accuracy. An orderly method of film analysis is required in all cases if diagnostic accuracy is to be increased. *The four basic pneumographic changes for diagnosis may be considered to be dilatation, displacement, deform-*

ity, and defective filling of the cerebrospinal fluid pathways.

Defective filling (nonfilling). Starting with the last of the tetrad, defective filling, it is known that this is not as reliable a finding as regards the lateral ventricles, as is the case with nonfilling (or incomplete filling) of the posterior fossa structures and third ventricle. In the group of patients studied by Davidoff and Epstein (1950), it was found that almost one-third of those examined by pneumographic methods did not have complete lateral ventricular filling on both sides. Under the circumstances of modern techniques previously described, it is thought that perhaps this incidence of unsatisfactory filling of the lateral ventricles is excessively high. It is also of interest that in the series studied by these authors, tumors of the frontal and temporal areas accounted for the majority of cases of defective filling of the lateral ventricles. Even patients with parietal tumors, however, may have good filling of one ventricle only. About 10 per cent of patients with occipital tumors will have full filling only of one ventricle, although defective filling is least common in the case of occipital lesions, a location that does not favor direct compression of interventricular communications.

The absence or incompleteness of filling of one lateral ventricle occurs usually, but not always, on the side of the tumor and presumably it is related to dislocation and distortion at the foramen of Monro. While defective filling is of lateralizing value, it is not of firm localizing significance because of the variety of possible locations of lesions just mentioned. When lateral ventricular filling inadequate for diagnosis occurs ipsilateral to the tumor, filling of the obstructed ventricle may be accomplished, in some cases, by the administration of urea. At other times, it may be advisable to proceed immediately with a complementary angiographic examination; repeated attempts to puncture a displaced or deformed opaque ventricle with a ventricular needle should be avoided.

Ventricular dilatation. Ventricular dilatation is another pneumographic change of cardinal significance. Although ventricular dilatation on the side opposite to the tumor is the more common event in the experience of most investigators (about 90 per cent of cases), homolateral ventricular dilatation is not uncommon. The causes of homolateral or contralateral ventricular dilatation are not well understood. In most instances, the presence of a dilated ventricle opposite the tumor serves as a compensatory mechanism to effect cerebral and cerebrospinal fluid homeostasis.

The finding of contralateral or homolateral ventricular dilatation is not, therefore, a sign of definite localizing value. The dilatation may be either obstructive or communicating; in the latter instance, it may be related to a generalized increase in intracranial pressure resulting from greater brain volume or increased chorioid filtration resulting in elevated ventricular pressure and volume.

Ventricular displacement (midline shift). The third finding in the pneumographic tetrad regarding supratentorial masses, ventricular displacement, refers most often to frontal views, and the relationship of hemispheric structures to the midline. In addition, the symmetry of relationships as seen normally in frontal projections is most helpful in pneumographic diagnosis.

Two midline structures, the septum pellucidum and third ventricle, may exhibit characteristic configurations as a result of displacement by space-occupying lesions. Dislocations (shifts) of the septum pellucidum and third ventricle may be placed in three general categories: (1) *straight (parallel, square or full)*, (2) *angular, and* (3) *curved shifts.* Each type of shift may be helpful in localizing a tumor within a hemisphere. By a *square or full shift* is meant one in which the shadow of the septum pellucidum remains as an essentially straight line in a sagittal plane of the body parallel to, but no longer in, the midsagittal plane (fig. 268). The superior portion of the third ventricle characteristically continues in the straight line established by the septum pellucidum in a parasagittal plane. In some cases, however, the third ventricle begins to return toward the midline immediately

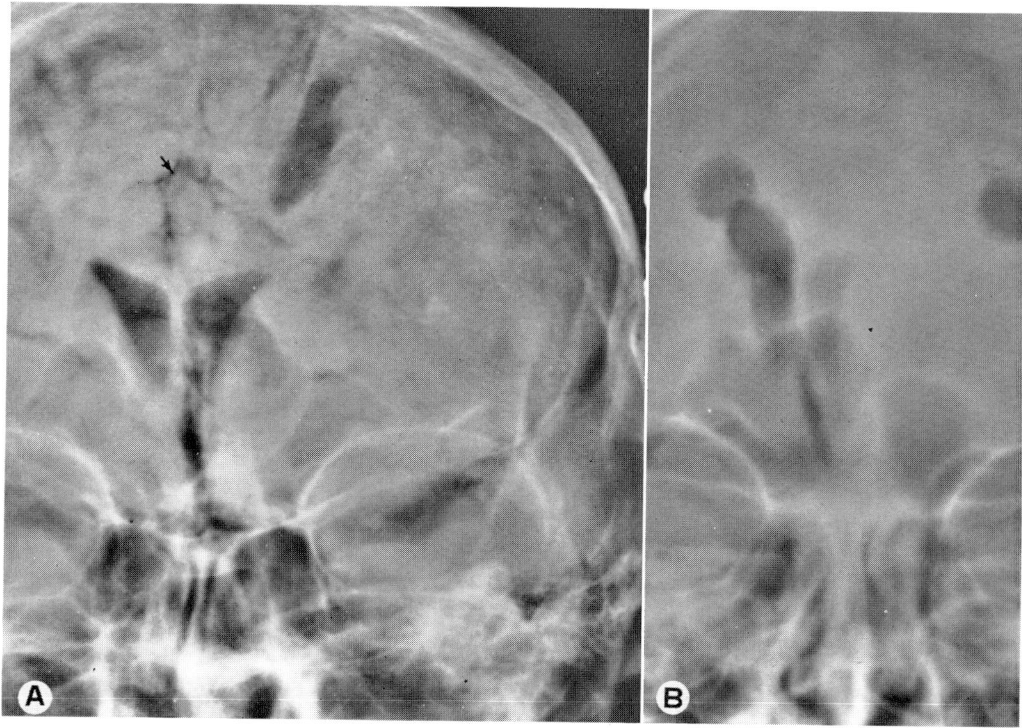

Fig. 268.—Straight Shift of the Ventricular System

When lateral displacement of the ventricular system occurs with the septum pellucidum parallel to its original position in the midsagittal plane, a straight or square shift is said to be present. The inferior portion of the third ventricle is relatively fixed, resulting in angulation or slight curvature of the third ventricular shadow in relation to its original midline position. The straight shift is not of localizing value since it may occur with a tumor in any portion of the hemisphere, or as a result of an extracerebral lesion, such as subdural hematoma. In the case shown in (B), an occipital tumor has compressed draining cerebral veins and produced hemispheric edema, resulting in herniation of the left lateral ventricle beneath the falx and a straight shift. In another case (A), the extent of a midconvexity tumor is shown by scattered neoplastic calcification and marginal dilatation of sulci. Subfalcial herniation of structures along the medial side of the hemisphere are well shown, the cingulate gyrus exhibiting maximum displacement, evidenced by the position of the cingulate sulcus (*arrow*). The septum pellucidum is well to the right of its normal position but remains straight.

below the septum; thus, the upper third ventricle may be slightly angular or curved. The inferior portion of the third ventricle must curve or be oblique toward the midline because of the relative fixation of the structures at the base, as compared with the telencephalic sections of the brain which are more free to move laterally beneath the falx. The square shift is often seen in the presence of posteriorly situated tumors and with frontal tumors; it may occur with any lesion that results in a general increase in volume of substance contained in one-half of the cranial cavity. In occipital and parieto-occipital lesions the cause appears to be a compression of the draining cerebral veins with generalized edema of one hemisphere. Subdural hematoma, a lesion which may produce relatively widespread pressure on the ventricular system laterally, frequently exhibits a square shift. Occasionally, a parietal tumor will produce a straight shift; in the majority of instances, however, a parallel dislocation appears to be associated with an equalized pressure throughout the hemisphere, such as results from edema ow-

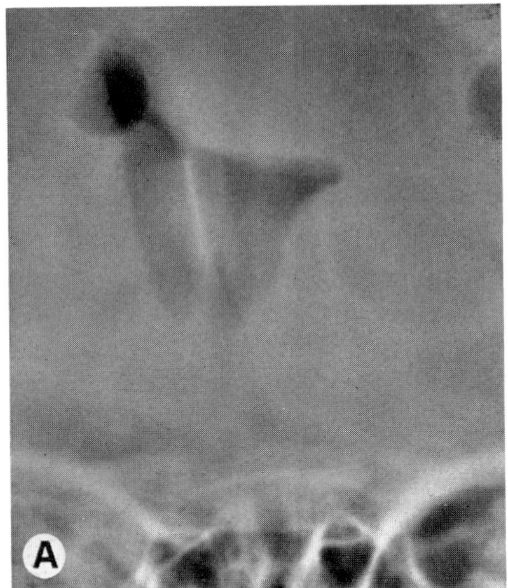

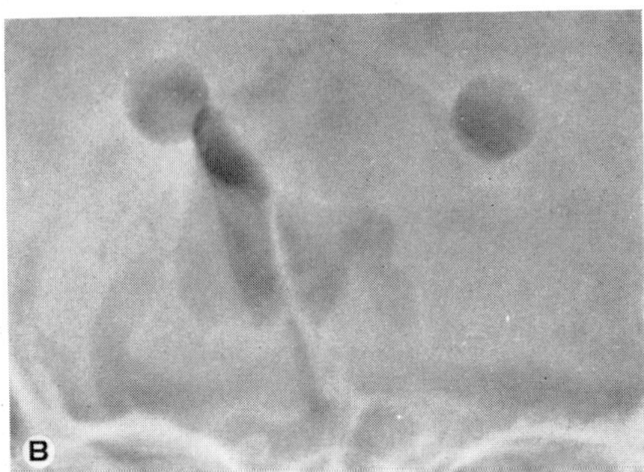

FIG. 269.—ANGULAR SHIFT OF THE SEPTUM PELLUCIDUM AND THIRD VENTRICLE

The frontal ventriculogram, shown in (A), exhibits a marked lateral dislocation of the lateral and third ventricles, the result of a parasagittal tumor. The top of the septum pellucidum is displaced more than its inferior margin and the top of the third ventricle, constituting an angular shift of these midline structures. In this instance, the medial half of the roof of the ipsilateral ventricle is flattened by subfalcial herniation; the lateral half of the roof is depressed more than the herniated portion, and the lateral angle is narrowed, owing to pressure from the tumor.

A tumor of the superior frontal (supramarginal) gyrus has produced an angular shift of the midline structures (B); in this instance also, the lateral portion of the roof and the lateral angle are lower than the medial angle. When the lateral angle is lower than the herniated portion of a ventricular roof, the tumor is above the ventricle. The figure illustrates rounding and dilatation of the lateral angle, which occasionally is found in these cases (see text).

ing to tumor, infection, infarction, trauma or whatever cause. The roof of one lateral ventricle may be flat, due to a large transverse herniation of medial hemispheric substance beneath the falx. If the septum pellucidum remains straight in the parasagittal plane, it forms a square or 90-degree angle at its junction superiorly with the ventricular roof. At other times, with less severe herniations, only the medial portion of the ventricular roof may be flat while the lateral, less deformed portion is angulated; still, the medial angle may remain square.

The second general type of displacement is angular. An *angular shift* is one in which the top of the septum pellucidum is displaced more than the base, with the result that the septum forms an angle with its original midline plane (fig. 269). The uppermost portion of the third ventricle again characteristically is in line with the septum pellucidum. The shadow of the inferior portion continues at an angle, or it may curve toward the midline. An angular shift is seen often in the presence of mass lesions situated above the transverse plane of the foramen of Monro, or even above the ventricles. Such lesions are most often midconvexity or low convexity in position in the coronal plane. Similarly, high convexity and parasagittal tumors often produce angular shifts. If the lateral angle of the involved ventricle is displaced downward to a greater extent than the more medial herniated portion of the roof, the tumor is almost always high convexity or parasagittal (above the ventricle). In such cases, the lateral angle may be either narrow or wide. More often narrowing

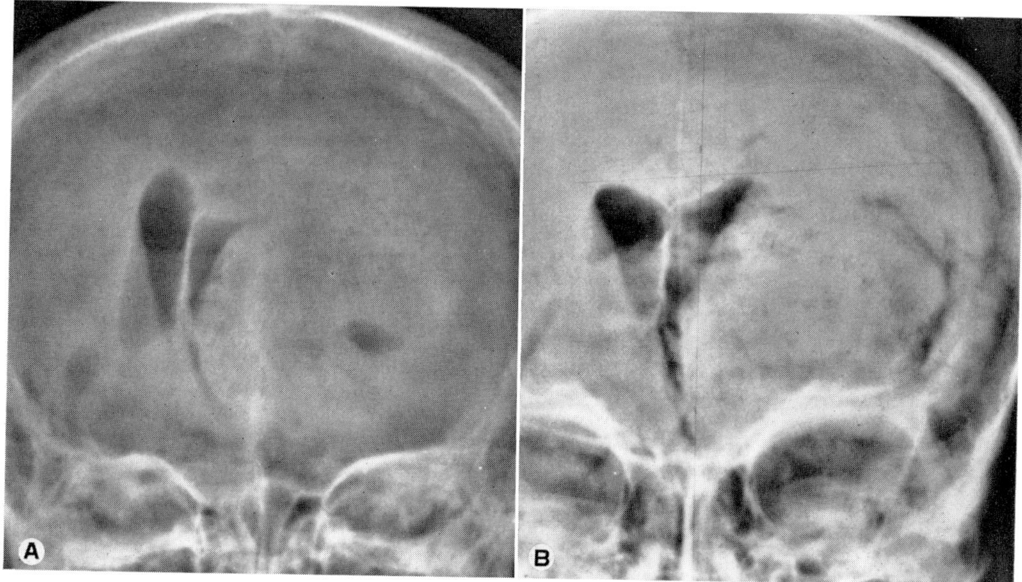

FIG. 270.—CURVED SHIFT OF THE VENTRICULAR SYSTEM

When the bottom of the septum pellucidum is shifted more than the top, a line constructed along the septum pellucidum and continued through the shadow of the third ventricle is a curve, concave toward the side of the tumor. Such displacements are caused by masses which are low, at, or beneath the level of the foramen of Monro. Tumors of the temporal lobe or the middle cranial fossa most often produce a curved shift. In the frontal pneumogram shown in (A), a sphenoid ridge meningioma has resulted in a 1.5 cm. contralateral shift of the top of the septum pellucidum and a 2 cm. shift of the inferior margin. The left temporal horn is elevated and displaced medially to a marked degree, and the left ventricular body and anterior horn are completely dislocated beneath the falx. In another case (B), an infiltrating temporal lobe tumor (glioblastoma multiforme) has produced a greater displacement of the bottom than of the top of the septum pellucidum.

occurs; in a minority, the angle is rounded, blunt, and widened (fig. 269).

Angular shifts, minimum in degree, may be associated with only slight depression of the ventricular roof. An angular shift may occur also with bulky or massive lesions situated in any portion of a hemisphere, if there is a resultant gross subfalcial dislocation of the ventricle. With severe subfalcial herniation, the top of the septum pellucidum is almost necessarily shifted more than the base; with such gross displacements, the angular nature of the shift is not of localizing value.

The third type of displacement of the septum pellucidum and third ventricle is the *curved shift*. A curved relationship of the septum pellucidum and third ventricle occurs when the lower end of the septum is displaced more than the upper end. This is just the reverse of the angular shift. A vertical line drawn downward from the upper edge of the septum pellucidum emphasizes the fact that a concavity toward the side of the lesion is produced (fig. 270).

The curved shift is seen as a result of tumors of the low convexity or of the temporal fossa. Such lesions are situated principally near or below the transverse plane of the foramen of Monro. The masses may be central or lateral to the temporal horn; thus, they may be of intracerebral or extracerebral origin (fig. 270).

The curved shift is the most specific of the three general types of displacement seen in the frontal view at pneumography. The lesions usually are either temporal or thalamic in position. If the temporal horn is visualized, it is possible to differentiate central from lateral tumors. Occasionally, however, a curved shift will be found with tumors in atypical locations.

Ventricular deformity. The nature of the dislocation of the septum pellucidum and third ventricle from the midline cannot be considered completely apart from deformity. In the case of the lateral ventricles, in particular, displacement and deformity almost always occur concomitantly. Deformity, generally, is a more sensitive parameter than displacement, unless the tumor is so located that edema is produced by vascular obstruction. Some tumors, particularly inflammatory lesions and metastatic tumors, may produce extensive edema and displacement, even though the primary mass is small; in such cases, only lateralization may be possible. In most instances, however, when deformity is absent, it is correct to say that a displacement is the result of diffuse changes, such as edema, rather than a focal mass (fig. 287). Deformities involving the lateral ventricles may be classified according to the segment of the ventricle that is involved, particularly as seen in lateral view; in this manner, tumors may be localized to segments of the brain as described previously in the discussion of radiologic anatomy (fig. 206).

Pneumographic Classification of Hemispheric Tumors

In the subdivision on "Anatomy," an attempt was made to integrate the anatomy of pneumography and angiography. It was suggested that three points of reference at pneumography be the foramen of Monro, the ventricular atrium, and the temporal horn. These locations provide points of cross reference with the center of the Sylvian triangle and the venous angle, the retro-Sylvian region, and the infra-Sylvian region, respectively (see figs. 204, 205, 206, and 367). On the basis of the anatomic points of reference listed, hemispheric tumors may be divided into the following categories: (1) preforaminal, (2) supraforaminal, (3) postforaminal, (4) periatrial, (5) temporal, and (6) thalamic. The preforaminal group may be divided into the straight anterior masses, the inferior lesions, and the superior tumors. The group corresponds to the anterior frontal tumor unit of angiography. Supraforaminal and postforaminal tumors correspond to the anterior and posterior supra-Sylvian lesions of angiography, while the periatrial tumors relate to the retro-Sylvian angiographic group. The latter may be subdivided into superior periatrial, posterior, and inferior periatrial masses. Temporal tumors may be related in a similar manner to the superior, anterior, and inferior masses of the infra-Sylvian angiographic class of tumors.

In the frontal pneumogram, a correlation between pneumographic and angiographic localization also may be made (fig. 432). Lesions high and medial in position may be either parasagittal or high convexity in origin. The former are along the medial aspect of the brain or face on midline structures. The latter exhibit very similar changes at pneumography in many instances but are situated predominantly on the convex surface of the hemisphere and usually are not attached to medial structures, even though the midline may be reached in the course of the tumor's growth. Lesions situated more laterally over the greatest arcing portion of the cerebral convexity may be referred to as midconvexity tumors. Lesions lower, but above the temporal region, may be termed low convexity tumors. Lesions situated more inferiorly and in the middle fossa are referred to as temporal. Thus, if a protractor is placed with its center at the foramen of Monro on the frontal film, lesions within 30 degrees of the midline may be termed high convexity or parasagittal, those of the more rounded convexity in the central third of the arc may be termed midconvexity, while those above the plane of the foramen but within 30 degrees of this plane may be called low convexity. Tumors of the temporal region may be either lateral or central to the temporal horn. Deep central tumors which arise in the midbrain or originate from any of the various supratentorial elements of the brain stem rostral to the midbrain are referred to as thalamic. The latter term is used in general clinical work even though structures outside of the strict anatomic limits

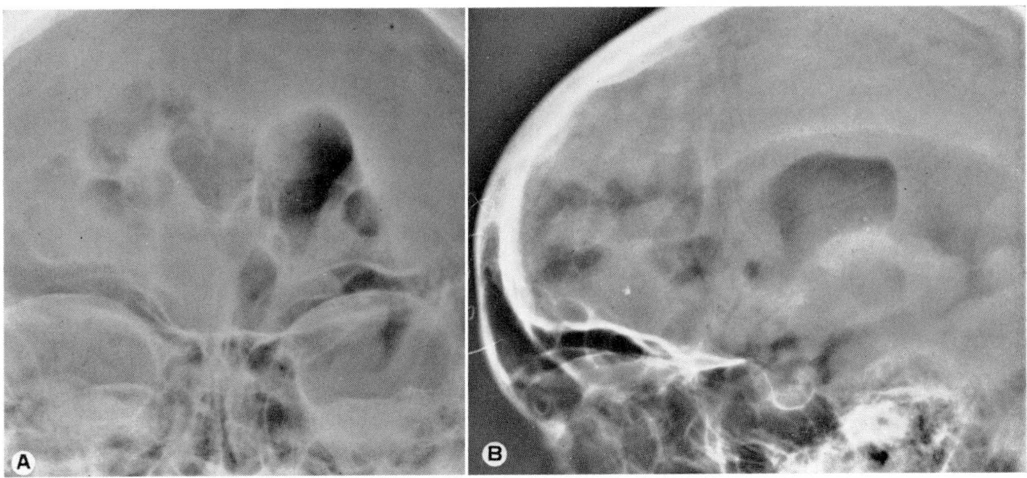

FIG. 271.—ANTERIOR PREFORAMINAL GLIOMA

A cystic glioblastoma multiforme has resulted in a straight lateral shift of the ventricular system, as shown in frontal view (A). The areas of cystic degeneration within the tumor, which communicate with the ventricular lumen, show the extent of the lesion and its relationship to the right lateral ventricle. The lateral ventriculogram (B) shows the anterior horn to be displaced backward and compressed. A nodular tumor projects into the ventricular lumen just anterior to the foramen of Monro. The bulk of the tumor extends straight forward from the foraminal region to the frontal pole of the brain.

of the thalamus are the areas chiefly involved.

Preforaminal Tumors

In order to be strictly anatomic in localizing lesions in the frontal lobe, one must draw the Taylor-Haughton lines or some other depiction of lobar divisions. For radiologic clinical description it probably is more satisfactory to consider cerebral localization of tumors according to the classification just given. The entire preforaminal area is, of course, in the frontal lobe territory. The preforaminal region, which is quite large, is subdivided into three general areas in the lateral view and three as regards its convex and medial surfaces in frontal projection.

Anterior preforaminal (frontal pole) masses. The frontal pole, or generally that part of the frontal substance forward of the tip of the anterior horn, constitutes the most anterior division. Tumors of the anterior pole may result in a combination of displacement and deformities which allow localization of tumors to this frontal segment. The most characteristic change is a foreshortening or truncation of the anterior horn due to pressure extending chiefly backward from the frontal tip. Tumors which lie slightly higher in the frontal pole may also exert an effect upon the roof of the anterior horn and cause it to be depressed slightly, but with the shortening predominant. Associated with these displacements are irregularities of contour due to indentation of the ventricular wall by the nearby tumor. Tumors which grow near the lumen of the anterior horn may produce a lobular irregularity (fig. 271), or with more extensive encroachment an occlusion of the lumen, while tumors growing more distantly forward will produce a foreshortening or telescoping of the frontal horn owing to transmitted pressure. All of these changes can be appreciated in the lateral view and most often to best advantage in the brow-up lateral projection.

In the frontal view, some loss of gas density of the normally sizable frontal horn usually can be appreciated. In addition, the lateral or central extension of a tumor in relation to the ventricle usually can be made

(Revised 1963)

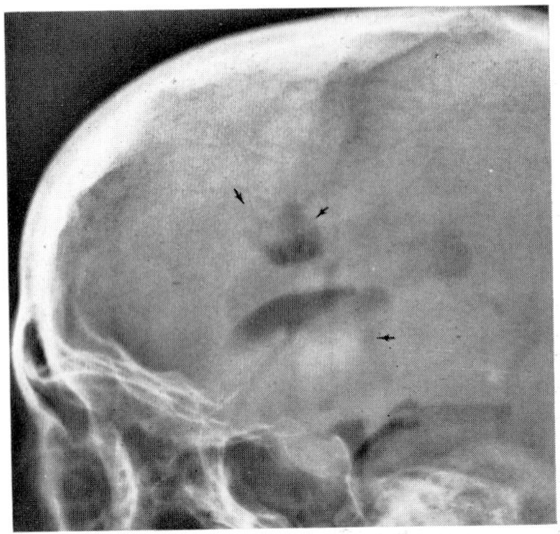

Fig. 272.—Superior Preforaminal Glioma

A tumor above the anterior horn has displaced this portion of the ventricle downward. The roof is depressed and the height of the lumen markedly narrowed. The anterior portion of the third ventricle is compressed by pressure above and forward of this structure. As in the previous figure, the relationship of the tumor to the ventricle is clearly shown by an area of cystic degeneration within the lesion (*upper arrows*) which gas has entered following ventriculography, thus allowing demonstration of the tumor location above and anterior to the foramen of Monro (*lower arrow*).

out. The superior or inferior spread of a frontal pole tumor is easily discerned. Deformity of the rounded lateral or inferior aspect of the frontal horn, for example, is most readily appreciated by slight relative flattening of the convex ventricular wall, when compared with the contralateral ventricular shadow. Medial displacement of the anterior horn may be seen in frontal pole lesions, probably as a result of increase in bulk of frontal lobe substance with tumor growth. The shift may be straight or angular, rarely curved. Dilatation is not a prominent feature of tumors confined to the frontal pole. There usually is no difficulty in filling the ventricles unless the tumor has extended to the interventricular foramen. The various changes are best seen in stereoscopic frontal films made with the patient supine, with either the straight, or sometimes the inclined, anteroposterior projection or the half axial view most advantageous. For the most part, however, tumors limited to the frontal pole do not have as extensive an effect on the side walls, roof, and floor of the frontal horn as is seen along the anterior wall in lateral projection.

Inferior preforaminal (subfrontal and inferior frontal) masses. Lesions affecting the subfrontal area in the region of the orbital gyri and gyrus rectus often are meningiomas or other extracerebral subfrontal masses. Intracerebral lesions in this general location may be more properly called inferior frontal, rather than subfrontal, to avoid confusion. Both exert effects upon the anterior portion of the ventricular system, either unilaterally or bilaterally. Tumors arising near the midline subfrontally often have eccentric growth, and the effect is usually more marked on one side even if the change is bilateral. Early in the growth of such lesions, the anterior horn may be encroached upon only from its inferior side, either with elevation of its floor or by indentation and narrowing of the ventricular lumen from below; the result is an anterior horn having a tapered appearance rather than a bulbous, smoothly rounded termination. When the tumor is larger, it may occlude one anterior horn almost entirely and through encroachment deform the other (fig. 273). Tumors of large size often exert an effect upon the body of one lateral ventricle and upon the anterior portion of the third ventricle as well, sometimes with obstruction at the foramen of Monro. If the tumor is a meningioma, the deformity of the lateral and third ventricles may be traced as a smoothly curved line convex superiorly and posteriorly; the curve parallels the margin of the tumor and, together with the bony floor of the anterior fossa, defines the size of the mass.

In frontal view the tumor is seen to elevate the floor of the anterior horn with obliteration of its smoothly oval or shieldlike configuration. If the lesion is central, as with olfactory groove meningioma, the medial portion of the ventricle may be elevated more than the outer, with the production of an angle rather than an even curve on the lateral side. Tumors originating more

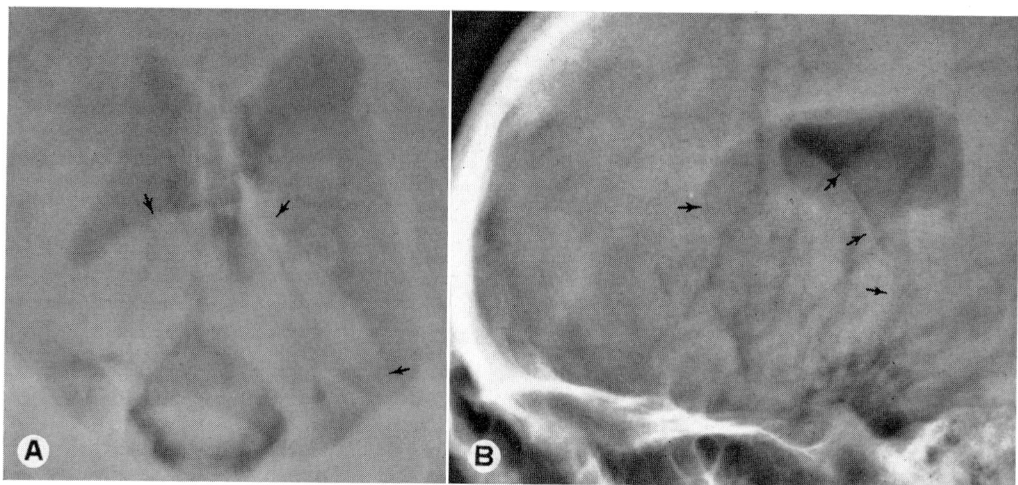

FIG. 273.—OLFACTORY GROOVE MENINGIOMA

An inferior preforaminal mass is present which, from the frontal view (A), is causing an impression on the inferior aspects of both frontal horns *(arrows)*. The medial aspects are encroached upon predominantly; the dilated lateral portion of the left anterior horn overlies the tumor *(inferior arrow)*. Because of the eccentric growth of the lesion, the opposite ventricle is encroached upon more, and the anterior segment of the right frontal horn is not visualized.

The lateral pneumogram (B) demonstrates a well rounded configuration of the anterior horn on the less involved side *(anterior arrow)*. The smoothly curved inferior aspect of the opposite ventricle *(upper posterior arrow)* demarcates the collapsed anterior horn. The foramen of Monro and anterior portion of the third ventricle are gas-filled and displaced backward *(lower arrows)*. The extent of the lesion is well defined; the smoothness on all sides indicates an encapsulated extracerebral tumor.

straight inferiorly, or inferiorly and laterally above the orbital roof, will have a converse effect. In general, it may be said that a subfrontal tumor affecting both frontal horns is most likely a meningioma. If only the inferior surface of one frontal horn is affected, the tumor may be intracerebral in location, or may still be a meningioma which arises in the subfrontal, parasagittal region.

Middle frontal tumors, usually gliomas arising lateral or lateral and inferior to the ventricle, constitute a large single group of preforaminal lesions. The surface projection is through the inferior frontal gyrus. Some tumors have their greatest mass at the level of the ventricle itself; often tumor growth is most conspicuous somewhat below, behind, or in front of the center of the anterior horn with the result that different changes can be expected with tumors situated at various points. The lesions may be considered together since they have a generally similar effect upon the anterior horn and anterior portion of the ventricular body, with variations depending upon the site of the bulk of the tumor. Lesions arising in the inferior frontal gyrus have more a directly lateral pressure effect upon the anterior horn of the ventricle than those arising above in the middle frontal gyrus, which have a downward, as well as a lateral, pressure effect upon the ventricular outline. The ventricle in the region of the anterior horn, as well as the cerebral substance surrounding it, is beneath the free edge of the falx, and subfalcial herniation occurs freely in this region; expanding lesions in this location often produce marked contralateral displacement of cerebral structures (fig. 268). When gross ventricular shifts occur (more than 1 cm.), ventricular deformities may be marked, up to complete occlusion of the ventricular lumen. The deformity often exhibits the composite effect of subfalcial herniation, direct pressure by the tumor,

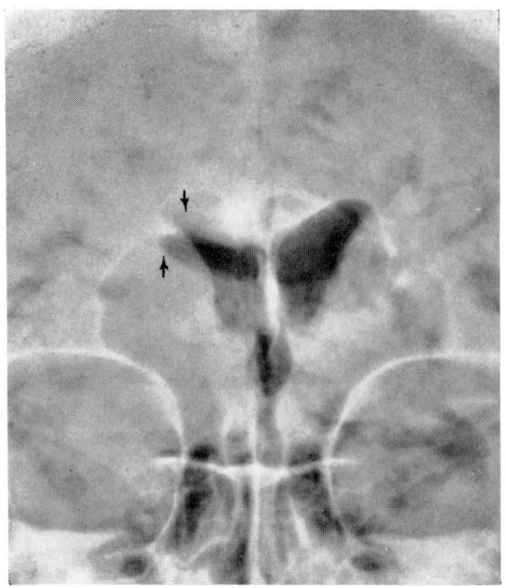

FIG. 274.—RIGHT PARASAGITTAL MENINGIOMA

The roof of the right lateral ventricle has a double contour, as seen in frontal projection. The lateral angle in the forward (preforaminal) portion of the lumen is partially preserved (*upper arrow*); the medial margin of the roof is less well defined. The more posterior portion of the ventricle, in the region of the body, exhibits another contour with the angle and roof (*lower arrow*) at a lower level. A straight shift of the septum pellucidum is shown. Such a double contour of the roof outline is indicative of a parasagittal mass with a sloping depression from before backward; confirmation usually is provided by the lateral view.

and generalized increase in frontal mass by neoplastic infiltration and edema.

In the lateral view, marked narrowing, or reduction in height, of the ventricular lumen is present, owing to the combined effect of encroachment by tumor and compression of the ventricular roof by the falx. In the frontal view, a large part of the involved ventricle may be across the midline. In these instances, there is usually marked flattening of the ventricular roof with the roof line essentially transverse, including the portion lateral to the line of the falx. There is usually marked narrowing of the space from the septum pellucidum to the side wall of the ventricle. In cases with less marked displacement and without true herniation, the width of the ventricular lumen still is narrowed as a result of medial displacement of the lateral ventricular wall. In such instances, the ventricles, in frontal projection, may appear tilted with increased slope of the roof line of the ipsilateral ventricle; almost always there is narrowing of the lateral angle. Many tumors, particularly those which are deeply seated, alter the contour of the lateral or inferior aspect of the anterior horn by flattening of the smooth curvature, as previously noted, without appreciable displacement of ventricular structures from their normal position. In the case of small preforaminal tumors, the replacement of fluid by gas for pneumography may introduce a slight ventricular shift which was not present in the fluid-filled state, or at least was not detectable on prior angiograms. Unfortunately, it is infrequent that patients with tumors present themselves with symptoms and signs requiring definitive evaluation at such an early stage of tumor growth.

Superior preforaminal masses. Lesions arising in the superior and middle frontal gyri, or extracerebral lesions at the same level, produce an effect which is maximum along the roof of the anterior portion of the lateral ventricle. In the lateral pneumogram, a depression and superior deformity is evident with narrowing of the ventricular lumen (fig. 272). The downward displacement is pronounced in the case of high convexity and parasagittal tumors. Such a deformity may also result from anterior ventricular herniation with more laterally situated lesions of the midconvexity. The roof deformity may be long and sweeping or it may be short and discrete in outline. The elongated sweeping deformities are most often seen in connection with tumors at some distance from the ventricle itself, usually meningiomas of the parasagittal area. The deformity has been likened to the shape of a dining fork. Gliomas arising near the cerebral surface produce an indistinguishable change. If, however, the roof depression and deformity is abrupt, lobular, steplike or shelving, or if there is a soft tissue shadow penetrating deeply into

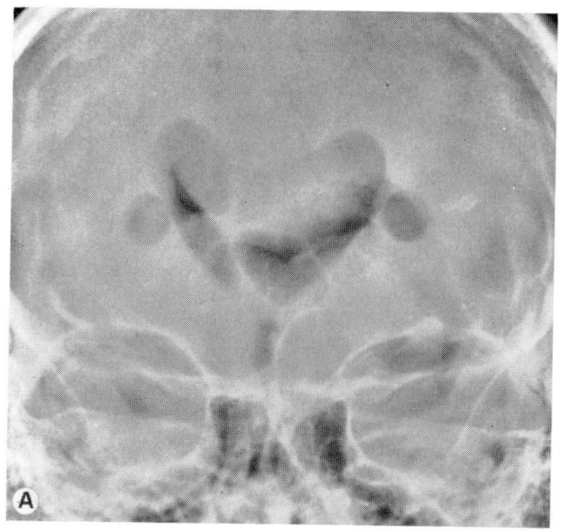

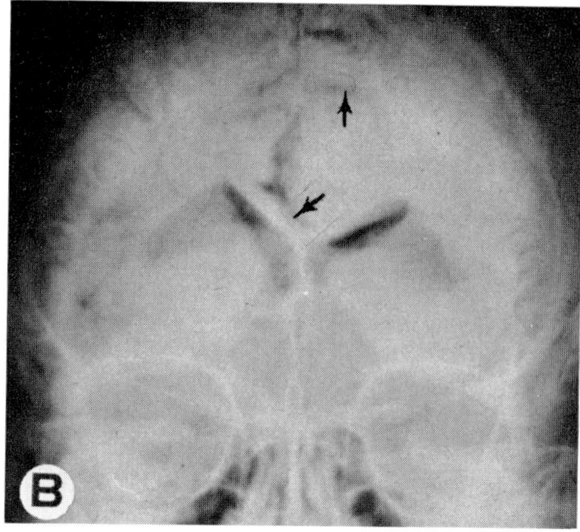

Fig. 275.—Parasagittal Tumor with Biventricular Deformity

Two types of tumors producing deformities of the roofs of both lateral ventricles are illustrated. An extracerebral tumor (falx meningioma) has produced marked depression of the ventricular roofs in the region of the bodies, almost occluding the lumen in this plane as a result of the size of the tumor (A). In another case (B), a glioma of the cingulate gyrus on the left has depressed the roof of the lateral ventricle and by subfalcial protrusion there is depression of the medial aspect of the right ventricular roof, increasing its slope. Were it not for gas in the callosal sulcus (*lower arrow*) and in the elevated cingulate sulcus (*upper arrow*), indicating that the tumor is between these structures, it would be difficult to distinguish the pneumogram from that associated with tumors of the corpus callosum or of the falx.

the ventricular lumen over a short segment, these findings are almost surely indicative of an intracerebral tumor and one not far removed from the ventricular wall.

In frontal view, flattening of the ventricular roof usually is conspicuous. Flattening is common even in the absence of significant lateral displacement. An early finding in superior preforaminal lesions again is narrowing of the lateral angle of the ventricle; as contrasted with lesions of the inferior preforaminal convexity, tumors arising in the superior frontal region will produce this narrowing by depression of the ventricular roof. The former (low lateral) lesions produce angle narrowing by medial displacement and elevation of the ventricular side wall. Even when pronounced subfalcial herniation occurs, owing to superior convexity or parasagittal lesions, depression of the lateral portion of the ventricular roof is usually prominent. Depression of the lateral angle below the level of the medial herniated portion of the ventricular roof is an indication of a tumor above the ventricle (fig. 269).

(Revised 1963)

Sometimes the lateral angle is rounded and dilated but still lower than the one on the opposite side. Tumors of the superior frontal area should be among the most readily diagnosed, through alterations in curvature and slope of the ventricular roof and a change in the lateral angle which is characteristic. In many instances, however, insufficient weight is given to minor changes; numerous cases have been brought to the attention of the authors in which a misinterpretation of dilatation on the contralateral normal side owing to atrophy was thought to be present rather than a recognition of the presence of a true constriction of the ventricle on the involved side.

Along the medial aspect of the frontal lobe, tumors arising in two specific segments, the cingulate gyrus and the corpus callosum, are of special interest since they give rather characteristic pneumographic appearances. Also occurring in this region are masses of extracerebral origin such as *meningiomas of the falx cerebri*. The latter lesions may simulate closely intraneural tumors of the superior frontal area. Meningiomas often produce a localized deformity of the ventricular roof; if the tumor arises from the inferior free edge of the falx, it is separated from the ventricle only by the corpus callosum. The depression and deformity usually are quite smooth and even, however, which is a helpful finding to differentiate meningioma from intracerebral lesions near the ventricular surface (fig. 275). The ventricular roof depression may be so marked in some instances that the ventricular lumen is virtually occluded. Both ventricular roofs may be affected by a falx meningioma; usually one side is depressed to a much greater extent than the other. Bilateral roof depression in most cases is the result of displacement of the falx itself by the tumor and the transmission of pressure to the roof of the opposite ventricle, altering its slope medially. Bilateral roof deformities may be associated with direct extension of the tumor through the falx to the opposite side.

Lesions may be seen occasionally which appear essentially localized to the *cingulate gyrus*. Without some gas along the superior longitudinal fissure and in its branch clefts, such discrete localization is not possible. In lateral projection, the changes appear much the same as those associated with lesions arising in the superior frontal gyrus, or more often resembling those arising even more inferiorly along the midline, such as a falx meningioma. Inability to localize the lesion in the cingulate gyrus itself in lateral view stems from the fact that sufficient gas usually is not present in the subarachnoid sulci above and below the expanded gyrus to define its bounds in lateral pneumograms. In frontal projection, however, the true nature of the lesion may be demonstrated if gas fills the superior longitudinal fissure and the callosal and cingulate sulci. In one such instance (fig. 275), the characteristic roof deformity was demonstrated and, in addition, subarachnoid gas delineated the superior, medial and inferior surfaces of the tumor about much of its circumference. The tumor is differentiated from one arising in or extending into the corpus callosum by visualization of the intact callosal sulcus inferior to the mass; the ventricular spreading characteristic of corpus callosum tumors is absent.

Tumors originating in or involving the *corpus callosum* itself are most readily recognized from the appearance of the frontal pneumogram. These tumors, arising immediately above the ventricle with no structure between to cushion the effect of pressure or retard invasion, grow downward to displace both lateral ventricles outward, as shown in Figure 258. More often, growth is asymmetrical, with one ventricle affected more than the other. There is sharp depression of the medial aspect of both ventricles in most instances along their roofs; encroachment upon the ventricular volume occurs from ventricular wall displacement on the superior and medial sides. As a result, the ventricles may even assume a narrow slitlike configuration extending at a wide angle from each other. If the lesion is at all advanced, extension downward into the septum pellucidum and further destruction of the ventricular wall is the rule. An inferiorly pointed wedgelike widening of the septum pellucidum occurs in many instances; in other cases, there is general widening throughout the vertical extent of the septum to the top of the third ventricle, such as is seen with tumors of the septum itself or with noncommunicating cysts.

Supraforaminal Tumors

Many of the lesions just described, occurring in the corpus callosum, cingulate gyrus, and even the posterior extremity of the superior frontal gyrus, may be in the coronal plane of the foramen of Monro. Masses that affect the anterior portion of the ventricular body or straddle the foramen, affecting also the anterior horn, may be classed as supraforaminal. The supraforaminal location correlates with the anterior supra-Sylvian group of tumors demonstrated by angiography.

The most characteristic changes found with supraforaminal tumors are seen in connection with those medially situated. High convexity or parasagittal tumors in the coronal plane of the interventricular

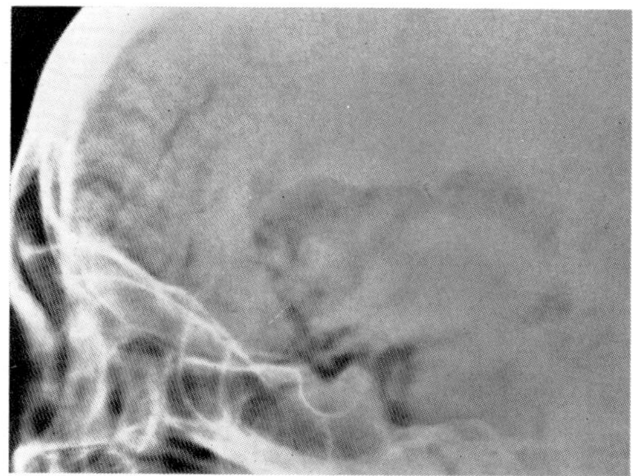

FIG. 276.—SUPRAFORAMINAL GLIOMA

The lateral pneumogram reveals a sessile mass that extends into the ventricular lumen from the roof of one ventricle. The mass extends longitudinally from the junction of the anterior and posterior portions of the frontal horn into the anterior portion of the ventricular body, the center of the mass being directly above the foramen of Monro. Such tumors are to be differentiated from the anatomic variants, in which a nick or rib may be found in this area owing to irregular radiations of the corpus callosum (see Fig. 225).

foramen produce first a flattening of the superiorly convex curve of the roof as seen in lateral view. With further growth, the lesion indents the ventricular roof from above and narrows the lumen, the point of greatest narrowing being above the foramen (fig. 276). The extent of the deformity indenting the roof depends to a significant extent on the distance of the neoplasm from the ventricular wall. Tumors arising in the wall or in the subependymal region result in discrete localized deformities; it is not uncommon for such tumors to grow downward from the ventricular roof and obstruct the foramen of Monro.

Tumors growing more laterally in the midconvexity or low convexity might well be termed periforaminal rather than supraforaminal. The differences occurring at pneumography are not sufficiently great in relation to the lesions growing slightly further forward to justify a separate category. The lesions occurring medially do differ from the medial superior preforaminal group in that the anterior as well as the posterior extent of supraforaminal masses is usually evident. In the case of preforaminal tumors, the anterior extent of the process frequently cannot be determined at pneumography. In some instances, a typical dining fork deformity with slight upward bowing of the roof of the anterior horn short of its termination will make it possible to state the point of greatest depression produced by an anterior tumor.

Tumors which are supraforaminal in location usually are situated entirely within the frontal lobe unless the tumor is very large or unless there is considerable distortion by displacement of ventricular structures. For this reason, the pneumographic diagnosis of a supraforaminal tumor has significance regarding surgical treatment of the case. This is particularly true of tumors located in the plane of the foramen but laterally, over the convexity, since the motor or premotor area usually is located in this plane.

Postforaminal Tumors

The neoplasms of the postforaminal area are rather closely related to those of the supraforaminal region. In a typical case, with a tumor situated medially, the deformity of the ventricular roof is quite similar to that just described, the only difference being the coronal plane of the maximum deformity of the roof. Postforaminal lesions may cause flattening or deformity of any portion of the roof of the ventricular body anterior to its junction with the atrium, or there may be flattening of the entire length of the roof (fig. 277). Small tumors located parasagittally above the ventricle may result only in straightening of the roof outline, owing to mild depression and flattening of its normal upward convexity. Large tumors may result in marked depression of the roof and obliteration of the ventricular lumen.

The frontal films usually will give good evidence regarding the relationship of a postforaminal tumor to the convexity. High convexity or parasagittal lesions characteristically produce a straight downward displacement of the roof shadow. In some instances, a double shadow is demonstrated in frontal projection, indicating that the

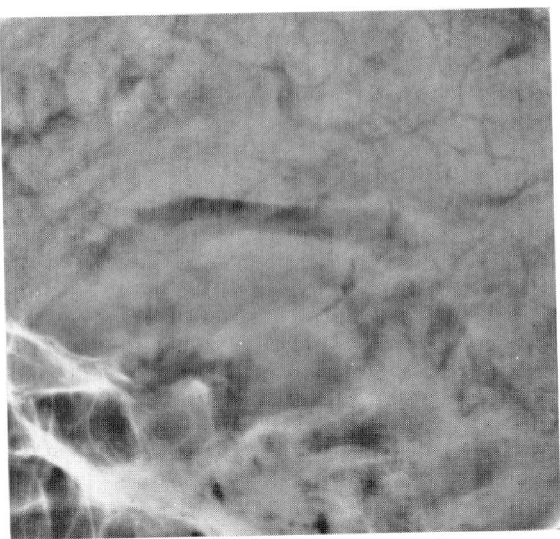

FIG. 277.—POSTFORAMINAL GLIOMA

An infiltrating tumor has resulted in flattening of the ventricular roof with reduction in height of the lumen of the ventricular body. The deformity extends from the region of the foramen of Monro to the junction of the ventricular body with the atrium. Postforaminal deformities may be produced by lesions either in the frontal or parietal lobes (see text).

roof is depressed posteriorly and that the ventricle is less deformed further forward (fig. 274). As with supraforaminal and preforaminal tumors occurring medially, it is not uncommon to see the lateral angle of the ventricle on the involved side displaced downward to a greater extent than the medial herniated portion of the ventricle. Here also, such a deformity indicates a mass above the ventricle. Tumors occurring in the midconvexity or low convexity tumors often produce a marked degree of ventricular deformity, owing to subfalcial herniation. The deformities resulting from herniation in the posterior plane of the ventricular body as a result of postforaminal tumors may be greater than those seen in connection with smaller tumors occurring further forward. The falx becomes wider and turns downward as it extends posteriorly, with the result that large portions of hemispheric substance may not shift as freely; the greatest pressure is exerted on medial structures near the ventricular walls, compressing them against the resistant edge of the falx.

The postforaminal tumors, like the supraforaminal group, have important lobar relationships. Tumors arising in either location may readily extend to the other and across the usual boundaries between the frontal and parietal lobes. Thus, supraforaminal tumors which extend posteriorly and many postforaminal tumors which extend forward, but not necessarily as far as the foramen of Monro, may be frontoparietal lesions. The postforaminal lesions which are of the high convexity or parasagittal type may be either frontal or parietal, or frontoparietal, because of the inclination of the Rolandic fissure in relation to the ventricular body. Postforaminal tumors of the midconvexity or of the low convexity are, for the most part, in the parietal lobe. When neoplasms occur, however, it is usually not possible to be certain of fissure boundaries since the fissures and sulci in the region of the tumor ordinarily do not fill with gas. A major fissure may be displaced away from the line constructed on a film with which it normally coincides. Even at the time of intracranial exploration it is not always possible to identify gyri deformed by underlying tumor with certainty without satisfactory electrical stimulation. For these reasons, it appears practical to localize tumors in relation to ventricular landmarks and their projection upon the bony and external surface, as has been done in this section, since attempts to classify tumors as frontal or parietal when they arise near the interlobar boundary may be meaningless or misleading. If, for some reason, it is considered desirable to continue designating tumors as frontal or parietal, it should be remembered that the posterior superior portion of the frontal lobe extends dorsally for a considerable distance, in fact, as far as the posterior third of the ventricular body, as explained earlier. The anterior inferior parietal margin is further forward due to the obliquity of the Rolandic fissure (fig. 207). For this reason, it is often necessary to use the term frontoparietal mass.

An important early finding with postforaminal tumors, as with lesions further forward, is narrowing of the lateral angle on the involved side. It is important to differ-

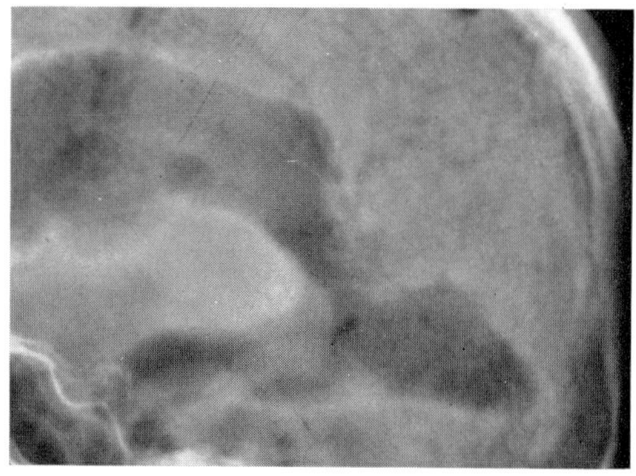

FIG. 278.—SUPERIOR PERIATRIAL GLIOMA

A deep tumor, situated near the ventricle, has produced a discrete indentation of the superior portion of the atrium and marked reduction in caliber of its lumen. The sharp definition of the tumor afforded in this case serves to illustrate the location of tumors of the superior periatrial class.

entiate narrowing resulting from tumor from that occurring with coarctation, as pointed out by Davidoff (1946). Coarctation usually occurs as an isolated pneumographic finding and is best seen on frontal films in the region of the ventricular body. Tomograms may be useful to demonstrate to best advantage the anatomic variant (fig. 225).

Periatrial Tumors

Space-occupying lesions about the ventricular atrium, or trigone, may arise in any one of three lobes of the brain, the parietal, occipital, or temporal. The intracerebral tumors often extend to involve portions of more than one lobe. Masses occurring in the periatrial area frequently are extracerebral and often they are massive. Some of the largest intracranial masses found and some of the most gross ventricular displacements encountered are the result of meningiomas arising in the posterior parietal area. The periatrial region corresponds to the general area of the brain lying behind the Sylvian triangle as seen in lateral view at angiography—the retro-Sylvian region. Tumors may occur above, behind, or below the atrium. The lesions also may be medial or lateral (convexity) in location.

(Revised 1963)

Superior periatrial masses. Tumors arising above the ventricular atrium are of parietal lobe origin. The statement is in sharp contrast to the discussion above concerning postforaminal lesions, many of which are parietal although many others are fronto-parietal or frontal. The parietal lobe is well defined on the medial cerebral surface but is not sharply demarcated from the occipital and temporal lobes on the cerebral convexity. Extension of tumors from the parietal region into the temporal and occipital areas occurs frequently; the ventricular appearance may be a composite of pressure from several different directions as a result of extraparietal extension. It is not always possible to designate such extensive deformities more definitely than to say that they are predominantly parieto-occipital or parieto-temporal in location.

The superior periatrial tumors affect principally the roof of this portion of the ventricle. Parasagittal tumors produce localized or sweeping depression of the roof, depending on the size of the mass and the distance of the tumor from the atrium (fig. 278). While the ventricle ordinarily is reduced in caliber, it is unusual for the atrial lumen to be obliterated. Laterally situated convexity tumors produce narrowing of the atrium, as seen in posteroanterior frontal films. When a parietal tumor extends deeply, it usually produces narrowing of the ventricular lumen in the transverse plane and the lateral angle may be elevated.

Posterior periatrial masses. The occipital lobe is the smallest major lobe of the cerebrum and harbors the least number of tumors, accounting for only 2 per cent of all primary brain neoplasms. The posterior lobe, however, is directly continuous with the parietal and temporal lobar divisions; many more tumors involve the occipital area than is indicated by the 2 per cent which originate in the occipital lobe. The occipital horn, if present, is involved by posterior periatrial tumors. To intensify the effect of occipital tumors on ventricular structures, the occipital lobe is bounded superiorly, laterally and posteriorly by bony walls and medially and inferiorly by the rigid falx and tentorium, respectively. The only direction, therefore, that occipital tumors can readily expand is forward.

The pneumographic diagnosis of occipital tumors is made almost exclusively from the lateral views, either the routine recumbent lateral films or the horizontal beam lateral views made with the patient in prone position. It is difficult to be certain that occlusion of a portion or all of an occipital horn has occurred, because of the great degree of anatomic variability of this structure. Apparent defective filling of an occipital horn, therefore, is not of diagnostic value. Dilatation does not occur often with occipital masses. The changes of greatest diagnostic value are deformity and displacement; the most common type of cornual displacement seen is an upward dislocation, owing to tumors in the inferior substance of the occipital lobe, or extracerebral masses arising from the tentorium. The degree of displacement depends on tumor size. In some instances, there may be only elevation of one portion of the occipital horn with obvious narrowing of its lumen as a result of compression. In other cases, the displacement may be marked, such as in the case illustrated by Figure 280, in which the occipital horn is erect.

The most frequent occurrence with occipital tumors is flattening of the atrium on its posterior aspect with resultant narrowing of the anteroposterior diameter of the atrial lumen. In some cases, the flattening results in widening of the atrial shadow in frontal view. After atrial flattening, and as the tumor grows, forward displacement of the posterior portion of the ventricular system occurs (fig. 279). In occasional instances, there may be marked forward displacement of the atrium. Other posterior parts of the lateral ventricle, including the body and temporal horn, are foreshortened; the ventricular contour often is remarkably well maintained. The prone lateral view may show that the anterior aspect of the atrium on the involved side is forward, in comparison to the other side. Such anterior displacement of the anterior wall may be seen even though the atrium is not collapsed by pressure from behind.

Occipital tumors, like those of the parietal lobe and in most other portions of the brain, may extend across conventional anatomic boundaries into the temporal and parietal regions and into deep structures as well. In such instances, the degree of forward displacement of the ventricular system may be extreme. It is of interest that even with 50 per cent foreshortening of the ventricle by forward displacement, the ventricular lumen may not be occluded completely in the atrial region, as contrasted with the earlier segmental occlusions which occur with tumors in other locations, particularly the temporal and frontal regions. Tumors near the lumen, however, are more prone to collapse the cavity than those far removed from the ventricle.

As previously mentioned, tumors occurring posteriorly frequently compress and obstruct draining cerebral veins; such an occurrence may be reflected by generalized hemispheric edema with ventricular shifts and occasionally severe herniations far forward of the location of the tumor itself. Such changes may be misleading in that they may suggest a tumor further forward than the true location of the mass, or multiple lesions may be suspected. As a general rule, the most posterior ventricular effect of a hemispheric lesion is most apt to give the best clue to the true position of a primary tumor.

The frontal views are useful to confirm observations made from the lateral projections. Displacement of the occipital horn without significant narrowing may be conspicuous in the posteroanterior view; this is suggestive of an extracerebral mass. An intact lumen, however, is not absolute evidence of a noninfiltrating tumor, since, in a number of cases seen with this finding, the tumor was within the occipital substance but situated at some distance from the ventricular lumen. More typically, occipital tumors produce indentations and irregularities along the lateral or medial aspect of the atrial wall which may be visible in posteroanterior projection. Tumors which extend

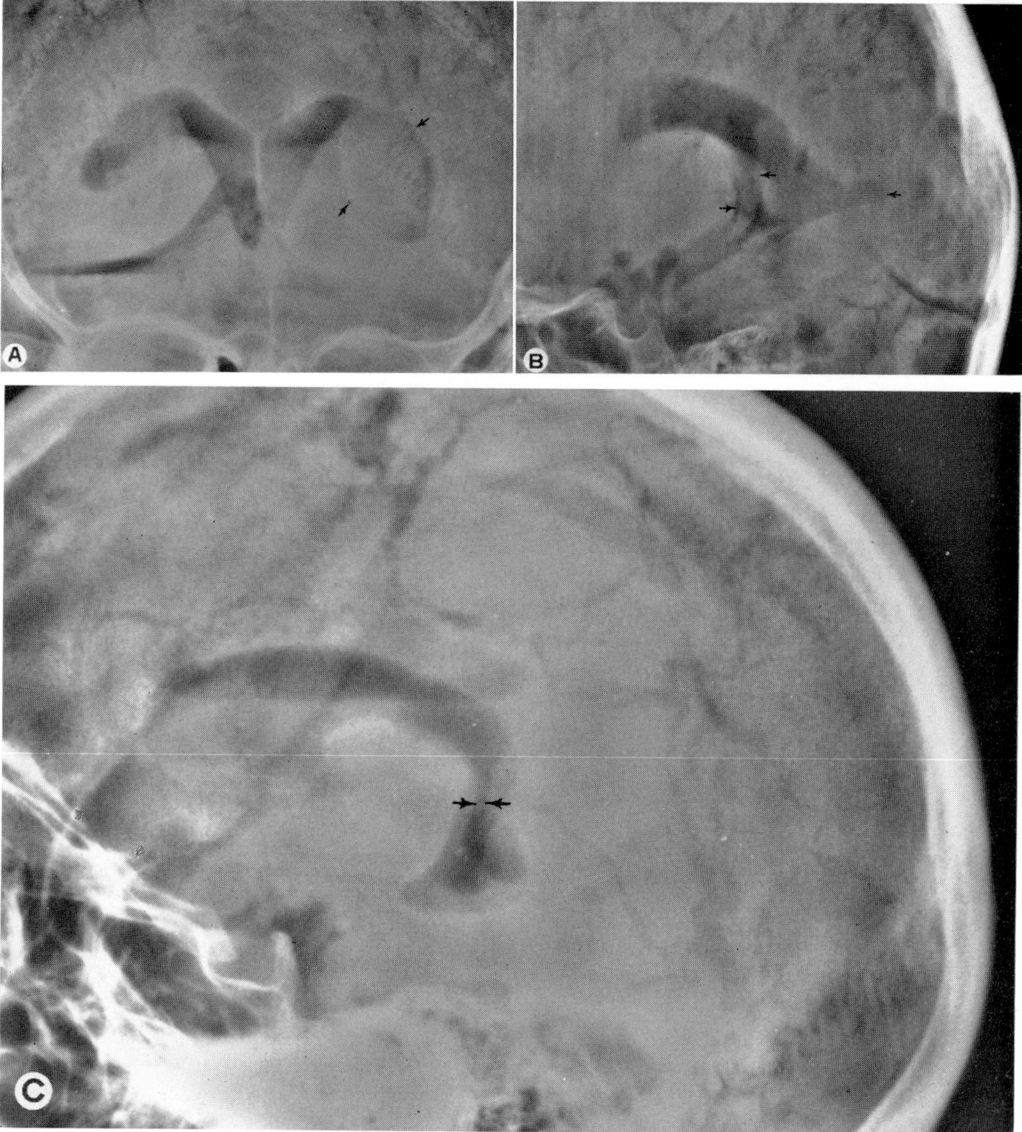

FIG. 279.—OCCIPITAL GLIOMA

An intracerebral tumor (astrocytoma) of the posterior periatrial region has produced a straight posterior filling defect in the atrial gas shadow (*middle arrow*) as seen in lateral view (B). The width of the atrial lumen is narrowed as a result of posterior encroachment. There is some forward displacement of the ventricle, as evidenced by the fact that the anterior margin of the atrium on the involved side is forward of its mate on the normal side in a straight lateral view. The retrothalamic cistern on the abnormal side also is displaced forward (*anterior arrow*). On the normal side, an atrium of normal contour is preserved, as is a well developed occipital horn (*posterior arrow*). If an occipital horn was present on the abnormal side prior to the development of the tumor, it has been collapsed by the mass. The frontal film (A) reveals flattening of the atrial portion of the ventricle (*arrows*) by encroachment of the tumor from the posterior aspect.

In another case (C), the same basic findings were present as shown in (A) and (B), but the tumor is larger. As a result of further growth, the atrium of the ventricle may be displaced far forward and may be very narrow or collapsed (*arrows*). Foreshortening of the entire length of the involved lateral ventricle may take place, as illustrated by the case shown.

(Revised 1963)

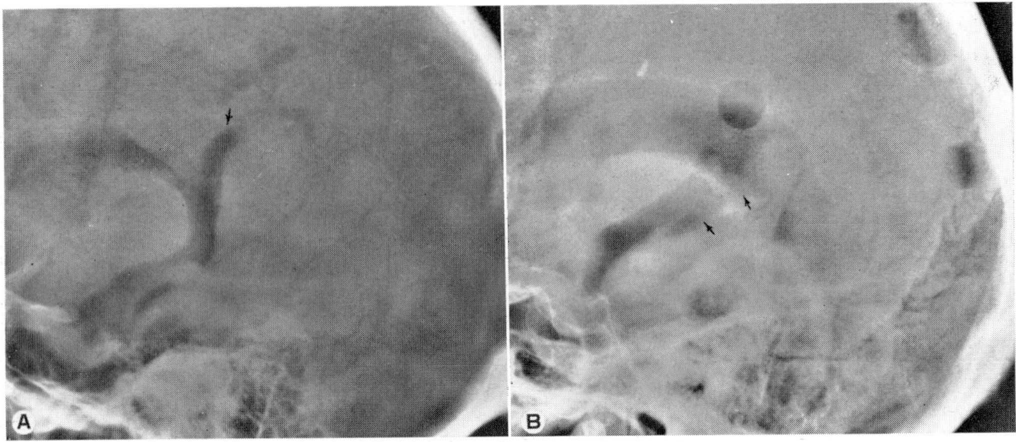

FIG. 280.—MENINGIOMA OF THE SUPERIOR SURFACE OF THE TENTORIUM

When a well developed occipital horn is present, it may be displaced, often straight upward (*arrow*), by tumors of the occipital region (A). Displacement rather than occlusion of the lumen of the occipital horn is seen most often as a result of extracerebral tumors. In addition, there is often also forward displacement of the atrium, with reduction in length of the lateral ventricle, similar to that shown in Fig. 279. There is also elevation of the posterior portion of the temporal horn, denoting the inferior periatrial position of the lesion.

Posterior temporal tumors (B) have their greatest effect in the inferior periatrial region. The atrium often is pushed forward and narrowed, and in addition the posterior portion of the temporal horn near its junction with the atrium is elevated (*arrows*).

deeply may produce flattening of the medial aspect of the atrium, in which case the space between the atria appears widened. Tumors extending into the temporal region may encroach upon the lateral aspect of the atrium. Frequently, forward extension is inferior, and the occipital horn and atrium are narrowed inferiorly, or elevated. Only occasionally, however, is the frontal view completely diagnostic of an occipital lesion; more often it is the lateral film that clearly indicates the diagnosis.

Inferior periatrial masses. Tumors arising along the posterior floor of the middle fossa, from the anterior and superior surface of the petrous bone or from the anterior margin of the tentorium, frequently produce their maximum effects upon the posterior portion of the temporal horn and the inferior part of the atrium. Similarly, lesions arising in the posterior part of the inferior temporal gyrus will affect the lower portion of the atrium along its inferior aspect. Usually there is a combined effect of ventricular narrowing and elevation of the posterior part of the temporal horn and of the lower atrium (figs. 280 and 281).

Tumors lateral and inferior to the posterior part of the temporal horn may produce considerable displacement before occlusion occurs. This is particularly true of extracerebral tumors which are situated posterolaterally opposite the atrium. Intracerebral lesions arising in the same region behave similarly in many instances. The frontal projection often is most useful for demonstrating the true extent of posterior temporal tumors; in typical cases, there is medial displacement and lateral narrowing of the atrial lumen. The changes may extend downward and lateralward for a considerable distance into the temporal lobe to affect the temporal horn further forward. The ventricular lumen often has an elongated or stretched appearance.

Posterior temporal tumors of the convexity may spread upward into the parietal region and produce downward displacement of the atrium. Severe lateral flattening of the atrium often results from such superior ex-

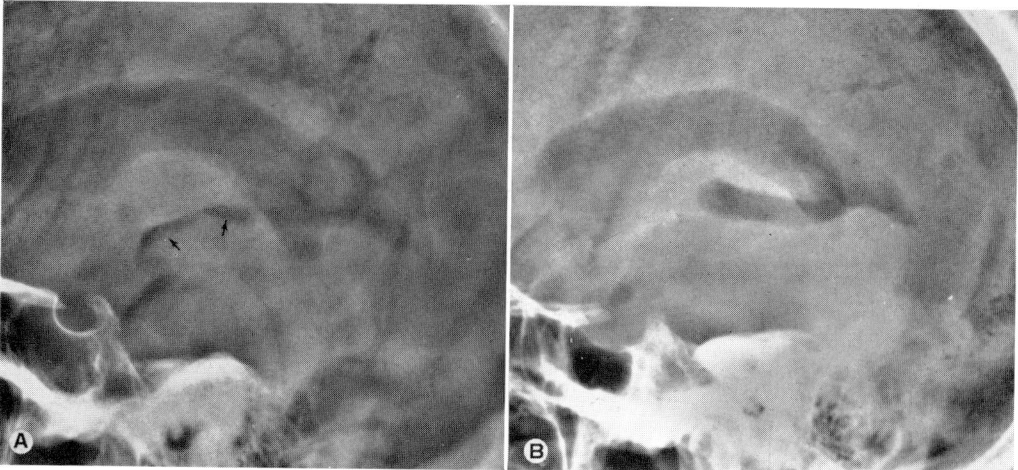

FIG. 281.—INFERIOR TEMPORAL TUMOR

Either tumors of the inferior temporal gyrus or extracerebral subtemporal tumors of the middle fossa may produce elevation of the temporal horn without occlusion of its lumen. In the case shown in (A), there is elevation of one temporal horn throughout its entire length and narrowing of the width of the lumen by encroachment from the inferior side (*arrows*). In the anterior portion of the involved temporal horn, the inferior margin is irregular, indicating the presence of the tumor near the ventricular wall. The normal uninvolved ventricle is shown terminating at its usual position and projected just behind the sella turcica.

In another case (B), the temporal horn is markedly elevated, but its lumen is relatively well preserved throughout by a glioma of the inferior temporal gyrus. Tumors arising in this gyrus and growing predominantly outward frequently exhibit features of subtemporal tumors rather than intracerebral masses which often occlude the adjacent ventricular lumen.

tension. If spread is to the occipital region, forward displacement of the atrium and elevation of the posterior part of the temporal horn will be more exaggerated than when the tumor is confined to the temporal lobe. Irregularities of the ventricular contour may be seen in addition to luminal narrowing and displacement, if the pathologic process is near the ventricle itself. With all of the inferior periatrial tumors, the anterior part of the temporal horn usually remains in an essentially normal position. As a result of increased brain bulk and edema, however, the anterior part of the ventricular body and even the anterior horn may be displaced to the contralateral side; in most instances, the midline structures usually exhibit a square shift. Tumors occurring medially in the inferior periatrial region will be given further consideration in the discussion of incisural masses.

(Revised 1963)

Temporal Tumors

Lesions of the temporal lobe and middle fossa affect principally the body of the temporal horn. Anterior tumors, and particularly extracerebral tumors of the forward portion of the middle fossa, such as sphenoid ridge meningiomas, affect the temporal tip. The temporal horn is situated slightly below the center of the temporal lobe proper in sagittal plane. In lateral view, the temporal horn is projected through the middle temporal gyrus; in frontal projection, the anterior tip and greater portion of the ventricular body are projected through the axis of the temporal lobe and are seen through the orbital cavities in inclined anteroposterior projections. Tumors arising in either the superior, middle, or inferior temporal gyrus, or arising lateral or deep to the ventricle, usually have a pronounced, and often characteristic, effect on the temporal horn.

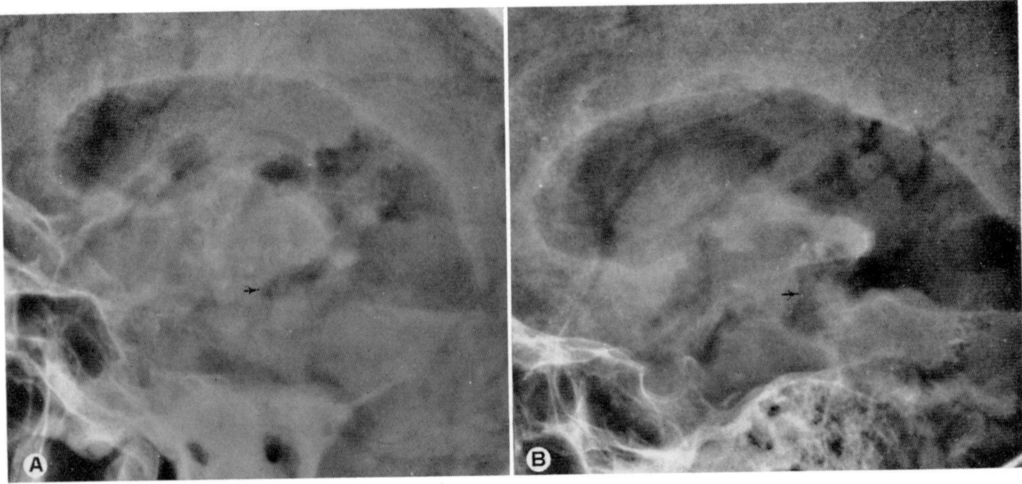

FIG. 282.—TEMPORAL TUMOR

The majority of infiltrating temporal tumors occlude the lumen and produce tapering toward the tip (A). The deformity is most often seen as the result of tumors near the horn and is the usual change with lesions of the superior or medial temporal gyrus. In some instances, the narrowing may extend over some length, while in other cases, the tapering may be abrupt (*arrow*). Tumors of the anterior temporal tip (B) may produce a truncation of the temporal horn without narrowing of the lumen proximal to the obstruction (*arrow*).

As mentioned in a previous section, the temporal horn is the highest point of the ventricular system with the head in lateral recumbent position; failure of the uppermost temporal horn to fill with gas in this position always must be explained. Defective filling is a common manifestation of temporal lobe tumors, particularly those arising in the middle temporal gyrus at the transverse level of the temporal horn (fig. 282). The point of ventricular occlusion usually provides a good indication of the most posterior extent of the tumor. Posterior tumors may result in failure of the temporal horn to fill at its point of junction with the atrium; masses near the temporal tip may produce only incomplete filling of the most anterior portion of the temporal horn. The point of ventricular occlusion may be sharp and straight but more often there is tapering of the lumen over a short segment. When ventricular occlusion occurs, the extent of the tumor and the location of its maximum effect on the temporal lobe cannot be ascertained by pneumography. Often, however, it is possible to find suggestions regarding some features of the unvisualized area by the nature of the deformity near the point of obstruction. When the temporal horn is cut off sharply, the cause most often is a tumor involving directly the ventricular wall, or even invading the lumen. Tumors of the middle temporal gyrus, for example, may encircle the temporal horn, compress it by adjacent growth, or penetrate the wall of the cavity. Tapering of the temporal horn to its point of occlusion indicates that the growth is predominantly on one side of the ventricle in some instances; at other times it denotes encirclement. Dilatation of the involved temporal horn is infrequent. The ventricle on the side contralateral to a temporal tumor very often is dilated, sometimes to a marked degree.

Superior masses. Tumors arising in the superior temporal gyrus usually produce first a narrowing of the lumen of the temporal horn. The narrowing may be maximum at one point in the lateral projection, indicating the coronal plane of the lesion. With the passage of time, the narrowing progresses to occlusion and most often the process has advanced to this point when pneumography is performed. In the preocclusive stage, there is usually very little, if any, downward displacement of a temporal horn. Depression of the ventricle is resisted by the nearby bony floor of the middle fossa. The pneumographic findings are the opposite of inferior temporal lesions since the latter masses characteristically elevate the temporal horn.

Early ventricular occlusion also occurs with tumor of the middle temporal gyrus. A temporal horn which tapers evenly in lateral view suggests a mass at the ventricular level, rather than one above or below. However, tumors above the temporal horn frequently spread into the middle temporal area, thus making it impossible to state where the lesion grew originally or, more important, where the bulk of the mass is located.

Frontal films are valuable to determine whether the mass is lateral or central to the temporal horn. The views are also most valuable to detect small lesions of the superior temporal area. Since a depiction of the opposite temporal horn is available for comparison, minor changes in shape or position are more readily detected than in the lateral films.

Inferior masses. Elevation of the temporal horn is a very common occurrence with tumors arising in the inferior temporal gyrus and tumors arising below the temporal lobe itself. Neoplasms of the inferior temporal gyrus may, of course, produce deformity and obliteration of the ventricular lumen, changes similar to those occurring elsewhere when tumors grow near the ventricle itself. The degree of temporal horn displacement that can occur through elevation, even with intracerebral lesions situated inferiorly, often is remarkable. Gross displacement often is not associated with occlusion or even with proportionate deformity or narrowing (figs. 281 and 283).

The marked elevation that can occur in the temporal region with extracerebral tumors is similar to that seen with posterior periatrial masses in the case of which the occipital horn may be turned at a right angle to its normal position (fig. 280). The various extracerebral tumors that arise along the floor of the middle fossa, particularly meningiomas, behave in a manner closely resembling tumors of the inferior temporal gyrus. The temporal horn is displaced through elevation, the plane of maximum elevation indicating the greatest bulk of the tumor. In such instances, again, there may be some ventricular deformity by narrowing, with the point of greatest narrowing conforming with the point of greatest elevation in most individuals. Complete occlusion may occur but is not the typical picture of a subtemporal mass; as with an inferior temporal gyrus tumor situated superficially, a buffer of cerebral substance is present between the tumor and the ventricle (fig. 281).

Comparison with the opposite side is most valuable for the detection of minor changes. The lateral supine or lateral prone pneumogram may be more useful than frontal views in the case of masses situated in the middle temporal area, as contrasted with those of the anterior temporal region. In some cases, only the midportion of the temporal horn will be elevated and slightly narrowed; the lateral pneumogram, in such instances, will reveal an upward bowing of the involved temporal horn with encroachment upon its lumen from the inferior side, the anterior temporal tip remaining in essentially normal position. More often, however, when the midportion of the temporal horn is elevated, the anterior portion also is high; this commonly occurs even though the bulk of a subtemporal mass is behind the temporal extremity. As a result, frontal pneumograms frequently show displacement of the temporal tip when the tumor is posterior to the coronal plane of this structure. The finding is reminiscent of the anterior horn and ventricular body deformities produced by posterior tumors, owing to edema (fig. 268).

Pneumographically, it is not possible to differentiate with certainty extracerebral subtemporal tumors from those confined to the superficial inferior temporal lobe substance. By and large, however, intraneural tumors are not limited to a superficial location when first recognized; rather, glial tumors usually have spread to other portions of the temporal lobe producing occlusion of the ventricular lumen, and other deformities primarily related to deep tumors. Because

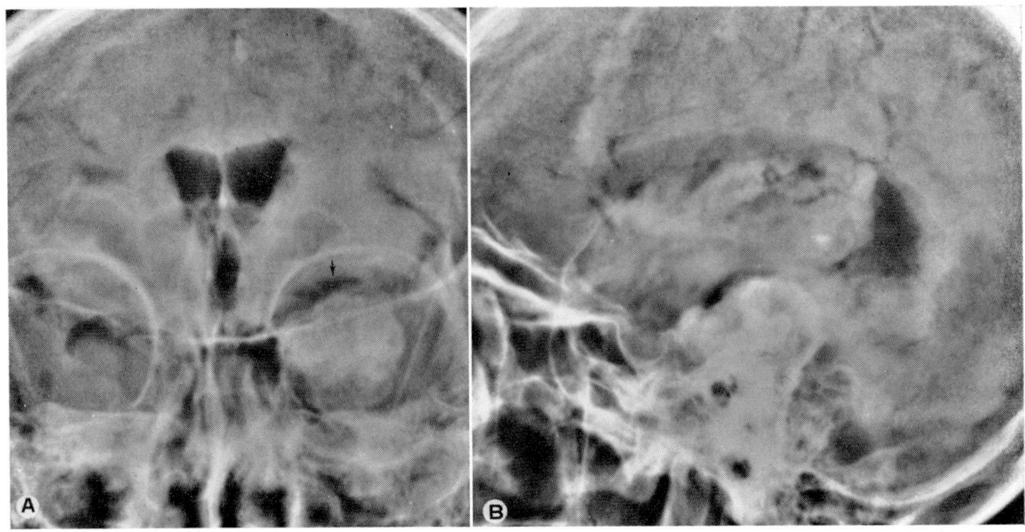

FIG. 283.—MENINGIOMA OF THE TEMPORAL FOSSA

The largely calcified tumor arising from the floor of the middle fossa has elevated the temporal lobe and displaced and deformed the left lateral ventricle without obstructing the temporal horn. The absence of obstruction is explained by the extracerebral position of the tumor and its slow growth. In frontal view (A), the left temporal horn is elevated and rotated (*arrow*) with the result that its curve parallels that of the normal shadow on the opposite side, rather than being a mirror image. The lateral film (B) demonstrates the relationship between the well delineated mass and the elevated temporal horn.

of the frequency of occurrence of middle fossa meningiomas (fig. 135), chondromas, and other masses (fig. 329), lesions which markedly displace, but do not primarily occlude, the temporal horn most often are extracerebral in origin.

Anterior masses. Those tumors arising at the anterior end of the middle cranial fossa near the temporal tip, particularly meningiomas of the middle and lateral thirds of the sphenoid ridge, result in a rather unusual and characteristic pneumographic appearance. There is almost always elevation of the temporal horn and in some instances the elevation may be marked. Frequently, the major part of the body of the temporal horn may be elevated rather than only the anterior extremity. Such tumors usually narrow the lumen of the elevated portion of the temporal horn; characteristically, however, it does not taper and become occluded. The temporal horn tip may appear foreshortened in lateral view, and occasionally it is occluded. The tip, rather than turning downward normally, often continues forward in line with the body of the temporal horn; at its termination there may be an area of irregular radiolucency as seen in the lateral film.

The *frontal pneumogram* in the case of a specific lesion, sphenoid ridge meningioma, is characterized by a medial turning of the anterior temporal tip. A segment of the anterior portion of the horn, sometimes 2 cm. in length, frequently is involved by such displacement. In some instances, the anterior part of the temporal horn body may abruptly change course, from its position along the central axis of the temporal lobe, to turn essentially at right angles and extend almost to the midline. At the most medial extent of the gas shadow, which is the anterior temporal tip, there is usually some down-turning, even when the deformity is marked. The mechanism of this marked alteration in the temporal horn produced by global meningiomas of the sphenoid ridge appears to be analogous to the action of extra-axial tumors of the cerebellopontine angle on the fourth ventricle described below. The tumor im-

(*Revised 1963*)

pinges upon and displaces slightly backward the anterior part of the temporal lobe; then the temporal horn is medially and superiorly rotated by further growth of the lesion. Thus, the tip of the temporal horn is sharply displaced inward and upward but the lumen is not occluded because of the cushion of brain substance between the temporal horn and the extracerebral mass.

The elevation that results in the presence of middle fossa tumors of extracerebral type is readily shown in frontal pneumograms by comparison with the opposite side (fig. 283). Narrowing of the ventricular lumen may be seen owing to pressure below. The encroachment is fairly even throughout, continuing through the abnormally sharp medial and downward turning of the anterior portion of the temporal horn. Even with marked narrowing, however, the temporal horn ordinarily can be followed to its tip, Not all temporal meningiomas produce characteristic findings, since some tumors are very large; associated changes may be present which cause occlusion of the anterior temporal horn. In these instances, therefore, the diagnosis of meningioma, or other extracerebral mass, cannot be made with certainty from the pneumographic changes alone; other findings in the total radiologic evaluation may give an indication of the true nature of the pathologic process.

Intrinsic tumors of the anterior temporal region behave in a manner similar to other lesions situated near the ventricle. The lumen is narrowed, often tapered, or sharply occluded by the adjacent tumor. Occlusion often results in a truncated appearance of the ventricle, as seen in lateral view. Frontal films, made following maneuvers to fill both temporal horns, find their greatest usefulness in the detection of small anterior temporal tumors. In addition, the location of the bulk of the mass, central or lateral to the temporal horn, is readily demonstrated.

While meningiomas of the sphenoid area often are associated with a frontal pneumographic picture quite characteristic of the type of tumor, other anterior temporal tumors infrequently invoke changes in the frontal pneumogram which are indicative of the identity of the mass. Localization, however, usually is afforded, as noted above. Temporal lesions frequently are associated with considerable shift of the septum pellucidum and third ventricle from the midline. A dislocation of 1 cm. is not unusual, in an average case; in some instances, the displacement may be very great, up to 2.5 cm. The configuration of the septum pellucidum and third ventricle typically is curved although it may be angular; the curved deformity may be associated with either intrinsic or extracerebral temporal lesions (fig. 270). Contralateral ventricular dilatation is the rule in the experience of most authors, although Davidoff and Epstein (1950) reported a lower incidence of dilatation than most writers. The ipsilateral ventricle usually is not dilated.

Elevation of the lateral angle of the lateral venticle, as seen in frontal projection, is one of the constant features of temporal masses, unless shift is severe (figs. 253, 270, and 283). The elevation involves usually the anterior and middle thirds of the body of the lateral ventricle. The floor of the same ventricle also may be slightly elevated. The lateral angle elevation, however, is more pronounced than that of the floor, a point which may serve to differentiate temporal changes from those seen with thalamic tumors.

When the temporal horn is cut off or truncated by the tumor, additional information from the temporal region itself concerning the type of lesion and the extent of spread is meager; conclusions often must be based on secondary effects found in the body of the lateral ventricle. When the temporal horn is displaced and visible, although narrowed, more precise evaluation is possible. If a temporal tumor is above or medial to the horn, and the ventricular lumen yet preserved, slight degrees of lateral or inferior displacement may be demonstrated; such displacement is never marked, however, since the rigid bony walls of the middle fossa confine the lobe. Displacement of one-half centimeter may occur fairly frequently, but lateral or downward displacement of 1 cm. is extraordinary; before this degree of displacement is reached, occlusion usually will take place. Tumors occurring deep to the temporal horn may displace this structure upward, as well as slightly outward. A somewhat dilated temporal horn, slightly outwardly and upwardly displaced, should suggest a tumor in the hippocampal area.

Other masses. Tumors may arise along the true temporal medial surface or the portion opposing the island of Reil. Similarly, lesions of this area may originate in the parietal or frontal operculum, or in the insular tissue itself. Visualization of the subarachnoid spaces of the island of Reil is inconstant, and failure of these spaces to be visualized is not necessarily of pathologic significance. It is somewhat unusual, however, to have gas outline the insular region if a tumor is present; often an early effect of tumor growth in this region is obliteration of the insular space. Occasionally, the growth of tumors is associated with atrophic changes about the tumor periphery; when gas fills these abnormally wide spaces, exact tumor localization is facilitated. Under such circumstances, as might be expected, the tumor outline is quite discrete and, although there is deformity and displacement of the ventricular system locally, there may be little general effect on the main portion of the ipsilateral ventricle. In some cases generalized ventricular enlargement, without evidence of significant encroachment upon the ventricular system, and associated marginal atrophy, suggest that the neoplasm has developed in cerebral tissue with a preexistent degenerative process.

The confluence of several cerebral lobes at the insula is an example of arbitrary anatomic divisions that are to be found in some areas of the brain, even with related function. Since most primary brain tumors are invasive, such arbitrary divisions serve as no obstacle to tumor extension from one portion to another. Because there frequently is bridging of tumor from one lobe to another, into the most deeply seated nuclei, and spread to the contralateral cerebral hemisphere, it usually is not possible to say at pneumography—or even at necropsy examination—where a moderately extensive tumor had its point of origin.

Temporal lobe epilepsy may be the principal manifestation of a temporal lobe tumor. In recent years, focal epilepsy of temporal lobe origin has been receiving increasing attention. In general, electroencephalographic changes, localizable to one temporal area of the brain, are detected in these cases; nevertheless, bilateral EEG abnormalities are common, even though the pathologic focus is unilateral. Temporal lobectomy has been advocated for the treatment of this condition; if accepted, it becomes necessary to decide which is the abnormal side.

Serial histologic sections of resected specimens disclose the presence of very slowly growing infiltrating gliomas in a fairly high percentage of cases. These infiltrating gliomas often do not produce typical findings of a mass lesion on the pneumoencephalogram. In fact, some pneumograms exhibit enlargement of the tip of the temporal horn without deformity; in other cases, the horn may be smaller than on the opposite side. In our experience, approximately one-half of the cases of temporal lobe epilepsy have been associated with some abnormality, usually slight, involving the temporal horn; often only slight enlargement is found. It is well to keep in mind that there may be as much as 3 cm. of temporal lobe tissue anterior to the tip of the temporal horn, and that an infiltrating tumor which replaces—rather than displaces—brain tissue cannot be expected to produce a gross deformity. For the same reason, and although the middle cerebral artery passes over this anterior portion of the temporal lobe, no abnormality ordinarily is visualized on the angiogram.

A review of a series of patients with temporal lobe epilepsy studied at the Neurological Institute by both angiography and pneumography has disclosed that usually negative results are yielded by the angiogram, whereas the pneumoencephalogram has demonstrated some abnormality of the temporal horn in 9 out of 18 cases (Goldensohn, 1962). The pneumogram often has been the procedure of greatest aid in deciding which temporal lobe is likely to be the abnormal one. Simple enlargement, in the absence of obstruction, is an indication of shrinkage of the mass of the temporal lobe; it may be primary atrophy, but also can be secondary to trauma, to inflammation, or to vascular disease. At other times, the pneumographic

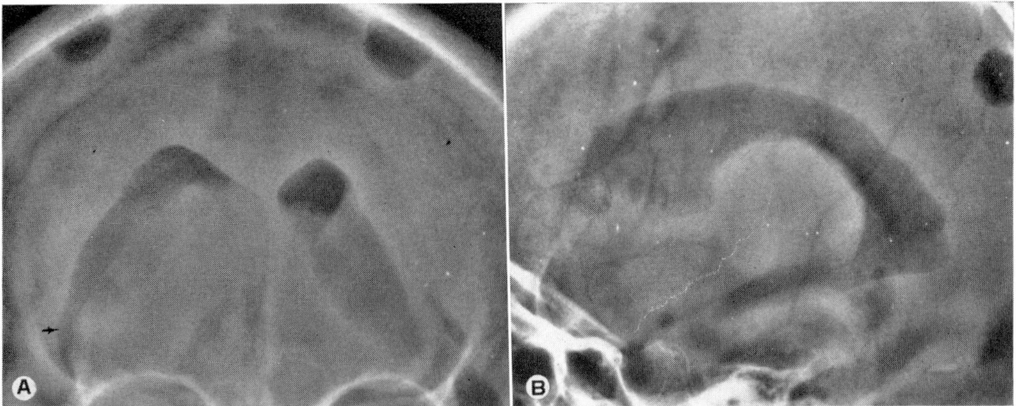

FIG. 284.—RIGHT THALAMIC GLIOMA

The frontal ventriculogram (A), made in prone position, reveals narrowing of the ventricular body, owing to elevation of the ventricular floor, and narrowing of the atrium by encroachment upon the lumen from the medial aspect. The midline structures are displaced to the contralateral side. The narrowing of the atrium extends into the temporal horn (*arrow*), which is very thin inferiorly and displaced laterally by the central mass, as compared with the opposite side. The deep structures bounded by the medial wall of the ventricle, the ventricular floor and the temporal horn are increased in height and width. The lateral film (B) reveals elevation of the floor of the body of the lateral ventricle extending from the foramen of Monro to the atrium. The posterior wall of the thalamus, bounded by the atrium, is prominent, and there is some narrowing of the superior and medial aspect of the temporal horn posteriorly.

findings have indicated the presence of a neoplasm. In all such cases, a painstaking and careful evaluation of the temporal horns, including anteroposterior laminagraphy, will often be rewarded by the finding of slight, but possibly important, deviations from the normal.

Thalamic Tumors

Tumors of the basal ganglia and thalamus, of the hypothalamus and of the posterior pathways in the peduncular region actually are tumors of the brain stem, inasmuch as these and associated structures constitute the supratentorial portion of the stem. Radiologically and clinically, however, neoplasms of these areas, with the exception of the peduncles and hypothalamus, are considered as deep hemispheric lesions according to most classifications. The hypothalamus may be regarded as a special area and considered in relation to the suprasellar lesions. Masses involving the peduncles usually are considered with the midbrain tumors, although they may sometimes originate in the thalamus. Other tumors of this region, such as colloid cysts and pinealomas, with a principal extension into the lumen of the third ventricle, are taken up in our discussion of the intraventricular tumors. Extraventricular tumors of the medial and inferior central hemispheric region are generally termed, as in this present description, *thalamic* tumors; no attempt is made to define at pneumography to which nuclei or substances of the general thalamic region the tumor is limited.

Since the thalamic tissues are situated inferior to the lateral ventricle, forming a large portion of the ventricular floor, and lateral to the third ventricle, forming the side wall, the early and principal effects of primary tumors in this region are on these structures which they bound. The frontal pneumogram is the most consistently helpful projection in the diagnosis of thalamic masses; generally, it allows the detection of lesions in this region earlier than the lateral projections. One of the earliest manifestations of a thalamic tumor is *elevation of the ventricular floor* on the involved side; it often is best appreciated by comparison of the position and contour of the ventricular floors on the two sides in frontal projection. In some instances, the lateral wall of the ventricular

(Revised 1963)

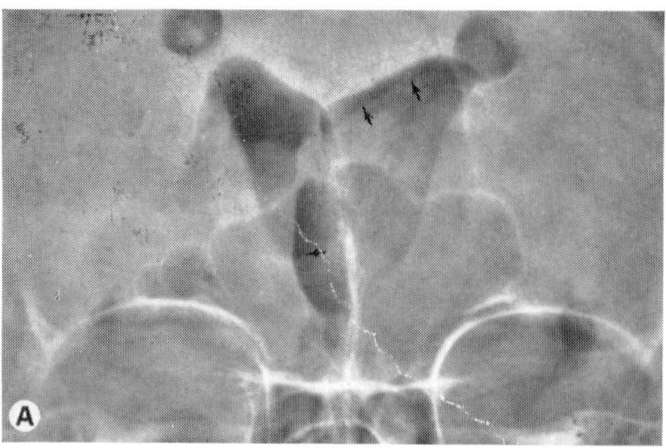

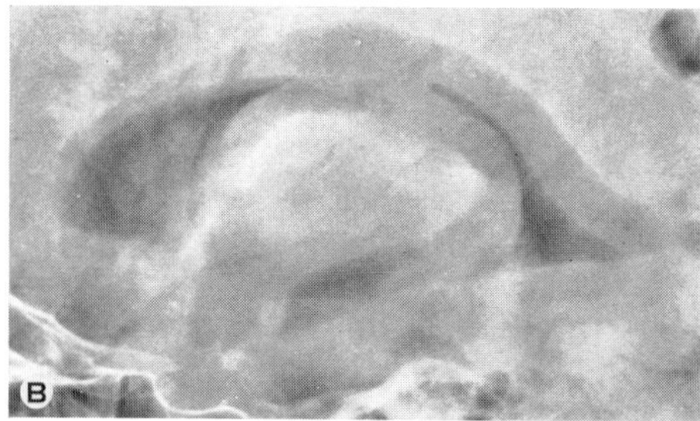

Fig. 285.—Left Thalamic Glioma

The frontal ventriculogram (A) reveals the lateral wall and floor of the ventricle to be markedly elevated, with only a thin linear gas shadow remaining over the elevated thalamus at the level of the ventricular body (*upper arrows*). The third ventricle is displaced to the right, and its wall on the side of the tumor is indistinct owing to projection of the thalamus into the third ventricular lumen in a curved manner (*lower arrow*). On the opposite side, the lateral wall of the third ventricle is seen on end and is sharply delimited. The central space between the temporal horn, ventricular body, and third ventricle is increased in volume, as are the linear measurements, by the tumor. The lateral film (B) reveals pronounced elevation of one lateral ventricular floor from the foraminal to the atrial region. The posterior portion of the third ventricle is not clearly visualized because the tumor obliterates the lumen by compression of one side wall against the other, accounting for the ventricular dilatation.

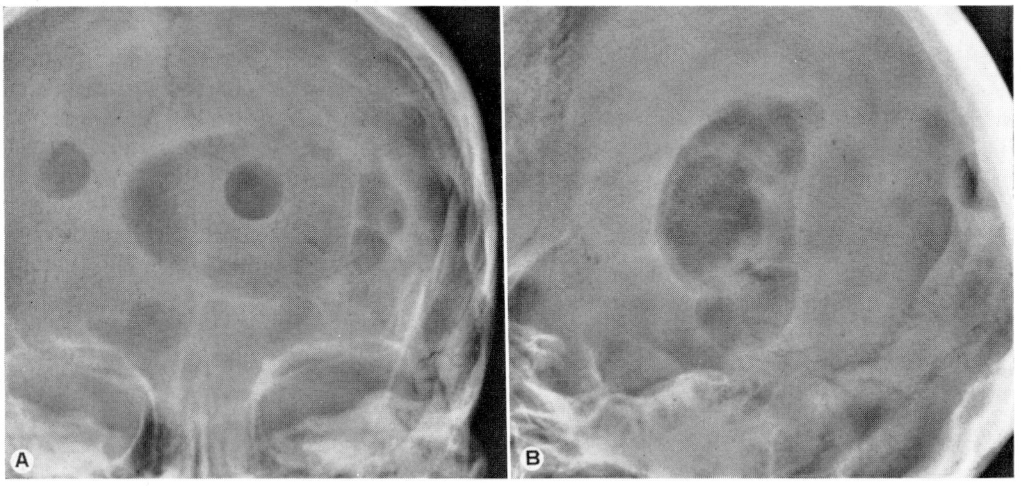

Fig. 286.—Cystic Glioma

The cavity of a tumor that had undergone gross cystic degeneration was tapped at the time of attempted ventriculography, and air was introduced to produce a cystogram (A) and (B). Such cystic tumors, which do not communicate with the ventricles, produce an isolated depiction of the interior of the tumor, allowing precise localization. Some portions of the cyst wall usually are smooth while others are irregular; the latter usually indicate the location of the bulk of the solid portion of the neoplasm.

body may be indented early; as the tumor grows, there is almost always a medial shift of the lateral ventricular side wall, as well as narrowing of the ventricular lumen from the inferior side by elevation of the lateral ventricular floor (fig. 284). In some advanced cases, the lumen of the ventricle may be occluded almost completely. When the elevation of the ventricular floor involves the posterior portion of the body and atrium, the posteroanterior half axial projection brings out the deformity most adequately.

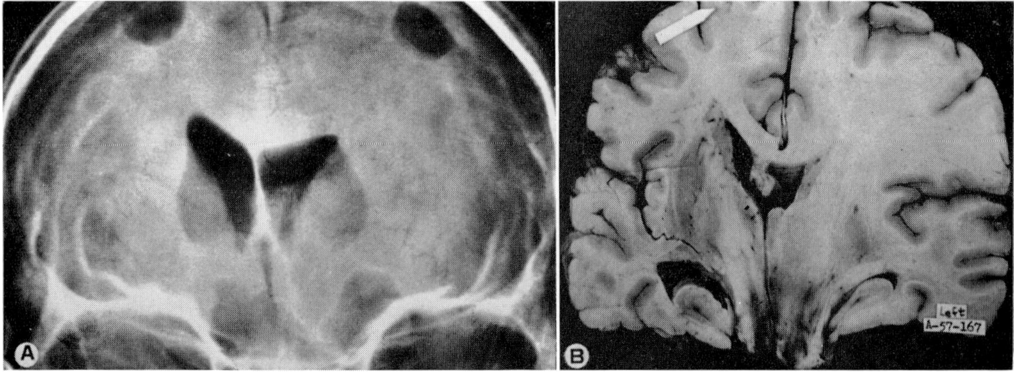

FIG. 287.—CEREBRAL INFARCTION SIMULATING BRAIN TUMOR

The ventriculogram (A) reveals lateral displacement of the ventricular system without localizing deformity. The coronal section of the brain (B) reveals extensive edema of the white matter of the left cerebral hemisphere. Edema usually is maximum 48 to 96 hours after occlusion of a major vessel.

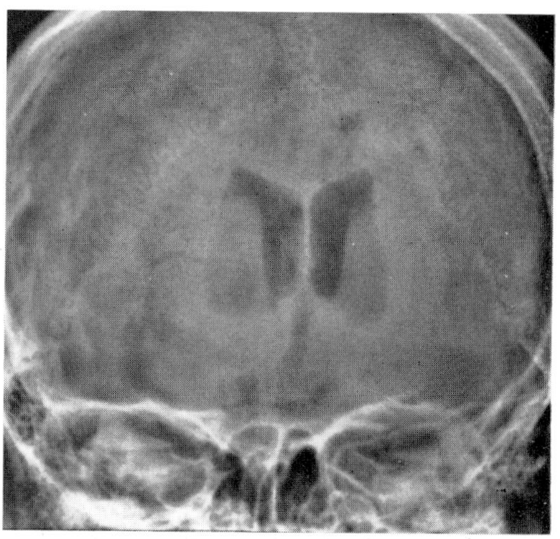

FIG. 288.—CEREBRAL ATROPHY WITH SHIFT OF MIDLINE STRUCTURES

The ventricular system is shifted to the left of its normal position. Slight widening of the lateral angle on the left side is present, but no other evidence of enlargement or deformity of the left lateral ventricle was found. The left half of the cranial vault was thicker than the right. The posterior portion of the sagittal suture and the crista galli deviate toward the left. Hemicerebral atrophy without more evidence of ventricular enlargement is unusual and may lead to the erroneous impression of a contralateral expanding lesion.

Slight ventricular dilatation on the contralateral side, on the involved side, or on both sides, may be present; this is more pronounced with tumors situated forward which are in a position to exert pressure at the foramen of Monro. In spite of fairly extensive involvement of one lateral ventricle, and the presence of ventricular dilatation of mild degree, both ventricles ordinarily are filled by gas, since the interventricular foramen usually is patent. The septum pellucidum is affected little, in early cases; larger lesions of this region may produce a curved shift of the septum pellucidum and third ventricle.

A second principal effect of thalamic tumors is on the *third ventricle*; it usually is seen early and is easily recognized. Flattening of the involved lateral wall, with alteration of the slightly oval or elongated contour of the third ventricle, usually is seen with tumors behind the foraminal plane. With larger lesions, flattening progresses to indentation, and eventually to the production of a concave rather than a convex wall. Thus, a semilunar or crescentic configuration eventually results. In some instances, there is a greater effect on the third ventricle than on the lateral ventricle; occasionally, there may be considerable contralateral displacement of the third ventricle with little lateral ventricular deformity. Ventricular occlusion by direct compression is seen occasionally, but usually only with advanced processes. Dilatation of the third ventricle is brought about more readily if the tumor is primarily in the posterior thalamic area, and if partial or complete occlusion of the posterior portion of the ventricular lumen is produced.

The third major area affected by thalamic

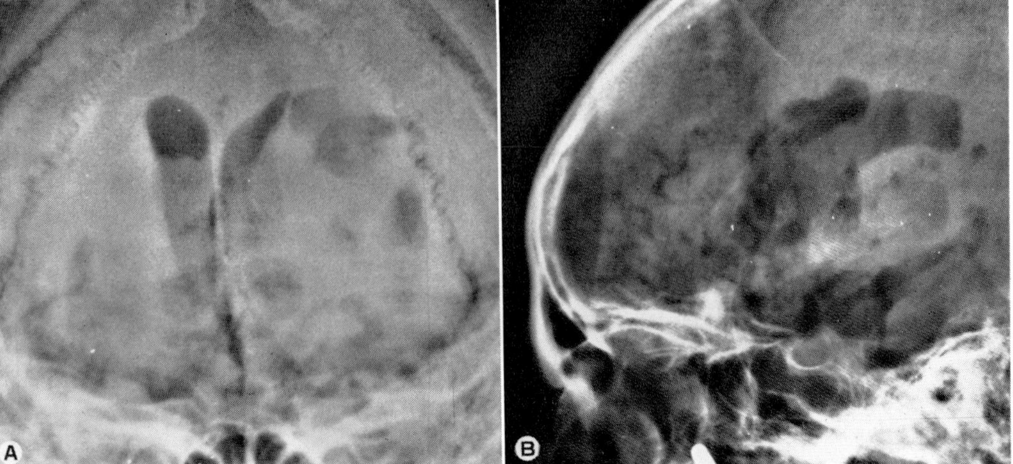

FIG. 289.—INTRACEREBRAL HEMATOMA WITH RUPTURE INTO LATERAL VENTRICLE

A spontaneous intracerebral hemorrhage, occurring deep in the frontal region, has caused displacement of the ventricular system and narrowing of the anterior horn and anterior portion of the ventricular body on the involved side (A). Through compression of adjacent cerebral tissue with subsequent necrosis and liquefaction, the hematoma has ruptured into the lateral ventricular lumen and gas has passed from the ventricle into the hematoma site at pneumoencephalography. The numerous intracerebral gas collections shown in the region of the caudate nucleus and lateral to it in frontal view are shown to be in and just anterior to the plane of the interventricular foramen in the lateral pneumogram (B).

tumors, as seen in frontal view, is the *temporal horn* of the ipsilateral side. The anterior portion of the temporal body and the temporal tip are displaced downward; usually, there is also slight lateral displacement. The degree of downward and lateral displacement ordinarily does not exceed 0.5 cm. and is best appreciated by comparison with the opposite side (fig. 284). Downward dislocation is more evident than lateral shift in the majority of instances. Compression and narrowing of the lumen may be found, particularly with anterior lesions. Unilateral dilatation of the anterior portion of the involved temporal horn may be seen with advanced posterior tumors; at this stage of development, however, other changes of a thalamic tumor usually are quite evident. In general, the temporal horn changes are more indicative of the extent of the tumor than of the basic locus of the lesion; that is, they are found in bulky masses only and not in the early cases.

The lateral pneumogram exhibits chiefly an elevation of the floor of the involved lateral ventricle. There may be a smooth elevation of the entire ventricular body, or it may be chiefly anterior or posterior. Lesions of the head of the caudate nucleus cause an elevation of the floor and narrowing of the anterior horn. Tumors of the posterior thalamic and pulvinar areas cause a narrowing of the atrium and an increase in its arc, as seen in lateral view, owing to encroachment from the anterior aspect. The lateral pneumogram is largely correlative, while the frontal pneumogram is essentially diagnostic.

In analyzing the frontal view changes, a triangular relationship of (1) the lateral wall and floor of the lateral ventricle, (2) the wall of the third ventricle, and (3) the temporal horn, may be considered as three key points. In advanced cases, there is spreading in all directions. The classical picture of a thalamic tumor shows (1) elevation of the lateral ventricular floor and medial displacement of the side wall, (2) indentation and displacement of the side wall of the third ventricle, and (3) downward and slight lateral dislocation of the temporal horn. There is usually a relative and absolute spreading of the lateral ventricular body and the temporal horn, and an increase in the distance

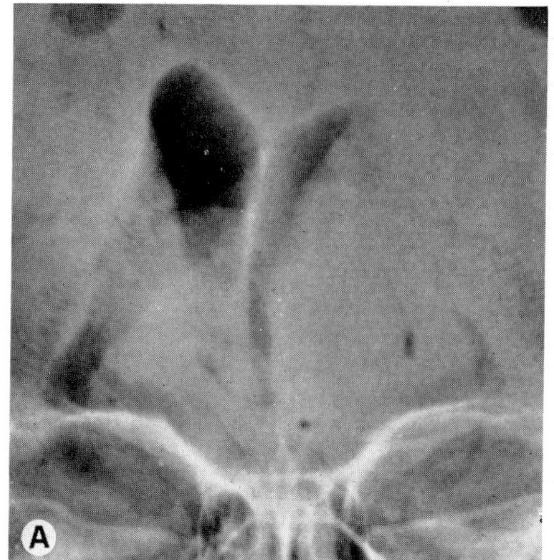

Fig. 290.—Brain Abscess

The frontal ventriculogram (A) reveals marked lateral displacement (curved shift) of the septum pellucidum and third ventricle, together with ventricular narrowing on the side of the mass.

A large brain abscess has been evacuated and filled with Thorotrast and air (B). Following taking of the film, the Thorotrast was aspirated from the cavity. A film made eight days later (C) shows contrast material still coating the periphery of the abscess cavity. The cavity is shown to be undergoing anticipated contraction with control of infection under antibiotic therapy.

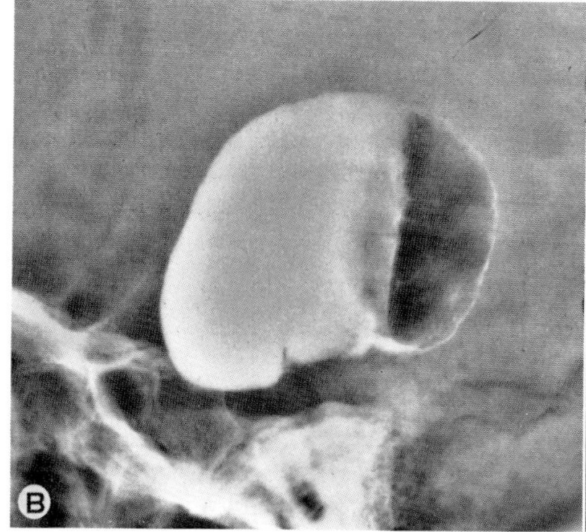

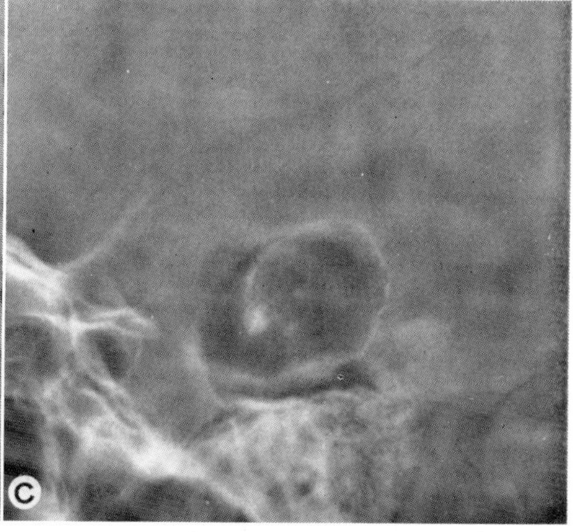

from the third ventricle to the temporal horn (fig. 285). There also may be a reduction in the measurement from the temporal horn to the inner table of the bony skull.

Thalamic tumors frequently extend downward into the hypothalamic region and affect the anterior portion of the third ventricle. Lateral displacement and occlusion of the hypothalamic third ventricle may be observed in such instances. Tumors that originate in the hypothalamus may spread upward into the thalamus. The latter lesions usually affect the anterior half of the third ventricle early in their development, because the ventricular lumen is very narrow, as are the related hypothalamic soft tissues. Tumors originating in the hypothalamus often extend primarily into the ventricular lumen with occlusion of the third ventricle; it is usually more important, therefore, to differentiate hypothalamic tumors from other anterior intraventricular masses than from a thalamic tumor that has spread downward. Primary hypothalamic tumors also must be considered in the differential diagnosis of extracerebral suprasellar and parasellar tumors; therefore, it probably is more germane to elaborate further concerning primary hypothalamic tumors under the discussion of suprasellar lesions.

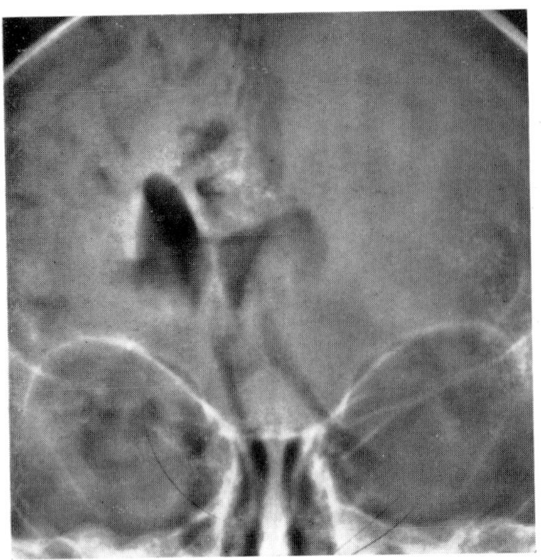

FIG. 291.—HERPES SIMPLEX ENCEPHALITIS

In some cases of viral infection, the cerebral inflammatory process may be localized rather than generalized. In the case illustrated, a unilateral cerebritis produced marked edema and encephalomalacia. Subfalcial dislocation of the ipsilateral ventricle was present, and there is absence of subarachnoid gas on the involved side.

Differential Diagnosis of Hemispheric Tumors

Throughout the section on intracranial pneumography, the relatively high degree of accuracy of the method for the detection and localization of space-occupying lesions is emphasized. The difficulty of accurate prediction of the pathologic identity of mass lesions, on the other hand, also is stressed. Intracranial tumors are considered in the broad sense; we have intended to make it clear that space-occupying lesions demonstrated by pneumography are not always neoplasms. In some instances, it is not possible to predict by all radiologic methods, or all other diagnostic methods short of intracranial exploration and pathologic study, the true nature of a space-occupying mass. Nevertheless, we include in the discussion of tumors located in various areas the characteristics not only of neoplasms of those regions, but also the common non-neoplastic processes which may be found. In addition to the changes strictly related to pneumograms, changes in the bony skull must be very carefully sought and evaluated to enhance the diagnostic accuracy of radiologic methods. It is the usual practice to carry out an objective film analysis, correlating plain film changes with pneumographic findings, and to go as far as possible in making a diagnosis as the first step. With the various diagnostic possibilities in mind then, the radiologist is in the best position for clinical consultation. A final opinion should be reached only after careful evaluation of clinical and laboratory data, and their correlation with the radiologic findings. By these steps a correct diagnosis should be reached in a high percentage of cases.

Non-neoplastic processes present as intracranial masses in the various areas which are considered. In the lateral ventricles, as discussed earlier, hematomas may pose as intraventricular tumors (fig. 250). Colloid cysts of the third ventricle (fig. 259) have been described at some length and in the fourth ventricle, the cysts of *Cysticercus cellulosae* may fill and obstruct the ventricular lumen, simulating an intraventricular neoplasm. Aqueduct stenosis may be caused by inflammation of various origins; in some cases stenosis is readily distinguished from a mesencephalic neoplasm, while at other times it is not (figs. 240 and 306).

Non-neoplastic processes presenting as supratentorial extraventricular masses, or hemispheric space-taking lesions, as discussed above, are multitudinous. In many instances, the true nature of the process is masked by a high degree of associated edema. Thus, acute infarction, resulting from occlusive vascular disease, commonly presents as an expanding intracranial lesion, both clinically and radiologically. Displacement of calcified structures on plain films, and midline shift of the ventricles at pneumography, may be found (fig. 287). Occlusive vascular disease of long standing is more commonly associated with atrophic changes at pneumography; it is not an uncommon finding in patients with bizarre clinical symptoms simulating neoplasm (fig. 288).

An intracerebral hematoma may resemble a brain tumor in every way (fig. 289). Such

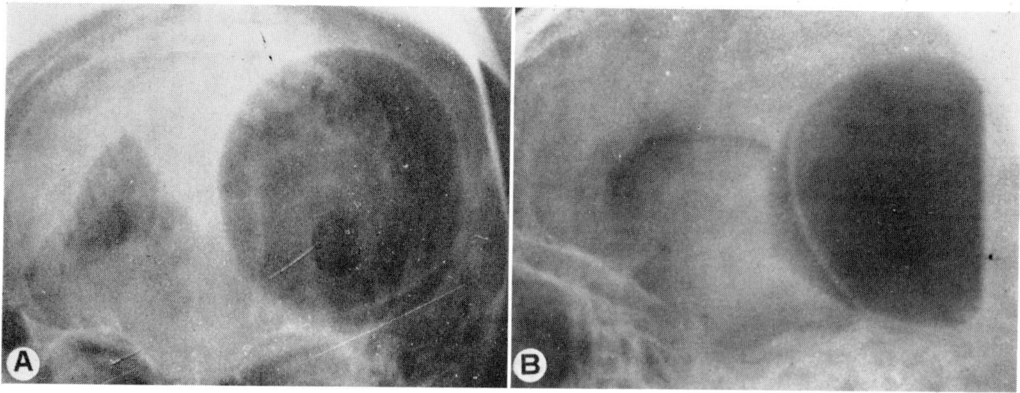

FIG. 292.—ECHINOCOCCUS CYST

The ventriculogram-cystogram reveals a very large, smooth-walled cavity in the left cerebral hemisphere. A portion of the cyst wall may be seen inferiorly in the posteroanterior view (A) and anteriorly in the supine lateral view (B). Just beyond the visualized portion of the cyst wall is a crescentic gas collection characteristically seen. The crescentic collection is visible when the contents of the cyst are removed and replaced by air under reduced tension, allowing partial collapse. (Courtesy of Dr. F. Garcia Cappuro, Montevideo.)

masses occur in various portions of the brain; they are frequently deeply seated in the frontal and temporal regions. The hemorrhagic mass and the edema of a hematoma ordinarily present as a solitary process and thus further mimic neoplasm.

Brain abscess, when solitary, also may be indistinguishable from a new growth (fig. 290). When multiple lesions are present, the correct diagnosis is more readily appreciated, although differentiation from metastatic neoplasm may be impossible. In these instances, plain film clues to the possible site of origin of an abscess, such as paranasal or mastoid sinus disease, may be invaluable for diagnosis, in cases in which there is no clinical or laboratory indication of the inflammatory nature of the process. Abscess is commonly accompanied by marked cerebral edema, which may cause further difficulty in precise localization and identification of the abnormality.

Nonsuppurative encephalitis occasionally manifests itself as a mass lesion of one cerebral hemisphere, as in the case of the cerebritis of *herpes simplex* infection (fig. 291). The acute inflammation, edema, and encephalomalacia accompanying such processes may make it impossible to arrive at a clinical and radiologic diagnosis, unless there is a high index of suspicion regarding the possibility of such a lesion. When *herpes simplex* encephalitis is regarded as a significant possibility, special cultures are required to substantiate the diagnosis.

Parasitic infestations may affect the brain in various ways, as exemplified by toxoplasmosis and hydatid disease. The acute phase of toxoplasmosis results in an encephalitis, which may be no more readily recognizable radiologically than other forms previously mentioned; the end results of toxoplasmosis, with atrophy and calcification, are more easily identified (fig. 175). Hydatid disease, on the other hand, may manifest itself by a large solitary cerebral mass lesion having a typical appearance when the cyst is filled internally with gas (fig. 292); otherwise, the cyst is indistinguishable from a neoplasm or other space-taking process at pneumography or angiography. It is not rare for patients with such infestation to have cerebral involvement, nor is it unusual for a hydatid cyst to be tapped inadvertently at the time of attempted ventriculography in such cases. Frequently, the cysts are very large, and owing to increased intracranial pressure which is produced, ventriculography is the procedure of choice. Clear fluid may be obtained and replaced

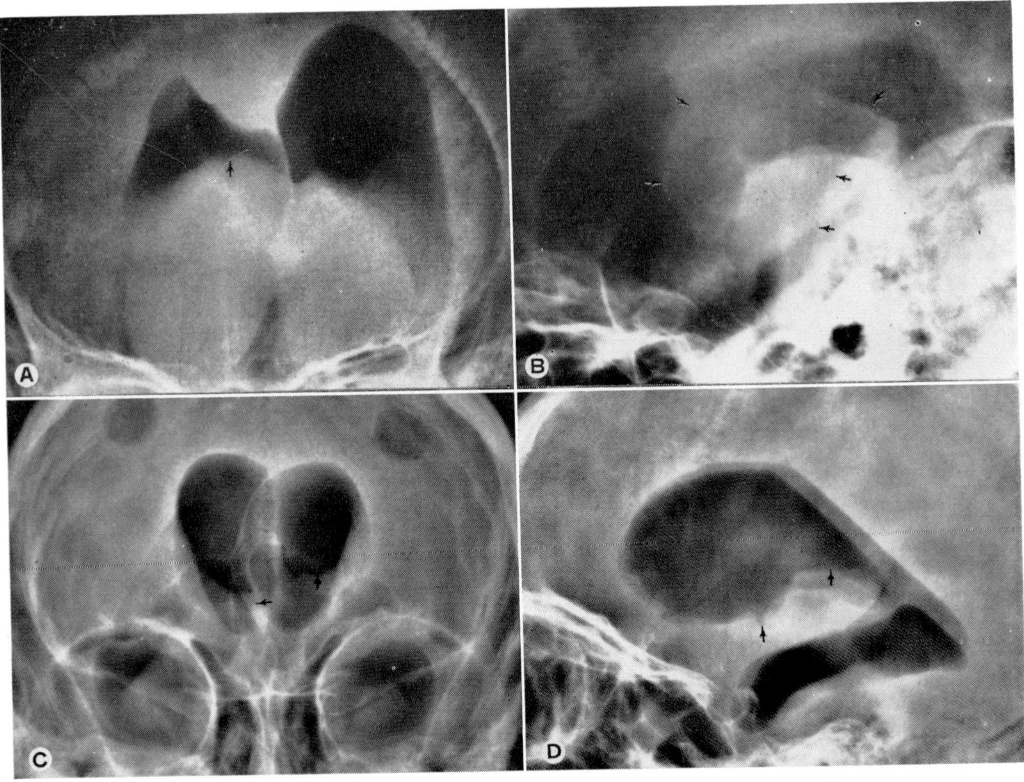

Fig. 293.—Granuloma of the Thalamus

A patient with multiple tuberculomas of the brain had a large lesion of the thalamus which produced elevation of the lateral ventricular floor (*arrow*), narrowing of the temporal horn, and contralateral displacement of the midline structures (A). There is obstruction of the posterior portion of the third ventricle (*lower arrows*) by compression of its side walls (B); the anterior part of the third ventricle is dilated, as are the lateral ventricles. The lateral ventricular body and anterior horn are deformed by the mass (*upper arrows*). Tuberculomas also were present in the parasagittal and convex portion of the same hemisphere and in the cerebellum.

A young woman with sarcoidosis, who had mediastinal lymphadenopathy and meningeal involvement, developed a right hemiparesis and signs of increased intracranial pressure. The frontal ventriculogram (C) reveals elevation of the floor of one lateral ventricle (*vertical arrow*) and contralateral displacement of the uppermost portion of the third ventricle (*transvese arrow*). The lateral film (D), made with the head in hyperextension (see Fig. 187), reveals an obstruction of the third ventricle just below the foramen of Monro (*anterior arrow*). Elevation of the lateral ventricular floor on one side by the thalamic mass (*posterior arrow*) also is shown in this projection.

by air. The interior of the cyst thus may be outlined. Ordinarily, the visualized internal portion of the cyst is smooth. Films made with the horizontal beam will show, in a typical case, a double contour superiorly, opposite the air-fluid level within the cyst (fig. 292). Presumably this results from replacement of fluid under tension by gas, and partial collapse of the cyst. Some gas must escape from the cyst through the needle hole into a pericystic space—or be injected into it directly—to account for the characteristic crescentic sign of hydatid disease. It is thought by some, in addition, that a degree of marginal atrophy may occur about the cyst, owing to brain pulsations, and this may contribute to the development of the peripheral gas collection. While cystography alone may cause dissemination, spread through subsequent surgical treatment is more probable, unless the cyst contents are sterilized by formalin. For this reason, it is highly important to recognize the diagnostic pneumographic appearance of cerebral hydatid disease (King and Couch, 1961; Dixon and Hargreaves, 1944; Obrador, 1948).

The granulomas often present at pneumography as intracranial masses indistinguishable from brain neoplasm. In the case of tuberculoma (fig. 293), the lesions may be multiple and thus provide a clue to the non-neoplastic nature of the disease. Solitary tuberculomas frequently are mistaken for true tumors. The granulomatous lesions of sarcoidosis may affect the brain, as illustrated by Figure 293, in which such a lesion occurred in the thalamus. Gummas are encountered rarely. In one instance, a xanthogranuloma (Hand-Schüller-Christian disease) simulated a neoplasm of the hypothalamus. While torulosis is restricted to a meningeal inflammation in the majority of instances, discrete space-occupying lesions within the brain may occur in some patients.

In contrast to the benign cysts, areas of cystic degeneration in neoplasms are irregular along the internal margins of their walls (fig. 286). The irregular outline denotes the location of solid mural masses of tumor. Wherever the margins of cystic cavities are irregular, a neoplasm should be suspected. The cystograms of tumors, like benign cysts, are obtained when such a lesion is tapped at attempted ventriculography. Cystic neoplasms usually contain yellowish fluid with a high percentage of protein, while benign cysts often contain clear fluid. Since the interior of the neoplasm is demonstrated, precise localization is afforded, as contrasted to the less exact localization resulting from secondary effects of masses on the ventricular system.

While it is axiomatic that a mass lesion of the brain must be considered a new growth until proven otherwise, the large number of pathologic processes that can simulate tumor make it imperative that every effort be made to identify mass lesions preoperatively. In the case of some non-neoplastic mass lesions, such as infarction, sarcoidosis, or even certain aneurysms, more harm may be done by surgical exploration than by the institution of nonoperative therapeutic measures. In other instances, intracranial surgical intervention is necessitated in any event; in some cases, a choice exists between surgical and nonsurgical treatment. The radiologist, through recognition of the diagnostic possibilities and an adroit evaluation of minor changes, may serve a most important role in clinical work, not only in diagnosis but in the proper direction of therapy.

INTRA-AXIAL POSTERIOR FOSSA TUMORS

Tumors of the cerebellum and of the caudal portion of the brain stem (excluding the thalamic areas) constitute approximately 30 per cent of all intrinsic brain tumors. Cerebellar tumors are second in frequency only to tumors of the frontal lobes. Between 70 and 80 per cent of brain tumors occurring in children are cerebellar tumors. In addition, it is well known that certain histologic types of neoplasms are more prone to occur in the posterior fossa and brain stem than elsewhere; medulloblastoma is the common midline cerebellar lesion in childhood, astrocytomas are common tumors of the cerebellar hemispheres in both childhood and adult life, and hemangioblastoma is the commonest primary cerebellar neoplasm of adult life. Polar spongioblastoma (astrocytoma) is the tissue type usually occurring in tumors of the brain stem in childhood; papillomas of the chorioid plexus and tumors of ependymal origin are found most frequently in the fourth ventricle. The occurrence of certain tumors by age group and by several sites of predilection in the posterior fossa enables the radiologist to anticipate preoperatively the character of the disease process in a high percentage of patients. In the majority of institutions, ventriculography is employed almost always when cerebellar tumors are suspected. On the other hand, lumbar pneumoencephalography is used when a brain stem or an extra-axial tumor of the posterior fossa is the probable diagnosis.

Neoplasms of the posterior fossa arising in the brain substance may be conveniently divided into cerebellar tumors and tumors of the brain stem, both clinically and radiologically. The presenting clinical features are quite different in the two types; at pneumography, cerebellar tumors are found posterior to the aqueduct and fourth ventricle, while brain stem tumors lie ventral to the posterior fossa ventricular structures. Cerebellar tumors may be subdivided into those that are in the midline, near the fourth ventricle itself in the vermis, and those that are in a cerebellar hemisphere, often at some distance from the fourth ventricle proper. Virchow (1864) described "hard gliomas" and "soft gliomas," and a similar terminology still is used occasionally in discussing tumors of the cerebellum. While Virchow's description probably was derived from histologic observations, solid tumors of the cerebellum grossly have the effect of a hard mass pressing on the ventricular system; the cystic astrocytomas, cystic hemangioblastomas and other soft tumors have a less intense effect on cerebrospinal fluid circulation. When ventricular occlusion is incomplete, more precise information may be gained from ventriculography than when the obstruction is complete; the rostral and caudal extent of a cerebellar tumor may be defined, as well as its lateral location, if the lesion is hemispheric and partially obstructive.

Cerebellar Tumors

Cerebellar tumors produce, in the majority of instances, increased intracranial pressure of varying degrees. The type and extent of radiologic changes are related to the duration and severity of intracranial hypertension. In the case of medulloblastoma, the rapidly growing tumor may produce symptoms of elevated intracranial pressure for only a few weeks, and yet plain film changes may be marked. A patient with cerebellar astrocytoma, on the other hand, may have a history of several years duration, and yet radiologic evidence of increased intracranial pressure may be absent or minimum.

In young children, there often is moderate or marked widening of the coronal and other major sutures; instances in which the frontal and parietal bones were separated more than 2 cm. at the coronal suture have been observed. Because of the decompression at the sutures, changes in the sella turcica are infrequent; however, increased convolutional markings of the inner table of the skull occur commonly (fig. 59).

Occasionally, cases are seen in which only a large head is present without other radiologic evidence of increased intracranial pressure. One such instance has been observed in which ventricular dilatation was quite marked as a result of a cerebellar medulloblastoma, and yet only megacephalus was found on the plain films. Some degree of progressive increased intracranial pressure must have been present for a considerable period of time in order that cranial enlargement without focal atrophy or suture widening was produced. In some instances, there may be enlargement of the posterior fossa itself, in the presence of long standing tumors. Such enlargement of the cerebellar chamber was emphasized as being of importance in clinical diagnosis by Dandy (1945). The enlargement, particularly in length, of the posterior fossa may be demonstrated in plain films as elongation and thinning of the horizontal portion of the occipital bone (fig. 67). In addition, the grooves of the lateral sinuses and the position of the internal occipital protuberance may be high in relation to the lambda, indicating enlargement of the vertical extent of the cerebellar chamber. Radiologically demonstrable calcification is rarely encountered with the more common tumors of the posterior fossa. Calcific deposits, however, may be demonstrated on plain films in the presence of dermoid or angiomatous tumors and in some cases of tuberculoma or abscess.

Ventriculography is the procedure of choice for the pneumographic examination of cerebellar tumors; pneumoencephalography usually results in nonfilling of the ventricular system. Symmetrical dilatations of the lateral ventricles of varying degree almost always is found. In occasional instances, there is slight asymmetry of the dilated lateral ventricles. Ventricular dilatation may vary from a mild to a marked extent, the transverse lateral ventricular measurement is above 10 cm. in some instances. The third ventricle is outlined readily and also exceeds normal measurements in most patients. Some tumors, particularly the cystic tumors of the cerebellar hemispheres, result in an incomplete obstruction of the fourth ventricle; in these cases the lateral ventricles may be only slightly enlarged.

The aqueduct of Sylvius frequently is the structure upon which diagnosis may depend. In the average case of cerebellar tumor, the upper aqueduct, or the portion above the tentorial incisura, is dilated but it is not displaced. The effect of the cerebellar tumor is seen ordinarily upon the portion of the aqueduct caudal to the tentorial notch. In the normal pneumogram, the aqueduct of Sylvius extends backward and downward in a smooth curve to join the posterior inferior angle of the third ventricle with the upper portion of the fourth ventricle. The caliber of the aqueduct should not exceed 2 mm. The distance from the aqueduct to the dorsum sellae is, on the average, 3.4 cm. with a minimum limit of 3 cm. (fig. 213).

Vermis masses. In the case of solid tumors of the cerebellar vermis, particularly medulloblastoma, the tumor obliterates the fourth ventricle, either by compression or invasion. Because the tumor encroaches upon the fourth ventricle from behind, it pushes the ventricular system and the brain stem forward as it grows. It is possible to follow the route of air injected at ventriculography through dilated lateral and third ventricles, and through a dilated short supratentorial segment of the aqueduct, to the level of the tentorial notch; caudal to this point, the iter and fourth ventricle, if visible, are displaced, deformed, and finally obliterated. *Angulation of the aqueduct* usually is found at or near the level of the tentorium, rather than the smooth curve of the normal aqueduct. The lower aqueduct is sharply bent and displaced forward; its distance from the dorsum sellae rapidly becomes less than the minimum 3 cm. (fig. 213).

Angulation and forward displacement of the lower aqueduct results in a configuration that has been termed a "hockey stick" deformity (fig. 294). The change is best brought out when a relatively long segment of the lower aqueduct is visualized, owing to a low position of the tumor in the vermis. In other instances, the aqueduct is sharply angulated forward; it tapers rapidly and the lumen is completely obliterated shortly after it passes through the incisura (fig. 294). When an unusually long segment of aqueduct appears to be present (more than 2.0 cm.), part of the upper fourth ventricle may be included. Usually, the displaced iter extends in a fairly straight line, following its forward angulation from a normal inclination; it narrows gradually and at its caudal extremity tapers to a point of complete occlusion.

The importance of making every attempt to visualize the fourth ventricle and aqueduct at ventriculography, if it is anatomically possible for these areas to fill, is apparent. The best opportunity for the posterior fossa segments of the ventricular system to fill is with the patient prone; a technically good lateral film made with the head in this position, using the horizontal x-ray beam, is essential in all cases.

Posteroanterior views, both straight frontal and half axial projections, usually give an indication of the side of the bulk of the growth by lateral displacement of the visualized segment of aqueduct. Lateralization, generally, is not as important with tumors of the vermis as in the case of a lesion of one cerebellar hemisphere. It is necessary, always, to appraise the configuration of the posterior aspect of the third ventricle in frontal projection. Some tumors may extend upward, or cause upward herniation, through the incisura. The posterior, inferior, and lateral margins of the third ventricle are affected; usually flattening of the inferolateral aspect of the third

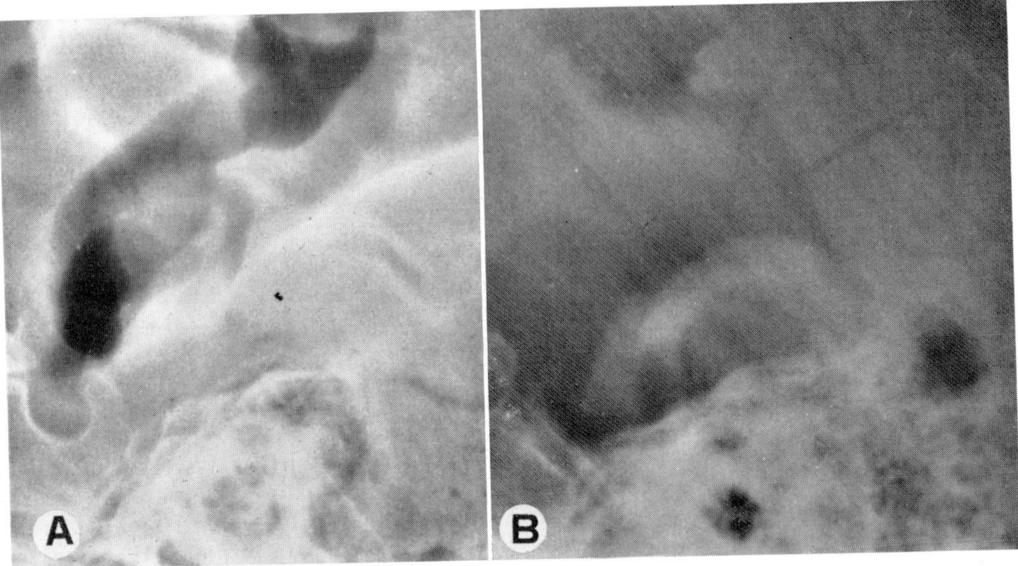

FIG. 294.—CEREBELLAR TUMOR

An astrocytoma has produced anterior displacement of the aqueduct of Sylvius, producing a deformity that resembles a hockey stick (B). The upper aqueduct is dilated, while the lower portion is narrowed. Anterior displacement of the subtentorial portion results in angulation at the incisura. The obstruction is incomplete, and gas passed through the fourth ventricle after injection via lumbar puncture.

In another case (A), an astrocytoma has produced marked anterior displacement of the cerebral aqueduct with occlusion of its distal portion. The upper aqueduct is sharply angulated and dilated, as is the ventricular system above.

ventricular outline in frontal view is the most apparent change (fig. 297). Symmetrical dilatation and bilaterally smooth lateral rounding of the third ventricle usually denote confinement of the tumor to the posterior fossa.

Tomograms should be used as required to visualize, in lateral view, the aqueduct and any portion of the fourth ventricle which is filled; also, frontal tomograms may be employed to demonstrate the posterior part of the third ventricle. Since many of the tumors of the cerebellar vermis occur in small children, it is highly desirable to obtain prone lateral roentgenograms after backward somersaulting; films can be made with the patient completely inverted. Such maneuvers give the greatest opportunity for good filling of the posterior ventricular structures. In older patients, leaving the patient prone for a period of time or somersaulting in a specially designed chair may serve the same purpose.

Since the fourth ventricle is compressed, deformed, and displaced by tumors of the cerebellar vermis, the point of maximum deformity and displacement may be used to determine precisely the location of the lesion. While deformity and forward displacement of the fourth ventricle often may be appreciated by inspection, it may be of help to apply measurements, as given in Figure 213, to the ventriculograms of some patients. The three measurements that have been most consistently helpful in the diagnosis of cerebellar tumor are: (1) the height of the fourth ventricle, as measured from the apex or fastigium to the floor, (2) the distance from the floor of the fourth ventricle to the dorsum sellae, and, less often, (3) the distance from the apex of the fourth ventricle to the base of the skull at the foramen magnum. In the case of cerebellar tumors, it is the minimum measurement of the first two distances that is of importance; the third measurement may be

(Revised 1963)

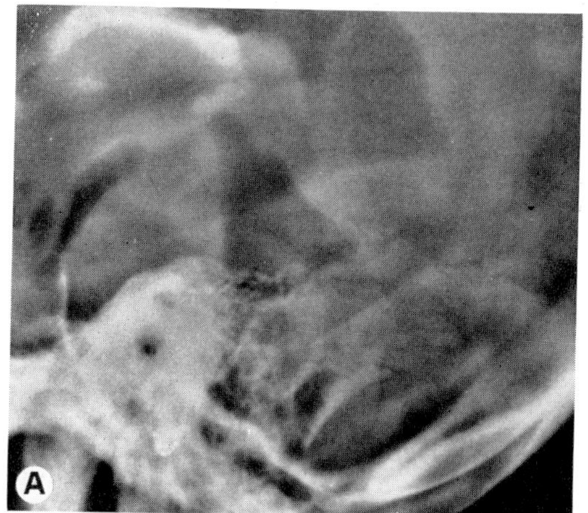

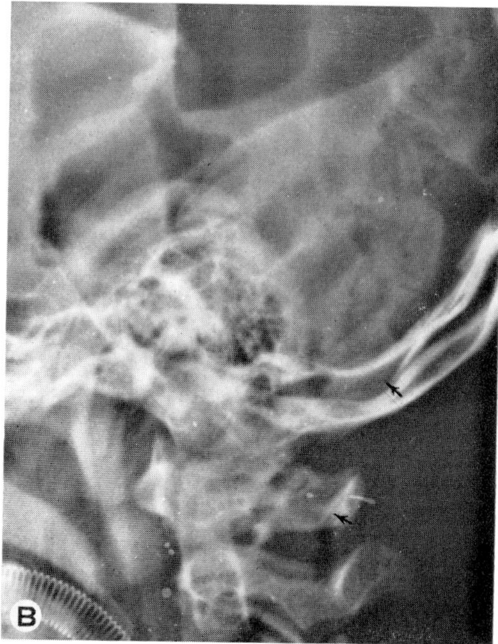

FIG. 295.—INFERIOR CEREBELLAR TUMOR

A tumor situated low in the cerebellum has elevated the fourth ventricle and displaced it forward producing subtotal obstruction of the outlet (A). The distance from the apex of the fourth ventricle to the rim of the foramen magnum is increased, while the distance from the floor of the fourth ventricle to the dorsum is reduced. The fourth ventricle and aqueduct are dilated to a greater degree than the lateral and third ventricles.

In another case (B), there is marked elevation of the fourth ventricle with foreshortening of the ventricle and of the aqueduct. There is marked forward displacement of the distal fourth ventricle, but the obstruction is not complete. Some gas escaped into the subarachnoid space. The subarachnoid space in the lower cisternal region and upper cervical region is obliterated posteriorly between the points marked by arrows, indicating tonsillar herniation.

increased or decreased by low or high tumors, respectively. As a substitute for measuring the distance from the floor of the fourth ventricle to the dorsum sellae, Twining's line may be drawn; the line of the floor of the fourth ventricle also may be extrapolated axially, and the relation of the extended line to the cervical spinal canal determined, as described earlier (see "Anatomy").

Small tumors in the lower portion of the cerebellar vermis, particularly in the region of the nodulus, will not always reduce the height of the fourth ventricle; they displace it forward and also may displace the fourth ventricle upward (fig. 295). The tumors often bulge into the inferior part of the fourth ventricle; there may be partial or complete obstruction at the ventricular outlet. Because the fourth ventricle is pushed upward by the tumor, it becomes foreshortened together with the aqueduct. The iter usually is dilated throughout its reduced length (sometimes called "ventricularization"); angulation, if present, ordinarily is not marked.

Tumors of the upper cerebellar vermis, in the region of the lingula, which do not completely obstruct, produce a generally opposite effect. In such cases, there is narrowing of the rostral half of the fourth ventricle in its anteroposterior diameter. There is also anterior displacement of the lower aqueduct and upper fourth ventricle (fig. 296). The combination of changes results in a forward bowing of these structures; frequently some degree of angulation is present at the level

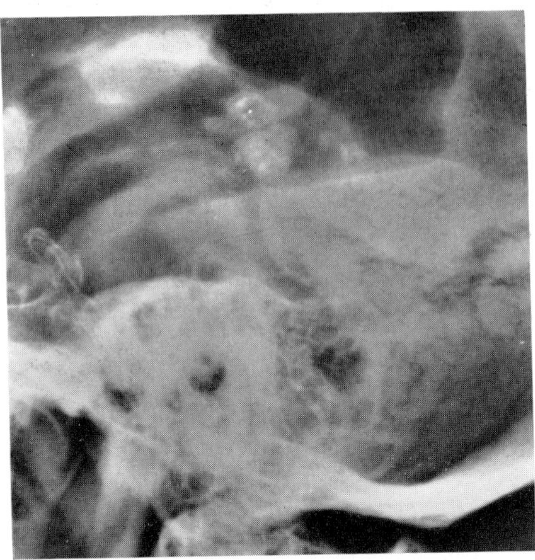

Fig. 296.—Superior Cerebellar Tumor

Masses originating high in the cerebellum produce effects on the aqueduct and fourth ventricle which are the opposite of those owing to inferior tumors. The apex of the fourth ventricle is displaced downward, and the distance from the apex to the foramen magnum is reduced. There is, however, also forward displacement of the fourth ventricle and of the aqueduct in its distal portion. If the aqueduct is not occluded, it may appear elongated and have a double curve. The height of the fourth ventricle usually is reduced.

of the tentorium, which Twining (1939) called abnormal kinking. Such tumors can, on occasion, actually push the fourth ventricle downward, with a reduction in the distance between the apex and the foramen magnum. When caudal displacement of the fourth ventricle occurs without the iter being completely occluded, the aqueduct is attenuated, and appears elongated and stretched (fig. 294). Thus, the common presentation of a vermis tumor develops, first through narrowing and displacement of the fourth ventricle, then displacement and thinning of the aqueduct, and finally, the very commonly encountered absence of the fourth ventricular shadow because of occlusion (fig. 297).

The straight posteroanterior and the posteroanterior half axial projections usually give minimum information in the presence of nonobstructing tumors of the cerebellar vermis. Localization usually is sufficiently precise from the lateral films alone. While a slight lateral predominance of the growth may be demonstrated in the frontal films, the marked lateral shifts occurring with tumors of the hemispheres are not ordinarily seen. Occasionally, some widening of the fourth ventricular shadow may be present as a result of flattening, owing to pressure from the dorsal aspect. Actual *invasion of the fourth ventricle* is common with medulloblastomas, and not too infrequent in cases of cerebellar astrocytoma.

Hemispheric masses. Tumors of the cerebellar hemispheres are chiefly astrocytomas and hemangioblastomas. Both tumors grow slowly and are compatible with many years of life. It is of interest that the natural course of untreated astrocytomas of the cerebellum is more than twice that of tumors of similar histologic type growing above the tentorium. The cerebellar hemispheric tumors have a tendency to undergo cystic degeneration; both astrocytomas and hemangioblastomas may become bulky, but remain "soft," if they are cystic.

Differentiation of astrocytoma from hemangioblastoma usually cannot be made radiologically with certainty, nor can these tumors be differentiated from other neoplasms of the cerebellar hemispheres, such as dermoids, ependymomas, or metastatic carcinomas; differentiation from non-neoplastic lesions, such as tuberculoma, abscess or intracerebellar hemorrhage also is difficult. Cerebellar hemangioblastomas are occasionally multiple and may be associated with angiomatous malformations. Hemangioblastoma of the cerebellum may occur with similar lesions in other organs, as well as with maldevelopments and different types of tumors of other organs. Lindau (1927) described a combination of hemangioblastoma of the cerebellum occurring in patients who had angiomatous malformations of the retina (Hippel's disease), as well as tumors of various other organs. This syndrome now usually is referred to as Lindau's disease and it presents some hereditary features. The ventriculographic findings in Lindau's disease are no different from those occurring

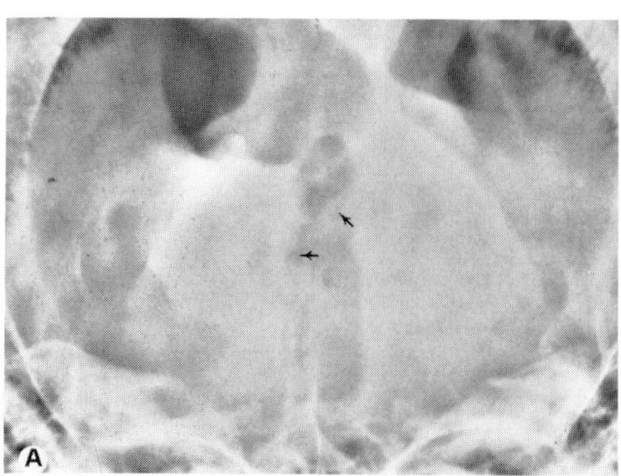

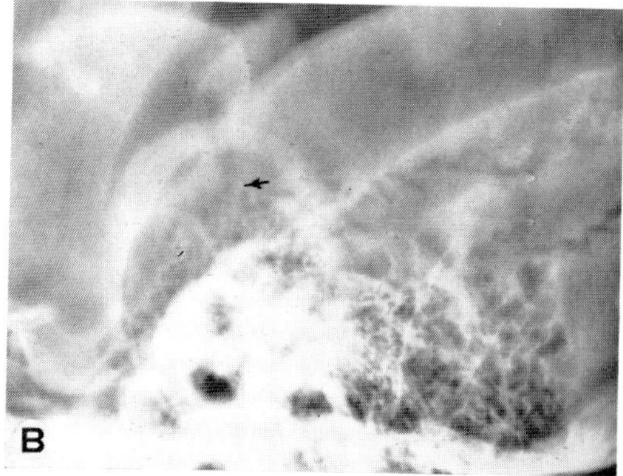

FIG. 297.—CEREBELLAR ASTROCYTOMA

A large cystic astrocytoma of a cerebellar hemisphere has resulted in lateral displacement and occlusion of the cerebral aqueduct (*lower arrow*), as seen in the frontal pneumogram (A). The posterior aspect of the third ventricle is tapered as a result of encroachment on the inferolateral side (*upper arrow*), owing to upward herniation at the incisura following ventriculography. The long, oval shadow of a markedly dilated anterior portion of the third ventricle is superimposed in the midline. In the lateral film (B), the aqueduct is displaced sharply forward and occluded (*arrow*). The inferior margin of one temporal horn is shown crossing the shadow of the aqueduct, the horn being elevated posteriorly by upward bowing of the tentorium produced by pressure of the large cerebellar hemispheric mass below.

with isolated hemangioblastoma of the cerebellum. Extraneural masses, such as meningiomas and posterior fossa subdural hematoma, may produce radiologic changes indistinguishable from intrinsic cerebellar tumors. Bony changes and calcification may occur with meningiomas arising in the posterior fossa, particularly those in the region of the torcular Herophili (fig. 149).

While the majority of the tumors just listed occur in a cerebellar hemisphere, occasionally they may be found in the midline; with some tumors it is not unusual for both hemispheres to be involved by extension. A mass of moderate or large size lying in a unilateral hemispheric location will produce a contralateral displacement of the fourth ventricle and of the iter; usually it is possible to demonstrate a shift of the structures in straight posteroanterior projection and in posteroanterior half axial views. Earlier there may be deformity of the lateral aspect of the fourth ventricle on the side of the tumor; the lateral recess may be preserved on the uninvolved side and obliterated on the diseased side. There may be rather marked lateral flattening and displacement in the frontal view, with a well preserved configuration of the fourth ventricle in the lateral projection (fig. 298). On the other hand, cases are encountered frequently in which only forward displacement of the aqueduct and fourth ventricle is demonstrated, even though there is a unilateral hemispheric tumor. We are inclined to agree with Davidoff and Epstein (1950) that when the aqueduct and fourth ventricle are displaced to either side, it indicates that the cerebellar tumor is located on the opposite side; when the aqueduct is displaced only forward, no conclusion can be reached as to the side of the cerebellum which the tumor occupies. Sometimes the aqueduct is difficult to visualize in frontal projection because it is superimposed on the third ventricle. Usually, however, the uppermost portion of the aqueduct is clearly visible as a dark spot superimposed on the third ventricle (fig. 217). Normally, this spot falls almost exactly in the middle of the transverse diameter of the third ventricle. Laterally placed tumors may shift even the upper portion to one side (fig. 299). Care should be taken not to confuse the dark spot produced by the aqueduct with the foramen of Monro, which can be superimposed on the third ven-

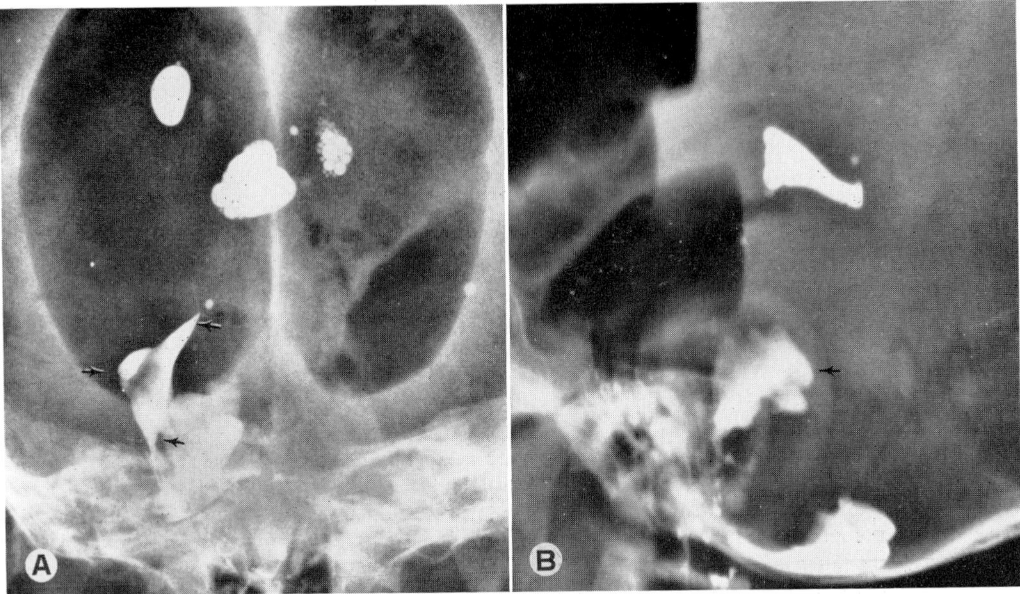

FIG. 298.—CEREBELLAR TUMOR

A large tumor of the left cerebellar hemisphere has produced gross displacement of the fourth ventricle toward the right (*arrows*) in the combined air-Pantopaque ventriculogram, as seen in frontal view (A). In the lateral view (B), the opaque material in the dilated and flattened fourth ventricle (*arrow*) shows this cavity to be displaced forward and elevated. In spite of the marked degree of displacement and deformity, the heavy opaque material passed out of the fourth ventricle promptly under fluoroscopic observation. In another case (C), with flattening of the fourth ventricle on the left side and displacement toward the right, the contrast material also entered the subarachnoid space readily from the ventricular system and is shown in the upper cervical subarachnoid space. Apparently the effect of gravity on the heavy contrast material causes it to pass through narrow channels which produce obstruction to gas (see text).

tricle in prone posteroanterior views if there is enough air to reach the level of this foramen.

In the ventriculogram, the degree of dilatation of the lateral and third ventricles varies with the degree of obstruction which is present, and its duration. Some degree of patency of the ventricular system often is present with hemispheric lesions, particularly hemangioblastoma; the tendency is to deform and displace rather than to block. A long standing cerebellar astrocytoma may result in a high degree of lateral and third ventricular dilatation, while in the case of cerebellar hemangioblastoma the ventricular dilatation is only slight in the majority of instances.

In lateral projection, the lower aqueduct and fourth ventricle usually are displaced forward, with reduction of the distance from the iter and fourth ventricular floor to the basisphenoid below the minimum limit (fig. 300). In some instances, as noted above, particularly those in which there is marked lateral displacement of the iter and fourth ventricle, forward displacement may be only minimum; the impression may be gained that there is only some straightening of these shadows. The measurement from the fourth ventricular floor to the dorsum sellae may remain within normal limits. The height of the fourth ventricle, however, is almost always reduced (fig. 213). Occasionally, hemispheric lesions may take on, in lateral view, some of the other features of cerebellar vermis tumors that have been described, such as bulging of the tumor into the superior or inferior aspect of the fourth ventricle pos-

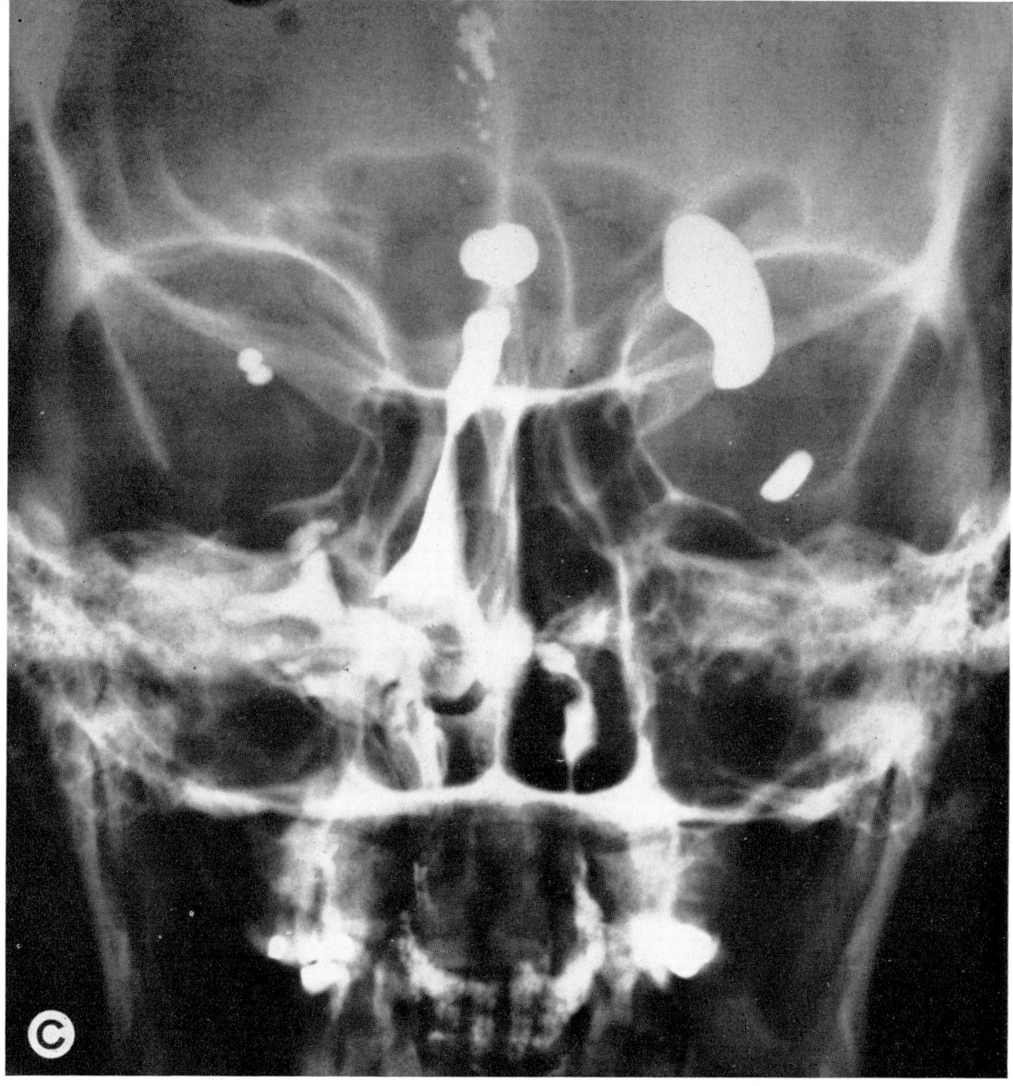

Fig. 298C

teriorly. Hemispheric tumors may produce upward herniation of posterior fossa structures through the tentorial incisura. The tentorium also may bulge upward on the side of the tumor, thus elevating the atrium and occipital horn of the lateral ventricle.

Gas in the subarachnoid space ordinarily is not seen in the case of a cerebellar tumor because ventriculography is used most commonly and some degree of obstruction is usually present. With only partially obstructing hemangioblastomas, some gas may enter the subarachnoid space and outline the basal cisterns. In most instances, pneumoencephalography in conjunction with ventriculography would be required to visualize the subarachnoid space well. While this is safer following ventricular puncture, it is indicated only infrequently. When there is difficulty in distinguishing an intraneural from an extra-axial tumor, a combined study may be necessary.

If air is injected by the lumbar route in a patient with a neoplasm of either the

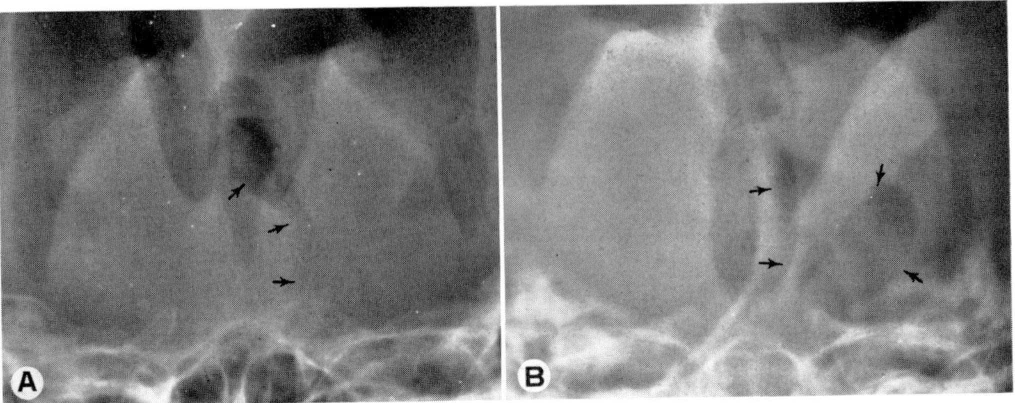

FIG. 299.—LATERAL POSTERIOR FOSSA TUMOR

The frontal ventriculogram (A), made with the patient prone, frequently shows sufficient gas in the posterior ventricular structures for lateralization, if a tumor is situated in one cerebellar hemisphere. High tumors, through upward transtentorial herniation, may produce flattening of the ipsilateral aspect of the posterior part of the third ventricle (*upper arrow*). The aqueduct of Sylvius may be displaced well away from the midline and may taper to a point laterally when completely obstructed (*lower arrows*).

In another case (B), a tumor lower in the cerebellum situated on one side produced marked flattening of the lateral aspect of the fourth ventricle on the side ipsilateral to the tumor (*medial arrows*). The entire fourth ventricle is displaced slightly to the contralateral side and it is markedly dilated (*lateral arrows*). The third ventricle, however, is not deformed posteriorly by upward herniation, although the aqueduct deviates from the midline away from the tumor.

vermis or a hemisphere, the cisterna magna usually is narrowed and may be obliterated (fig. 197). Frank herniation of the cerebellar tonsils into the upper cervical area may be evident (fig. 295). More often there is only partial herniation, and in some instances only prominence or low position of the tonsils. The tonsils may be asymmetrical normally, but enlargement of one cerebellar tonsil, with displacement of the vallecula, is indicative of an intracerebellar tumor. The cisterna pontis, when visualized, is narrowed or nearly obliterated. A reduction in width below the normal minimum of 0.5 cm. is found in almost all patients with cerebellar tumor; in the great majority of patients the pontine cistern is very narrow. Subarachnoid gas over the hemispheres is observed infrequently in the presence of a cerebellar tumor. Sometimes frank upward transtentorial herniation is present affecting the quadrigeminal cistern and the retrocallosal air shadow.

With the recent more extensive use of vertebral angiography, *cerebellar angiomas* are being diagnosed radiologically with increasing frequency. (The role of vertebral opacification studies in the diagnosis of posterior fossa tumors is discussed in the section on angiography.) Angiomas may cause compression of the fourth ventricle because of the bulk of their vascular mass. At other times hemorrhage occurs into the cerebellar substance, into the subarachnoid space, or both.

In pneumograms, a *cerebellar hematoma* most often resembles a tumor of one cerebellar hemisphere. Occasionally, a hematoma may extend into the contralateral hemisphere; in such cases the "butterfly" or "saddle" hematoma exerts pressure on the ventricular system from two posterolateral aspects and thus mimics a straight posterior lesion. Obstructive hydrocephalus may develop with surprising rapidity after a cerebellar hemorrhage.

Many cerebellar hematomas are not caused by the bleeding of angiomas but develop spontaneously. Intracerebellar and posterior fossa subdural hematomas also occur owing to trauma. A cerebellar hematoma may rupture into the fourth ventricle,

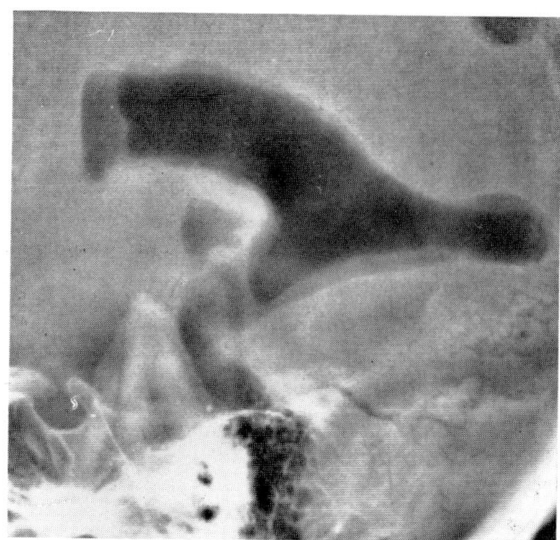

FIG. 300.—HEMANGIOBLASTOMA OF THE CEREBELLUM

A lateral ventriculogram reveals the aqueduct to be displaced far forward of its usual position, and the fourth ventricle to be reduced in height and also to be displaced forward, partially obscured by the mastoid. In spite of the marked displacement, there is not complete occlusion, which often occurs with soft cystic tumors, and only mild ventricular dilatation is shown.

although such extension is seen more often secondary to medullopontine hemorrhage. Metastatic tumors may simulate either hematomas, in their acute development, or more slowly growing primary cerebellar neoplasms.

Brain Stem Tumors

Tumors of the brain stem, in the usual sense, comprise those which arise in the medulla oblongata, in the pons varolii, in the midbrain, and in the cerebral peduncles. Anatomically, the brain stem includes also the supratentorial portions, principally the thalami and basal ganglia. The latter have been included in the section dealing with hemispheric tumors, since it is in this context that they must be considered in differential diagnosis.

Medullopontine gliomas. Brain stem tumors are infrequent but not rare lesions; in the experience of the authors, they occur more frequently than the 1 per cent incidence given by Davidoff and Epstein (1950). The great majority of the tumors are found in children and young adults. Pathologically, a large number of tumors originating in the brain stem are polar spongioblastomas (piloid astrocytomas). Tumors of this type respond favorably, even though temporarily, to radiation therapy; because of the location of the lesion in an inoperable vital structure, and because surgical relief of increased intracranial pressure usually is not necessary, the majority of patients are treated with radiation alone. For this reason definitive radiologic diagnosis is very important. Recurrent brain stem tumors are more resistant to treatment and at autopsy it is found frequently that the principal cell type is glioblastoma multiforme, more malignant metaplasia presumably having taken place with tumor recurrence.

(Revised 1963)

Typically, the tumors arise unilaterally in the medullopontine portion of the brain stem and give rise to ipsilateral cranial nerve palsies and contralateral hemiparesis. It is not infrequent, however, for several cranial nerve nuclei, situated close together, to be involved on both sides of the midline at the time the patient first is seen. Extensive cranial nerve involvement may occur from relatively small tumors because of the clustering of cranial nerve nuclei in a relatively small area. Ordinarily, impaired neural function causes the patient to seek attention when the tumor is still small and also before increased intracranial pressure has developed. It is rather unusual to have patients with brain stem tumors exhibit radiologic evidence of increased intracranial pressure at the time of their first examination.

Since the clinical manifestations are often so characteristic, and because intracranial hypertension usually is absent or mild, the majority of patients are examined by pneumoencephalography. This is advantageous, since it is important to differentiate intraneural brain stem tumors from extra-axial tumors and aneurysms; visualization of the subarachnoid space is essential for identification of the latter lesions. Ventriculography performed alone often leaves the radiologist with only a diagnosis of a tumor anterior to the fourth ventricle. Ventriculography is a

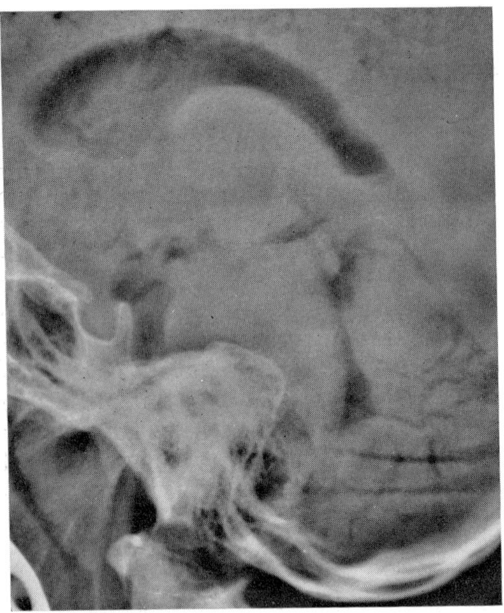

Fig. 301.—Brain Stem Glioma

The lateral pneumoencephalogram reveals enlargement of the shadow of the brain stem, owing to a nonobstructing intraneural tumor in a child. The pontine portion of the brain stem exhibits the greatest enlargement, which is predominantly dorsal in this case. The height of the fourth ventricle is markedly reduced by encroachment from the ventral side due to backward bowing of the expanded brain stem. The ventral outline of the pons, however, is well preserved, and the cisterna pontis does not appear narrowed.

useful adjunct following pneumoencephalography, however, if visualization of the ventricular system is not as complete as required; the combined procedure occasionally should be carried out.

At pneumography, the first films made during the filling phase give an isolated and often the best visualization of the fourth ventricle and the basal cisterns of the posterior fossa. In lateral projection, the fourth ventricle and aqueduct are displaced backward, with an increase in the distance from the floor of the fourth ventricle to the basisphenoid. The average measurement of 3.6 cm. is almost always exceeded, except as noted below, and the maximum normal distance of 4 cm. is exceeded very often. The height (floor to fastigium) of the fourth ventricle is correspondingly reduced. The height is diminished by backward displacement of the ventricular floor with narrowing of the lumen from the ventral aspect. The configuration of the roof of the fourth ventricle frequently is preserved, including a sharply outlined apex. As a result of the changes of displacement and ventral encroachment, the fourth ventricle and aqueduct appear bowed backward; a striking concavity toward the basiphenoid, rather than the normal straight line of the ventricular floor, is produced. Even when the ventricle is appreciably reduced in size in the sagittal plane, with the result that it may appear as a curvilinear shadow, the ventricular pathway usually will remain patent. Obstruction, when it does occur, may be either at the foramina of the fourth ventricle, owing to distortion by stretching, or it may result from extension of the tumor cephalad into the midbrain with occlusion of the iter.

Some tumors of the pontine region will not produce backward displacement of the fourth ventricle beyond the normal measurement. They can be diagnosed, however, because of the *increase in the sharpness* of the air shadow outlining the floor of the fourth ventricle and because of the slight diminution of the height of the fourth ventricle. The increase in the sharpness is secondary to stretching of the floor produced by the tumor, which causes the normal elevations present in this region to disappear (fig. 301).

When the center of the tumor is situated in the pons, the floor of the fourth ventricle will exhibit maximal displacement; if the tumor center is higher, involving the midbrain, the aqueduct will show the greatest displacement. If the tumor center is in the medulla, the region of the foramen of Magendie will be affected to the maximum (fig. 302). Extension into the upper cervical cord is not unusual, and this will be manifested in the pneumogram as enlargement of the spinal cord shadow.

The patency of the fourth ventricle, although it is markedly deformed and reduced in height as seen in lateral view, is better understood when the frontal view is

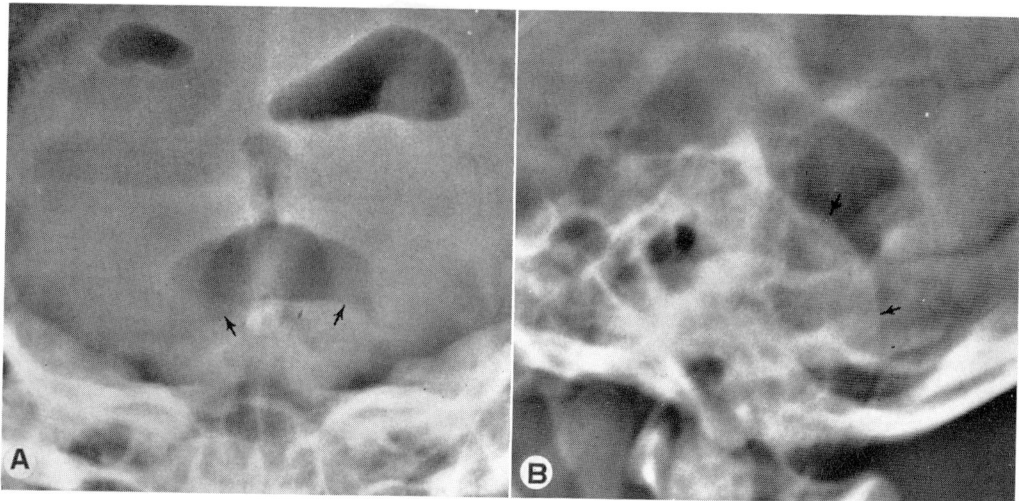

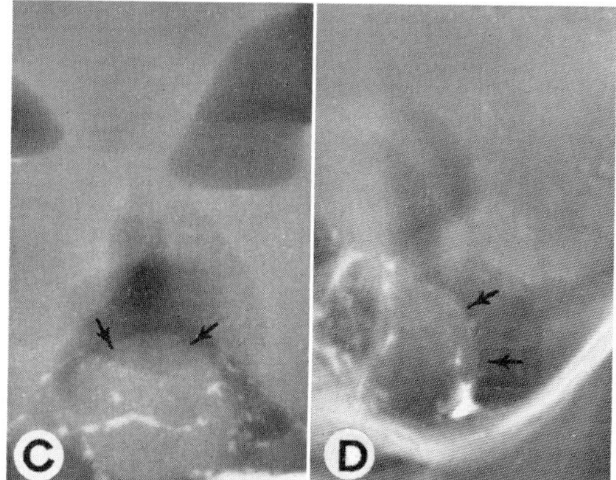

FIG. 302.—TUMORS OF THE MEDULLA OBLONGATA

The lateral pneumogram (B) reveals partial obstruction of the fourth ventricular outlet resulting from a mass encroaching upon the lumen of the fourth ventricle from the ventral side in its caudal half (*upper arrow*). Gas in the vallecula outlines the posterior tumor surface inferiorly (*lower arrow*). The frontal pneumogram (A) reveals enlargement of the fourth ventricle laterally, with the superior margin of the intramedullary tumor well outlined by gas (*arrows*).

A smoothly rounded mass (lipoma) extends backward from the shadow of the caudal portion of the medulla oblongata into the cisterna magna (D). The mass (*arrows*) elevates and partially obstructs the outlet of the fourth ventricle, and a partial obstruction also is present at the foramen magnum. The frontal film (C) reveals the rounded shadow of the tumor (*arrows*) as outlined by cisternal gas. Residual Pantopaque is from earlier myelogram for study of the foramen magnum region.

examined. In the average case *the fourth ventricle is widened in the coronal plane* by the flattening from the ventral aspect. The tumors characteristically remain confined within the substance of the brain stem and do not invade and occlude the fourth ventricle proper. Therefore, what is seen, in essence, is an extrinsic pressure effect upon the ventricle along the ventral side.

Since most of the brain stem tumors occur at the pontine level, it becomes necessary to differentiate intraneural tumors of the brain stem from the extraneural masses, particularly the extra-axial tumors which can simulate pontine glioma clinically. The lesions which must be considered in differential diagnosis are the midline anterior extra-axial tumors, and the cerebellopontine angle tumors arising anterolaterally. When there is any difficulty in distinguishing an intra-axial from an extra-axial mass, either clinically or radiologically, fractional selective filling and multiple filming techniques described earlier are very useful.

Good visualization of the posterior fossa cisterns is the greatest single aid in differentiating intramedullary from extra-axial masses. Medullopontine tumors expand the brain stem in all directions, ventrally as well as dorsally. Thus, the cisterna pontis will be narrowed below the minimum meas-

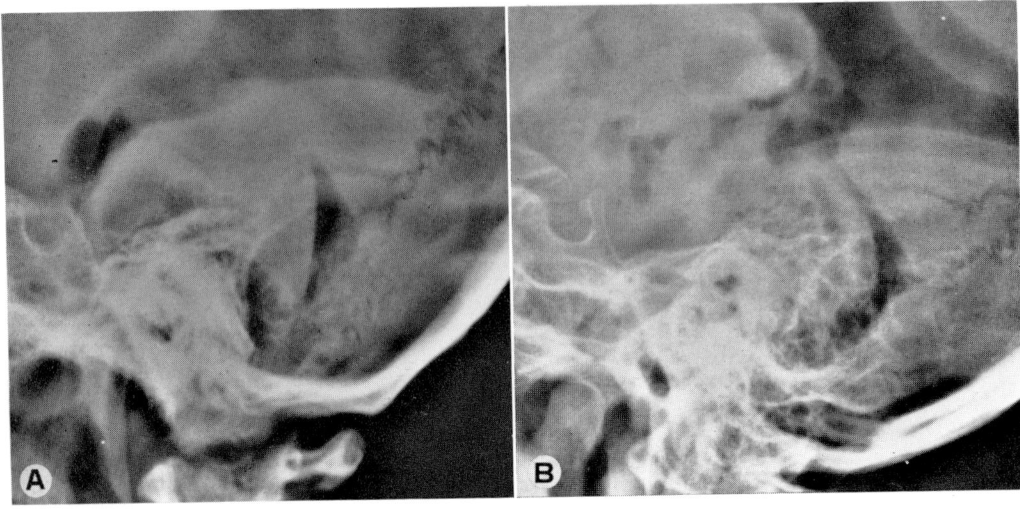

FIG. 303.—BRAIN STEM GLIOMA

Lateral ventriculograms of two patients with intraneural tumors that produced partial obstruction are shown. In one instance (A), both the pons and medulla oblongata are markedly enlarged, and the fourth ventricle is displaced far backward and downward from its normal position. The fourth ventricle is greatly reduced in height, owing to encroachment from the ventral aspect, and the dorsal contours being fairly well preserved. The cisterna pontis is markedly narrowed. In another case (B), the fourth ventricle is displaced backward and its floor bowed backward into the ventricular lumen, reducing the ventricular height. The aqueduct also is displaced posteriorly. Gas which escaped into the subarachnoid space reveals narrowing of the cisterna interpeduncularis, owing to enlargement of the midbrain between this cistern and the aqueduct, and obliteration of the cisterna pontis, owing to marked transverse enlargement of the brain stem at the pontine level.

urement of 5 mm. Frequently, the cisterna pontis is markedly compromised, measuring only 1 to 2 mm. from the ventral aspect of the pons to the bony structure of the basisphenoid. In addition, the ventral curve of the pons may be altered, owing to elongation and flattening. The effect on the cisterna pontis is not unlike that occurring with cerebellar tumors. Extra-axial tumors, on the other hand, and particularly those which are in the midline anteriorly, produce a widening of the cisterna pontis; the brain stem is pushed backward by the tumor, but the tumor may fill this cistern completely so that no air is visible anterior to the pons. Gas flowing anteriorly into the enlarged ventral cisterns may, in other cases, partially surround an extra-axial tumor and demonstrate it to be a mass apart from the brain stem (figs. 308 and 316).

The effect on the fourth ventricle by pontine and midline anterior extra-axial tumors is qualitatively the same but quantitatively different. Intra-axial tumors cause a much greater posterior displacement of the fourth ventricle and more flattening than is usually seen with extra-axial lesions. There is not the degree of smooth curvature of the fourth ventricle and aqueduct with extra-axial tumors as is seen with pontine gliomas. The latter effect might be expected since the medullopontine gliomas are closer to the ventricular lumen (figs. 303 and 304).

It is characteristic of intrinsic tumors of the pons to produce a straight backward displacement of the fourth ventricle. Such displacement occurs, even though pontine tumors frequently grow predominantly on one side of the brain stem. Since the tumor growth is confined within the brain stem, and the growth tends to occur axially, a spindle-like enlargement of the pons results. We have not observed frequently cases in which there is a significant shift of the fourth

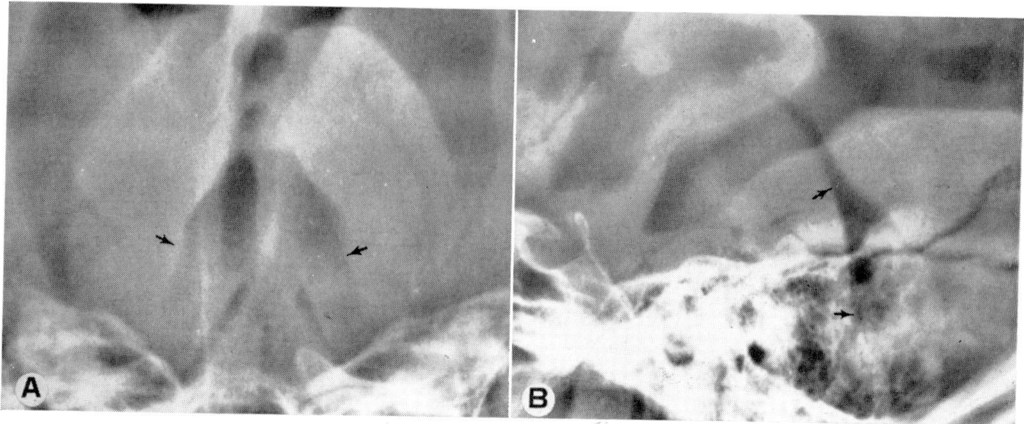

Fig. 304.—Brain Stem Glioma

The frontal film (A) shows marked widening of the fourth ventricular shadow (*arrows*) in a symmetrical manner. The lateral film (B) shows that the widening of the frontal view is the result of flattening, owing to ventral encroachment upon the air shadow of the fourth ventricle by the dorsally expanded pons and medulla (*arrows*). Cephalic extension of the medullopontine growth has produced also posterior displacement of the upper aqueduct which is narrow at its outlet from the third ventricle. The third ventricular floor is elevated, and the vertical height of the third ventricle reduced.

ventricle from its midline position in frontal view; some cases of this type have been encountered and a larger number have been reported. It is typical, also, for brain stem gliomas to widen the fourth ventricle, but for its angles and general geometric configuration to be preserved in the frontal projection. The same findings apply to extra-axial tumors which are midline anterior in relation to the brain stem; direct posterior displacement of the fourth ventricle is of no assistance in differentiating the two groups. However, extra-axial tumors which arise anterolaterally do change the appearance of the fourth ventricle and often displace the fourth ventricle and aqueduct of Sylvius from the midline. After some encroachment upon the brain stem and slight displacement, the tumors of the cerebellopontine angle rotate the brain stem, causing a striking alteration in depiction of the fourth ventricle in frontal projection (fig. 311). The absence of a rotary effect in the frontal and lateral views may be helpful in the diagnosis of a medullopontine intra-axial tumor. The deformity of specific cisterns, such as the cerebellopontine cistern and partial delineation of the tumor itself by cisternal gas aid in the identification of anterolateral extra-axial tumors, as described below.

(Revised 1963)

Distant effects of brain stem tumors are seen in the size of the lateral ventricles and in the appearance of the third ventricle. Medullopontine tumors ordinarily produce only slight dilatation of the lateral ventricles. Acoustic neurinomas and various other extra-axial tumors often result in moderate, and sometimes marked, ventricular dilatation by the time pneumography is carried out.

When pneumography does not provide a clear differentiation between medullopontine and extra-axial tumors, vertebral angiography often is helpful in separating the two. A significant percentage of extra-axial tumors are aneurysms, and will be demonstrated directly by arterial injection of contrast material. Typically, midline anterior prepontine tumors, such as meningiomas, chordomas, and epidermoid tumors, displace the basilar artery backward. Intramedullary tumors of the brain stem displace and compress the basilar artery forward against the clivus, as do the majority of cerebellar tumors. Some extra-axial tumors, such as the meningiomas and epidermoid tumors, may grow behind the basilar artery

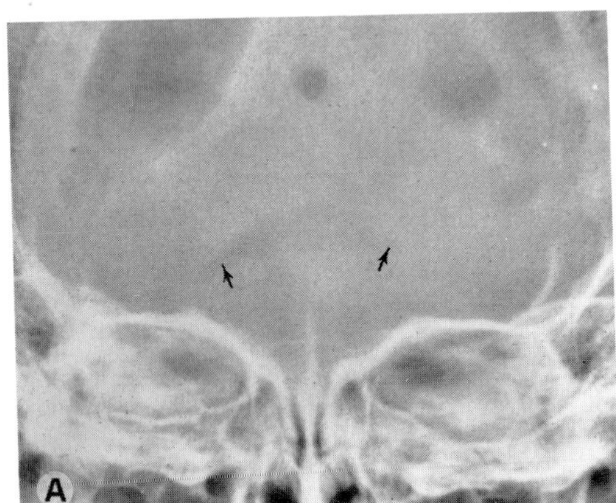

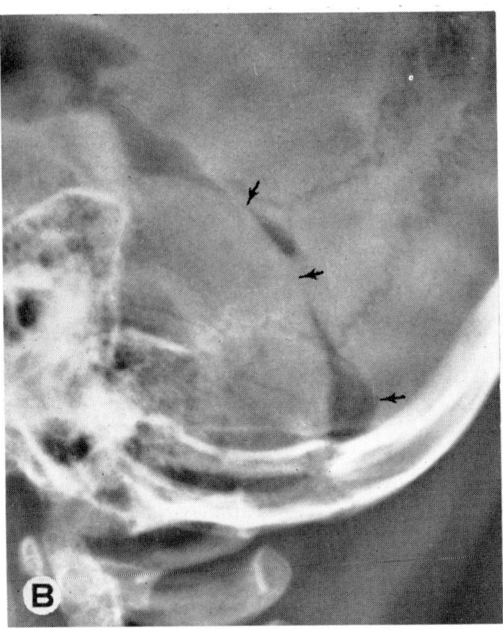

FIG. 305.—SYRINGOBULBIA

Extreme enlargement of the medullopontine portion of the brain stem is present. The frontal film (A) exhibits a narrow transverse gas shadow outlining the superior margin of the symmetrically enlarged brain stem (*arrows*). The lateral view (B) reveals dilatation of the third ventricle and iter, indicating partial obstruction. The fourth ventricle is stretched and displaced backward to a marked degree of posterior expansion of the brain stem (*arrows*). The apex of the fourth ventricle is displaced far backward and downward (*lowest arrow*). The smooth surface of the mass indicates the intramedullary location of the tumor. A tumor of such large size in an area containing vital centers favors a benign, noninvasive process.

and in front of the pons, although fortunately rarely; in these instances, angiography does not provide adequate differentiation. Angiography also will serve to demonstrate angiomas of the brain stem. Intra-axial hematomas secondary to such lesions, or occurring as primary hemorrhages, may simulate a tumor radiologically. The rapid development of acute obstructive hydrocephalus may be observed, with or without extension of a hematoma into the fourth ventricle. At other times, the axial dissection of a hematoma beside the fourth ventricle, aqueduct, and third ventricle can mimic a brain stem glioma in every way. Metastatic tumors also cause radiologic findings simulating primary masses.

Syringobulbia. Syringobulbia usually results from an extension of the lesions of syringomyelia cephalically into the medulla oblongata. Rarely, syringobulbia may be isolated. The condition is considered to be congenital in origin; because of the nature of the cellular lining of the cystic cavities, it has been postulated that the malformation results from intraneural displacement of pial tissue during embryonic development of the nervous system. The cysts of syringobulbia may be numerous and very large, resulting in mammoth enlargement of the medulla oblongata and pons varolii.

The basic pneumographic disturbance of syringobulbia is the same as in the case of medullopontine glioma. The process is confined within the brain stem anterior to the fourth ventricle, and causes backward displacement and compression of the ventricle. When brain stem enlargement is gross, a benign process is suggested by the large size of the intraneural mass. In one instance,

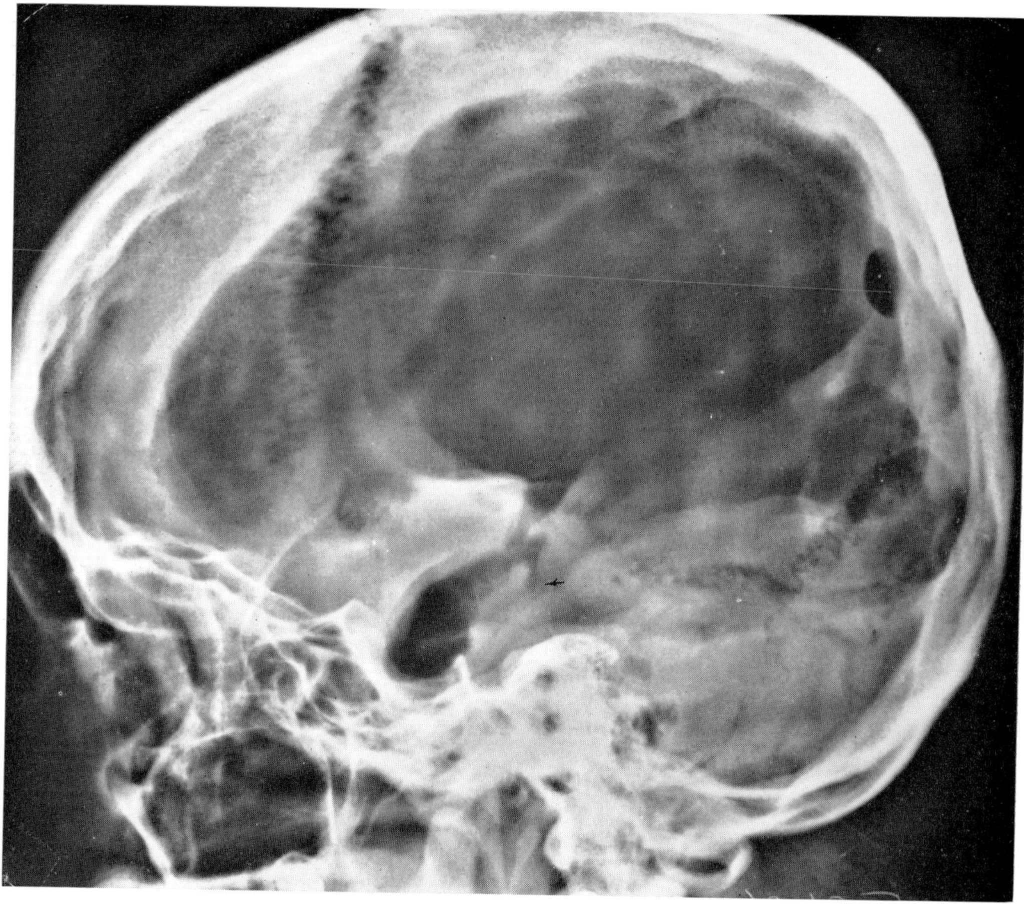

FIG. 306.—MIDBRAIN ASTROCYTOMA

A glioma growing in the region of the quadrigeminal plate has produced obstruction and sharp forward displacement of the aqueduct of Sylvius (*arrow*). The tumor was a slowly growing fibrillary astrocytoma, resulting in long standing obstruction of the iter and extreme ventricular dilatation reminiscent of the findings with benign aqueduct occlusion (see Fig. 240); with benign aqueduct stenosis, there is no dislocation of the visualized portion of the cerebral aqueduct.

the compressed fourth ventricle was displaced so far posteriorly in lateral view that it was mistaken initially for gas in the cisterna magna (fig. 305). It is doubtful that a new growth could attain the great size often seen with syringobulbia without destruction of vital centers; with syrinx, tracts and nuclei may be compressed, but are not extensively destroyed by the soft cysts.

Aside from the quantitative differences, the pneumographic changes of syringobulbia resemble those of intra-axial glioma. In the frontal projections, the fourth ventricle is almost always found to remain in the midline. The general configuration is preserved, but there is marked widening as a result of flattening from the ventral side.

Midbrain gliomas. Tumors may *originate in the midbrain,* may extend into it from below, having arisen in the pons, or may spread downward from above, after originating in the thalamus. When midbrain tumors extend into the cerebral peduncles, deformity of the floor of the posterior portion of the third ventricle usually is present. When the tumor is confined to the midbrain, the pneumographic findings often are indistinguishable from benign aqueduct stenosis. Tumors originating in the midbrain are, for the most part, astrocytomas; angiomas are found not infrequently. Because of the slow growth and their strategic position for blockage of the aqueduct of Sylvius, a high degree of obstruction may be present for a prolonged period of time.

Since increased intracranial pressure often is a prominent clinical finding, the patients ordinarily are examined by ventriculography. Marked symmetrical dilatation of the lateral ventricles and corresponding enlargement of the third ventricle usually are present (fig. 306). If the tumor is limited to the midbrain, the third ventricle is markedly dilated but not otherwise deformed; the prone lateral view will show obstruction at the third ventricular outlet, but there is no characteristic configuration.

Tumors *originating in the quadrigeminal area* produce a similar picture of obstruction, but with these lesions there is more often deformity of the posterior portion of the third ventricle simulating pinealoma. If the subarachnoid space should be outlined by the lumbar injection of air, it is found that small tumors of the collicular region obliterate or deform the quadrigeminal cistern. Tumors ventral to the aqueduct frequently extend into the cerebral peduncles, and result in elevation of the posterior third ventricular floor and reduction in height of the third ventricle. In these instances, the differentiation to be made is often from extra-axial tumors of the posterior fossa in the incisural region, as described below; the ventriculographic appearance often is strikingly similar. While clinical and plain film radiologic findings, especially in the way of calcification and bony erosion, should be of help in recognizing the extra-axial tumors, as opposed to the tumors involving the peduncles, vertebral angiography may be valuable in some instances. The opacification of an aneurysm or deformity of the basilar artery and its branches may serve to differentiate the extraneural masses from peduncular tumors.

The use of Pantopaque injected into a lateral ventricle has been mentioned elsewhere as an occasionally helpful procedure. When other attempts at localization of an obstruction and visualization of narrow cerebrospinal fluid pathways fail, the use of a few cubic centimeters of Pantopaque, with the flow directed under fluoroscopic guidance, often facilitates diagnosis. It has been found that rapid filming, even the use of cinefluorography, is valuable in problem cases, since Pantopaque may pass through channels that are impervious to air. The use of Pantopaque, after lumbar injection, to visualize various cisterns and posterior ventricular areas has been advocated by some—Malis (1958) and others—but the authors have found this technique of limited usefulness; ordinarily, it is not superior to air properly directed (figs. 192 and 219).

EXTRA-AXIAL POSTERIOR FOSSA TUMORS

Extra-axial tumors of the posterior fossa may be divided into two groups, those which arise below the incisura of the tentorium, and those which arise at the tentorial notch itself. The majority of the tumors that arise in these areas may be localized by deformities that they produce in the cisterns, the fourth ventricle, and the aqueduct. Recognition of defective filling of various anatomic fluid spaces by gas also is important in diagnosis; frequently dilatation of cisternal and ventricular areas will give a clue to the presence of the lesion.

In the vast majority of instances, carefully performed selective pneumoencephalography, carried out under radiographic control, is the procedure of choice for diagnosis. Ventriculography usually is unsatisfactory for complete localization, since the cisternal visualization necessary for diagnosis usually is not accomplished by ventricular air injection. Angiography may be a valuable adjunct to diagnosis in some instances; it is invaluable if a lesion of vascular origin is present. Ordinarily, however, angiography does not allow the precise

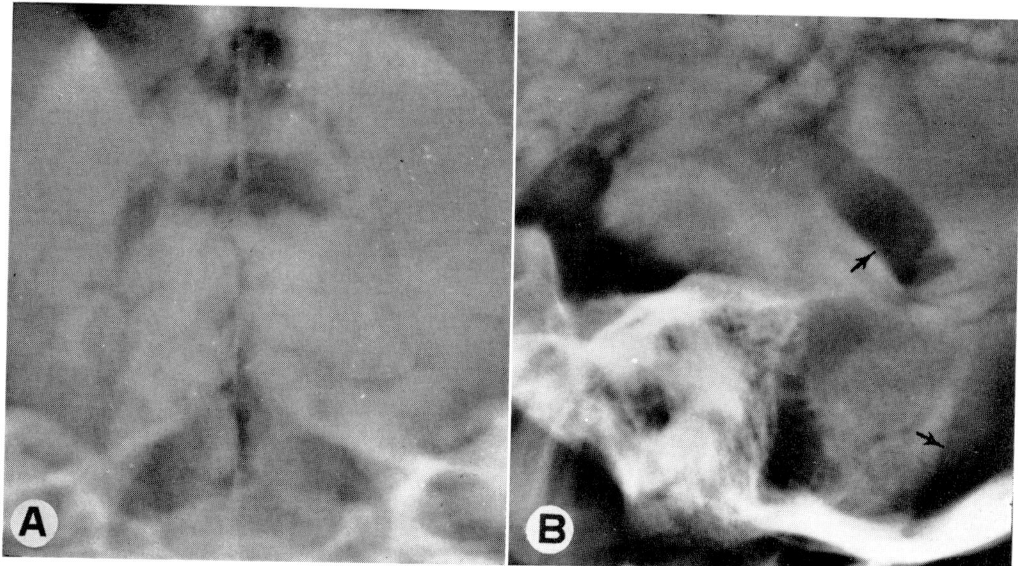

FIG. 307.—PREMEDULLARY EPIDERMOIDOMA

An epidermoid tumor, growing ventral to the medulla oblongata, has displaced the brain stem far backward. The lateral film (B) shows an increase in the width of the cisterna pontis and of the medullary cistern containing the tumor, obscured by overlying mastoid structure. The fourth ventricle is displaced backward and upward with encroachment chiefly upon its caudal portion from the ventral aspect (*upper arrow*). The cisterna magna is also narrowed anteriorly by backward bowing of the medulla (*lower arrow*). In the frontal film (A), the fourth ventricle is widened and flattened; the gas seen in the posteroanterior half axial view is in the preserved dorsal portion of the fourth ventricular lumen, which is seen on end.

preoperative localization desired in cases of subtentorial tumors, but only a pre- or postbasilar artery designation. Angiography may be very valuable in diagnosis of those tumors arising at or near the tentorial incisura.

Infratentorial Tumors

All subtentorial extra-axial tumors and those arising at the tentorial incisura may be divided into midline anterior, anterolateral, straight lateral, posterolateral, and straight posterior, in their relation to the brain stem. The most common lesions are those in anterolateral location, which include the entire cerebellopontine angle group, particularly the neurinomas arising from the sheath of the eighth cranial nerve and the meningiomas. Dermoid, vascular, and other unusual tumors also may be found in the cerebellopontine angles on occasions.

Midline anterior masses. The anterior midline tumors of the lower portion of the cerebellar chamber, or prepontine tumors, often are meningiomas, epidermoid tumors, or aneurysms arising from the basilar artery; occasionally, a large aneurysm arises from a vertebral artery (figs. 307 and 308). This also is a common place for chordomas to occur; frequently chordomas may be diagnosed by plain film changes in the region of the clivus (fig. 309).

Prepontine tumors usually can be differentiated readily from masses in the pons (and cerebellopontine angles), if gas flows anteriorly into the cisterns and partially surrounds the tumor. Filling may be facilitated when widening of the cisterna pontis occurs, because the brain stem is pushed backward by the tumor; demonstrable enlargement of the cisterna pontis alone also favors the diagnosis of a prepontine lesion. Ventricular filling usually occurs; in the average case, there is no dilatation owing to obstruction. The fourth ventricle, and often

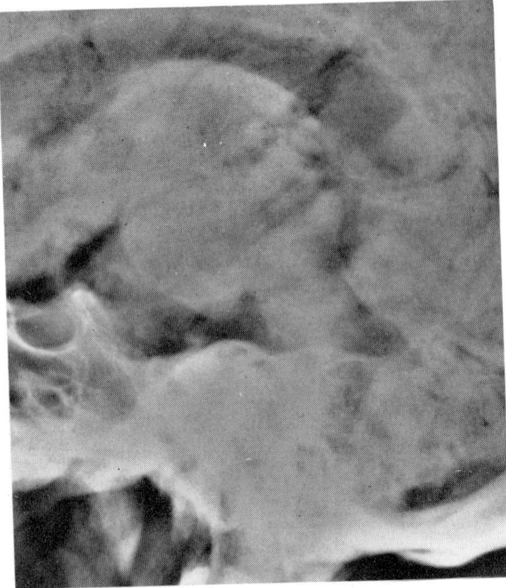

FIG. 308.—BASILAR ARTERY ANEURYSM

The lateral pneumogram reveals the brain stem to be markedly displaced backward and the fourth ventricle displaced and narrowed by encroachment from the ventral side. The ventral aspect of the pontine shadow is displaced upward and backward. Between the pons and the dorsum sellae and clivus, a soft tissue shadow is present in the widened prepontine cistern, which is a part of the aneurysmal mass. The medullary cistern is grossly widened, owing to elevation and backward displacement of the brain stem.

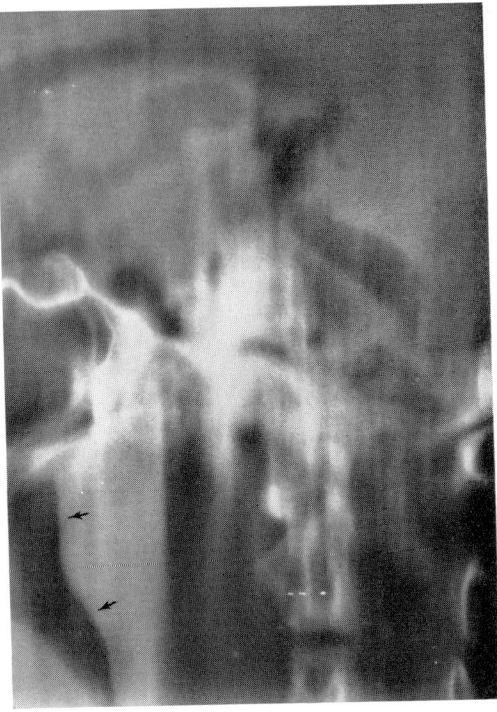

FIG. 309.—CHORDOMA

The basiocciput exhibits irregular destruction and is flattened. A large soft tissue mass is present in the nasopharynx (*arrows*) from which a biopsy was made. The pons and medulla are displaced backward by intracranial extension of the tumor. Similar displacement of the fourth ventricular floor is present, and the height of the fourth ventricle is reduced.

the distal aqueduct, are displaced posteriorly. There is usually not the marked flattening of the fourth ventricle from the anterior aspect that is characteristic of intramedullary gliomas, and the increase in width due to stretching, usually seen in the frontal projection, is not observed. The tumor may imbed itself in the pontine tissue, which acts as a cushion between the mass and the fourth ventricle; an unusual shape of the anterior aspect of the pons may be demonstrated (figs. 307 and 308).

Vertebral angiography is preferred by some to differentiate between prepontine and pontine tumors. Typically, *in the presence of a prepontine tumor, the basilar artery and some of its branches are displaced backward*; with a pontine glioma, the basilar artery is displaced forward. However, any tumor arising posterior to the basilar artery will displace it forward, and in some rare instances extra-axial tumors may grow behind the basilar artery and in front of the pons.

Cerebellopontine angle masses. Tumors that arise *anterolaterally* are very common and of great importance in pneumographic diagnosis because they usually are benign and amenable to surgical treatment. For practical purposes, these lesions may be thought of as comprising largely tumors of the eighth cranial nerve and meningiomas arising in the angle, although tumors of other types occasionally are found (fig. 310). It is now generally held that air studies can be performed by the

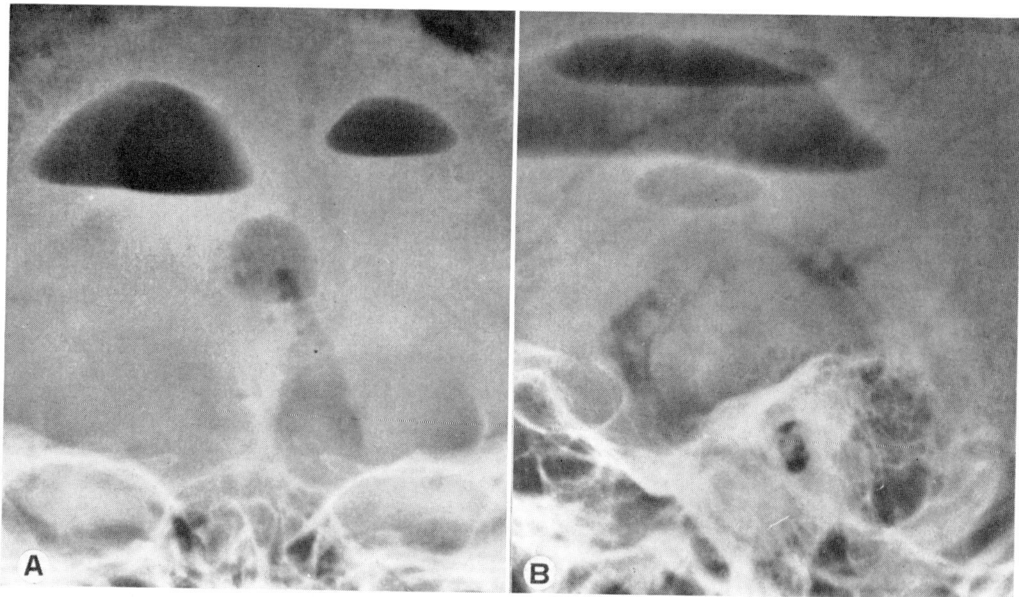

Fig. 310.—Posterior Fossa Meningioma

An extraneural tumor arising anterior and lateral to the brain stem has displaced the aqueduct and fourth ventricle well to the left of the midline (A). In the lateral film (B), the dilated aqueduct is posterior to its usual position, but the fourth ventricle is not well seen because of overlying mastoid shadows. The cisterna pontis is partially obscured, and the posterior margin of the clivus is not well demarcated, but the cistern is not widened.

lumbar route with safety in the presence of cerebellopontine angle tumors, and that pneumoencephalography is the most satisfactory method of establishing the diagnosis. Ventriculography is very rarely satisfactory, and angiography is needed infrequently.

A very common finding at pneumography in cases of tumors situated in the cerebellopontine angle is posterior and lateral displacement of the fourth ventricle and aqueduct of Sylvius. Individual tumors may grow in different directions; if the tumor becomes large and grows more ventrally than elsewhere, there is greater posterior displacement of the fourth ventricle and the lower portion of the aqueduct than dislocation in other directions. On the other hand, if the tumor grows more laterally then contralateral displacement of the fourth ventricle, with little and sometimes no posterior displacement of this structure and the aqueduct, is observed. Visualization of the fourth ventricle is an essential part of the pneumographic diagnosis of cerebellopontine angle tumors and every effort must be made to make sure that the pneumoencephalogram is adequate to demonstrate this structure; visualization must be accomplished in the frontal as well as in the lateral projection. Repeated injections of small quantities of air may be required in order to see the fourth ventricle in frontal views. In almost all instances of cerebellopontine angle tumors, there is more displacement of the fourth ventricle than of the aqueduct. This is in contrast to the incisural group of extra-axial posterior fossa tumors which will be described subsequently.

Not only displacement but a decrease in the width of the fourth ventricle usually is found in frontal films. The reduction in width of the ventricle may be very striking, even when displacement of the fourth ventricle is minimum. The deformity of the ventricle, usually seen in straight frontal views may be misleading unless it is realized that the ventricle is not markedly compressed without being displaced, but that

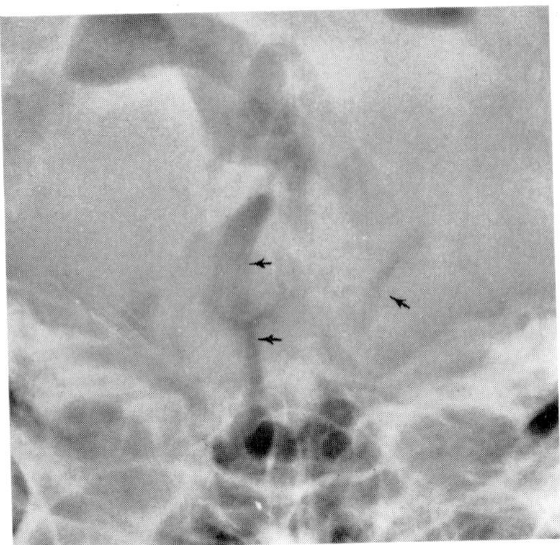

Fig. 311.—Acoustic Neurinoma

The fourth ventricle is displaced away from the midline and rotated, with the result that in the posteroanterior half axial view, its configuration resembles a banana (*upper medial arrow*). The vallecula also is displaced from the midline (*lower medial arrow*). The cerebellopontine recess is elevated and displaced medially (*lateral arrow*) owing to a mass at the internal auditory meatus, while on the opposite side, the gas shadow of the recess remains normally related to the petrous pyramid.

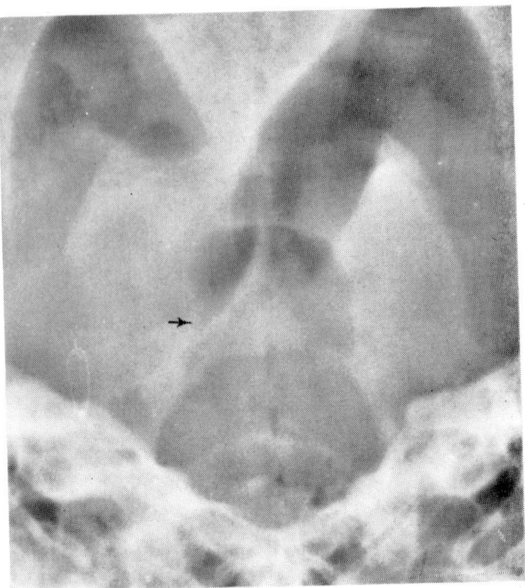

Fig. 312.—Acoustic Neurinoma

The fourth ventricle is obstructed, and the ventricular system is moderately dilated. The fourth ventricle is quite large with well rounded borders, except on one side where a shallow indentation is shown (*arrow*). With more advanced lesions, the secondary ventricular dilatation tends to obscure the primary deformity and only minor changes may be found that denote the true nature of the process, as in this case.

the ventricular plane has been changed. This is brought about by rotation of the ventricle, as the tumor grows. After some posterior displacement of the brain stem, the tumor imbeds itself often deeply in the pons, since it is relatively fixed by bony and meningeal structures, and the cerebellar substance (fig. 311). It would be unusual for a mass not adjacent to the ventricle, but exerting its pressure through a cushion of neural substance, to produce collapse of the lumen without producing maximum displacement. If desired, oblique films may be made which frequently will reveal the configuration of the fourth ventricle to be intact in one oblique projection; at the same time, straight frontal views will show the lateral aspect of the fourth ventricle on the involved side to appear flat, or even indented and curved away from the tumor. The fourth ventricle often has a shape resembling a banana. Such a configuration on frontal films, especially if seen at ventriculography when there is inadequate filling of the cisterns, should suggest the diagnosis of cerebellopontine angle tumor. Rather than subject these patients to supplemental procedures, such as the lumbar injection of air following ventriculography, 45-degree oblique films may be used to show with certainty that there is rotation of the ventricle, and not obliteration of the ventricular lumen.

In addition to the characteristic deformity and displacement of the fourth ventricle described above, changes in the posterior fossa cisterns are found at pneumoencephalography. Cisternal changes may be the first evidence of a tumor when the lesion is still small (fig. 220). Lumbar pneumoencephalography is superior to other methods for detecting early changes and for identification of the lesion, as well. The cerebello-

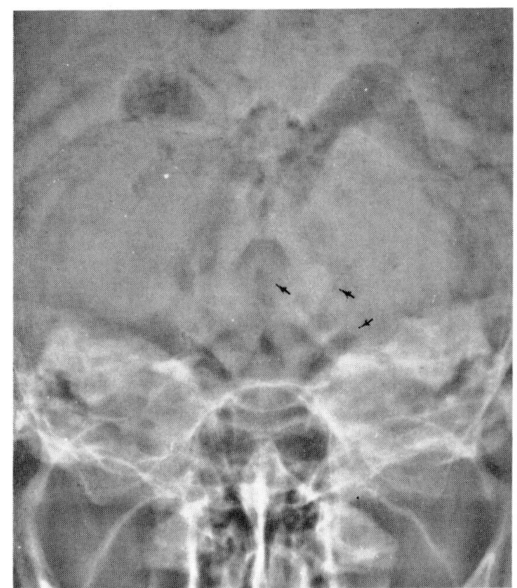

FIG. 313.—ACOUSTIC NEURINOMA

The value of carefully performed posterior fossa pneumoencephalography is illustrated. The fourth ventricle is not displaced or obstructed but exhibits a slight indentation on its ventrolateral aspect (*upper medial arrow*). The cerebellopontine extension is elevated (*upper lateral arrow*), and the main portion of the recess obstructed by the margin of the tumor (*lower arrow*). On the opposite side, there is dilatation of the cerebellopontine recess and of the communicating cistern extending laterally around the brain stem.

pontine recess most often is elevated. This is best demonstrated in a film made in posteroanterior half axial projection, which often depicts a normal and an abnormal cerebellopontine recess for comparison (figs. 311 and 313). Obstruction of the cerebellopontine fluid space may result in unilateral dilatation of the space, or in nonvisualization. Dilatation may be associated with the demonstration of a mass producing the obstruction (fig. 314); nonfilling is unsatisfactory, and may be resolved only by supplemental gas injection and re-examination, as described below. In some patients, elevation of the cerebellopontine recess may be accompanied by unilateral lifting of a lateral communicating channel and encroachment upon the quadrigeminal space.

It is important not to mistake a crural cistern for a displaced cerebellopontine recess. If there is good bilateral filling of the cerebellopontine or the crural cisterns, then a false identification is not likely. When there is unilateral filling, however, with no opportunity for comparison, mistaken identity may occur, since the angle of the crural cistern may be identical to that of a cerebellopontine recess displaced by tumor. Frequently a tumor interferes with filling of the cerebellopontine fluid space. Stereoscopic films may be helpful in determining the relationship of an unidentified cisternal shadow to the petrous pyramid.

In lateral projection, the fourth ventricle and aqueduct may be normal in appearance when the tumor is small. In the presence of an eighth nerve tumor or meningioma which grows laterally and posteriorly, the cisterna pontis may be partially obliterated. Because there is gas in the contralateral side of the cisterna pontis, this structure may appear normal in the lateral view (fig. 310). Even bilateral eighth nerve tumors may show a large, well filled prepontine cistern. Tumors that become very large may produce other changes. The posterior portion of the third ventricle may be elevated by a massive growth. When this occurs, differentiation from an intra-axial tumor must be made, particularly gliomas that spread into the supratentorial segments of the brain stem. In the latter cases there is a true deformity of the fourth ventricle, with encroachment by a mass directly adjacent to the lumen, rather than rotation of the ventricle.

When the fourth ventricle is large, the typical findings of a cerobellopontine angle tumor may not be present. After dilatation, characteristic rotation of the ventricle usually does not occur. Such cases are often examined by ventriculography; in these instances, good visualization of the fourth ventricle in frontal projections is essential. Slight *lateral flattening* is all that may be seen in some instances in the presence of fourth ventricular dilatation (fig. 312). Extreme degrees of dilatation of the fourth ventricle occasionally occur out of all proportion to the hydrocephalus; this almost always masks the deformity. On careful scrutiny, it may be noted in such cases that one side of the fourth ventricle is less

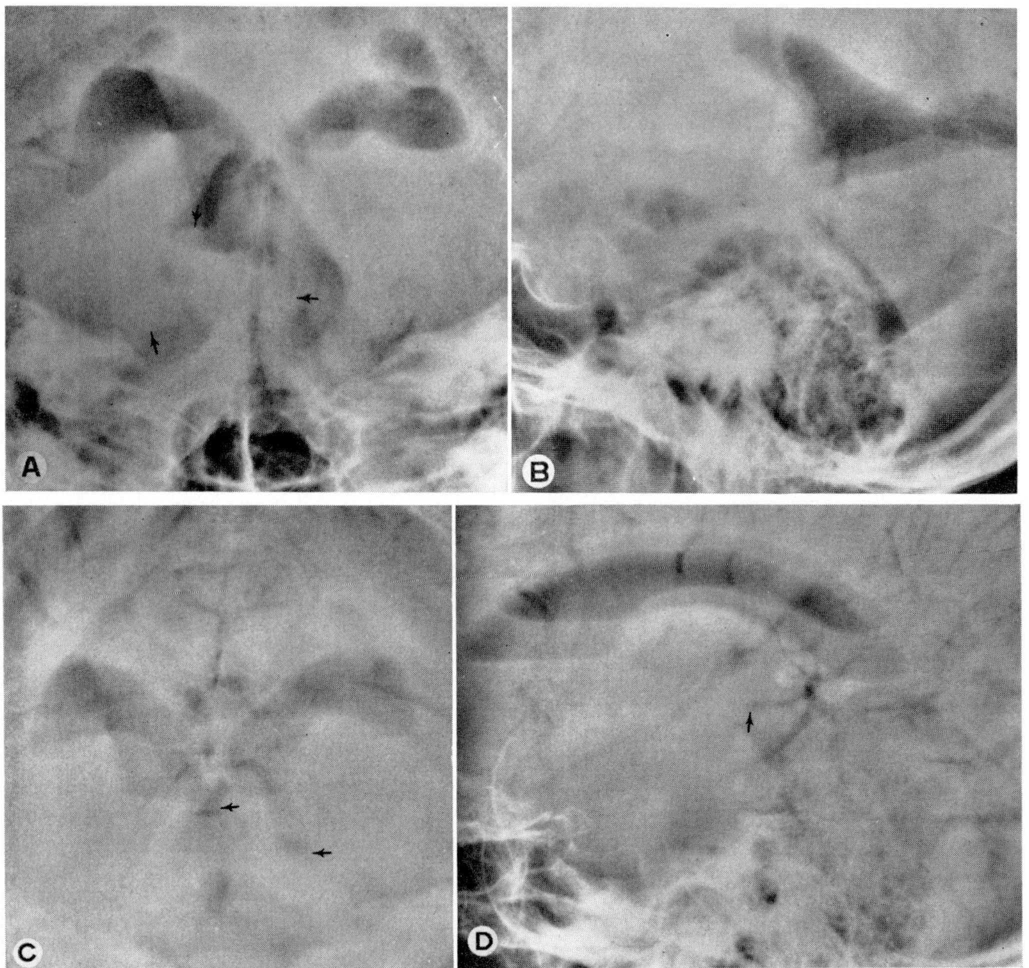

FIG. 314.—ANTEROLATERAL EXTRA-AXIAL TUMOR

In (A) and (B), a neurinoma of the fifth cranial nerve has displaced the fourth ventricle lateralward and far backward and produced partial obstruction. The fourth ventricle in frontal view is rotated, simulating that shown in Fig. 311, with the margin on the side of the lesion (*central arrow*) indented and indistinct. The cerebellopontine recess is obstructed by the tumor (*lower arrow*) and dilated (compare with opposite side). The superior extent of the mass is shown by gas in the dilated lateral communicating cistern (*upper arrow*).

A meningioma extending posteriorly from the middle cranial fossa is shown in (C) and (D). In the frontal film (C), the aqueduct is shown to be displaced lateralward (*upper arrow*), while the fourth ventricle is not greatly affected because it is in a different plane. The lateral communicating cistern on the involved side is dilated and obstructed at the edge of the tumor (*lower arrow*). In the lateral view (D), the retrothalamic extension of the quadrigeminal cistern is elevated on the involved side and obstructed (*arrow*). The shadow of the normal retrothalamic space on the opposite side is shown below and behind the deformed structure.

radiolucent than the other, owing to the fact that it is compressed on the side of the tumor. The lateral view often discloses a normal contour of the fourth ventricle, aside from enlargement. Neurinomas arising from the fifth cranial nerve may, on ordinary pneumograms, resemble eighth nerve tumors; in these cases, however, the cerebellopontine recess does not show the characteristic elevation, but it may be dilated and obstructed (fig. 314). A banana-like configuration of the fourth ventricle may be present (fig. 311).

Tumors other than those arising from the eighth cranial nerve may produce erosion of the petrous pyramid. Preservation of the internal auditory canal and radiolucent defects in other portions of the petrous bone suggest the possibility of such processes. While meningiomas may produce some sclerosis, a pure osteolytic change may be found. Instances of bone destruction by cholesteatoma in the posterior fossa have been encountered; tumors of the fifth cranial nerve may produce an erosion of the tip of the petrous bone, as well as the cranial floor, with a relatively intact internal auditory canal (Lindgren, 1941; Jefferson, 1955; Holman, Olive, and Svien, 1961). Cholesteatomas and the other tumors do not usually produce elevation of the cerebellopontine recess, as noted above.

When the cerebellopontine recess on the suspected side does not fill, it becomes necessary to rule out a technical artifact, if no other abnormalities are present. This may require repeating the usual maneuver to fill the cerebellopontine spaces two or three times (extension of the head during injection of 5 cc. of gas, followed by flexion 10 to 15 seconds later). If one cerebellopontine recess does not fill, for example, the right side, the head should be tilted slightly to the left upon flexion.

Lateral and posterior masses. Tumors situated laterally, posterolaterally, and posteriorly usually are indistinguishable from cerebellar tumors, in our experience. Varying degrees of lateral and anterior displacement of the fourth ventricle and lower aqueduct take place, depending on the relationship of the tumor to the ventricular pathways. Because of the relative rarity of extra-axial tumors in these locations, as compared with cerebellar tumors, the possibility of the former type of lesion usually is not suspected. In occasional cases, the frontal films may reveal asymmetry of the communicating cisterns. Dilatation of a cistern, or cisternal

(Revised 1963)

recess, on one side should always arouse suspicion concerning a tumor on the same side, owing to obstruction. Unilateral dislocation and deformity also may be observed. Many patients, however, are examined by ventriculography and visualization of the cisterns is not afforded. Since some of the masses are aneurysms or meningiomas, vertebral angiography often is of advantage in establishing a diagnosis; the potentiality of vertebral angiography in the evaluation of of posterior fossa masses has not been thoroughly explored (see "Angiography").

In summary, straight posterior displacement of the fourth ventricle and of the distal aqueduct, with no lateral deformity or rotation of the fourth ventricle, is found with midline anterior prepontine lesions. A wide cisterna pontis and the outlining of a margin of the tumor by cisternal air serve to differentiate prepontine from intra-axial neoplasms. When a vertebral angiogram is done, anterior displacement of the basilar artery usually indicates a pontine or cerebellar lesion, while posterior displacement of the basilar artery indicates a ventral extra-axial lesion.

Lateral and posterior displacements of the fourth ventricle suggest an anterolateral or cerebellopontine angle tumor. This must be differentiated from a lesion in the brain stem itself, involving predominantly one side of the stem. Oblique views show that the frontal deformity usually results from rotation of the ventricle rather than from flattening by an adjacent mass. Elevation of the cerebellopontine recess on the suspected side at selective pneumoencephalography will serve to identify the lesion as one arising from the region of the internal auditory meatus. Dilatation of the fourth ventricle, with flattening on one side, and elevation of the posterior portion of the third ventricle indicate a tumor of large size. Lateral and posterior tumors resemble cerebellar lesions in their effects on the ventricular system.

Incisural Tumors

The second group of extra-axial tumors of the posterior fossa are those that arise in the neighborhood of the incisura or notch

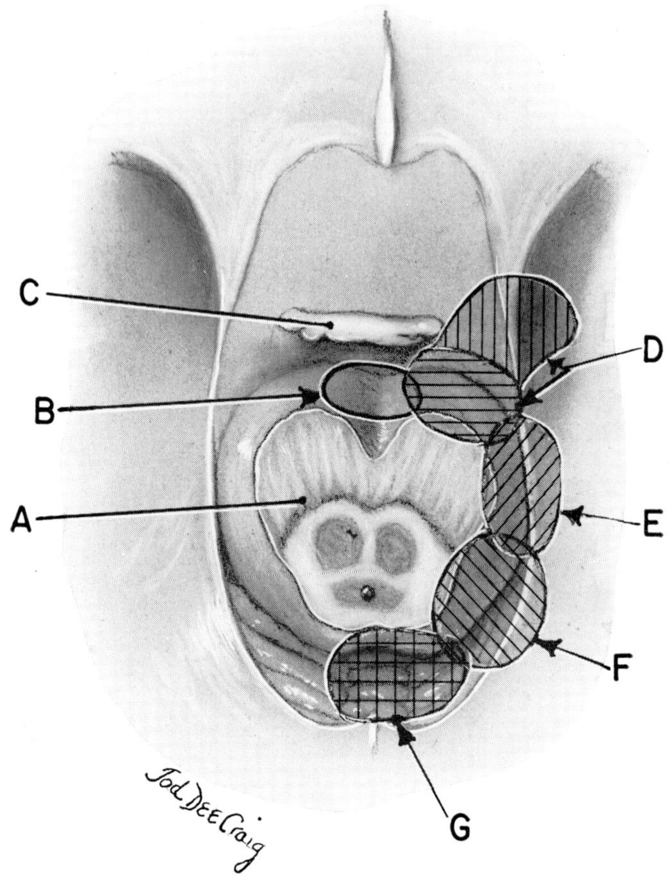

FIG. 315.—EXTRA-AXIAL TUMORS OF THE TENTORIAL INCISURA

A drawing of the incisura viewed superiorly shows the location of extraneural tumors occurring in relation to the midbrain (A). The anterior masses (B) are situated between the brain stem and the dorsum sellae (C). The location of anterolateral lesions (and the frequent site of saddle tumors) is shown at (D). Tumors also may be found in lateral position (E), in posterolateral location (F), or they may be posterior (G).

of the tentorium. Since these tumors are higher than those described above, they have their principal effects upon the aqueduct of Sylvius and the third ventricle (fig. 315). Lesions arising in this area are less common than those occurring in the cerebellopontine angle; the incidence of tumors of various types found at the incisura also is different, with the majority being meningiomas. A sizable number of incisural lesions are vascular in origin and may arise from the basilar artery, the posterior cerebral artery, or the vein of Galen. Tumors arising in the pineal gland may occasionally cause confusion in diagnosis. Incisural tumors also can arise from cranial nerves, such as the third nerve or fifth nerve, and congenital epidermal rests may occur in this region. The sketch in Figure 315 indicates the various locations of extra-axial masses occurring at the incisura of the tentorium. As in the case of the more caudal lesions described above, it is important to determine the relationship of incisural tumors to the brain stem in cross section, and to recognize whether a tumor is anterior, posterior, lateral, or intermediate in location.

Midline anterior masses. The straight

anterior incisural masses most frequently originate from aneurysmal changes in the basilar artery. Characteristic features are elevation of the posterior portion of the third ventricle, and posterior displacement of the aqueduct of Sylvius. These displacements do not allow differentiation between a pontine and a prepontine lesion. If, however, there is sufficient air in the cisterns of the posterior fossa, gas may partially encompass the extra-axial mass. Occasionally, gas may be present between the mass and the anterior margin of the pons indicating the prepontine nature of the lesion. In other instances, gas collections about the cerebral peduncles may outline anterior lesions in the rostral segment of the notch. When vascular, the lesions may be either arterial or venous in origin (fig. 316).

Because of the high frequency of vascular lesions occurring among extra-axial masses which are directly anterior to the brain stem, vertebral angiography or a substitute is indicated in the majority of instances, preoperatively, unless the clinical differentiation between an aneurysm and a solid tumor is quite clear. If the tumor is a solid mass, backward displacement of the basilar artery will be found at angiography in most cases.

Because of the large size of some masses, poor filling of the pontine and other ventral cisterns may occur. In some instances, gas may enter only a narrow angle between the inferior margin of the lesion and the basisphenoid. There is, however, almost always elevation of the floor of the third ventricle posteriorly which is demonstrable either by lumbar pneumoencephalography or ventriculography. Aqueduct displacement, while common, may not be shown because of obstruction; if there is associated atrophy of the brain stem, the aqueduct may fill but not be displaced backward.

In cases of basilar artery aneurysm situated along the distal course of the vessel, or at its bifurcation, some gas may pass anterior to the aneurysmal sac because of the backward bending of the vessel in its distal segment. A portion of a rounded mass may be clearly visible by gas inferior and anterior to the lesion. The finding, if present, is helpful in differentiating aneurysms from anterior incisural lesions arising from the basisphenoid or tentorial margin, either chordomas or meningiomas. In the latter conditions, cisternal gas is found dorsal to the mass. It is common, also, to find bone destruction in the region of the clivus, together with calcification in a mass, with chordoma; if tumor calcification alone is present, or if sclerotic changes in the sphenoid bone accompany the calcification, the lesion most often is a meningioma.

(Revised 1963)

Anterolateral masses. The masses that are *anterolateral* in their relationship to the midbrain may be divided, in turn, into two groups: (1) the solitary anterolateral masses and (2) the dumbbell, or saddle, tumors. The majority of the tumors falling into the first category are meningiomas that arise from the free edge of the tentorium, or from the medial end of the petrous bone. Neurinomas of the fifth cranial nerve also may occur in this location; they are more commonly of the dumbbell variety. Large cerebellopontine tumors can bulge through the incisura, and produce secondary effects that resemble anterolateral incisural masses.

Because the tumors are anterior and lateral to the brain stem, the pressure effect is chiefly on the aqueduct and the posterior part of the floor of the third ventricle. The curve of the ventricular floor is exaggerated, or there may be indentation and elevation of the posterior portion. Tumors that are truly incisural have their greatest effect upon the aqueduct of Sylvius, which is maximally displaced in a lateral direction; there usually is a backward displacement also, although frequently this is not prominent. Large tumors may displace the fourth ventricle.

The lateral displacement of the aqueduct of Sylvius is due not only to the center of the mass being high, at the level of the iter, but also a frequent absence of occlusion owing to transmitted pressure. In the average case, there is bowing of the aqueduct in frontal projection with the third ventricle and fourth ventricle approaching normal midline position. The deformity of the aqueduct results in varying degrees of ventricular obstruction, but in most cases moderate

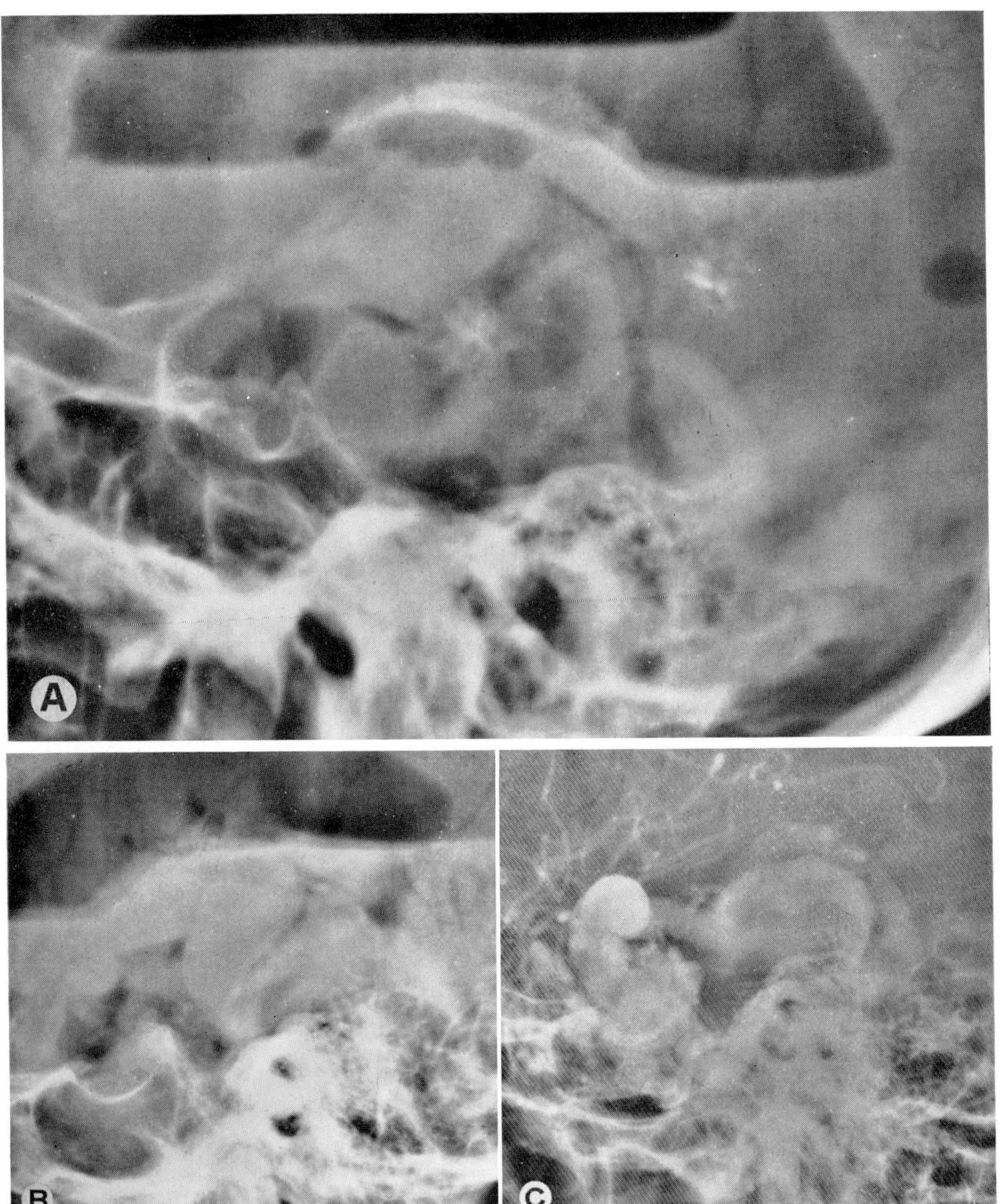

Fig. 316.—Anterior Vascular Masses

A lateral pneumogram (A) reveals posterior displacement of the aqueduct of Sylvius with partial obstruction and hydrocephalus. The fourth ventricle is dislocated to a less marked degree than the iter. A mass is present in the cisterna interpeduncularis and in the upper portion of the cisterna pontis partially outlined posteriorly and separated from the shadow of the displaced brain stem by a crescentic shadow of cisternal gas. The lesion proved to be an arterial aneurysm of the upper portion of the basilar artery. Rather marked asymmetry of the calcified chorioid glomera is shown, one being mobile and descending into the temporal horn with the patient upright.

In another case (B), a mass in the cisterna interpeduncularis is less well defined, but there is widening of the basal cisterns. An anteriorly convex shadow projecting into the cistern is not a markedly displaced pontine margin but a vascular mass (C). The other structures noted in the cisterns in the pneumogram are shown to be elements of an arteriovenous malformation by the angiogram.

(Revised 1963)

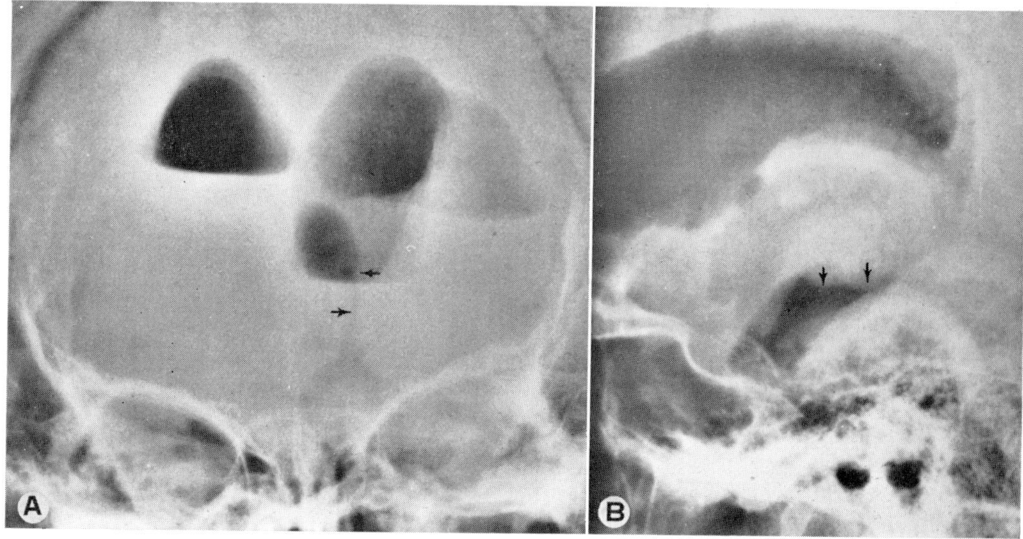

FIG. 317.—TENTORIAL MENINGIOMA

A mass arising from the anterolateral edge of the tentorium shows the aqueduct to be displaced sharply laterally (A) between its outlet (*upper arrow*) and the distal portion (*lower arrow*). The high position of the lesion at the tentorial edge is denoted by the greater displacement of the aqueduct between the arrows than pertains to the lowest portion of the aqueduct and the fourth ventricle. The lateral view (B) reveals elevation of the posterior portion of the third ventricle and a bilobular indentation of the margin of one temporal horn (*arrows*), owing to supratentorial extension of a tumor.

dilatation of the ventricular system is found, due to long standing narrowing. The majority of the patients are examined by pneumoencephalography, and ventricular filling usually is successful. Direct visualization of the tumor owing to subarachnoid gas in contact with a segment of the lesion is not a common feature of tumors arising in an anterolateral location; it is more often seen in connection with lesions arising in a midline anterior position. Subarachnoid cerebrospinal fluid circulation at the incisura is impaired, and dilatation of subtentorial cisterns often results.

The second subgroup (*saddle tumors*) of anterolateral incisural masses comprises mainly meningiomas and neurinomas (usually of the fifth cranial nerve) which extend both into the posterior fossa and into the middle cranial fossa. Some bone destruction of the petrous tip may be observed, either with neurinomas or meningiomas; cases have been seen in which sclerosis in the region of the dorsum sellae and clivus, as well as calcification in the tumor, was present.

At pneumography, the ventral indentation of the posterior aspect of the third ventricle and the lateral and posterior displacement of the aqueduct characteristic of single masses in this region is found. In addition, some deformity of the temporal horn may be demonstrated as a result of the supratentorial, middle fossa extension of one lobe of the lesion (fig. 317). Vertebral angiography, in addition to air studies, may be required to establish a diagnosis.

It is necessary, in considering anterolateral lesions, to differentiate them from intrinsic tumors of the brain stem or peduncular region. At ventriculography, elevation of the floor of the posterior portion of the third ventricle frequently suggests first the possibility of an intra-axial tumor deforming this area. The most important clue to the correct diagnosis is visualization of the aqueduct of Sylvius, which exhibits prominent lateral displacement, with or without blockage (fig. 318). Intrinsic tumors more often oc-

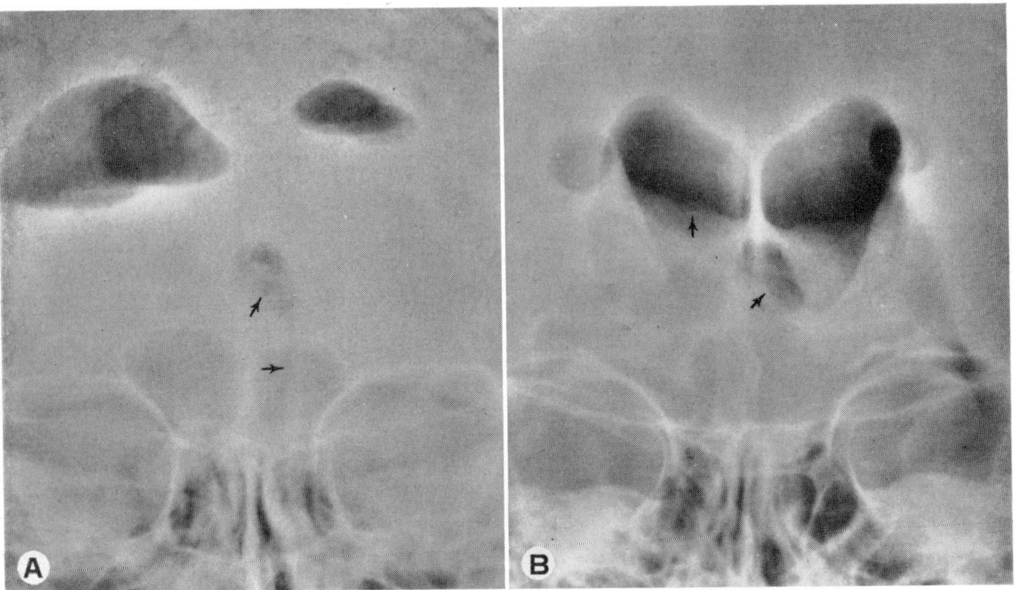

FIG. 318.—TENTORIAL MENINGIOMA

An anterolateral meningioma (A) has produced indentation of the posterior inferior aspect of the third ventricle (*upper arrow*). The aqueduct as far caudad as its distal portion (*lower arrow*) is sharply displaced. Downward extension of gas into the fourth ventricle shows that this structure returns almost to the midline. In another case (B), an anterolateral saddle meningioma, the third ventricle is dilated and indented on the inferolateral aspect (*lower arrow*). The floor of the lateral ventricle on the corresponding side is markedly elevated (*upper arrow*). At the time of operation, a large meningioma was found in the middle cranial fossa, accounting for the deformity shown even on the anteroposterior view, and the tumor extended through the incisura, from which it arose, into the posterior fossa. Two cases illustrate different stages: (A) the preocclusive state with the aqueduct patent, and (B) the postocclusive stage.

clude the aqueduct of Sylvius before marked lateral displacement can occur.

Lateral and posterolateral masses. Tumors lying *lateral* to the midbrain are less common than those arising further anteriorly. Occasionally, a tumor, particularly a meningioma, taking origin from the lateral aspect of the free tentorial edge, may compress the brain stem from one side without anterior or posterior extension (fig. 319). In these cases, as in those just described, inferior indentation of the posterior portion of the third ventricle is found. The aqueduct of Sylvius usually is visible and exhibits sharp lateral displacement; varying degrees of obstruction and ventricular dilatation are encountered.

Tumors arising *posterolaterally* may be meningiomas of the tentorium, or aneurysmal masses originating from the posterior cerebral artery. The lesions encountered in this area ordinarily do not deform the third ventricle. Instead, a deformity of the posterior communicating channels occurs. The retrothalamic space of the quadrigeminal cistern may be displaced forward and become concave posteriorly (fig. 320). The posterolateral masses may displace the aqueduct of Sylvius laterally and also may deform the medial aspect of the atrium of the lateral ventricle through upward extension. The fourth ventricle usually is not affected.

Midline posterior masses. Posterior central incisural masses are more common than those laterally situated. Most often the tumors originate as meningiomas of the posterior angle of the tentorial notch, or as

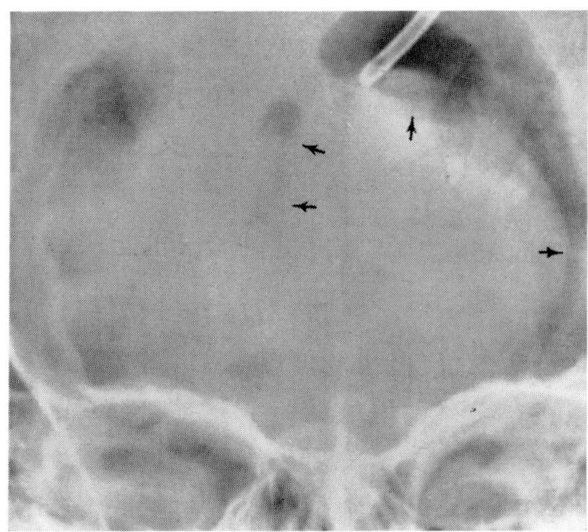

Fig. 319.—Lateral Incisural Meningioma

A mass situated straight laterally in relation to the midbrain and arising from the tentorial edge has deformed the posterior inferior margin of the third ventricle (*upper central arrow*) and displaced the aqueduct laterally (*lower central arrow*). A partial obstruction of the iter has resulted. In addition, there is elevation of the ventricular floor in the region of the atrium and narrowing of the lumen of the posterior portion of the temporal horn by pressure on the medial side (*lateral arrows*). Except for the displacement and obstruction of the cerebral aqueduct, the findings are strongly suggestive of a thalamic tumor; the possibility of supratentorial extension of a benign, operable incisural lesion should be considered in the differential diagnosis of deeply seated lesions.

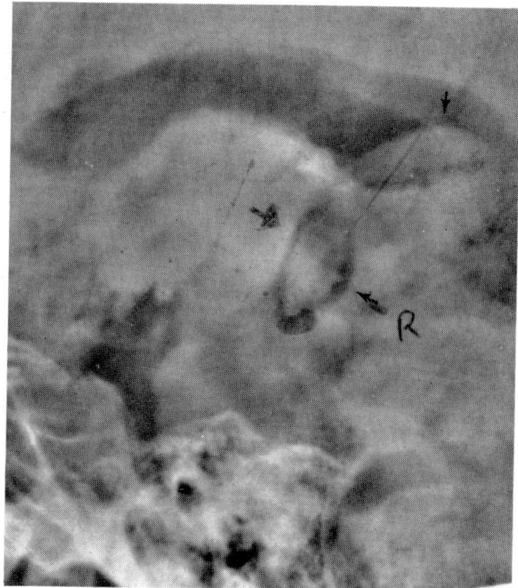

Fig. 320.—Posterolateral Incisural Mass

An aneurysm of the posterior cerebral artery has produced a discrete filling defect in the atrium of the left lateral ventricle (*upper arrow*). The retrothalamic extension of the quadrigeminal cistern on the same side exhibits a reversal of its curve (*anterior arrow*). The same structure on the opposite side (labeled R with *arrow*) has a normal configuration. Intracranial exploration revealed that the mass was an aneurysmal sac filled with thrombus.

vascular lesions arising from the vein of Galen or its tributaries. Pinealomas growing strictly outward and downward occur; more often their extension is into the ventricular lumen.

The midline posterior incisural masses frequently manifest themselves by deformity or obliteration of the cistern over the quadrigeminal plate. There is often forward displacement and indentation of the quadrigeminal cistern, if it is visible. Ordinarily, anterior displacement of the aqueduct of Sylvius is present. In some instances, there may be encroachment on the upper portion of the fourth ventricle from behind and above; when present, the deformity usually occurs without displacement.

Masses, particularly meningiomas, arising posteriorly in the midline at the angle of the tentorium, may exhibit the distinguishing feature of *spreading* of air-filled structures. When the midbrain is flattened from behind, there may be spreading of the retrothalamic spaces, as seen in frontal projection (fig. 321). Tumors which grow predominantly upward may result in a widening of the space between the lateral ventricles posteriorly, together with indentation of the medial portions of the atria (fig. 322). In such cases, the vertebral angiogram may demonstrate marked displacement of the posterior cerebral arteries, usually elevation and separation; the spaces between the superior cerebellar arteries and the posterior cerebral arteries are widened.

Posterior tumors may present problems in differential diagnosis because pineal tu-

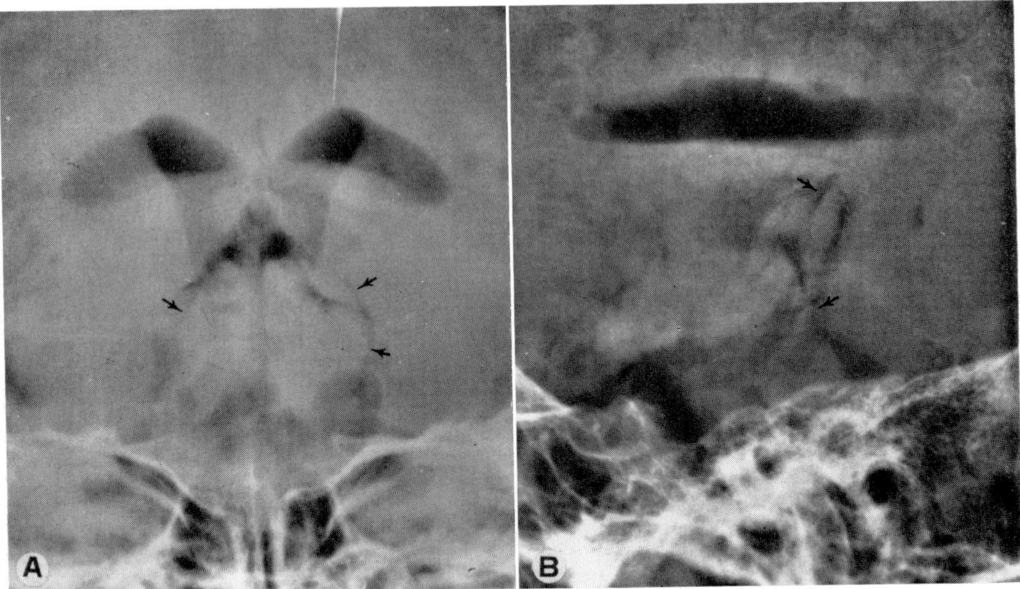

FIG. 321.—POSTERIOR INCISURAL MENINGIOMA

A meningioma arising straight posteriorly from the tentorial edge has compressed the midbrain from the posterior side, causing widening of the shadow as a result of flattening. The lateral communicating channels, marked with *arrows*, are narrowed and bowed lateralward on the side toward which the bulk of the slightly eccentric growth has extended (*two arrows*), as seen in the frontal view (A). In another case (B), a malignant meningioma, arising straight posteriorly from the incisural edge, has produced forward bowing of the cerebral aqueduct with partial obstruction (*lower arrow*). One retrothalamic extension of the quadrigeminal cistern (*upper arrow*) is displaced forward and upward, is straightened, and is occluded in its lower portion. The dark linear shadow projected slightly below and behind the indicated shadow is the deformed contralateral retrothalamic extension.

mors may grow downward, as previously stated, and because tumors of the posterior incisural angle may grow upward and forward toward the pineal region. The latter tumors may indent the posterior aspect of the third ventricle, with deformity and dilatation similar to that produced by pinealoma. If angiography is carried out, deformity of the deep veins may be demonstrated; downward and forward displacement of the vein of Galen and of the posterior portion of the internal cerebral vein may be found. Some of these lesions are aneurysms of the vein of Galen, and because of this, it obviously is advisable to recommend that angiography be carried out prior to surgical procedures in this region, chiefly to differentiate vascular masses from meningiomas. In some instances, upward herniation of posterior fossa structures through the tentorial incisura, owing to an intra-axial posterior fossa tumor, may simulate the changes of an extra-axial incisural mass (fig. 323).

Considering the extra-axial incisural tumors as a whole, it is usually possible to arrive at a correct diagnosis by roentgen methods. In the majority of instances, pneumoencephalography is the procedure of choice. Cisternal filling through pneumoencephalography is highly desirable for accurate identification of the lesion as being extra-axial; when carefully performed, the lumbar injection of gas does not appear to be a hazardous procedure in the presence of extra-axial lesions. In the occasional cases in which a high degree of ventricular obstruction exists, as reflected by clinical evidence of increased intracranial pressure, ventriculography should be carried out, followed by the lumbar injection of gas if

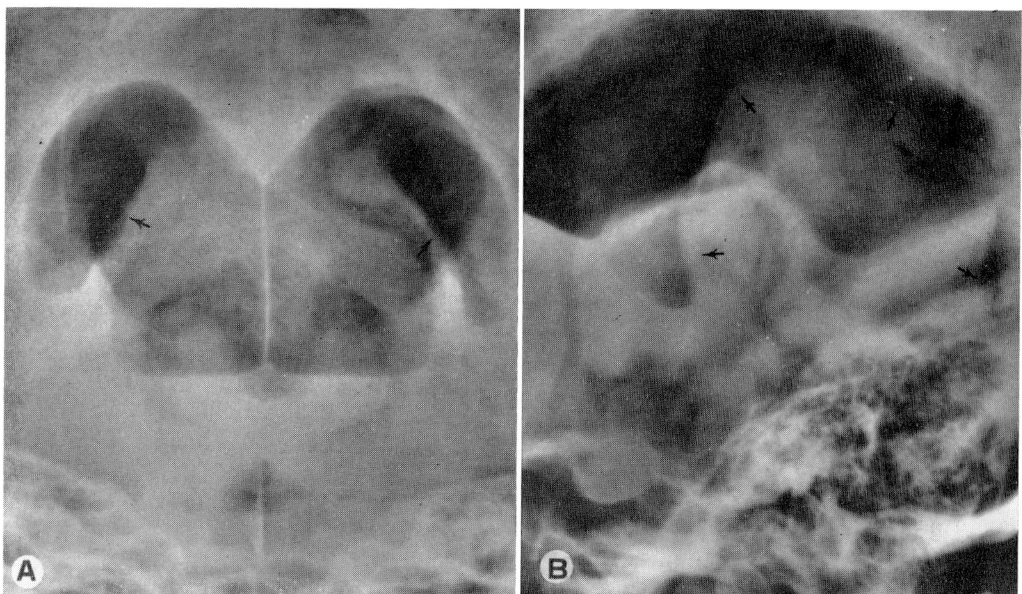

FIG. 322.—STRAIGHT POSTERIOR TENTORIAL MENINGIOMA

A large midline meningioma, growing chiefly upward and forward from the anterior aspect of the tentorium, has produced obstruction by encroachment on the posterior portion of the third ventricle (*anterior arrow*), as seen in lateral view (B). There is also deformity of the atrial portions of the lateral ventricles, the superior extent of the large tumor being shown by gas in these structures (*upper arrows*). There is also downward bowing posteriorly and inferiorly, depressing the gas outline of the superior subarachnoid space over the surface of the cerebellum (*posterior arrow*). The small amount of subarachnoid gas present was introduced by lumbar puncture. In the frontal view (A), medial encroachment by the midline tumor on the atrial shadows is shown, spreading the atrial shadows (*arrows*) or widening the space between these structures.

necessary. On other occasions, ventriculography may be employed when pneumoencephalography is nondiagnostic.

The consideration of extra-axial tumors arising in the region of the incisura becomes important whenever there is partial obstruction and deformity of the outlet of the third ventricle. In general, elevation of the posterior portion of the third ventricular floor is associated with tumors lying anteriorly and laterally, while deformity of the posterior end of the third ventricle is owing to masses arising dorsally at the incisural angle. Elevation of the posterior third ventricular floor may be found also with intra-axial brain stem tumors. Lateral displacement of the aqueduct of Sylvius favors an extra-axial lesion; intrinsic brain stem tumors rarely grow entirely laterally, and more often produce compression and posterior displacement of the aqueduct. Lateral pressure upon the cerebral aqueduct, with little or no deformity, favors the presence of a high posterior fossa lesion of true incisural origin. The diagnosis of extra-axial tumor is best made by gas in the subarachnoid cisterns around the tumor; by means of gas outlining a segment of the lesion itself, the mass is separated from the brain stem. The masses situated anteriorly and posterolaterally frequently are vascular in origin; vertebral angiography should be performed routinely.

EXTRA-AXIAL SUPRASELLAR TUMORS

Suprasellar tumors comprise a group of lesions that are properly considered together because of the associated clinical manifestations. Among the various lesions there is overlapping of the clinical changes characteristic of each; in addition, the similarity of location, size, and shape of the masses at pneumography may result in radiographic images among which it is difficult to distinguish. The structures most often damaged are the pituitary gland itself, the optic chiasm, the optic and other cranial nerves, and the hypothalamic portion of the third ventricle. Large tumors often affect more remote structures. The masses most frequently presenting in the suprasellar cistern are pituitary adenomas, craniopharyngiomas, aneurysms, meningiomas, and optic gliomas, generally in that order of frequency. Tumors of the hypothalamic portion of the third ventricle often encroach upon the suprasellar cistern and occasionally cause difficulty in diagnosis. Chordomas originating in the superior portion of the sphenoid bone, or extending there from the region of the clivus, occasionally are encountered; suprasellar extension of other basal tumors may occur. Metastatic deposits from tumors of distant organs, or the direct spread of nasopharyngeal tumors, may involve the sphenoid bone and the pituitary gland itself.

Because of the variety of lesions occurring in the suprasellar area, it is important to have as accurate a preoperative identification as possible; this sometimes taxes all clinical,

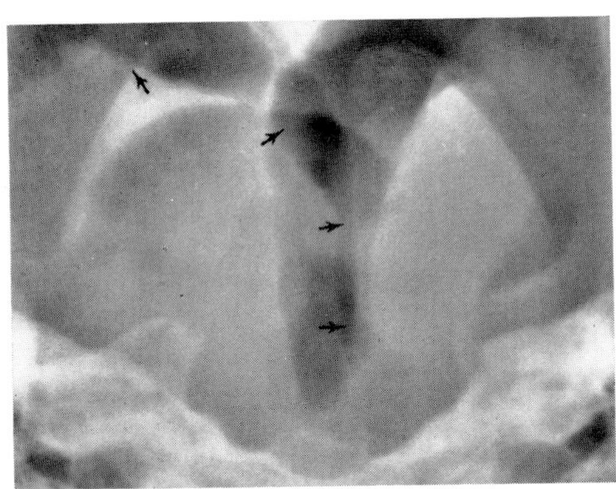

Fig. 323.—Upward Herniation Simulating Incisural Tumor

The frontal pneumogram reveals elevation of the floor of the atrium and some encroachment upon the shadow of the temporal horn from the medial side (*lateral arrow*). The posterior portion of the third ventricle is tapered away from the side of the lesion (*upper central arrow*). The rounded shadow of the outlet of the third ventricle is well shown. The marked lateral displacement of the cerebral aqueduct and upper fourth ventricle (*lower medial arrows*) indicates that the bulk of the mass is below the tentorium. Without the latter evidence, the atrial and third ventricle deformities might be mistaken for changes associated with an incisural tumor, rather than upward herniation of posterior fossa contents following ventriculography. The erosion of the dorsum sellae, as visualized in frontal projection, is well demonstrated.

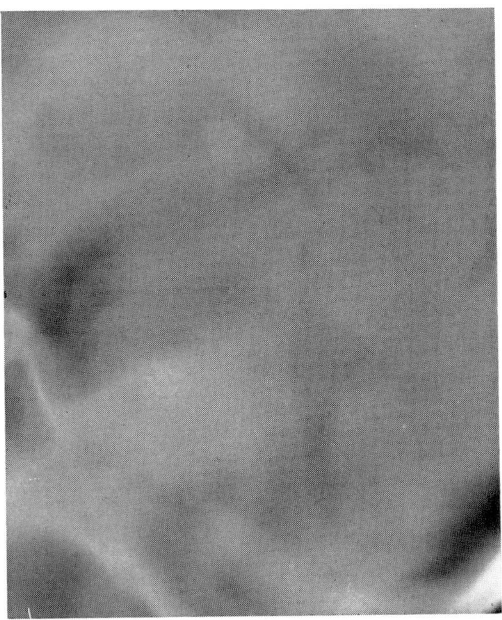

Fig. 324.—Quadrigeminal Cistern Simulating Displaced Aqueduct

When the aqueduct of Sylvius is not gas filled, care must be exercised not to mistake other gas shadows for this structure. In the midsagittal tomogram shown, gas in the quadrigeminal cistern and its cerebellomedullary extension appears to be continuous with the suprapineal recess above and the rostral end of the fourth ventricle below. The unusual demonstration occurred in connection with a normal pneumographic examination.

(Revised 1963)

radiologic, and laboratory resources. Among the radiologic methods, plain film findings play an important role; changes of bone destruction, bone production, and abnormal calcification, either produced in the tumor itself or imbedded in the tumor as a result of sequestration, deserve heavy emphasis. Demineralization of various portions of the sella turcica, enlargement of the optic foramen, and basal erosion are a few of the more common changes that have been described in detail earlier. While the contrast studies serve well to show the size and extent of a tumor, and often to diagnose it with certainty, as in the case of an aneurysm at angiography, the pneumographic configuration is not always of an identifying nature; considerable reliance on plain film changes, in conjunction with pneumographic findings, often is necessary.

Pituitary Tumors

Pituitary adenomas have been a subject of interest since the days of Pierre Marie (1886); because tumors of the hypophysis are quite common, in addition to being of unusual interest, medical literature contains an enormous amount of writing on the subject. A classic description of the clinical findings of pituitary adenomas, and of the sella turcica changes observed at operation and at autopsy, was given by Cushing in 1912. Schüller (1912) early obtained successful radiographs of the normal and abnormal sella turcica. Jefferson (1940) emphasized the information that pneumography can provide concerning the extrasellar extension of pituitary tumors; the fact that cisternal deformities could be demonstrated had been mentioned by Dyke and Davidoff (1935) and even earlier in isolated reports by others.

Tumors may originate from any of the glandular or supporting elements of the anterior lobe of the hypophysis. The vast majority of primary tumors of the pituitary gland are benign adenomas which may be classified as follows: (1) chromophobe, (2) chromophil, either eosinophilic or basophilic (rare), and (3) mixed chromophobe and chromophil tumors. In addition, the possibility of primary carcinoma of the pituitary

must be considered with lesions which exhibit extensive destruction, but the incidence of malignant primary hypophyseal tumors is less than 1 per cent.

Chromophobe adenoma. In the great majority of patients, certainly more than 80 per cent, the sella turcica is enlarged, measuring near or above the upper limits of normal. There is rounding of the interior of the pituitary fossa in most instances; the feature termed "ballooning" is often more striking with eosinophilic adenoma than with other types. The adenomas often grow asymmetrically, with corresponding asymmetry of the sella enlargement, particularly of the sella floor; a "double floor" appearance is thought to be a valuable diagnostic finding in favor of pituitary adenoma (Sosman, 1927). In almost all instances there is some pressure erosion of the walls of the sella turcica by the expanding intrasellar mass, resulting in thinning and discontinuity of the cortical boundaries. In most cases, the dorsum sellae is thin and demineralized; it is usually found that the inner cortical boundary of the dorsum exhibits the earliest and often the greatest change. As has been described earlier, the posterior sellar boundary may be relocated behind its original position. Along the floor of the pituitary fossa the weakest point appears to be posteriorly near the dorsum where often there is a notch-like defect in the basisphenoid, usually with irregular margins. The cause of the vulnerability of this area is not clear, but it may be related to the fact that the bone here often is cancellous in type, rather than compact, as is the case above the pneumatized sphenoid sinus. However, any portion of the sella floor may exhibit thinning or a loss of compactness of its cortical boundary. Anteriorly, there may be pressure erosion in the region of the tuberculum; the pressure atrophy here, together with erosion of the inferior aspect of the anterior clinoid processes, results in an appearance termed "undercutting," a characteristic finding of pituitary adenoma, when present. Inferior erosion and apparent pointing of the anterior clinoids above the transverse plane is seen in some cases of aneurysm but occurs commonly with adenoma.

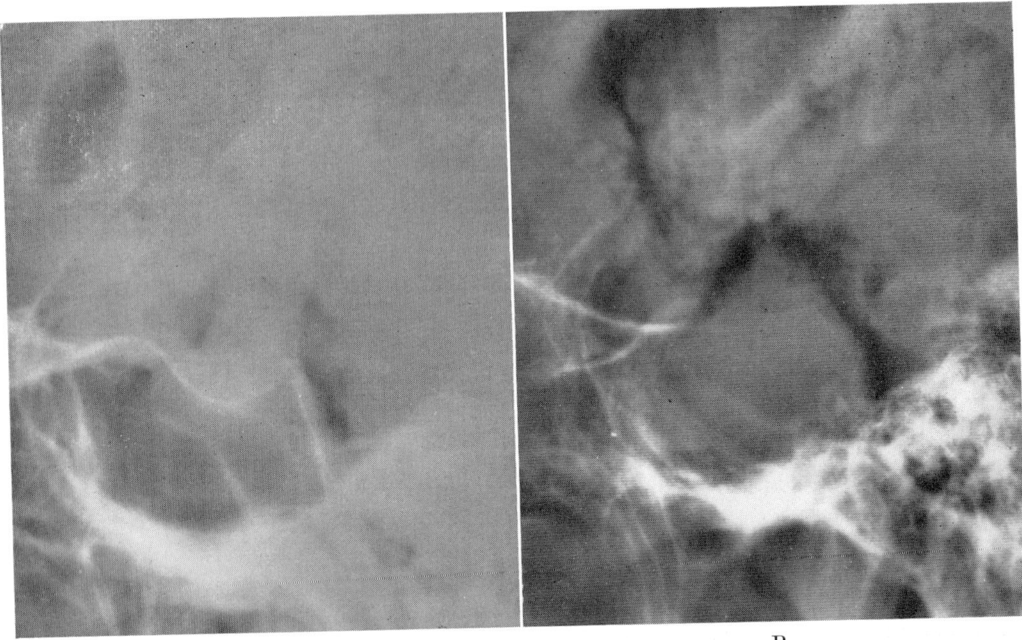

FIG. 325.—PITUITARY ADENOMA WITH SUPRASELLAR EXTENSION

A lateral pneumogram, with the patient supine, made after the injection of only 10 cc. of gas (A), reveals a sheet of tumor tissue extending upward above an open sella turcica into the postchiasmatic portion of the suprasellar cistern, which is obliterated. In some instances, a small amount of gas may give a more accurate impression of the size of the extrasellar extension than pneumograms made after larger replacements, since in the latter, gas lateral to the sella and superimposed upon the suprasellar tumor may give a false impression of an upward extension of smaller size than actually exists. (Cases have been encountered in which an erroneous interpretation of no suprasellar extension was made when actually a large suprasellar mass existed.) In a case such as that shown, it would be desirable to have some gas in the anterior portion of the third ventricle as well as is the basal cisterns, and this can be accomplished by using small quantities of gas and a somersaulting technique.

In the second case (B), a larger pituitary adenoma is present. There is gross enlargement of the sella turcica, indicating a large component in the pituitary fossa, and the tumor extends straight upward, having a bulblike configuration. The main suprasellar cistern is obliterated. Because of the size of the tumor, there is narrowing of the cisterna interpeduncularis. With the patient in a slightly hyperextended position, adequate opportunity for the hypothalamic portion of the third ventricle to fill was afforded, but this compartment is compressed and largely obliterated.

It has been suggested by some that anterior and posterior clinoids which are separated more than average (open sella), prior to the development of a pituitary adenoma, favor upward or extrasellar extension of a pituitary tumor. Contrariwise, clinoids that are close together (closed sella) are said to favor confinement of the growth within the pituitary fossa. When there is marked ballooning of the sella turcica, the clinoids often are relatively spared and close together; when the bulk of the tumor is suprasellar, and the size of the sella turcica relatively normal, the clinoids often are widely separated. How much, if any, the original shape of the sella turcica determines the confinement or direction of the tumor's growth is not clear. Contrary to the statements of many other investigators, we have observed calcification in pituitary adenomas on a number of occasions, particularly a shell-like calcification in the capsule.

Lumbar pneumoencephalography is the pneumographic procedure of choice for the diagnosis of pituitary adenomas and other suprasellar masses. While the third ventricle is deformed in a high percentage of patients with pituitary adenoma, ventriculography will fail to outline small lesions unless sufficient air is injected for a significant quantity to enter the subarachnoid space. It is undesirable, however, to overfill the ventricular system, particularly the lateral ventricles, when the cisternal areas are the sites of chief interest; gas in the temporal horns may obscure important cisternal abnormalities, especially if the horns are dilated. Likewise, angiography is not as ideal a method of investigation as might be expected, since those adenomas which grow backward, as well as upward, may produce no discernible deformity of the circle of Willis.

In the past, there has been some reluctance to carry out pneumoencephalography routinely, since it was known that occasional patients with pituitary insufficiency, even at the subclinical level, did not tolerate pneumoencephalography well. With the advent of substitution hormonal therapy, and the use of smaller amounts of gas, the objection appears to have been largely overcome. We do not agree, therefore, with those who have stated that the diagnosis of pituitary adenoma seldom requires confirmation by contrast study. Rather, it appears highly important to try to obtain all information possible concerning the characteristics of such a tumor, particularly if surgical treatment is to be carried out. It is also extremely helpful to have the lesions well defined if radiation therapy is to be administered; a second pneumogram after treatment is helpful to assess the results of radiation therapy, and acts as a valuable baseline in case of recurrence. As more knowledge is gained about these lesions, it is appreciated more fully that their growth is not always typical; visual field and other clinical examinations may be a crude and even inaccurate method of estimating the tumor's size and its regression after treatment. The visual difficulties may persist although the tumor has shrunken in size, owing to irreversible damage of the optic pathways. The appearance of the sella turcica on plain films usually does not give a satisfactory idea of the bulk of the tumor or of the direction of extrasellar growth. After radiation therapy the size of the sella turcica may be reduced and its boundaries become recalcified, but the process usually requires many months. The sella turcica often remains large after the tumor shrinks.

Selective pneumoencephalography, with direction of part of the gas into the anterior cisterns, is desirable; partial filling of the ventricular system also should be accomplished in order to visualize the anterior portion of the third ventricle. Several of the various views taken in connection with the routine examination give useful information; lateral and frontal films, taken with the patient supine, usually are the most informative. If a sizable amount of gas has entered the lateral ventricles, or is disposed laterally in the subarachnoid space, stereoscopic supine lateral films may be invaluable; of great diagnostic aid, in some cases, is sagittal autotomography with the head hanging.

Occasionally, as previously described, a small downward projection of the main suprasellar cistern below the level of the diaphragm of the sella turcica is present; rarely a large intrasellar extension of the subarachnoid space may occur normally. When a pituitary adenoma of significant proportions develops, the intrasellar extension is obliterated. Since it is usually not known that an intrasellar extension did exist prior to the time of the examination, the information is of limited diagnostic value. On the other hand, in the case of a large sella turcica of unknown significance, extension of cisternal gas into the pituitary fossa indicates that the enlargement is not due to an actively growing tumor. Upward bulging of the diaphragma sellae usually is the earliest definable evidence of a pituitary adenoma. If the superior boundary of the sella turcica is convex superiorly, and if its dome extends above the level of the interclinoid line, the change is indicative of an expanding lesion within the sella turcica.

In most cases, the growth pattern of a chromophobe pituitary adenoma follows along one of three general lines: (1) it may be predominantly upward and forward, (2) extension may be upward and backward, and (3) growth may be predominantly lateral in direction. *Upward and forward growth*, or

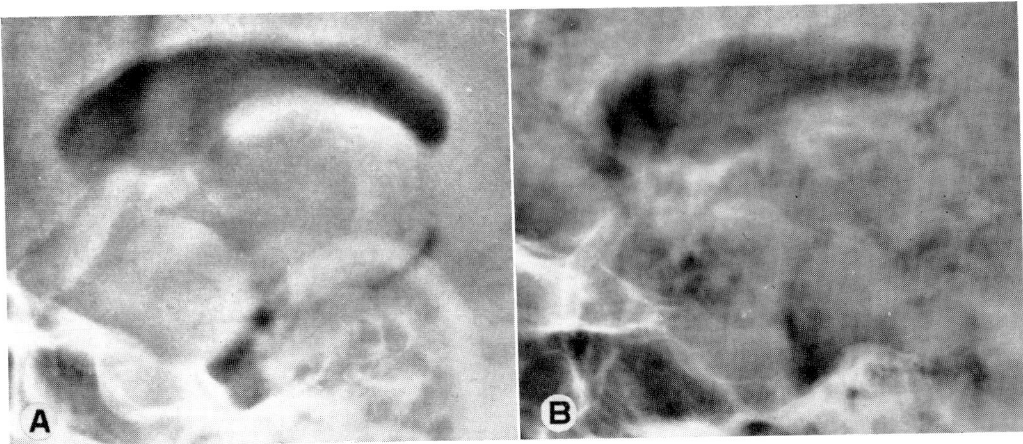

Fig. 326.—Pituitary Adenoma with Third Ventricular Deformity

The suprasellar cisterns are obliterated by a globular tumor based upon a moderately deformed sella turcica (A). The hypothalamic portion of the third ventricle is compressed and invaginated by the tumor; gas in the third ventricle outlines sharply the dome of the rounded adenoma. The posterior rim of the mass bulges into the cisterna interpeduncularis. In another case (B), the sella turcica is larger and the suprasellar component is not as globular. The top of the suprasellar extension, however, invaginates the anterior portion of the third ventricle, and gas in this structure again defines well the superior extent of the tumor.

growth straight upward, first obliterates the main suprasellar cistern and impinges upon the optic pathways (fig. 325); thereby the soft tissue density of the pituitary gland becomes continuous through the tumor with that of the optic chiasm and nerves. As the tumor grows, further elevation and compression of the chiasm occurs. The tumor also bulges forward, anterior to the optic chiasm and between the optic nerves. The prechiasmatic portion of the suprasellar cistern, as well as the postchiasmatic portion, then is narrowed or occluded. The optic and infundibular recesses of the third ventricle are blunted, elevated, and then obliterated; in many instances, the tumor later invaginates the hypothalamus, with obliteration of part or sometimes all of the anterior third ventricular cavity (fig. 326). In other instances, the third ventricle appears elevated but not appreciably deformed.

The suprasellar extension of a chromophobe pituitary adenoma is usually dome shaped, round or lobulated. The rounded configuration of the tumor may be masked by air situated beside it in the lateral aspects of the suprasellar cisterns, and in the region anterior and medial to the temporal lobe on each side. This gives the tumor an apparent pyramidal shape (fig. 325). Sometimes air is seen anterior to the tumor, and the true rounded configuration can then be appreciated (figs. 202 and 327). Too much gas in the suprasellar cistern will tend to obscure a tumor; in general, the injection of more than 5 cc. of gas with the head extended prior to filming should be avoided. If, after seeing the film, more air is desired, it can be added then.

Approximately 25 per cent of all pituitary adenomas, and the majority of large adenomas growing upward and forward, produce a deformity of the inferior aspect of the anterior horns of the lateral ventricles (fig. 327). In the lateral pneumoencephalogram, there may be only incomplete distention of the inferior aspects of the anterior horns, or both horns may be significantly narrowed by encroachment from below, with a superiorly convex configuration of their floors. In most instances, the deformity of the lateral ventricles produced is fairly symmetrical. Rarely, an obstruction occurs at the foramen of Monro; to produce this a pituitary tumor has to be very large, although it may be seen in a neglected case. Foraminal ob-

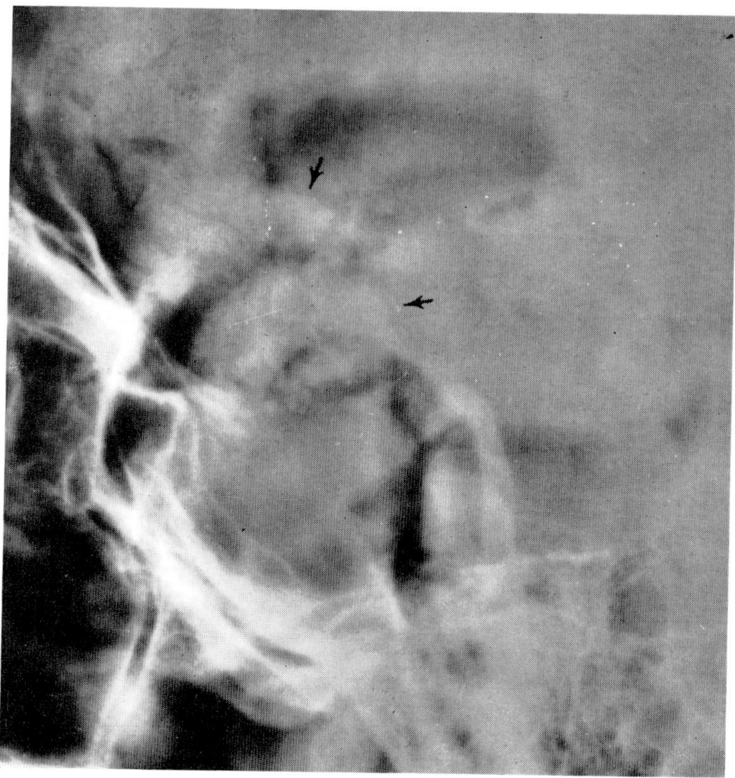

FIG. 327.—PITUITARY ADENOMA DEFORMING LATERAL VENTRICLES

An unusually large pituitary adenoma has extended well above the markedly eroded sella turcica. Subarachnoid gas and gas in the deformed hypothalamic portion of the third ventricle (*lower arrow*) outlines well the extrasellar extent of the tumor in lateral view. The inferior margins of the frontal horns are elevated and convex superiorly (*upper arrow*), with reduction in height of this portion of the ventricles, owing to pressure by the tumor below.

struction occurs much more often with other types of suprasellar masses.

The principal direction of growth in some cases is *upward and backward*. In these instances, the main suprasellar cistern is again invaded early. In the lateral pneumogram, a rounded shadow of soft tissue density, based upon the top of the sella turcica, extends toward, or to, the tuber cinereum. As in the case of the more anterior lesions just described, the rounded surface of the adenoma may be masked by subarachnoid gas beside the tumor. Under these circumstances, the mass may appear somewhat triangular, rather than globular (fig. 328). In some instances, if the tumor is small, a narrow gas space may be preserved between the anterior extremity of the tumor and the optic chiasm. More often, however, the chiasm is reached and forms the anterior margin of the suprasellar soft tissue shadow. The posterior margin is formed by the capsule of the tumor proper, which is continuous with the posterior margin of the eroded dorsum sellae; posteriorly and superiorly, the shadow may be continuous with the diencephalon (fig. 328). Thus, the cisterna interpeduncularis is encroached upon or obliterated. Large tumors may invaginate the floor of the third ventricle, and examples of obstruction of the aqueduct of Sylvius have been reported. Such tumors, with a predominantly backward extension, are said to "spill over" into the posterior fossa. Downward or retrosellar extension, with filling of the cisterna pontis, may occur rarely

(*Revised 1963*)

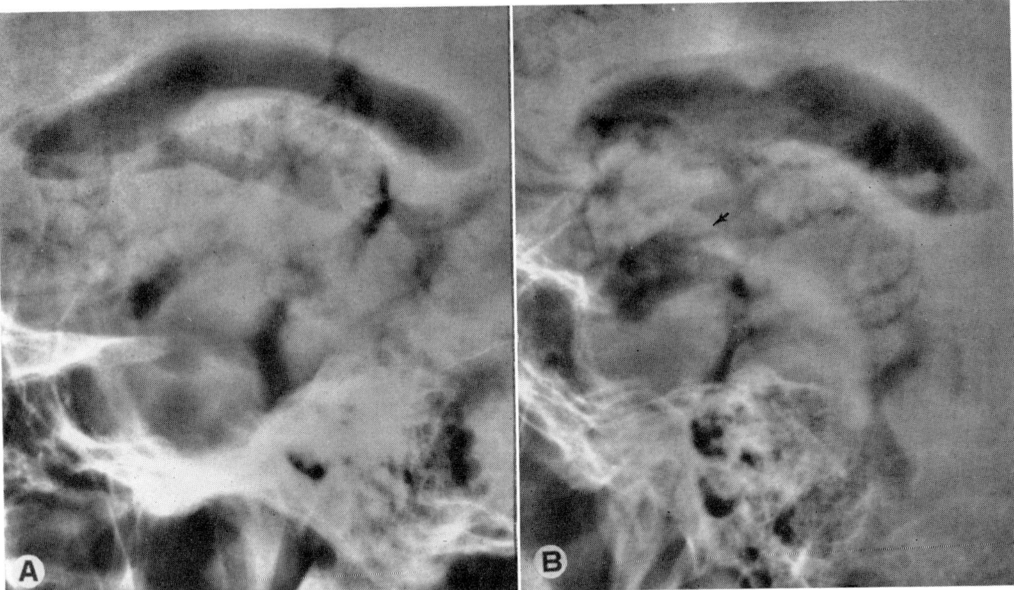

FIG. 328.—RETROSELLAR EXTENSION OF PITUITARY ADENOMA

A pituitary tumor, having a large suprasellar component, is shown in (A). The posterior inferior margin bulges into the cisterna interpeduncularis, displacing the brain stem slightly backward and widening the cisterna pontis, although measurements remain within normal limits. The entire third ventricle is elevated, with the greatest elevation anteriorly in the infraforaminal area, indicating that the greatest suprasellar extension is in this plane. Subarachnoid gas situated laterally is projected above the anterior clinoid processes but should not be mistaken for gas anterior to the tumor, a mistake that is avoided by stereoscopic examination.

In another case (B), there is more marked retrosellar extension inferiorly, apparently as a result of complete erosion of the dorsum and significant growth of the tumor backward into the posterior fossa cisterns. The brain stem is displaced backward, and there is backward bowing of the cerebral aqueduct and the floor of the fourth ventricle. The upward extent of the lesion is again shown by the anterior third ventricular deformity (*arrow*) and slight elevation of the floor of the anterior horn is shown. Gas situated laterally again is projected through the suprasellar region, which might give a false impression of the size of the neoplasm. A better impression of the true size of the suprasellar extension may be gained when smaller quantities of gas are used and directed in a manner which will outline the immediate perisellar region and the hypothalamic portion of the third ventricle (see Fig. 325).

and there may be backward displacement of the brain stem.

Occasional chromophobe pituitary adenomas grow predominantly *toward the side*, rather than upward. In these cases, the tumor spreads outward into the middle fossa and usually beneath the temporal lobe. Tumors in this area may attain appreciable size. Their presentation at pneumography, often ventriculography, is chiefly as a temporal or subtemporal mass (fig. 329). Elevation and deformity of the temporal horn is found; the third ventricle and floor of the lateral ventricular body are compressed on one side. In frontal view, the pneumogram may resemble the presentation of a thalamic tumor, except that the temporal horn is elevated infrequently by thalamic lesions. The lateral view, demonstrating elevation of the anterior portion of the temporal horn, usually defines the subtemporal location of the mass. Because ventriculography often is carried out with this group of adenomas, the subarachnoid cisterns ordinarily are not visualized. For this reason, correlation of the plain film findings in the region of the sella turcica with the ventricular changes is of increased importance for correct diagnosis.

(*Revised 1963*)

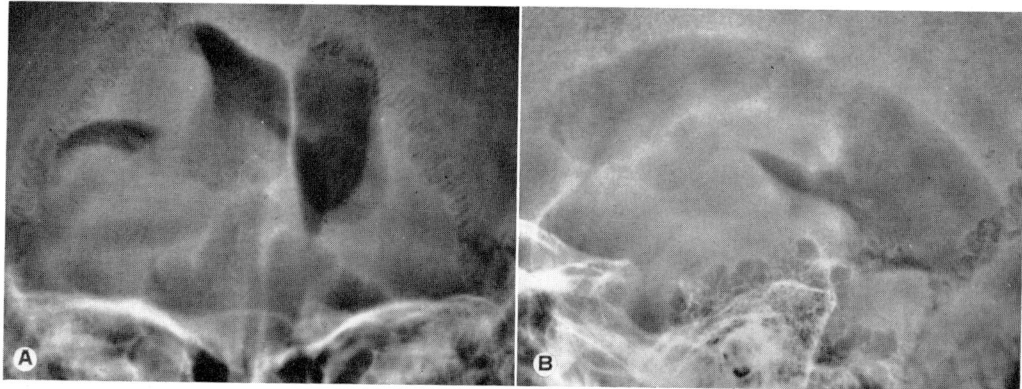

Fig. 329.—Pituitary Adenoma Beneath the Temporal Lobe

A large pituitary adenoma has grown predominantly into the middle fossa beneath the temporal lobe. The temporal horn is grossly elevated, as seen in frontal view (A); the floor of the lateral ventricle is elevated and displaced medially, and the lateral and third ventricles are dislocated toward the contralateral side. In the lateral view (B), the temporal horn is elevated throughout its length and tapers forward to a point of complete occlusion toward its tip in a plane just behind the sella turcica.

Additional hypophyseal lesions. As noted above, the majority of pituitary adenomas that extend outside of the sella turcica, and therefore are subjected to pneumography, are chromophobe tumors. By the time the normal portions of the gland are compressed sufficiently to produce endocrine deficiency detectable clinically, the tumor frequently has grown outside of the sella turcica. However, pituitary function usually is impaired prior to the development of visual changes. On the contrary, the active secretory nature of the cells involved in *eosinophilic adenomas* causes their early clinical recognition; only in the minority of instances is their size a problem. Occasionally they do become large, and there is a tendency to develop cystic changes which may add to their bulk. The majority, however, do not extend outside of the sella turcica. Eosinophilic adenomas may have a spontaneous arrest of growth, with regressive changes, including the development of calcification (fig. 160). In most instances, the sella turcica is more rounded or ballooned with eosinophilic adenoma than with chromophobe adenoma; erosion, on the other hand, is not often as prominent. Lack of erosive changes may be related to slow growth, or cessation of growth, but an enlarged sella turcica frequently is found with well mineralized boundaries (fig. 330). The diagnosis of eosinophilic adenoma is facilitated by the clinical presence of growth and other hormonal disturbances; the skull films which show the abnormal sella turcica also reveal frequently enlargement and elongation of the mandible. In the adult, acromegalic changes may be demonstrable in films of the hands, feet, vertebral column, and other bones.

Basophilic adenomas are almost always very small, often microscopic in size. Attention usually is called to their presence by the strong secretory activity of the cells. Any change in the appearance of the sella turcica usually is incidental to the generalized demineralization of the bones and not the result of pressure atrophy by tumor. Only rarely is a true basophilic tumor found which is large enough to erode the sella. The *mixed tumors* have been considered by some to be variants of eosinophilic adenomas.

Carcinoma of the pituitary may occur primarily, or may be the result of malignant metaplasia in a benign adenoma. One case that was encountered by the authors is thought to be an example of the latter form of origin, since in this instance the radiologic changes suggestive of a large benign pituitary adenoma were well developed (fig. 330). As might be expected, pituitary carcinoma is found in older patients and exhibits a rapid

(*Revised 1963*)

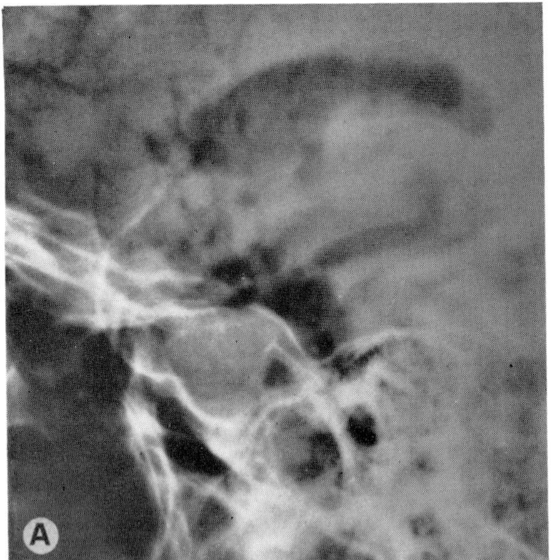

FIG. 330.—LESS COMMON TUMORS OF THE SPHENOID REGION

An eosinophilic pituitary adenoma has enlarged the sella turcica with considerable downward extension, but the basal cisterns and ventricular extensions are not deformed (A).

An adenocarcinoma of the pituitary gland (B) has produced extensive erosion of the basal bony structures and extended into the nasopharynx (*lower arrows*), from which a biopsy was obtained. Extensive intracranial extension also was present, including spread into the middle fossa on one side with elevation of one temporal horn (*upper arrow*).

A chordoma (C) has extensively destroyed the sella turcica and basisphenoid; fragments of sequestrated bone can be seen within the mass. The upward extent of the tumor is visible, owing to gas in the basal cisterns and anterior third ventricle (*anterior arrow*). There is also extensive retrosellar spread with backward displacement of the brain stem and posterior dislocation of the aqueduct (*upper posterior arrow*) and the fourth ventricle (*lower posterior arrow*).

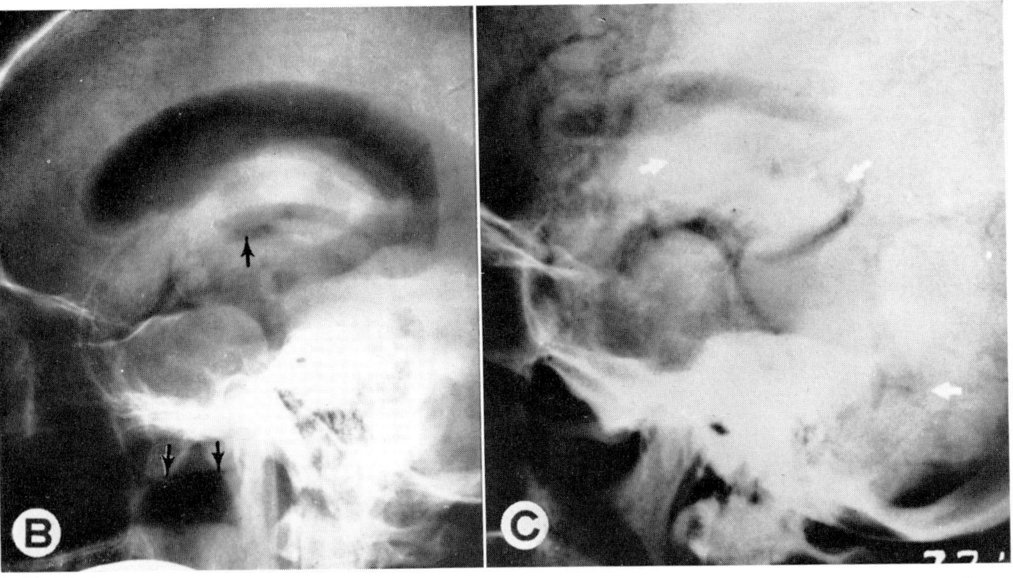

and often extensive growth. Local bone destruction usually is prominent. Extension into the nasopharynx led to the diagnosis in one case encountered by the authors. *Metastatic tumors* of the pituitary do not present a radiologically characteristic appearance. No changes may be present in some instances, while in others there may be diffuse destruction of the basisphenoid. In one case encountered, there was destruction of the pituitary gland by a blood-borne metastasis, and focal erosion of the dorsum sellae by an adjacent metastatic deposit in the bone. In some cases, there has been upward extension with a domelike soft tissue shadow projected above the sella turica in the pneumogram. In another patient, the third ventricle was elevated with blunting and deformity of the hypothalamic recesses; in this instance there was nothing to indicate the malignant nature of the lesion, and it could not be distinguished from a benign suprasellar tumor.

Craniopharyngioma

Rathke's pouch tumors (suprasellar cysts) are epithelial neoplasms arising from cellular remnants of the craniopharyngeal canal. Their pathology and general growth characteristics have been described earlier, since a high percentage (70 to 80 per cent) of such tumors contain calcium. The majority of patients develop clinical manifestations in childhood, although the authors have encountered one patient who had an onset of symptoms at the age of 62 years.

As in the case of pituitary adenoma, the plain film appearance of the sella turcica may be an important part of radiologic diagnosis; bony changes and the nature of pathologic calcifications, when present, strongly complement the pneumographic findings for correct identification of the lesion. Some craniopharyngiomas have a significant intrasellar component, or even grow entirely within the sella turcica. In such instances, identification may depend largely on the presence of calcium. More characteristically, however, the lesions are suprasellar cysts with only a rudimentary attachment in the pituitary fossa. Under these circumstances, sellar changes result from direct pressure by the contiguous neoplasm. The clinoid processes, particularly the posterior clinoids, often are poorly developed and the dorsum is short. The entire sella turcica often is shallow; in some instances, there may be thinning or depression of the sellar floor (figs. 158 and 331). In many cases the mineral content of the sella turcica appears to be well preserved, suggesting a maldevelopment rather than pressure erosion, possibly as a result of the long standing presence of the tumor. In other patients, particularly those with obstruction at the foramen of Monro, there may be sellar changes indicating generalized increased intracranial pressure.

(Revised 1963)

In the average case, the lateral pneumogram will reveal obliteration of the main suprasellar cistern and the prechiasmatic space; the hypothalamus usually is invaginated. Tumors of small size are not often examined by pneumography; frequently the masses are enormous when the patients are first seen. Cisternal gas usually outlines only the dorsal aspect of the tumor, which frequently is well defined along its posterior convexity (fig. 333). The posterior margin of the tumor may extend backward and upward from the top of the sella turcica into the cisterna interpeduncularis to obliterate the anterior portion of the cistern. Deformity of the third ventricle usually is smooth and sharp, because gas in the anterior part of the third ventricle outlines the superior convexity of the tumor through only a thin mantle of interposed hypothalamic tissue. By means of visualization of the superior surface of the mass by third ventricular gas, of the posterior surface by subarachnoid gas, and delimitation of the inferior aspect by the sella turcica, a reasonably accurate impression of the size of the lesion is afforded at pneumography (fig. 332).

In many instances, the tumor not only obliterates part or all of the hypothalamic portion of the third ventricle, but also produces an indentation of the inferior margins of the frontal horns. The deformity resembles that found with pituitary adenomas which grow upward and forward; it is seen much more frequently with cystic craniopharyngiomas because the tumors often are of such large size. In approximately one-third of patients, there is a sufficient increase in intracranial pressure to require ventriculography rather than pneumoencephalography; hypertension usually is caused by an obstruction at the foramen of Monro.

In the frontal pneumograms, the normal midline slitlike configuration of the anterior part of the third ventricle usually is not seen, because the hypothalamic portion is compressed and obliterated. In some cases, however, the hypothalamus is not elevated, but displaced laterally by tumors which grow predominantly to one side of the midline. Under these circumstances, the anterior portion of the third ventricle may be dis-

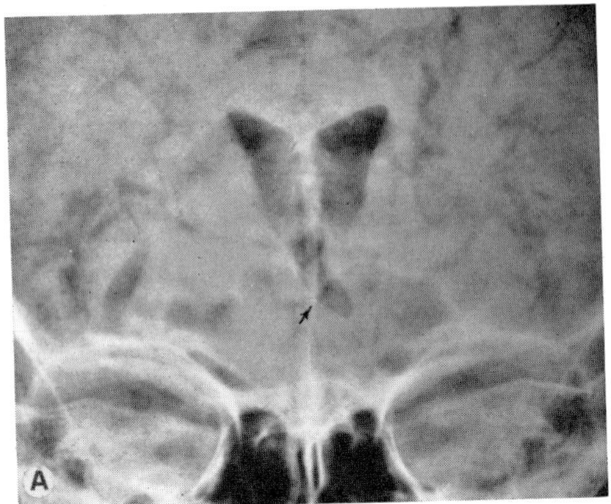

Fig. 331.—Optic Glioma and Craniopharyngioma.

The hypothalamic portion of the third ventricle has deviated sharply from its midline position (*arrow*) in a frontal pneumogram made with the patient supine in this case of optic glioma involving the chiasm. (A).

(B) and (C) are a craniopharyngioma. Through a burr hole made near the pterion, a large cystic craniopharyngioma was tapped and Thorotrast was injected. The extent of the lesion in frontal view (B) is shown by a curvilinear shadow of opaque material outlining the cyst wall (*arrows*). The mass projects well upward but predominantly to one side of the midline. Both the frontal and lateral (C) projections show a dense collection of contrast material which has passed from the cyst into the sella turcica where the lesion is rooted. Contrast material has also escaped into the subarachnoid space.

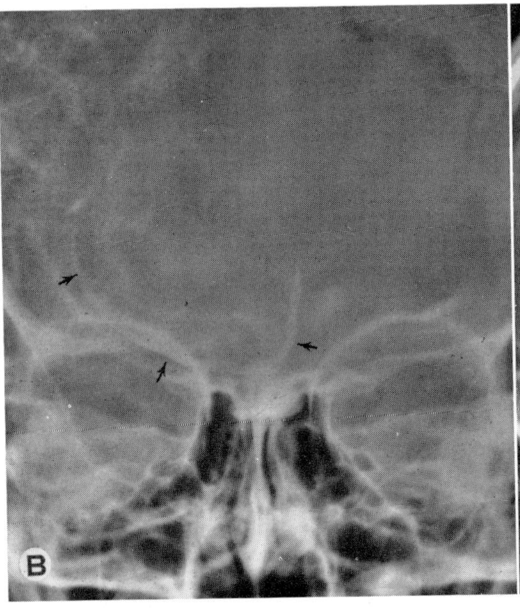

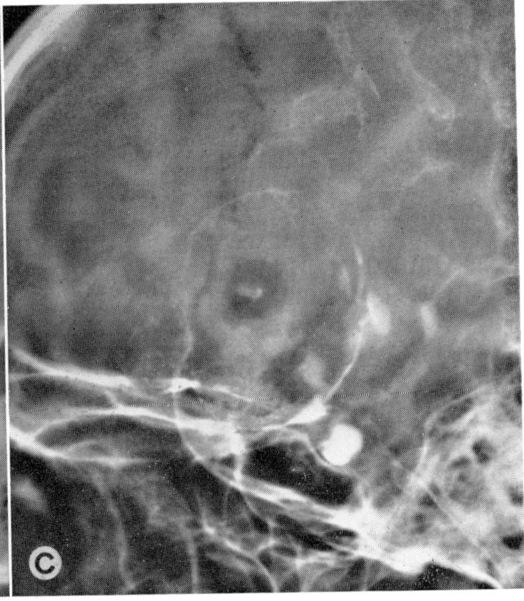

located to one side, narrowed, but not occluded. Owing to elevation of the floor of the anterior horn medially, the inferior medial angle of the horn is deformed. In most cases, the shape of the floor of each anterior horn is fairly symmetrical, since the suprasellar mass usually is central. Symmetry of the lateral ventricular deformity, as seen in frontal films, usually is a point in favor of the diagnosis of craniopharyngioma (fig. 333). On the other hand, many of the cases described by Davidoff and Epstein (1950) had asymmetrical dilatation of the lateral ventricles; the authors also illustrated a case in which a craniopharyngioma extended into one of the lateral ventricles, and could not be distinguished from an intraventricular tumor.

Suprasellar *midline epidermoid cysts* are not rare. Pathologically they are often called craniopharyngiomas, although they do not seem to have the usual intrasellar connections of craniopharyngiomas and can be

(Revised 1963)

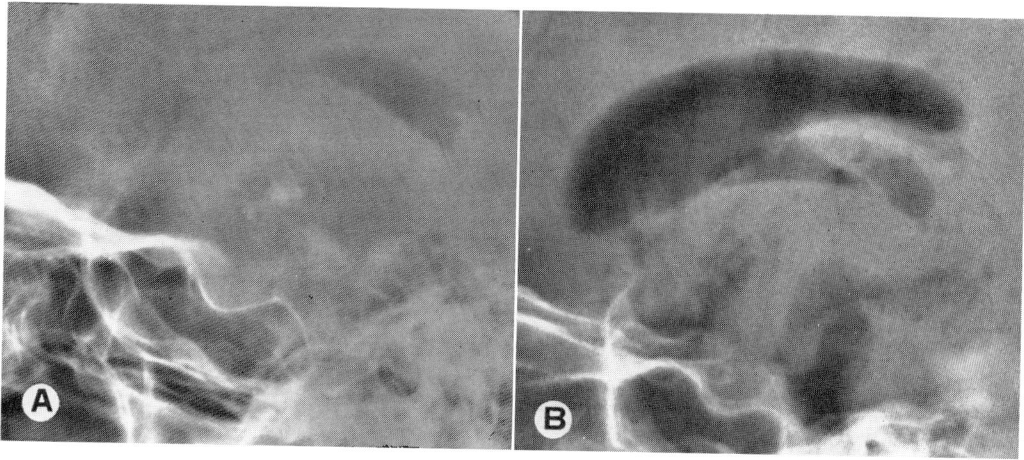

FIG. 332.—CRANIOPHARYNGIOMA

Films made after the installation of a small amount of gas shows satisfactorily the extent of a partially calcified suprasellar tumor (A); the gas outline of the third ventricle, which is encroached upon inferiorly to a marked degree, is unobscured by other gas shadows. In another case (B), a somewhat similar deformity of the third ventricle is present. Gas in the subarachnoid space lateral to the anterior and posterior margins of the lesion suggests that the tumor has a mushroom rather than a globular configuration. While craniopharyngiomas can extend through the suprasellar area on a stalk, this feature is not ordinarily demonstrated by pneumography.

completely removed surgically. The majority are located just above the dorsum sellae, and the sella turcica usually is normal in appearance.

Aneurysm

Saccular aneurysms of the internal carotid artery, arising either from the cavernous portion or from the immediately supraclinoid portion of the main trunk, may attain considerable size. Such lesions frequently present as perisellar masses. The supraclinoid aneurysms of the main carotid trunk characteristically grow backward and a surprising number are found to occupy a midline position immediately above the sella turcica (figs. 163 and 334). Aneurysms arising at the points of origin of branch vessels do not very often attain sufficient size to present as tumors. While aneurysms are almost always readily identified by angiography, it happens not infrequently that pneumography is performed first, because a suprasellar aneurysm may simulate clinically a pituitary adenoma, craniopharyngioma, meningioma or other perisellar neoplasm. A saccular aneurysm must always be considered in the differential diagnosis when a suprasellar mass is found at pneumography; from time to time, diffuse dilatation and elongation of the carotid siphon owing to atherosclerosis may cause filling defects in the basal cisterns.

Aneurysms of the cavernous portion of the carotid artery often cause changes on plain films that suggest the nature of the lesion and help in choosing the correct contrast procedure, angiography, for confirmation of the diagnosis. Erosion of the sphenoid bone is the change most commonly encountered, especially a unilateral destruction of the sella turcica. The posterior clinoid processes and dorsum sellae are affected in the great majority of patients, perhaps as high as 90 per cent (fig. 572). Ipsilateral erosion of an anterior clinoid process along the medial side is seen with almost equal frequency (fig. 89); the anterior clinoid may be short and pointed and even "elevated" in some cases. Destruction of the sella floor simulating the double floor occurring with a pituitary adenoma is unusual. Widening of the superior orbital fissure is found in three-fourths of the cases, and erosion of the inferior and lateral wall of the optic canal is often seen in special films of this structure.

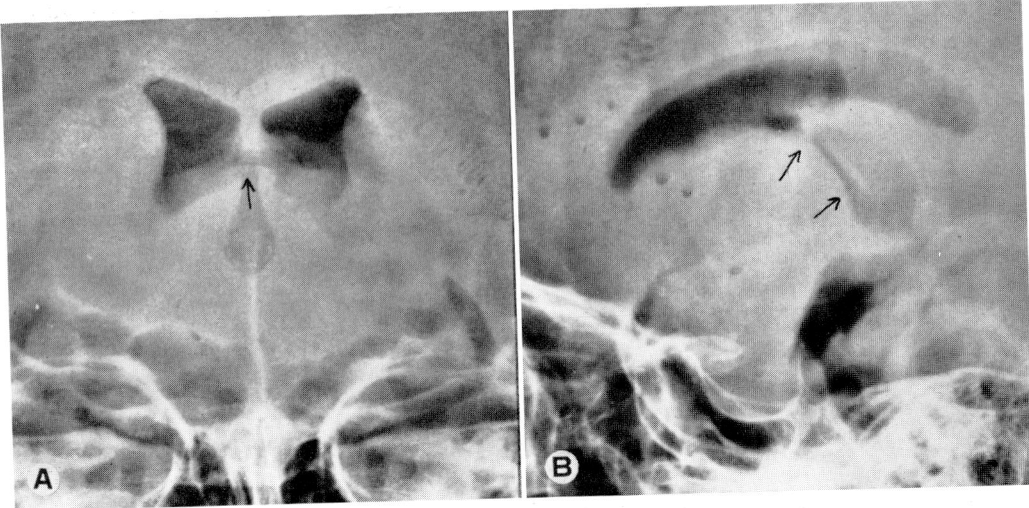

FIG. 333.—CRANIOPHARYNGIOMA

A large mass has extended upward to compress the ventral aspects of the anterior horns (A). The lesion is essentially midline, with the dome of the mass well shown (*arrow*), as contrasted with the case shown in Fig. 331. Only the posterior portion of the third ventricle is visualized in the frontal film, even with the patient supine. The lateral view, also made supine (B), shows that the third ventricle is obliterated from its anterior extremity to its midportion (*arrows*).

In somewhat less than half of all patients with a cavernous aneurysm, calcification is visible in the wall of the lesion on plain film examination (fig. 164).

Pneumoencephalography serves to demonstrate the presence of a mass, and to reveal its size, in cases of suprasellar aneurysm. The smoothly rounded configuration is the most characteristic feature of an aneurysm at pneumography; the appearance is not diagnostic, however, since smoothness and roundness may be seen with craniopharyngioma, meningioma, and pituitary adenoma. The main suprasellar cistern usually is obliterated. The posterior aspect of the mass may be defined by subarachnoid gas in the cisterna interpeduncularis. Occasionally, a small amount of gas may be present in a partially preserved prechiasmatic portion of the suprasellar cistern, to determine the anterior extent of the lesion. Superiorly, the aneurysm often invaginates the hypothalamus, as do other lesions extending into this area; it may present as a smoothly rounded, superiorly convex deformity of the hypothalamic portion of the third ventricle (fig. 334). Larger lesions deform the inferior aspects of the frontal horns; one unusual aneurysm seen by the authors presented as a colossal mass between the frontal lobes of the brain (fig. 162).

In the average case, an aneurysm does not obstruct the foramen of Monro, but it may interfere with the anterior circulation of cerebrospinal fluid in the subarachnoid space. It is stated by most authors that enlargement of the lateral ventricles does not occur with aneurysm. We have noted, however, that often in the absence of obstruction, there may be ipsilateral ventricular enlargement, apparently owing to atrophy. In some instances, there is corresponding enlargement of the cerebral sulci. The degree of atrophy varies greatly, but significant changes may be seen even with small aneurysms that clinically have not bled.

Meningioma

Meningeal tumors arising along the superior surface of the sphenoid bone may exert pressure on the optic pathways when they are still relatively small. The majority of such tumors arise in the region of the planum sphenoidale and some may grow principally backward. Meningeal tumors also arise from the diaphragma sellae. Tumors

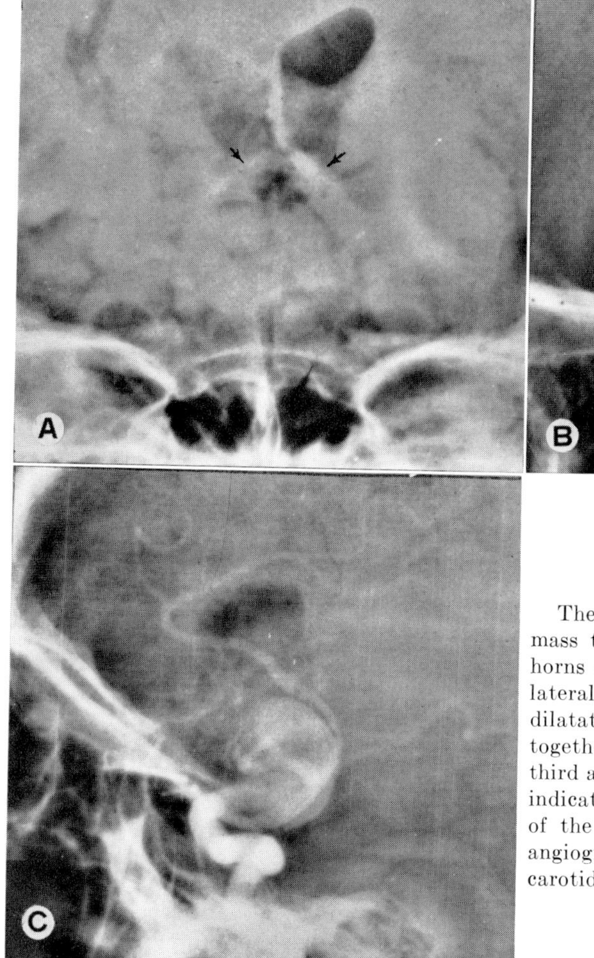
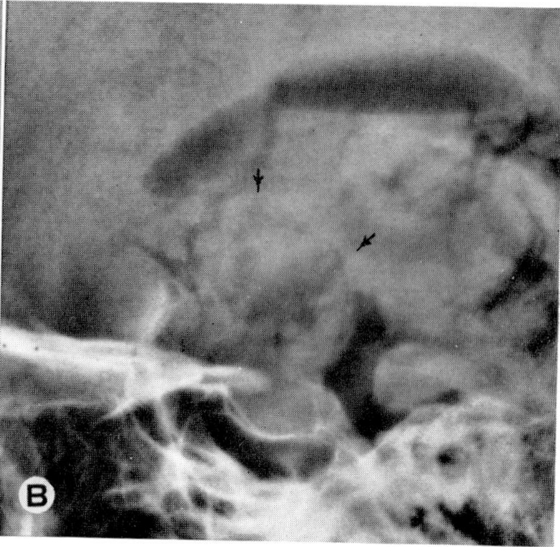

Fig. 334.—Suprasellar Aneurysm

The pneumograms reveal an essentially midline mass that elevates and compresses the anterior horns (*arrows*) on their ventral aspects (A). The lateral pneumogram (B) reveals obstruction and dilatation of the interpeduncular cistern which, together with gas in the anterior portions of the third and lateral ventricles (*arrows*), gives a good indication of the extent of the mass. The nature of the lesion, however, is revealed only in the angiogram (C), in which a large aneurysm of the carotid artery is disclosed.

arising in this region often are referred to also as tuberculum sellae meningiomas.

Changes may be found in plain films consisting of hyperostosis and "blistering" in the region of the planum (fig. 144). Calcification may be present in the tumor itself; in some cases, the calcification represents only a small portion of the mass, while in others essentially the entire lesion is calcified (fig. 148). The extent of damage to the sella turcica is variable and pituitary insufficiency usually is absent. The tumors not infrequently produce a partial blockage of cerebrospinal fluid circulation in the subarachnoid space; intracranial hypertension of low grade may be present for a long period of time and then pressure atrophy of the sella turcica often is evident. In some instances, the anterior clinoid processes appear short and the pituitary fossa may be shallow, a finding somewhat similar to that occurring with craniopharyngioma.

In the pneumoencephalogram, suprasellar meningiomas appear as oval or rounded masses, varying greatly in size; the majority are relatively small, because visual disturbances are produced early. Some meningiomas of the planum sphenoidale present as global masses that measure several centimeters in diameter and resemble the tumors that occur further forward in the region of the olfactory groove. In the average case, the basal cisterns are visualized but are deformed, particularly the prechiasmatic portion of the

(*Revised 1963*)

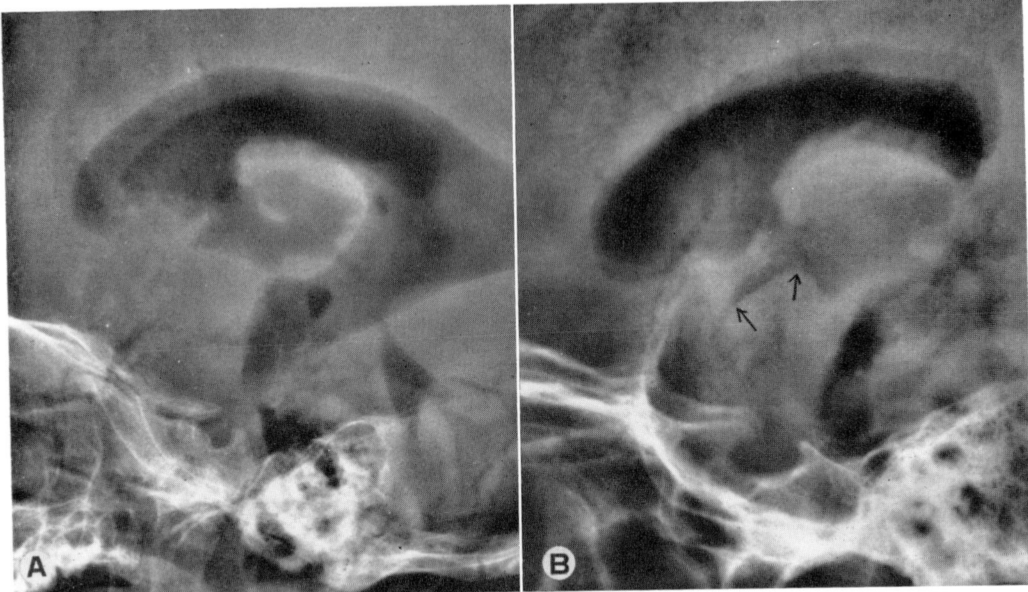

FIG. 335.—OPTIC CHIASM GLIOMA

A large mass is present above the sella turcica, which has elevated the third ventricle and obliterated its hypothalamic extension. The sella turcica has a J, gourd, or mandolin shape, a configuration that is encountered in some young patients with optic glioma. At operation, a large spongioblastoma was found, the tissue type most commonly present in optic glioma. (Courtesy of Dr. Everett Hurteau, Akron, Ohio.)

In another case (B), an optic glioma occurring in an older child has invaginated the third ventricle in an uneven manner (*arrows*).

suprasellar cistern. The posterior margin of the lesion may cover the suprasellar area, encroaching upon the postchiasmatic space and occasionally extending slightly behind the posterior clinoids into the cisterna interpeduncularis. The posterior margin usually is convex backward, but may not be as smooth as in the case of the cystic and aneurysmal masses occurring in this region. When still small, the tumors deform the hypothalamic portion of the third ventricle by elevation and indentation; further growth often is more to one side of the midline than central. Some tumors encroach primarily upon the anterior aspect of the third ventricle, displacing it backward and indenting the anterior portion in the region of the lamina terminalis. In such instances, the prechiasmatic space and cisterna lamina terminalis are not visualized. The parolfactory spaces, if visible on the pneumoencephalogram, can be distorted by any midline mass just anterior to the sella. When such forward extending meningiomas become very large, they then are indistinguishable from the subfrontal tumors of the olfactory groove (fig. 273).

Optic Glioma

Primary glial tumors of the optic chiasm, optic nerves, or optic tracts are found chiefly in young patients, principally children. It has been suggested by some that the tumors develop prior to birth, although they often do not clinically manifest themselves until later; some of the bony changes are most consistent with alterations during the formative period of the base of the skull (Dyke, 1941). On the other hand, the visual loss produced is often rapidly progressive and it seems probable that the tumor growth is no different from other neoplasms of similar histologic type. The optic gliomas usually are astrocytomas of the unipolar spongioblastic

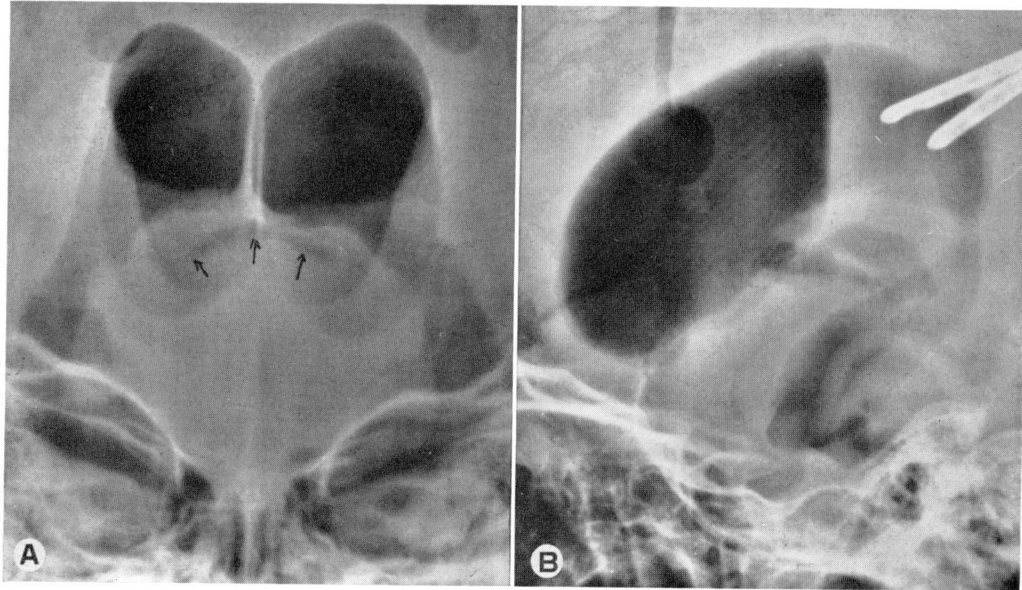

FIG. 336.—OPTIC GLIOMA

A tumor of the optic chiasm and nerves presents as a symmetrical midline lesion in frontal view (A) elevating the gas shadow of the superior portion of the third ventricle (*arrows*). The lateral film (B) reveals the hypothalamic area to be occluded with the dome of the tumor presenting at the dilated foramen of Monro. The lateral film shown was made following operation, at which time only a biopsy of the tumor was carried out, revealing it to be a spongioblastoma. The child, who was almost completely blind at the time of the ventriculogram, regained essentially normal vision following radiation therapy.

variety. In the majority of instances, the tumors remain confined to the optic pathways, even when they attain large size (fig. 335); some optic gliomas produce obstruction of the foramen of Monro (fig. 336).

In pneumograms, optic gliomas ordinarily present no distinguishing features which are of great aid in diagnosis. The changes are those commonly encountered with other suprasellar tumors. The prechiasmatic area is almost always obliterated, and frequently there is a soft tissue mass invading or occluding the main suprasellar cistern. There may be encroachment upon the cisterna interpeduncularis. The anterior portion of the third ventricle is deformed, as a result of invagination of the hypothalamus by the tumor. A significant number of patients are examined by ventriculography, because it is not rare for the lesions to produce some degree of ventricular obstruction, usually at the foramen of Monro. In these instances, a large part of the third ventricle will be compressed and obliterated, and there may be an inferior indentation of the anterio horns (fig. 336).

The correct diagnosis may not be suspected clinically if the tumor has not advanced along one or both optic nerves to be visible in the nerve head by funduscopic examination. Plain films often give the most important clues to diagnosis. Many years ago (1923), Martin and Cushing reviewed a group of cases of optic glioma and emphasized the gourd-shaped or pear-shaped sella turcica commonly found. It is recognized also that this is not a rare appearance of the sella turcica in young children, and it is not always associated with disease. When seen, however, the possibility of optic glioma should be considered, and the presence of such a lesion excluded by clinical and further radiologic examination, as required. Enlargement of one or both optic foramina occurs in a high percentage of patients; calcification is not a feature of optic glioma. Whenever possible, it is important to make

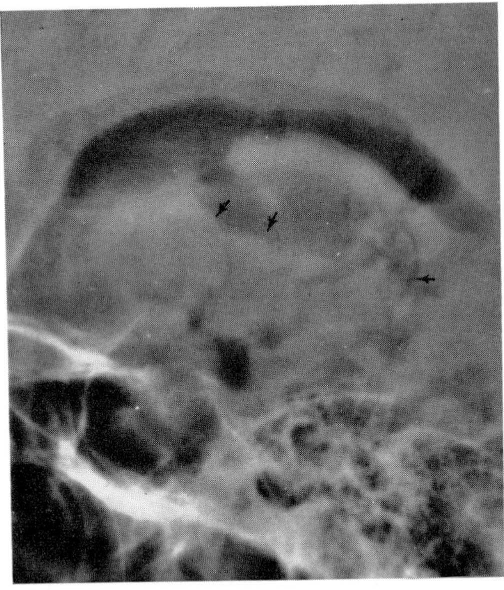

FIG. 337.—HYPOTHALAMIC GLIOMA

A primary glioma of the hypothalamus has compressed and occluded the anterior portions of the third ventricle. The lobular superior surface of the tumor presenting in the ventricle is sharply delineated (*anterior arrows*). The glioma, which originated in the hypothalamus, is extending into the thalamus, predominantly on one side; the retrothalamic extension of the quadrigeminal cistern is displaced backward unilaterally (*posterior arrow*).

the correct diagnosis early; many of the tumors are remarkably radiosensitive, and complete restoration of vision may occur following radiation therapy.

Other Tumors

In addition to the five more common types of suprasellar tumors that have been described in this section, several other neoplasms may be encountered occasionally. These include chordomas and other tumors arising from the bony floor of the skull, epidermoid tumors, ependymomas, metastatic tumors, and tumors of the hypothalamic portion of the third ventricle. *Chordomas* occur more characteristically in the retrosellar region along the clivus, and have been considered in connection with prepontine tumors. They may occur, however, along the midline as far forward as the olfactory groove and are encountered in the suprasellar and parasellar regions. Basal erosion of the skull and the incorporation of sequestrated bone in the tumor substance are findings of importance for diagnosis (fig. 330).

It is important not to mistake one or a combination of the numerous normal structures occurring in the suprasellar cisterns for a tumor. The carotid siphon in some instances may interfere with complete filling of the suprasellar subarachnoid space, and a false impression of an extraneous mass in this region may result. An elongated tortuous basilar artery not infrequently produces incomplete filling of the cisterna interpeduncularis; the artery also produces an indentation of the posterior part of the third ventricle, owing to elevation of the floor. The deformity may resemble changes resulting from either a suprasellar or retrosellar tumor.

Hypothalamic tumors must be considered in the differential diagnosis of suprasellar neoplasms. The majority of the tumors are gliomas arising in the thalamus or hypothalamus, which form the side walls of the third ventricle. Some arise from the third ventricular floor, particularly in the region of the tuber cinereum. As with the optic gliomas, the majority are astrocytomas and some may be of the unipolar spongioblastic variety and may be cystic. An occasional hypothalamic granuloma may be encountered and the authors have seen such a case in a patient with diffuse reticuloendotheliosis—probably of the Hand-Schüller-Christian type. Ordinarily, however, the lesions in this area, associated with Hand-Schüller-Christian disease and diabetes insipidus, are not demonstrable on pneumoencephalography.

Hypothalamic gliomas that grow downward must be differentiated from other suprasellar masses at pneumoencephalography. The gliomas encroach upon the main suprasellar cistern from above, and the margin of the tumor may be visible projecting into the cisterna interpeduncularis. The hypothalamic tumors tend to extend more posteriorly than into the anterior cisternal regions; often the prechiasmatic spaces are preserved.

Hypothalamic tumors are a diagnostic problem at pneumography more often owing to upward extension and obstruction at the foramen of Monro than in connection with their infrequent suprasellar extension. The majority of tumors of this type are examined by ventriculography, since there is obstruction to the flow of cerebrospinal fluid through the third ventricle. In many cases, there are sella turcica changes resulting from generalized increased intracranial pressure or a direct pressure effect upon the sella turcica by the tumor. In some instances there is complete obstruction at the foramen of Monro, and the tumor may extend into a lateral ventricle. Under these circumstances, there may be some difficulty in differentiating a hypothalamic tumor from a colloid cyst. In the typical case of colloid cyst, the differentiation is made by the presence of an oval cystic mass, which is sharply outlined in more than 75 per cent of patients. When a hypothalamic glioma protrudes into a lateral ventricle, it usually presents an irregular configuration, often multilobular; failure of gas to pass anterior to the tumor and into the forward portion of the third ventricle is commonplace with a glioma, but unusual in the case of a colloid cyst.

When the foramen of Monro is patent, the anterior portion of the third ventricle, and sometimes the greater portion of the third ventricle, does not fill with gas when a hypothalamic glioma is present. Gas in the ventricle may outline the irregular margin of a hypothalamic mass (fig. 337). In some instances, only the anterior inferior portion of the third ventricle does not distend well. Tumors arising slightly higher, along the lateral wall of the third ventricle but not strictly hypothalamic, displace rather than occlude the third ventricle. The distance of a new growth from the lateral wall of the third ventricular cavity will determine whether the lumen is occluded early or late in the growth of the neoplasm.

Of the various suprasellar tumors described, the pituitary adenoma is encountered most commonly; it also is the tumor which most often is accompanied by characteristic plain skull and pneumographic changes. In the majority of instances, a craniopharyngioma is identified by its calcification and its growth characteristics as seen in pneumograms are usually different from those of a pituitary adenoma. On the contrary, pneumographic differentiation of craniopharyngioma, aneurysm, meningioma, optic glioma, and some of the less common tumors occurring in this region is more difficult. Plain film changes are relied upon heavily to provide a high degree of diagnostic accuracy. Pneumoencephalography is the procedure of choice for the diagnosis of the average suprasellar tumor; ventriculography, although less informative, is necessitated in some instances. Reliance on angiography alone is increasing, but the authors consider angiography to be complementary to pneumoencephalography, its greatest usefulness in cases of extra-axial suprasellar tumors being for the identification of aneurysms.

ANGIOGRAPHY

Egas Moniz was not only the originator of carotid angiography, but with his colleagues, Almeida Lima and others, he laid down the anatomic and pathologic foundations of the method.

At a history making soire of the Neurological Society of Paris in 1927, he described in detail his successes and also his earlier failures in attempting to opacify the brain and the carotid blood vessels. In the beginning Moniz used percutaneous puncture for injection of the carotid artery, but his extensive clinical success was with the open method, following exposure of the artery in the neck after a skin incision. The technique of percutaneous carotid angiography, using Thorotrast, was introduced by Loman and Myerson of Boston in 1936. In Europe, Shimidzu (1937) described his experience with the percutaneous method, using water soluble as well as colloidal contrast media; at the same time he recommended techniques of injecting the vertebral and subclavian arteries. For the current popularity of carotid angiography, however, credit is due to the Scandinavian school for establishing percutaneous carotid puncture, employing water soluble contrast media, as a more or less routine radiologic procedure (Engeset, 1944). Many techniques of carotid and vertebral angiography involving percutaneous arterial puncture, are now in wide use and today it is only infrequently that direct exposure of the vessel is required.

Contrast Media

The search for the ideal contrast medium for all angiography and particularly for cerebral angiography still continues. In his initial trials Moniz used strontium bromide but soon changed to sodium iodide which was employed for several years. In 1931 Moniz and Lima began to use Thorotrast, which is a 25 per cent colloidal suspension of thorium dioxide. This is a good medium because it is nonirritating to the endothelium of the vessels. Unfortunately, it is slightly radioactive and, being a colloidal suspension, it is picked up by the cells of the reticuloendothelial system where it is permanently fixed. Cases of hepatoma and of bone sarcoma have been reported many years after the administration of Thorotrast. In addition, if extravasation of this substance outside of the arteries in the neck takes place, considerable fibrosis results, causing pain that is often disabling to the patient. Soft tissue sarcomas have also been observed in the area of a long-standing Thorotrast granuloma.

Diodrast (35 per cent) was used for many years to perform cerebral angiography with satisfactory results. Later 30 per cent Urokon was tried with almost equally satisfactory results. In the 1950's the diatrizoate drugs (Hypaque and Renografin) became available, and these have been found to be preferable to the earlier drugs. Hypaque and Renografin are slightly more viscous than Diodrast or Urokon; Renografin is more viscous than Hypaque because it has a significant percentage of the methylglutamine salt, but for cerebral angiography, this is not a disadvantage. By warming the solutions, the viscosity is decreased. Fifty per cent Hypaque and sixty per cent Renografin both have been used extensively at the Neurological Institute. The latter drug has been found to be slightly better in that it produces less head pain during the injection. Broadridge and Leslie (1958) found few differences in 60 cases where one side was performed with Hypaque and the other was examined with Renografin. Twenty-three patients found the media equal, 24 preferred Renografin, and 13 preferred Hypaque. Broman and Olsson (1949) and Basset *et al.* (1953) found that the fundamental effect on the cerebral circulatory system is one of alteration of the endothelial capillary membrane or the blood brain barrier. The extent of the change is proportional to the concentration of the test substance in contact with the capillary endothelium, and the time during which the application prevails. They have found that repeated fractional doses have a cumulative effect which is enhanced if the interval between the individual injections is too short. Broman, Forssman, and Olsson (1950) found that the damage to the endothelium of the vessels is increased not only by repeating injections, but also by retarding the circulation in the brain which tends to prolong the application time. In addition, latent vascular disease of the brain may be aggravated and may become manifest by the injection of a contrast medium. The alteration of the vessel walls leads to an increase in their permeability which breaks down the "blood brain barrier."

At least some of the injurious effects of these contrast substances are due to their hypertonicity. Some of the physiologic effects of Diodrast have been produced experimentally in animals by hypertonic saline solution (Weatherall, 1942). Kagstrom *et al.* (1960) have demonstrated an increase in cerebral blood flow consistently after the injection of these contrast substances. The effect is most marked with compounds of the acetrizoate type (Urokon). The drugs of the diatrizoate type (Hypaque) produced only moderate increase. There was 2 to 4 times greater increase in blood flow in cats when the former compounds were used as compared with the latter ones. Moreover, the duration was 12 minutes in the former on the average, as against 2 minutes when the latter compounds were used. They also found that sodium diprotrizoate (Miokon) had the same effects as the diatrizoate drugs. There appears to be agreement that the injection of contrast substances is followed by a vasodilatation lasting a variable period of time, although some contradictory opinions have appeared in the literature.

Technique

A painstaking technique is most important in obtaining the optimum results in cerebral angiography. To obtain examinations of consistent and superior quality requires the services of a radiologist particularly interested in neuroradiologic problems. It is probably best for the neuroradiologist to carry on the entire procedure, including the insertion of the needle, the taking of the proper radiographs, the modifications of the technique which become necessary in the course of the examination, and the interpretation of the films. This has been done for many years in many centers in Europe and this fact may be considered responsible for the superiority of the technical developments of the past years in Europe as compared to the United States. The production of superior radiographs under all circumstances must be based on a thorough knowledge of all of the factors involved. It cannot be expected that a clinician who is not trained in this field could solve these problems under all manner of difficult circumstances encountered during examinations. It is not necessary for the neuroradiologist to insert the needle himself, but he must supervise every phase of the examination. Therefore it seems wasteful of manpower to have a second person just to insert the needle, and this method is only justifiable when other physicians are being trained to perform these procedures.

CAROTID ANGIOGRAPHY

Preparation of the Patient

The patient should be psychologically prepared to undergo the examination. It is usually advantageous to see the patient the day before the examination and explain part of what will be done. On the day of the examination, before the injection is made (but after the insertion of the needle), it is helpful to explain to the patient that he may have head pain or a hot feeling in the face or behind the eyes at the time the injection is made, but that it will only last a few fleeting seconds. The patient should be premedicated lightly for the examination. We advocate simple barbiturates and atropine; others add scopolamine. Demerol in an average dose of 50 mg. may be used about 30 minutes before the examination, particularly in apprehensive patients. Intravenous Demerol in doses of 10 mg. is used occasionally during the examination, particularly in extremely apprehensive patients. Demerol may be injected into the tube of a constant intravenous drip. In children and in some extremely nervous patients, it is necessary to use general anesthesia. In children it is necessary to use endotracheal anesthesia. A morphine analogue (phenazocine) has been proposed by some (Sugar, 1961). This material is given intravenously and causes the patients to be quiet, to sleep, and to recall virtually nothing of the procedure. Unfortunately, it produces depression of the respiratory center.

More recently all diagnostic procedures in infants and children have been performed under sedation without general anesthesia. For this purpose a combination of sodium Seconal, Thorazine, Demerol, and atropine at dosage levels to be varied according to the age and weight of the child is recommended. For a child up to 4 years of age the dosage

(*Revised 1963*)

levels have been 8 to 10 mg. of Seconal per kg., 1.5 mg. of Thorazine per kg., 1.5 mg. of Demerol per kg., and 0.1 to 0.2 mg. of atropine. From 4 to 8 years of age the dosage has been 6 to 8 mg. of Seconal per kg., 1.0 mg. of Thorazine per kg., 1.0 mg. of Demerol per kg., and 0.3 mg. of atropine. Over 8 years the dosage levels have been 4 to 6 mg. of Seconal per kg., 0.75 of Thorazine per kg., 0.75 mg. of Demerol per kg., and 0.4 mg. of atropine. The medication is usually given one hour before the beginning of the examination. The basic medication has to be varied somewhat depending upon the case; usually Demerol is not employed for pneumoencephalography but is used for cerebral angiography. More medication may be added if necessary. Usually a small amount of intravenous sodium Seconal (10 mg.) may quiet the child if he does not seem to be sufficiently well sedated.

It has not been our custom to use antihistaminics prior to the examination, although it has been pointed out that this may decrease or eliminate the possibility of allergic reactions from the contrast substances. Intravenous and intradermal test injections of contrast substance are used prior to the examination and if the patient shows a marked sensitivity, the procedure is cancelled or, in older individuals, Thorotrast (thorium dioxide) is used. One-tenth of a cubic centimeter of contrast substance is injected intradermally, and if a wheal of 1 cm. in diameter forms and persists, the test reaction is considered positive. Simple reddening without a papule is not considered significant. One cubic centimeter of contrast substance is injected intravenously and if the patient shows urticarial wheals or nausea and vomiting, the test reaction is considered positive. In one case of an older child who presented evidences of a positive reaction to the test with the contrast substance, it was decided to perform the examination because it was considered essential (the patient had an arteriovenous malformation), and because the patient was a child, it was not considered wise to use Thorotrast. Simultaneous anteroposterior and lateral serialograms were made, and only a single injection of contrast substance of 8 cc. was necessary. The patient developed respiratory difficulties which were thought to be due to laryngeal edema, but recovered. Other than this one, no "allergic" reaction to the drug has been encountered in our practice, but it has been our custom not to perform the procedure with that substance. Rather we use another iodine contrast agent or Thorotrast when the initial tests are positive.

Positioning of the Patient

The patient is placed in the supine position on a well padded table. The head is extended and placed over a very thin pad of foam rubber or polyurethane, preferably the latter to prevent any shadows on the x-ray films. An inflatable rubber bag is placed under the patient's shoulders; this bag can be inflated at will to elevate the shoulders and increase the extension of the head (fig. 338). By elevating the shoulders with a rubber bag it becomes unnecessary to move the patient later in order to remove the pillows or sandbags that might be used for the same purpose. Excessive extension of the head should be avoided because it tends to make the feeling of pulsations of the artery more difficult. The elevation of the chin beyond that which is produced by simple extension of the head should be avoided because this tends to make the skin taut and to stretch the platysma. Once the head is extended by dropping it to a level lower than the shoulders, further extension of the chin upward does not help in stretching and fixing the carotid artery. A strap is placed across the patient's knees, which are slightly flexed over a pillow, and both wrists are fixed by padded straps to prevent motion of the extremities at an inconvenient time.

Insertion of the Needle

The skin is first prepared with local antiseptic and towels are draped over the lower portion of the neck below the site of puncture. Local anesthesia is performed by injecting a small amount (1 cc.) of 2 per cent procaine intradermally; the subcutaneous tissues and the deeper tissues are infiltrated

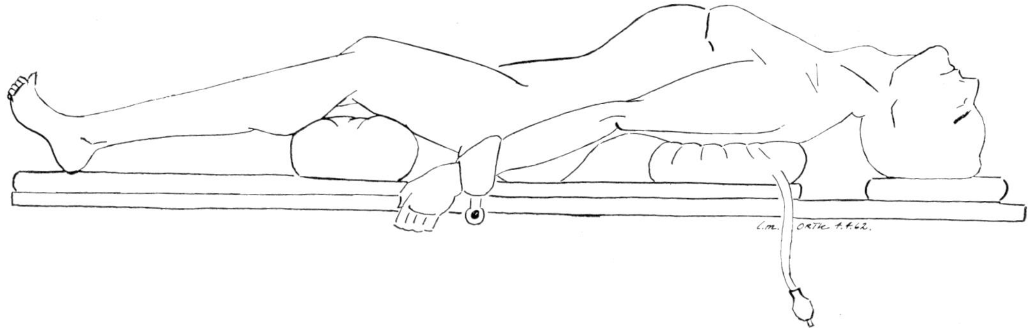

FIG. 338.—POSITION FOR CEREBRAL ANGIOGRAPHY

The diagram represents the usual position for cerebral angiography. A pad is placed under the knees, and the forearms are tied to the sides of the table. An inflatable bag is placed under the shoulders, and after the needle is inserted, the bag can be deflated. A thin pad is placed under the patient's head for comfort.

with local anesthetic, making sure that none goes into the bloodstream. A total of 6 to 8 cc. of anesthetic is sufficient. The injection of an excessive amount of local anesthetic is discouraged because this would be equivalent to producing edema of the tissues, which makes palpation of the vessels more difficult. The injection of most of the local anesthetic behind the artery is advantageous because it tends to push the artery forward.

The artery is then palpated and the area is massaged to spread the local anesthetic. There should be a pause of a few minutes until the anesthesia is fully effective. The artery is then fixed with the second and third fingers of the left hand. With one finger the anterior margin of the sternocleidomastoid muscle is displaced laterally. An attempt is made to displace the jugular vein laterally so that the anterior wall of the artery is uncovered as much as possible (fig. 345). When inserting the needle, one should not forget that the artery is surrounded by many structures, as explained in Figure 345. An important reference point is the superior margin of the thyroid cartilage. At this level, the bifurcation of the common carotid artery usually takes place. Therefore, if it is decided to inject the common carotid artery, the puncture of the skin should be made as low as possible. If it is decided to puncture the internal carotid artery, this should be done near the bifurcation of the common carotid at the origin of the internal carotid artery. It is the custom at the Neurological Institute to puncture the common carotid artery because when serialograms are taken, the superimposition of branches of the external carotid is not bothersome, and by injecting 10 cc. instead of 8 cc. of contrast substance, one obtains a sufficient distention of the internal carotid branches. In addition, puncture of the common carotid makes it possible to diagnose partial and complete occlusions of the internal carotid artery at its origin, the most common site of occurrence, a finding which may not be suspected clinically. The region of the bifurcation of the common carotid artery is the most frequent place for arteriosclerotic plaques which may be dislodged by the needle; this tends to increase the incidence of complications. There are, however, definite indications for the performance of selective angiograms in which the internal carotid artery is punctured separately from the external carotid. If the puncture is not made too high above the origin of the internal carotid artery, it is often possible simply to withdraw the needle and to change its direction somewhat without removing it from the artery in order to opacify the external carotid on the second injection.

The type of needle to be used is a matter for individual consideration. For most cases we prefer the Cournand-Greenough. This

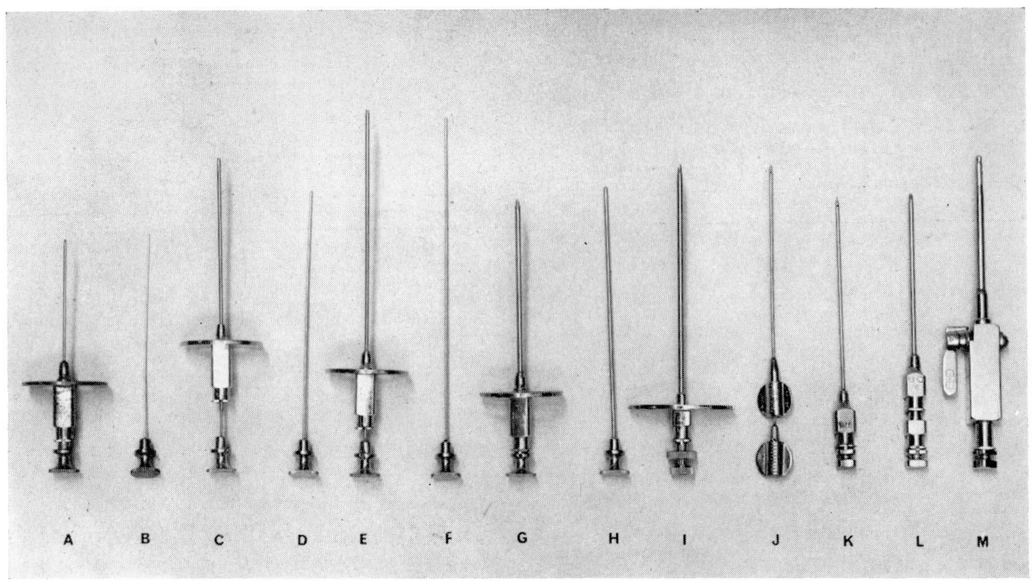

Fig. 339.—Needles

(A) Cournand fitted cannula, 20 gauge, 1½″ (baby)—carotid. (B) stylet, blunt (for (A))., (C) Cournand fitted cannula, 18 gauge, 2³⁄₆₄″ (adult)—carotid. (D) stylet, blunt (for (C)). (E) Cournand fitted cannula, 18 gauge 3″—subclavian. (F) stylet, blunt (for (E)). (G) Cournand fitted cannula, 17 gauge, 2³⁄₆₄″—brachial retrograde, percutaneous. (H) stylet, blunt (for (G)). (I) Seldinger, 17 gauge, 3″—brachial. (J) Swan modification of Sheldon's needle, 19 gauge, 2½″—vertebral. (K) Whitacre, 18 gauge, 2½″—vertebral. (L) modified Lindeman, 16 gauge, 2″—brachial. (M) Kuhn cannula, 12 gauge, 1⅜″—brachial retrograde, open method.

needle has the advantage of a blunt stylet which may be inserted after the removal of the sharp stylet. Through use of the blunt stylet it is possible to advance the needle in the arterial lumen without much danger of perforating the posterior wall (fig. 339). There is a flange at its base which tends to keep the needle steady after it has been inserted, but it does not permit the operator to rotate the needle if he desires to change the direction of the bevel. A needle without a flange is lighter and makes it easier to feel the arterial pulsations when the tip is resting on the anterior wall of the artery during the puncture. Another needle used is a simple 2.5-inch spinal needle which should be of 19 or 18 gauge in order to permit a rapid injection. In children, smaller needles are necessary. The advantage of this needle is that it may be rotated 90 or 180° if necessary. An ordinary thin walled, 18-gauge, 2.5-inch short bevel intravenous needle may be used without a stylet. The advantage of such needles is that they are inexpensive and a new needle can be used each time which will assure a very sharp point and, therefore, reduce tearing of the arterial wall. This type of needle also facilitates puncture through providing for the escape of blood immediately after it enters the lumen, and this helps avoid damage to the posterior wall of the vessel. A sharp needle is preferable to one that has been blunted by usage because even a slightly blunted needle tends to slip off the anterior wall of the artery. A disadvantage of a sharp, cutting needle, as against a Cournand type needle is that it increases the incidence of hematomas; it can actually tear the arterial wall in inexperienced hands.

It has been our custom to place the needle directly into the artery and, once it is in the arterial lumen, to connect to it a plastic tube which has been previously filled with physiologic saline solution. An alternate method is to connect the plastic tubing to the needle and to fill both with saline, leaving a syringe connected to the plastic tubing until the needle, without stylet, is pushed through the skin and subcutaneous tissues. The syringe is then removed but the plastic tubing is left connected to the needle. If the artery is entered, blood will promptly displace the saline. This makes it unnecessary to connect the tubing after the needle is in place, a maneuver which might, on occasion, dislodge the needle.

It may be necessary to have another person hold the patient's head during the manipulations leading to the arterial puncture, particularly in apprehensive or uncooperative patients.

During the actual puncture the artery is first fixed firmly by the first two fingers as explained above. The fingers should be placed approximately 1 cm. above the point where the needle tip will actually puncture the artery. It is usually better not to go too obliquely toward the artery because this tends to strip the adventitia. By going more nearly vertical, one can be sure to go through the arterial wall with least damage to the wall. Two methods of puncture have been advocated, one in which the artery is perforated and the other in which it is only penetrated. In the first the artery is impaled, the needle going through both the anterior and the posterior walls. At this point the needle is slowly withdrawn (after removing the stylet) until blood begins to spurt. An attempt is then made to thread the needle in a cephalad direction while leaving the stylet out and permitting blood to flow to confirm the correct position of the needle within the artery. Others advocate the use of the blunt stylet during advancement of the needle. With the latter, blood cannot be seen to escape from the needle while it is advancing, but the bluntness of the stylet usually assures that the needle will remain in the arterial lumen.

The second method of approach employs a needle without a stylet and through puncture of the anterior vessel wall, an attempt is made to enter the lumen of the artery with the bevel pointing downward. The posterior wall is not intentionally pierced, and the needle usually can be advanced within the lumen with relative ease. For this type of puncture the needle should be slightly more oblique than when the first technique is used. Advancing the needle in the lumen of the artery should be done slowly to prevent injury to the posterior vessel wall. For the actual injection the needle may be turned 180° to bring the stream of contrast substance more nearly into the mainstream of blood flow.

When the lumen of the artery is satisfactorily entered, a vigorous pulsating stream of blood is seen to escape from the hub of the needle. If the jugular vein is entered instead, the stream of blood is not very forceful. In order to make certain during the insertion that the needle has actually reached the anterior wall of the artery, transmitted pulsations should be felt. In addition, the force of the arterial pulsations may be obliterated by exerting some downward pressure with the needle which will indicate that it is actually resting on the artery. At the time of actual puncture of the artery the two fingers used to fix the vessel should be pressed firmly on each side of the artery to try to prevent its slipping or rolling. In spite of this, some arteriosclerotic vessels often escape the needle.

Injection and Filming

Once the needle has entered the artery and is securely in place, it is connected to the long saline-filled plastic tube, unless this has already been done prior to the insertion of the needle. In order to remove any air bubbles that might still remain within the tube, one should allow the blood to push some of the saline out before connecting the syringe. It is important to inject enough saline to displace all of the blood so that the entire length of the lumen of the needle is filled with saline solution. This is necessary to prevent clotting. The end of the plastic tube near the needle may be fixed with towel clips to prevent side motion. When an automatic injector is used, it is necessary to have a tube at least 20 inches in length and a 26-inch tube is more convenient. The actual arrangement for use of one type of automatic injector is illustrated in Figure 340. The *injection time* should be short to prevent undue dilution of contrast substance. When given by hand, the injection should

(Revised 1963)

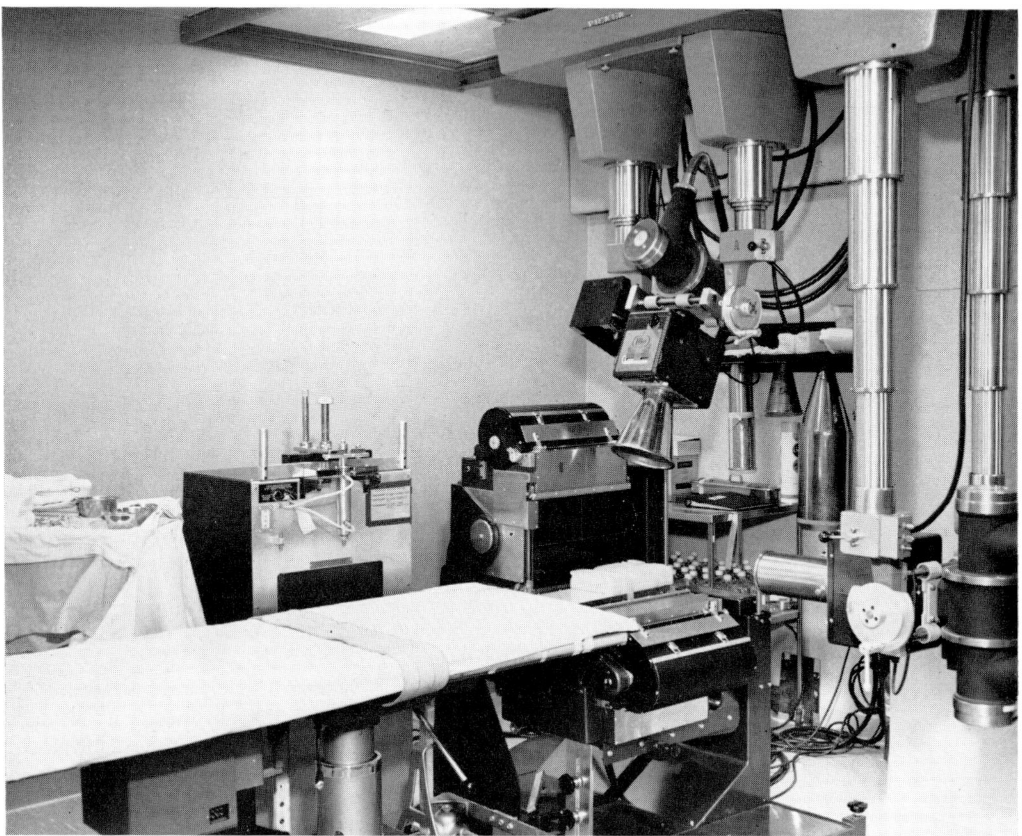

FIG. 340.—LAYOUT OF ROOM FOR BIPLANE SIMULTANEOUS CEREBRAL ANGIOGRAPHY USING AN AUTOMATIC INJECTOR

The automatic injector is set slightly behind the lateral serial film changer, and for this reason requires the use of a polyethylene tube as long as necessary (usually about 28″) to connect the needle to the syringe.

be as forceful as possible. With an automatic device, the injection time is more constant and may be made longer or shorter as desired. In an average case the injection time for 8 cc. of contrast material should be approximately one second.

It is our practice to inject 1.5 to 2.0 cc. of contrast substance and expose a single film to visualize the position of the needle in relation to the lumen of the artery. If the needle is not in a correct position, it is modified and another scout film is taken. When the position of the needle is considered to be correct, the injection of 8.0 cc. is made if the needle is in the internal carotid artery. A smaller amount of contrast substance (6 cc.) sometimes is used, but when bi-plane simultaneous serial angiograms are made, the full amount of 8 cc. becomes necessary to obtain better contrast, since some film fogging cannot be avoided. If the needle is situated low in the common carotid and, particularly, if the patient has tortuous vessels, an additional 2 or even 4 cc. of contrast substance are added so that 10 cc. or sometimes 12 cc. of contrast substance are injected. This tends to maintain approximately the same concentration in the intracranial vessels in all cases, even if some of the material is diluted in dilated tortuous vessels and some is lost in the external carotid artery branches. The "scout film" referred to above is taken after the injection of two cc. of contrast substance, with the use of a *Polaroid* cassette, 0.5 second exposure time, and high speed special paper which is ready for viewing in one minute. It is a lateral view centered at the needle, which permits us to see the relationship of the tip of the needle to the arterial walls, particularly the posterior wall which is the usual site of injury. An anteroposterior view is also made, simultaneously, which will show the relationship of the needle with the artery in the transverse plane. Sometimes subintimal blebs are demonstrated only in the anteroposterior film.

After the films are exposed, developed, and viewed, a decision is made as to necessary additional films. With a bi-plane simultaneous radiographic arrangement it is possible to do the entire examination with one single injection of 8 to 10 cc., following the taking of the "scout film" with 1.5 to 2 cc. If a second injection becomes necessary, a period of about 10 to 12 minutes has elapsed by the time the films are available, and it is safe to inject again. At least 10 minutes should be permitted to elapse between any two injections of the full amount of contrast substance. It has been shown in animals (Broman et al., 1950) that there is a cumulative effect of the contrast substances; if two injections are made too close together, damage to the brain may take place (see "Morbidity and Complications").

At the end of the examination the needle is removed and compression of the area of puncture in the neck is maintained for approximately ten minutes to prevent the formation of a hematoma. The pressure should be moderately firm and over a long area, made not with one or two fingers but with the four fingers to prevent direct occlusion of the arterial lumen. It is most important to check the patient after every injection for possible paralysis or weakness of the extremities. The same applies to testing the patient's ability to speak and possible weakness of the extremities after the removal of the needle and compression.

As the patient is returned to his room it is usually advisable to place an ice bag around his neck and to order analgesics such as codeine and aspirin. Two to three hours after the examination the patient is again checked for any evidence of neurologic sequelae which might be attributed to the angiogram, and if there are none, the patient may be considered discharged. It is rare to see complications arising after two to three hours.

VERTEBRAL ANGIOGRAPHY

The performance of angiography involving the vertebral system is more difficult than that of the carotid system. The caliber of the vertebral artery is smaller than that of the carotid, and it is contained within a bony canal, namely the foramen transversarium of the vertebrae. Significant danger of damage to neighboring structures, especially the spinal cord, also exists. The most satisfactory way of obtaining a good vertebral angiogram is still a direct percutaneous puncture of the artery. This may be performed with a short-beveled spinal needle, or the Sheldon or Swann needle may be used. The puncture may be performed in the mid-cervical region or in the suboccipital region. If this is not possible, a retrograde vertebral angiogram after the injection of the right carotid artery may be tried, but this is only successful in about 30 per cent of the cases. A direct percutaneous puncture of the subclavian artery is more satisfactory and is relatively easy to perform. The brachial artery also may be punctured if desired (see below).

A technique for the percutaneous puncture of the vertebral artery was first described by Sugar *et al.* (1949) and by Lindgren (1950), who developed the techniques independently. They are quite similar. A later modification by Sjögren (1953) is preferable. The technique consists in the insertion of the needle (18 gauge, 2.5-inch spinal needle) not too low in the neck and as close to the midline as possible after displacing the trachea medially and the carotid artery laterally. The needle is inserted between the two, directed upward

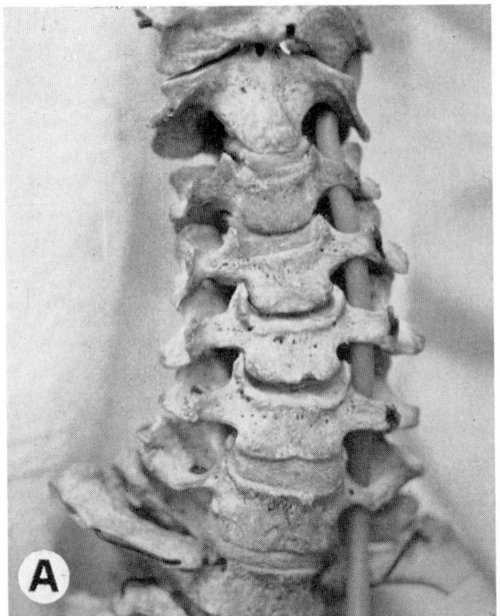

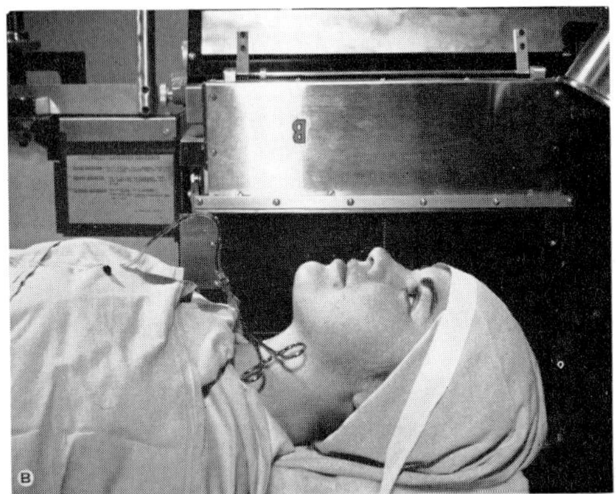

FIG. 341.—(A) FRONTAL VIEW OF THE CERVICAL SPINE WITH THE VERTEBRAL ARTERY PASSING THROUGH THE FORAMINA TRANSVERSARIA. (B) POSITION FOR VERTEBRAL ANGIOGRAPHY FOLLOWING THE INSERTION OF THE SWAN-SHELDON NEEDLE.

It is necessary to hold the needle down with a forceps because any movement will tend to dislodge it from the lumen of the artery. In addition, when the injection is made, the reverse-jet tends to pull the needle out. Usually the left side is punctured.

and slightly laterally in order to avoid entrance of the spinal canal, which was often the case with the first techniques described by Sugar *et al.* and by Lindgren. The tip of the needle passes along the anterolateral aspect of the vertebral body; it will hit the anterior aspect of the transverse process directly or it may slide under or over it. If it slides above, it will then go under the anterior aspect of the transverse process of the next vertebra. The abutment of the anterolateral aspect of the vertebral body and the transverse process tend to fix the needle in the direction of the foramen transversarium. An effort should be made at the time that the common carotid artery is displaced laterally, to feel the anterior tubercle of the transverse processes. This is an important reference point; if the fingers are placed on this point, the needle then may be directed very slightly medial to it. A similar technique to that described by Sjögren was also described by Ecker (1951). It is probably advantageous to connect the needle to a polyethylene tube and syringe after filling the entire system with saline with or without added heparin. This will permit the removal of the stylet prior to the puncture; the blood will be seen in the tube as soon as the artery is pierced.

Local anesthesia well applied to this area down to the prevertebral region is important, otherwise the patient will not cooperate because of pain. General anesthesia is necessary in children and in apprehensive adults. The percentage of success of percutaneous vertebral angiography by this method is between 80 and 90 per cent (Ruggiero, 1959). In inexperienced hands, however, the percentage of failure is rather high.

The method described by Sheldon (1956) is based almost exclusively on the special needle he devised and its modification (Swann, 1958). Another modification of the Swann needle consists in a round pencil point instead of a squared point (fig. 339). It appears that the "pencil point" needle is less traumatic to the arterial wall but is more difficult to position because it tends to be deviated by the fascial planes and liga-

(Revised 1963)

ments, whereas the cutting edge of the Sheldon needle and the Swann modification is not so deviated. The Sheldon technique is based on a puncture perpendicular to the skin and to the artery. After locating the anterior tubercle of the transverse processes with the fingers, the needle is directed to a point just medial to it (fig. 341). The greatest difficulty with the use of this and the other percutaneous techniques is the maintenance of the needle within the artery. In the ordinary technique, the needle is very often dislodged by the recoil force of the injection; this is minimized by the use of the Swann needle. Great care is needed to maintain the needle in position; if the patient turns his head or coughs or swallows, the needle may be dislodged. The use of a thin walled polyethylene tube is preferable to that of a wider tube that might be too heavy. A shorter needle, 2.0 to 2.25 inches, is recommended. With the Sheldon technique, our percentage of success has been about 90 per cent and the number of complications has been negligible.

We have not used extensively the method of puncturing the vertebral artery between the atlas and the occipital bone as recommended by Maslowski (1955) and by Krayenbühl and Richter (1952).

If the percutaneous method fails, we prefer a retrograde percutaneous brachial or a direct puncture of the subclavian artery as recommended originally by Shimidzu. Others recommend the use of the technique described by Radner (1951) which consists of the introduction of a catheter into the radial artery and advancing its tip until it reaches the vertebral artery origin from the subclavian artery. The catheter may then be introduced directly into the vertebral artery. This method gives good results, but it has the disadvantages which go with any catheterization, and the radial artery must be ligated following the procedure. A catheter also may be introduced into the brachial artery after exposing the vessel surgically. This does not require the ligation of the vessel, but it often results in a diminution of the pulse and a cold hand which may last for a while. The catheter method is less desirable, also, because examination is preferably performed on the right side and if any complications arise as a result of the injury to the vessels, it involves the patient's right hand. The catheter may also be introduced percutaneously into the brachial artery using the Seldinger technique. A simpler approach appears to be the direct puncture of the subclavian artery or the retrograde injection of the brachial artery first described by Gould, Peyton, and French (1955) and later popularized by Kuhn (1960).

SUBCLAVIAN ANGIOGRAPHY

The first description of percutaneous puncture of the subclavian artery was given by Shimidzu (1937). It escaped attention for a number of years until it was adopted by numerous workers (Barbieri and Verdecchia (1957), Crawford *et al.* (1959), and Baker (1960)). More recently, however, it has lost popularity. The technique is rather simple; it consists in the insertion of the needle through the triangle formed by the anterior scalenus muscle, the omohyoid muscle, and the upper margin of the clavicle. The pulsations of the artery may be felt by flexing the head slightly to relax the neck muscles. The needle is directed downward, backward, and medially, and the artery is entered at or just medial to the anterior extremity of the first rib. A 17- or 18-gauge needle 3 inches in length is necessary. Baker introduced a modification of the technique. He advised introduction of the needle more medially in order that the artery actually can be threaded with the needle. The most common complication of subclavian angiography is a pneumothorax which occurs in approximately 10 per cent of the patients, according to Crawford *et al.* (1959). Using Baker's modification, pneumothorax occurs less frequently because the needle is directed medially instead of toward the apex of the pleural cavity. It is necessary to inject at least 20 cc. of contrast substance (60 per cent Renografin, 50 per cent Hypaque, etc.) as rapidly as possible. A blood pressure cuff should be placed on the arm to prevent flow in this direction which will divert some of the contrast substance. The puncture may be performed on the right side where filling of the vertebral and of the common carotid artery are obtained. If done on the left side, only the vertebral artery is filled, but it should be remembered that in approximately 6 per cent of the cases, the vertebral artery on the left side arises directly from the aorta (Radner, 1951). The filling of the intracranial vessels by this method is not as good as that obtained by direct puncture of the vertebral artery. However, demonstration of the origin of the vertebral artery is only possible in all instances by a method which involves visualization of the junction of the vertebral with the subclavian artery. It is, therefore, imperative to use this or a similar method when surgery to correct occlusion or stenosis of extracranial arteries is considered. If the needle is large enough, it is possible to insert a thin polyethylene catheter through the needle and to remove the needle part way to prevent injury to the arterial wall.

It is also advisable to use a Rochester needle which has a Teflon sleeve around it. The needle can be withdrawn and the Teflon sleeve will remain in place. More recently, a technique for infraclavicular puncture of the subclavian artery has been described (Amplatz and Harner, 1962). This avenue of approach has the advantage of eliminating the pneumothorax which is a frequent complication when the supraclavicular approach is employed. The injection can be made directly through the needle or a catheter may be inserted by the Seldinger method.

BRACHIAL ANGIOGRAPHY

Retrograde brachial angiography was first proposed by Gould, Peyton, and French (1955) and has been popularized by Kuhn (1960). It is performed by exposing the artery in the lower half of the arm and by inserting a cannula 3 inches in length into the artery. The cannula should be wide enough to permit a rapid injection of contrast substance (12 or 13 gauge). A small gauge needle is not recommended. Kuhn uses a special cannula which permits the partial withdrawal of the stylet and before blood escapes, the stopcock can be closed (fig. 339). It is necessary to inject 30 cc. of 50 per cent Hypaque (60 per cent Renografin is probably too viscous for this purpose) to obtain a satisfactory filling. This is usually done on the right side but, like the subclavian puncture, it may also be done on the left side where only filling of the left vertebral artery is obtained. The injection of contrast substance is somewhat painful to the patient, more so than subclavian puncture. Percutaneous puncture of the brachial artery may also be performed (Pygott and Hutton, 1959) and the results can be as satisfactory as those of the cut-down method. Immediately after the injection, the arteries should be flushed with 50 cc. of saline solution.

Percutaneous brachial angiography is becoming increasingly popular. The needle may be inserted just above the antecubital fossa or it may be inserted anywhere up the arm to the axilla. It is advantageous to start the puncture just above the elbow because if the needle cannot be inserted at this level it is possible to go at a higher level. The collateral circulation seems to be adequate in case any complications arise as a result of the lower puncture. In the higher punctures it is also probable that there would be sufficient collateral circulation. The authors have not encountered any difficulties in several hundred brachial angiograms with punctures of the brachial artery at any level except for an occasional lowering of the pulse pressure which only lasts for a few hours or days. A Cournand-type needle is usually employed, 17-gauge, and the needle should be well threaded in the artery. A satisfactory dose was 30 cc. of 50 per cent Hypaque followed on the same syringe by 15 to 20 cc. of saline injected as rapidly as possible under a pressure of 525 lbs. The saline flotation method described above produces much better filling of the carotid and vertebral arteries and also diminishes the arm pain because the contrast material is only in contact with the arm vessels for a short period of time and is immediately washed away by the saline. The saline is floated on top of the Hypaque and does not mix with the Hypaque as long as the syringe is maintained in the vertical position. This method can only be used in mechanical injectors which keep the syringe in the vertical position and which inject downwards so that the contrast material is injected first. The needle should be well fixed to the skin to prevent recoil during the forceful injection. Recoil of the needle is often responsible for the intramural injections. With a well-threaded, well-fixed needle it is rare to make any intramural injection. The puncture may also be made in the axillary artery, but in this case it is advisable to insert a catheter by the Seldinger method because it facilitates filming (Newton, 1963). In spite of the fact that the axillary artery is surrounded by the branches of the brachial plexus it is possible to puncture it by using a gentle technique without any injury to the nerve trunks.

During the taking of the films, whether a retrograde percutaneous angiogram or a catheter method is used, it is possible to move the patient down rapidly between the second and the third seconds for a distance of 4 to 6 inches. This maneuver permits, with a single injection on biplane serial angiography, to visualize the neck arteries and after 2.5 seconds to visualize the intracranial arteries. The downward movement of the patient should be rapid and can be performed by hand after a little practice but a mechanical arrangement would be more satisfactory. Our usual programming for percutaneous brachial angiography as well as for those cases where a catheter is placed in the subclavian artery, is two films per second for the first second, four per second for the next two seconds and one film per second for four seconds.

FEMORAL CATHETERIZATION

This technique, as originally described by Seldinger (1953), is chiefly used for aortography and angiocardiography. It can be applied to cerebral angiography because it has the advantage of showing the origin of all of the major vessels satisfactorily. Unfortunately, superimposition of the shadows of all of the vessels of the brain is not desirable for accurate diagnosis of intracranial lesions. It is more applicable to the diagnosis of extracranial vascular lesions. The catheter can, however, be placed at the origin of the vertebral artery according to the technique described by Lindgren (1956), in which case selective visualization of the vertebral artery may be obtained. With a good technique and by injecting a sizable amount of contrast substance, the results are fairly good even for the intracranial vessels (Giencini and Ecker, 1960).

SUPERFICIAL TEMPORAL CATHETERIZATION

This technique was originally proposed by Weiner *et al.* (1958) and consists in the introduction of a thin catheter by way of the superficial temporal artery following surgical exposure of this vessel in the pre-auricular region. The catheter can be introduced caudally into the common carotid artery and even into the aortic arch. Difficulties may be encountered in threading the catheter in arteriosclerotic individuals. It also is objectionable because it requires surgical exposure which will leave a scar, but it may be kept in mind in dealing with special situations.

INTRAVENOUS ANGIOGRAPHY

This procedure consists in the simultaneous injection of as much as 100 cc. of a highly concentrated contrast substance (90 per cent Hypaque or 70 per cent Urokon), usually divided into two equal doses injected into each arm simultaneously while holding the arms up above the horizontal to facilitate the rapid passage of contrast substance into the great veins (Steinberg and Evans, 1961). The recommended dosage is 1.0 cc. per kg. of body weight. Serialograms are made starting 4 or 5 seconds after the beginning of the injection, usually while rotating the patient slightly toward the right side, that is, lifting the left shoulder to open up the aortic arch and visualize the origin of the neck vessels more clearly. This method results in a faint visualization of the arteries in the neck. Thus far it has not been considered satisfactory to demonstrate the presence of partially obstructing lesions of the extracranial and intracranial vessels. A complete obstruction in the cervical region as well as a narrowing in a favorable proximal position may be detected with this technique. Perhaps further advances will produce better results.

Radiographic Technique

It is a well accepted fact that at least two radiographs taken at right angles, that is, a lateral film and a frontal film, are needed in every cerebral angiogram. In the majority of instances, multiple films in each projection are required for satisfactory diagnosis and localization of abnormalities. In addition to these two views, however, some other films may be required to study special problems.

In order to produce films of good quality, it is essential to immobilize the head; otherwise the patient will move at the time of the injection. The simplest method is to place an adhesive band over the forehead and bring it around the headrest firmly. Another adhesive band is placed over the chin, which is brought around the board where the patient's head is resting. This has been found to be reasonably satisfactory. Other methods of head holding usually interfere with the taking of the lateral view because they cast a shadow.

Lateral View

The lateral view is taken with the patient in the supine position and the film is placed alongside the head of the patient. *For best results, the film should be against the side of the head being injected.* It is recognized, of course, that every physical layout will not allow such an arrangement, either because of restricted space or limitation of equipment available. More complicated equipment such as bi-plane apparatus, may improve many aspects of the examination but make it more difficult to provide the simple geometric arrangement of the shortest object-film distance possible. If necessary, good work can be done with the film away from the side being injected. This requires, however, constant vigilance on the part of the technician, for the most accurate positioning of tube, film, and patient. The radiologist must be constantly aware of the possible existence of distortions, and he must make allowance for technical variations in his interpretation. Notwithstanding, instances will be encountered in which it is impossible to give proper weight to the interpretation of minor changes and the distortion and magnification which results will make it impossible ever to compare the two sides. For these reasons, lateral filming on the side injected is strongly recommended whenever feasible.

A distance of at least 36 to 40 inches between the target and the film is desirable. *The head should be as close to the film as possible* (short object-film distance) whether or not lateral filming on the side injected is carried out. When the film cannot be placed close to the head, distortion and magnification result which are very undesirable. For some compensation, however, increasing the

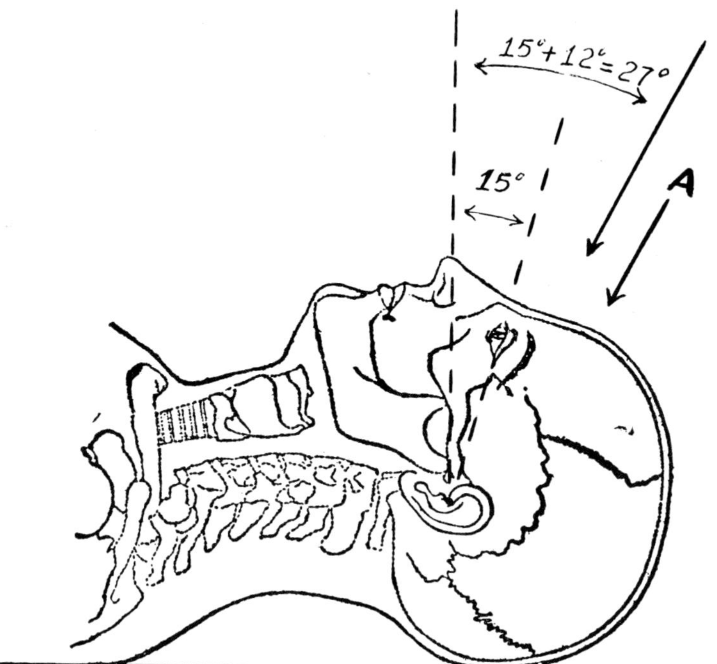

FIG. 342.—ILLUSTRATION OF THE METHOD USED TO OBTAIN THE CORRECT DEGREE OF ANGULATION

First the angle of the orbitomeatal line with the vertical is determined, and to this angle, 12° are added. In the case shown in the illustration, a total angulation of 27° would be used. The central beam would be placed below the hairline at (A), and passed at or just above the upper margin of the pinna of the ear.

target film distance may improve the results when it is necessary to have a long object-film distance, which cannot be avoided when certain serial film changers are used. However, this requires a more powerful piece of equipment, at least 500 milliamperes and 125 KV peak. More powerful equipment (1000 milliamperes or higher) may be required for optimum results to make possible the use of a long target film distance. In selecting the apparatus for angiography, one should, therefore, select a cassette or changer which will permit the placing of the head as close to the film as possible.

The taking of lateral radiographs with the vertical x-ray beam and turning the head to the same or to the opposite side of that being injected, is to be discouraged. It is not possible to obtain good straight lateral views when the head has to be turned to the side. On the other hand, it is relatively easy to obtain good, straight, reproducible

(Revised 1963)

lateral views with the patient in the supine position.

Frontal View

The anteroposterior view is made using the vertical x-ray beam. The angulation of the tube varies with the results that one wishes to obtain. Our *standard frontal angiographic projection* consists in angling the tube 12° toward the feet from the orbitomeatal line. First, the angle of the orbitomeatal line with the vertical is determined and, to that angle, 12° are added. The central beam enters approximately at the hairline and passes just above the upper margin of the pinna of the ear (fig. 342). Using this projection, the upper margin of the orbits and that of the petrous pyramids are usually either superimposed or almost superimposed upon each other in the majority of cases. In the remaining cases, depending on the configuration of the head, either the orbits or the petrous pyramids may be projected slightly above or below one another. It is important to use the same projection in all cases in order to acquire a mental image of the angiographic picture.

Special Views

In certain instances a greater degree of angulation, as much as 30 or even 35 degrees, is indicated to study special problems. At other times, no angulation of the tube is required or even a slight degree of angulation cephalad (25° caudocephalad from orbitomeatal line) is used. This projects the orbits squarely through the middle of the cranial cavity, and the bifurcation of the internal carotid artery and the proximal portion of the anterior and middle cerebral vessels are seen through the orbits. This projection is usually taken in cases of aneurysms and sometimes in suprasellar tumors. Depending on the degree of angulation, the configuration of the middle cerebral vessels as seen in the frontal projection will vary.

Sometimes *oblique views* are necessary. In order to take an oblique projection, it is best to start by rotating the head between 25 and 35 degrees to the *opposite* side of that being injected. The angulation of the tube should be decreased by 5 degrees, if the standard angiographic angulation (12 degrees caudad) is being used. Occasionally an oblique view taken with the head rotated to the same side as the injection is necessary. It is usually possible to decide which oblique to take first by observing the direction of an aneurysm as seen in the preliminary lateral and frontal films. For instance, if an aneurysm of the internal carotid artery at the junction of the posterior communicating artery seems to be directed posteriorly and medially in relation to the carotid siphon, in order to visualize the neck of the aneurysm, the head should be rotated to the same side as that being injected. On the other hand, if the aneurysm projects posteriorly and laterally, the head should be rotated to the opposite side of that being injected.

An *off-lateral* projection may be needed to show an aneurysm or to rule out an aneurysm as seen in the lateral projection. The head may be rotated 10 degrees to either side. With bi-plane simultaneous angiographic equipment, it is possible to take both a frontal oblique and an off-lateral film at the same time with one injection.

In studying the vertebral circulation, it is usually desirable in taking the lateral view to center the tube slightly more posteriorly than is usually done for carotid angiography. In addition, the routine frontal films should be in half axial projection, that is, a film with 30-degree angulation caudad from the canthomeatal line. In addition, *basal views* may be required in certain instances. The usefulness of this view, however, is quite limited. Ecker (1951) recommends this view for the study of intrasellar masses. We have found this view not to be necessary in these cases, since the information is available on the standard lateral and frontal angiogram films (Chase and Taveras, 1962).

Filming Procedure

The use of serial films is highly recommended in a routine manner both in lateral and in frontal projection. In this way, all of the phases of the angiogram, as the contrast substance passes from the arteries to the capillaries to the veins, are recorded on films. The use of simultaneous frontal and lateral views is also desirable because it is possible to get all of the necessary films with a single injection.

In taking serialograms, it is also desirable to take films more rapidly than one per second during the arterial phase. During the venous phase, films at one per second are adequate. Our routine consists of the taking of 6 films at two per second following which the speed of the film changer is shifted to one per second for an additional 4 films. This will cover 7 seconds of circulation time. The first exposure is made at the start of the injection. In patients who may have a slow circulation time due to increased intracranial pressure clinically recognizable, or if cerebral thrombosis is suspected, the routine is varied in that 6 films at one per second are taken instead of four. This covers 9 seconds of circulation time. Only rarely is it necessary to repeat the serial study in these instances because the venous phase was not properly recorded.

(Revised 1963)

From the technical point of view, it is easier to produce radiographs of good quality when only a single serialogram in frontal or in lateral projection is made. When simultaneous frontal and lateral views are made, a certain loss of contrast occurs due to cross fogging. This is unavoidable, but it can be minimized to a great extent. The use of cross-hatch grids in the lateral projection helps in eliminating lateral film fogging. In the frontal projection a cross-hatch grid cannot be used because of the beam angulation which is necessary. We have found that by using a high ratio grid—at least a 12 to 1 or, preferably, a 16 to 1 ratio grid—it is possible to obtain almost complete elimination of frontal film cross fogging. This is further aided by the use of very small cones, just large enough to cover the desired area.

At the present time we are using simultaneous frontal and lateral serialograms with a stereoscopic shift of the tube in the lateral film so that simultaneous serials in the frontal and lateral projections as well as stereoscopic laterals are obtained with a single injection. Again this introduces some difficulties which can be overcome. The major difficulty is that a slightly larger cone is required to take the lateral view since the tube must oscillate for about 2.5 to 3 inches to produce alternating stereoscopic images. It is possible to move the table top instead of the tube to obtain three-dimensional images. It is also possible to use a double focus tube or to turn the head rhythmically very slightly.

The use of an automatic injector is highly desirable in order that the technique can be reproduced in every instance. In addition, reproducible techniques on the same patient may be provided if a repeat examination is required. The value of automation in eliminating radiation exposure to personnel is obvious.

The kilovoltage used can be as high as needed, particularly for the frontal projection. However, the higher the kilovoltage, the greater the amount of cross fogging obtained in simultaneous bi-plane angiography. For this reason it is desirable to lower the kilovoltage as much as possible, compensating by increasing the milliamperes. The use of high speed, high detail film and high speed intensifying screens also helps in maintaining a lower kilovoltage. The exposure time should be short, not longer than $\frac{1}{10}$ of a second, and $\frac{1}{20}$ of a second is preferable.

The use of closed circuit television as a technical adjunct in diagnostic roentgenology has been described recently (1963) by Holman. In cerebral angiography such an electronic system, when applied to subtraction radiography, appears to have distinct advantages over the photographic method. Two television cameras operate simultaneously, one picking up the image of the angiogram while the other records an early film of the serialogram exposed before contrast material arrived in the cranium. The image of the plain film is reversed electronically, and the signals from both cameras applied to a television monitor through a synchronized supply. Thus, the final image produced is of the contrast material alone, the bone and soft tissue shadows being largely erased. The method provides considerably improved detail of the contrast outline of structures, many small vessels being visible that are not discernible from ordinary angiograms; the image also may be magnified. Closed circuit television is an expedient solution for the previously difficult and time consuming problems of subtraction radiography.

Morbidity and Complications

MORBIDITY

A certain morbidity always accompanies cerebral angiography, including neck pain following the puncture, sometimes slight elevation of temperature, and headache. Occasionally slightly more undesirable reactions occur, such as a local hematoma at the

(Revised 1963)

site of puncture, petechiae in the distribution of the external carotid and sometimes in the territory of the ophthalmic artery, vomiting, transitory dilatation of the pupil, transitory recurrent laryngeal nerve paralysis (rare), and convulsions. The administration of barbiturates is advisable before any angiogram because it tends to diminish the incidence of convulsions. The patient should not eat or drink for several hours before the examination in case vomiting occurs, which might result in aspiration of some of the material, and in dislodging of the needle. In a study of cerebral angiography in children, Poser and Taveras (1957) found that the morbidity is approximately the same when one compares angiography with pneumoencephalography. At least in children, some of the morbidity is apparently due chiefly to the general anesthesia except for the local reactions which are attributable to the puncture.

COMPLICATIONS

The true complications of angiography are those which involve the central nervous system, namely, hemiplegia, aphasia, unilateral sensory disturbances, and hemianopsia. A certain number of patients in all the series reported developed a transient paralysis or aphasia or both, hemisensory syndrome, or hemianopsia, the incidence of which has varied usually between 0.2 and 4.5 per cent, and for which even higher figures have been given (Frovig and Koppang (1953), Dimant *et al.* (1956), and Kaplan and Walker (1954)). Most if not all of the reports appearing in the literature are retrospective studies which involve the review of cases performed within a certain period of time. If the information is not available on the patient's chart, it is usually assumed that the patient fared well, but this is not necessarily correct. The true incidence of morbidity and complications of cerebral angiography is therefore not known because of the lack of a study involving a large consecutive series performed in a prospective fashion. Undoubtedly there is a considerable difference in the morbidity and complication rate depending on the experience of the operator. The complication rate is lower in the cases that are performed by a small, experienced, well supervised team of physicians. A clean arterial puncture without any difficulties is apt to contribute to a lower morbidity rate than one that may have to be performed several times with stripping of the adventitia and other arterial tissues and some tearing of the arterial wall, intramural injection of saline and of contrast substance, etc. Crawford (1956) has published an excellent study of the pathologic effects of cerebral angiography in 75 autopsy cases. He found that in two patients, false aneurysms developed at the site of the puncture and 9 had small dissecting aneurysms varying from 0.5 to 4 cm. in length. Five autopsies revealed multiple cerebral infarcts thought to be due to multiple emboli. In these cases, the only possible site of origin found was the location of carotid puncture. It is the opinion of the authors that the mechanical trauma consequent to the performance of the arterial puncture and the maintenance of the needle in the correct position are the most important causative factors in the development of complications at cerebral angiography. In a retrospective study of approximately 2000 cerebral angiograms at the Neurological Institute, the incidence of transient neurologic complications was 2.0 per cent. In this series of cases there appears to be little difference in the complication rates when Diodrast 35 per cent is compared with 30 per cent Urokon, 50 per cent Hypaque and 60 per cent Renografin. It is likely, therefore, in view of the fact that the latter two compounds are presumably less irritating or damaging to the cerebral blood vessels, that the main factor in the morbidity and complication rate is the method of performance of the examination. The number of injections and the total amount of contrast substance injected also apparently are clinically important. It may be said without fear of error that the least amount of contrast substance and the smallest number of injections compatible with a satisfactory cerebral angiogram constitute the most desirable technique. This is one reason in favor of bi-plane simultaneous serialograms in frontal and lateral projection in all cases, although a slight sacrifice in film contrast may occur in this type of radiographic arrangement.

Deaths in connection with cerebral angiography are always difficult to evaluate because most of these patients are acutely ill before the angiogram is performed. In most instances autopsy demonstrates an adequate cause for the patient's death other than the cerebral angiogram. Whether the angiogram is capable of precipitating death in some of these desperately ill patients is another matter. Undoubtedly some deaths are directly linked to the cerebral angiogram. In some of the deaths reported in the literature (Utterback and Haymaker, 1952) an excessive amount of contrast substance has been used (up to 120 cc. in a single sitting). For this reason it has been our custom for many years to limit the amount of contrast substance to be used to a maximum of 50 cc., including both sides of the brain, in any one sitting. Of Thorotrast the maximum amount is 25 cc. in any one sitting. It is known that Thorotrast can precipitate a bleeding tendency owing to interference with the blood clotting mechanism. One case of severe bleeding in multiple body systems was seen in our series in a patient who received approximately 50 cc. of Thorotrast, inadvertently, in one sitting. The patient recovered. In our series at the Neurological Institute, which comprised well over 5000 cerebral angiograms, only one death is directly attributable to the angiogram. This was in a patient who received Thorotrast; the material apparently flocculated and produced capillary block followed by immediate hemiplegia which did not clear and led to death within several days. Autopsy demonstrated multiple small Thorotrast emboli. This type of complication from Thorotrast has been previously reported (Northfield and Russell, 1937). Apparently it is common to find at necropsy particles of thorium dioxide in capillaries of the brain even when a considerable period of time has elapsed following Thorotrast angiography. Infarction does not always take place and in only a very small percentage of patients do neurologic disorders appear.

(Revised 1963)

The incidence of complications in patients with carotid thrombosis is higher than in patients with other conditions. In the first 66 cases of internal carotid thrombosis seen at the Neurological Institute, 3 patients developed permanent hemiplegia, an incidence of 4.0 per cent. On the other hand in a review of approximately 2000 cases, in which the patients with thrombosis of extracranial vessels were excluded, not a single case of permanent hemiplegia was seen. One patient developed a monoparesis of the foot which lasted approximately 2 weeks but had cleared almost completely by the time the patient left the hospital.

Vertebral angiography has a higher complication rate than carotid angiography. One annoying complication of percutaneous vertebral angiography is brachial neuritis. Injury to the spinal cord has been reported. An unusual complication was seen in one of our cases; the patient developed respiratory paralysis and quadriparesis and had to be placed in a respirator for several weeks. She recovered completely. The indication for the angiogram was a peculiar posterior fossa syndrome and it is possible that at least part, if not all, of the symptoms described above were due to a myelitis, particularly in view of the fact that the patient did not develop respiratory difficulty until 24 hours after the vertebral angiogram was performed. Bilateral cortical blindness occurred in another patient, who also recovered completely.

Treatment of Angiographic Complications

It has been our custom to have the patient inhale 5 per cent carbon dioxide in oxygen as soon as a complication is recognized. We have not used papaverine intra-arterially or intravenously. Cervical sympathetic block had been done in most of the patients prior to 1960 and in at least one case, the patient improved from the hemiplegia each time that a sympathetic block was carried out; this improvement happened

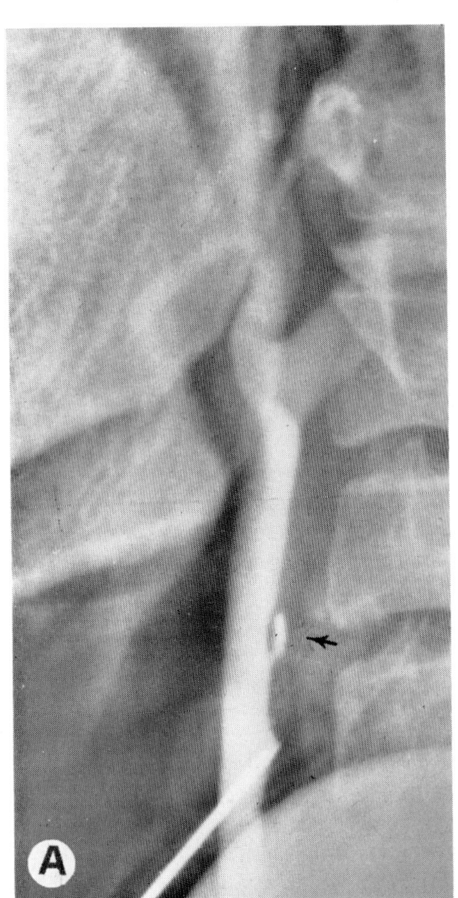

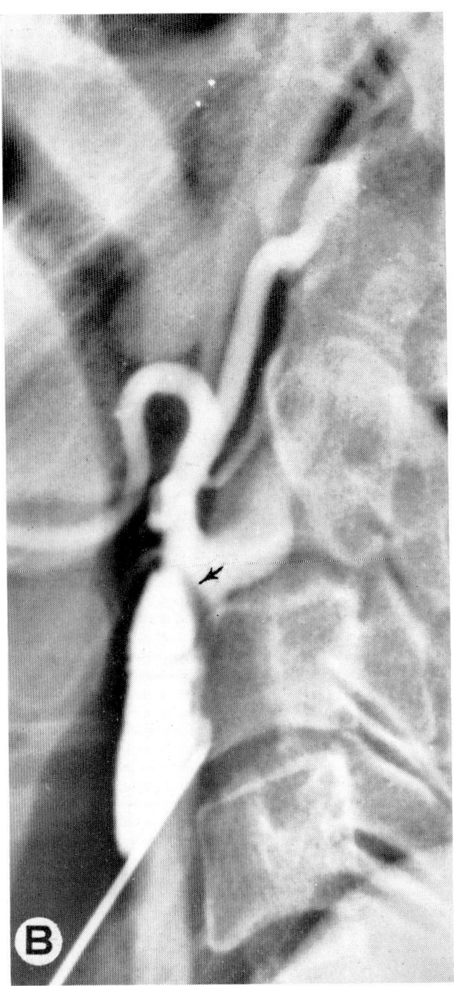

FIG. 343.—TECHNICAL COMPLICATIONS OF CAROTID ANGIOGRAPHY

In (A), an intramural injection of the contrast material has been performed. A small projection on the posterior wall represents a previous attempt at needling of the artery. In (B), a large intramural bleb has been formed and the wall of the artery is visible as a radiolucent line separating the denser bleb from the surrounding contrast substance in the arteries (*arrow*).

two or three times in this patient who eventually recovered. If the blood pressure is low, vasopressor agents should be administered, such as ephedrine, 25 mg. intravenously, which may be repeated if necessary. In cases of respiratory difficulties, the advisability of performing a tracheostomy should be considered. Tracheostomy should not be delayed and should be performed in any case where there is a question about the ability of the patient to maintain an adequate airway. In case of laryngospasm, which occurs sometimes in children, tracheal intubation may be lifesaving. For this purpose an intubation kit is kept in the angiographic room at all times.

As mentioned above, routine testing of the patient with the contrast substances to be used, both intravenously and intradermally, is carried out, and in case of a positive reaction to the test dose of each of the available contrast agents, the angiogram is not performed. It is only rarely, however, that an angiogram is cancelled for

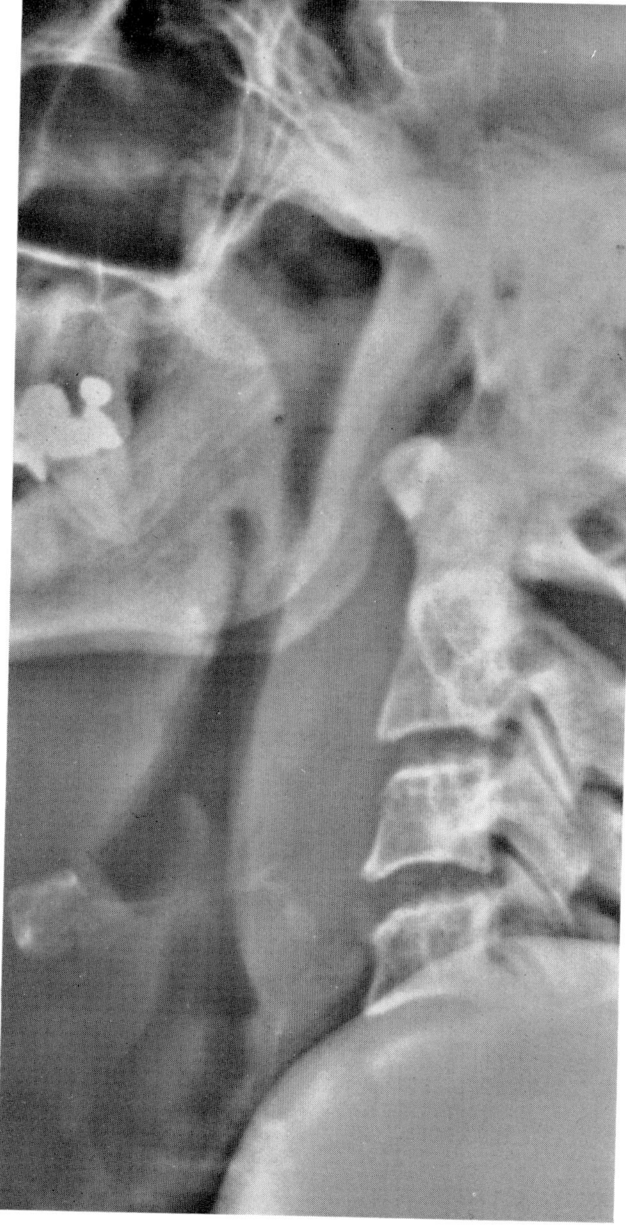

Fig. 344.—Prevertebral Soft Tissue Swelling Following Carotid Angiography
Soft tissue swelling is present in a certain percentage of patients after percutaneous carotid puncture.

this reason. The routine use of antihistaminics to prevent allergic reactions might be advisable in patients who show any signs of sensitivity to the contrast substance or any history of severe allergies.

Technical Complications

As explained under morbidity of cerebral angiography, injury to the arterial wall is only slight when a clean puncture is performed. If the needle is placed partly in the lumen and partly underneath the endothelium, an intramural injection will take place. A bleb of contrast substance may be introduced within the arterial wall, which will tend to block the flow of contrast substance temporarily (fig. 343) and will simulate a thrombosis. The contrast substance may

(Revised 1963)

dissect upward for a considerable distance. When a subadventitial injection is made, some of the contrast substance escapes into the surrounding tissues.

In cases where a subintimal bleb is produced at the time of the injection, the upward flow is blocked and the contrast substance will then regurgitate and be lost via the subclavian artery or aorta. Some of the contrast substance which remains in the common carotid artery, however, will, after the end of the injection, be pushed upward by the bloodstream and a partial filling of the intracranial vessels will be obtained.

It is common to see prevertebral soft tissue swelling following cerebral angiography of both the carotid and vertebral systems. In a series of 100 cases where a lateral film of the neck was taken following cerebral angiography, 28 exhibited an increase in the thickness of the prevertebral tissues as outlined by air in the upper respiratory tract. In some cases it was only slight while in other patients it was very marked (fig. 344). It is obvious that the degree of swelling in this region is dependent on the amount of trauma which accompanies the angiogram. In children this swelling may be partly responsible for the respiratory difficulties encountered in some of them (a 5 per cent incidence in the cases reported by Poser and Taveras, 1957), because a child has a soft, compressible trachea. Endotracheal intubation for anesthesia is another factor.

Anatomy

CAROTID SYSTEM

The common carotid artery arises, on the left side, directly from the aortic arch; on the right side it is one of the two branches resulting from the bifurcation of the innominate artery (brachiocephalic artery). The common carotid bifurcation is usually situated at the level of the upper portion of the thyroid cartilage (fig. 384) approximately at the upper portion of the body of the 4th cervical vertebra. The level of bifurcation may be higher and sometimes lower than usual. The common carotid artery is rarely absent. When absent the internal and external carotid arteries arise directly from the aorta. On the contrary, anomalous origin of the common carotid is fairly frequent. In our own autopsy series (Stein, McCormack, Rodriguez, and Taveras, 1961) the left common carotid originated from the (right) innominate artery in 9 out of 130 cases. The right subclavian artery originated as the last branch of the aortic arch and had a retroesophageal course in two instances. In these cases the right common carotid may originate directly from the aorta. Multiple anomalies are frequent in the same subject.

In order to appreciate the relationship of the neck arteries to the various structures, careful study of Figure 345 is advised.

Internal Carotid Artery

The internal carotid artery may be divided into four segments: cervical, intrapetrosal, intracavernous, and supraclinoid.

Cervical portion. From the bifurcation of the common carotid, the internal carotid artery is directed laterally, dorsally, and upward (fig. 346). When the artery is tortuous, the lateral swing is more pronounced. The intrapetrosal segment begins as the internal carotid artery enters the carotid canal in the petrous bone. This segment can be recognized in the frontal projection because of its horizontal direction, which ends in an upward curve (fig. 349). The cervical portion has no branches. Anomalies are occasionally found, however, and communication between the carotid and vertebral systems may be found (see p. 1.534). In the distal portion, buckling of the vessel upward and forward may be seen frequently, apparently related to elongation and dilatation with loss of elasticity.

Intrapetrosal portion. In the lateral projection, the intrapetrosal segment is partly obscured by the heavy density of the

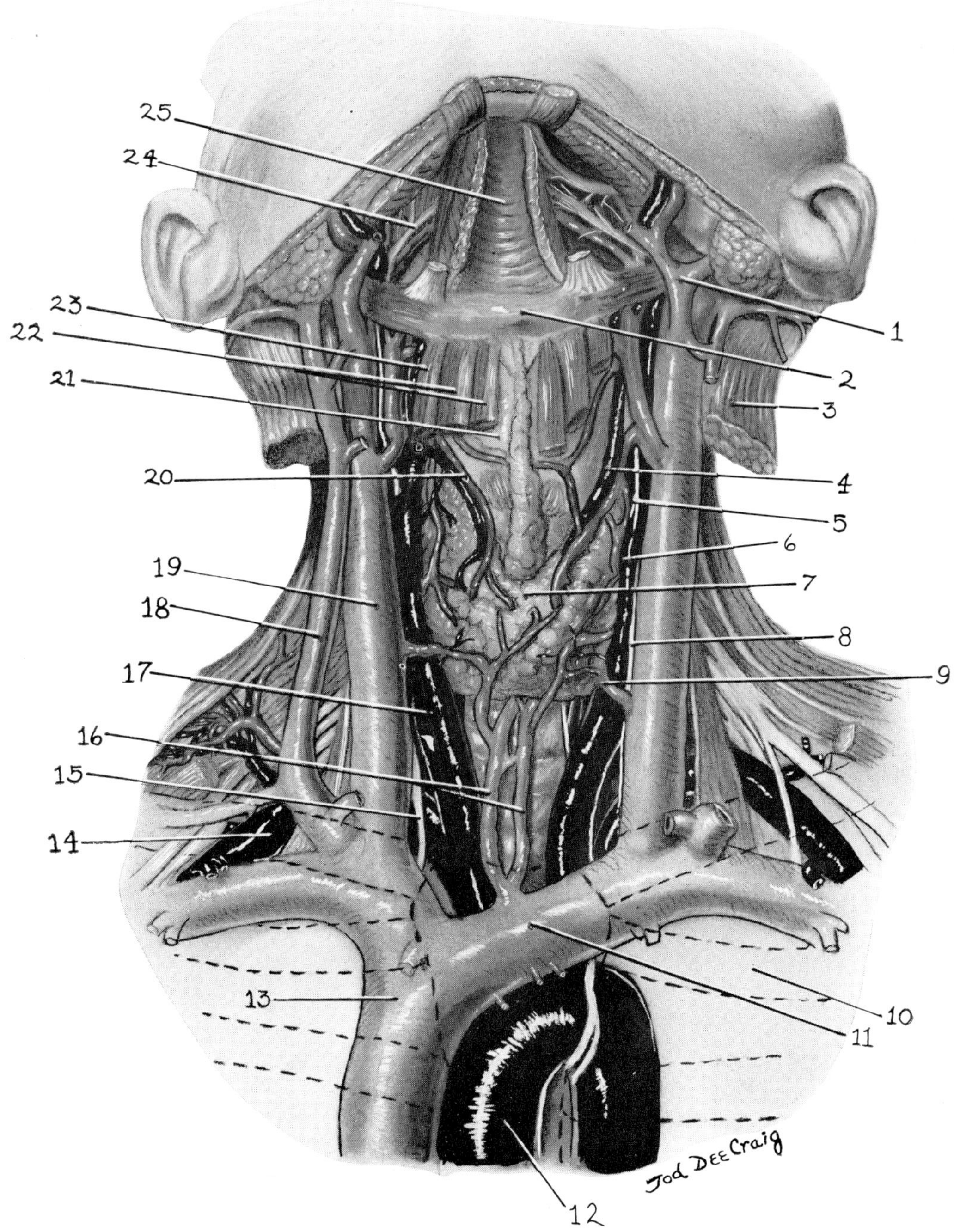

FIG. 345.—DIAGRAM TO ILLUSTRATE THE RELATIONSHIP OF THE CAROTID ARTERIES WITH OTHER STRUCTURES IN THE NECK, ANTERIOR VIEW

The diagram is intended to indicate the fact that the carotid arteries are surrounded by many structures which should be kept in mind when doing carotid punctures: (1) facial vein. (2) hyoid bone. (3) sternocleidomastoid m. (4) superior thyroid a. (5) XII nerve (ansa cervicalis). (6) common carotid a. (7) thyroid gland. (8) X nerve (vagus). (9) middle thyroid v. (10) first rib. (11) innominate v. (12) aorta. (13) vena cava. (14) subclavian a. (15) X nerve (vagus). (16) inferior thyroid v. (17) common carotid artery. (18) external jugular v. (19) internal jugular v. (20) superior thyroid v. (21) thyroid cartilage. (22) sterno-hyoid m. (23) omohyoid m. (24) XII nerve (hypoglossus). (25) milo-hyoid m.

(Revised 1963)

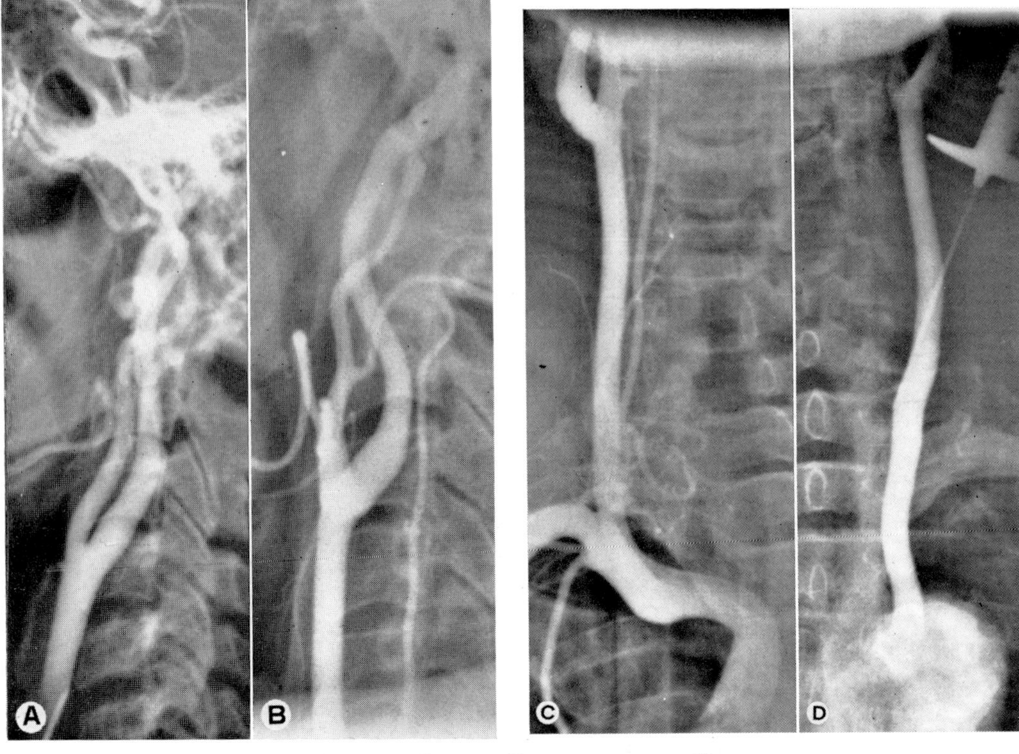

FIG. 346.—NORMAL COMMON CAROTID AND ITS BIFURCATION

In (A) there is no evidence of tortuosity; in (B) there is a moderate degree of tortuosity. The internal carotid artery is always directed upward and backward. In (C) and (D) the direction of the internal carotid following bifurcation of the common is seen in anteroposterior projection. It is usually directed upward and outward. (D) represents a retrograde common carotid arteriogram showing filling down to the origin of this artery from the aorta.

petrous bones; the most medial portion of this segment is recognizable as the artery turns up to emerge from the carotid canal at the petrous tip, thus entering the cranial cavity. The artery is contained for a short distance in a variable space of areolar tissue, extradurally, which permits the vessel to become tortuous. Shortly thereafter the artery enters the lumen of the cavernous sinus (fig. 347). As it enters the cavernous sinus, the artery sometimes presents a circular constriction which should not be confused with pathologic narrowing (fig. 348).

Intracavernous portion. Within the cavernous sinus, the internal carotid artery lies near the medial wall of the sinus.

As seen in the lateral view, the intracavernous segment is roughly horizontal, but a certain degree of tortuosity is common; sometimes marked tortuosity is present even in the absence of arteriosclerosis (fig. 375). The intracavernous segment is usually at or just above the floor of the sella turcica.

In the *frontal projection*, the *intracavernous portion* is superimposed on itself, but by following the artery up, it is easy to define the posterior aspect, and by following the intracranial portion of the artery down, the anterior aspect of the intracavernous segment can be defined. For our purpose, the intracavernous segment ends at the lower margin of the anterior clinoid process. Usually the posterior aspect is either superimposed upon or slightly medial to the anterior aspect (fig. 349).

Supraclinoid segment. This portion begins as the artery emerges from the

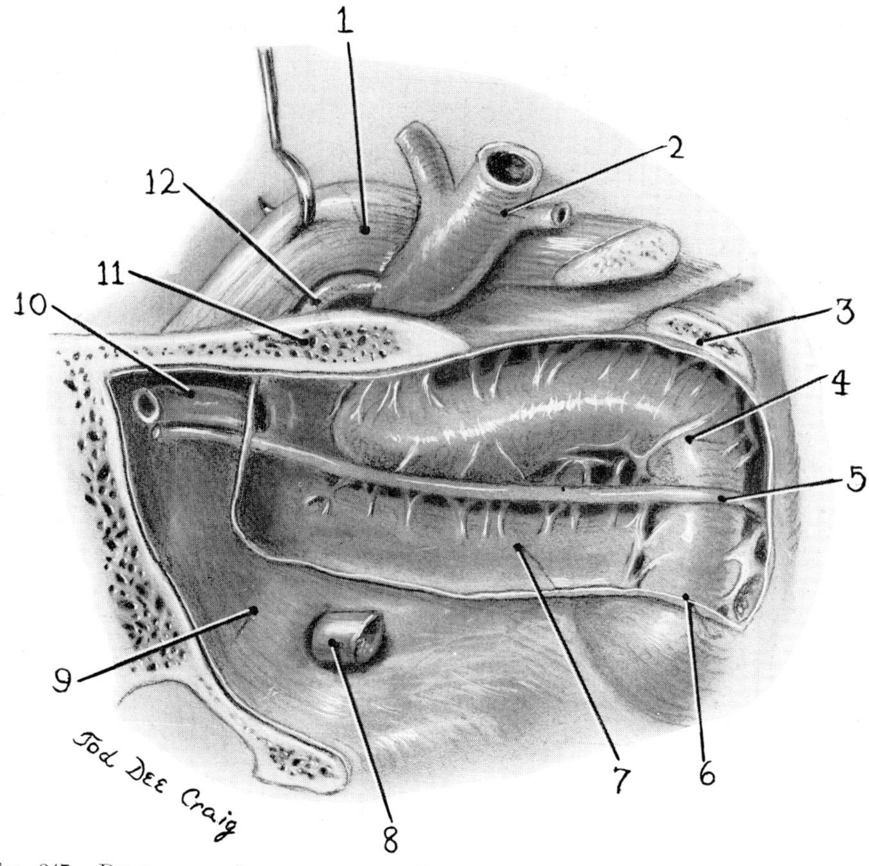

FIG. 347.—DIAGRAM OF INTRACAVERNOUS PORTION OF THE INTERNAL CAROTID ARTERY
(1) Optic nerve. (2) internal carotid artery. (3) posterior clinoid process. (4) internal carotid artery. (5) sixth nerve (abducens). (6) internal orifice of carotid canal. (7) cavernous sinus. (8) superior maxillary nerve. (9) floor of middle fossa. (10) ophthalmic vein. (11) anterior clinoid process. (12) ophthalmic artery.

cavernous sinus, after passing under and medial to the anterior clinoid process. As the artery emerges, it usually extends upward and backward. It may continue upward and backward to its bifurcation, or it may turn forward and upward, or straight up, before dividing (fig. 350). The point of bifurcation is often difficult to see on lateral films due to superimposition of anterior and middle cerebral arteries. By following the anterior cerebral artery downward, however, it is usually, although not always, possible to determine the exact point at which bifurcation takes place. It is important to determine this point because in abnormal cases it may be displaced backward, upward, forward, etc. Unfortunately, variations are common, but usually the point of bifurcation falls on the posterior half of the intracavernous segment if a perpendicular to the plane of the diaphragma sellae is dropped from the bifurcation. (See discussion on suprasellar tumors.) Because of the shape of the intracavernous and supraclinoid segments of the internal carotid artery, Egas Moniz coined the term "carotid siphon" to refer to this portion of the internal carotid artery.

In the *frontal projection*, the supraclinoid segment of the internal carotid artery is directed upward and lateralward up to the bifurcation. The apparent lateral inclination of the supraclinoid portion of the internal carotid artery varies with the projection used to take the anteroposterior view.

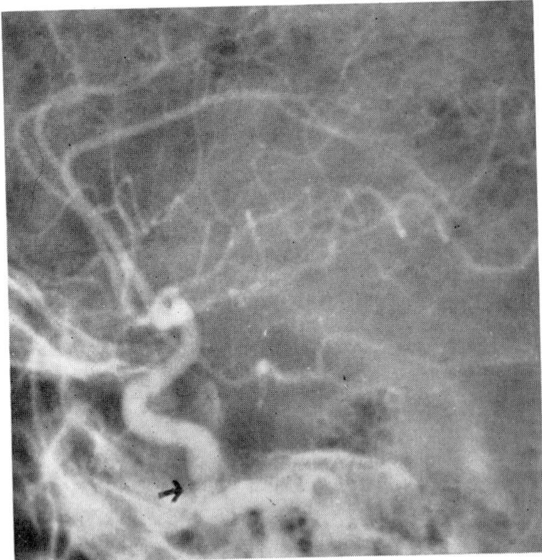

Fig. 348.—Normal Carotid Angiogram, Lateral View

There is constriction in the precavernous portion of the internal carotid siphon, probably at the entrance of the wall of the cavernous sinus. The Sylvian triangle is very well outlined in this case.

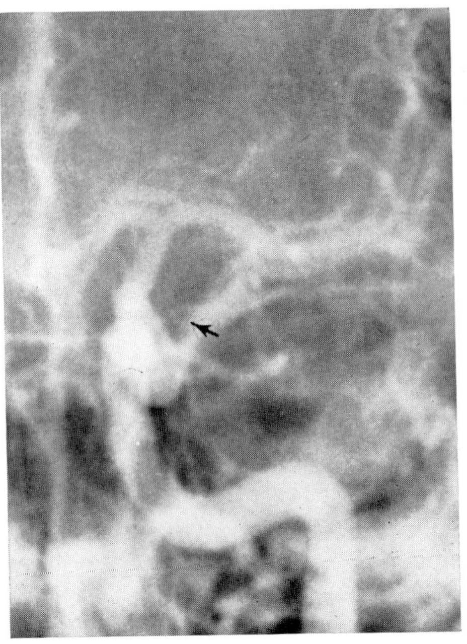

Fig. 349.—Anteroposterior View, Normal Carotid Angiogram

The figure demonstrates the fact that the posterior portion of the intracavernous segment of the internal carotid artery is slightly more medial than the anterior portion. This can be ascertained by following the cervical portion of the internal carotid artery upward, for the posterior portion, and the supraclinoid portion of the artery downward for the anterior portion. The anterior clinoid process is marked by an arrow.

As noted in "Radiographic Technique," a standard angiographic projection will give to the siphon the appearance shown on Figure 351; an orbital view will produce a much sharper lateral swing of the supraclinoid portion (fig. 351). A half axial view will make the lateral swing appear more gradual.

Minor branches of the internal carotid artery. All of the major branches of the internal carotid artery arise from the supraclinoid portion of the vessel. However, small branches arise from the intrapetrosal and intracavernous portions which are not usually visible on the angiogram. These branches are: (1) the *caroticotympanic*, which leaves the internal carotid artery in the carotid canal to supply part of the tympanic

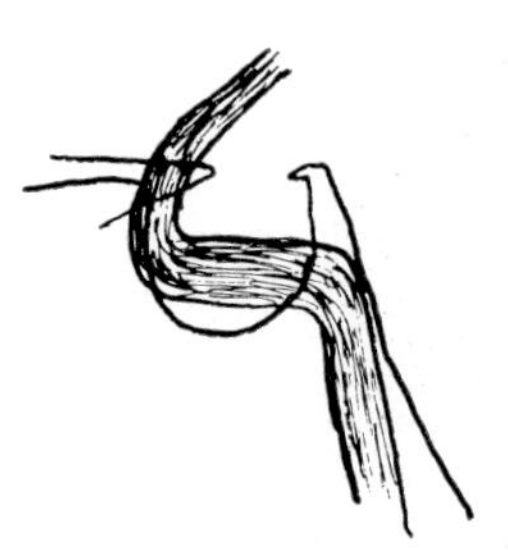

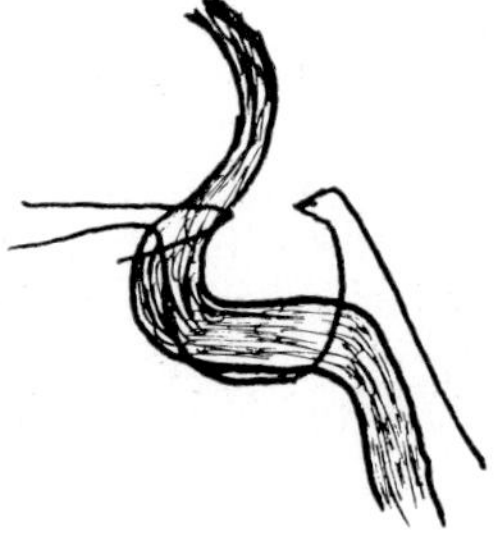

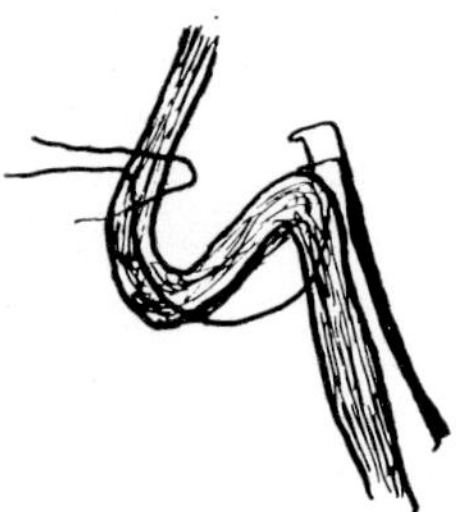

Fig. 350.—Common Configurations and Relationships of Internal Carotid Siphon with Sella Turcica in Intracavernous and Supraclinoid Portion

(Revised 1963)

cavity; (2) the *cavernous branches,* which are many small vessels supplying the wall of the sinus as well as that of the inferior petrosal sinus; (3) the *semilunar branches,* which are small branches to this ganglion; (4) an *anterior meningeal branch,* which together with a meningeal branch of the ethmoidal, supplies the dura of the anterior cranial fossa; (5) the *branches to the Gasserian ganglion* which supply also the dura of the middle cranial fossa. The caroticotympanic branch and the cavernous sinus branches anastomose with small branches of the internal maxillary and of the middle meningeal arteries which in turn arise from the external carotid artery. Rarely do these branches become visible on the angiogram, but potentially they represent a source of collateral supply between the external and internal carotid artery. Some may be enlarged in richly vascular meningiomas. The authors have seen a case of carotid-cavernous fistula which, following ligation of the internal carotid artery in the cervical as well as in the

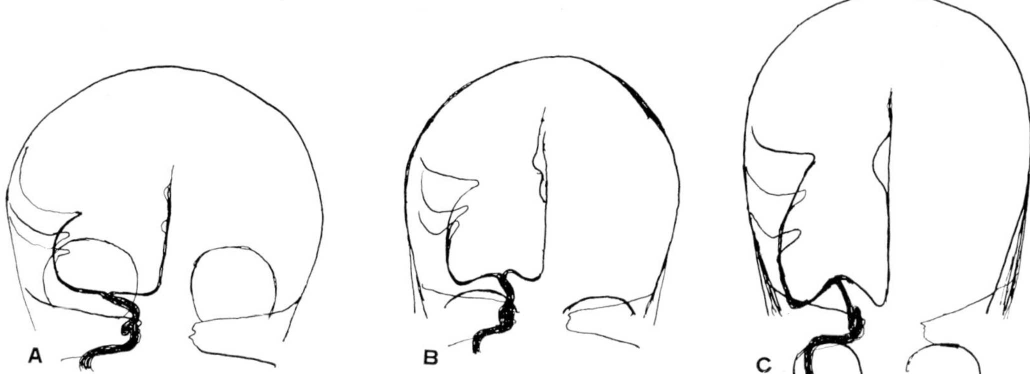

FIG. 351.—APPEARANCE OF THE INTERNAL CAROTID ARTERY AND ITS BRANCHES ACCORDING TO PROJECTION

(A) Orbital view; (B) standard angiographic anteroposterior projection; (C) half axial projection.

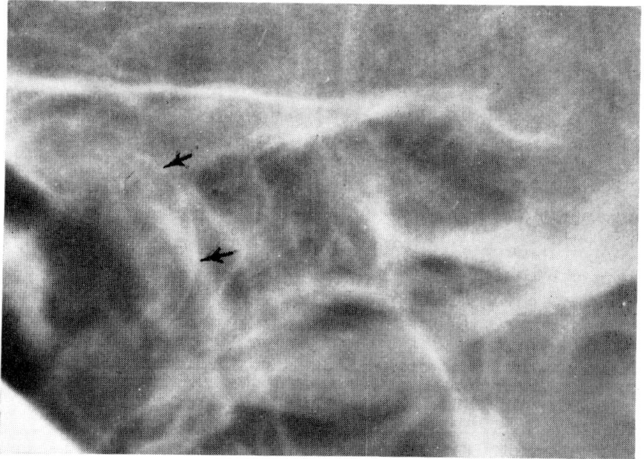

FIG. 352.—CHORIOID-RETINAL BLUSH IN A NORMAL PATIENT

The curvilinear dense shadow marks the posterior margin of the globe, and it is possible to determine the presence of exophthalmus by this means. In addition, it may be possible to follow the results of therapy for conditions causing exophthalmus. Although this is a graphic means of showing this, the morbidity of carotid angiography precludes its use in routine cases.

(Revised 1963)

intracranial segment, including the ophthalmic artery, still showed slight filling of the fistula (Mount and Taveras, 1957). This probably occurred by way of the carotid branches to the wall of the cavernous sinus which anastomose with branches of the middle meningeal artery. Small branches have been described between the two internal carotid arteries across the floor of the sella turcica.

Major branches of the internal carotid artery. The major branches of the internal carotid artery, those which can be seen on the cerebral angiogram, follow.

Ophthalmic artery. The ophthalmic arises from the internal carotid artery immediately after it leaves the cavernous sinus, medial to the anterior clinoid process. It enters the orbit through the optic foramen below and lateral to the optic nerve (fig. 384). The artery then turns upward and medially passing over the nerve to reach the medial wall of the orbit. Its *main branches* are the *lacrimal*, which proceeds along the lateral

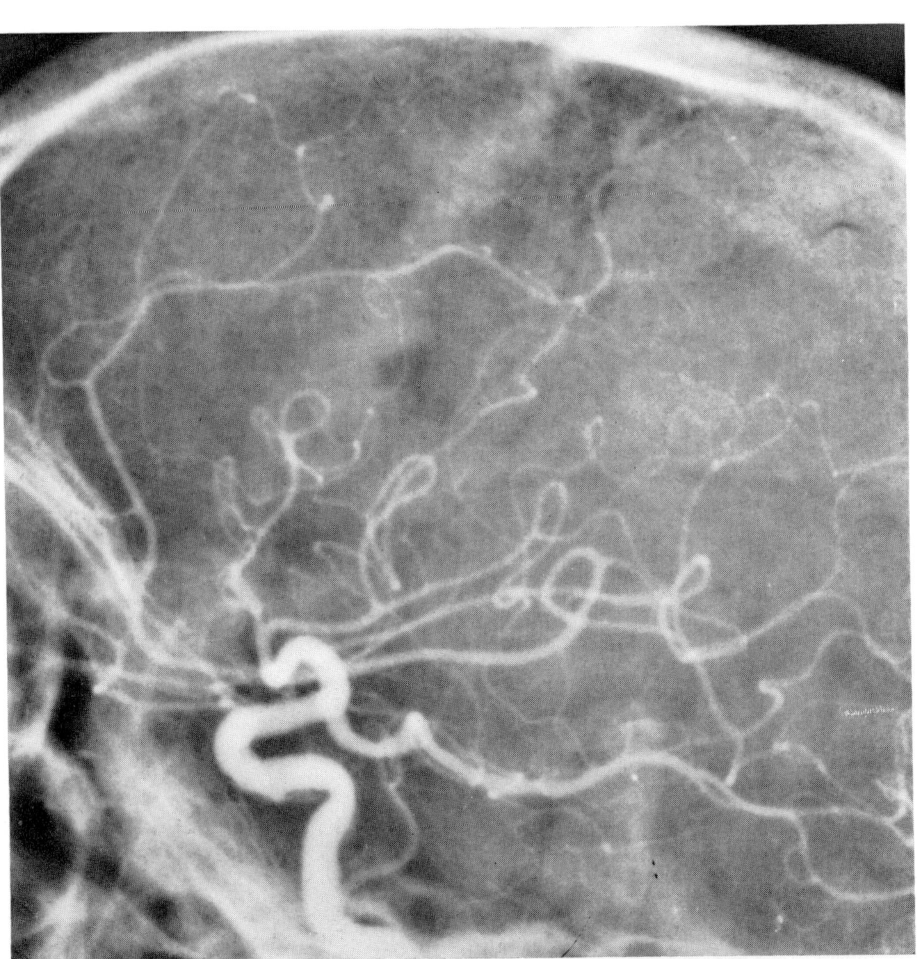

FIG. 353.—NORMAL CAROTID ANGIOGRAM, LATERAL VIEW

The posterior communicating is well shown and its characteristic upward curvature as it joins the posterior cerebral artery is well demonstrated. Just above the posterior communicating artery is the anterior chorioidal. The anterior cerebral artery demonstrates one of its normal variants, namely, the callosomarginal artery is arising from early bifurcation of the anterior cerebral artery and both pericallosal arteries filled from the opposite side. An appearance such as this may sometimes mislead the observer because it suggests ventricular dilatation.

(Revised 1963)

wall, and the *supraorbital*, which courses approximately in the center of the orbit above the globe. The *main trunk* of the ophthalmic artery continues along the medial orbital wall giving off the ethmoidal and the palpebral branches which, except in some pathologic cases, are usually not visible on the angiogram. In the lateral view, the ophthalmic artery trunk can easily be seen but superimposed bone shadows and superimposition of the three branch vessels of the artery make identification difficult or impossible within the orbit. In order to visualize the artery and its branches to better advantage, an orbital view is necessary, and a stereoscopic view is preferable in order that the branches of the ophthalmic may be separated from the intracranial arteries. The central retinal artery is not visible on angiograms, but the arteriolar and capillary blush of the chorioid and retina are visible in the late arterial and capillary phases. They are identified readily owing to the concave appearance of the posterior aspect of the globe (fig. 352), and this can be used to locate accurately the posterior aspect of the eyeball. The "retino-chorioid blush" is normally 2 to 4 mm. posterior to the anterior margin of the frontozygomatic border of the orbit on the corresponding side. If it is anterior to this, exophthalmus may be present. In a straight lateral view, the anterior margin of the lateral orbital border of the side against the film projects dorsal to the one away from the film.

Posterior communicating artery. This vessel arises from the dorsal aspect of the carotid siphon and proceeds posteriorly and medially. It is approximately 1.5 cm. in length. At its dorsal extremity, it joins the posterior cerebral artery approximately 1.0 cm. distal to the bifurcation of the basilar artery (fig. 387E). Its configuration is somewhat vari-

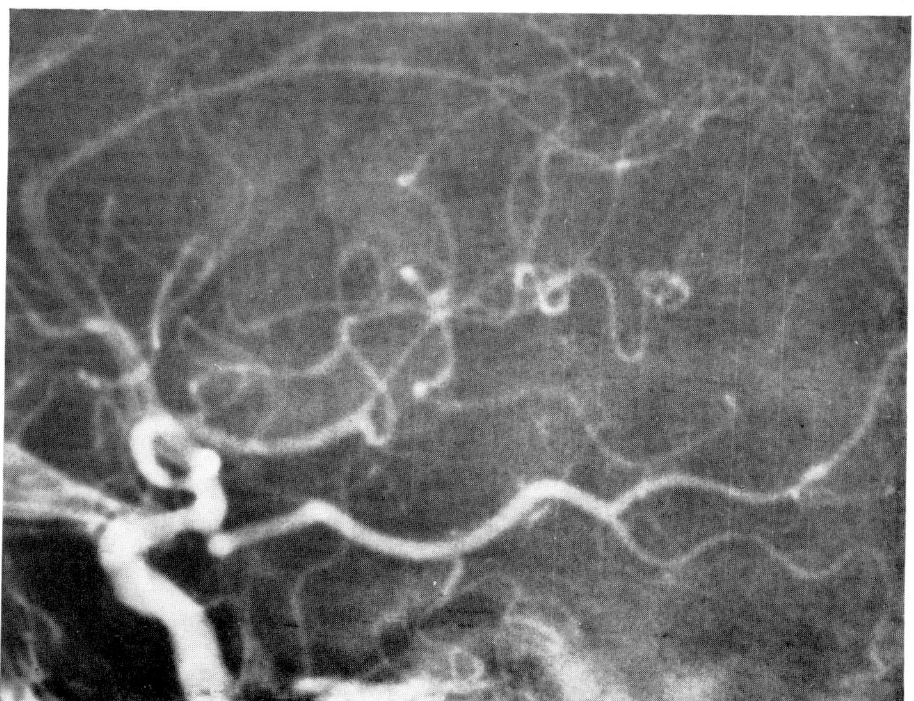

FIG. 354.—CAROTID ORIGIN OF THE POSTERIOR CEREBRAL ARTERY

There is no change in the caliber of the posterior communicating artery when it joins the posterior cerebral artery; in fact, the posterior communicating is slightly larger than the posterior cerebral artery, indicating that the blood supply to this artery is coming from the carotid system. This is the lateral view of the same case shown in Fig. 389.

(Revised 1963)

able. In the *lateral view* it usually describes a slight curve concave upward (fig. 353). Sometimes it is almost straight and its junction with the posterior cerebral artery cannot be seen on the films. The latter appearance usually denotes carotid origin of the posterior cerebral artery (fig. 354). The posterior communicating and posterior cerebral arteries fill completely or incompletely in a high percentage of cases depending on the location of the needle and other technical factors. According to Saltzman (1959) it filled in 48 to 49 per cent of internal carotid punctures and in 26 to 30 per cent of common carotid puctures. They may fill on one side and not on the other, and one side may be larger than the other. At the junction of the posterior communicating artery with the carotid siphon, there is often a slight dilatation which we have come to call "junctional dilatation" and should not be confused with an aneurysm. The shape of this dilatation may be triangular or round (fig. 355) with the posterior communicating usually joining the dilatation at its apex. We have had the opportunity to obtain an autopsy specimen in a case of junctional dilatation and histological sections revealed that all of the arterial layers were present. More recently Hassler and Saltzman (1961) have described several cases in which anatomic defects were found in the infundibular or junctional portion of the vessel, similar to those found in aneurysms. The dilatation should be considered as a possible aneurysm only when it measures more than 3 mm. in diameter, or when the posterior communicating artery does not join the dilatation at its apex. Whether or not this represents a "pre-aneurysmal" lesion has not been established, but is suggested by the findings of Hassler and Saltzman. One recent case seen at the Neurological Institute appears to confirm these findings.

In the *frontal projection*, the posterior communicating artery is partly superimposed on the supraclinoid portion of the internal carotid. The posterior portion usually projects medial to the carotid artery (fig. 356). This is a relatively constant relationship and deviation should be regarded as probably pathologic.

From the dorsal segment of the posterior communicating artery arise a number of small branches which supply the medial surface of the thalamus and the wall of the

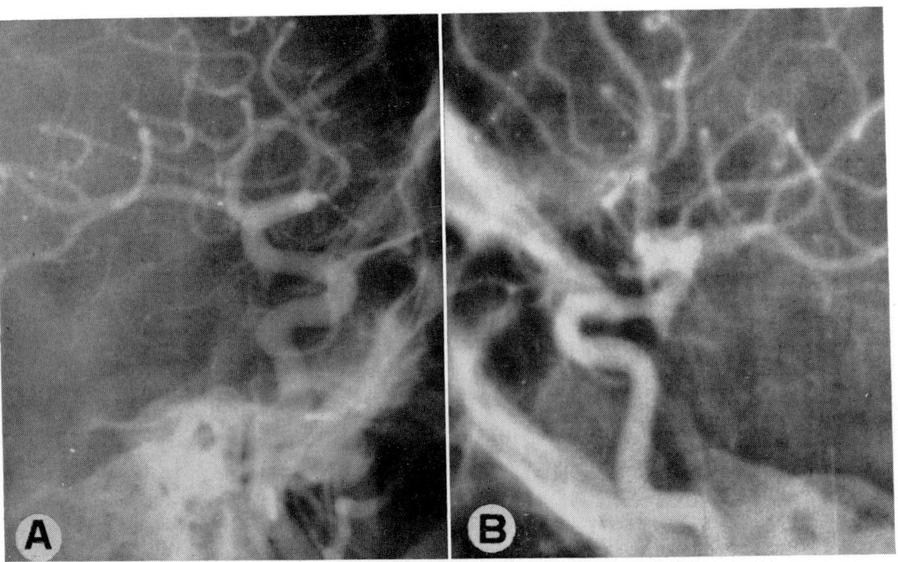

Fig. 355.—Two Cases of "Junctional Dilatation" at Junction of Posterior Communicating with Internal Carotid Artery

(A) Rounded type; (B) funnel shape.

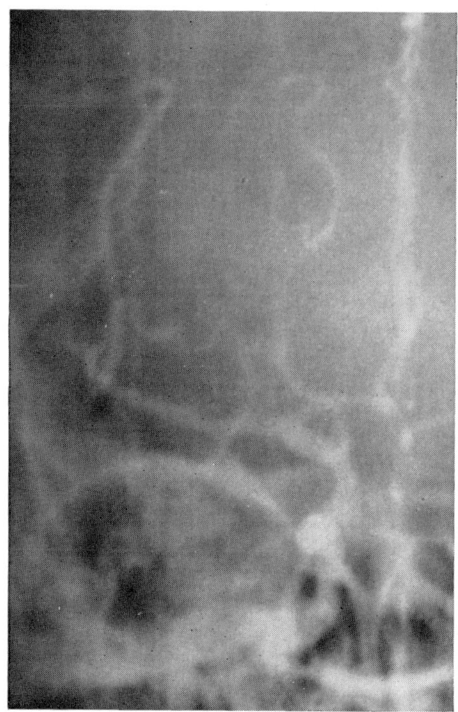

FIG. 356.—CAROTID ANGIOGRAM, NORMAL, SHOWING FILLING OF POSTERIOR COMMUNICATING AND POSTERIOR CEREBRAL ARTERIES

The posterior communicating artery is directed backward and slightly medially, and after joining the posterior cerebral artery, it follows the course of this artery around the brain stem.

third ventricle, but these usually are not visible in the angiogram unless they are enlarged (fig. 393).

Anterior chorioidal artery. A small but important branch of the internal carotid artery, the anterior chorioidal, arises just distal to the origin of the posterior communicating artery in three-fourths of cases. Carpenter and co-authors (1954) found that it arose from the middle cerebral artery in 7 of 60 dissections, from the posterior communicating artery in 4, and from the bifurcation of the internal carotid artery at the junction of the anterior and middle cerebral arteries in 2 cases. In one of the 60 dissections it was absent; it may be double. Sjögren (1956) was able to identify it in 93 per cent of 100 normal angiograms.

Although in 90 per cent of the cases, the anterior chorioidal is the first branch immediately above the posterior communicating artery, one, two, or even three branches may arise from the carotid siphon before the origin of the anterior chorioidal. These are usually perforating arteries which enter the anterior perforated substance together with the lenticulostriate vessels (Carpenter and co-authors).

After its origin from the posterior aspect of the internal carotid artery, the anterior chorioidal is directed posteriorly and slightly medially as it crosses the cisternal space in the parasellar region. This segment has been called the cisternal portion by Sjögren and is about 1.0 cm. in length. The artery, passing laterally, then reaches the medial surface of the tip of the temporal lobe, extends around the uncus, and swings laterally and dorsally to enter the temporal horn through the chorioidal fissure. Within the temporal horn it supplies the chorioid plexus. The latter has been called the plexal portion (Sjögren) and can usually be identified because the shadow of the artery gets broader at this point (fig. 357). A capillary "blush" is sometimes seen in this region representing the chorioid plexus. The anterior chorioidal artery supplies, in addition to the chorioid plexus, the hippocampus, and the basal ganglia.

In the *lateral view* the anterior chorioidal artery is directed backward and slightly downward for a short distance; then it curves upward and backward, describing a gentle curve with a superior convexity (figs. 357 and 358), but this is variable. The usual length of the anterior chorioidal artery is approximately 3 cm. as seen on the films. When longer than 3 cm. the artery may be pathologically elongated and enlarged, although this is not necessarily so. Enlargement of the anterior chorioidal artery may indicate the direct blood supply of an intracerebral tumor by this artery, but it may also be enlarged in cases of increased intracranial pressure produced by a tumor in any location. Under these circumstances, enlargement evidently is related to the abnormal pressure and may be caused by a need for increased production of cerebro-

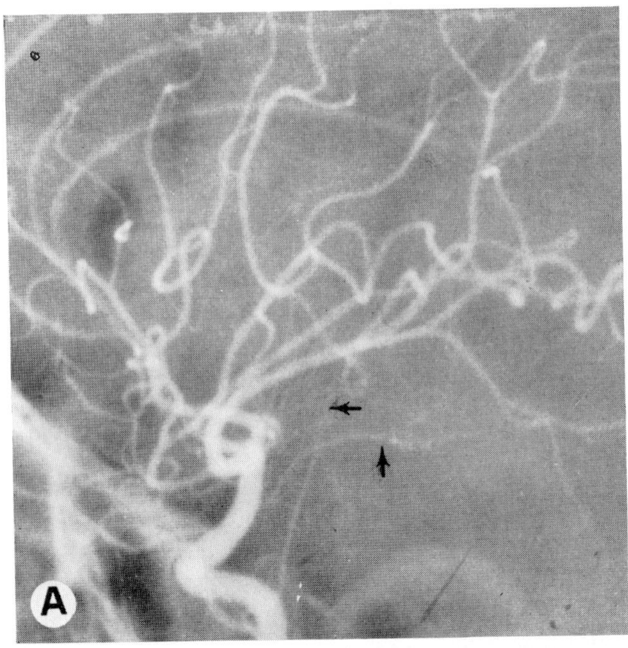

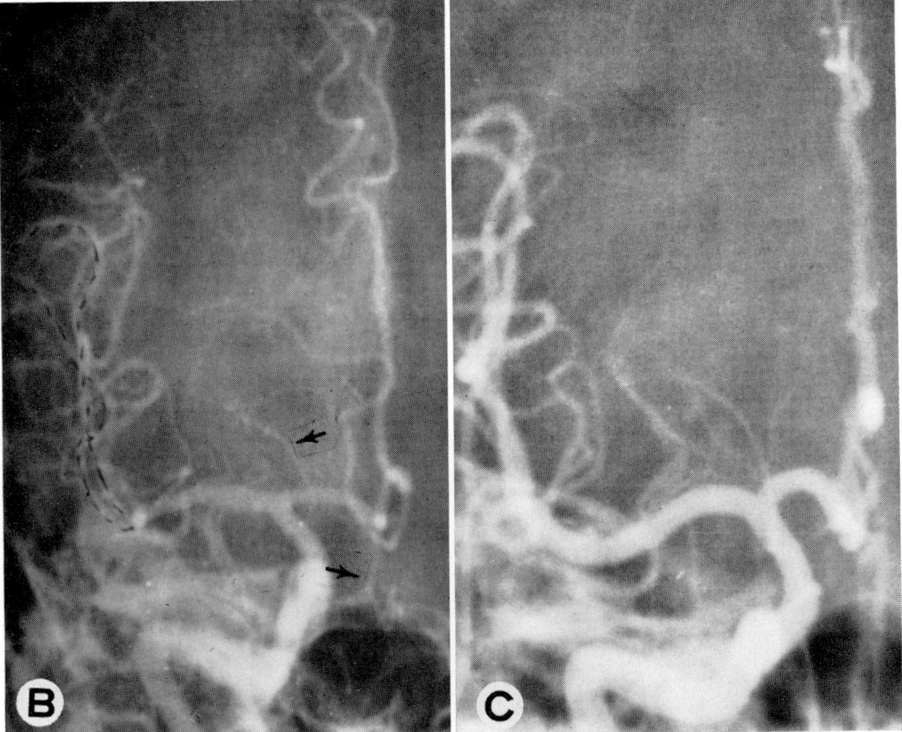

FIG. 357.—NORMAL FRONTAL AND LATERAL CAROTID ANGIOGRAMS

The lateral view (A) shows the anterior chorioidal artery (*lower arrow*). The upper arrow points to the lenticulostriate arteries seen in the lateral view. They form a fanlike group of thin vessels with the apex downward, which is usually obscured by the branches of the middle cerebral artery. The Sylvian triangle

(Revised 1963)

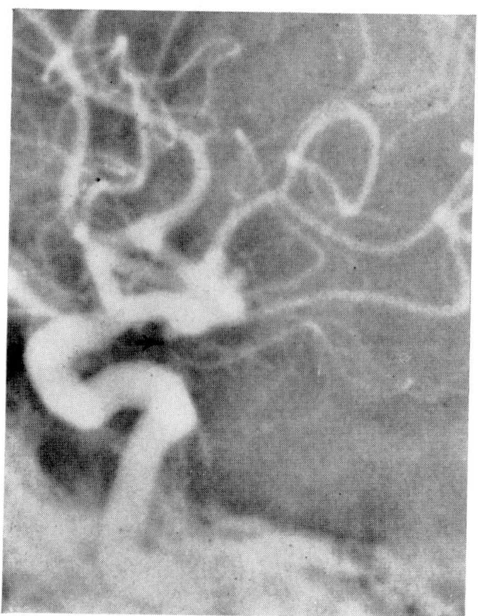

FIG. 358.—NORMAL CAROTID ANGIOGRAM, JUNCTIONAL DILATATION AT ORIGIN OF ANTERIOR CHORIOIDAL ARTERY

The carotid siphon presents a very slight irregularity on its posterior aspect, and at the origin of the anterior chorioidal artery (*arrow*) there is a junctional or infundibular dilatation.

spinal fluid as well as supplying vital areas of the brain. The artery may also be enlarged in cases of middle cerebral thrombosis (figs. 553 and 557). A junctional or infundibular dilatation at the origin of the anterior chorioidal from the internal carotid is sometimes seen (fig. 358).

In the *frontal projection*, the anterior chorioidal artery is seen to arise from the internal carotid and to proceed upward and medially for a short distance, after which it turns laterally. After completing its turn around the medial portion of the tip of the temporal lobe, it enters the temporal horn and soon disappears from sight in the angiogram. The curve described by the anterior chorioidal artery depends on the projection used. The greater the caudal angulation of the central beam used to make the exposure in relation to the canthomeatal line, the broader is the curve described by the artery (fig. 359), and vice versa.

The shadow of the artery becomes slightly broader as it forms the chorioid plexus (fig. 357), and it is often possible to see the chorioid plexus as an area of slightly increased density immediately above the artery (chorioid blush). At times the artery can be followed high along its course in the temporal horn. When visible in this manner it may indicate that an abnormal condition is present, as explained above. In its posterior portion, the artery anastomoses with the posterior chorioidal artery which supplies the greater portion of the chorioid plexus. The anastomotic pathway is sometimes seen in cases of thrombosis with collateral circulation (fig. 565).

Anterior Cerebral Artery

The anterior cerebral artery has its origin at the bifurcation of the internal carotid artery at the medial aspect of the Sylvian fissure. It has a horizontal and a vertical segment. In its horizontal portion the artery passes medially and forward above the optic nerve or chiasm until it reaches the anterior communicating artery. At this point the artery bends fairly sharply to proceed directly forward and upward along the interhemispheric fissure. It courses beside the anterior aspect of the corpus callosum to the genu, where it turns dorsad. The latter turn may be called the genu or the "knee" of the anterior cerebral artery. The artery continues along the medial surface of the hemisphere directly backward as the pericallosal artery and finally anastomoses with a branch of the posterior cerebral artery.

In the region of the anterior communicating artery, the anterior cerebral artery is usually convex downward initially, then it

is well shown. The frontal view (B) shows the normal curvature of the anterior chorioidal in this projection (*upper arrow*). The lenticulostriate arteries are also shown just lateral to the anterior chorioidal artery. The lower arrow in the midline indicates the frontopolar artery which, because of projection, is thrown downward. The frontal view is not of the same patient as the lateral view. (C) is another frontal view that illustrates the course of the anterior chorioidal artery. Its curvature is broader owing to greater angulation of the tube.

(Revised 1963)

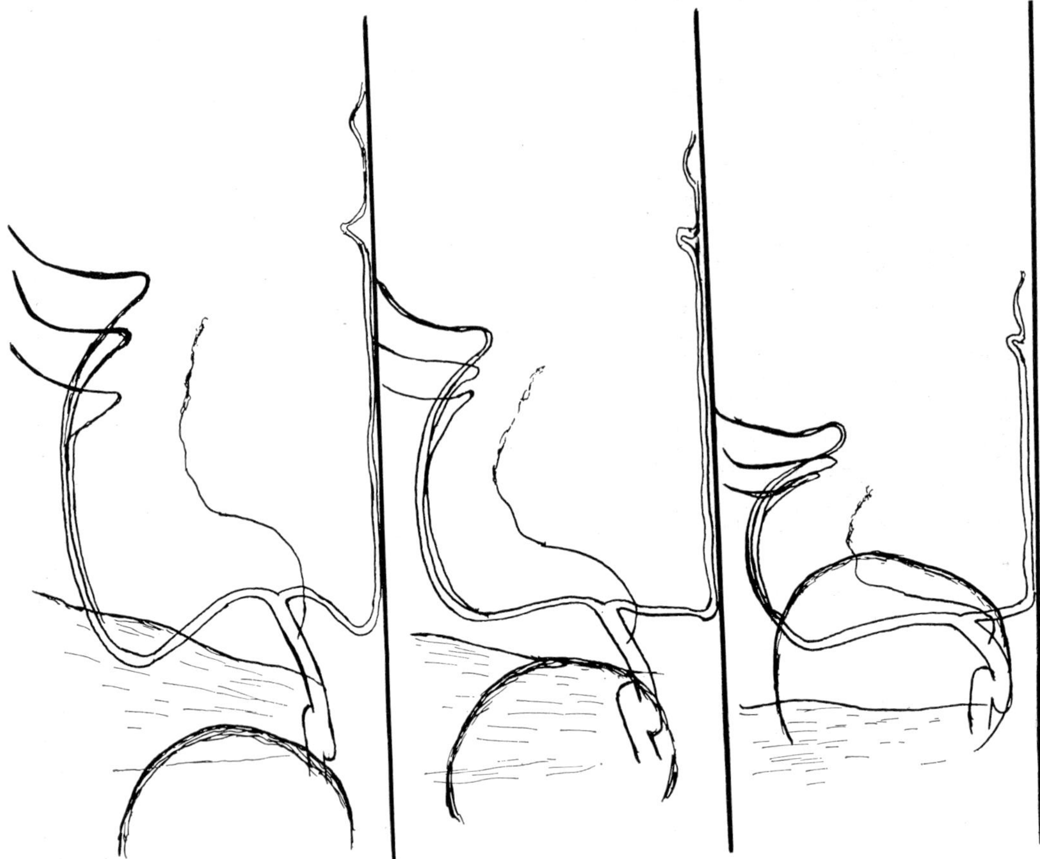

FIG. 359.—DIAGRAM TO EXPLAIN THE DIFFERENCES IN THE CURVATURE OF THE ANTERIOR CHORIOIDAL ARTERY AND IN THE CONFIGURATION OF INSULAR CURVE OF MIDDLE CEREBRAL ARTERY WITH DIFFERENT PROJECTIONS

reverses to describe a slight curve concave downward followed by another convex forward curve (fig. 360). In children and in younger individuals these curves are less pronounced than in the older age group, owing to increased tortuosity. Throughout their course in the interhemispheric fissure, the anterior cerebral and pericallosal arteries are fairly close to the corpus callosum, but this relationship is variable. The normal tortuosity of the vessels, which sometimes is quite pronounced in normal individuals, tends to separate the anterior cerebral vessels from the corpus callosum at intervals.

The anterior cerebral artery gives off many branches. From its horizontal portion, tiny branches emerge which pierce the brain at the anterior perforated space and supply the rostrum of the corpus callosum, the head of the caudate nucleus, and the septum pellucidum. Heubner's artery also arises from this segment proximal to the anterior communicating artery. None of these branches is visible on the angiogram except for a rare case in which Heubner's artery is visible. The latter vessel arises from the anterior cerebral artery close to the origin of the anterior communicating artery. From this point it passes laterally along the horizontal portion of the anterior cerebral and of the middle cerebral, until it reaches the origin of the lenticulostriate arteries. At this point the artery swings upward to penetrate the brain through the anterior perforated substance, together with the medial lenticulostriate arteries. Because of its course, Heub-

(*Revised 1963*)

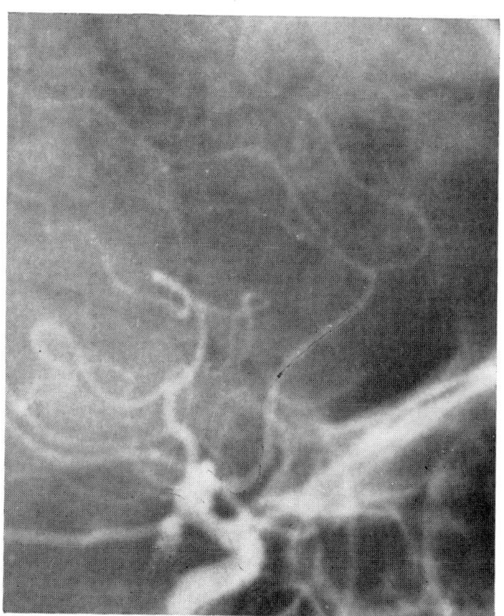

FIG. 360.—NORMAL CAROTID ANGIOGRAM, LATERAL VIEW

The anterior cerebral artery presents a downward convex curve in its proximal portion followed by a downward concave curve, after which it turns around the corpus callosum. These curvatures are usually less pronounced in children than in adults.

ner's artery may also be called the *recurrent lenticulostriate* artery. Functionally it is considered an important vessel because it supplies the anteromedial aspect of the head of the caudate nucleus and adjoining putamen, part of the septal nucleus, and cells in the rostro-lateral area of the olfactory trigone. The artery of Heubner anastomoses with the lenticulostriate arteries, and also with surface branches of the anterior and middle cerebral arteries (Kaplan, 1958). The recurrent artery of Heubner is only occasionally seen on angiograms.

In studying the branches of the major cerebral arteries, it should be kept in mind that variation is the rule.

Orbital branch. The orbital branch or branches (sometimes two or three in number) are the first to arise from the ascending portion of the anterior cerebral artery. They extend forward and downward to supply the orbital surface of the frontal lobe. These branches are usually not too conspicuous on the angiogram but often can be detected if sought. They may be displaced by subfrontal tumors, thus providing a clue to the extracerebral location of the mass (fig. 361). The orbital branch anastomoses with the orbitofrontal branch of the middle cerebral artery.

Frontopolar branch. The branch usually arises from the anterior cerebral artery *proximal* to the maximum bend (knee) of this vessel, but it may arise from the callosomarginal branch of the anterior cerebral artery. From its origin, the artery passes forward and usually upward to reach the region of the anterior pole of the frontal lobe. It ordinarily divides into two or three branches which surround the anterior border of the frontal lobe and then turn laterally to reach the convexity of the hemisphere.

The origin of the frontopolar artery from the anterior cerebral as seen in the anteroposterior view is an important reference point to the remainder of the vessel. The relative position of the origin of the vessel depends on the projection used to take the anteroposterior film; if more angulation is used, the point of origin is projected lower; in turn this can be transferred to the lateral view to determine corresponding segments in the two projections (fig. 357).

Callosomarginal artery. The major branch of the anterior cerebral artery is the callosomarginal. It usually arises distal to the origin of the frontopolar artery. The callosomarginal artery passes backward and upward and gives off the *anterior, middle,* and *posterior internal frontal branches* (fig. 361), terminating in the *paracentral* branch around the paracentral lobule. Sometimes the anterior internal frontal branch arises directly from the anterior cerebral; at other times the middle and posterior internal frontal branches may arise directly.

The callosomarginal artery is usually contained during part of its course in the callosomarginal sulcus, but as it courses dorsad, it may leave this sulcus to course over the cingulate gyrus only to enter the same or another sulcus further back. This causes the artery or its branches to separate themselves from the midline when entering a sulcus, and to return to the midline when over a gyrus (fig. 362). When the internal frontal and the paracentral branches reach

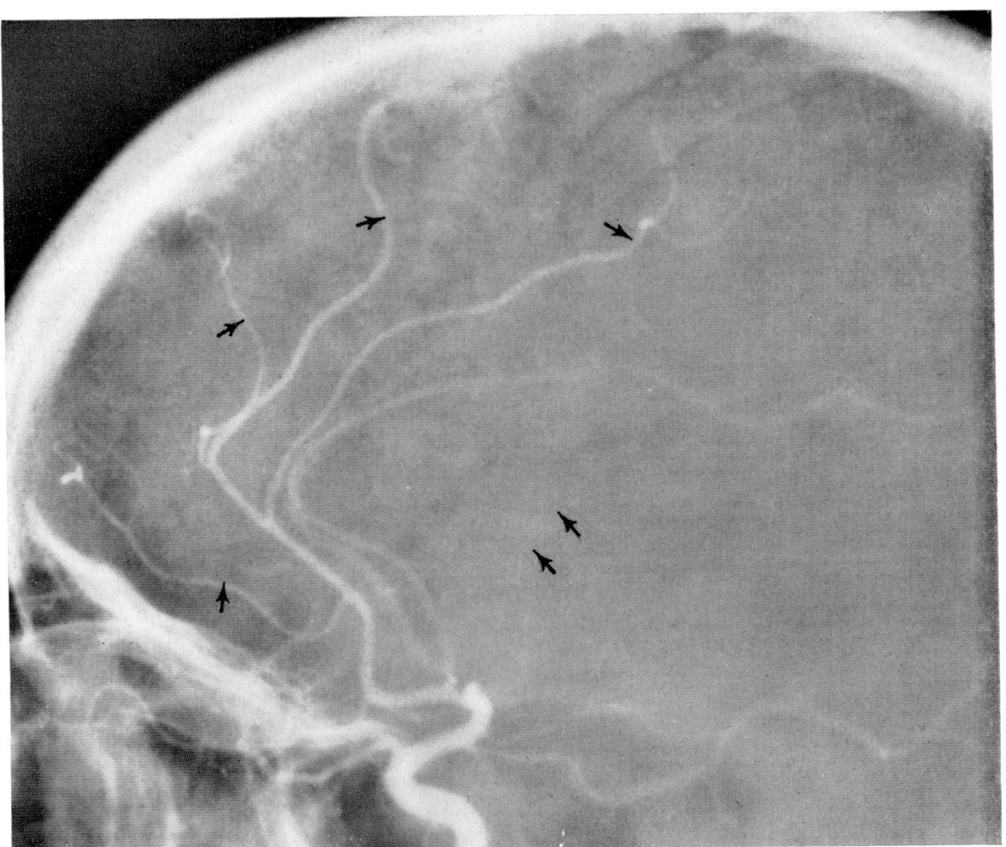

FIG. 361.—LATERAL CAROTID ANGIOGRAM TO DEMONSTRATE THE BRANCHES OF THE ANTERIOR CEREBRAL ARTERY IN A PATIENT WITH THROMBOSIS OF THE MIDDLE CEREBRAL ARTERY

There is early bifurcation of the anterior cerebral artery. The callosomarginal artery arises at the origin of the anterior cerebral, and it gives off the anterior, middle, and posterior internal frontal branches (*three upper arrows*). The frontopolar is the first branch coming off the callosomarginal artery (*lower arrow*). There was flash filling of the opposite anterior cerebral artery. The anterior chorioidal and the posterior communicating and cerebral arteries also fill. There is a fine ascending branch in the region of the lenticulostriate arteries which (*two arrows*) is often seen in cases of thrombosis of the middle cerebral artery. It evidently represents an enlarged lenticulostriate branch which could arise either from the middle cerebral trunk or from the anterior cerebral artery.

the upper margin of the hemisphere, they go over the top and turn out over the convexity of the hemisphere where they anastomose with pre- and post-Rolandic branches of the middle cerebral artery (fig. 363).

The callosomarginal artery may originate just distal to the anterior communicating artery. In the latter case it ascends more or less parallel with the main anterior cerebral artery which in this case should probably be called pericallosal artery. It sweeps around parallel to the pericallosal artery but describes a wider arc. Under these conditions, the callosomarginal artery gives off not only the anterior, middle, and posterior internal frontal branches, but the frontopolar branch as well (fig. 361). In the latter cases, it will be found, not infrequently, that both pericallosal arteries fill from one side only. If an angiogram of only the opposite side from which bilateral filling takes place is done, a false impression of ventricular dilatation may be gained (fig. 364).

Pericallosal artery. The pericallosal

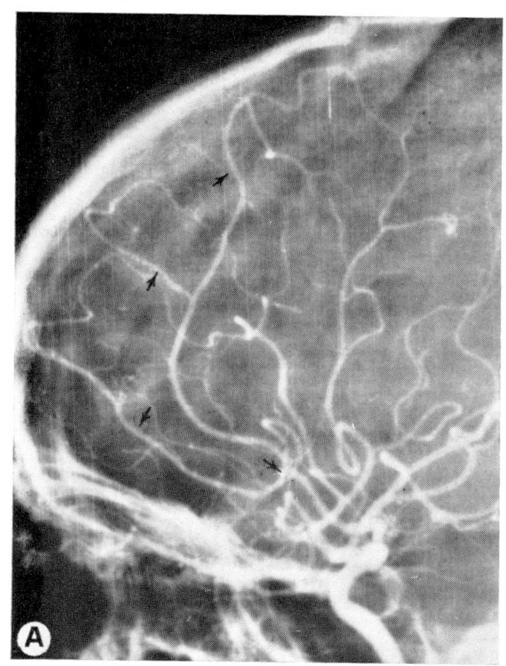

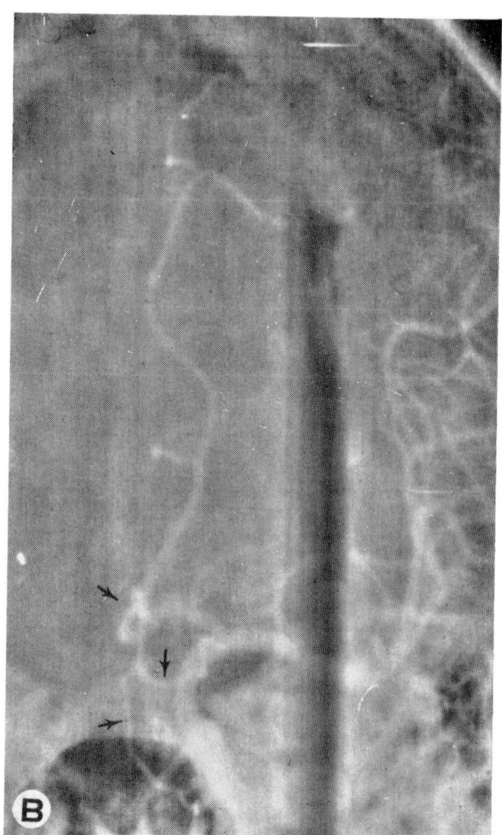

FIG. 362.—ANATOMICAL VARIANT OF ANTERIOR CEREBRAL ARTERY

The lateral projection (A) shows a branch of the anterior cerebral artery, the callosomarginal artery from which arise the frontopolar and the anterior and middle internal frontal branches *(arrows)*. The pericallosal artery did not fill from this side but filled from the opposite side when the other carotid was injected. The frontal projection (B) shows that the callosomarginal separates from the midline, probably because it entered the cingulate sulcus, thus giving the impression of a midline shift. The frontopolar artery and its branches are outlined by the *three arrows*.

artery may be called the terminal branch of the anterior cerebral. It is usually fairly close to the outer surface of the corpus callosum except when tortuosity is present. Ordinarily it gives off the *paracentral branch* which may, however, arise from the callosomarginal. The pericallosal artery terminates as the *precuneal branch*, which supplies the precuneus, or as a *posterior callosal* branch, which supplies the corpus callosum.

Anatomical variants. In addition to the variant just described above, others may be encountered. The initial portion of the anterior cerebral artery is usually horizontal, as seen in frontal films, or it may turn downward (fig. 360). Sometimes, however, it is directed upward, giving a false impression of upward displacement such as may be produced by a suprasellar mass. The latter configuration is found more frequently in children than in adults (fig. 365).

The horizontal portion of the anterior cerebral artery may be hypoplastic on one side as compared with the other. Absence of this segment, however, is extremely rare; Riggs (1937, 1953) did not find it totally absent in a single case out of 1647 dissections of the circle of Willis. Therefore the lack of filling of the trunk of one anterior cerebral artery, even with compression of the opposite

(Revised 1963)

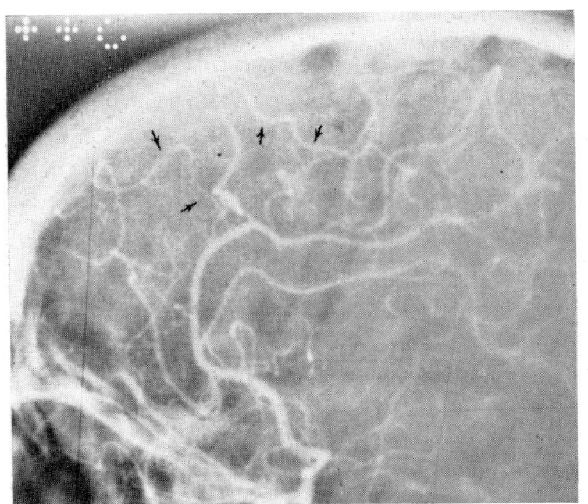

Fig. 363.—Branches of Anterior Cerebral Artery Going Over the Upper Surface of the Hemisphere and on to the Outer Surface of the Hemisphere

side during injection of the contrast substance, indicates that the segment is probably hypoplastic and not absent or thrombosed. Moreover, this hypoplastic segment usually is capable of dilating if partial or complete occlusion of the opposite internal carotid artery occurs. Spasm may also cause the anterior cerebral artery trunk to be thinner on one side.

There may be a common trunk of the anterior cerebral arteries. In these cases, both horizontal segments join at the midline and thereafter ascend as a common trunk until reaching the falx. At this point they may separate into two groups of branches, one on each side of the falx. Rarely, it may continue as a single pericallosal artery giving branches to both sides (Vander Eeken and Adams, 1953). A branch from the right pericallosal artery may supply an area on the left hemisphere after crossing the midline, and vice versa. This was found in 12 of 90 specimens studied by Vander Eecken (1961). The latter arrangement is found normally in the horse.

The anterior communicating artery is usually not clearly visible on the films. It may be single or multiple.

As seen in the lateral view, the proximal segment of the ascending portion of the anterior cerebral artery may present a fairly deep curve concave downward which should not be confused with a suprasellar tumor. More distal, another curve concave upward may to be found normally just proximal to the knee (fig. 360). Further dorsad, the pericallosal artery may present a flat seg-

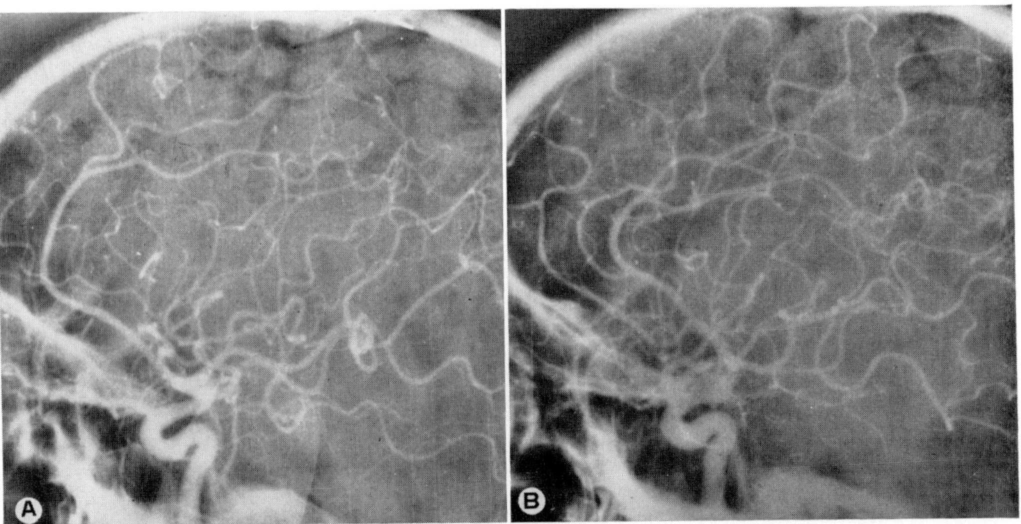

Fig. 364.—Normal Carotid Angiogram, with both Pericallosal Arteries Arising from One Side and Simulating Ventricular Dilatation on the Opposite Side

The first side was examined and it showed an apparently wide sweep to the anterior cerebral artery, which suggests ventricular dilatation. The second side (B) was then injected and showed a normal pericallosal curve; the pericallosal arteries are almost completely superimposed on each other.

(Revised 1963)

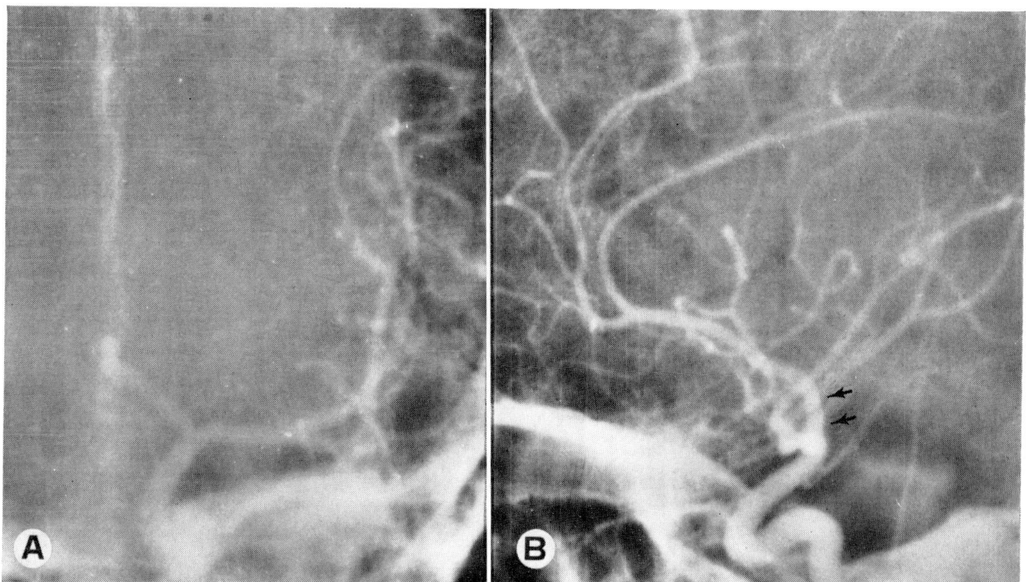

FIG. 365.—NORMAL CAROTID ANGIOGRAM

The frontal projection (A) shows that the anterior cerebral artery goes upward and medially instead of straight across or slightly downward. In the lateral projection (B) there is also an upward course to the anterior cerebral artery in its proximal portion (*arrows*). This appearance is more commonly observed in children than in adults, and it is not rarely seen in arteriosclerotic older individuals where the arteries are somewhat stiff.

ment which corresponds to the same configuration of the pericallosal sulcus found in some cases (fig. 366). The segment may even present an upward concavity. Such appearances, when present alone, should not be interpreted as indicative of a parasagittal mass.

Middle Cerebral Artery

The middle cerebral artery is a continuation, or the main branch, of the internal carotid artery. It is almost never absent. When the anterior cerebral artery does not fill, the internal carotid artery extends onward uninterrupted directly laterally to become the middle cerebral artery. Its origin usually is at the medial aspect of the temporal lobe. The proximal portion of the middle cerebral artery is horizontal in its course as it passes laterally and slightly forward. It often extends laterally, forward and slightly downward (as does the anterior cerebral artery); only occasionally does it extend laterally and upward in a normal case. As seen in the *lateral view*, this initial segment is foreshortened by virtue of its lateral direction. Although short, it should be sought since it is usually present except in children, where it may not be discernible. If the segment is not visible in a *straight* lateral view, posterior displacement of this portion of the artery may be present (fig. 365). The actual extent of the lateral and forward direction of this segment of the middle cerebral artery may be best shown on a basal view (fig. 367).

As the middle cerebral artery extends laterally from the bifurcation, it is situated between the temporal lobe and the lower aspect or the insula or island of Reil (fig. 368). The middle cerebral artery and its branches then turn up around the lower aspect of the island of Reil to continue their course upward and backward in the deepest portion of the Sylvian fissure, between the outer surface of the island of Reil and the medial surface of the temporal lobe (fig. 369). By this time the middle cerebral artery has given off several branches which will be described presently.

(*Revised 1963*)

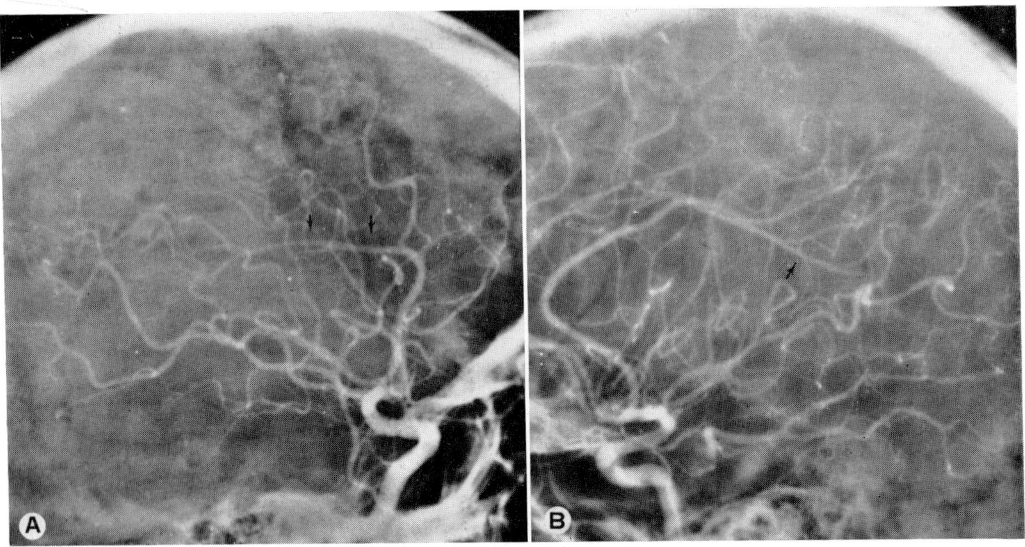

Fig. 366.—Normal Carotid Angiogram

(A) shows flattening of the anterior portion of the pericallosal artery in a normal case. (B) illustrates flattening of the posterior portion of the pericallosal artery (*arrows*).

Variation in the way in which the middle cerebral branches originate from the common trunk as well as in the number of the branches is the rule. However, it is best to consider the middle cerebral as bifurcating or trifurcating at or just before reaching the end of its horizontal segment. From these branches, other divisions arise which are all contained initially within the Sylvian fissure and which leave the fissure at various levels from its anterior to its posterior extent.

Lenticulostriate arteries. The horizontal portion of the middle cerebral artery gives rise to the *lenticulostriate vessels.* These are represented by two groups of 2 to 4 small branches, the medial and the lateral lenticulostriate arteries, which ascend from their origin in the middle cerebral artery to penetrate the brain through the anterior perforated substance. The medial group passes on the inner side of the lentiform nucleus to supply this nucleus, the caudate nucleus, and the internal capsule. The lateral lenticulostriate group passes on the lateral side; it supplies the caudate nucleus and the thalamus. The lenticulostriate arteries describe an S-shaped curve on the right side and a reversed "S" on the left (figs. 368 and 370) as the observer faces the patient. That is, they pass upward and medially for about 0.5 cm. and then describe an arc concave inward as they ascend further for a distance of about 2 cm. The lenticulostriate arteries are usually visible if looked for in radiographs of good quality. Some of these arteries may arise directly from the internal carotid artery or from the trunk of the anterior cerebral artery. The lenticulostriate arteries may be enlarged in cases of thrombosis and in neoplasms associated with increased intracranial pressure, particularly if the neoplasm is partly supplied by these vessels.

Andersen (1958) has attempted to establish normal measurements of the distance from the midline to the most medial and the most lateral of these arteries. He found that the distance to the most medial artery measured at the apex of the concave curve was 26 mm. in normal cases; and to the most lateral artery, it was 38 mm. These measurements have not been used by the authors and no opinions can be given as to their practical value. On the lateral projection, the lenticulostriate arteries are more difficult to visualize; they usually overlie the region of the internal carotid bifurcation. Actually they, or the areas which they supply, have a fan

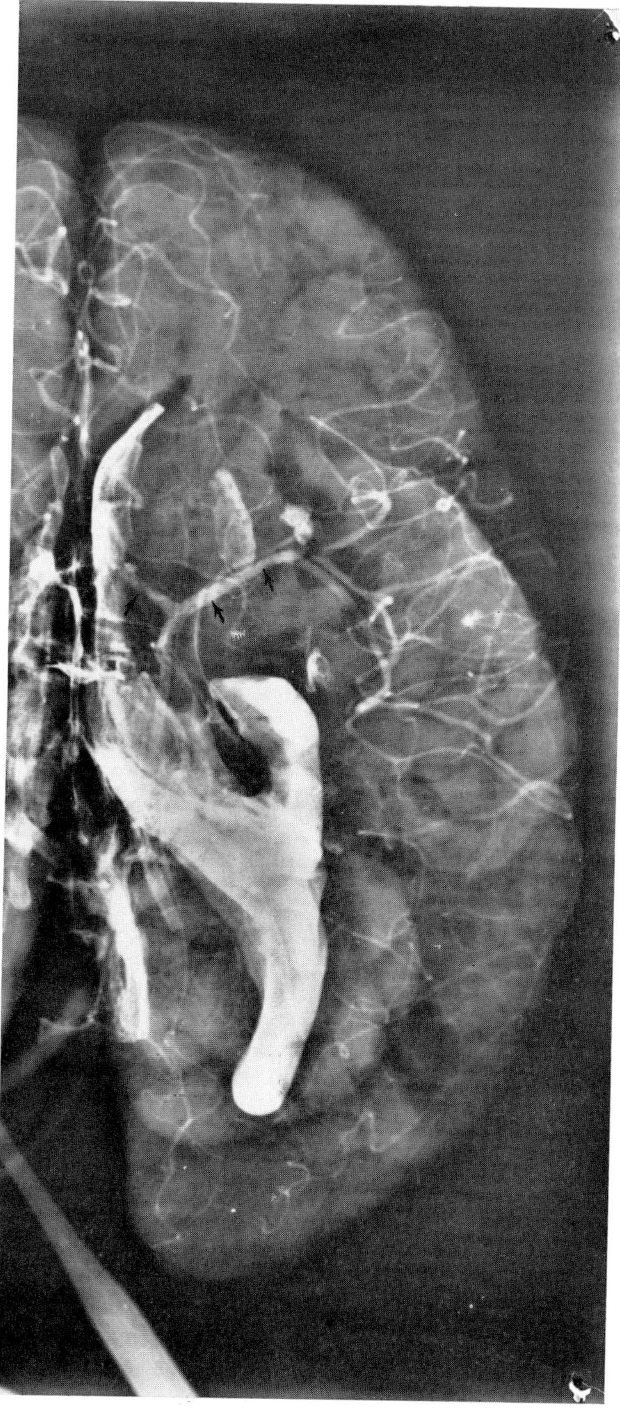

FIG. 367.—SPECIMEN ANGIOGRAM IN BASE PROJECTION WITH INJECTION OF THE VENTRICULAR SYSTEM

The bifurcation of the internal carotid artery is shown and its position in relation with the ventricles is seen. The middle cerebral artery describes a curve concave backward. The anterior cerebral artery is directed forward and medially (*arrow*).

(Revised 1963)

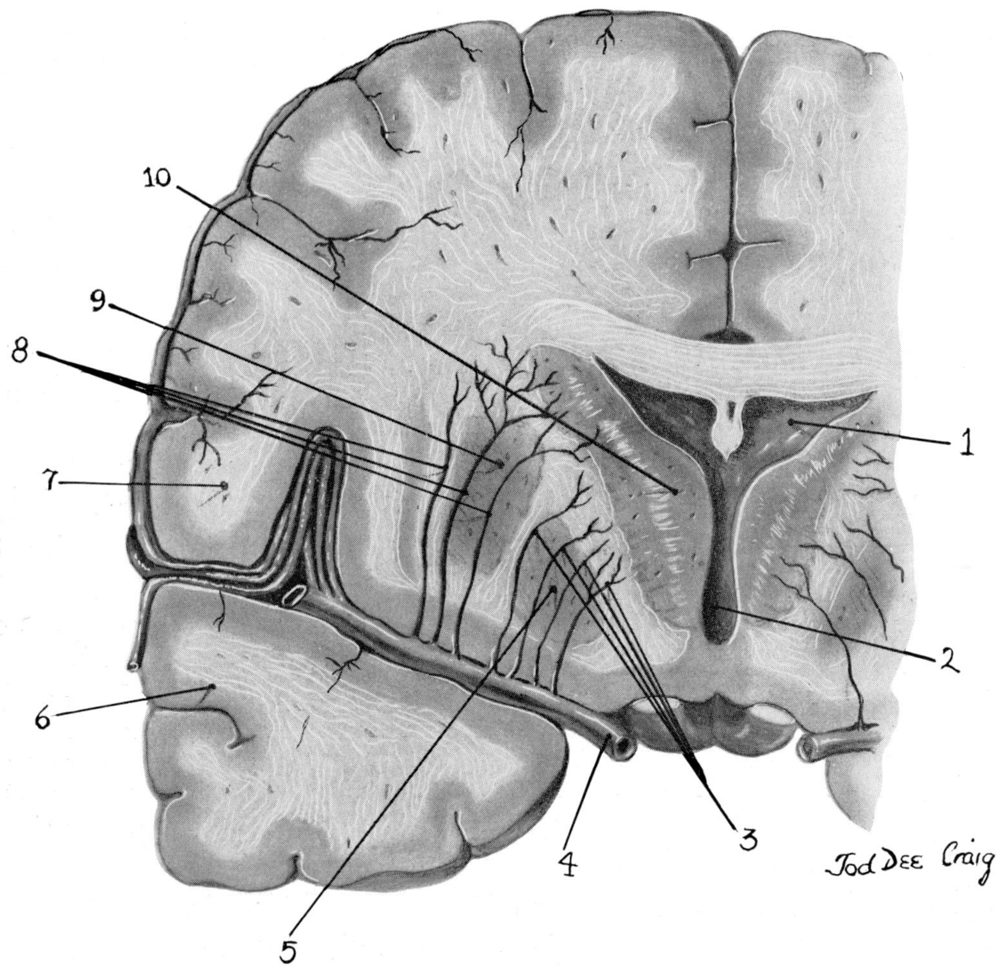

FIG. 368.—CORONAL SECTION OF THE BRAIN PASSING THROUGH THE ANTERIOR TEMPORAL REGION, DIAGRAMMATIC REPRESENTATION

The diagram shows the branches of the middle cerebral artery as they go upward to the top of the Sylvian fissure and then downward before emerging from the Sylvian fissure. (1) lateral ventricle. (2) third ventricle. (3) medial lenticulostriate arteries. (4) middle cerebral a. (5) globus pallidus. (6) temporal lobe. (7) frontoparietal operculum. (8) lateral lenticulostriate arteries. (9) putamen. (10) caudate nucleus.

shape with the apex downward as seen in the lateral view (fig. 370). The artery of Heubner ascends with the medial lenticulostriate arteries.

Anterior branches. After the lenticulostriate vessels, the first branches to arise from the middle cerebral artery are the *anterior temporal* branch, which passes downward on the outer surface and near the tip of the temporal lobe, and the *orbitofrontal branch*. The latter comes out of the Sylvian fissure anteriorly and distributes itself along the lateral portion and the undersurface of the frontal lobe. The orbitofrontal frequently anastomoses directly with the frontopolar branch of the anterior cerebral artery. The anterior temporal anastomoses with the anterior temporal branch of the posterior cerebral artery. The orbitofrontal and anterior temporal branches may arise from a common trunk.

After the two most anterior branches,

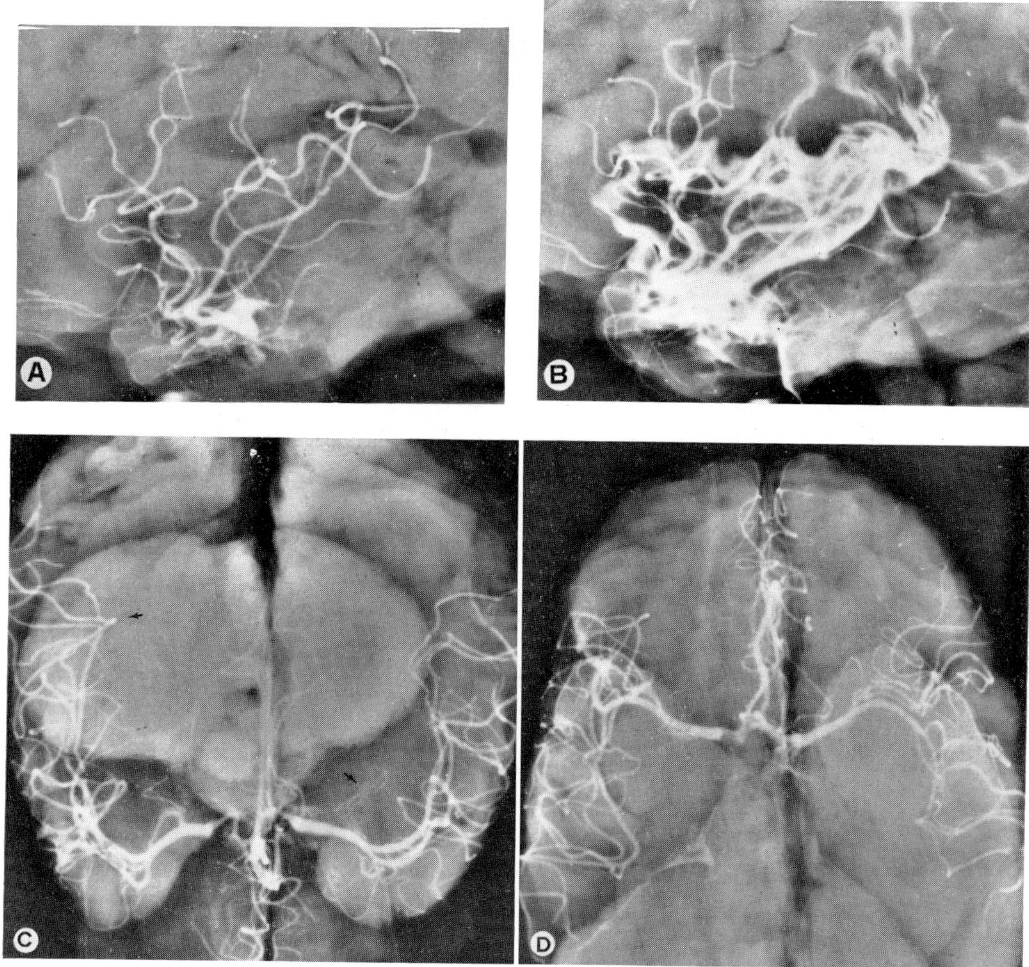

Fig. 369.—Postmortem Injection of the Arteries of the Brain in a Normal Case

(A) Lateral view after injection of the middle cerebral artery. The Sylvian triangle can be visualized but becomes much more clearly shown after injecting the Sylvian fissure with radiopaque material as shown in (B). (C) is an anteroposterior view of the middle cerebral vessels on both sides demonstrating the configuration of the middle cerebral branches around the insula. The more anterior branches are the lower ones, and the most posterior one forms the angiographic Sylvian point (*upper arrow*). The lenticulostriate arteries are very well shown (*lower arrow*). The base view (D) shows the normal configuration of the middle cerebral vessels in this projection. The anterior cerebral and the anterior communicating arteries are also shown. (Courtesy of Dr. R. J. Nahon, Veterans Administration Hospital, East Orange, New Jersey.)

which are often not too conspicuous in the angiogram, come a series of three or more branches which we have been in the habit of calling *ascending branches* of the middle cerebral artery (they include one or two pre-Rolandic branches, a Rolandic, and an anterior parietal or post-Rolandic branch). The term ascending frontoparietal branch should be avoided because it denotes that only one major branch is found here. While this is true in some cases, the majority will not present this arrangement. The term *candelabra* has also been applied to these branches. Sometimes an appearance suggestive of candelabra may be noted in connection with one or two of the vessels.

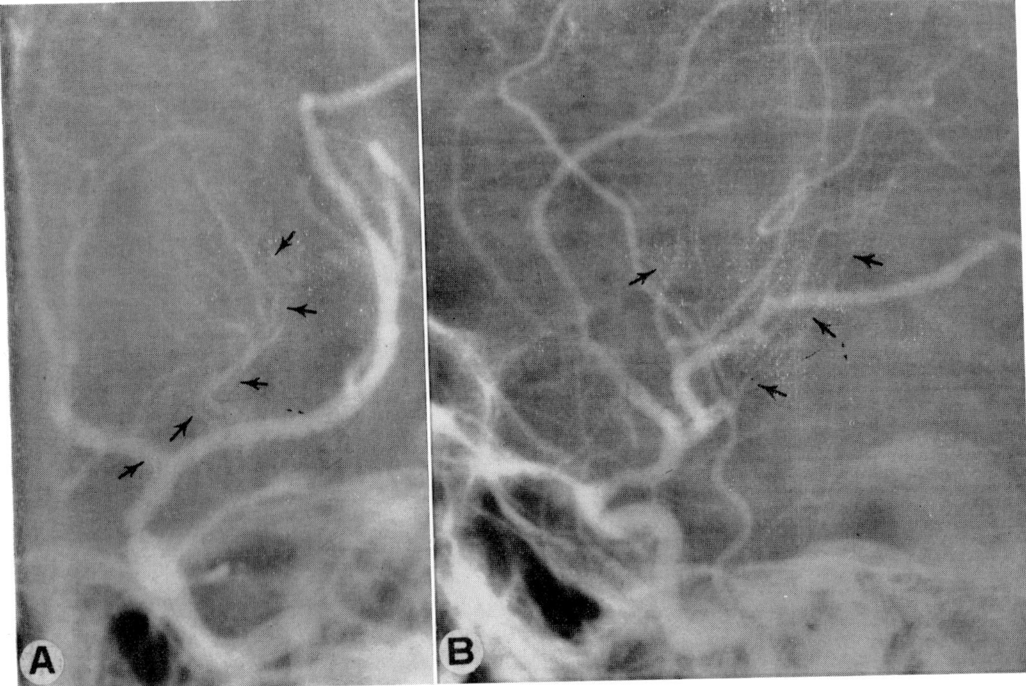

FIG. 370.—LENTICULOSTRIATE ARTERIES IN FRONTAL AND LATERAL PROJECTION

The anteroposterior view (A) shows the lenticulostriate arteries arising from the horizontal portion of the middle cerebral artery (*arrows*). They describe an S-shaped configuration. In this patient they are well developed, actually enlarged, because this 8-year-old child had an old thrombosis of the middle cerebral vessels and evidently the lenticulostriate arteries enlarged to provide some collateral supply. The anterior chorioidal artery (*lower arrow*) is well shown. There is slight irregularity of the initial portion of the middle cerebral artery also extending into the two major branches seen on the films due to the old thrombosis, possibly with recanalization. The lateral view (B) of the same patient shows the lenticulostriate branches unusually well and distributed in a triangular configuration with the apex at the middle cerebral artery (*arrows*). The irregularity of the arteries of the carotid siphon and the middle cerebral artery is even more conspicuous in the lateral view than in the frontal view, due to the old thrombosis.

Since this is less common than other arrangements of these arteries, it serves no purpose and will not be used here. The most posterior or terminal branches of the middle cerebral artery have been called, after Moniz, posterior parietal, angular, and posterior temporal arteries. These branches are variable, as are all of the other branches, and it is often difficult to designate them in a given case.

Sylvian segments. It is essential to consider in some detail the *middle cerebral artery branches in the Sylvian fissure*. In order to facilitate the interpretation of cerebral angiograms, it is basic to have a thorough understanding of the relationship of the branches of the middle cerebral artery to the Sylvian fissure, with each other, and with the surrounding brain *in three dimensions*.

The brain is narrower in its transverse diameter anteriorly than it is posteriorly. Therefore, the surface of the anterior portion of the brain is usually projected more medially than the posterior aspect. The discrepancy between the widths of the anterior and the posterior portions is exaggerated in the posteroanterior projection as against the anteroposterior projection, due to uneven magnification. Angiography is

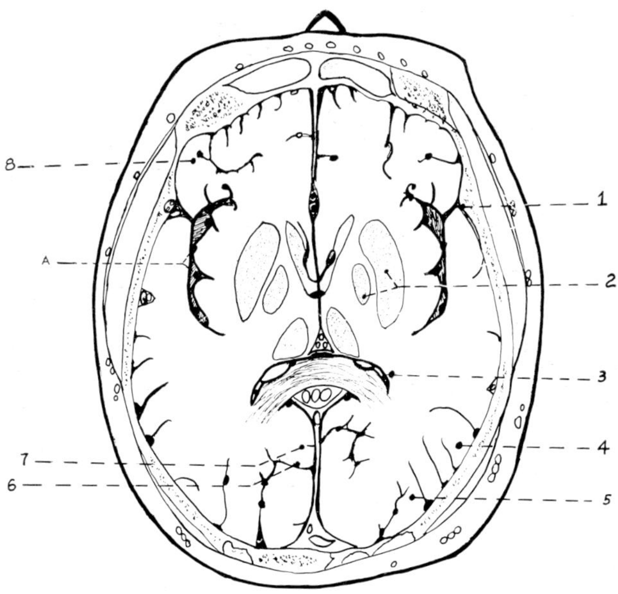

FIG. 371.—HORIZONTAL CROSS-SECTION OF BRAIN

The drawing indicates the configuration of the Sylvian fissure and lateral surface of the insula. The anterior aspect of the insular surface is further medially than the posterior aspect. (1) lateral aspect of the Sylvian fissure. (2) lenticular nucleus. (3) chorioid plexus of lateral ventricle. (4) angular gyrus. (5) lateral occipital gyri. (6) parieto-occipital sulcus. (7) precuneus. (8) inferior frontal gyrus (pars orbitalis). (A) shows the middle cerebral artery in Sylvian fissure.

usually performed in the anteroposterior projection so that the distortion due to magnification is lessened but not eliminated. The insula or island of Reil is closer to the midline in its anterior aspect than in its posterior aspect (fig. 371). Actually, on a horizontal cross section, the insula on its outer surface describes an arc slightly convex outward so that the anterior end as well as the posterior end are more medially placed than its center (fig. 371). The outer surface of the insula is hidden by the opercular portions of the frontal, parietal, and temporal lobes (fig. 374). As the branches of the middle cerebral artery enter the Sylvian fissure, they are situated against the outer surface of the insula. Some of them (the more anterior ones) are directed straight upward and most of them are directed upward and backward. As they reach the uppermost portion of the outer surface of the insula, they do not perforate the brain but, rather, they reverse their course and are directed downward to the lower margin of the fronto-

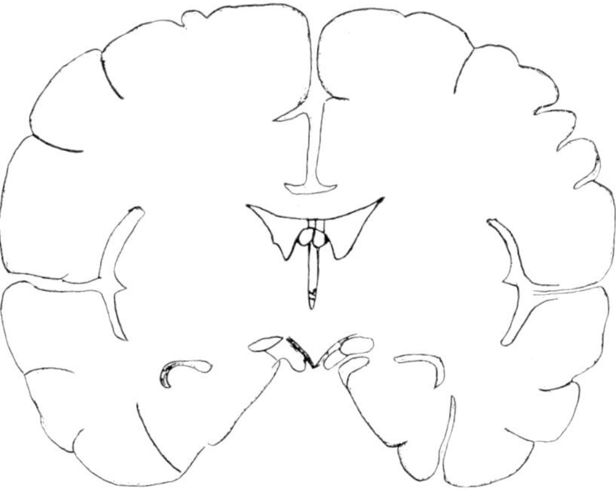

FIG. 372.—DIAGRAM OF A CORONAL SECTION OF THE BRAIN TO SHOW THE RELATIONSHIPS OF THE OUTER SURFACE OF THE INSULA TO THE PARIETAL AND TEMPORAL OPERCULA

parietal operculum. At this point, they are directed laterally to emerge from the Sylvian fissure. Immediately after emerging, the majority of the branches go upward or up-

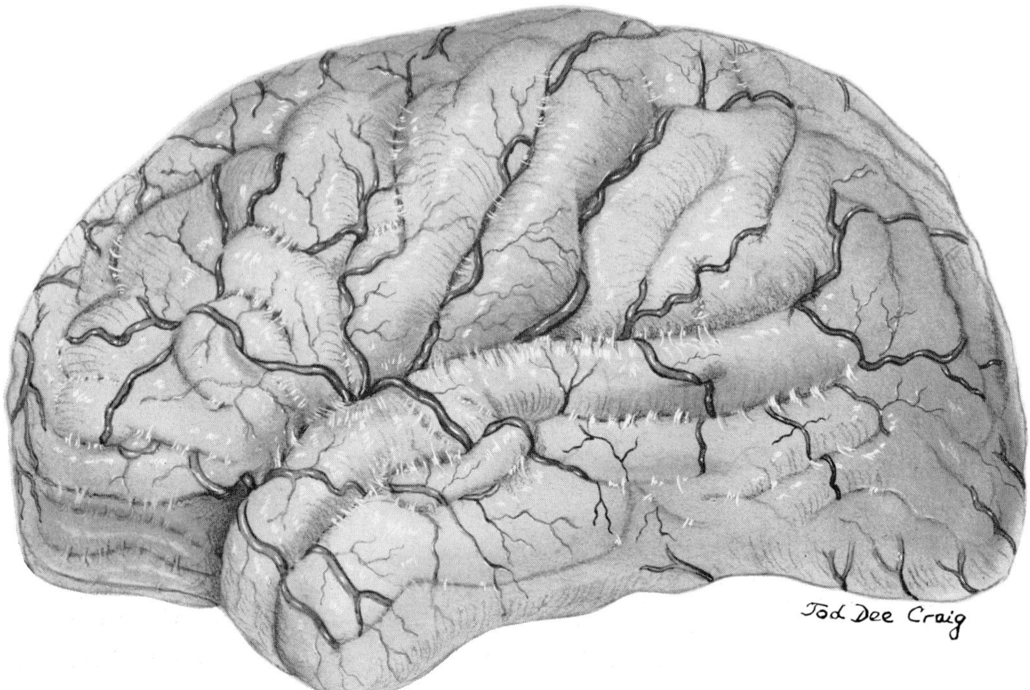

FIG. 373.—LATERAL SURFACE OF BRAIN

The cerebral arteries are situated on the surface of the brain, either on the outer surface or on the medial surface of the hemisphere. They go in and out of the sulci very frequently. Sometimes they are entirely within a sulcus and at other times they emerge only to enter the sulcus again.

ward and backward on the outer surface of the hemisphere (fig. 373). If the frontoparietal operculum is removed, it is noted that the superior margin of the insula is horizontal in position, since the outer surface of the central lobe is roughly triangular in configuration (fig. 374).

In all there are five to eight branches of the middle cerebral artery on the outer surface of the insula which, in "fanlike" fashion, reach the deepest portion of the sulcus formed at the junction of the insula and the frontoparietal operculum. As they reach this area they must change direction and proceed caudally for a short distance before emerging from the Sylvian fissure. For this reason, if one looks carefully, it is possible to pick the point at which reversal of the course of each artery takes place and a straight line can be traced from the most anterior to the most posterior portion of the insula. This straight line is the upper margin of what will be called from this point on the *Sylvian triangle*. It is possible that one of the branches may not reach its highest point within the Sylvian fissure in its initial course before reversing, and one of them may perhaps penetrate slightly deeper into a sulcus so that it actually goes higher than the others. These are normal variations which are of no pathologic significance unless there is a trend in one direction, involving several branches which appear to be displaced upward or downward. The first reference in the literature to the term Sylvian triangle was that of Schlesinger (1953).

The last branches to emerge from the Sylvian fissure posteriorly are recognized because they produce a dense dot of contrast substance. This represents the most posterior point of the Sylvian fissure. As can be easily realized, the opercular portion of the brain has a greater vertical dimension anteriorly than it has posteriorly, where it finally disappears at the posterior end of the

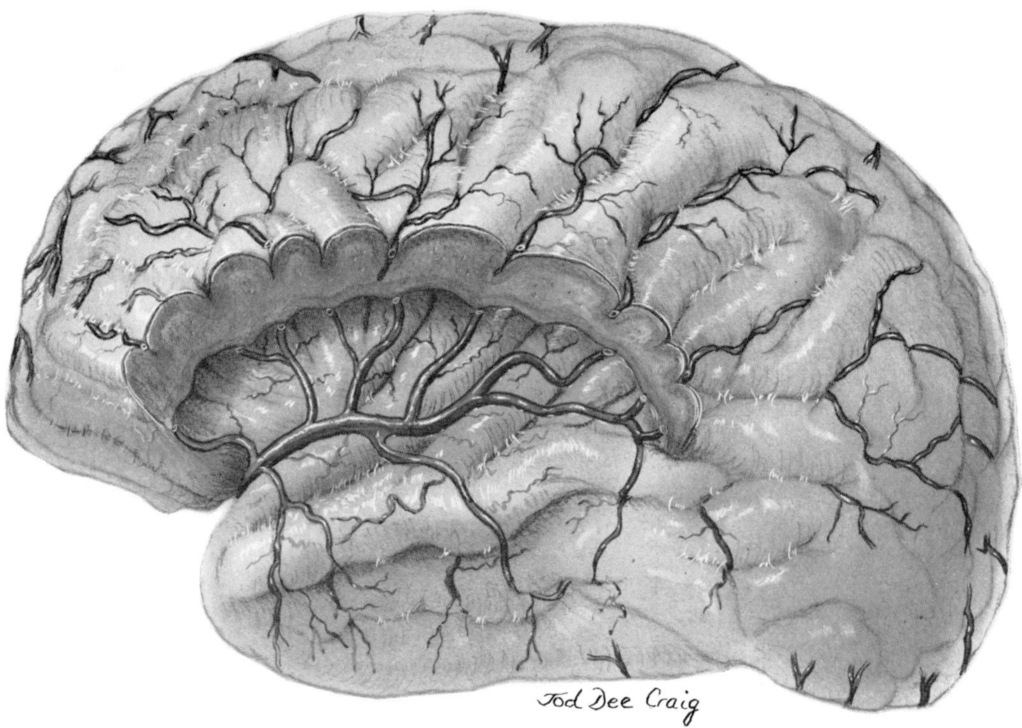

FIG. 374.—LATERAL SURFACE OF BRAIN WITH FRONTOPARIETAL OPERCULUM CUT

The diagram shows the middle cerebral branches over the surface of the insula after the frontoparietal operculum has been cut and the temporal lobe pulled downward. The outer surface of the insula has a triangular configuration which is not brought out on the diagram because the operculum was sectioned in a curved manner.

insula. Therefore, the last branch or branches (they may be two or three in number) would not have an up and down course as the more anterior branches do, but they simply come out of the Sylvian fissure to distribute themselves over the surface of the brain. A glance at Figure 375 will clarify this concept.

The inferior margin of the Sylvian triangle, for our purpose, is formed by a line starting at the posterior point of the Sylvian fissure, which we shall call the *angiographic Sylvian point,* and extending along the lower branches of the middle cerebral artery to the anterior extremity of this vessel as seen in lateral view. The anterior aspect of the Sylvian triangle can now be traced from this point up to the first opercular branch within the Sylvian fissure, that is, the most anterior one (fig. 375). The description just given applies to the lateral view and it is now necessary to translate this into the anteroposterior projection.

In order to understand the anatomy of the middle cerebral vessels as seen in the *frontal projection,* one must realize that the Sylvian fissure is inclined backward and upward on the brain. Therefore, in a film made with the standard frontal angiographic projection (12 degrees cephalocaudad from the canthomeatal line), the central ray forms an angle with the plane of the Sylvian fissure (fig. 376). Therefore, the anterior branches of the middle cerebral artery are thrown downward and the posterior branches are thrown upward. One easy way to remember this point is by remembering that *anterior moves down, posterior moves up.* The same applies to the deep veins of the brain which will be studied later.

For the sake of clarity, it should again be mentioned that the branches of the middle

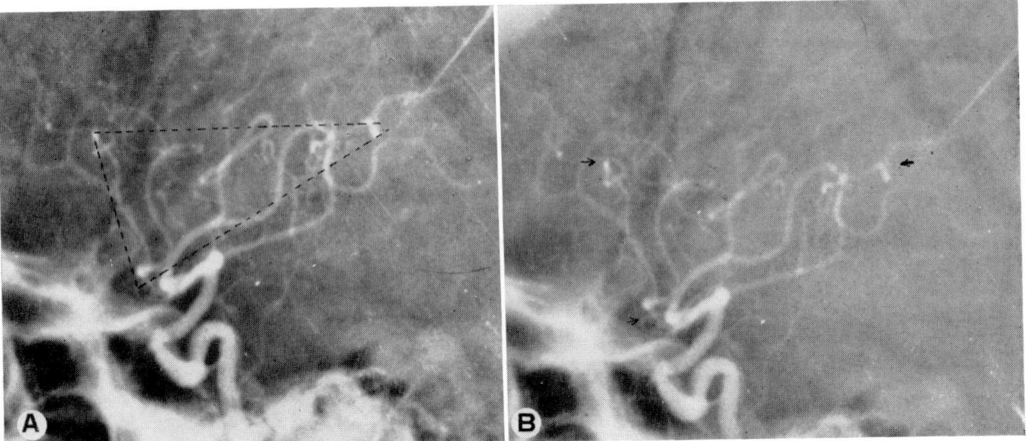

FIG. 375.—ARTERIOGRAPHIC DEMONSTRATION OF THE SYLVIAN TRIANGLE

Normal arteriogram, lateral view. The authors' method of determining the Sylvian triangle is indicated by *dotted lines* (A). The *horizontal arrows* (B) demonstrate the limits of the triangle. The anterior superior aspect of the Sylvian triangle is marked by the first identifiable opercular branch; the anterior inferior aspect of the Sylvian triangle is represented by the most anterior portion of the trunk of the middle cerebral artery or the inferior aspect of the first opercular branch if this is visible, as shown in the figure.

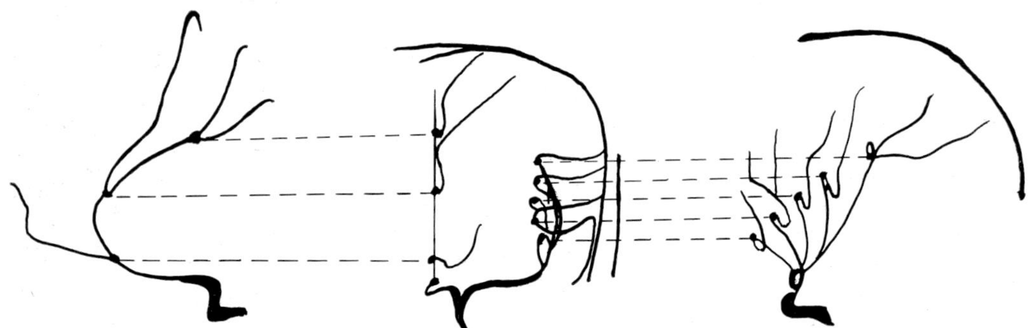

FIG. 376.—DIAGRAMMATIC REPRESENTATION OF THE PROJECTIONS OF THE MIDDLE AND ANTERIOR CEREBRAL ARTERIES AND THEIR RELATIVE POSITIONS ACCORDING TO THE ANGULATION OF THE CENTRAL BEAM OF X-RAY

In both the middle and anterior cerebral diagrams, the head has been tilted with the chin down.

cerebral artery first ascend against the outer surface of the insula in the Sylvian fissure, descend still within the Sylvian fissure, and then are directed laterally to emerge from the fissure. There will be an interlacing of these branches in the frontal view, produced by the projection. However, they could still be followed individually if desired. The more anterior branches may project more medially than the more posterior branches due to the fact that the brain is narrower anteriorly (fig. 371). Although the anterior branches may not extend further medially than the posterior branches, they are projected medial to the lateral aspect of the insula (fig. 376). If the frontal angiographic view were made in posteroanterior projection, the anterior Sylvian branches would nearly always project medial to the posterior branches, but because anteroposterior films are used, the appearance is that explained in the diagram of Figure 376. The last branch to emerge

Revised 1963)

from the Sylvian fissure often describes a perfect arc which is sometimes suggestive of a tumor. This is a perfectly normal appearance (fig. 377). The medial aspect of the last branch to emerge from the fissure is called the angiographic Sylvian point and corresponds to the same point in the lateral projection. On a film with the degree of magnification produced by a target film distance of 40 inches and with the head approximately 1.5 inches from the film, the deepest portion of this last Sylvian vessel is usually up to 43 mm. from the inner table of the skull. The minimum distance encountered in a large group of normal cases was not less than 30 mm.

Angiographic Sylvian point. As has been described in the preceding paragraphs, the last vessel or vessels, branches of the middle cerebral artery, which emerge from the Sylvian fissure usually mark the most posterior (and the highest) point of the Sylvian fissure. This can be seen, if looked for, in the lateral as well as in the frontal projection. In the lateral projection, this point marks the posterior limit of the Sylvian triangle and is recognizable because at least one, two, or more vessels are seen

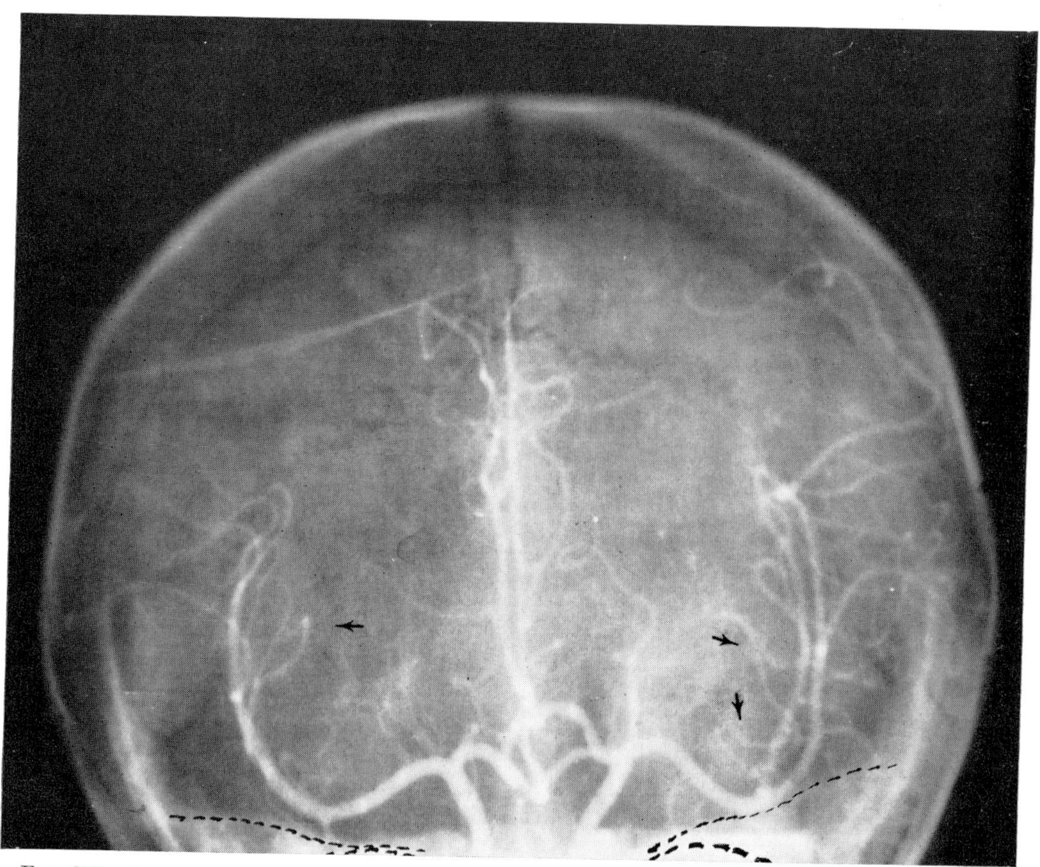

FIG. 377.—ANTEROPOSTERIOR ANGIOGRAM IN A TWO-YEAR-OLD CHILD MADE WITH COMPRESSION OF THE OPPOSITE SIDE DURING INJECTION

It demonstrates that both angiographic Sylvian points are almost exactly in the same position in height. One point is slightly more medial from the inner table than the opposite side, but the difference is very minimum. The anterior branches of the middle cerebral artery (*arrows*) are slightly more medial in position than the posterior branches; that is, they project more medially than the angiographic Sylvian point above. The top of the Sylvian vessels as they emerge may have a concave configuration.

(Revised 1963)

end on as a rounded dense dot. In the frontal projection, the last artery to emerge usually describes a curve concave upward as it reaches the outer surface of the hemisphere. The medial end of this vessel is the angiographic Sylvian point in the frontal projection.

The Sylvian point in the frontal angioraphic projection is situated close to the center of the distance from the upper margin of the petrous pyramid (or the roof of the orbit, whichever is lower) to a horizontal line drawn tangential to the inner table of the vertex of the skull. If the groove of the superior longitudinal sinus is deep, the internal lateral margin of the bony sinus walls should be used (fig. 378). In a film made in the standard frontal angiographic projection, this point is up to 9 to 10 mm. below the center of the distance. If more of the orbits show, that is, if the petrous pyramids are lower, it tends to be a little lower; in half axial anteroposterior projections, the point is closer to the center. The Sylvian point is usually symmetrical when the right side is compared with the left in normal cases (fig. 377).

Another important relationship is to be noted. The distance from the angiographic Sylvian point to the inner table of the skull in the temporoparietal region measured horizontally varies from 30 to 43 mm. in films made with a 40-inch target film distance, with the head approximately 1 to 1.5 inches from the film. A slight increase over the 43 mm. upper limit may be seen in patients with very tortuous vessels, particularly of arteriosclerosis. But usually a distance over 43 mm. is abnormal. The above measurements do not apply when there is magnification due to a short target-film distance or to a long object-film distance.

The Sylvian point may also be localized in the lateral projection, as mentioned above, because at this point one, two, or more vessels may be seen end on as they are directed straight out parallel to the x-ray beam in order to emerge to the surface. Fairly frequently, however, no dense dots can be seen but rather dense, short loops are present because the x-ray beam did not catch the vessels end on. The exact Sylvian

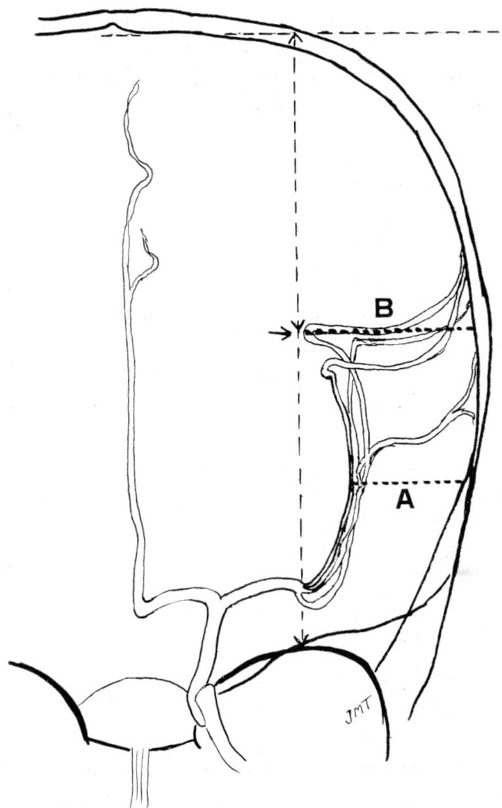

FIG. 378.—THE DIAGRAM ILLUSTRATES THE METHOD THAT THE AUTHORS HAVE USED TO DETERMINE THE POSITION OF THE ANGIOGRAPHIC SYLVIAN POINT

The arrow in this particular case is almost in the center of the vertical distance from the highest point of the skull to the upper margin of the orbit. Distance (A), to the medial aspect of the most medial vessel outlining the lateral margin of the insula, varied from 20 to 30 mm. Distance (B), from the medial margin of the most medial vessel in the region of the Sylvian point to the inner table, varied from 30 to 43 mm.

point is more difficult to recognize in those cases, but a good approximation is always possible. If it is kept in mind that the Sylvian point is the apex of the Sylvian triangle, the upper margin of this triangle can be followed to the point where it meets the major middle cerebral branches (fig. 375).

The *exact position of the Sylvian fissure* can be approximated in the lateral view by tracing a line along the points where the opercular vessels turn to go cephalad after

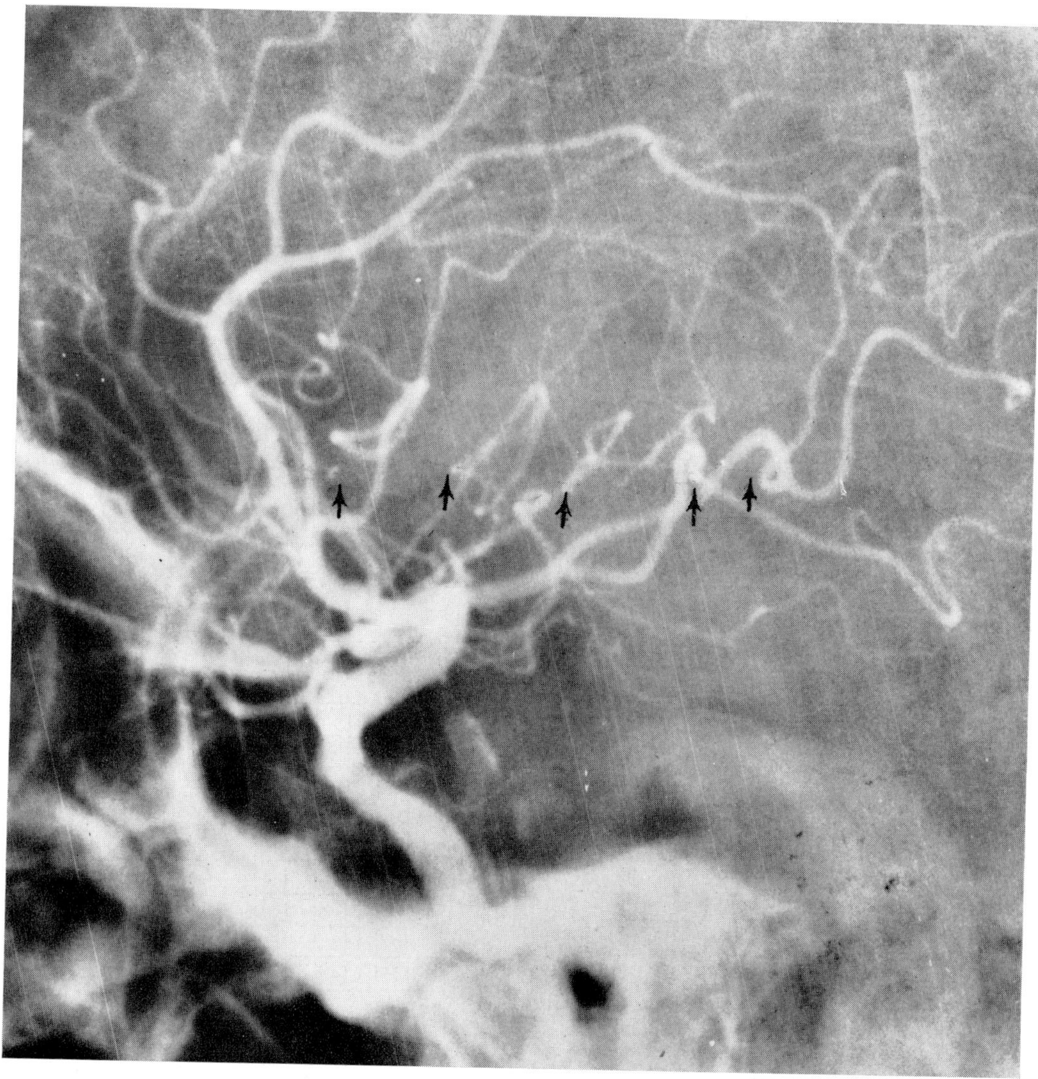

FIG. 379.—NORMAL LATERAL CAROTID ANGIOGRAM

The figure illustrates how it is possible to trace the actual position of the Sylvian fissure with a fair degree of accuracy by taking the lower portion of the branches of the middle cerebral artery as they return downward and extend laterally to emerge from the Sylvian fissure. Absolute accuracy is not possible because the artery may be either on the gyrus or in the sulcus.

having descended a little. However, it should be kept in mind that as the opercular branches turn, some may be deep within a sulcus whereas others may be on the surface of a gyrus (fig. 379).

Clinoparietal line. A line traced in the lateral view from a point 2 cm. above the lambda to the anterior clinoid process is usually situated at or just below the lower major branches of the middle cerebral artery (fig. 380). Occasionally the line is just above the lowest major branch in the adult. In children, the major middle cerebral branches are always above the clinoparietal line (fig. 380). The actual measurments encountered in a group of normal children varying in age from 5 months to 13 years and in adults are given in Figure 381. In the adult and some-

(Revised 1963)

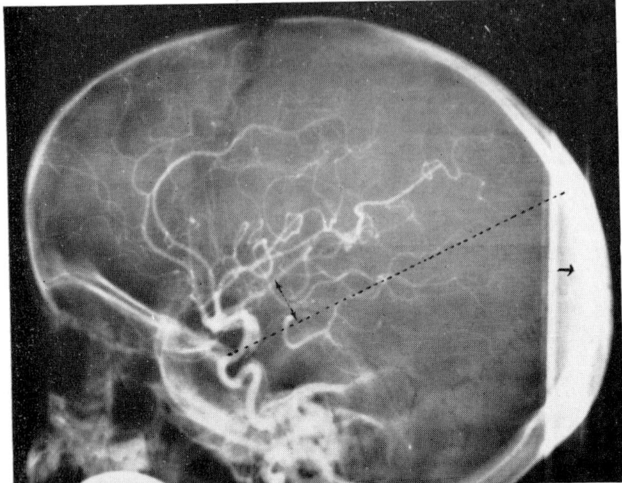

FIG. 380.—CLINOPARIETAL LINE

The dotted line was traced from a point 2 cm. above the lambda (*indicated by arrow*) to the anterior clinoid process. In the original radiograph of this two-year-old child, the distance from this line to the lowest major branch of the middle cerebral artery, measured 2 cm. behind the carotid siphon, was 1.4 cm.

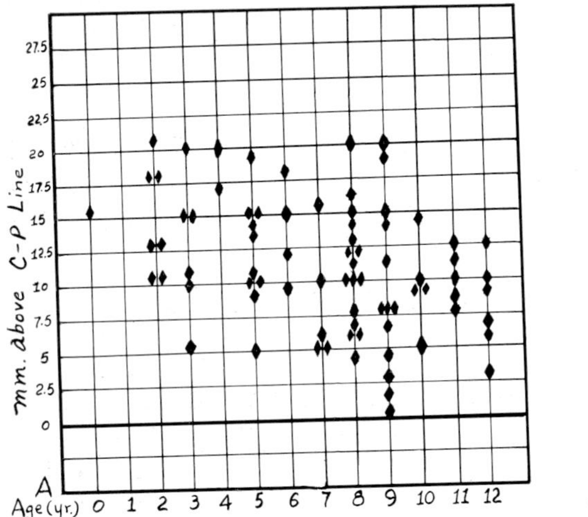

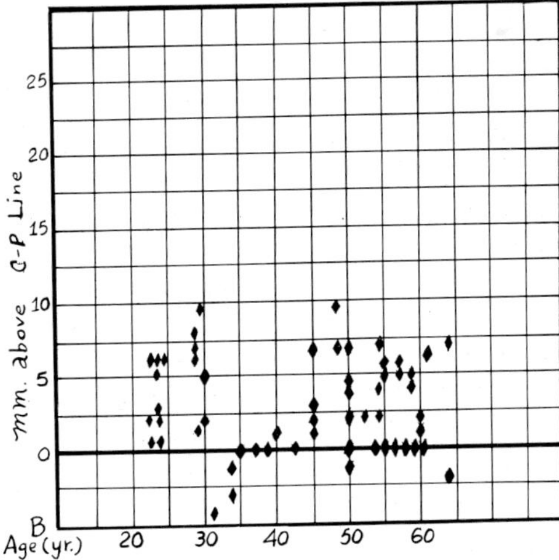

FIG. 381.—RELATION OF MIDDLE CEREBRAL ARTERY TO CLINOPARIETAL LINE

The graphs indicate the relationship of the lower main branch of the middle cerebral artery to the clinoparietal line in children and in adults. The middle cerebral branches seem to become lower with advancing age, as indicated in (A), but remains stationary after growth is completed (B).

times in older children, the lambda is not clearly visible on the films. In these cases a point on the inner table 9 cm. above the internal occipital protruberance is taken as the point from which to trace the line (Taveras and Poser, 1959). It may be noted in Figure 381A that in younger children the distance from the clinoparietal line to the

FIG. 382.—LATERAL VIEW OF A CEREBRAL ANGIOGRAM IN WHICH THERE WAS NO FILLING OF THE ANTERIOR CEREBRAL VESSELS, PRESUMABLY DUE TO HYPOPLASIA OF THIS VESSEL

(A) demonstrates the initial stage of filling, approximately 0.75 second after the beginning of the injection, and (B) was taken 0.5 second later. In (A) the filling of the middle cerebral branches has extended just beyond the Sylvian triangle, and the fanlike distribution is easily appreciated. In (B) the filling has extended to the terminal branches of the middle cerebral artery. The branches of the middle cerebral artery do not extend to reach the uppermost portion of the hemisphere. On the other hand, the anterior cerebral vessels usually come down for a certain distance on the outer surface of the hemisphere after reaching the upper margin at the midline (see Fig. 363).

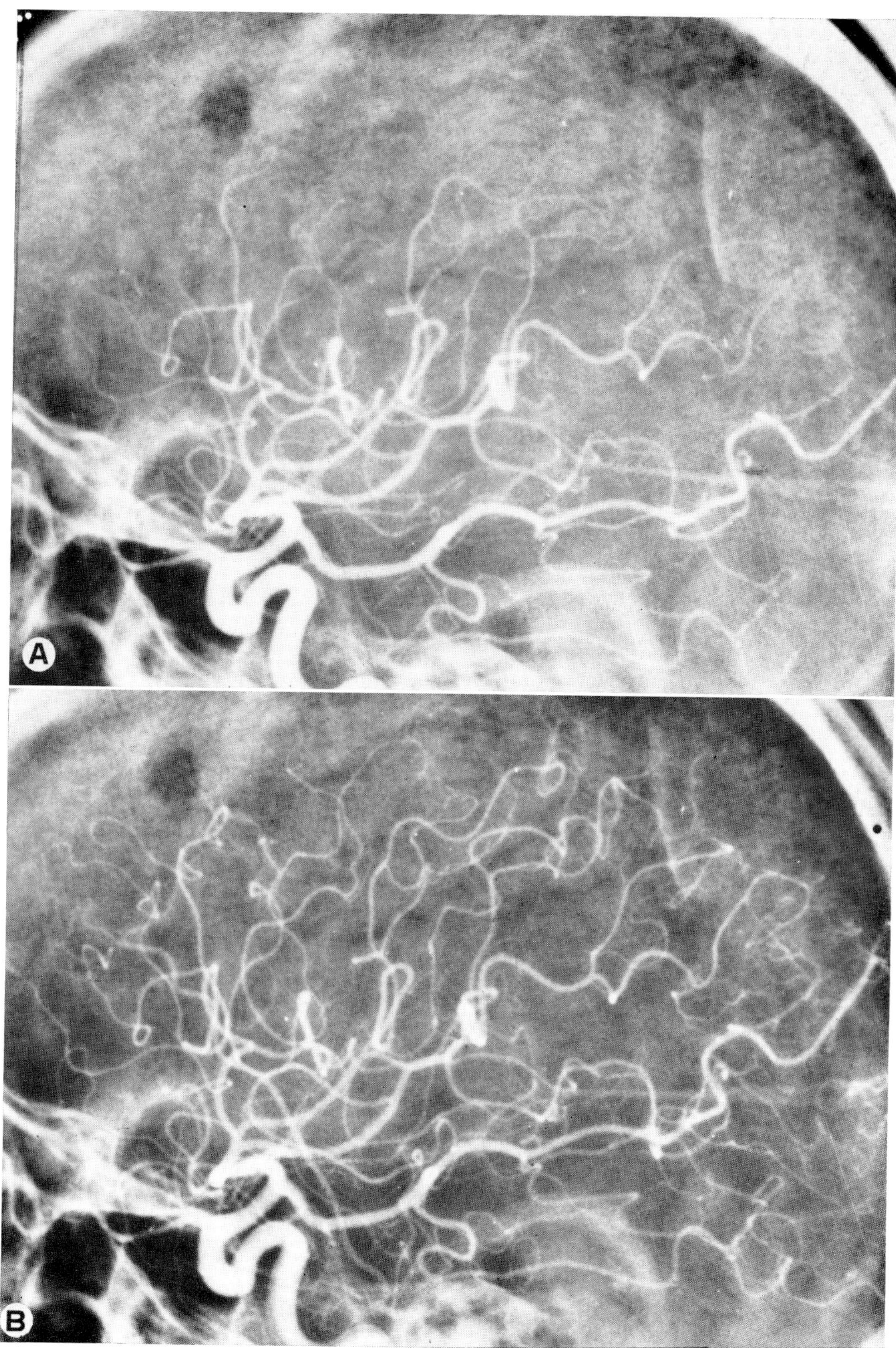

Fig. 382

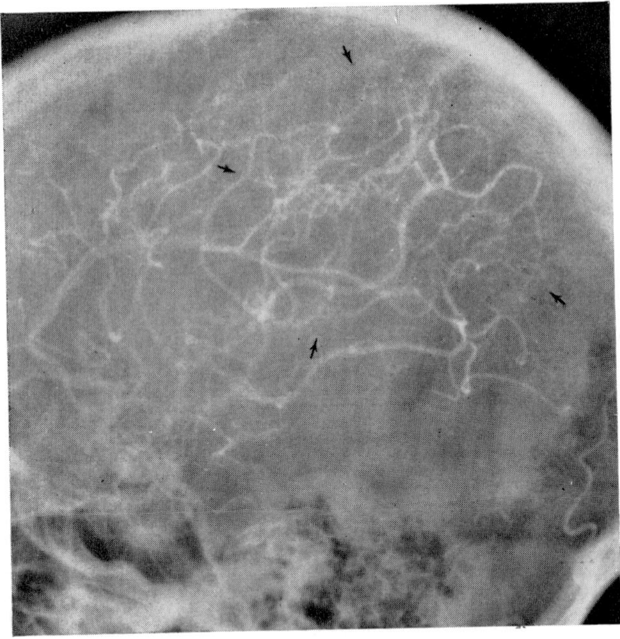

FIG. 383.—INCREASED VASCULARITY IN THE PARIETAL REGION IN A NORMAL CAROTID ANGIOGRAM

The overlying branches of the middle cerebral artery over the anterior cerebral artery branches often give the impression of increased vascularity in the parietal region, which should not be mistaken for a tumor.

lowest major branch of the middle cerebral artery, measured 2 cm. behind the carotid artery siphon, is greater than in older children; the distance decreases with advancing age to approach the relationship found in the adult. This is evidently related to brain development.

Ascending branches. As the various branches of the middle cerebral artery emerge from the Sylvian fissure they turn directly upward or, in the case of the more posterior ones, they are directed upward and backward. The most anterior ones may be directed upward and forward. The distribution of the middle cerebral group over the convexity of the hemisphere may be compared with the outstretched hand where the thumb is placed in the direction of the Sylvian fissure following the three major branches (posterior parietal, angular, and posterior temporal arteries). The other four fingers of the outstretched hand represent the ascending branches of the middle cerebral artery (the one or two pre-Rolandic, the Rolandic, and the anterior parietal or post-Rolandic arteries). In some instances the distribution is much more irregular. Sometimes the branches present only a few undulations, while at other times they are more tortuous. Within their tortuosity, however, they still preserve a certain organization. On glancing at an injected specimen of these branches one can readily observe that these arteries are sometimes on the convolutions where they are clearly visible, and sometimes they penetrate into the sulcus where they disappear from view (fig. 373), only to emerge again perhaps a little higher.

In the arteriogram, the branches of the middle cerebral artery usually fill well to the superior portion of the convexity of the hemisphere where they become quite thin and usually disappear by branching and by simply losing their density, that is, the contrast substance fades away. This is very easy to appreciate in the cases in which the anterior cerebral artery does not fill from one side (fig. 382). Of course, it is known that many of these branches of the middle cerebral artery anastomose end to end directly with branches of the anterior cerebral artery (see collateral circulation of the brain, p. 1.707). However, these anastomoses do not function unless there is a difference in pressure between the anterior and middle cerebral arterial systems, such as may be found in thrombosis.

As the posterior branches of the middle

cerebral artery ascend and pass backward, they are superimposed upon the branches of the anterior cerebral artery, which are in a different plane, on the medial surface of the hemisphere. The latter include the pericallosal artery and its branches and the callosomarginal artery and its branches. If these happen to be prominent in their distribution and in their filling with contrast substance, an artifact is produced which always suggests increased vascularity and the possible presence of a tumor (fig. 383). Another artifact which is often seen in the middle cerebral distribution is that of a "pseudocloud" in the region of the Sylvian triangle; this is produced by the very rich vascularity present in this region and is a normal finding.

In trying to evaluate the relative position of the ascending branches of the middle cerebral artery, one should think of them as each one following a sulcus or a gyrus (one of the sulci or gyri of the Rolandic region). We know, however, that this is not the case in most instances; the artery may be on the gyrus at one point and in the sulcus at the next turn. Nevertheless it is helpful in appreciating what may be taking place in a given instance to imagine each artery as belonging to a sulcus when the vessels are displaced by a mass. When the artery is bowed, so the sulcus and the adjacent gyrus are also probably bowed by the mass. This will be studied in detail in the section dealing with diagnosis of intracranial masses.

The branches that go to the anterior and middle thirds of the temporal lobe are often inconspicuous although they can be seen if looked for. They are usually thinner than the other branches and are sometimes superimposed on the region of the anterior chorioidal and posterior communicating vessels, making identification of these arteries difficult. When there is elevation of the middle cerebral branches by temporal masses, these branches become much more conspicuous.

VERTEBRAL BASILAR SYSTEM

Vertebral Artery

The vertebral artery originates in the neck and is the first branch of the subclavian artery on each side. From its origin, the artery is directed upward and medially to enter the foramen transversarium of the 6th cervical vertebra. Here the artery ascends on each side contained within the foramina transversaria until it reaches the 2d cervical vertebra. It emerges from the foramen transversarium of the 2d cervical vertebra and passes laterally to enter the foramen transversarium of the atlas, which is more laterally placed; then posteriorly to wind itself behind the superior articular process of the atlas. At this point it may be surrounded by a complete ring of bone forming a foramen, which is visible on the plain films in the lateral projection. Most often, however, only a ligament is present behind the artery. Sometimes an incomplete ring of bone is present. The artery then proceeds forward, upward, and medially to pierce the dura as it enters the foramen magnum (fig. 384). It continues forward, medially, and upward to reach the posterior surface of the clivus where it unites with the opposite vertebral artery at the lower border of the pons, thus forming the basilar artery.

The vertebral artery may sometimes arise from the common carotid artery, from the inferior thyroid artery, from the innominate artery, or directly from the aorta. The anomalous site of origin may be on either side. The left vertebral artery arises directly from the aorta in 6 per cent of cases (Radner, 1951; Stein *et al.*, 1962). In reference to the course of the vertebral artery within the foramina transversaria, it may not penetrate the foramen transversarium of the sixth cervical, but it may start at the fifth cervical vertebra. Occasionally it has been seen to emerge from its bony canal between the third and the second cervical vertebra to go back in the foramen transversarium at the atlas. In the rare cases in which the right vertebral artery comes off the aorta, behind the left subclavian artery, the vertebral artery passes behind the esophagus as it goes

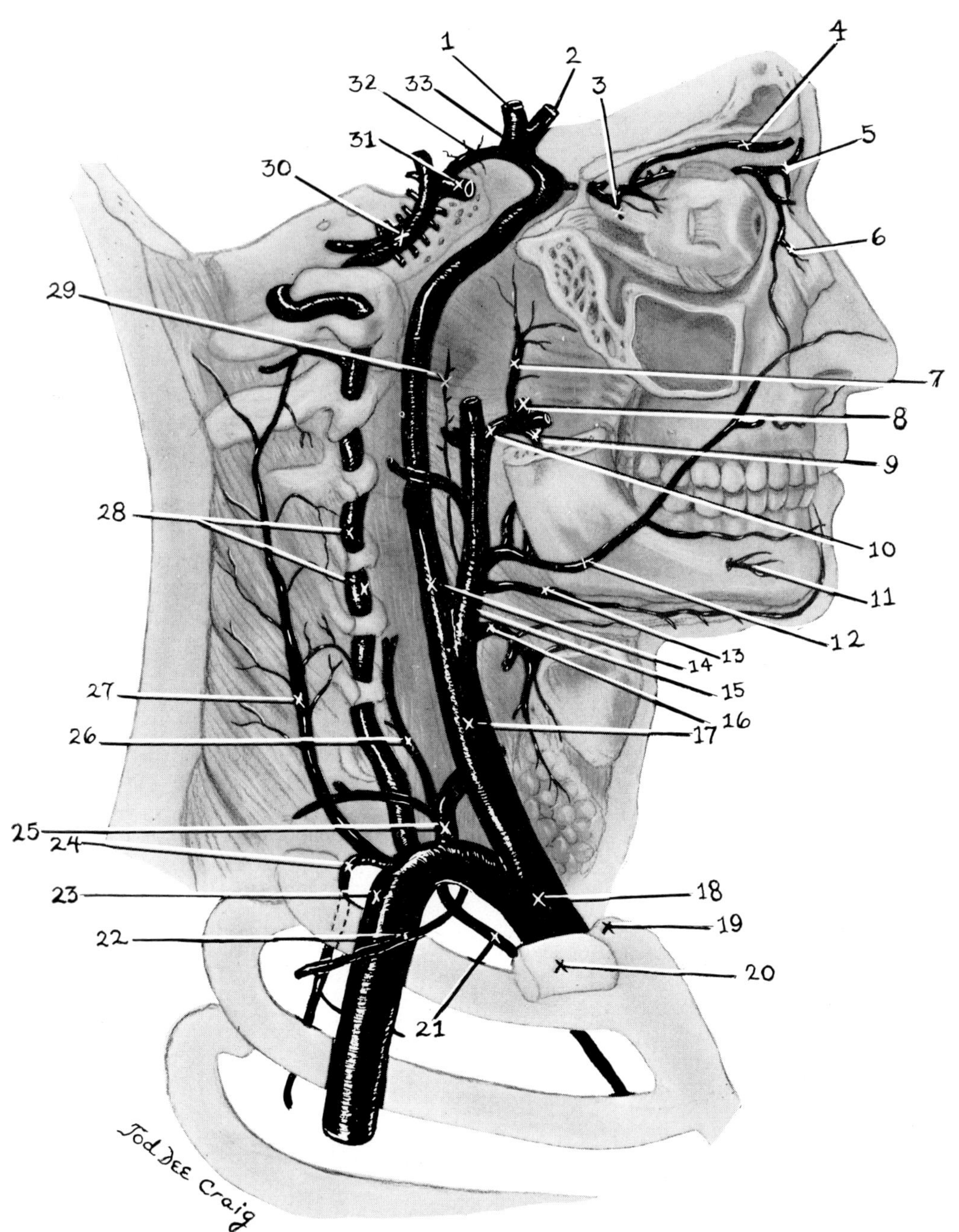

FIG. 384.—DIAGRAM OF THE VERTEBRAL ARTERY AS WELL AS OF THE SUBCLAVIAN AND COMMON CAROTID ARTERIES AND THEIR BRANCHES

(1) Middle cerebral artery. (2) anterior cerebral artery. (3) lacrimal branch of the ophthalmic artery. (4) supraorbital artery. (5) frontal artery. (6) dorsal nasal artery. (7) ascending palatine artery. (8) middle meningeal artery trunk. (9) inferior alveolar artery. (10) internal maxillary artery. (11) mental artery. (12) external maxillary (facial) artery. (13) lingual artery. (14) internal carotid artery. (15) external carotid artery. (16) superior thyroid artery. (17) common carotid artery. (18) brachiocephalic trunk. (19) sternum. (20) clavicle. (21) internal thoracic (internal mammary artery). (22) suprascapular a. (23) subclavian a. (24) superior intercostal a. (25) thyrocervical trunk. (26) ascending cervical a. (27) cervical profundis a. (28) vertebral a. (29) ascending pharyngeal a. (30) basilar a. (31) posterior cerebral a. (32) posterior communicating a. (33) internal carotid a.

(Revised 1963)

laterally to enter the foramen transversarium of the sixth cervical vertebra (Testut, 1930).

The left vertebral artery is larger than the right in a higher percentage of cases (42 per cent), the right and left vertebral arteries are approximately of the same caliber in 26 per cent, and the right side is larger than the left in 32 per cent of the cases (Krayenbühl and Yasargil, 1957). One vertebral artery, usually the right, may be hypoplastic. The anatomical relationships of the cervical portion of the vertebral artery are illustrated in Figure 384. Within the foramina transversaria of the cervical vertebrae, as it ascends to the skull, the vertebral artery is surrounded by a plexus of veins which in their lower portion, come together and form the vertebral vein which emerges from the foramen transversarium of the sixth cervical vertebra and accompanies the vertebral artery for a short segment.

Cervical branches. In the *cervical portion*, the vertebral artery gives rise to spinal and muscular branches. The spinal or radicular branches are thin. They enter through the intervertebral foramina and supply the meninges; some anastomose with the anterior and posterior spinal arteries and supply the spinal cord. The muscular branches supply the paraspinal muscles; they anastomose with branches of the occipital artery and the ascending pharyngeal arteries which also supply the muscles.

Intracranial branches. The *intracranial portion* gives rise to the posterior inferior cerebellar artery, the anterior and the posterior spinal arteries, and a posterior meningeal artery. The *posterior inferior cerebellar artery* is present bilaterally and is of the same caliber on both sides in approximately 25 per cent of cases (Krayenbühl and Yasargil, 1957). In the remaining 75 per cent of cases, it is asymmetrical. Sometimes both arteries are very small, one or both may be absent, or they may arise from the basilar artery.

The posterior inferior cerebellar artery arises on each anterolateral aspect of the medulla (fig. 387). From its origin, the artery passes upward and laterally around the medulla describing a curve concave downward as it reaches the posterolateral aspect of the medulla (*cephalic curve*). At this point the artery is close to the posterior aspect of the outlet of the 4th ventricle. The artery then describes another curve concave upward which is in fairly close relationship with the cerebellar tonsils (*caudal curve*). The artery may be displaced downward in cases where the cerebellar tonsils are displaced downward (fig. 385). The lower portion of this curve brings the artery to about the level of the foramen magnum or just above it. In some normal cases the artery can descend to the level of the arch of the atlas or even lower (fig. 386). The posterior inferior cerebellar artery supplies the chorioid plexus of the 4th ventricle. It divides into a medial (vermis) branch and a lateral (tonsilohemispheric) branch (figs. 385 and 387). The medial branch may anastomose directly with a branch of the superior cerebellar artery over the vermis. The lateral branch describes a third curve concave downward as it passes laterally along the inferolateral surface of the cerebellar hemisphere. The various curves of the posterior inferior cerebellar artery are extremely variable.

Basilar Artery

The basilar artery proceeds upward against the posterior surface of the clivus and separated from it by only two to three millimeters until it nears its final bifurcation. The bifurcation of the basilar artery is usually situated behind and at or slightly above the tip of the dorsum sella. Sometimes it is just below the level of the tip of the dorsum sella. If the basilar artery is tortuous, it may wind around toward one side or the other in normal cases. This should not be considered abnormal. When the artery is arteriosclerotic, the point of bifurcation may be considerably higher than normal and it may produce an indentation of the floor of the third ventricle which is clearly visible on air studies (fig. 388). The higher and lower bifurcations of the basilar artery produce a different configuration of the posterior cerebral and superior cerebellar arteries as seen in frontal projection, which is illustrated in Figure 387 *B* and *C*.

Minor branches. The basilar artery gives

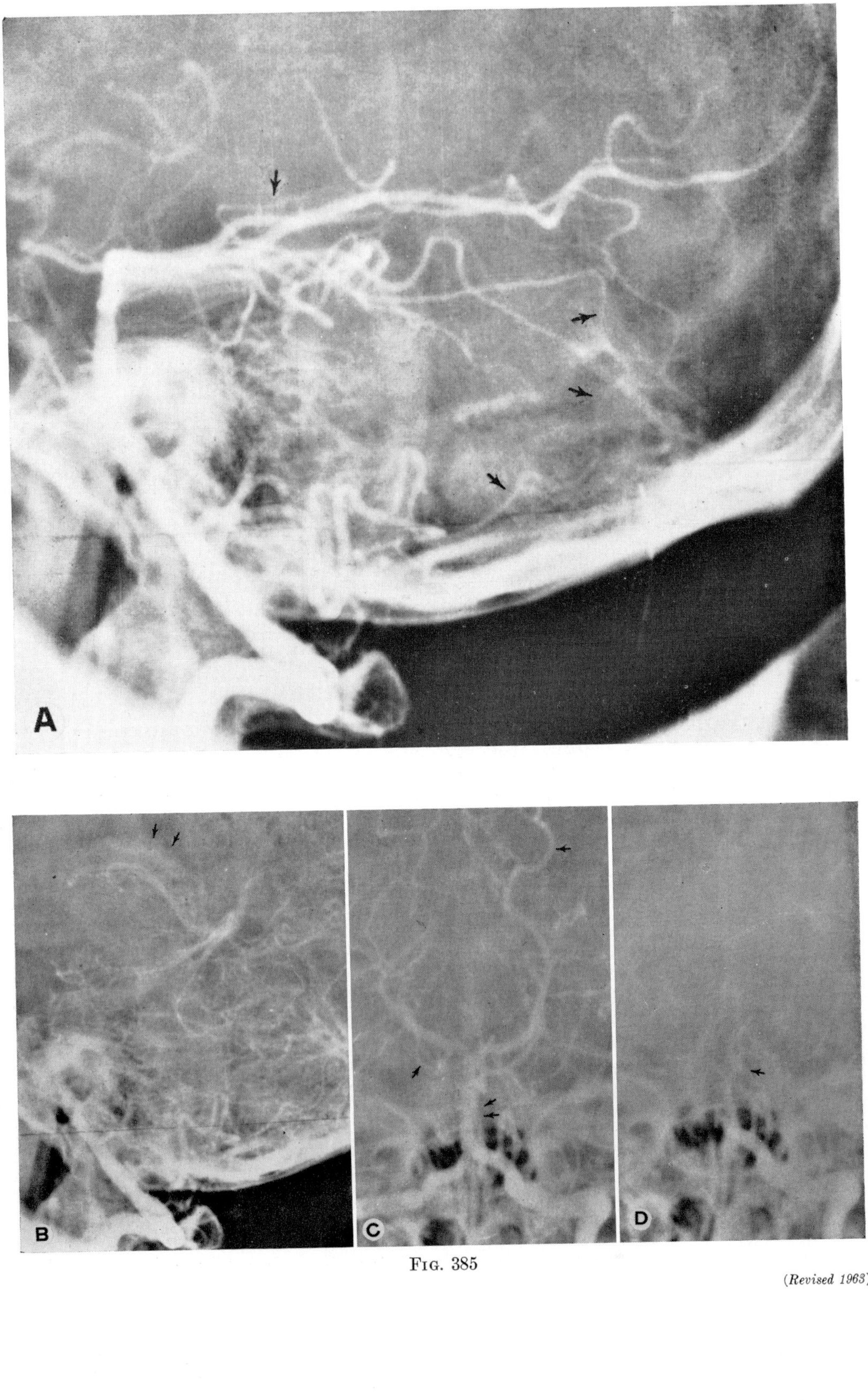

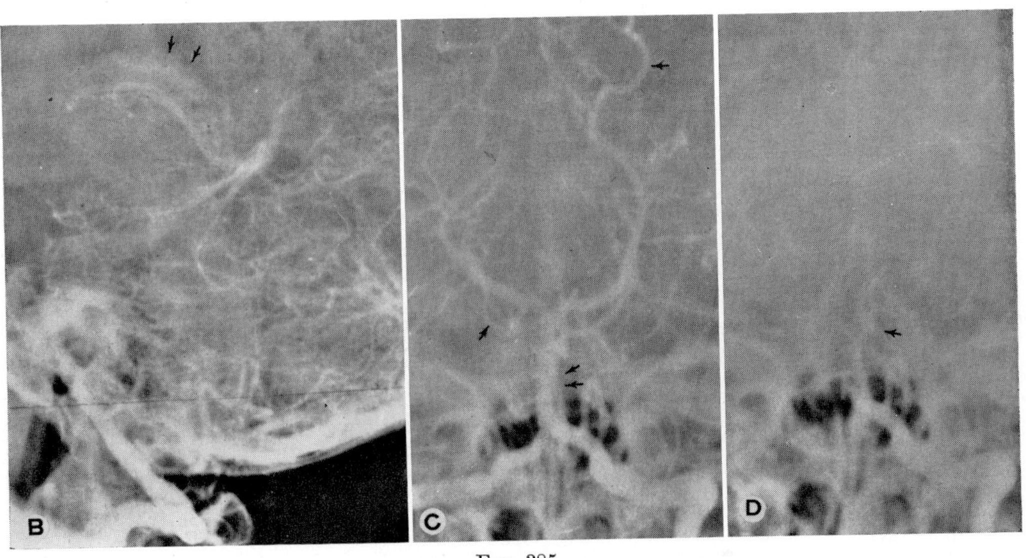

Fig. 385

(*Revised 1963*)

off many branches, most of which are small and supply the pons (fig. 387). The anterior inferior cerebellar artery is large enough to be seen on vertebral angiograms. However, this area is obscured by the heavy bone of the petrous pyramids, and it is difficult to visualize in detail. The most important branches are those resulting from the bifurcation of the basilar artery. These are the posterior cerebral and the superior cerebellar arteries.

Superior cerebellar artery. The superior cerebellar arteries first pass laterally and slightly downward as they go around the midbrain, describing a curve concave upward as seen in the lateral view (fig. 393). After going one-third the distance, they reach the posterolateral aspect of the midbrain, lateral to the quadrigeminal plate. Continuing dorsad, they reach the upper surface of the cerebellum where they divide into several branches, some of which anastomose with branches of the inferior cerebellar arteries (fig. 385). They describe a broad curve concave downward over the top of the cerebellum. The dome of this curve should be below the medial branch of the posterior cerebral arteries. If the dome is above it, cerebellar tumor or upward cerebellar herniation is suspected (fig. 390).

Posterior Cerebral Artery

The posterior cerebral arteries are the terminal branches of the basilar artery. Their point of origin from the basilar artery is only slightly above that of the superior cerebellar arteries, almost from a common trunk (fig. 387). On a review of over 200 vertebral angiograms, Saltzman (1959) found that both posterior cerebral arteries filled in 88 per cent of cases, one only filled in 10 to 11 per cent of cases, and in 2 per cent none filled (fig. 389 and 390). In the latter cases it is presumed that the initial segment of the posterior cerebral artery is hypoplastic or, rarely, absent. The posterior cerebral artery passes laterally and turns around the cerebral peduncles to the posterolateral aspect of the midbrain (fig. 393). As it turns around the midbrain, the artery often makes a downward swing (concave upward); as it swings down, occasionally it comes in contact with the anterolateral aspect of the pons which has normally a

---

Fig. 385.—Normal Vertebral Angiogram

The lateral projection (A) shows the upper portion of the vertebral artery and its curve around the atlas. The basilar artery has a normal relationship with the clivus and separates as it goes upward in its upper portion. The bifurcation of the basilar artery takes place at or just below the top of the dorsum sellae (low bifurcation). The posterior inferior cerebellar artery is seen to describe its cephalic and caudal curves. The lower portion of the caudal curve is at the margin of the foramen magnum. The medial branch of the posterior inferior cerebellar artery is shown (*posterior arrows*). It seems to anastomose directly with a branch of the superior cerebellar artery. The medial posterior chorioidal artery is well outlined and can be traced forward to a considerable extent because it lies just above the posterior cerebral arteries (*upper arrow*). In the venous phase (B), the vertebral artery is still filled but the basilar artery is not. Because the vertebral artery is still filled, the posterior inferior cerebellar artery is also outlined. The chorioid plexus is seen (*upper arrows*) just above the internal cerebral vein. In the frontal projection (C), regurgitation into the opposite vertebral artery is noted. The posterior inferior cerebellar artery is seen on the left side (the side of the injection). Its cephalic and caudal curves are well seen and the medial branch is seen to ascend parallel to and partly superimposed on the basilar artery (*two arrows*). As it goes upward, it produces a dense shadow just below the bifurcation of the basilar artery which could easily be confused with an aneurysm. However, the fact that it is still visible at the end of the serial when the basilar artery is empty and the posterior inferior cerebellar artery is filled indicates that it is not an aneurysm arising from the superior cerebellar artery. The configuration of the posterior cerebral and superior cerebellar vessels is that seen in cases where the bifurcation of the basilar artery is low. Compare with Fig. 387B. The posterior communicating artery is seen on the right side. The right superior cerebellar artery seems to be double (*arrow*). The parieto-occipital (*upper arrow*) and the posterior temporal branches of the posterior cerebral arteries are well shown on both sides. In the venous phase (D), the posterior inferior cerebellar artery is still filled. The medial or vermis branch is well shown and the appearance suggestive of an aneurysm is still visible (*arrow*). However, no aneurysm is seen in the lateral projection, and the increase in density is due to superimposition of segments of the artery.

(*Revised 1963*)

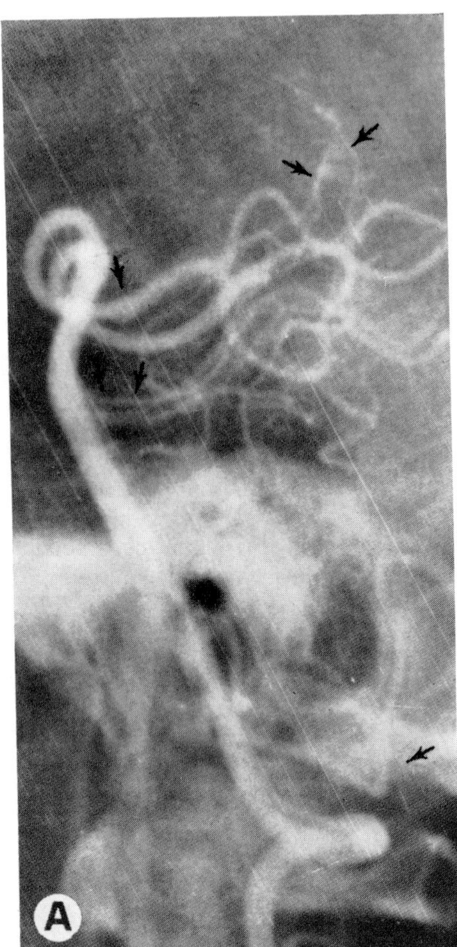

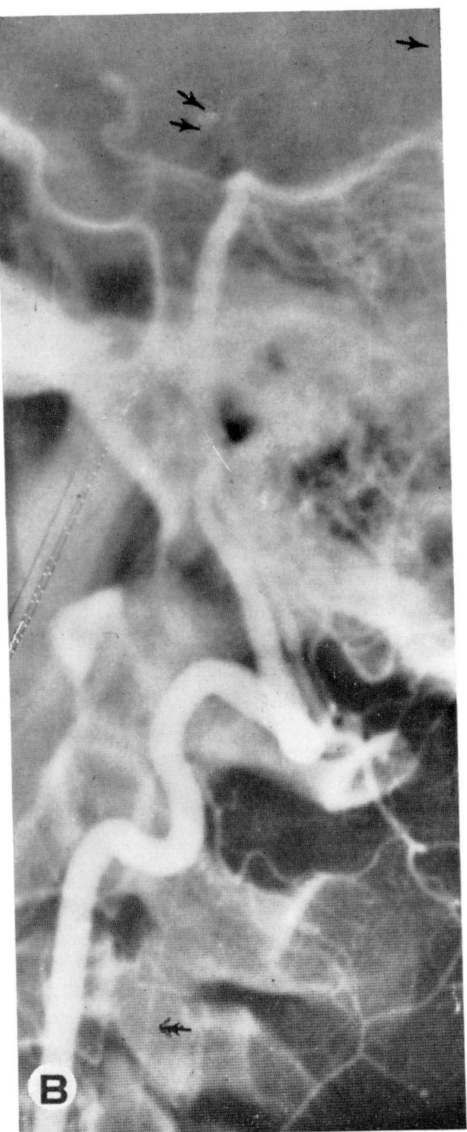

Fig. 386.—Normal Lateral Vertebral Angiogram

The posterior inferior cerebellar artery (*lower arrow*) shown in (A) extends below the margin of the foramen magnum but does not indicate tonsillar herniation. The two posterior cerebral arteries are symmetrical (*upper left arrow*). The superior cerebellar arteries describe their usual downward curve (*left double arrows*). The upper right arrows point to the posterior chorioidal arteries. The film shown in (B) also reveals a slight downward curvature of the posterior inferior cerebellar artery below the foramen magnum. The lower arrow points to the anterior spinal artery. The upper left arrow points to the thalamic branches arising from the posterior communicating arteries which supply the anterior inferior aspect of the thalamus. The upper right arrow indicates a posterior chorioidal artery. See also Fig. 393C.

broader curve. The resultant asymmetry as seen in the frontal projection may be confusing. The artery is contained within the *tentorial incisura* and actually follows the medial edge of the tentorial slit. As it continues its course dorsally, it goes above the tentorium to run on the medial aspect of the undersurface of the temporal lobe. Here the pos-

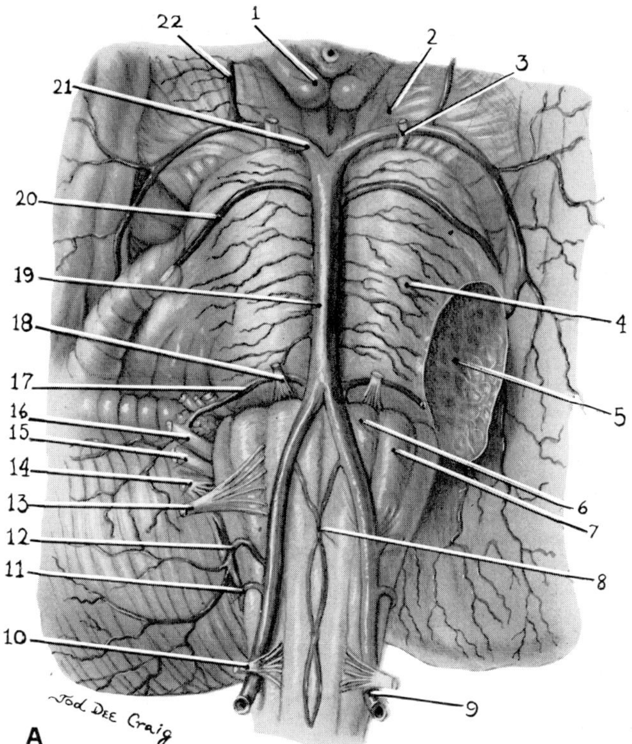

FIG. 387.—DIAGRAM OF VERTEBRAL AND BASILAR ARTERIES AND THEIR BRANCHES

Frontal view of the pons and medulla showing the branches of the vertebral and basilar arteries. (1) Mammillary body. (2) cerebral peduncle. (3) III nerve (oculomotor). (4) pons. (5) cross-section brachium pontis (middle cerebellar peduncle). (6) pyramid of medulla. (7) olive. (8) anterior spinal artery. (9) vertebral artery (10) first cervical nerve root. (11) posterior spinal artery. (12) posterior inferior cerebellar artery. (13) XII nerve (hypoglossus). (14) XI nerve (spinal accessory). (15) X nerve (pneumogastric). (16) IX nerve (glossopharyngeal). (17) anterior inferior cerebellar artery. (18) VI nerve (abducens). (19) basilar artery. (20) superior cerebellar artery. (21) posterior cerebral artery. (22) posterior communicating artery (after Testut).

FIG. 387 (cont.).—NORMAL VERTEBRAL ANGIOGRAMS, ANTEROPOSTERIOR VIEW

The appearance of the vessels in half axial projection is shown in (B). The depiction in a standard anteroposterior angiographic projection (C), similar to that employed for carotid angiography, is foreshortened; it usually is not desirable to use such a position in vertebral angiography except for the demonstration of specific lesions. In a less inclined view (D) at vertebral angiography the appearance is entirely different; such a projection may be helpful to demonstrate certain small aneurysms that arise at the basilar artery bifurcation. In (E), a symmetrical appearance of the bifurcation of the basilar artery with the posterior cerebral and superior cerebellar arteries is shown; these arteries arise almost from a common trunk. The arrow points to one posterior communicating artery which is seen to arise about 1 cm. from the origin of the posterior cerebral artery. (F) shows the appearance in patients with a low bifurcation of the basilar artery. See FIG. 387 (cont.) on next page.

terior cerebral artery divides into two main branches, the *posterior temporal* (or temporo-occipital) and the *internal occipital* branches. The posterior cerebral artery also gives off an anterior temporal branch which supplies part of the anterior portion of the temporal lobe. The latter branch is inconspicuous on the angiogram; it often anastomoses with the anterior temporal branch of the middle cerebral artery. The temporo-occipital branch supplies the undersurface of the posterior portion of the temporal lobe (fusiform and lingual gyri). The internal occipital branch bifurcates into two divisions, the *calcarine* and the *parieto-occipital arteries* which supply the medial aspect of the occipital lobe and the precuneus (fig. 393).

As seen on the lateral projection, it should be remembered that these arterial branches are first on the undersurface of the temporal lobe which is slanted downward and laterally to conform to the configuration of the tentorium. Therefore, the posterior temporal branch which is directed laterally and posteriorly also passes slightly caudally. For this reason, on the angiogram the artery and its branches overlie the superior cere-

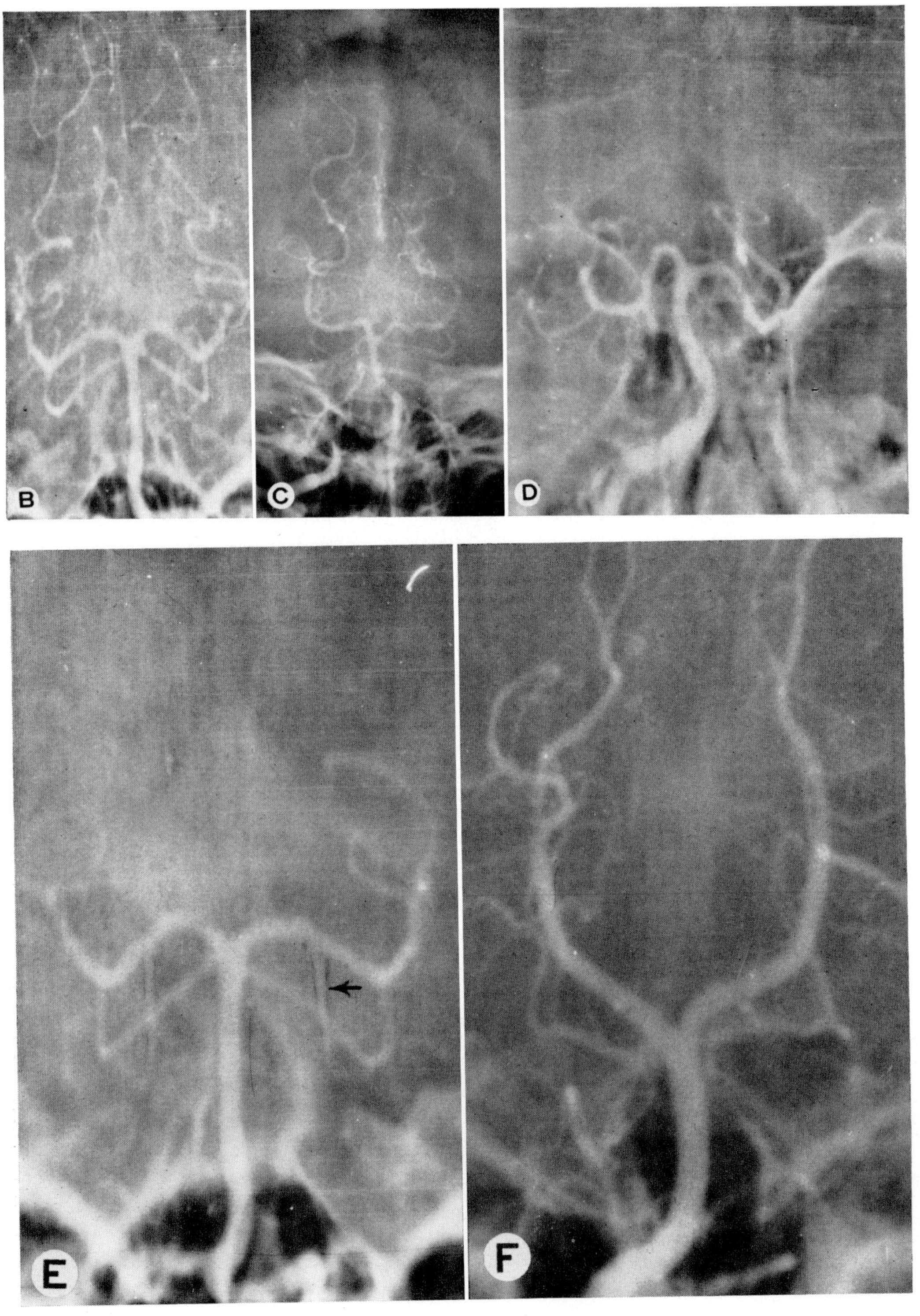

Fig. 387 (cont.)

(Revised 1963)

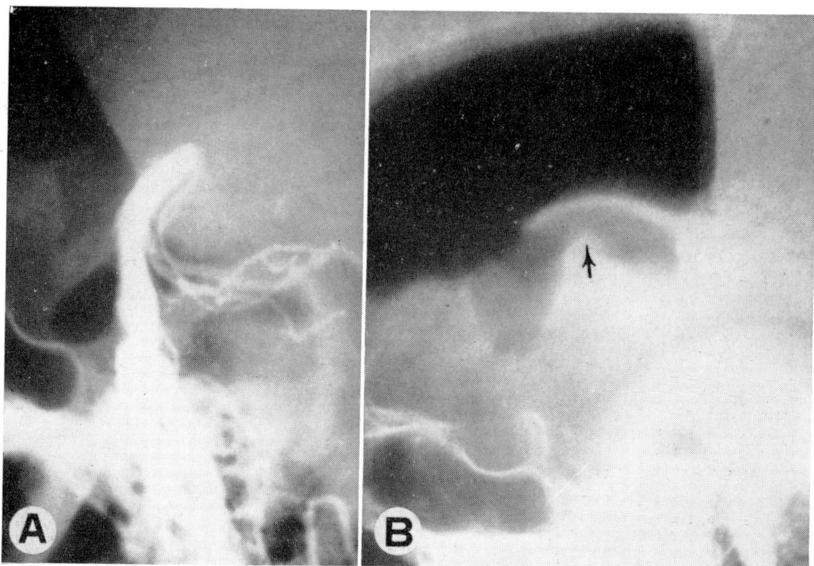

FIG. 388.—INDENTATION ON LOWER ASPECT OF THIRD VENTRICLE PRODUCED BY LONG TORTUOUS BASILAR ARTERY

The basilar artery is markedly elongated (A), and the air study (B) demonstrates the indentation on the lower aspect of the third ventricle produced by this tortuous elongated artery (*arrow*).

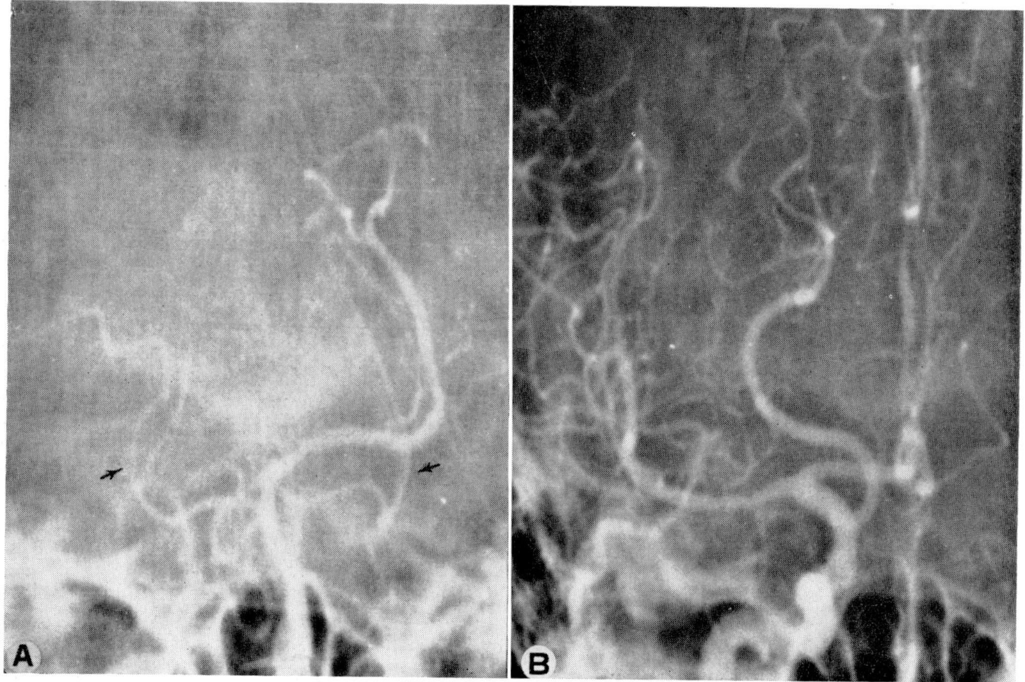

FIG. 389.—NORMAL VERTEBRAL ANGIOGRAM

The anteroposterior view (A) shows that the posterior cerebral artery does not fill on one side. Both superior cerebellar arteries fill and are slightly asymmetrical (*arrows*). A carotid angiogram on this patient (B) disclosed carotid origin of the posterior cerebral artery on the side that does not fill on the vertebral angiogram.

(Revised 1963)

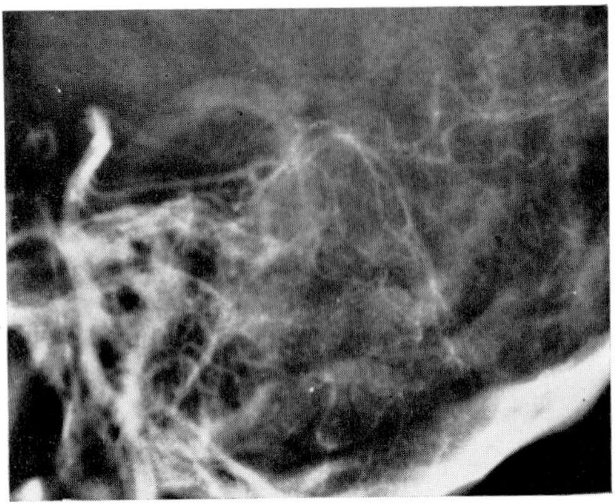

FIG. 390.—NONFILLING OF POSTERIOR CEREBRAL ARTERIES FROM BASILAR ARTERY

The lateral view shows that none of the posterior cerebral arteries fills. For this reason the upward convexity of the branches of the superior cerebellar arteries is clearly seen without any overlying branches of the posterior cerebral artery. In these cases, the appearance always suggests a tumor of the cerebellum.

bellar arteries which are beneath the tentorium (figs. 385 and 386).

Posterior communicating artery. The posterior communicating artery joins the posterior cerebral about 1.0 cm. from its origin (fig. 387E). The proximal segment of the posterior cerebral artery, between the basilar and the posterior communicating, is often hypoplastic on one side and sometimes on both sides (fig. 395). In the latter cases there is bilateral carotid origin of the posterior cerebral arteries. The angiographic appearance of the posterior communicating artery has been described under minor branches of the internal carotid artery.

Posterior chorioidal arteries. The posterior chorioidal arteries arise from the posterior cerebral arteries on each side. There are a medial and two or more lateral arteries (Galloway and Greitz, 1960). The *medial posterior chorioidal artery* arises from the posterior cerebral just lateral to the bifurcation of the basilar artery. It goes around the midbrain together with and usually obscured by the posterior cerebral artery. It reaches the posterolateral aspect of the midbrain where it ascends describing a double arch (figure of "3") and passes just lateral to the pineal body to reach the midline. It enters the tela chorioidea of the 3d ventricle, following along the roof of this ventricle (figs. 385 and 391). The *lateral posterior chorioidal arteries* (at least 2 in number) arise on each side from the posterior cerebral arteries as these vessels go around the brain stem, in the crural cistern and further posteriorly. They usually penetrate the chorioidal fissure almost immediately describing a curve concave forward, as they ascend, corresponding to the posterior aspect of the thalamus (fig. 391). They can be differentiated from the medial posterior chorioidal artery because they describe a smooth concave curve, whereas the medial posterior chorioidal artery describes a double curve

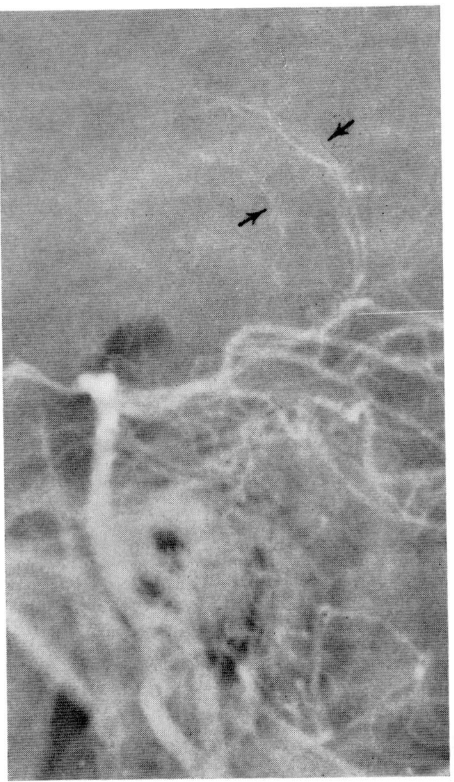

FIG. 391.—NORMAL LATERAL VERTEBRAL ANGIOGRAM

The film demonstrates the medial and the lateral posterior chorioidal arteries. The posterior chorioidal arteries (*posterior arrow*) are superimposed on each other, and the same is true of the medial posterior chorioidal arteries.

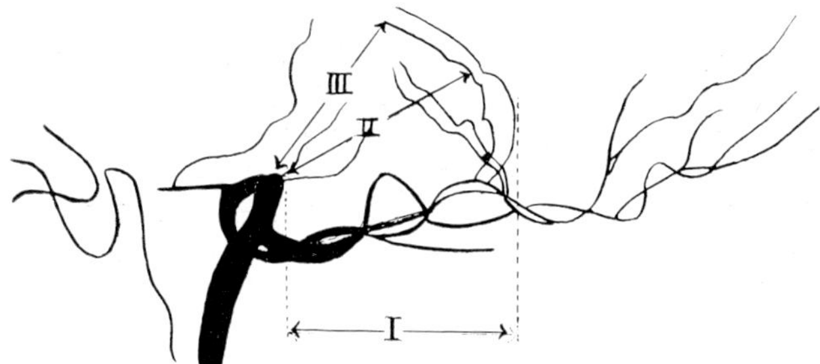

FIG. 392.—DIAGRAM OF LÖFGREN TO INDICATE THE MEASUREMENTS THAT HE FOUND TO APPLY TO THE POSITION OF THE NORMAL POSTERIOR CHORIOIDAL ARTERIES, AS EXPLAINED IN THE TEXT.

and is usually slightly more anterior than the lateral posterior chorioidal vessels. On stereoscopic films, the medial posterior chorioidal vessels are near the midline, on each side. The posterior chorioidal arteries usually are not visible on frontal angiographic films.

Measurements of chorioidal vessels were made by Löfgren (1956) in 100 normal vertebral angiograms. He found that the origin of the posterior chorioidal vessels as seen on the angiogram is 1 to 2 cm. posterior to the basilar artery. He took three measurements of the arc of the posterior chorioidal arteries as shown in Figure 392. The measurements found by him were as follows:

I = 30 to 45 mm. (95 per cent between 33 and 42)
II = 30 to 45 mm.
III = 25 to 37 mm.

Thalamic tumors usually increase the width of the curve and stretch the chorioidal vessels on one side, whereas pineal tumors

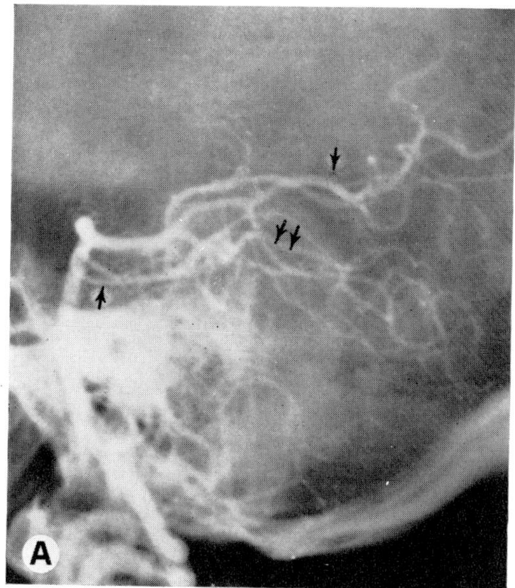

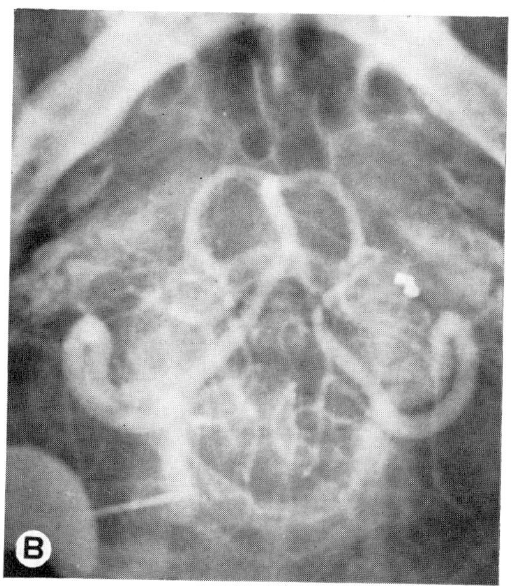

FIG. 393.—NORMAL VERTEBRAL ANGIOGRAM, LATERAL AND BASE VIEWS

The lateral view (A) shows the short perforating branches supplying the midbrain and the thalamus, which arise from the anterior portion of the posterior cerebral arteries. There was considerable downward regurgitation of the contrast substance into the opposite vertebral artery. The *upper posterior arrow* points at the internal occipital artery. The *double arrows* indicate the posterior temporal branches. The anterior arrow shows the superior cerebellar arteries. The base view (B) shows the normal appearance of the posterior cerebral and superior cerebellar arteries as they go around the brain stem. The appearance is often less regular than is present in this case when, in normal instances, the vessels are tortuous.

(Revised 1963)

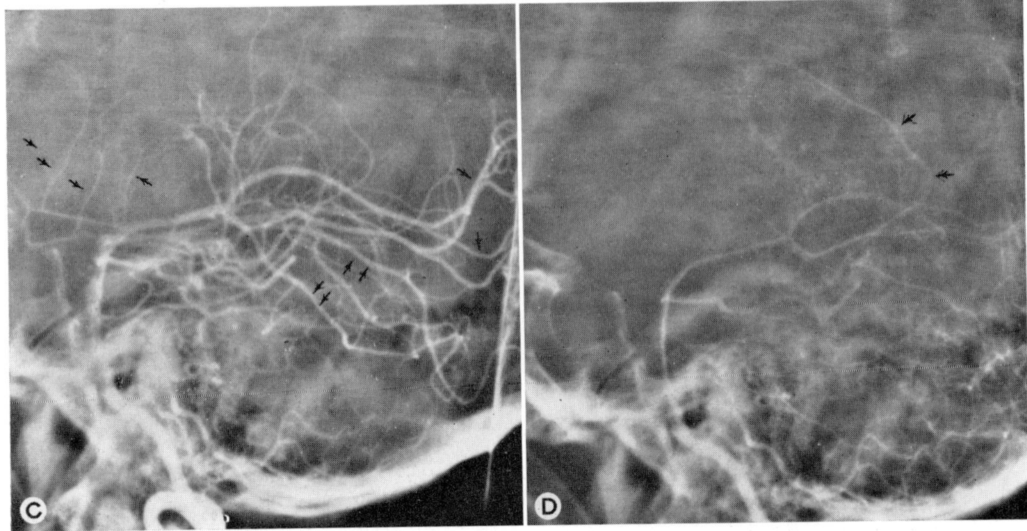

FIG. 393 (*Cont.*).—LATERAL VERTEBRAL ANGIOGRAM IN CHILD WITH TEMPORAL TUMOR

The internal occipital branch of the posterior cerebral arteries with the two branches resulting from their bifurcations on each side are shown by the posterior arrows. The right and left sides are partly superimposed. The *two double arrows* point at the posterior temporal branches of the posterior cerebral arteries which are always directed caudally and overlie the superior cerebellar arteries. There are numerous branches in the region of the posterior chorioidal vessels which show an unusual prominence and length, probably because they are supplying the posterior portion of the neoplasm. There is also enlargement and prominence of the thalamic branches arising from the proximal portion of the posterior cerebral artery and from the posterior communicating arteries (*anterior arrows*). (D) shows the same case as (C) at 2.5 seconds after injection. The enlarged posterior pericallosal artery is now outlined completely (*arrows*).

may cause stretching on both sides, involving usually the medial chorioidal arteries only (see under pineal and thalamic tumors).

Other branches. There are many small perforating branches which arise from the posterior cerebral artery trunk. These branches supply the cerebral peduncles and other vital structures in the midbrain (fig. 393). In addition, the thalamic branches arise from the posterior cerebral artery and supply the anterior thalamus (figs. 386 and 393). Some thalamic branches also arise from the posterior communicating artery. These branches are only occasionally seen on the angiogram unless they are dilated in cases of neoplasm and in thrombosis. The rest of the thalamus is supplied by the lateral posterior chorioidal arteries. A posterior pericallosal (or artery of the splenium) is seen in some normal cases but is not commonly seen unless it is enlarged to serve as collateral supply in cases of vascular occlusions and in neoplasms (figs. 393D and 565).

ARTERIAL VARIANTS AND ANOMALIES

Carotid System

The left common carotid artery arose from the (right) innominate artery in 9 out of 130 cases examined by Stein and co-authors (1961). The right subclavian artery, in the same series, originated as the last branch of the aortic arch and had a retro-esophageal course in two instances. In the latter cases, the right common carotid artery may originate directly from the aorta.

The site of bifurcation of the common carotid artery, which usually takes place at about the level of the upper margin of the thyroid cartilage, may be higher or lower. Occasionally the internal carotid artery may be altogether absent. In one instance,

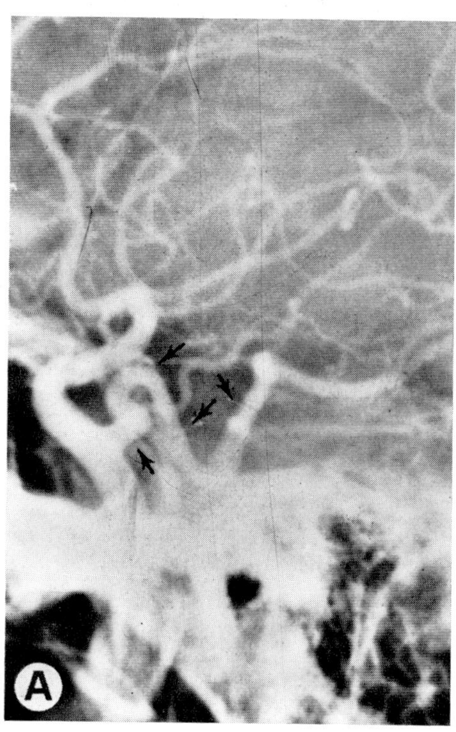

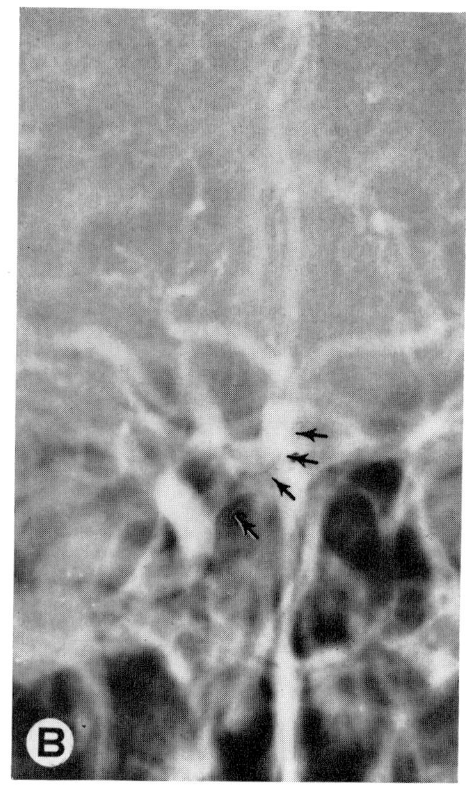

FIG. 394.—PERSISTENT PRIMITIVE TRIGEMINAL ARTERY

The lateral view demonstrates the origin of this vessel from the posterior portion of the intracavernous segment, or just before the artery enters the cavernous sinus. It has a tortuous course and joins the basilar artery after passing through the anterior and anterolateral aspect of the tentorial incisura. The frontal projection (B) demonstrates the course of the artery (*arrows*) and the filling of both posterior cerebral and superior cerebellar arteries.

the cranial portion of the internal carotid artery was replaced by two branches coming off the internal maxillary artery entering the skull through the foramen rotundum and foramen ovale joining intracranially to form a single vessel (Gray).

In cases of absent internal carotid arteries the opposite internal carotid may provide the blood supply by way of a transverse collateral arising from the intracavernous portion of the internal carotid artery. Of 24 such cases reported in the literature, there were 4 with aneurysms of the anterior communicating artery, and in 1 case there was cranial nerve involvement due to pressure by tortuous basilar artery (Turnbull).

Carotid-basilar anastomoses may exist at three levels. These anastomotic channels are the result of persistent arteries encountered during embryologic development (Padget, 1944). (1) The persistence may be seen with greatest frequency just proximal to the intracavernous portion of the internal carotid artery. This is called the *persistent primitive trigeminal artery* and joins the trunk of the internal carotid artery and of the basilar artery directly. Under certain circumstances, the anomaly can be a very important anastomotic channel (fig. 394). In fact, it is the authors' impression that this persistent artery is seen with greater frequency when other anomalies such as saccular aneurysms are present. (2) The *persistent primitive acoustic artery* is in a slightly lower position than the trigeminal artery and arises from the intrapetrosal portion of the internal carotid artery. (3) The third is the *persistent hypoglossal artery*. This communicates the

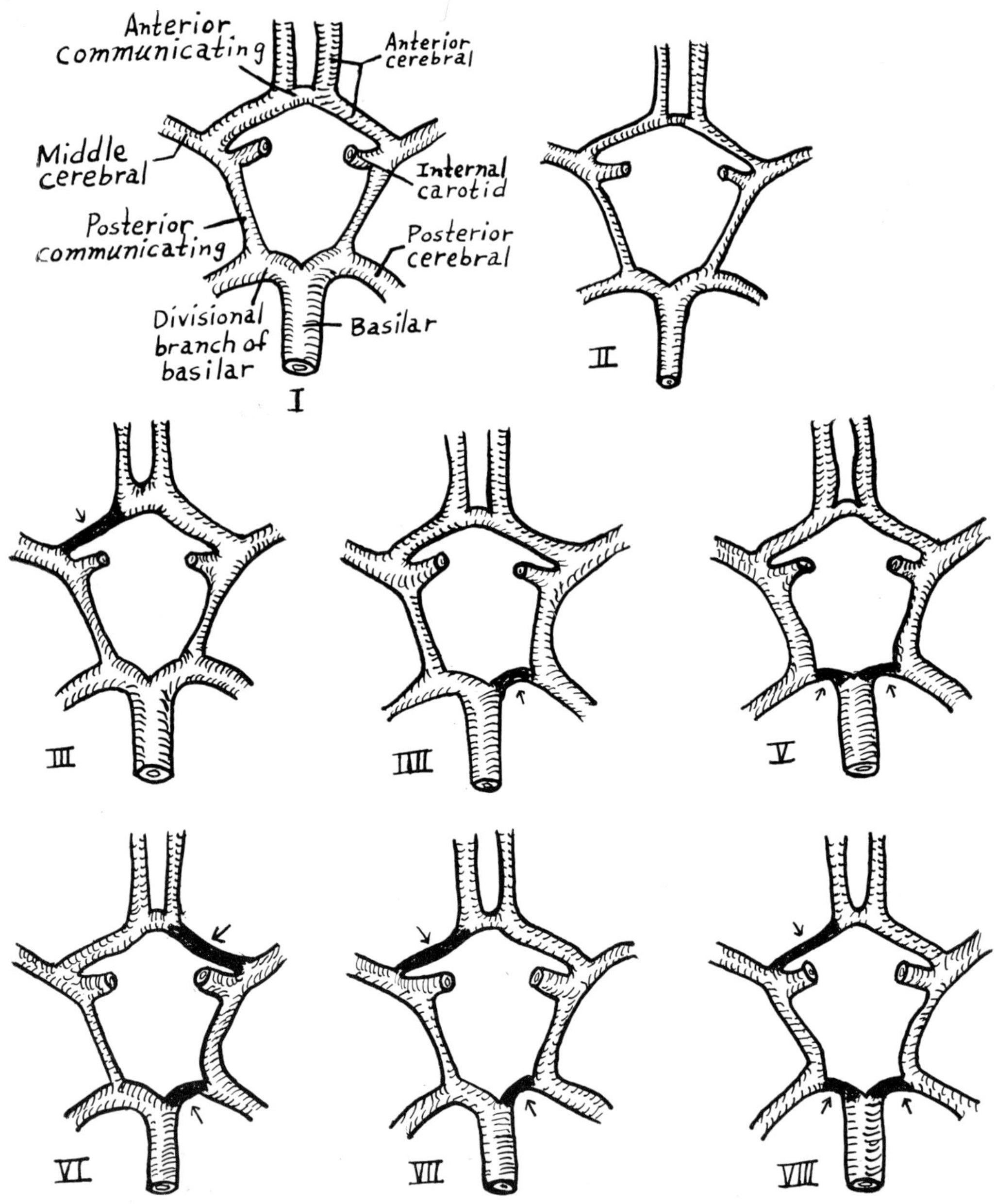

FIG. 395.—ANATOMICAL VARIANTS OF THE CIRCLE OF WILLIS ACCORDING TO HODES *ET AL.*
Type 1 represents a symmetrical circle of Willis and is present in 18 per cent of cases. Type 2, 6 per cent incidence; type 3, 25 per cent; type 4, 16 per cent; type 5, 11 per cent; type 6, 8 per cent; type 7, 8 per cent and type 8, 8 per cent. The hypoplastic segments are indicated by *solid lines*. Type 2 is a symmetrical circle of Willis but with all of the components rather small.

cervical portion of the internal carotid artery with the vertebral artery. It is extremely rare. This persistent artery should not be confused with dilated anastomotic channels that occur after thrombosis of the internal carotid and vertebral arteries and sometimes after thrombosis of the common carotid artery. These anastomotic channels exist between the external carotid (and not the internal) and the vertebral system. The latter is illustrated in Figure 559. Some variations of the cerebral arteries that involve the anterior chorioidal, anterior, and middle cerebral arteries as well as the posterior cerebral arteries are mentioned when these arteries are described.

Vertebral System

The vertebral artery originates directly from the aorta on the left side in 6 per cent of the cases (Radner, 1951; Stein and co-authors, 1961). The vertebral artery may arise directly from the common carotid artery, from the inferior thyroidal artery, or from the innominate artery. These latter anomalies are less common. The vertebral artery may not penetrate the foramen transversarium of the sixth cerebral vertebra, but it may start at the fifth cervical vertebra. It has been seen to come out of the foramen transversarium between the third and the second cervical vertebrae and to go back in the foramen transversarium of the atlas. Other details on anatomical variations of the vertebral arteries have been given on page 1.523.

Circle of Willis.

Originally described by the author whose name it bears (Willis, 1684), the circle of Willis is an important anatomic structure. Its constant configuration is an indication of its relative physiologic importance. Nevertheless, it is extremely common to find asymmetrical development of the various components. According to Riggs (1953) only 18 per cent of specimens of circle of Willis were found to be normal; that is, none of the components of the circle was hypoplastic, and the circle was symmetrical. Based on a study of 1647 specimens removed at autopsy, the distribution of the various anatomical variants in percentages are shown in Figure 395. Riggs found complete absence of a component of the circle of Willis to be very rare. Even though one component is extremely hypoplastic, usually tiny arterial branches can be seen to bridge the area between the two vessels.

The circle of Willis apparently is important in cases of occlusion in the neck of the major arteries that supply the brain. The relative sizes of the components of the circle of Willis have, no doubt, some bearing on the ability of a patient to withstand occlusion of a major artery either by surgical ligation of the vessel or by spontaneous occlusion due to thrombosis or embolism. Mount and Taveras (1960) have tried to evaluate on pre-operative angiograms the significance of the collateral circulation of the brain by way of the circle of Willis in order to determine whether the patient will be able to withstand surgical ligation of the internal or of the common carotid arteries (see under "Arterial Saccular Aneurysms. Post-operative Evaluation, p. 1.732).

CEREBRAL VEINS

Superficial Cerebral Veins

The superficial cerebral veins are extremely variable in their configuration. Most of these veins run upward to end in the superior longitudinal sinus (*superior cerebral veins*). The great majority ascend upward and backward, but as they reach the superior convexity of the brain, they turn rostrad and enter the superior longitudinal sinus against the flow of the bloodstream. Only one or two of the anterior frontal veins join the longitudinal sinus in the direction of the bloodstream. Blood flow in these veins is toward the sinus. The largest of these veins is the *vein of Trolard*, the position as well as the size of which is variable. The vein of Trolard anastomoses with the *vein of Labbé* which is directed downward and backward to end in the lateral sinus. Together they form an important venous anastomotic pathway. Like the vein of Trolard, the vein of Labbé is quite variable in position, size, and configuration (figs. 396 and 403).

Another of the descending veins is the superficial *middle cerebral vein* or veins; they

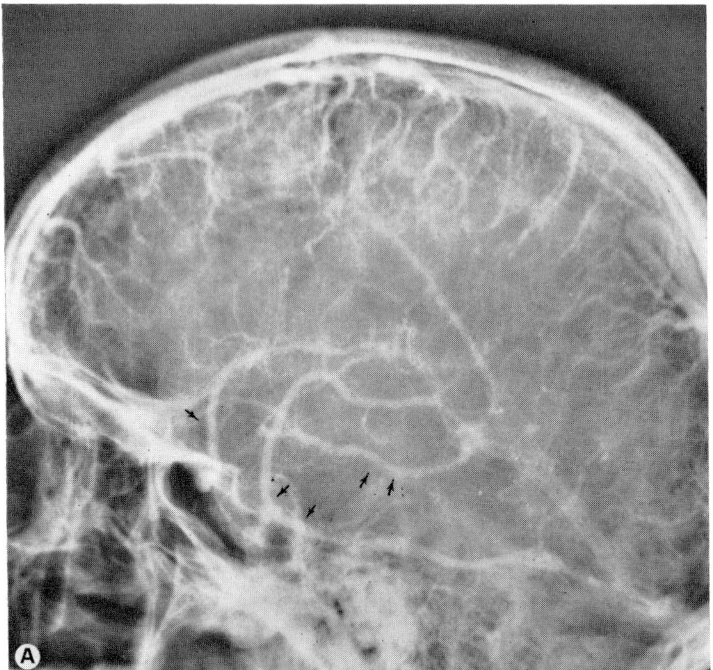

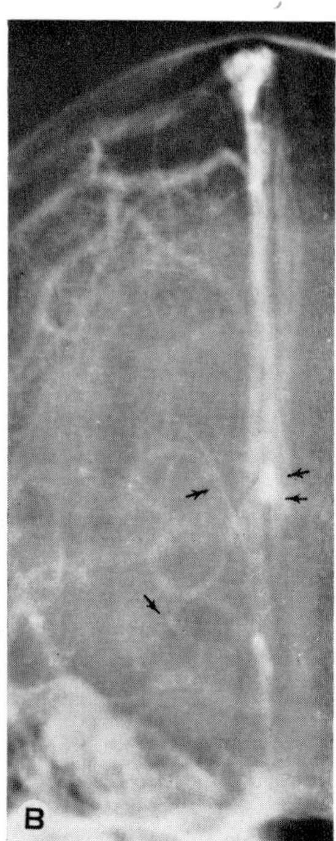

FIG. 396.—NORMAL VENOGRAM

The lateral view (A) shows the superficial superior cerebral veins curve rostrad to join the superior longitudinal sinus. The superficial veins in the lower half of the brain usually drain downward by way of the superficial middle cerebral or Sylvian vein (*anterior arrow*) and by way of the vein of Labbé, a variant of which is illustrated in this venogram (*lower arrows*). The basilar vein is well filled and shows a relatively typical configuration (*upper two arrows*). The inferior longitudinal sinus is well shown and its change in caliber following junction with the deep veins to become the straight sinus is well demonstrated. (B) Anteroposterior view of venogram showing superficial cerebral veins as well as the deep veins. The thalamostriate vein is indicated by the *upper arrow* and the basilar vein by the *lower arrow*. The internal cerebral vein is indicated by the *double arrow*. It is often possible to confuse the superficial veins with the deep veins, particularly if no serialogram is available which will usually show persistence of the deep veins, whereas the overlying superficial veins, usually in the frontal region, would have disappeared in the later phases.

may be two in number. These veins run in the Sylvian fissure, downward and forward and then medially along the sphenoid ridge to end in the sphenoparietal sinus or directly in the cavernous sinus.

The inferior cerebral veins drain the undersurface of the hemispheres. The veins under the temporal lobe join the middle cerebral and basal veins; those on the orbital surface of the frontal lobe join the superficial frontal veins and empty into the superior sagittal sinus.

On the angiogram the frontal veins fill slightly before the posterior frontal and parietal veins. Actually if a serial study is made, it is observed how, in very rapid succession, the frontal veins appear first very faintly, and shortly thereafter the parietal veins fill. The deep veins, which we will describe promptly, are usually the last ones to fill and they frequently remain filled longer than the superficial veins (at least with sufficient concentration of contrast substance to be well visualized).

Deep Cerebral Veins

The deep cerebral veins are more important than the superficial veins from the angiographic point of view. The important ones to consider are the internal cerebral

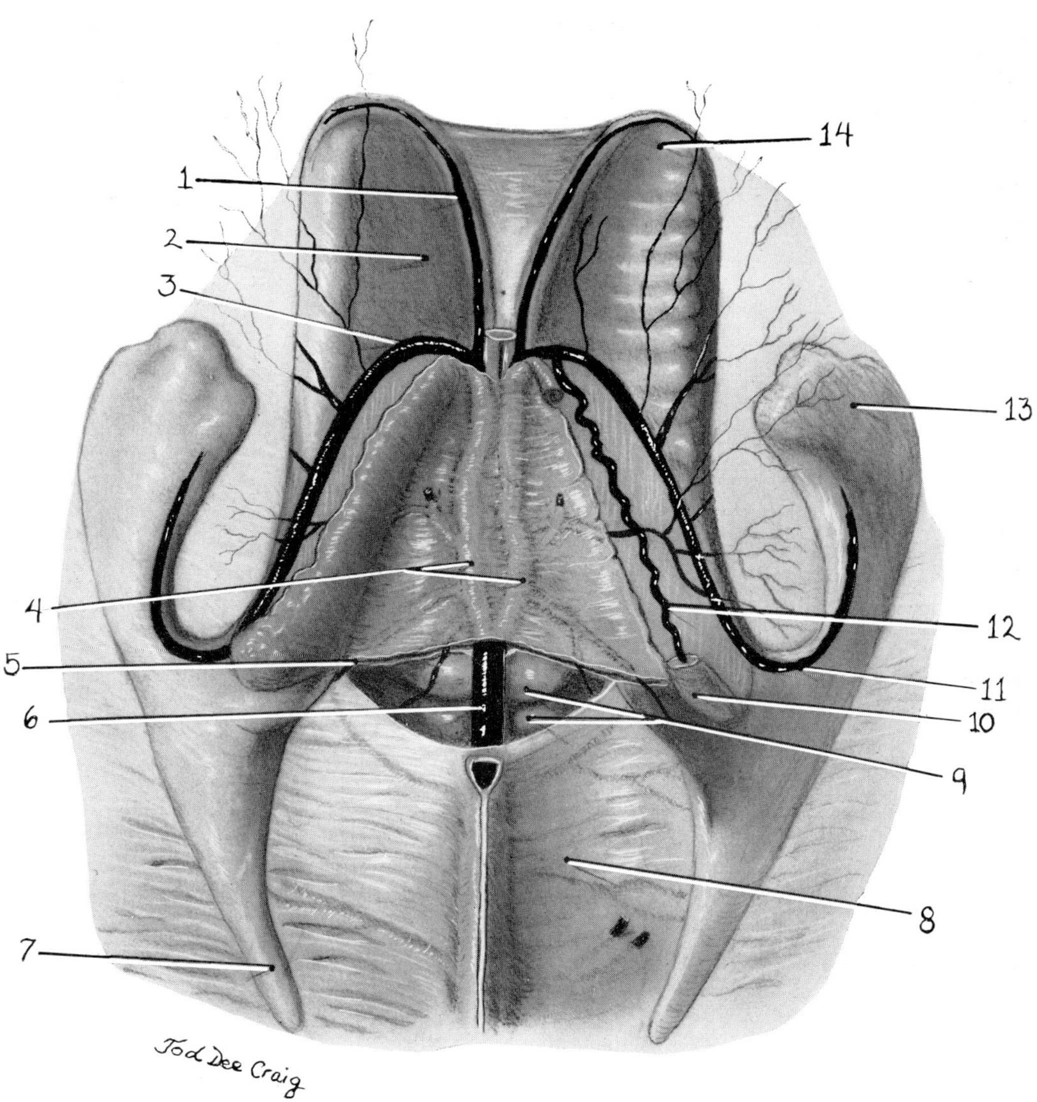

FIG. 397.—DIAGRAMMATIC REPRESENTATION OF THE DEEP CEREBRAL VEINS

The two thalamostriate veins are seen to join the septal vein to form the internal cerebral vein on each side. The internal cerebral veins are contained within the velum interpositum and join posteriorly to form the vein of Galen. The chorioid plexus was removed on the right side to show the chorioid vein. The thalamostriate vein is drawn to the temporal horn. This is seen sometimes but is by no means a constant feature. Variation in the configuration of the veins is, of course, the rule.

(1) Septal vein. (2) anterior horn at the junction with the body of the lateral ventricle. (3) thalamostriate vein. (4) internal cerebral veins. (5) the two leafs of the velum interpositum. (6) vein of Galen. (7) occipital horn. (8) tentorium. (9) quadrigeminal tubercles. (10) chorioid plexus. (11) initial segment of the thalamostriate vein or terminal vein. (12) chorioidal vein. (13) temporal horn. (14) frontal horn of the lateral ventricle. See also Fig. 401.

Medial to the thalamostriate vein is the thalamus and anterolaterally is the caudate nucleus.

(Revised 1963)

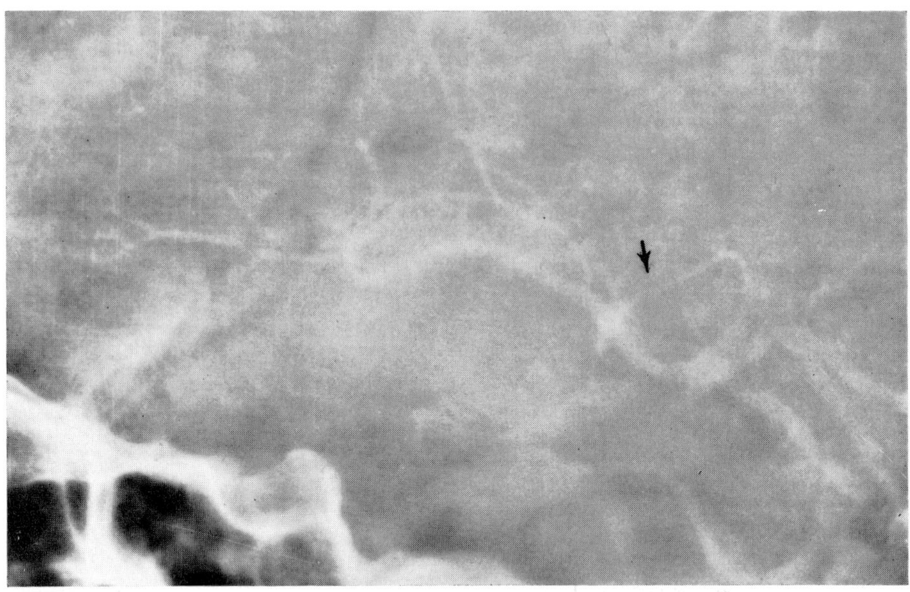

FIG. 398.—NORMAL VENOGRAM, LATERAL VIEW

The septal vein is well shown and it is seen to end at the thalamostriate vein just above the curve at the foramen of Monro. The thalamostriate vein also receives the anterior and posterior caudate veins and the terminal vein. The callosal vein (*arrow*) is also shown. Its position at the junction with the internal cerebral vein marks the splenium of the corpus callosum. The basilar vein is only faintly outlined. Usually the basilar vein fills earlier in the angiogram and empties in the later phases of the angiogram, when this film was made (4.5 seconds after the injection). The visible end of the septal vein and of the anterior and posterior caudate veins marks the approximate size of the lateral ventricle.

veins and their branches, the basilar vein (vein of Rosenthal), and the vein of Galen.

Internal cerebral veins. The vessel is paired and the two veins are situated just off the midline so that they are, for their greater extent, placed one against the other. They are at the roof of the third ventricle in the tela chorioidea (fig. 397). Their configuration is that of the roof of the third ventricle as seen in the lateral projection. The veins begin at the foramen of Monro and extend slightly upward and backward, and after reaching their highest point gradually descend backward and downward forming a fairly regular, semicircular, or somewhat parabolic, curve. *The anterior slope of the curve is approximately equal in lenth and configuration to the posterior slope*, but variations are fairly common. The internal cerebral veins leave the roof of the third ventricle just above the suprapineal recess and enter the upper portion of the quadrigeminal cistern where they join to form the great vein of Galen. The vein of Galen describes a curve concave upward and ends as it joins the straight sinus (fig. 398).

The main branch of the internal cerebral vein on each side is the *thalamostriate vein* or *terminal vein*. This vein is itself formed by tributaries running on the wall of the lateral ventricle and it also receives the *chorioid vein* which runs along the chorioid plexus of the lateral ventricle. From its junction with the internal cerebral vein, the thalamostriate vein extends backward and slightly upward in the groove formed by the caudate nucleus and the thalamus (fig. 397). The vein is, therefore, situated on the inferolateral aspect of the ventricular wall and actually outlines the approximate size of the lateral ventricle (fig. 396). If the ventricle has become enlarged, the arc, concave upward, described by the thalamostriate vein would become much wider (fig. 474). If the ventricle is narrowed, such as may be produced when there is medial displacement by a mass, the arc will be quite sharp or actually nonexistent (fig. 467).

The *venous angle* (Krayenbuhl and Richter, 1952) is the point of junction of the thalamostriate vein with the internal cerebral vein. At this point usually the *septal vein*, which comes from the frontal horn of the lateral ventricle on each side, joins the internal cerebral vein. This point is usually situated at the foramen of Monro (fig. 397). It may be found, however, that the thalamostriate vein does not join the internal cerebral vein at the foramen of Monro, but behind this point (fig. 398). This anatomical variant is fairly common and has been referred to as "false venous angle" by Lin *et al.* In some cases the usual arc of the internal cerebral vein is completed by the septal vein. In other cases the septal vein joins the thalamostriate vein directly and if the thalamostriate vein joins the internal cerebral vein more posteriorly than usual, the usual arc of the internal cerebral vein is not completed. In the latter cases, the appearance is always suggestive of upward displacement of the internal cerebral vein, even in a normal case (fig. 399). One can usually judge that this is an anomaly and not a displacement because the foramen of Monro is usually situated directly above or a little behind the dorsum sella (fig. 396), whereas in the cases of a false venous angle, the junction takes place considerably behind the sella turcica and, therefore, too far back to represent the foramen of Monro. Likewise if, in a given case, the venous angle was in normal position and later backward displacement of the foramen of Monro occurred (such as in frontal pole tumor), the arc of the internal cerebral vein would be deeper—the vein is "humped," Figure 426. In the cases of a false venous angle, the arc is flatter or no arc is present (fig. 399).

There are numerous veins in the depths of the cerebral hemispheres distributed in radial fashion and draining into the deep cerebral veins (Kaplan, 1959). These veins, however, are not visible on the angiogram except when they are pathologic. The deep veins *become visible only as they reach the ventricular wall* and from that point to their junction with the internal cerebral vein or thalamostriate vein, they are well shown (fig. 397 and 398). This makes it possible to outline the ventricular surface on the lateral angiogram fairly accurately and enlargement of the ventricle can be seen readily in this way (fig. 478).

A small vein is often seen which joins the anterior portion of the vein of Galen just behind the junction of the two internal cerebral veins. This small vein is the *posterior callosal vein*; it extends around the splenium of the corpus callosum before it joins the vein of Galen. Actually the vein of Galen approximates the position and shape of the splenium of the corpus callosum, but its relationship with this structure is variable. The posterior callosal vein (vein of the corpus callosum) is seen in a fairly high number of cases if looked for carefully. Ring (1959) found it in over 95 per cent of 100 normal cases. Occasionally, however, the vein is absent. Presumably the junction of this vein with the posterior aspect of the internal cerebral vein or the vein of Galen indicates fairly accurately the position of the inferior margin of the splenium of the corpus callosum.

Attempts have been made to determine the normal position of the internal cerebral vein by measurement. At least three different methods have been proposed to determine the position of the foramen of Monro based on the venous angle. Because of the variations in the point at which the internal cerebral vein and thalamostriate vein join, this determination by angiography is not too accurate. The simplest methods to use are those proposed by Wolf *et al.* (1955) and by Laine and co-authors (1956). In a comparative study of the methods proposed by Wolf and by Laine, Ring found that the method proposed by Laine to estimate the position of the foramen of Monro is slightly more accurate. The method proposed by Wolf *et al.* is also of help in determining the presence of upward or downward displacement of the middle and posterior portions of the internal cerebral vein.

Like all biological measurements, only gross separations from the normal fall outside the usual limits in all cases. Slight displacements may fall within accepted limits,

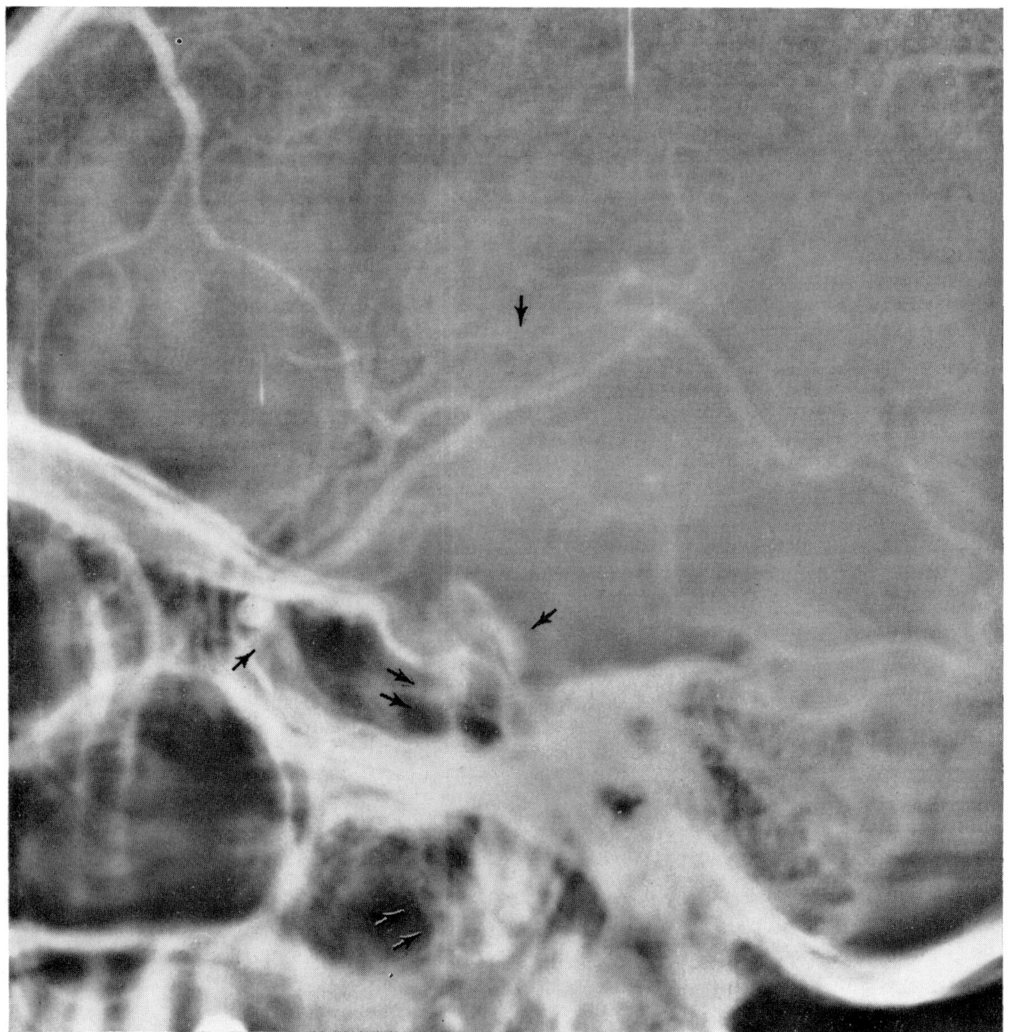

FIG. 399.—NORMAL CAROTID VENOGRAM

The superficial cerebral veins are well outlined. The internal cerebral vein shows that the junction of the thalamostriate vein with the internal cerebral vein (venous angle) is farther back than usual ("false" venous angle). However, the septal vein joins the internal cerebral vein (*arrow*) which continues forward to complete its normal curve. Sometimes the septal vein joins the thalamostriate vein directly, and in this case the internal cerebral vein gives the appearance of being elevated. Branches of the thalamostriate vein are also visible. The ventricular outline extends forward as far as the anterior tip of the septal vein because the deep veins do not become visible until they reach the ventricular wall. The superficial middle cerebral veins are also visible and also a portion of the sphenoparietal sinus (*lower arrow*). The shadow behind the sella turcica may be produced by the basilar plexus or the petrosal sinus (*posterior lower arrow*). In this case there is a large vein (emissary) crossing the sphenoid sinus (*double arrow*) and a prominent pterygoid plexus (*lower double arrow*).

and vice versa, normal veins may sometimes fall outside of the usual limits. Ring found that at least 19 per cent of patients present a false venous angle. In the majority of these cases, it is easy to determine that a false venous angle is present. In many cases, however, it is not realized that this anatomical variation is present and, therefore,

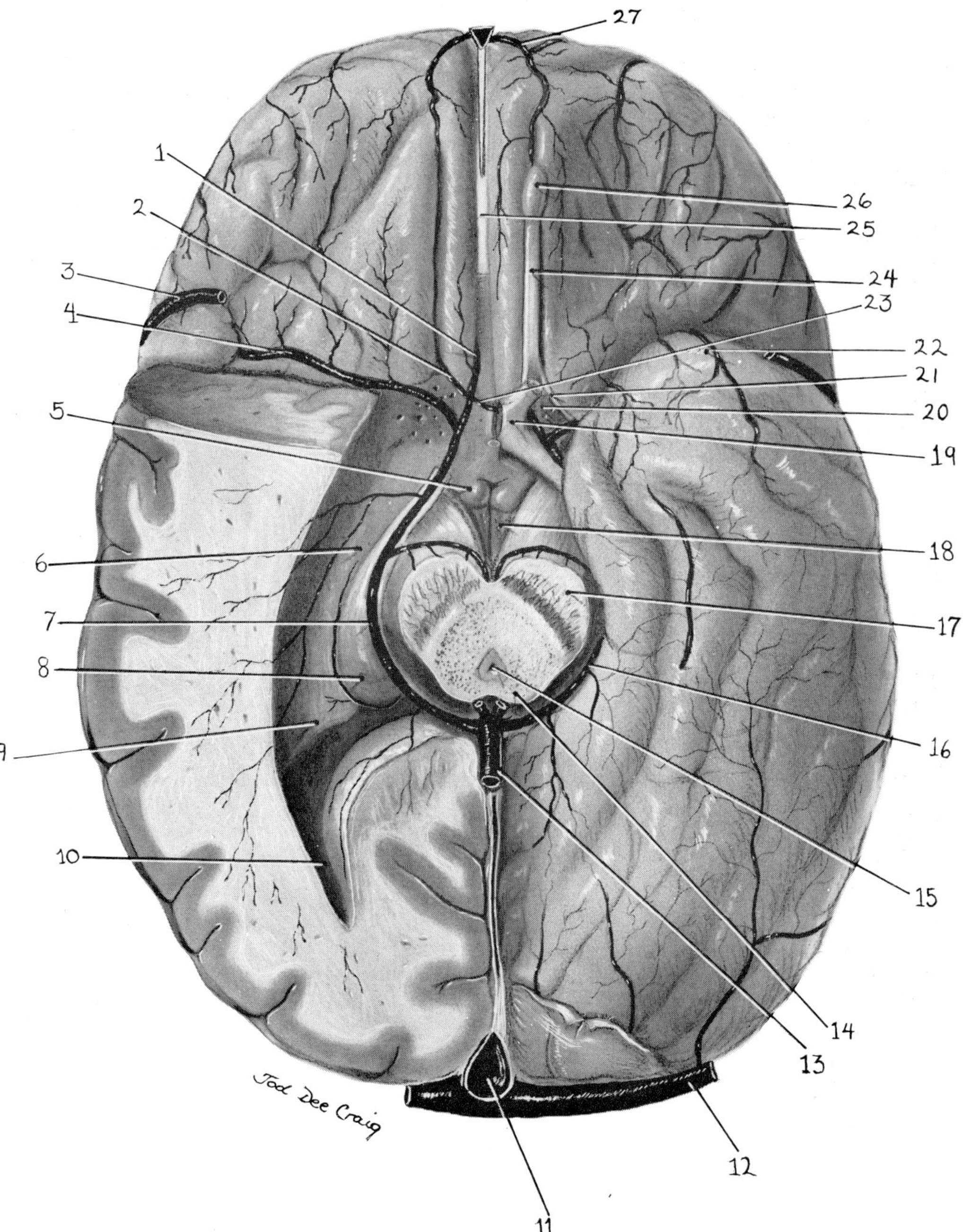

FIG. 400.—DIAGRAM DEPICTING THE BASAL VEIN, ITS ORIGINS AND RELATIONS WITH THE MIDBRAIN

The tip of the temporal lobe on the right side has been removed and a horizontal cross section of the temporal and occipital lobes has been done to open the temporal horn, occipital horn, and atrium of the ventricle. (1) anterior cerebral vein. (2) olfactory vein. (3) superficial middle cerebral vein. (4) deep middle cerebral vein. (5) mammillary body. (6) temporal horn of the lateral ventricle. (7) basilar vein. (8) hippocampus major. (9) collateral eminence. (10) posterior horn of the lateral ventricle. (11) superior sagittal sinus joining (12) transverse sinus. (13) vein of Galen. (14) quadrigeminal plate. (15) Aqueduct of Sylvius. (16) basilar vein. (17) cerebral peduncle. (18) posterior perforated substance. (19) optic chiasm. (20) anterior perforated substance. (21) lateral olfactory striae. (22) anterior tip of the temporal lobe. (23) anterior communicating vein. (24) olfactory tract. (25) longitudinal (interhemispheric fissure). (26) olfactory bulb. (27) superficial cerebral vein.

(Revised 1963)

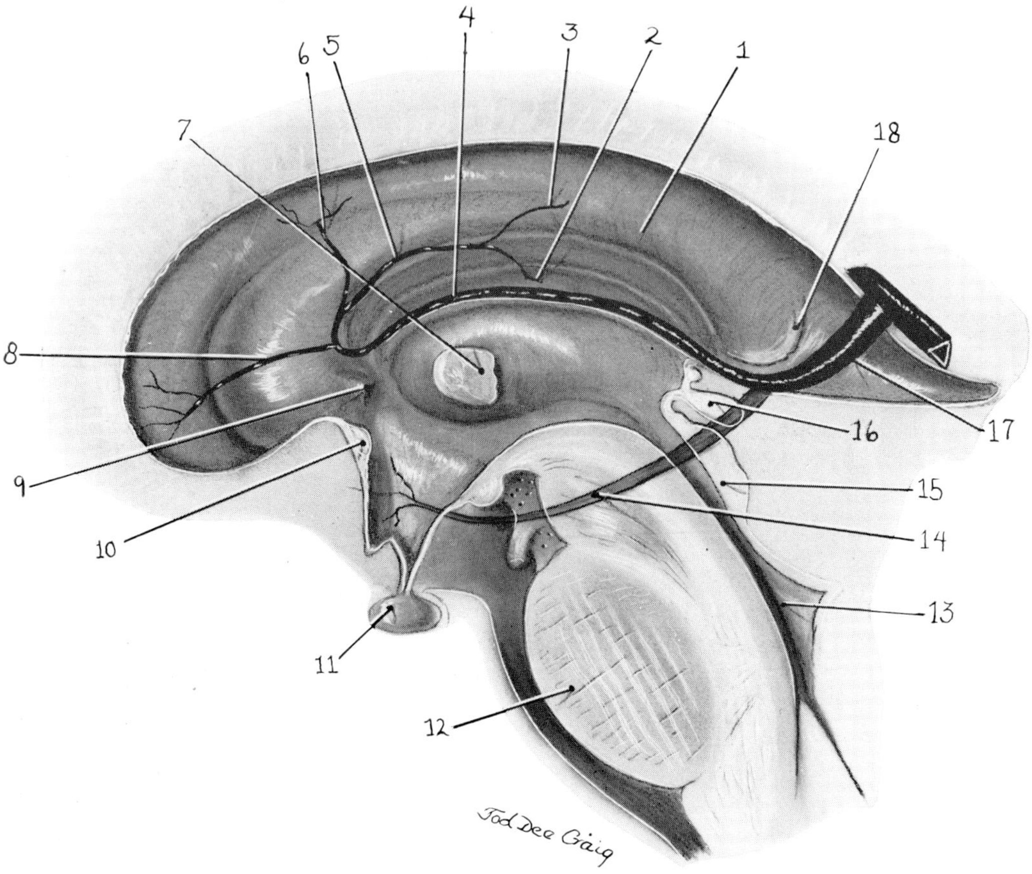

Fig. 401.—Diagrammatic Representation of the Deep Cerebral Veins and Their Relation with the Adjacent Brain Structures in Lateral Projection

(1) Lateral ventricle. (2) terminal branch of thalamostriate vein. (3) posterior caudate veins. (4) internal cerebral vein. (5) thalamostriate vein. (6) anterior caudate vein. (7) massa intermedia. (8) septal vein. (9) foramen of Monro. (10) anterior commissure. (11) hypophysis. (12) pons. (13) fourth ventricle. (14) basilar vein passing schematically behind the midbrain. (15) quadrigeminal plate. (16) pineal. (17) vein of Galen. (18) splenium of corpus callosum.

a false conclusion could be reached. With experience one may be able to eliminate this possible source of error, but this anatomic variant tends to decrease the accuracy of any method of locating the posterior aspect of the foramen of Monro based on angiograms.

The configuration of the arc of the internal cerebral vein differs with the shape of the head. In a patient with a dolichocephalic head, the arc of the internal cerebral vein is flatter than in a patient with a brachycephalic type of head. In the latter case, the vein describes a deeper arc.

Basilar vein. The basilar vein (*vein of Rosenthal*) originates at the level of the medial aspect of the anterior portion of the temporal lobe by tributaries arising from the medial surface and the temporal horn. It also receives veins coming from the hippocampal gyrus, the interpeduncular fossa, and the mid-brain. The basilar vein receives a small *anterior cerebral vein*, which passes laterally with the anterior cerebral artery, and the *deep middle cerebral vein* (fig. 400). It also receives many fine branches, the *inferior striate veins*, which leave the corpus striatum at the anterior perforated substance. From

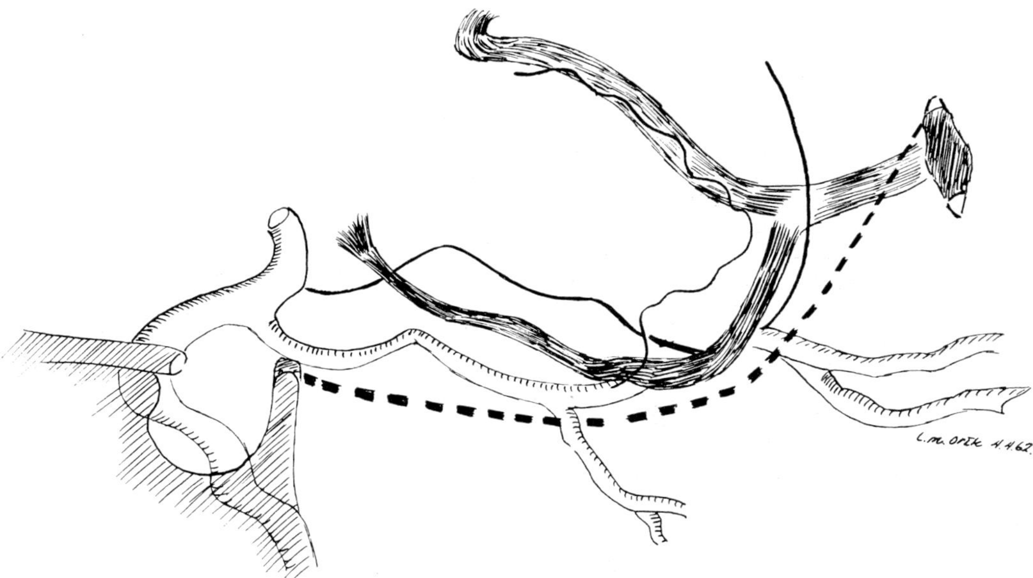

Fig. 402.—Diagram Representing the Relationship of the Posterior Cerebral Artery and the Basilar Vein, with the Tentorial Incisura, the Posterior Chorioidal Arteries, and the Anterior Chorioidal Artery

these origins the basilar vein passes backward and goes around the brain stem as it extends upward to join the two internal cerebral veins immediately before they fuse to form the vein of Galen. Variations from this usual confluence are very common. The basilar vein may not join the internal cerebral vein at the vein of Galen but may end directly in the straight sinus. It may join the vein of Galen just before this great vein enters the straight sinus.

The basilar veins are somewhat similar in their configuration to the posterior cerebral arteries but are situated slightly higher. These relationships are explained in Figure 402. Because the basilar vein is higher in position than the posterior cerebral artery, it does not behave in a manner identical with the artery when displaced by various pathological processes. When seen in the lateral projection, the basilar vein originates above the sella turcica and from its origin it first passes slightly downward before going upward and backward (fig. 401). The degree of downward curve from its origin is slightly variable, and care should be taken not to consider the anterior portion of this vein to be displaced upward unless it is a definite change. The anterior portion is usually considered elevated if the change in curve takes place far posteriorly instead of approximately 1.5 cm. above and behind the sella turcica, the usual point where the curve changes (fig. 403).

The appearance of the internal cerebral vein as seen in the *frontal projection* is that of a band of increased density in or near the midline. The length of the vertical band of increased density in the midline produced by the internal cerebral vein varies, depending on the degree of angulation of the x-ray tube used to make the radiograph. The greater the degree of angulation, the longer the internal cerebral vein will appear to be in the frontal projection. The inferior portion of the shadow represents the anterior portion of the vein in the latter cases. If the projection is such that the orbits are high up on the film, the vein is either completely telescoped on itself or the posterior portion may be lower than the anterior portion. This latter projection is rarely used by us to show cerebral veins and is only occasionally used to diagnose aneurysms or for suprasellar tumors where the internal cerebral vein is not important. The curves described by the

(Revised 1963)

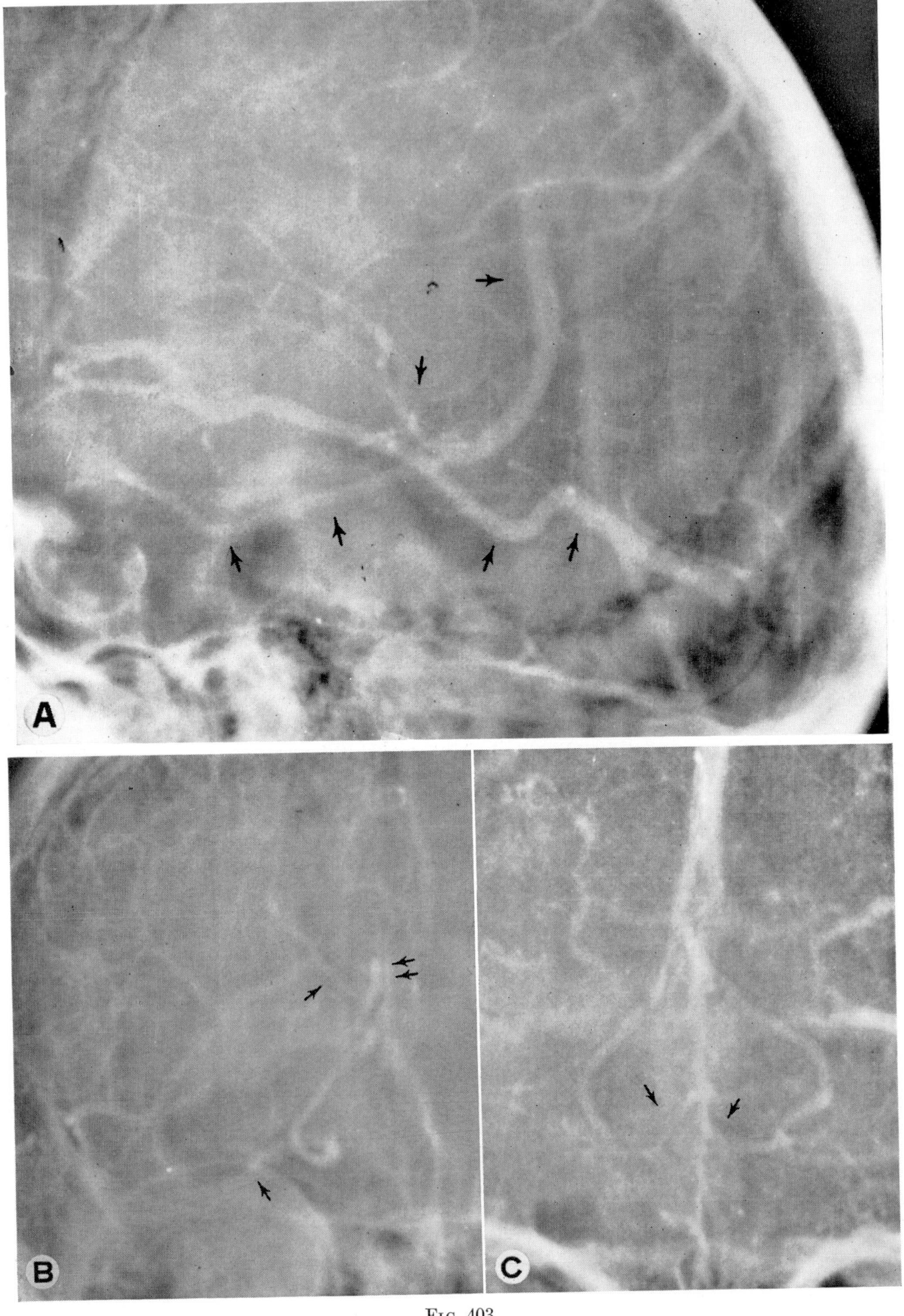

Fig. 403

(*Revised 1963*)

thalamostriate and the basilar veins are best shown on a very good reproduction of an angiogram or on a diagram (figs. 401 and 403). The curve of the basilar veins is again related to the angulation of the tube; the greater the angulation, the wider the sweep would be. The septal vein is difficult to visualize on frontal angiograms. In half axial projection, the septal veins are sometimes well shown.

Dural Sinuses

The *superior longitudinal sinus* is seen in a discontinuous manner because only part of the blood draining into the sinus is opacified with contrast substance in unilateral angiography. If it is desired to outline the superior longitudinal sinus, compression of the opposite side during injection of a larger amount of contrast substance (12 cc.) may be used. To show the superior longitudinal sinus, the lateral projection is useful and also a half axial projection taken with slight rotation of the head toward one side to prevent superimposition of the anterior on the posterior aspect of the sinus. The *lateral sinuses* are often quite well shown on the anteroposterior projection. One sinus (the right) is usually larger than the other, and sometimes practically all the contrast substance drains on one side. It should be kept in mind that "streaming" or "laminar flow" is the rule in the superior longitudinal and lateral sinuses so that it is possible, if only one side is injected, that the contrast substance would turn toward the lateral sinus on the same side, unless this sinus is smaller than the opposite side. Drainage of contrast substance through the lateral sinus on the side of the injection, therefore, does not mean that the opposite side is hypoplastic or obstructed.

The posterior portion of the superior longitudinal sinus is often situated off-center even in perfectly aligned anteroposterior films (fig. 404). This is a normal variant. Sometimes it is extremely laterally placed and instances are known in which it was so laterally situated that upon placing a burr hole for ventriculography, the outer sinus wall was pierced with resultant fatal bleeding. In these extreme cases, the sinus is probably lateral to the attachment of the falx.

The *inferior longitudinal sinus* is not always shown in angiograms (fig. 396). On the other hand, the *straight sinus* which receives the vein of Galen, is shown almost constantly, although opacification may be very faint. The vein of Galen joins the straight sinus, usually at the junction of the falx and tentorium, but sometimes they may join

Fig. 403.—Normal Carotid Venogram, Lateral View

(A) The basilar vein (lower anterior arrows) shows its typical configuration, with its downward and forward course and then formation of an angle upward and forward just behind the dorsum sella. In most instances, the angle is less well marked than the one shown in this case. The figure also illustrates an anomaly of the vein of Galen which joins the inferior longitudinal sinus very high up (*upper arrow*). The vein of Labbé (*lower posterior arrows*) does not join the lateral sinus, as is the case usually, but extends posteriorly apparently to join an eccentrically placed superior longitudinal sinus. The vein of the splenium is seen to join the internal cerebral vein before this vein joins the basilar vein (*upper anterior arrow*). Other variants of the veins are illustrated in the same figure, namely tributaries ending in the internal cerebral vein posterior to the foramen of Monro. The anteroposterior view (B) of an angiogram from another patient shows the normal configuration of the basilar vein. In its anterior (lower) end, the vein turns medially at the same time that it turns slightly upward. The deep middle cerebral vein is prominent (*lower arrow*). The thalamostriate vein is seen (*upper arrow*) to describe an arc with convexity upward which usually indicates the approximate size of the lateral ventricle. The internal cerebral vein is seen as a small band of increased density. This configuration should be compared with that seen in Fig. 396, which was taken with a slightly greater angulation of the x-ray tube, closer to a half axial projection. (C) The anteroposterior film shown in (C) demonstrates bilateral filling of the basilar veins because compression of the opposite side was made during injection and a slightly greater amount of contrast material was used. The configuration of the basilar veins in their anterior portion demonstrates their position around the midbrain. The branches coming from the interpeduncular fossa are clearly demonstrated (*arrows*).

(Revised 1963)

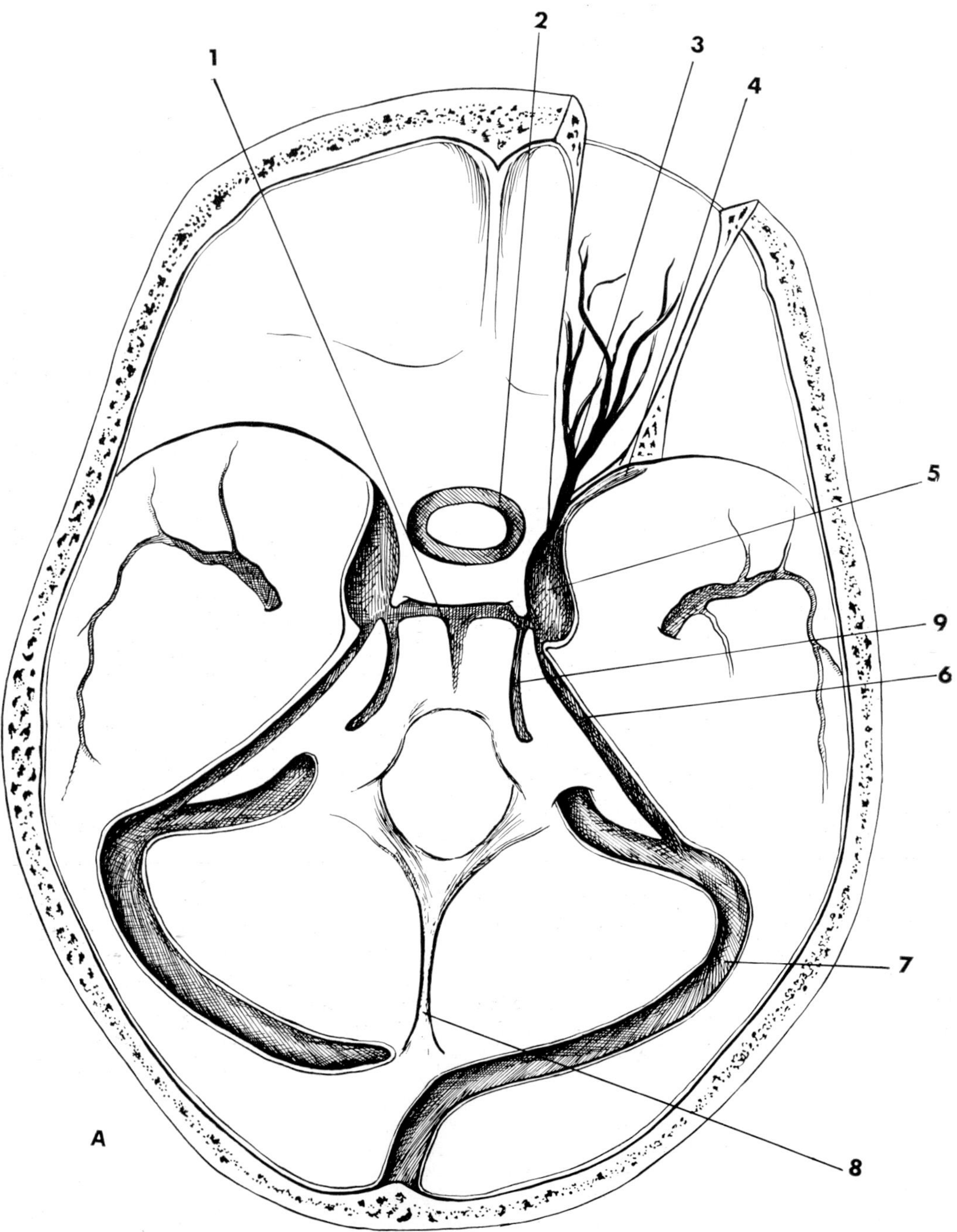

FIG. 404.—(A) DIAGRAM OF DURAL SINUSES

(1) Basilar plexus. (2) circular sinus. (3) superior ophthalmic vein. (4) sphenoparietal sinus. (5) cavernous sinus. (6) superior petrosal sinus. (7) transverse sinus. (8) occipital sinus. (9) inferior petrosal sinus.

(*Revised 1963*)

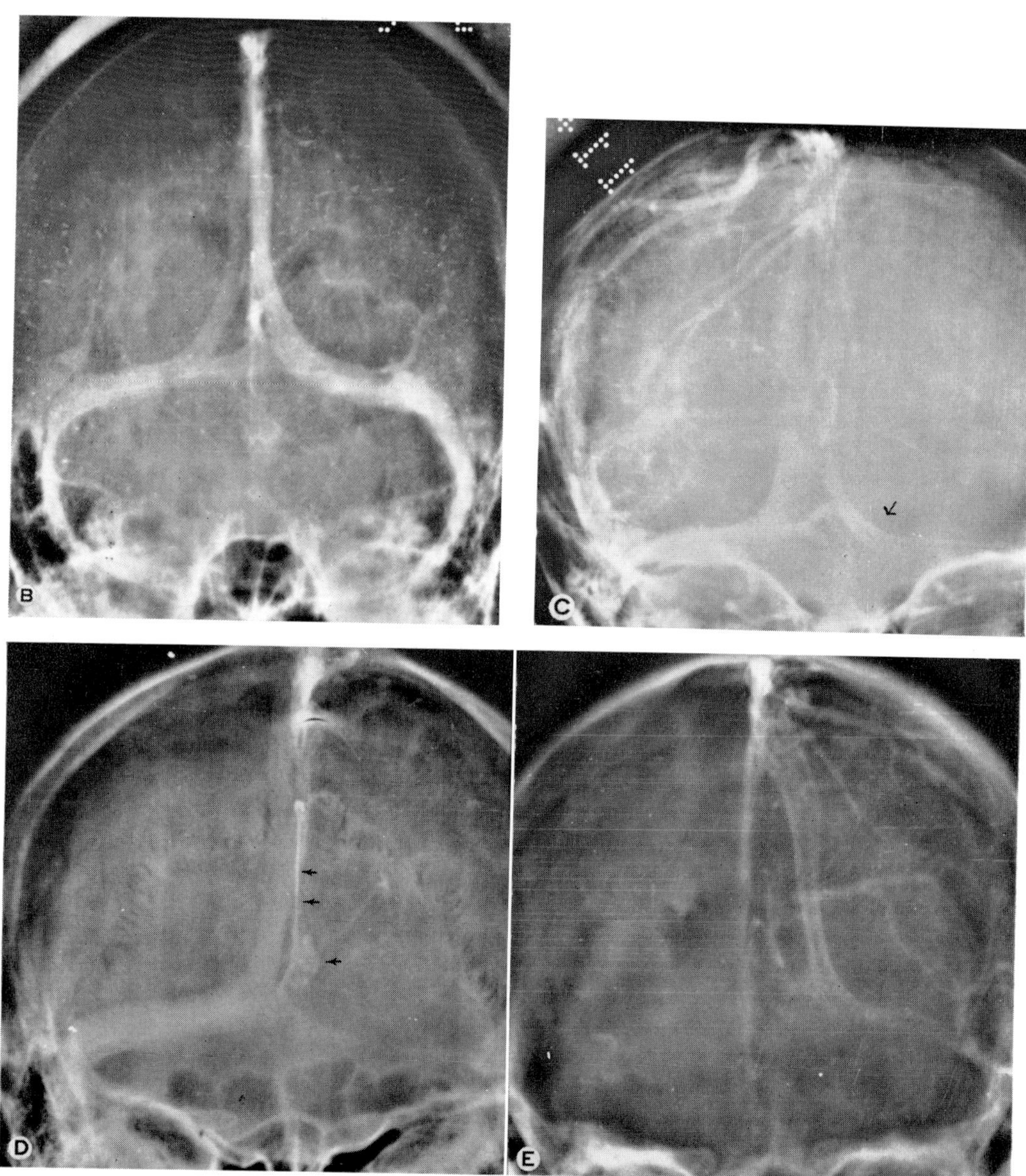

FIG. 404 (*Cont.*).—VARIATIONS OF THE SINUSES IN THE REGION OF THE TORCULAR HEROPHILI

In (B), the superior longitudinal sinus divides into two branches which are then connected by a transverse component. In (C), the right transverse sinus is much larger than the left. The left transverse sinus filled even though this was a right carotid angiogram, and it is a smaller sinus. In (D) the posterior portion of the superior longitudinal sinus is deviated to the right of the midline and all of the contrast substance drains on the right side, even though this was a left carotid angiogram. The thalamostriate vein is shown coming down to join the internal cerebral vein (*arrow*). The inferior longitudinal sinus outlines the position of the free edge of the falx (*two arrows*). (E) demonstrates an anomaly of the superior longitudinal sinus which in its posterior portion is markedly off center in position. The deviation is almost always toward the right side and rarely to the left.

(*Revised 1963*)

higher along the posterior edge of the falx, or at least it would so appear in some angiograms (fig. 403). The height of the anterior margin of the tentorium also is variable.

The *sphenoparietal* sinus which runs on the inferior aspect of the sphenoid ridge is often shown on the angiogram. Sometimes a slight area of increased density can be seen adjacent to the sella turcica; this is produced by the cavernous sinus. The *petrosal sinuses* (*superficial* and *deep*) are shown fairly frequently, particularly the deep ones. The deep petrosal sinuses are seen just behind the dorsum sella and cannot be distinguished from portions of the basilar plexus (fig. 399). The torcular Herophili is usually seen at the inferior portion of the superior longitudinal sinus where this joins the straight sinus. Its anterior aspect often presents a rounded configuration. Variations of the confluence of the sinuses are frequent (fig. 404). From this point the lateral sinuses arise and are often seen in the lateral projection as a band of increased density. The lateral sinus may be equal on both sides, but in the majority of cases the right sinus is larger, and occasionally the left lateral sinus is absent (fig. 404). The various sinuses join and form the jugular vein which is often visualized on the films in the later phases of the serialogram. The jugular vein is usually wider than the internal carotid artery.

Cerebellar Veins

The cerebellar veins are on the surface of the organ. They are divided into two groups, the superior and the inferior cerebellar veins. Some of the superior veins are near the midline, where they pass forward over the vermis to join the internal cerebral veins and the straight sinus. Others are laterally placed and end in the transverse sinus and in the superior petrosal sinus. The inferior venous group end in the transverse sinuses, in the occipital, and in the superior petrosal sinuses.

Physiology

GENERAL CONSIDERATIONS

Some of the observations that can be made regarding the physiology of cerebral circulation by angiography may not be entirely accurate for various reasons. Two factors that may cause a change in the preexisting physiologic status are: (1) a needle has been placed in the artery in the neck and this may cause local spasm, and (2) it is possible that there is a temporary increase in intra-arterial pressure at the time of the injection. The latter factor has never been adequately demonstrated. However, it is a fairly common observation that some regurgitation of the contrast substance into the basilar artery occurs, particularly in children and young adults. Bilateral filling of the anterior cerebral arteries also is common when the anterior cerebral trunk on the opposite side is not hypoplastic, and in the absence of hypotension on the opposite side. To explain this phenomenon, it is necessary to postulate that there was a temporary increase in pressure in the system that was being injected. The same is true when vertebral angiography is performed. Regurgitation proximally into the opposite vertebral artery, sometimes all the way down to its origin or near its origin, is a common observation. It would be difficult to explain this fact if one did not postulate that a temporary increase in pressure occurs.

It is, of course, one thing to produce a local increase in pressure in the major vessels and another to have this wave of increased pressure transmitted to the smaller branches over the surface of the brain. It is possible, therefore, that measurement of the intra-arterial pressure in a relatively small branch over the surface would not reflect the short peak of increased pressure which might have been produced by the injection of the artery in the neck. Another consideration is that if the patient has arterial hypertension, it is likely that a local increase in pressure over the systolic pressure due to the injection in this individual would be less significant than

(Revised 1963)

added pressure in a patient who has a relative hypotension. This is particularly true in children. Since the injection is usually made with the same force in all patients, it is easier to produce a temporary increase in pressure in children than in an adult or in a patient who has hypertension.

Two other factors that should be considered are: (1) the amount of contrast substance injected, and (2) the speed with which the injection is made. If a large amount of contrast substance is injected, a relative increase in intra-arterial pressure on the side being injected may result in reversal of flow through the circle of Willis and filling of the posterior cerebral system or of the contralateral anterior cerebral system. For this reason, physiologic observations made on injections of large amounts of contrast substance (over 8 cc.) are probably not accurate. The other factor, that of the speed with which the injection is made, is very important. In order to obtain reproducible angiograms, the injection time should be constant. We use an automatic injector and the injection time varies between 1.0 and 1.25 seconds. Eight cubic centimeters of contrast material are usually injected if the needle is at or near the origin of the internal carotid artery. If the needle is low in the common carotid or if the vessels are large and tortuous (as seen in a preliminary film made after the injection of 2 cc. of contrast substance to determine the position of the needle), a volume 2 or 4 cc. greater is injected. That is, 10 or 12 cc. may be used in these cases because some is lost in the external carotid artery.

VASCULAR PHASES

As the contrast substance is observed passing through the brain it is customary to refer to three phases in the arteriogram, as originally suggested by Moniz (1934). These are the *arterial* phase, the *intermediate*, capillary, or mixed phase, and the *venous* phase.

Arterial Phase

The arterial phase lasts approximately 1.5 seconds. It varies between 1.0 and 2.5. A circulation time greater than 2.5 seconds should be considered abnormal if one can eliminate a technical artifact, such as poor positioning of the needle or a prolonged injection time. The arterial phase, of course, cannot be shorter than the injection time. Therefore, one cannot speak about prolonged arterial phase unless the injection time is controlled. Actually, as the arterial phase is observed on the serialogram, one can see first the proximal arteries filling; as the serial proceeds, the distal arteries become well filled while the carotid siphon and proximal anterior and middle cerebral arteries begin to empty and then the emptying proceeds gradually toward the periphery. Actually, therefore, there are *arterial filling* and *arterial emptying* phases. It is important to observe in the serialogram the arterial filling phase because this is very often a clue to the presence of a neoplasm as well as of arterial occlusion. The arterial emptying phase is important in cases of multiple small emboli, and when there has been damage to the perforating vessels which arise from the larger arterial branches and give the brain its blood supply. (For greater detail, see the section on cerebral thrombosis.)

The average arterial circulation time is 1.5 seconds. An arterial circulation time longer than 2.5 seconds is usually considered abnormal. The arterial circulation time is much faster in the internal carotid artery system than in the external carotid system. In fact, the arterial circulation time is nearly twice as fast in the internal as in the external carotid artery in the average case. For this reason it is possible to inject the common carotid artery and in almost every instance, in the normal case, there is no interference with visualization of the intracranial vessels. This relationship may change under certain conditions, such as the presence of increased intracranial pressure and vascular thrombosis. (See below.)

Intermediate Phase

The *intermediate or mixed phase* (so-called capillary phase) is not very well defined. It

(Revised 1963)

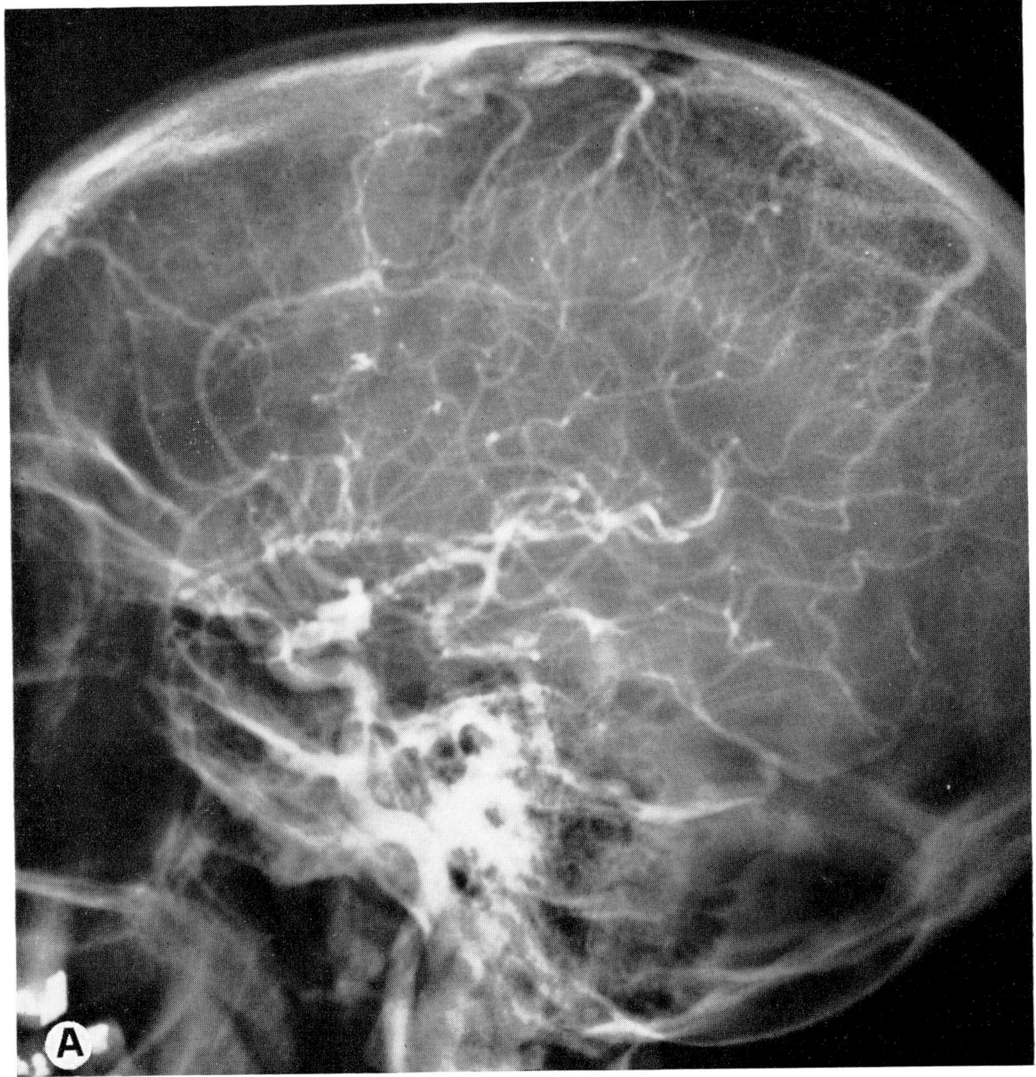

FIG. 405.—(A) MIXTURE OF PHASES IN A NORMAL CEREBRAL ANGIOGRAM DUE TO PROLONGED INJECTION TIME

The internal carotid artery as well as the branches of the anterior and middle cerebral artery are filled at the same time that the cerebral veins are also shown. Such an angiogram might occasionally bring out details that may not be seen otherwise. However, it will obscure the anatomical details of the vessels, and for that reason it is undesirable. Serial filming is much more satisfactory.

corresponds to the period of time when the terminal branches of the arteries are seen and perhaps nothing else aside from very faint visualization of the origin of some of the frontal veins. Occasionally, a true capillary phase exists in that no arteries and no veins are visible. This phase lasts between 0.5 and 1.0 second, but is quite variable. In many normal cases, it is so poorly defined that the terminal branches of the arteries are seen followed immediately by the filling of the veins without any intermediate stage.

Venous Phase

The *venous phase* begins when the first branches of the superficial cerebral veins are

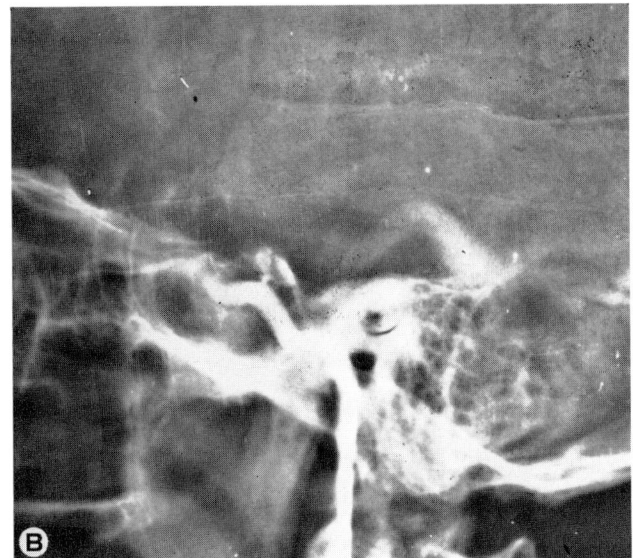

FIG. 405 (*Cont.*).—(B) ANGIOGRAM IN PATIENT DURING ACUTE STAGE OF TRAUMA SHOWING ARREST OF CONTRAST SUBSTANCE AT CAROTID SIPHON

This film was made 13 seconds after injection, and the needle was in good position within the lumen of the artery. The arrest was presumed to be due to extremely high intracranial pressure. The patient died several hours later.

visualized and lasts possibly 4 or 5 seconds. Of course, the venous phase actually continues until all of the contrast material is out of the veins, which is a variable length of time. It is somewhat dependent on the speed of the injection and on the amount of the contrast material injected. In fact, it may be difficult to determine when all of the veins are completely empty. The so-called venous circulation time is of little importance clinically.

The frontal veins usually fill just before the parietal veins. This probably is related to the distance that the contrast substance has to travel in the arteries; that is, the arteries supplying the frontal lobe are a little shorter and, therefore, the contrast substance reaches the capillary stage and the veins a little sooner than in the parietal and occipital regions. The same is true of the arterial filling phase where the frontal arteries may be completely filled whereas the parietal arteries are not. If the parietal veins fill before the frontal veins, an abnormal condition may exist; this could indicate either that there is a slowing of circulation in the frontal region, or there is an increase in the speed of circulation in the parietal region. The former may be seen in neoplasms or in thrombosis. The latter may be seen in certain neoplasms, in arteriovenous malformations, and very rarely in thrombosis where collateral flow becomes established.

It is usually noted that the deep cerebral veins fill later than the superficial cerebral veins. Occasionally, the deep cerebral veins fill at the same time as the superficial ones, but whenever this is noted, one should consider the possibility of an abnormal increase in the speed of circulation through the deep veins. Likewise, the deep cerebral veins remain filled to a greater extent in the later stages of the venous phase than do the superficial cerebral veins. The late films in the serialograms are usually the best for study of the deep veins without overlying surface veins.

LAMINAR FLOW

The current of blood through a vessel is faster in the center of the vessel than it is in the periphery near the walls. Where two arteries come together carrying blood, such as the two vertebral arteries forming the basilar artery, the current of blood opacified with contrast substance can be followed usually along the same side of the vessel, and nonopacified blood will continue on the other side for variable distances. Sometimes one can see a change of the opacified flow from one wall to the other, but still remaining separated from the current of non-opacified blood coming from the other vertebral artery. This is a very important phenomenon because there is a tendency to call abnormal a basilar artery which appears narrow (fig. 406). This narrowing may be simply a manifestation of incomplete filling. A basilar artery cannot be considered as completely filled unless sufficient regurgitation into the opposite vertebral artery for

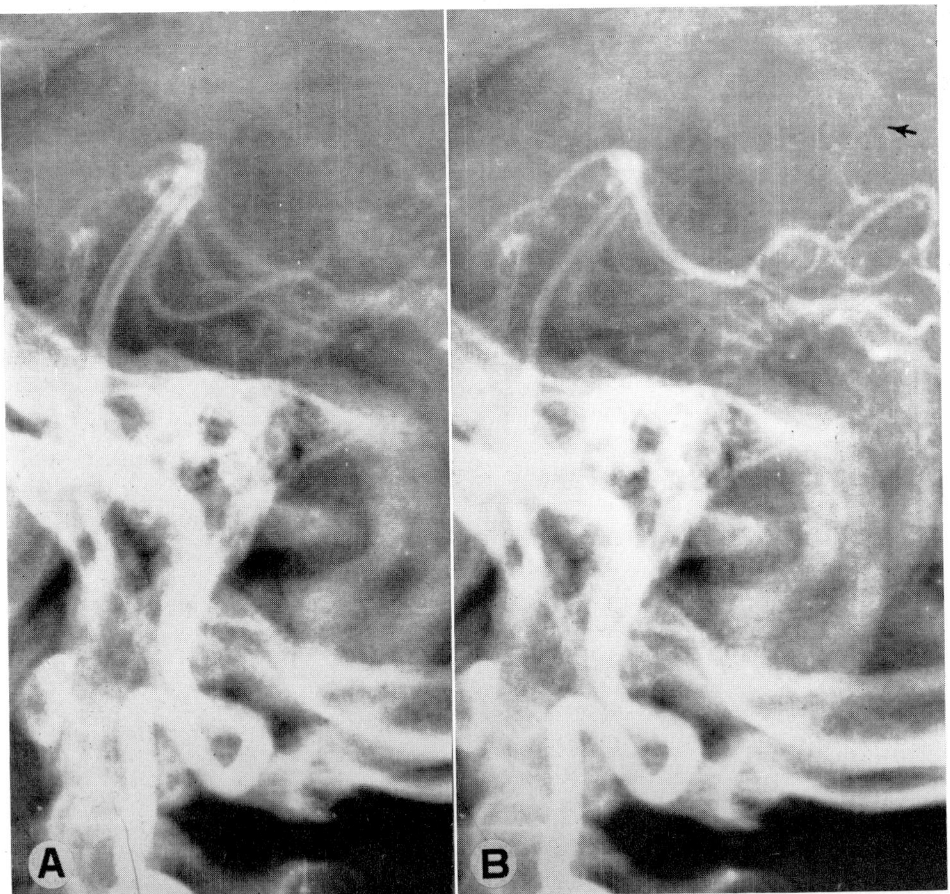

Fig. 406.—Laminar Flow in the Vertebrobasilar System and in the Arteries of the Neck

The films shown in (A) demonstrate a double column of contrast substance in the basilar artery with a radiolucent center. This may be due to spiraling of the contrast substance as it ascends unmixed with blood from the other vertebral artery. The film in (B) was taken 0.5 second later, and it already shows that the basilar artery is very thin. Had we not had the film in (A), a diagnosis of narrowing of the basilar artery might have been entertained. The medial posterior chorioidal artery is extremely well shown in (B) (*arrows*).

(Revised 1963)

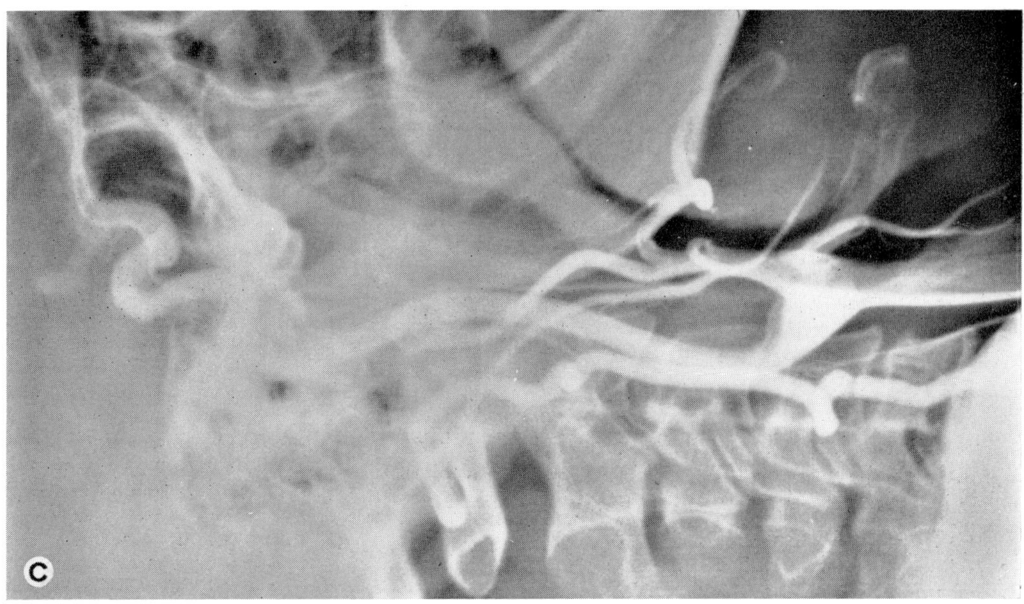

FIG. 406 C

The brachial angiogram (C) in another patient shows how the contrast substance ascends on the posterior, the most dependent, side of the vessel up to the common carotid bifurcation. At this point, turbulence causes the contrast substance to mix with the nonopacified blood. However, still a thin radiolucent line against the anterior wall of the vessel can be followed up for a certain distance in the internal carotid artery. It is also to be noted that the anterior branches of the external carotid artery are not nearly as well opacified as the posterior branches of this same vessel.

mixing is obtained during the injection. In this case, contrast substance is washed up toward the basilar artery from both sides, and filling should be complete.

It is common to observe that when the internal carotid artery is injected, the contrast substance is washed along by the bloodstream in the entire artery except toward the most dependent wall. That is, the contrast substance, being heavier than the blood, tends to remain for a longer period of time along the most dependent side of the artery (fig. 406). The slower the flow of blood is, the greater the chance of having the heavier contrast substance lag along one wall of the vessel. A similar phenomenon also is observed frequently in the veins. It is not uncommon to see that the posterior sides of the veins, as the patient lies in the supine position, are denser than the rostral sides of the veins.

Something to consider in studying angiograms is that it is possible for one of two branches to opacify less well than the other following bifurcation of an artery. Observations in the frog mesentery reported by Kniseley and co-authors (1960) indicate that at the point of bifurcation of a vessel the blood cells may continue together in one branch and only plasma may continue in the other. It is also possible that contrast substance may fill better, with the help of gravity, the more dependent of two branches of a cerebral artery (fig. 406). With increases in the speed of flow, increased turbulence is produced at the point of bifurcation, and this condition tends to mix the radiopaque substance with the nonopacified blood. However, if flow is relatively slow, the chances of occurrence of the above described phenomenon are enhanced.

The actual calibre of the arteries as seen in the angiographic pictures may be greater when the injection is made in the internal carotid artery than when it is made in the common carotid artery. This is probably a manifestation of a more complete filling when the injection is made directly into the internal carotid. Owing to the flow tending to be in the center of the vessel, if the vessel is not completely and rapidly filled with contrast substance, the periphery of the vessel never becomes completely opacified; therefore, it appears narrower in the angiogram. Additional factors may influence the progress of contrast substance in the smaller vessels. In making physiological observations on arteriograms, it is, therefore, of the utmost importance to consider the factors of laminar flow, injection time, the position of the needle, and the amount of contrast substance injected. Other factors, which cannot be controlled, are arteriosclerosis, speed of blood flow in a given patient, the presence of anomalies in the circle of Willis, status of intracranial pressure, systemic blood pressure, and arterial spasm.

FACTORS INFLUENCING CIRCULATION TIME

Increased Circulation Time

The arterial circulation time is frequently increased in the presence of increased intracranial pressure. Generalized increased intracranial pressure may produce a generalized increase in the arterial circulation time. Lengthening of the arterial end arteriovenous circulation time is found in about half the cases of intracranial hypotension.

The presence of a neoplasm or another type of space-occupying mass, such as an abscess, may produce a *local slowing of the circulation time*. The arteries in the region of the mass may fill slower than elsewhere and the veins then would also fill more slowly. Local slowing of the arterial circulation time as well as slower filling of the veins are more commonly observed angiographically in tumors situated in the frontal and parietal regions, regardless of whether the tumor mass is intracerebral or extracerebral in location (Leeds and Taveras, 1963).

Arterial thrombosis is a frequent cause of slow circulation time locally in the region of the thrombosed vessel. Whether slowing of the circulation time is also seen in the prethrombotic stage associated with severe arteriosclerosis, cannot be stated at the moment. There is no significant difference in cerebral blood flow in older patients up to the sixth decade as compared with younger adults in the absence of arteriosclerosis (Nylin, 1961). In later ages there is a reduction in cerebral blood flow, but this is felt to be due to arteriosclerosis and not to aging per se (Sokoloff, 1961).

It has been reported that a marked increase in intracranial pressure may actually prevent the contrast substance injected into the internal carotid artery from proceeding beyond the intracavernous portion of the artery. This has been observed several times by other individuals (Pribram, 1961, Horwitz and Dunsmore, 1956). The authors have seen this phenomenon a number of times; it may be associated with trauma or with intraventricular bleeding. It is possible that the taking of routine serial films in every case would show that the contrast substance eventually gets into the cerebral vessels, whereas if only a few films are taken, there would be insufficient time for the contrast substance to enter the cranial cavity. In one instance the ventricles were tapped and the injection repeated and on the second injection following the tap, the contrast substance entered the intracranial portion of the vessels promptly (Pribram, 1961). This would tend to confirm the belief that the intracranial pressure had some influence in the lack of filling of the intracranial vessels. It should be mentioned in regard to this type of case that all of these patients have died, and the possible existence of some type of pre-agonal condition leading to spasm of the vessels should be considered (fig. 405).

It is hard to conceive of the intracranial pressure being higher than the blood pressure for a period of time; presumably, irreversible chemical changes that eventually lead to death could produce a degree of generalized cerebral edema resulting in an intracranial pressure actually higher than the systolic blood pressure. We have had occasion to see at least one patient in whom an arteriogram was performed while the patient was moribund. The serialogram simply showed stasis within the arteries so that throughout the serialogram, which covered a period of approximately 6 to 7 seconds, no filling of the veins was observed, the arteries being filled even on the last film. It is obvious that at such a stage there had been great slowing of circulation in the brain, possibly as a result of sludge formation in the capillaries. In a recent case, an extreme slowing of the circulation was noted. The patient had had an acute episode suggesting subarachnoid hemorrhage. The injection was repeated, and this time the first film was taken at 6 seconds after the injection. A serial study was continued for 15 additional seconds and the last film still showed distal arteries filled. There were also a few superficial veins poorly outlined; the deep veins were never seen. This patient died several hours later and was found to have intraventricular bleeding, a large clot in the region of the incisura and under the temporal lobe. It is felt that sludge formation in this patient prevented normal flow by blocking the capillaries. The first films made at 6, 7, and 8 seconds showed only filling of the cervical portion of the internal carotid artery to the siphon. Had we not taken any more films we would have concluded, with Pribram, that marked increased pressure prevented entrance of contrast substance intracranially.

A block at the level of the capillaries has been observed under two other circumstances at the Neurological Institute. The first case was a patient in whom the arteriogram showed only an extremely prolonged arterial phase, and in 7 seconds the arteries were still fully filled, although some contrast substance had passed beyond the arteries into the capillaries. Autopsy demonstrated the presence of numerous microscopic tumor emboli from a carcinoma of the lung. The second instance was in a patient who had an arteriogram with the use of Thorotrast, in which the colloidal suspension precipitated and produced a generalized blockage of the capillaries. The films made throughout the serialogram up to 9 seconds did not show passage of the contrast substance beyond the distal arterial branches. Autopsy showed obstruction of arterioles and capillaries by Thorotrast emboli. This type of complication from injection of Thorotrast was reported by Northfield and Russel (1937). Another possible cause is sludge formation just discussed above. One of the authors has examined several patients in whom Thorotrast was used for angiography and who died at a later time because of brain tumor. Traces of Thorotrast were found along the walls of small cerebral vessels as long as three weeks after angiography. As far as could be determined, the patients' clinical course was not altered by these occurrences. (Further details on changes in circulation time in cerebral thrombosis are given in the section on vascular thrombosis.)

A *prolonged injection time* may cause an increase in the arterial circulation time but will not cause an increase in the intermediate and arteriovenous circulation time. Because arteries and veins are seen on the same films, it is possible to tell that this is an artifact produced by a prolonged injection time (fig. 405A).

Decreased Circulation Time

An increase in the speed of circulation may be caused by tumors that shunt the blood such as glioblastoma multiforme, metastatic carcinoma, and a few other neoplasms. Also, it may be produced by an arteriovenous malformation or arteriovenous fistula, such as in the cavernous sinus. Inhalation of 5 to 8 per cent carbon dioxide decreases circulation time. (For further details see under "Diagnosis of Intracranial Masses by Abnormal Circulation." Also see under "Arteriovenous Lesions.")

Arteriovenous Circulation Time

Greitz (1956) has proposed the following method of measuring the circulation time. The progress of the contrast material in the serialogram is studied and the film selected, which shows the greatest beginning concentration in the carotid siphon. The error here in picking the right film is probably no more than 0.25 second. Then the maximum concentration of the contrast material in the parietal veins is determined. This, again, is not too difficult to detect in a serialogram.

(Revised 1963)

The first film that shows a *decrease* in the contrast substance in the parietal veins as compared with the previous one indicates that the maximum concentration has been passed. The time that it takes from *maximum concentration of the contrast substance in the carotid siphon to maximum concentration of the contrast substance in the parietal veins is called the circulation time.* We would propose the name *arteriovenous circulation time* when this method is used to differentiate it from the circulation time as measured in the arteries, in the intermediate phase, and in the veins, as described above. The mean arteriovenous circulation time is 4.13 seconds according to Greitz, with a standard deviation of plus or minus 0.74 second. If greater than 6.0 seconds, the arteriovenous circulation time is considered to be definitely prolonged.

In a group of normal children the average *arteriovenous circulation time* was 3.3 seconds; that is, slightly shorter than in adults (Taveras and Poser, 1959).

Diagnosis of Brain Tumors

The word tumor as applied here indicates a localized space-occupying mass, be it a neoplasm, a hematoma, an abscess, or an area of localized cerebral edema. Just which one of these conditions is to be suggested on the basis of the angiographic findings depends on the clinical history in the individual case as well as on observations made from the angiogram. The importance of a careful evaluation of the history before offering a final opinion based on the angiographic findings cannot be overemphasized.

General Manifestations of Intracranial Tumor

The general or nonspecific signs of intracranial tumors are: cerebral herniations, including shift of the midline structures, stretching or straightening of the cerebral arteries, and changes in the circulation time.

Cerebral Herniations

The most commonly observed herniation is a displacement of the cerebral structures across the midline, the subfalcial herniation or so-called *midline shift.* Cerebral dislocation under the falx can be very minimum or it can be extremely marked with complete herniation of the cingulate gyrus and even of a greater portion of the medial aspect of the hemisphere.

Transtentorial herniations, most commonly consisting of a hernia of the hippocampal gyrus through the incisura of the tentorium, are very frequently found at autopsy; they are often a prime cause of death owing to compression of, and hemorrhage into, the upper portion of the brain stem. The hemorrhage may be venous or arterial or both. According to Johnson and Yates, arterial bleeding may be seen in the more acute cases; it is due to sudden elongation of the arteries with rupture of the vessels as a result of lateral flattening of the midbrain with consequent increase in anteroposterior diameter.

The hernia may be anterior involving only the uncus and anterior portion of the hippocampus, or it may be posterior (fig. 407). Anterior and posterior herniations may combine to form a complete downward herniation (Azambuja *et al.*, 1956). The herniation may sometimes be bilateral but usually is only on the side of the mass lesion (fig. 198).

The presence of transtentorial herniations does not necessarily indicate a fatal outcome. On the contrary, the majority of patients recover, following simple surgical removal of the causative factor or simple decompression. Sometimes removal of the herniated portion of brain or sectioning of the tentorial edge may have to be performed.

Lateral displacement of the upper brain stem (midbrain) is often present in association with a midline cerebral dislocation, especially in connection with masses involving the lower portions of the hemisphere, the deep tumors, temporal lobe masses, and subdural hematomas. When a marked

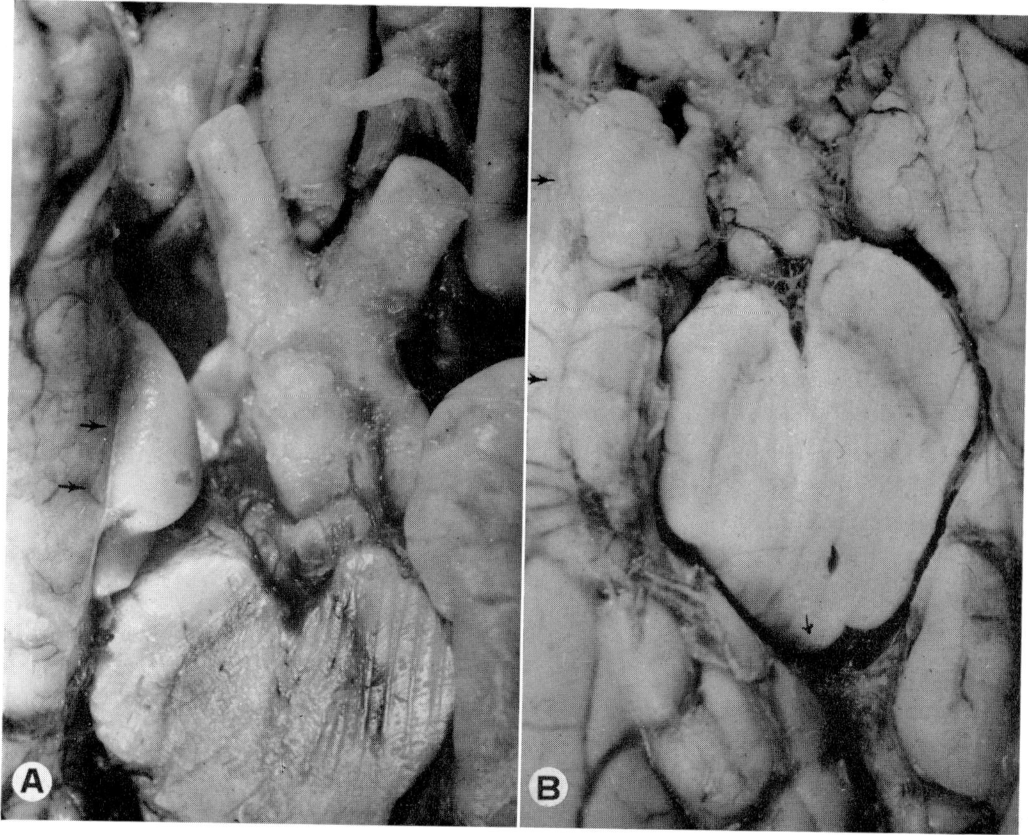

Fig. 407.—Hippocampal Herniations

In (A) there is an anterior hippocampal herniation which is, however, not producing any compression of the brain stem. There is no deformity of the peduncles on the side of the herniation as compared to the opposite side. In (B) there is a larger anterior herniation and there is involvement also more posterior than the uncus (*arrows*). There is deformity and flattening of the corresponding cerebral peduncle and asymmetry of the quadrigeminal tubercules; the tubercle on the side of the herniation is more posterior than the one on the other side. (Courtesy of Dr. Abner Wolf.) A severe posterior herniation is shown in Fig. 198.

lateral displacement of the midbrain exists, this structure may be compressed against the side of the tentorium opposite the tumor, thus producing ipsilateral neurologic signs. Any case in which a marked midline shift is present is a candidate for transtentorial herniation of the hippocampus. These cases should, therefore, be handled with great care to prevent a potential or a small hernia from becoming a large one.

Other cerebral hernias that may be encountered are: (1) a hernia of the gyrus rectus behind the tuberculum sella, (2) the base of the frontal lobe behind the sphenoid ridge, (3) the anterior temporal lobe over the sphenoid ridge, and (4) central incisural herniations.

Upward herniations of the contents of the posterior fossa, usually the cerebellum, through the tentorial incisura may occur in connection with masses involving the posterior fossa. They usually occur behind the quadrigeminal plate, in which case the brain stem is displaced forward against the clivus. Herniation may be posterolateral in location, on one or both sides.

Foramen magnum herniations involve the cerebellar tonsils. They occur more frequently in the presence of posterior fossa tumors, particularly those involving the cerebellum, but may also occur with supratentorial masses and in cases of pseudotumor cerebri. In severe downward herniations through the foramen magnum, the cerebellar tonsils as well as the adjacent portions of the biventral lobules of the cerebellum protrude through the foramen magnum. Death may be caused by cerebellar tonsilar herniation when it is severe enough to produce compression of the medulla. In the great majority of cases, however, this is not a fatal herniation.

Radiologic Manifestations

Subfalcial Herniations

The main structures that evidence such herniations in the angiogram are: (1) the anterior cerebral artery and its branches, and (2) the internal cerebral vein and the vein of Galen.

Because the anterior cerebral artery and its branches are situated more forward, their position may be changed readily by rotation of the head at the time that the frontal film is made. On the other hand, the internal cerebral vein is not changed appreciably in position by rotation of the head because it is situated approximately in the center of the skull. In every case, both the venous and the arterial clues should be looked for not only because one checks the other, but also because it is possible to determine that a tumor is more posteriorly or more anteriorly situated by the degree of displacement of the artery as compared with the vein. Deep tumors, for instance, will produce a greater displacement of the vein and little or no displacement of the anterior cerebral artery and its branches. It is for this reason that it is important to obtain biplane serialograms to record the venous phase in the frontal as well as in the lateral projection.

In order to understand the mechanism of shift of the anterior cerebral artery and its branches as seen in the frontal angiogram, it is necessary to recall the relationship of the pericallosal, the frontopolar, and the callosomarginal arteries and their subdivisions with the edge of the falx. A glance at Figure 408 suffices to clarify the fact that the falx is thinner in the frontal region and gets progressively wider in its vertical diameter as it extends backward. It becomes quite thick in the parieto-occipital region where it joins the tentorium. Brain herniation across the midline occurs easily anteriorly, but cannot occur posteriorly because the falx is too thick and finally joins the tentorium. The brain can herniate under the falx, but the falx is such a rigid structure that it cannot itself be displaced proportionately to the opposite side by the forces generated. Therefore, the vessels dislocate beneath the falx but return toward the midline as they reach the edge of the falx. Therefore, the pericallosal artery, which is situated almost entirely under the edge of the falx, may be displaced throughout its entire extent except for its terminal branch. The frontopolar artery as it passes forward first is displaced and then returns to the midline as it reaches the edge of the falx in its forward course to the frontal pole. The callosomarginal artery, depending upon its configuration is displaced in its more proximal portion, and in its more distal portions it returns to the midline. The same applies to branches of the callosomarginal artery. For this reason, a "step" is often visualized where an artery suddenly changes direction to reach the midline. The presence of a "square step" is almost always an indication of a true shift and not produced by either rotation of the head at the time that the film was made or by excessive tortuosity of the vessels.

The shift of the anterior cerebral vessels may involve the proximal portion, the central portion, or the distal portion. It may also involve the entire course of the vessels. It may be worthwhile mentioning again at this time a statement made under "Anatomy" in the description of the anterior cerebral artery: "anterior is down, posterior is up." That is, in the frontal angiogram an anterior shift is one in which the inferior or proximal portion of the anterior cerebral vessels is displaced. In a posterior shift, the upper or distal portion of the anterior cerebral vessels is displaced. The way in which

(Revised 1963)

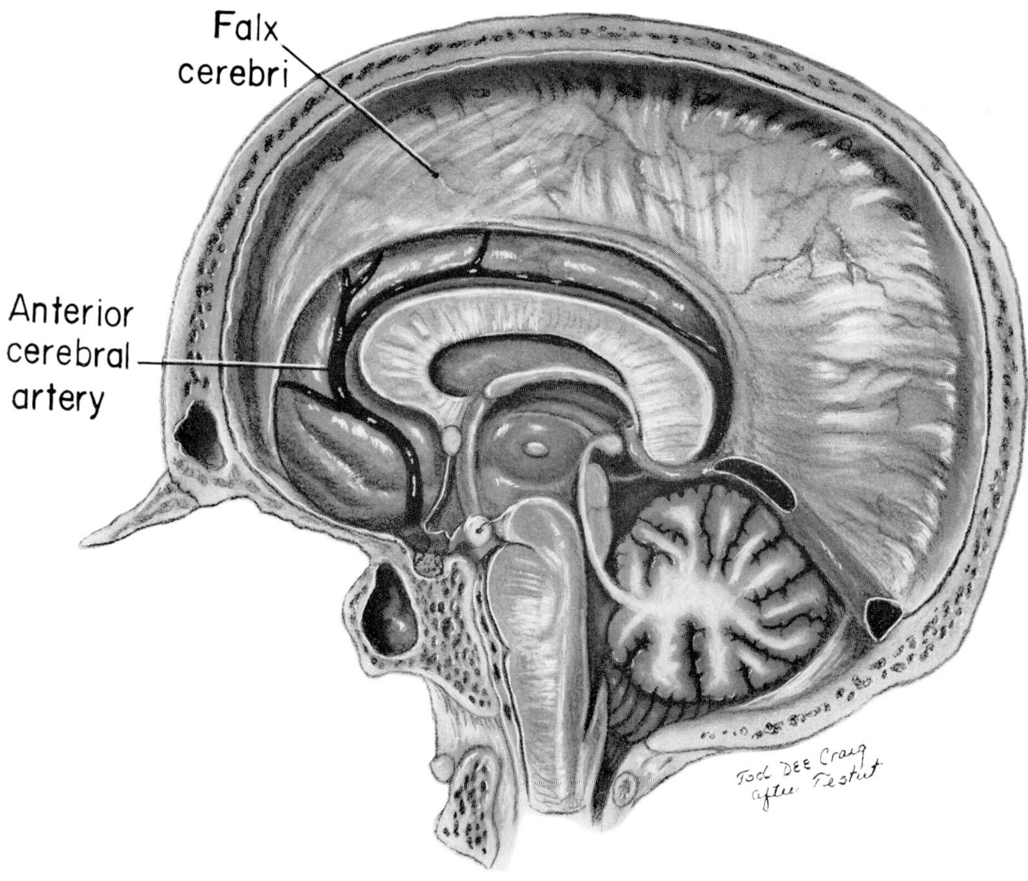

FIG. 408.—DIAGRAM OF LONGITUDINAL SECTION OF SKULL AND BRAIN

The falx is much thinner on its anterior aspect and becomes thicker as it goes posteriorly to join the tentorium. The anterior cerebral artery gives off branches which, as they extend peripherally, go beyond the edge of the falx. Therefore, when these arteries are displaced, they must return to the midline as they reach the falx edge.

the artery is shifted is quite important and very often permits us to locate the tumor in a general manner, even before looking at the lateral view. Shift of the anterior cerebral vessels may be divided into several categories.

Rounded shift. The anterior cerebral artery and its branches form an arc as they are displaced across the midline. This is typical of frontal tumors. It indicates that the center of the tumor is probably at or near the level of origin of the pericallosal artery in its anterior portion (fig. 409). Therefore, it displaces the pericallosal artery as well as the origins of the frontopolar and the callosomarginal arteries.

(Revised 1963)

Square shift. In this type of shift there is a very well defined step beneath the falx. As the anterior cerebral artery is followed proximally, it is seen to descend straight downward forming a fairly square angle at the lower portion of the artery. This type of shift indicates that the tumor is situated behind the anterior portion of the pericallosal artery (fig. 410).

Proximal shift. The inferior portion of the anterior cerebral artery is displaced across the midline and then the artery ascends obliquely to reach the midline as it ascends without forming a step under the falx. This usually indicates that the tumor is inferiorly located. It is often seen in tem-

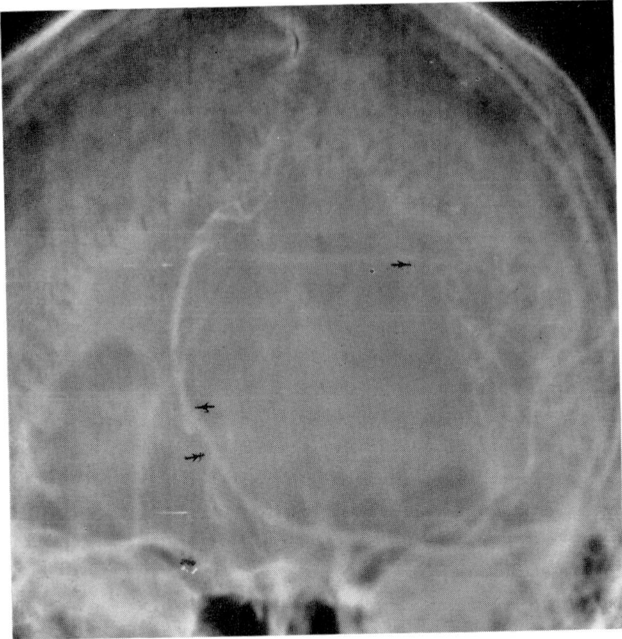

FIG. 409.—ROUND SHIFT PRODUCED BY AN ANTERIOR FRONTAL LOBE TUMOR

The rounded configuration indicates that the tumor is situated in the anterior half or two-thirds of the frontal lobe. The origin of the frontopolar and of the callosomarginal arteries (*arrows*) are displaced to the same extent as the pericallosal artery. The Sylvian point (*upper arrow*) is in normal position.

poral lobe tumors or in lesions situated subfrontally or in the inferior frontal region, but not large enough to produce a rounded shift (figs. 445 and 448).

Distal shift. In these cases there is a well defined step under the falx where the vessels are displaced across the midline, but the anterior cerebral artery is situated in the midline in its inferior portion. Thus, the vessel is oblique in a direction opposite to that seen with proximal shift. This is typical of tumors situated in the superior convexity of the hemisphere or in the parasagittal region (figs. 436 and 437).

The so-called *frontopolar sign*, as described by Fischer (1938), is produced when the anterior cerebral artery is shifted and the frontopolar artery is also displaced in its proximal portion. As the distal portion of the frontopolar artery reaches the falx anteriorly, it returns to the midline. Upon doing this it appears to pull the pericallosal artery slightly toward the midline, thus producing a checkrein effect. The frontopolar sign indicates that the tumor is behind the level of the knee of the pericallosal artery. The sign is observed infrequently, and in standard anteroposterior views the check-rein effect is not produced by the frontopolar but by the callosomarginal artery (fig. 411).

In order to evaluate the significance of arterial shift, the observer should first glance at the other vessels and try to appreciate the general tortuosity of the anterior cerebral artery and its branches. The shift of these vessels should be estimated in the proximal and in the distal portions of the artery. The central portion, the knee of the pericallosal artery, often presents an additional bulge to the opposite side or to the same side, which is normal (fig. 412). In fact, in some instances where there is a definite shift to the opposite side, the central portion or knee of the pericallosal artery returns to the midline (fig. 412). The reason for this is not clear to us, but it is possible that the larger frontal horn on the side opposite the tumor tends to bulge a little toward the midline and, thus, pushes the vessel. However, this explanation does not fit all cases. Another possible mechanism is that the artery reaches the edge of the falx in its forward curve and thus returns to the midline in that region; still another explanation is that the artery

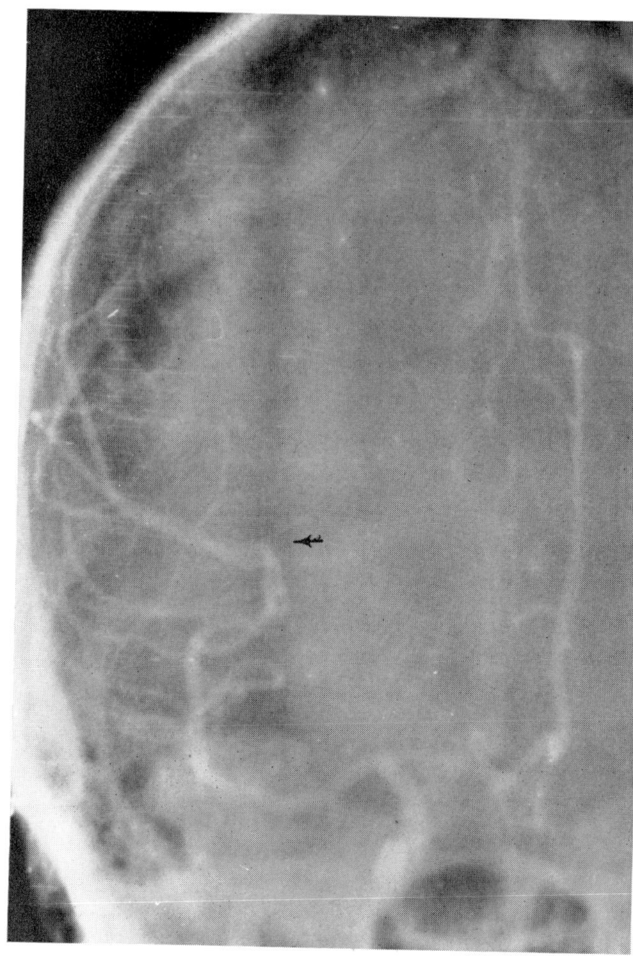

Fig. 410.—Example of a Square Shift Produced by a Posteriorly Placed Tumor

The presence of a square shift indicates that the tumor is situated behind the anterior two-thirds of the frontal lobe. The proximal as well as the distal portions of the anterior cerebral artery, usually the pericallosal artery, are equally displaced. The angiographic Sylvian point (*arrow*) is markedly displaced downward, indicating that the tumor is posteriorly placed. Compare the Sylvian point with that of Fig. 409.

may be contained within a sulcus on the side of the tumor during part of its course.

A measured shift of the anterior cerebral artery of 3 mm. or more might be considered significant, but a conclusion should be reached with care because of the normal wavy tortuosity of the vessels. If the head is rotated toward the side opposite the injection, the anterior cerebral artery and its branches acquire a slightly rounded shape without the formation of a step at the edge of the falx. Rotation to the same side as the injection would produce a curve in the opposite direction to that just described. It is possible to estimate the degree of displacement due to rotation of the head by using the distance from the temporal bone, as shown in the anteroposterior film, and the zygomatic process of the frontal bone, and comparing this distance on both sides. The orbital process of the frontal bone is not too far removed from the knee of the anterior cerebral artery. Since this bony process is almost always visible in the angiogram, it serves as a good landmark for deciding whether the vessel is shifted or rotated. By this it is meant that if the orbital process is turned, so is the knee of the anterior cerebral artery, and to about the same extent. (See Figure 413 for further explanation.) The malar bone and the ascending ramus of the mandible may also be used to evaluate head rotation in films that include the facial bones. By comparing the measurement

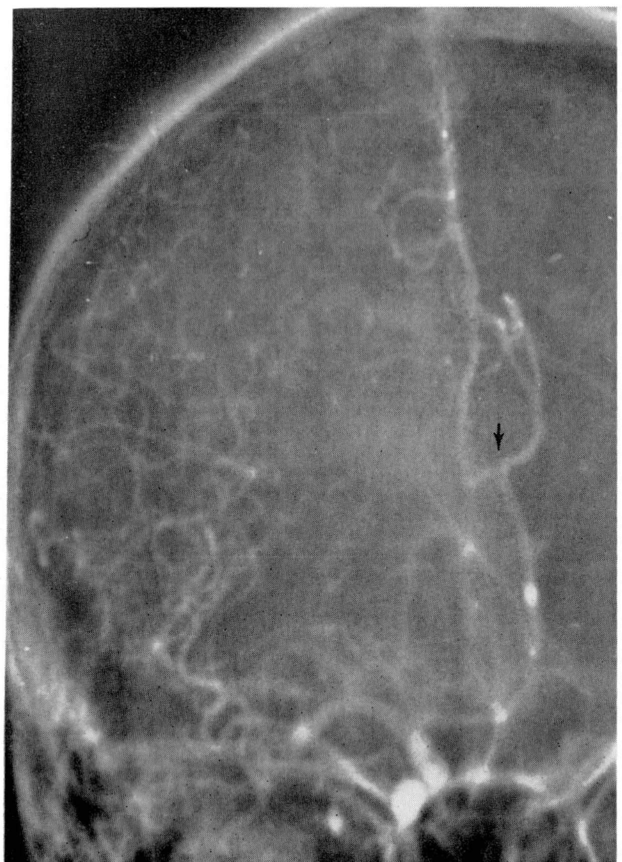

Fig. 411.—Shift of the Anterior Cerebral Artery with "Checkrein" Effect (Frontopolar Sign)

This patient had a large retro-Sylvian mass and the anterior cerebral vessels are shifted, but there is a pull at the origin of the callosomarginal artery (the frontopolar artery is lower) which has been mentioned in the text as the "frontopolar sign."

between the most lateral point of the malar bone and the mandible ramus on the right side with that on the left side, one can easily determine the degree of rotation. By dividing the difference between the two measurements in half, it is possible to predict the deviation of the anterior cerebral vessels from the midline (fig. 413). This measurement is especially useful in half axial projection or a modification of this view.

Study of the *midline veins* also is important in the evaluation of shift. As mentioned previously, the internal cerebral vein is approximately in the center of the head and therefore may be shifted in a manner similar to the pineal calcification. Its displacement is not affected by rotation nearly as much as the anterior cerebral vessels (fig. 414). The point that should be selected to obtain a measurement of the position of the internal cerebral vein is the center of this vein, which is also the highest point of the vein. The internal cerebral vein should not be confused with the vein of Galen. The posterior portion of the vein of Galen, which is the highest point of this vein, is fixed in position as it joins the straight sinus and therefore cannot shift from the midline. The internal cerebral vein can be recognized by tracing the thalamostriate vein to the anterior portion of the internal cerebral vein and then going up to the highest point of this vein. In most instances, if there is no rotation of the head, the vein appears as a vertical dash (figs. 396 and 403). When there is rotation of the head or if there is displacement from the midline (figs. 414 and 415), the vein will be partly uncoiled.

Generally, altered position of the internal cerebral vein is a more reliable sign of shift than a similar change of the anterior cerebral

(Revised 1963)

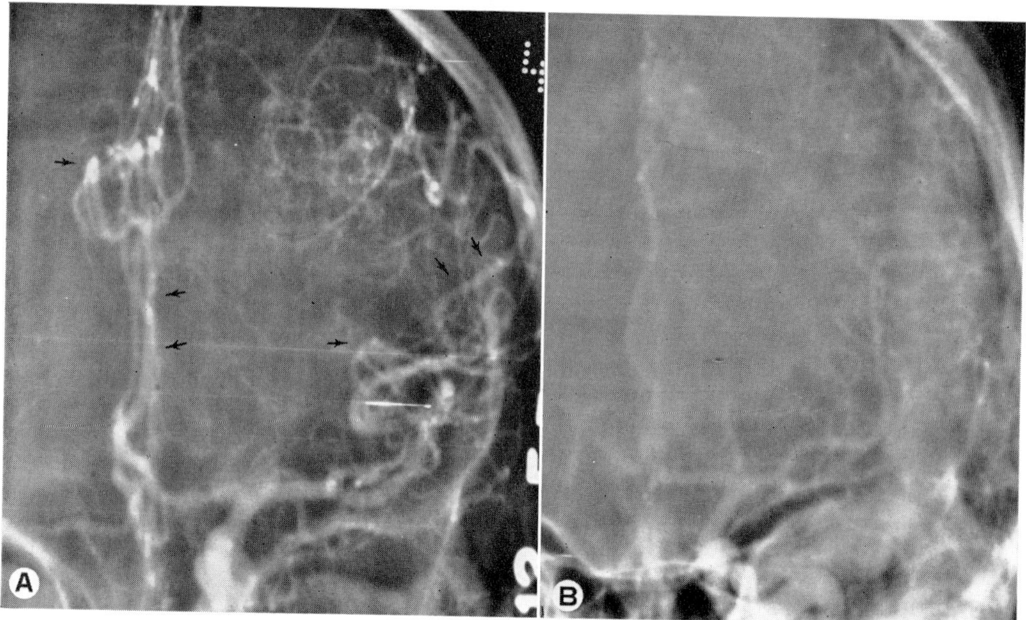

Fig. 412.—(A) High Convexity Meningioma Producing a Distal Shift and Herniation of the Cingulate Gyrus

Although the distal portion of the anterior cerebral vessels are markedly displaced across the midline, the central portion of the anterior cerebral artery returns almost to the midline (*arrows*), but the proximal portion is again shifted across the midline. This may be due to greater dilatation of the contralateral frontal horn, or the vessels may be within a sulcus instead of on the gyrus, and therefore they would not be displaced as far across the midline. There is marked downward displacement of the angiographic Sylvian point with the last emerging vessel extending upward and lateralward. This is because the center of the neoplasm is higher up in the convexity, and although it is a meningioma, the sloping skull surface brings the center of the tumor more medially.

(B) Normal Carotid Angiogram Showing Apparent Displacement of the Knee of the Pericallosal Artery across the Midline. This condition is often seen in normal patients, particularly when there is tortuosity. It is probably due to the artery going into the callosal sulcus for a short distance.

vessels, in the questionable cases. This is true because of the central position of these veins and because there is no tortuosity of these veins such as is present in the anterior cerebral artery. Therefore, this vein should always be measured very accurately. It is our custom to measure from the outer table to the medial side of the vein and from this point to the outer table of the opposite side of the skull (fig. 414B). Inasmuch as the internal cerebral vein is a paired midline structure, the midline is usually between the two veins and thus the measurements should be to the venous margin opposite to that side of the head which was injected.

If the internal cerebral vein is shifted and the anterior cerebral artery is not, it usually indicates that the tumor is deeply situated in the posterior frontal region or in the thalamic region. If the internal cerebral vein is displaced more than the anterior cerebral vessels, the mass is probably posteriorly situated, and vice versa.

Complete herniation of the cingulate gyrus can be suspected on the angiograms from the appearance of the callosomarginal branches. The vessels are displaced to the opposite side and after reaching a certain level extend down, that is, pass caudad to go under the edge of the falx to reach the midline again (fig. 412). Complete herniation of the cingulate gyrus is most commonly pres-

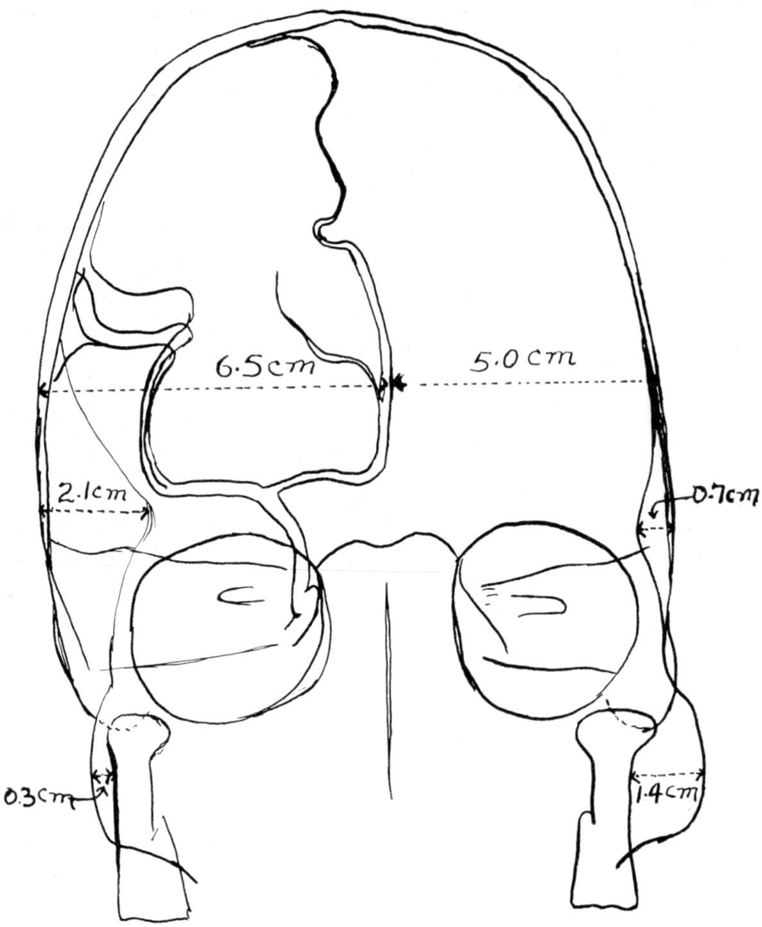

Fig. 413.—Diagram Illustrating the Method Used by the Authors to Evaluate Rotation of the Head and its Influence on the Resulting Shift of the Anterior Cerebral Vessels

As explained on the diagram, the distance from the zygomatic process of the frontal bone to the lateral margin of the skull on the left side is 0.7 cm. and on the right it is 2.1 cm. The difference between the two distances is 1.4 cm. Dividing this distance by 2, the result is 0.7 cm., and therefore an apparent displacement of the anterior cerebral vessels of this magnitude would be considered within normal limits. Of course, exact measurements of the anterior cerebral vessels cannot be made because the artery is slightly wavy. Measurements should be taken at the lower portion and at the upper portion of the artery as explained in the text. In the diagram, the measurement of the anterior cerebral artery, for the purposes of illustration, was taken slightly higher than is our custom. The presence of a "step," as explained in the text, is a more important sign of a midline shift than slight differences in measurement.

ent with a parasagittal tumor but may be present in any large neoplasm, subdural hematoma, or abscess.

As in the case of intracranial pneumography, angiographic findings may be present in connection with non-neoplastic processes that result in vascular displacement. Thus, degenerative changes on one side of the brain may cause a midline shift which may, on superficial inspection, be thought to be the result of displacement by mass rather than loss of substance. Such changes are found most frequently in cases of hemiatrophy of the brain resulting from early cerebral damage, either traumatic or interference with normal growth. Such

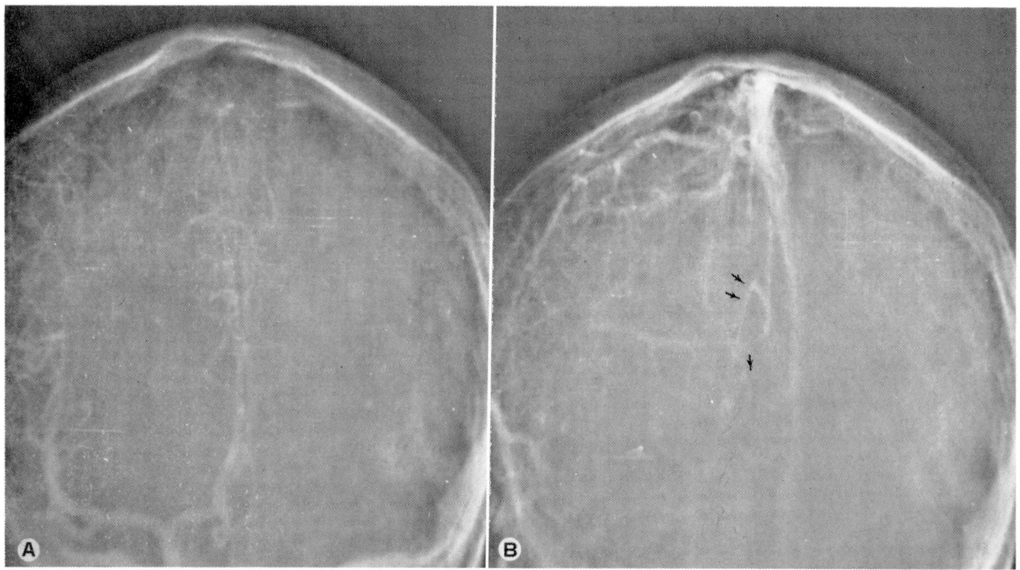

FIG. 414.—NORMAL ANTEROPOSTERIOR ANGIOGRAM TAKEN WITH A SLIGHT ROTATION OF THE HEAD

(A) Rotation of the head to the opposite side of that injected produces a generally rounded configuration to the anterior cerebral vessels, but there is no "step" outlined at the upper portion of the anterior cerebral vessels where they would return to the midline after being shifted in abnormal cases.

(B) The venous phase demonstrates that although there is rotation, the point usually selected for measuring to determine shift is exactly in the center of the skull. This point is the medial margin of the uppermost portion of the internal cerebral vein (*arrow*). The medial margin should be measured because there are two veins and, presumably, the midline is between the two veins. The internal cerebral vein should not be confused with the inferior longitudinal sinus which is situated a little higher and also has a curved configuration with an "up" and a "down" portion and an area of increased density which represents the highest point of this sinus (*two arrows*).

marked midline shifts as are seen in Figure 415 occur only when interference with brain growth occurs early in life. In these instances, the injured side fails to develop while the normally developing brain occupies part of the contralateral cranial space, thus carrying vessels with it. In the majority of instances, clues from plain films, which have been discussed earlier, may provide an obvious indication of the correct diagnosis. In other instances, careful clinical correlation may be necessary.

Transtentorial Herniations

In the majority of cases, herniation of the hippocampal gyrus through the tentorial incisura may be diagnosed or at least strongly suspected on the basis of the angiogram. In addition, upward herniation of posterior fossa structures through the incisura may be demonstrated, especially by vertebral angiography. Caudal hippocampal herniations may be subdivided into those occurring principally anterior or posterior to the brain stem.

The vascular structures that may help us in evaluating the presence of transtentorial herniations are: (1) the anterior chorioidal artery, (2) the posterior communicating and the posterior cerebral arteries, (3) the basilar artery, (4) the basilar vein, and (5) the vein of Galen. In some cases the superior cerebellar and the posterior chorioidal arteries may assist in arriving at a diagnosis.

Anterior herniations involving the uncus and adjacent portion of the temporal lobe may affect the anterior chorioidal artery as seen in the *frontal angiogram*. Inasmuch as the anterior chorioidal artery surrounds the medial aspect of the uncus of the hippocampus, it may be displaced medially when the

(*Revised 1963*)

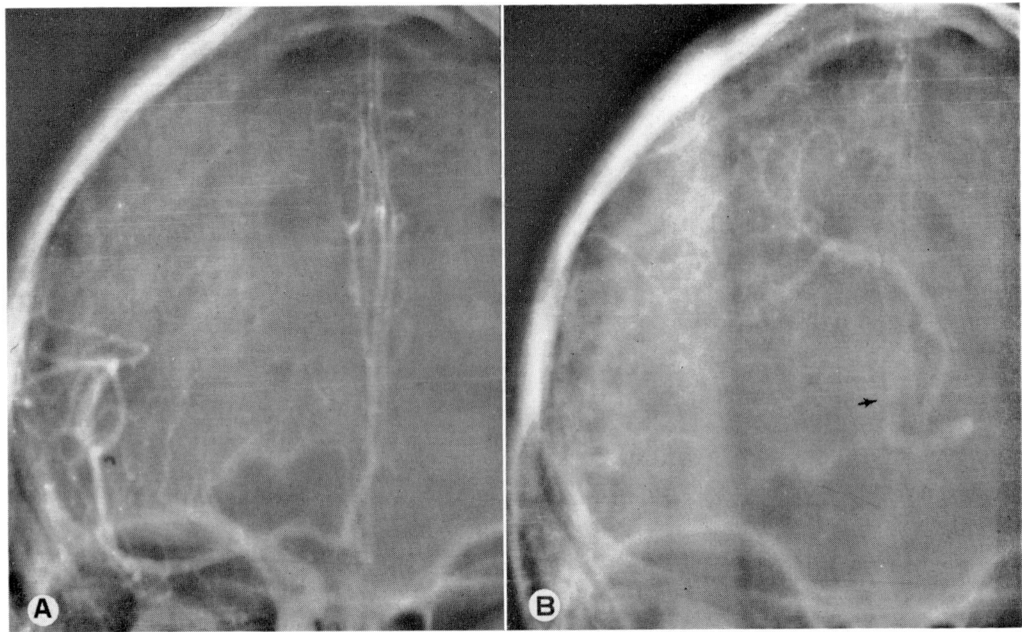

FIG. 415.—RIGHT CEREBRAL NEOPLASM SHOWING NO SHIFT OF THE ANTERIOR CEREBRAL VESSELS AND MARKED SHIFT OF THE INTERNAL CEREBRAL VEIN

(A) arterial phase. (B) venous phase. Deeply placed tumors often do not displace the anterior cerebral artery but almost always would displace the veins. An abnormally draining vein is seen to empty into the thalamostriate vein, which is markedly displaced and in turn drains into the internal cerebral vein. At least the posterior portion of the vein of Galen is in normal position (*arrow*).

uncus moves toward the midline. The latter movement usually precedes the herniation. The artery may actually reach or even go beyond the midline. *Medial displacement of the anterior chorioidal artery is the most important finding in anterior hippocampal herniations;* it is difficult to make a diagnosis angiographically unless this is present. At the same time, the curve or arc of the anterior chorioidal artery becomes wider (Azambuja *et al.*, 1956) (fig. 416). The evaluation of the arc (convex medially) described by the anterior chorioidal artery should be made according to the angulation used to make the frontal film. The greater the angulation of the tube, the wider is the curve of the anterior chorioidal artery (fig. 359). In the standard radiographic projection for anteroposterior films (12° caudad from the orbitomeatal line), the curve of the anterior chorioidal artery is about equal to the circumference of a U. S. 5-cent coin, a circle approximately 2.0 cm. in diameter. The most medial portion of the convexity of the curve is usually about 1.2 to 1.5 cm. from the midline. Widening of the curve of the anterior chorioidal artery without significant medial displacement should not be taken as conclusive evidence of anterior hippocampal herniation. It may be produced by "swelling" or infiltration of the hippocampus by tumor, particularly if the tumor is temporal in location (fig. 455). The posterior communicating artery may be displaced medially in some severe or extensive herniations (fig. 417), but it is more commonly displaced downward, and this is better shown in the lateral view.

The anterior chorioidal artery as seen in *lateral view* is usually stretched and straighter than usual, and often horizontal in position (figs. 416 and 447). It may also be displaced downward or even upward depending on how the medial portion of the temporal lobe shifted or rotated prior to the occurrence of actual herniation (fig. 417). The anterior

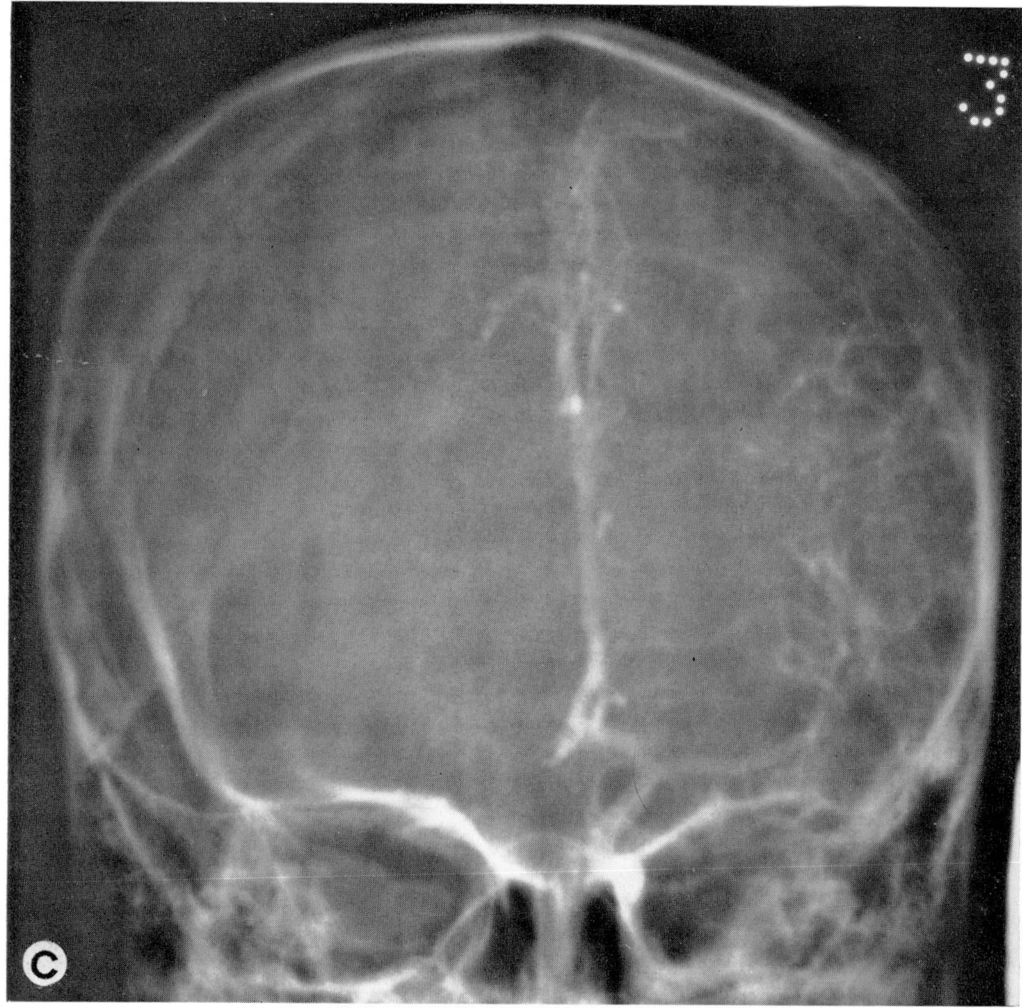

Fig. 415 (*Cont.*).—(C) Marked Off-Center Position of Anterior Cerebral Vessels in Patient with Cerebral Hemiatrophy

The anterior cerebral artery ascends straight up and down and it is off-center almost 2 cm. in the original film. The asymmetry of the skull is plainly visible, the convexity of the skull on the left side, the side of the angiogram, is much less than that on the opposite side.

chorioidal artery is often larger than normal in these cases.

The posterior communicating artery may be found to be displaced downward. However, the posterior communicating and proximal portion of the posterior cerebral artery are often low in position in normal cases, and care should be taken not to misinterpret this normal configuration. In true herniations, the posterior communicating artery approaches a vertical direction, and its distal (posterior) aspect dips below the top of the dorsum sella. The adjacent portion of the posterior cerebral artery is also displaced downward. It is not uncommon to see evidence of anterior hippocampal herniation by means of changes in the anterior chorioidal artery, with a normal appearance of the posterior communicating and posterior cerebral arteries.

In vertebral angiograms, the bifurcation of the basilar artery may be displaced down-

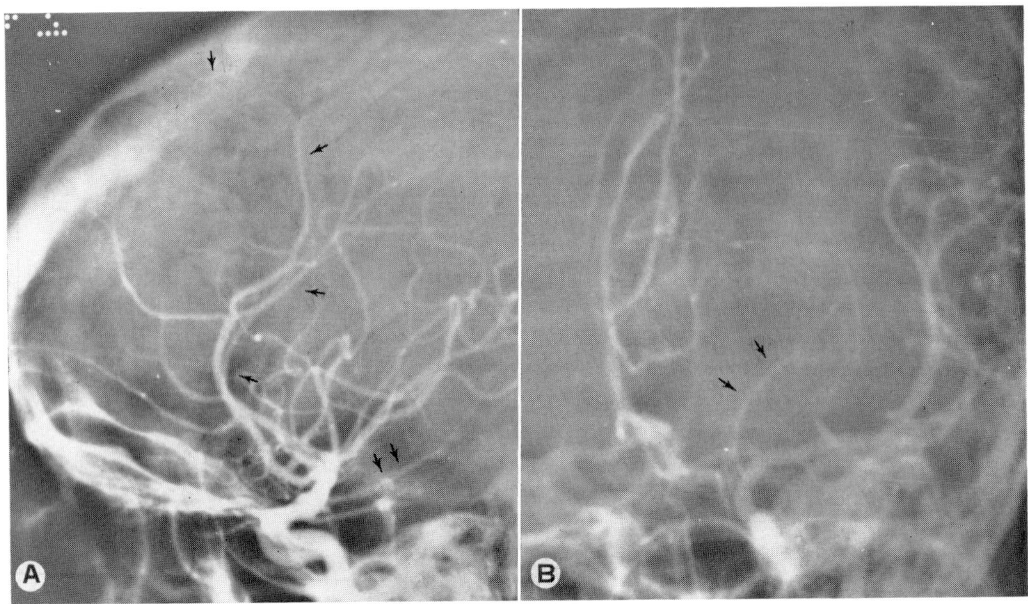

FIG. 416.—UNCAL HERNIATION IN A PATIENT WITH A FRONTAL LOBE TUMOR

The frontal projection (B) shows an increase in the length of the arc described by the anterior chorioidal artery, which is at the same time slightly displaced medially. The tumor was frontal in location, and the increase in the curvature of the anterior chorioidal artery cannot be ascribed to infiltration of the medial portion of the temporal lobe by tumor. The typical configuration of the rounded midline shift usually associated with anterior frontal tumors is present. The lateral projection (A) shows disruption of the branches of the anterior cerebral artery, which are stretched, and the curve of the pericallosal artery, which is blunted (*arrows*). The anterior chorioidal artery is stretched and enlarged (*two arrows*). The enlargement of the anterior chorioidal artery does not necessarily imply that there is blood supply of the tumor by the anterior chorioidal artery but is a phenomenon observed in patients with intracranial tumors in any location.

ward and the artery may be buckled, particularly in bilateral complete hernias. Similar changes may also be produced by a mass involving the 3d ventricle or by extreme dilatation of this ventricle (fig. 482).

The displacements and other changes in the vessels described above may be present in cases where an actual hernia has not occurred, but they indicate that at least great danger of herniation exists. In temporal lobe tumors, the anterior chorioidal artery is often displaced to the midline, and its curve widened, but it is possible that downward hernia does not exist in all of these cases. Likewise, the degree of medial displacement in the latter cases is not necessarily related to the severity of the herniation.

Posterior herniation of the hippocampus affects principally the posterior cerebral artery as it passes around the brain stem and it is displaced medially in *frontal view* (fig. 417A and B). This is the most important sign of posterior herniation and can be seen in carotid angiograms when the posterior cerebral artery fills, or on the vertebral angiogram. The basilar vein in its posterior portion is also displaced medially.

In *lateral view* the posterior cerebral artery is displaced downward and the main vessel or its branches present a "step" upward as they reach the edge of the tentorium (fig. 417). The basilar vein may be displaced downward, thus widening the space between it and the internal cerebral vein. When there is *complete anterior* and *posterior* herniation, signs of both types of herniation may be present on the angiogram (figs. 417C, D, and E, and 443).

(Revised 1963)

Central transtentorial down herniations. This term is here applied to the downward herniations occurring through the center of the tentorial slit due to midline masses, (bifrontal tumors, corpus callosum, and intraventricular masses within the 3d ventricle). The central structures are considerably displaced backward and downward, thus shifting the brain stem and cerebellum in a caudal direction. The angiogram shows downward displacement of the internal cerebral and basilar veins, and of the vein of Galen (fig. 431). The basilar artery is displaced backward and downward and is "buckled on itself" (fig. 482). The anterior chorioidal arteries, on the contrary, are displaced laterally (fig. 431).

Upward transtentorial herniations may be shown particularly on angiograms. The bifurcation of the basilar artery is usually displaced forward because these herniations are most frequently posterior or posterolateral in location. The vein of Galen and posterior portion of the basilar vein are displaced upward against the splenium of the corpus callosum. The posterior cerebral arteries are usually displaced upward and spread apart in their posterior portion where they ordinarily approximate each other, in symmetrical posterior upward herniations (fig. 495). The superior cerebellar arteries may be elevated on one or both sides as they go over the upper portion of the cerebellum and are seen to project above the posterior cerebral arteries (fig. 494). The most important findings are probably elevation of the vein of Galen and the posterior portion of the basilar vein.

Other Herniations

Three other herniations may be discovered at angiography.

(1) Herniation of the orbital portion of the frontal lobe behind the lesser wing of the sphenoid may be suspected when there is backward displacement of the anterior opercular branches of the middle cerebral artery.

(2) Gyrus rectus herniation into the sella turcica theoretically should produce posterior and downward displacement of the anterior cerebral artery and possibly lateral displacement of the carotid siphon. However, in two cases which at autopsy were found to have gyrus rectus herniation, the angiogram failed to reveal any changes in this region. It is possible that herniation occurred before death subsequent to the performance of the angiogram. On the other hand at least one case of gyrus rectus herniation has been seen where pneumoencephalography demonstrated bowing of the cisterna chiasmatis. An angiogram was not performed in this case.

(3) Herniations of the cerebellar tonsils and adjacent portions of the biventral lobules may be suspected when there is downward displacement of the posterior inferior cerebellar artery. Its caudal curve is pushed down to a level below the posterior arch of the atlas or even lower (fig. 494). In some normal cases, the posterior inferior cerebellar artery may present a long downward curve difficult to differentiate from cerebellar tonsillar herniations.

Straightening and Stretching of Cerebral Arteries

The cerebral vessels are normally undulated as they follow the cerebral sulci and convolutions. They are less tortuous in children than in adults. Loss of these normal undulations is a frequent finding in cerebral tumors. Several factors enter into the production of this nonspecfic change.

If *local edema* affects two adjacent gyri, the artery situated in the sulcus between them loses its normal undulations because the sulcus between the two gyri becomes straighter. This occurs because whenever two elastic surfaces (*e.g.* 2 rubber balloons) press against each other, the result is a straight plane if the tension is equal in the two; or a *smooth* curved plane if the tension is unequal. In the latter case, the curve is concave toward the side with the greater tension. The greater the amount of edema (*i.e.* tension) in two adjacent gyri, the straighter is the course of the vessel. When the edema is less pronounced, the straightening is less marked (fig. 418). Local edema can extend for a certain distance beyond the cen-

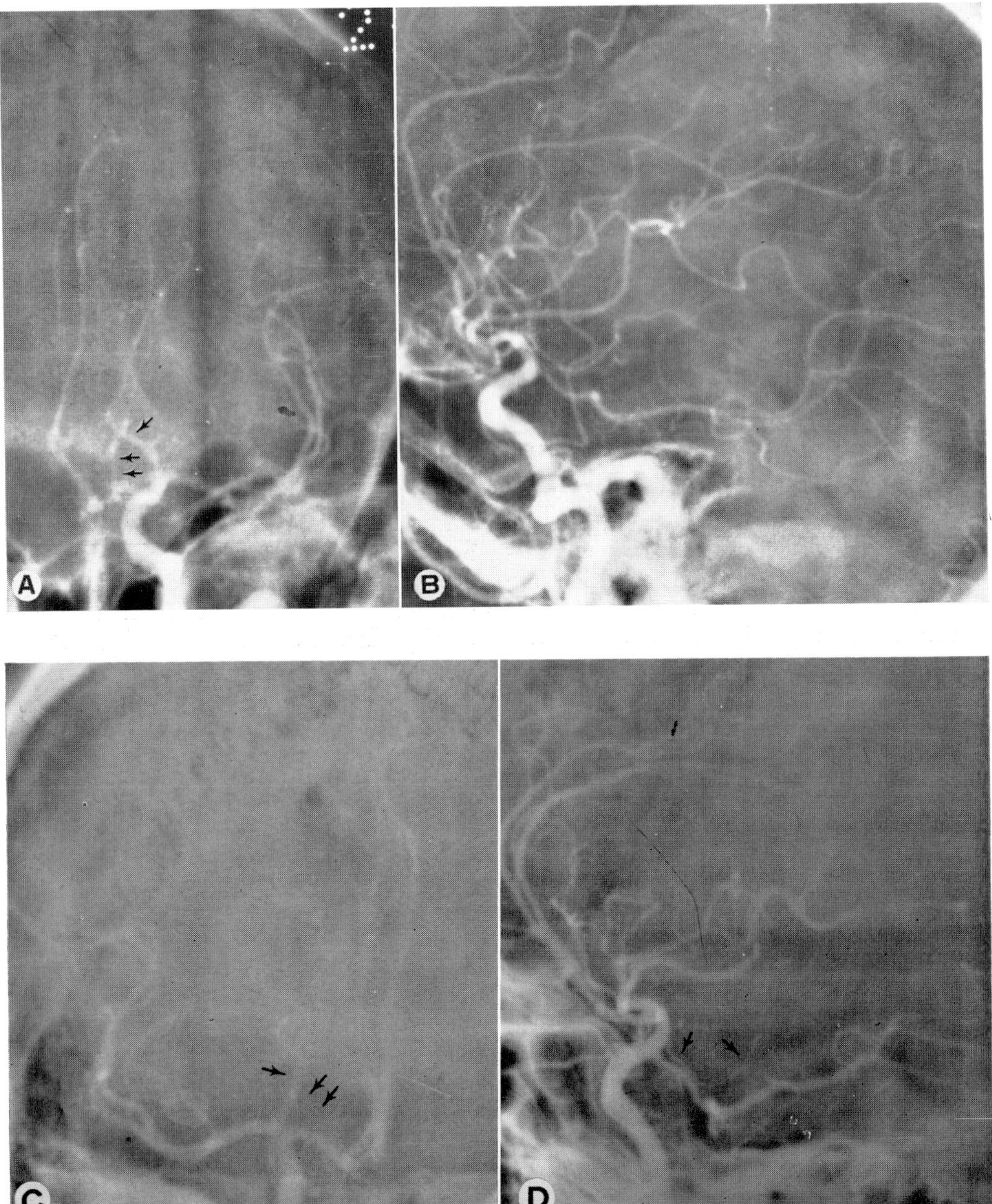

Fig. 417.—Posterior Hippocampal Herniation in Patient with a Posterior Temporal Mass

The frontal projection (A) shows medial displacement of the posterior cerebral artery in its posterior portion at the completion of its curve around the brain stem (*arrow*). The anterior chorioidal is displaced medially (*double arrows*). The lateral view (B) demonstrates downward displacement of the posterior communicating artery and of the anterior portion of the posterior cerebral artery. The posterior portion of this artery, however, is markedly displaced downward and demonstrates a step upward to go over the edge of the tentorium.

(*Revised 1963*)

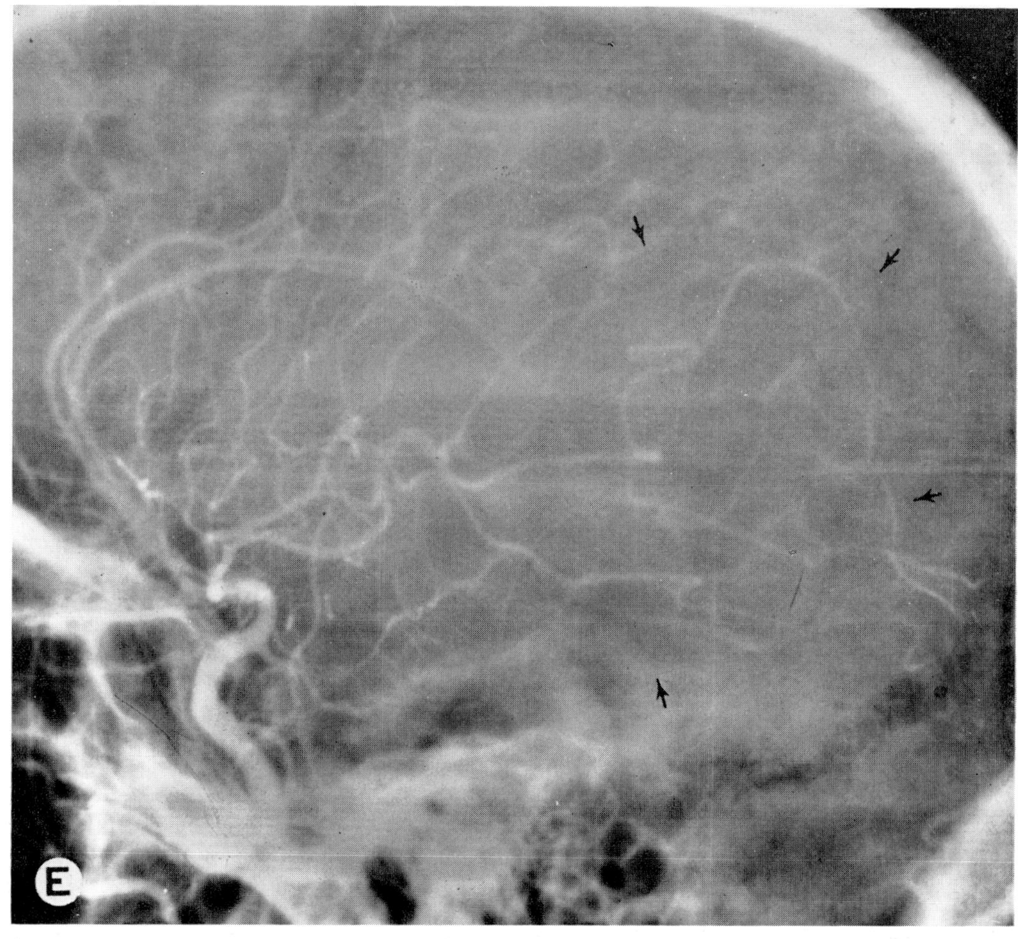

Fig. 417 (*Cont.*).—Anterior and Posterior Hippocampal Herniations (Complete Herniation)

A retro-Sylvian (parieto-occipital) mass was present in a second case. The frontal projection (C) shows medial displacement of the posterior cerebral artery in its posterior portion at the completion of its curve around the brain stem (*arrow*). The anterior chorioidal artery is crinkled and also slightly displaced medially (*double arrows*). The lateral view made at one second (D) demonstrates the marked downward displacement of the posterior communicating artery and of the anterior portion of the posterior cerebral artery. The posterior cerebral artery then goes backward and slightly upward to go over the edge of the tentorium. There is also extremely marked downward displacement of the anterior chorioidal artery (*arrows*). A film made at three seconds (E) discloses an abnormality in the vessels in the retro-Sylvian region (*arrows*), indicating the position of the tumor.

tral disturbance and cause loss of normal undulations of the arteries (fig. 419).

The same type of local change can occur when there is infiltration of convolutions by a neoplasm. It should be pointed out that edema is an extremely important factor in the production of the changes seen on the angiogram. Tumor infiltration without edema may produce no changes. Even a tumor as large as 4 cm. in diameter can go undetected in spite of its large size, if there is no significant cerebral edema; not so if it is accompanied by marked swelling. The same point also is particularly apparent in the case of relatively slowly growing tumors that calcify. Many of these tumors would go

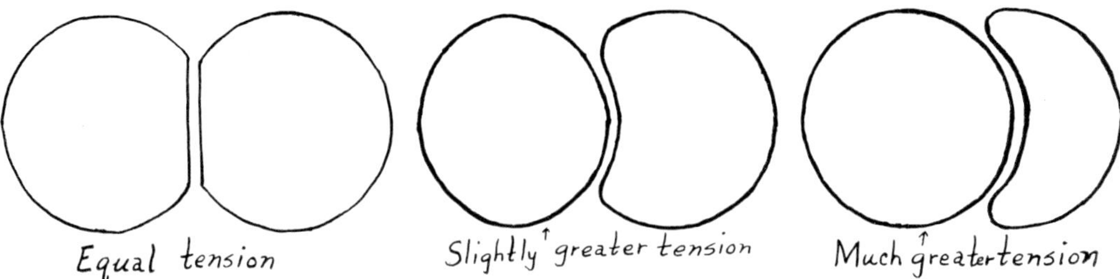

FIG. 418.—DIAGRAM ILLUSTRATING THE RESULTING SURFACES WHEN BALLOONS OF EQUAL AND UNEQUAL TENSION ARE PRESSED AGAINST EACH OTHER

With equal tension, the result is a straight surface; with slightly increased tension on one balloon as compared with the other, the result is a slightly curved surface; and with a much greater tension on one balloon, the result is a markedly curved surface. Similar conditions are felt to exist in the gyri of the brain when they are involved by neoplasm or by edema.

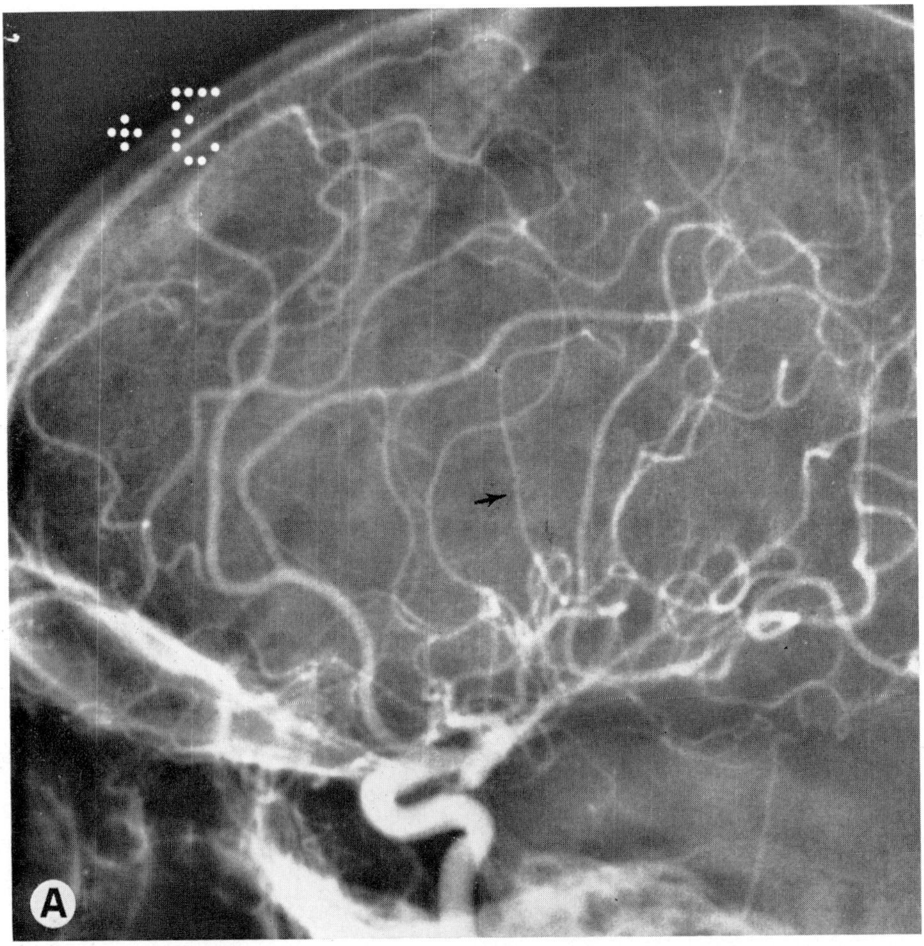

FIG. 419.—STRAIGHTENING OF ARTERIES IN THE FRONTOPARIETAL REGION SECONDARY TO INTRACEREBRAL MASS LESION

In (A), all of the posterior frontal and parietal branches of the middle cerebral artery show loss of their normal undulations. Some are almost straight, probably those in the region of the center of the mass (*arrow*). The arteries toward the periphery of the mass show bowing with incomplete loss of their undiagnosed were it not for the presence of calcification seen on the plain films, since frequently there is no associated edema (fig. 121). The same considerations regarding the important role of edema in diagnosis apply to pneumoencephalography.

When there is *generalized edema* of the convolutions, other factors may modify the above described changes since the gyri cannot expand as they do in local edema. The result is that some degree of loss of the normal undulations of the arteries takes place, but this is difficult to ascertain in many instances.

A tumor may produce *stretching* of adjacent arteries and veins. The artery loses all of its undulations and may become straight (figs. 419 and 420). In some cases the artery describes an arc around the circumference of the tumor and the actual size of the tumor at that point may be estimated from this curve. Care should be taken in trying to estimate tumor size from the curve of a single vessel since it is difficult to be sure that the central beam is perpendicular to the plane of the vessel. A vessel may be near the pole of an oval tumor and its curve not fully indicative of tumor size (fig. 442). Some of the arterial changes in a given tumor may be those of stretching and displacement by a neoplasm, while others are simple loss of the normal tortuosity due to edema.

An extreme degree of *ventricular dilatation* produces stretching with loss of undulations of the cerebral arteries. The stretching of the vessels is easily explainable in children, because the head grows and so the convolutions are actually stretched over the enlarged ventricles (fig. 473). In adults the streching of the convolutions is slight; loss of the normal undulations of the vessels occurs, but it is often difficult to ascertain. A more accurate

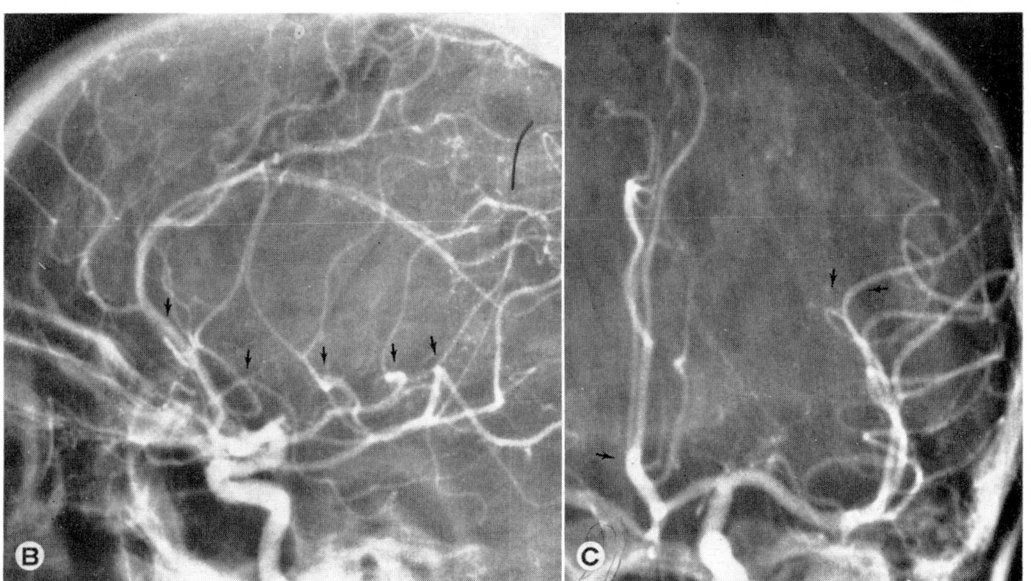

Fig. 419 (*Cont.*)

normal undulations. The exact anterior and posterior extent of the tumor cannot be ascertained. The mass was a spontaneous intracerebral hematoma.

(B) represents an anterior supra-Sylvian tumor in another patient. There is straightening and spreading of the ascending branches of the middle cerebral artery over the frontoparietal operculum. There is bowing of the upper margin of the Sylvian triangle (*arrows*) which is typical of anterior supra-Sylvian tumors situated in the lower convexity. The area occupied by the spreading is much more circumscribed than in (A), indicating that the mass is more localized. The frontal projection of the same case (C) shows a shift of the anterior cerebral artery which is slightly more pronounced in the proximal (*arrow*) than in the distal portion. The angiographic Sylvian point (*arrow*) is displaced medially but not significantly downward (*arrows*).

(*Revised 1963*)

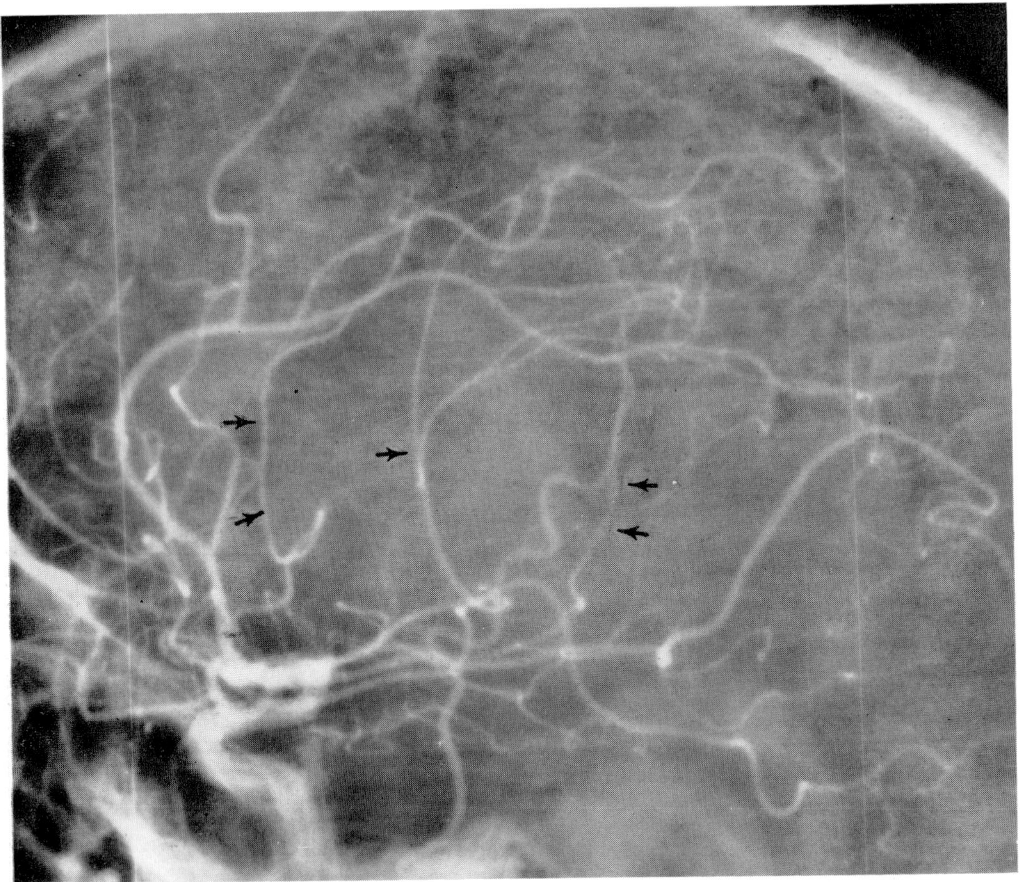

FIG. 420.—STRAIGHTENING AND BOWING OF ARTERIES IN A FRONTOPARIETAL TUMOR

The arteries are spread apart in the region of the frontoparietal operculum. The vessel marked by the *single anterior arrow* shows bowing with loss of undulation. The vessel shown by the *double anterior arrow* shows bowing without complete loss of undulation. It is likely, therefore, that the vessel marked by the *single arrow* is closer to the center of the mass, which is probably situated just behind this vessel. On the posterior margin of the tumor, there is also evidence of bowing of the vessels in an opposite direction (*posterior arrows*). Vessels further posteriorly also show loss of undulations, indicating that the edema, or possibly infiltrating tumor, extends further backward. The patient had an intracerebral glioma.

FIG. 421.—FRONTO-PARIETAL PARASAGITTAL TUMOR SHOWING LOCAL CIRCULATORY CHANGES (SLOW CIRCULATION IN INTERMEDIATE PHASE)

The arterial phase (A) shows a slight disruption of the branches of the anterior cerebral artery in the high fronto-parietal convexity or parasagittal region (*arrows*). However, variations in the distribution of the branches of the anterior cerebral artery are common and should be interpreted with caution. The branches of the middle cerebral artery do not reveal any significant abnormalities. The intermediate phase (B) shows a paucity of vessels in the same region (*arrows*), with evident bowing of the sulci outlined in this intermediate phase, both in the area immediately adjacent to the avascular area and in those further away. The appearance indicates slowing of the circulation in the intermediate phase. In the venous phase (C), the appearance is essentially normal in the parasagittal region. However, there is some flattening of the internal cerebral vein (*arrow*). The basilar vein is also displaced downward.

(*Revised 1963*)

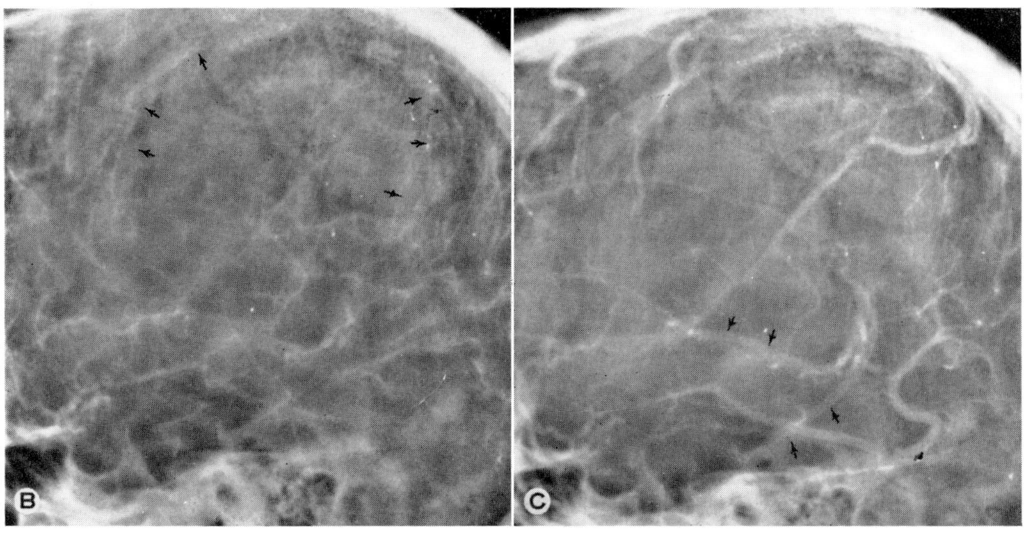

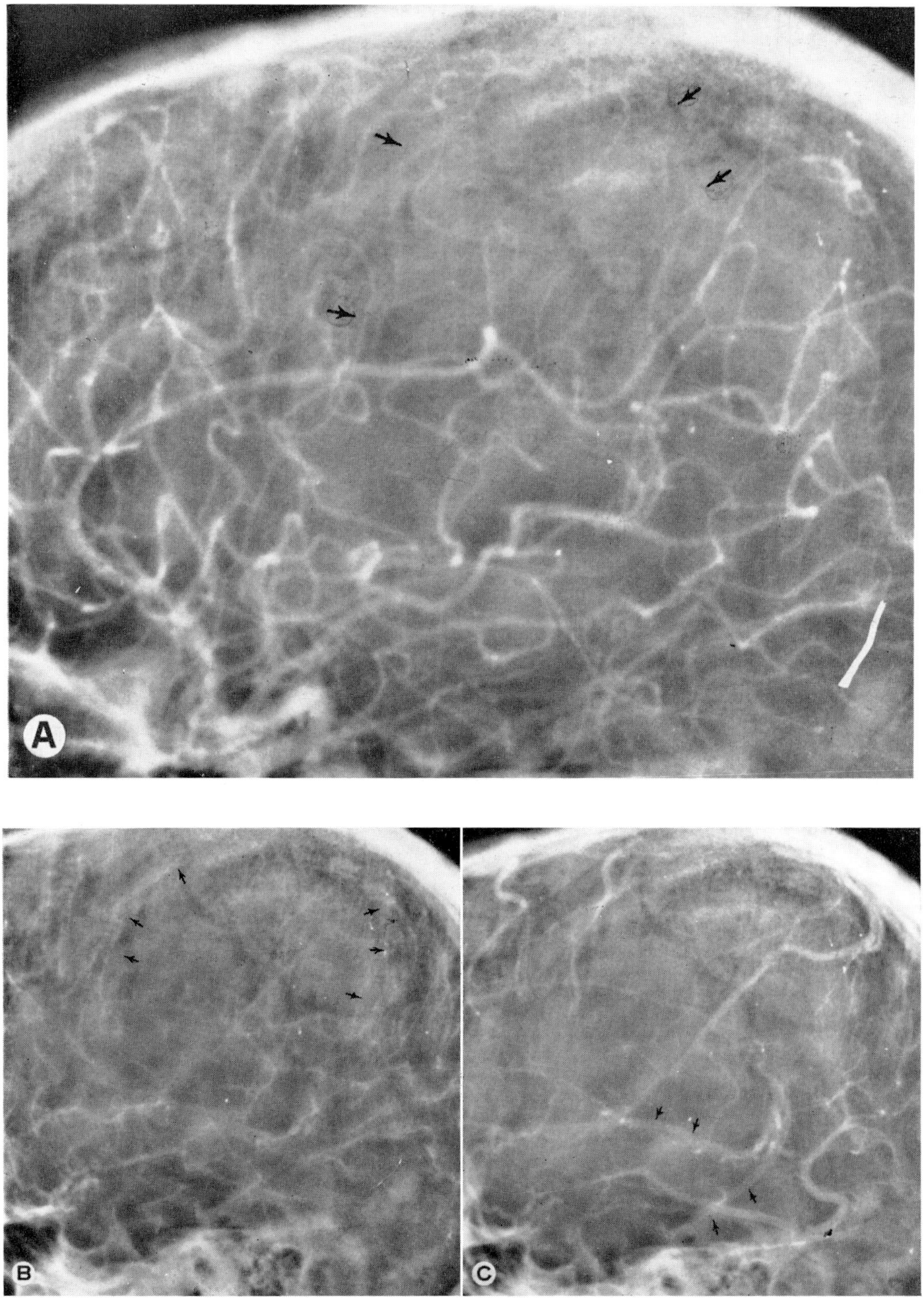

FIG. 421

evaluation of ventricular dilatation is made by other means (see "Ventricular Dilatation").

Cerebral vessels become *bowed* although the tumor is situated beneath the surface of the brain because the gyri over the tumor become edematous and wider, thus bowing the adjacent sulci (fig. 420). The deeper portions of the sulci may be bowed to a greater degree than the superficial aspects. Thus, the deeper an artery is situated in a sulcus, the more it will be bowed. The bowing may be associated with stretching and loss of undulations of the artery, in which case it is easily recognizable. Bowing, however, may be present without loss of the normal undulations, and under these circumstances it is not obvious and may be overlooked (fig. 433). Bowing without loss of undulation is a very important sign of tumor in posterior frontal and parietal locations.

In the late arterial and intermediate phases, bowing of the sulci often becomes more conspicuous and is easier to recognize (fig. 421).

While the arteries frequently show bowing, the veins are usually not so affected. This is partly because the veins tend to be on the surface, between two convolutions, rather than deep in the sulci as the arteries frequently are, at least during part of their course. Also, bowing is characteristically seen over the mid-convexity of the brain and is less often found in the upper convexity and parasagittal region. The branches of the middle cerebral artery are best seen over the convexity and taper as they ascend, which causes them to exhibit the bowing which is described. On the other hand, the veins originate in the convexity of the brain, usually by several branches, and become larger and more conspicuous as they approach the superior longitudinal sinus, which is the area where bowing is less frequently observed in the cerebral convexity. For this reason the veins show these local changes less frequently.

Changes in Circulation Time

There may be *local* changes in the circulation time with an increase in the speed of circulation through the tumor (usually malignant tumor). Slowing (lengthening) of the circulation time also may be found in the neighborhood of a tumor. The local lengthening involves usually the arteriovenous circulation time (fig. 421), but the circulation time of some of the arteries may also be slowed in some cases; this is, however, less common. If the tumor causes increased intracranial pressure, generalized slowing or lengthening of the circulation time may be encountered. These findings have been described in detail under "Factors Influencing Circulation Time," page 1.556.

ANGIOGRAPHIC CLASSIFICATION OF TUMOR LOCATION

The Sylvian fissure is used as the reference point to classify the various locations of supratentorial tumors. It is relatively easy to locate with accuracy the angiographic Sylvian point which represents the highest, deepest, and most posterior point of the Sylvian fissure (see under discussion of the anatomy of "Middle Cerebral Artery"). Likewise within the Sylvian triangle, and a little below the upper margin of this triangle, the true line of the Sylvian fissure itself can be approximated. Therefore, it seems reasonable to use these landmarks as reference points and to relate the location of various space-occupying masses to these key structures.

The masses of the anterior frontal region do not produce sufficiently well defined changes in the Sylvian group of vessels and deserve consideration separately. The same applies to suprasellar tumors, and subdural hematomas situated in unusual positions.

One tumor classification which has been found pathologically satisfactory and clinically practical follows and is illustrated by Figure 422.

I. Supratentorial tumors
   1. Anterior frontal
   2. Supra-Sylvian (posterior frontal and parietal). This group also includes the parasagittal masses in the posterior frontal and parietal areas.

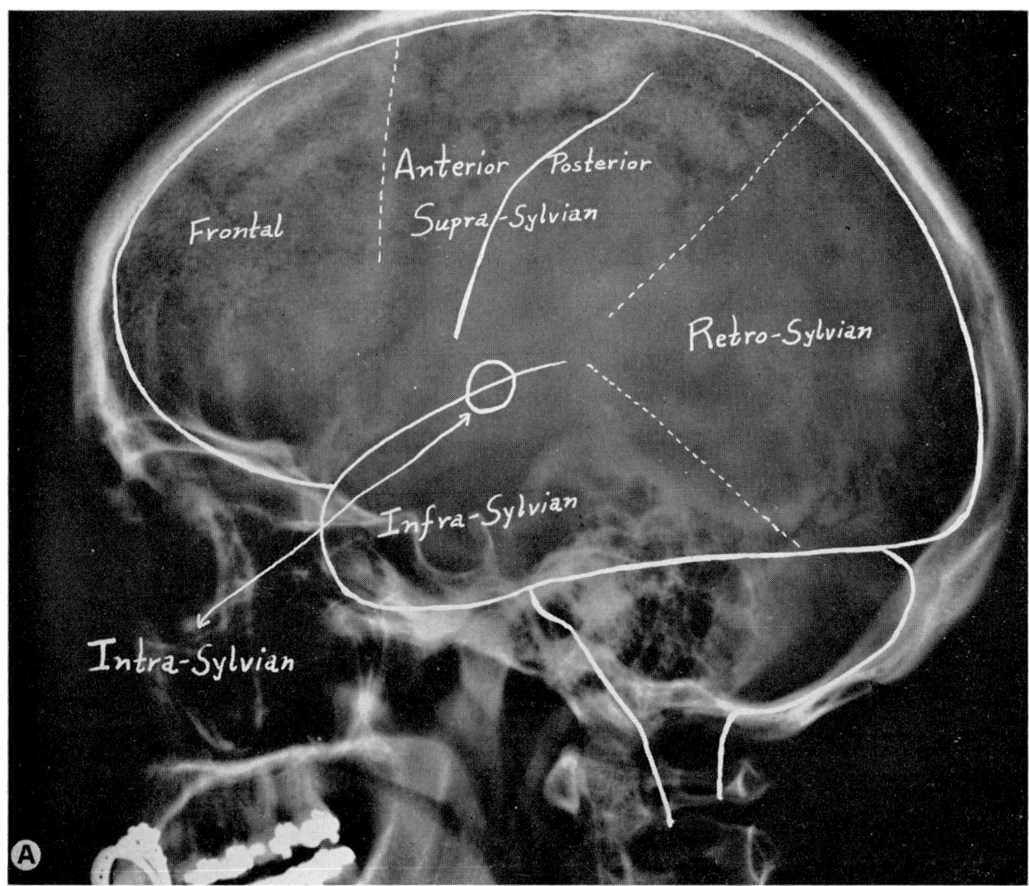

FIG. 422.—ANGIOGRAPHIC CLASSIFICATION OF BRAIN TUMORS

The angiographic classification proposed here for brain tumors is, as explained in the text, based on the Sylvian fissure, the Sylvian triangle, and the angiographic Sylvian point. The subdivisions correspond fairly well to those used in the localization of intracranial masses when diagnosed by pneumography (Fig. 206). The frontal tumors have to be subdivided into various subgroups, and in addition the supra-Sylvian, retro-Sylvian, and infra-Sylvian masses have to be subdivided, depending on the location of the mass in relation to the brain. In (B) the masses are classified again according to whether they are lateral or medial to the Sylvian fissure.

3. Infra-Sylvian (temporal)
4. Retro-Sylvian (temporoparietal, temporo-occipital, and parieto-occipital masses, as well as true occipital masses)
5. Intra-Sylvian (masses situated between the lips of the Sylvian fissure)
6. Latero-Sylvian (usually parietotemporal or frontotemporal extracerebral masses, including subdural hematomas in this location)
7. Centro-Sylvian (thalamic and deep posterior frontal)
8. Ventricular dilatation (unlocalizable tumors and other lesions resulting in hydrocephalus)
9. Miscellaneous (deep tumors of intraventricular, interventricular, and periventricular structures)
10. Suprasellar and parasellar

II. Infratentorial tumors

III. Incisural tumors

(Revised 1963)

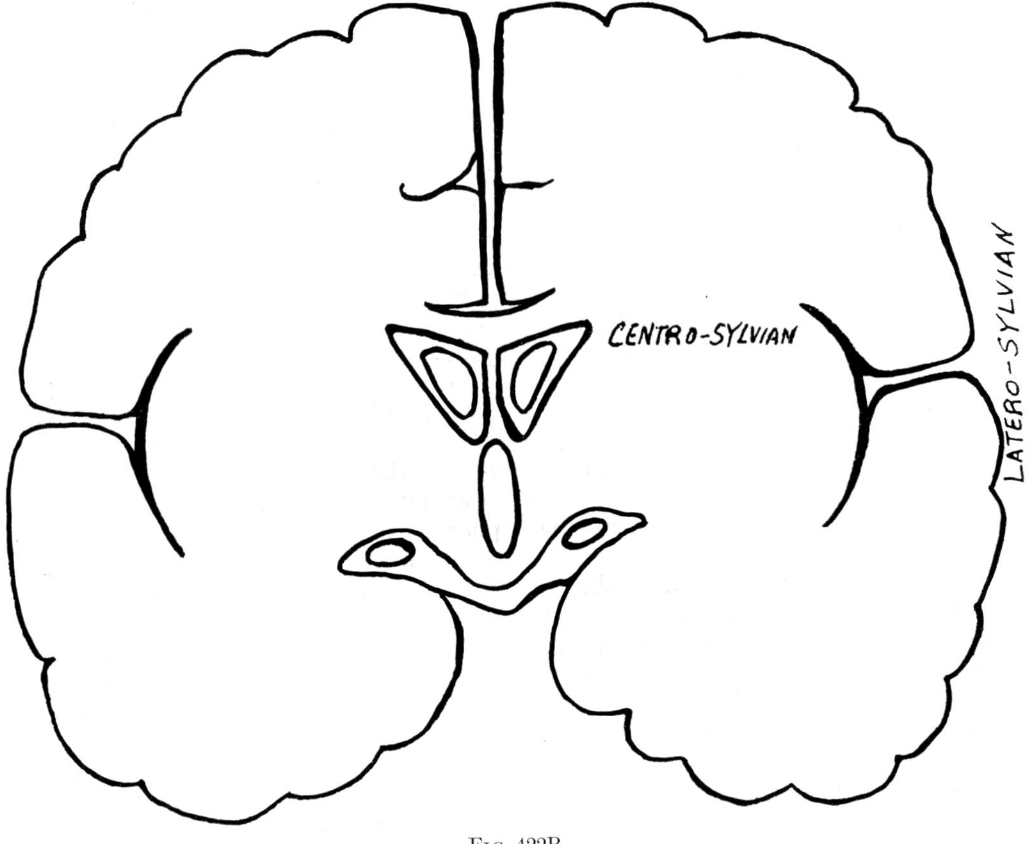

FIG. 422B

DIAGNOSIS OF INTRACRANIAL MASSES BY VASCULAR DISPLACEMENT

Anterior Frontal Tumors

Since the frontal lobe is so large, it is desirable to subdivide it into several portions for more precise designation of tumor location. The same procedure was followed in connection with intracranial pneumography. While overlapping terminology is preserved whenever possible, angiographic anatomy does not correspond sufficiently well with pneumographic anatomy in all areas to allow a free interchange of terminology as regards the sub-lobar designation of tumor sites. Such a difference pertains to the intracerebral tumors of the frontal lobes which fall into three general displacement patterns. Therefore, under anterior frontal tumors will be included the frontal masses, which are situated in the anterior half or two-thirds of the frontal lobe, anterior to the coronal suture. The masses situated behind the coronal suture are posterior frontal or frontoparietal and are considered as supra-Sylvian masses. The deep posterior frontal masses usually produce diffuse swelling of the central structures and are considered with the centro-Sylvian masses. The anterior frontal tumors, therefore, include:

(1) Subfrontal (extracerebral), (2) inferior frontal (intracerebral), (3) frontal pole, (4) parasagittal, (5) midfrontal (lateral), and (6) midline. This classification is justifiable from the point of view of angiography because each location produces specific displacements in the angiogram.

General manifestations. The anterior frontal tumors tend to produce certain signs in the angiogram in the majority of cases, depending on the actual size of the mass or the degree of the accompanying edema. Tumors may be intra- or extracerebral. The general signs of anterior frontal tumors may be listed and briefly described as follows.

(1) The shift of the anterior cerebral artery may be rounded in configuration (figs. 409 and 416).

(2) The carotid siphon is displaced downward (closing of siphon) (figs. 426 and 431).

(3) The carotid bifurcation may be displaced backward, so that a line drawn through it perpendicular to the plane of the anterior fossa falls behind the intracavernous portion (fig. 426).

(4) The bifurcation of the internal carotid artery as seen in the frontal projection, often acquires a "T"-shaped configuration due to stretching of the horizontal portions of the anterior and middle cerebral arteries (fig. 427E).

(5) There is usually widening of the "U loop" formed by the anterior and middle cerebral arteries as seen in the frontal projection. This, however, is often more apparent than real and is due to the shift of the anterior cerebral artery, unless the tumor (or edema) extends deep posteriorly to push the insular vessels outward.

(6) The foramen of Monro, *i.e.* the anterior portion of the internal cerebral vein, is shifted contralaterally and usually backward, thus increasing the depth of the curve ("humping") of the internal cerebral vein (figs. 426 and 427). In the more rostral frontal tumors, the anterior cerebral artery is displaced across the midline to a greater extent than the internal cerebral vein.

(7) Depression of the anterior portion of the Sylvian triangle may be present. This, like some of the other signs, is dependent upon the size of the tumor (figs. 428 and 429).

(8) Depression of the anterior portion of the middle cerebral artery branches as seen in the lateral view is frequently observed, particularly with large tumors (fig. 431). If the temporal horn is dilated due to obstruction, the middle cerebral group may even be elevated in some cases.

(9) Large anterior frontal masses tend to produce a rotation of the brain along a horizontal axis that passes through the midbrain, as well as a posterior and downward shift that favors the production of incisural herniation. This may be appreciated particularly in the venous phase by the position of the internal cerebral and basilar veins and their junction with the vein of Galen. The vein of Galen is often markedly displaced backward and downward, with the result that it becomes nearly vertical in position (figs. 426, 431).

Subfrontal masses. Such tumors are extracerebral in origin and usually are meningiomas arising from the olfactory groove or from the planum sphenoidale. Therefore, they usually involve the midline, although they frequently extend more toward one side or the other. An occasional extremely large pituitary adenoma or cystic craniopharyngioma may produce some of the signs of a subfrontal tumor. They will also produce signs of a suprasellar mass and, therefore, can be differentiated from the meningiomas on the basis of plain films and angiography. It is understood that, in each instance, the plain films are scrutinized first for any local changes.

The most characteristic angiographic evidence of a subfrontal extracerebral mass, at or slightly off the midline, is elevation of the anterior cerebral artery and its branches. The arteries are pushed and stretched upward above the floor of the anterior fossa, usually describing an arc. The size of the arc indicates the size of the tumor at that point (fig. 423). The anterior cerebral artery and its branches may remain in the midline in well centered tumors, or they may be displaced off the midline; the degree of displacement depends on how much of the main tumor mass is lateral to the midline. Often the anterior cerebral artery appears angulated in the frontal projection (fig. 423).

The carotid siphon is closed due to downward displacement of the artery, and in addition, the point of bifurcation of the internal carotid artery is displaced backward (fig. 423B). The ophthalmic artery usually supplies these tumors at least partially, and even when no discernible "tumor cloud" is present, the artery is enlarged. In order to be considered abnormal, the ophthalmic artery should give rise to visible branches extending

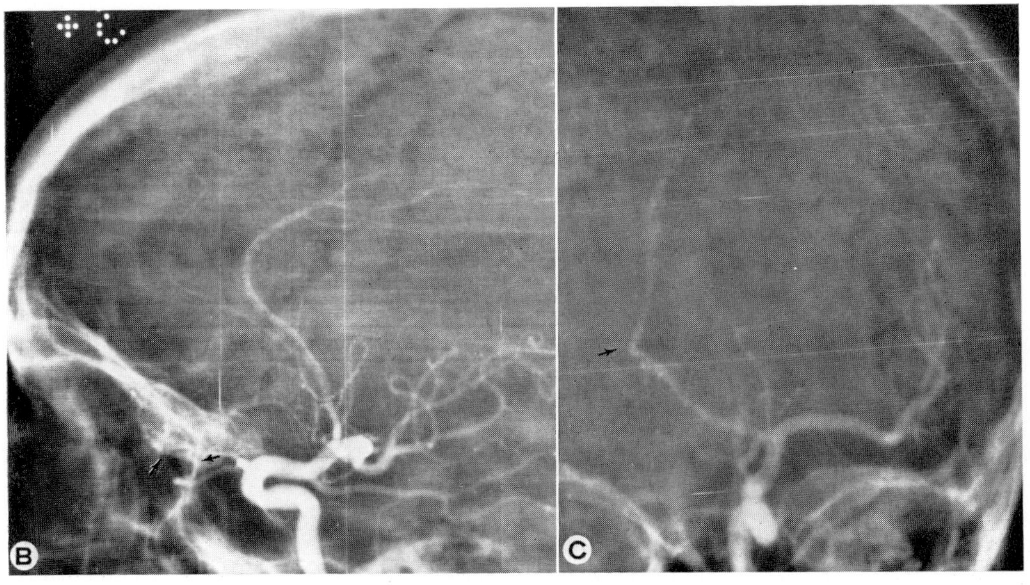

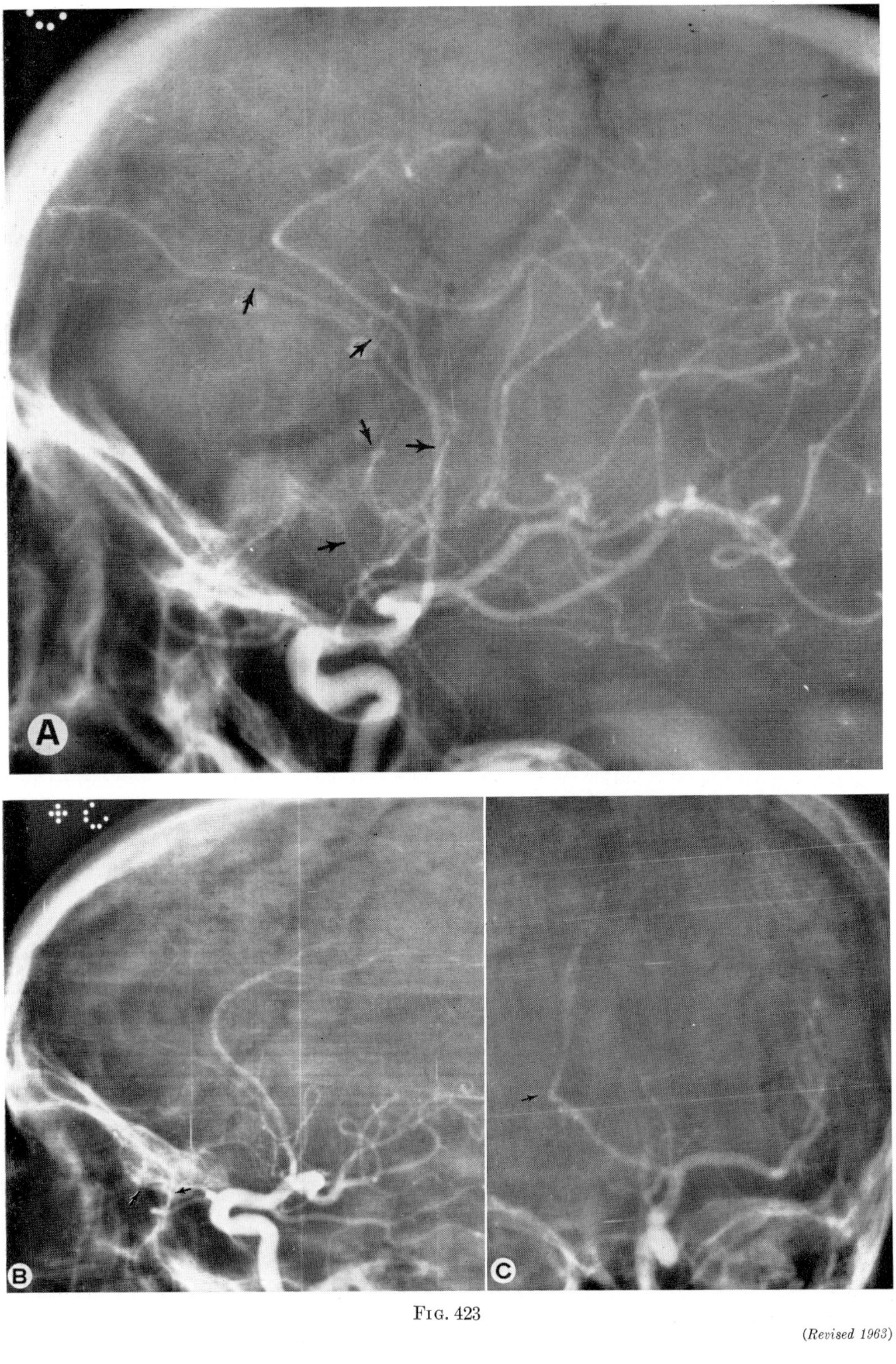

Fig. 423

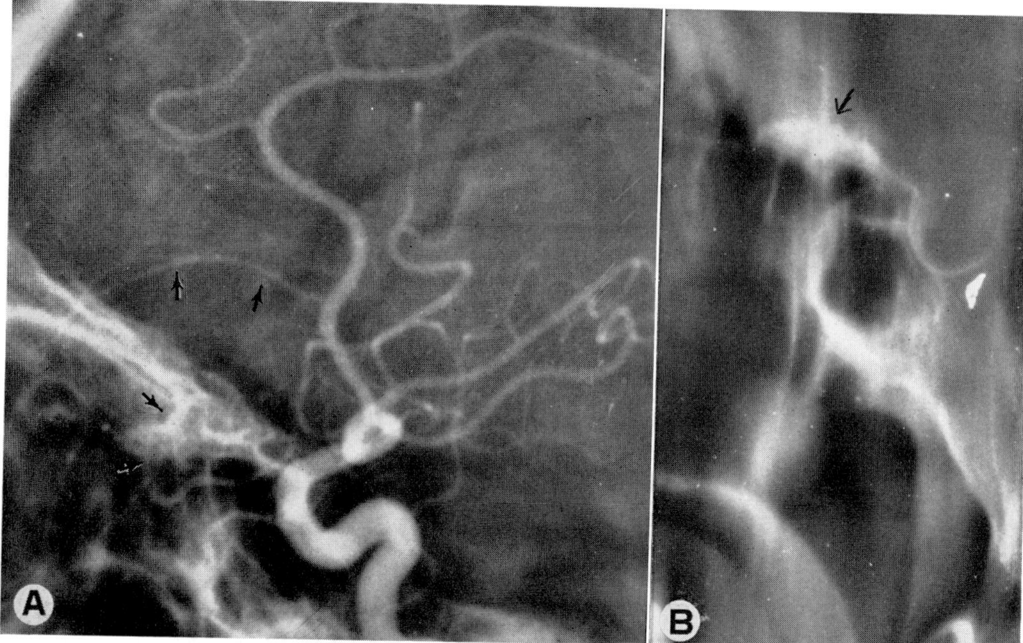

FIG. 424.—SUBFRONTAL MENINGIOMA ARISING IN THE PLANUM SPHENOIDALE

The plain film of the skull (B) shows the presence of spongy sclerotic bone in the region of the planum sphenoidale (*arrow*). The lateral angiogram (A) discloses elevation of the proximal branches of the anterior cerebral artery with bowing and downward concavity. No branches of the anterior cerebral artery are seen within the area of the tumor, but the middle cerebral branches are projected over the area, as in the previous figure. The ophthalmic artery gives off branches which can be seen in the area of the tumor (*arrows*).

to the roof of the orbit (fig. 424). Branches of this artery anastomose directly with branches of the meningeal arteries through the orbital roof, but these anastomoses are not seen on the angiogram under normal circumstances. The abnormally prominent ophthalmic artery branches may be brought out by the subtraction method (fig. 508) (Ziedses des Plantes, 1934, 1961). The septal vein is displaced upward, and the anterior portion of the internal cerebral vein may be pushed backward and its curvature may increase. These changes vary according to the size of the tumor.

Laterally situated subfrontal masses would not affect the anterior cerebral artery and its branches in a characteristic manner. They would produce signs of a midfrontal mass (see below), but in addition would lift the orbitofrontal and anterior opercular branches of the middle cerebral artery (fig. 425).

Inferior frontal masses. This denomina-

FIG. 423.—SUBFRONTAL MENINGIOMA

There is elevation of the pericallosal artery and of the frontopolar arteries, which have a generally concave downward curve typical of subfrontal tumors. The arterial branches seen in the area of the tumor are mostly those of the middle cerebral arteries (the anterior opercular branches and the orbitofrontal branch overlie that area (*arrows*)). The ophthalmic artery is well shown, and on the original film, there seemed to be branches extending upward toward the planum sphenoidale, which is characteristic of subfrontal meningiomas.

(B) This lateral view of another subfrontal tumor illustrates the blood supply from the ophthalmic artery (*arrows*). The figure also illustrates the marked posterior displacement of the carotid bifurcation and closing of the siphon. The frontal projection (C) of the same case shows the angular shift often observed in subfrontal tumors.

(Revised 1963)

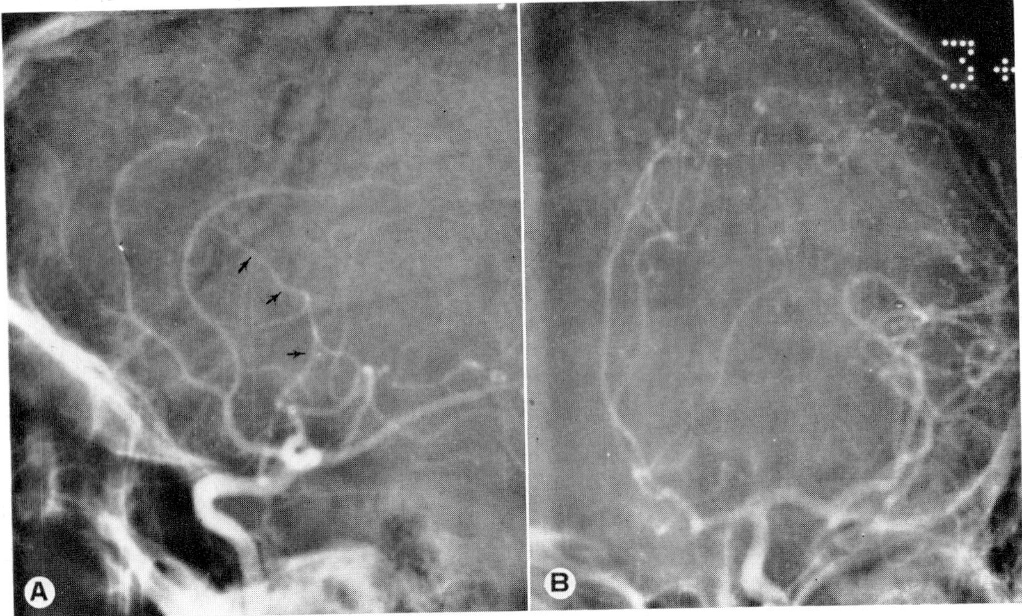

Fig. 425.—Lateral Subfrontal Mass (Meningioma)

The frontal projection (B) has the appearance of a frontal tumor in that the shift has a generally rounded configuration. The Sylvian point is in normal position. In the lateral projection, taken in the early arterial phase (A), it is noted that the anterior cerebral artery can be visualized to its origin from the internal carotid artery, which occurs when the middle cerebral artery is displaced backward by frontal tumors. The carotid bifurcation is displaced backward and the supraclinoid portion of the siphon is slightly displaced downward. The more anterior opercular branch of the middle cerebral artery shows a bowing without complete loss of undulation (*arrows*). This type of displacement is produced by tumors situated on the lateral aspect in the subfrontal region, possibly arising from the outer third of the sphenoid ridge on its superior aspect and not extending into the floor of the middle fossa to a significant degree. The latter extension would have produced elevation of the horizontal portion of the middle cerebral artery.

tion refers to masses that are low and involve the undersurface of the frontal lobe but are intracerebral in location. The chief point of difference between inferior frontal and subfrontal masses is that not all of the branches of the anterior cerebral artery are displaced upward away from the floor of the anterior fossa by the tumor. It is possible for the tumor to grow and to involve the inner aspect of the lobe and to protrude medially, across the midline, in such a way as to lift the anterior cerebral artery, similar to the growth of subfrontal masses. However, the branches of the anterior cerebral artery going to the orbital surface of the frontal lobe would not be so affected (fig. 426). These tumors usually produce a well defined lateral shift (fig. 427) which may be more pronounced in the proximal (inferior) portion of the anterior cerebral artery. Otherwise, they may produce angiographic signs similar to those outlined under subfrontal masses, such as closing of carotid siphon, posterior displacement of carotid bifurcation, and elevation of septal and anterior cerebral veins. However, the ophthalmic artery is not enlarged and does not send visible branches to the roof of the orbit.

Frontal pole masses. Tumors of the anterior frontal extremity may be intracerebral, usually gliomas, or extracerebral (meningiomas or subdural or epidural hematomas). There is usually a sharp, rounded shift of the anterior cerebral artery. The knee of the pericallosal artery may be flattened due to posterior displacement (fig.

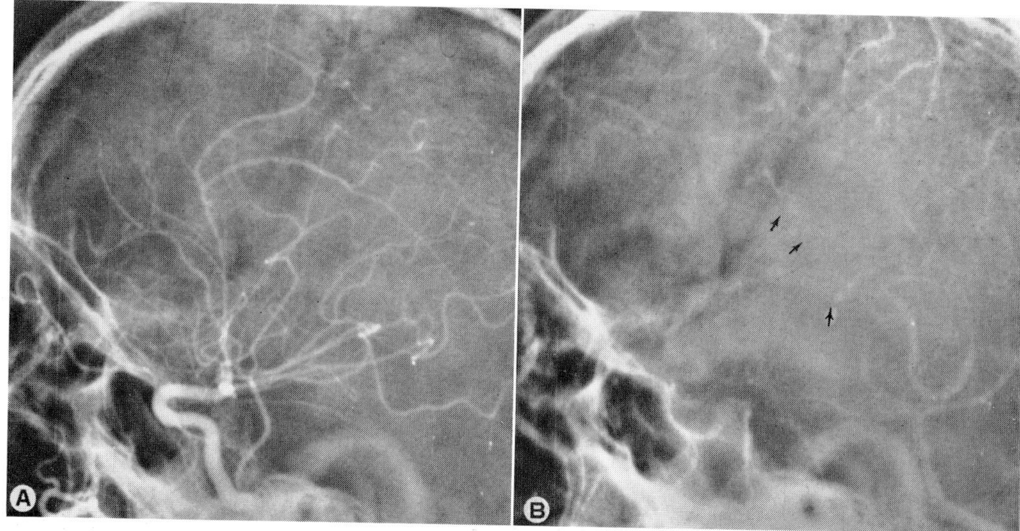

FIG. 426.—INFERIOR FRONTAL (INTRACEREBRAL) TUMOR SIMULATING A SUBFRONTAL MASS
The lateral view (A) shows elevation of the proximal portion of the pericallosal artery similar to that shown in the previous figure. There is even one branch of the anterior cerebral, the frontopolar artery, which shows a perfect bowing very suggestive of a subfrontal mass. In these cases it is extremely difficult to differentiate the two. The configuration is produced by protrusion of the tumor across the midline below the vessels, thus elevating some of those branches. It is always possible in these cases to see some fine vessels supplying the undersurface of the frontal lobe which normally arise from the anterior cerebral artery. However, similar vessels may be seen sometimes in subfrontal tumors as well, and under these circumstances it is not possible to differentiate between the two in the absence of typical abnormal vascularity. The venous phase (B) shows posterior displacement of the venous angle (*arrow*) and "humping" of the internal cerebral vein, which is typical of anterior frontal tumors. There is elevation of the septal vein (*double arrow*) which confirms the inferior frontal location of the mass.

429). It should be pointed out, however, that the knee of the pericallosal artery may give the appearance of backward displacement owing to a marked degree of lateral shift by a tumor which is not in the frontal pole.

The internal cerebral vein presents an increased curvature (humping of the internal cerebral vein), and the venous angle is displaced backward. Other general signs of frontal tumors may be present (see above). In subdural and epidural hematomas, the anterior cerebral artery branches do not reach the inner table of the skull as they do normally (fig. 609).

Parasagittal frontal masses. Tumors of the anterior parasagittal area can be intra- or extracerebral. Characteristically they produce depression of the anterior portion of the pericallosal artery, but it is common to find no significant depression (fig. 428). At the same time they may produce a distal (upper) shift of the anterior cerebral artery. Care should be taken not to confuse a normal downward curve, often present behind the knee of the pericallosal artery, with a true depression. The presence of a distal lateral shift, even though minimum, is of great help in evaluating these cases. A minimum shift of the pericallosal artery is sometimes very inconspicuous, but it can be discerned because the artery makes a short horizontal "V" as it goes over and back under the falx.

In addition to pericallosal artery changes, other general signs of frontal tumors may be present. The internal cerebral and septal veins may be displaced downward. For greater detail and discussion see "Supra-Sylvian Tumors."

Midline frontal masses. Again, the tumors may be extracerebral, such as meningiomas of the falx cerebri, or intracerebral in location. The extracerebral falx

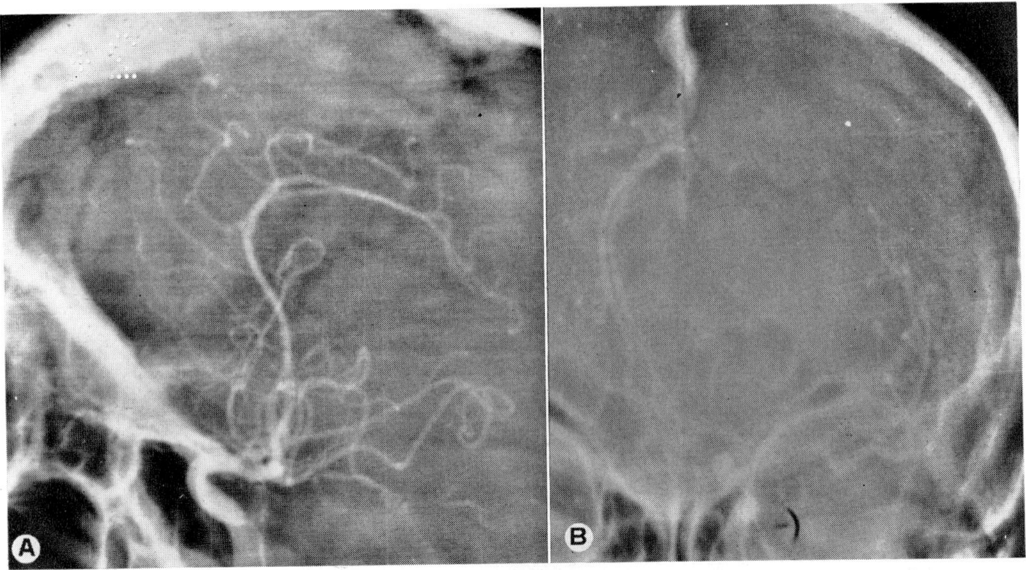

FIG. 427.—INFERIOR FRONTAL TUMOR (INTRACEREBRAL) SIMULATING A SUBFRONTAL MASS

The lateral view (A) shows elevation of the proximal portion of the anterior cerebral artery extending up to the knee of the pericallosal artery. However, the branches that normally extend rostrad to supply the inferior aspect of the frontal lobe are not displaced. The carotid bifurcation is displaced backward. The frontal film (B) shows a typical rounded configuration of frontal lobe neoplasms. The Sylvian point is not displaced downward.

meningiomas produce downward displacement of the pericallosal artery, and lateral bowing of the anterior cerebral artery branches normally situated on the inner surface of the frontal lobe, but sometimes surprisingly little distortion of these vessels is present (fig. 429). The intracerebral masses are usually in the anterior portion of the cingulate gyrus. They often produce spreading of the pericallosal and callosomarginal arteries (fig. 430). General signs of frontal tumors may also be present. The internal cerebral vein may be sharply displaced backward, depending on the size of the mass (fig. 431).

The midline frontal masses often grow posteriorly to invade the corpus callosum. From the corpus callosum they can grow into the medial aspect of the frontal lobe on the opposite side. These are referred to as *bifrontal* or "butterfly tumors." The angiographic picture depends on whether the tumor is symmetrically invading both frontal lobes, or whether it is larger on one side than the other. If it is symmetrical, there may be no midline shift. Bilateral angiography may be necessary to arrive at a diagnosis (fig. 431), but pneumography gives a more complete picture of the extent and exact location of the bifrontal tumors.

FIG. 427 (*Cont.*).—INFERIOR FRONTAL INTRACEREBRAL TUMOR

This case represents an example of a moderately difficult localization which, nonetheless, can be made accurately on the basis of the angiogram. The lateral view in the arterial phase (C) shows an essentially normal appearing angiogram. The siphon is not depressed and the pericallosal arteries are normal in position. This is not uncommon in frontal tumors. The lateral view in the venous phase (D) shows "humping" of the internal cerebral vein and elevation and prominence of the septal vein (*arrows*). The frontal projection (E) shows a fairly typical, generally rounded configuration of the shift of the anterior cerebral vessels to the opposite side. There is a T-shaped configuration of the bifurcation of the internal carotid artery. The lenticulostriate arteries are prominent.

(*Revised 1963*)

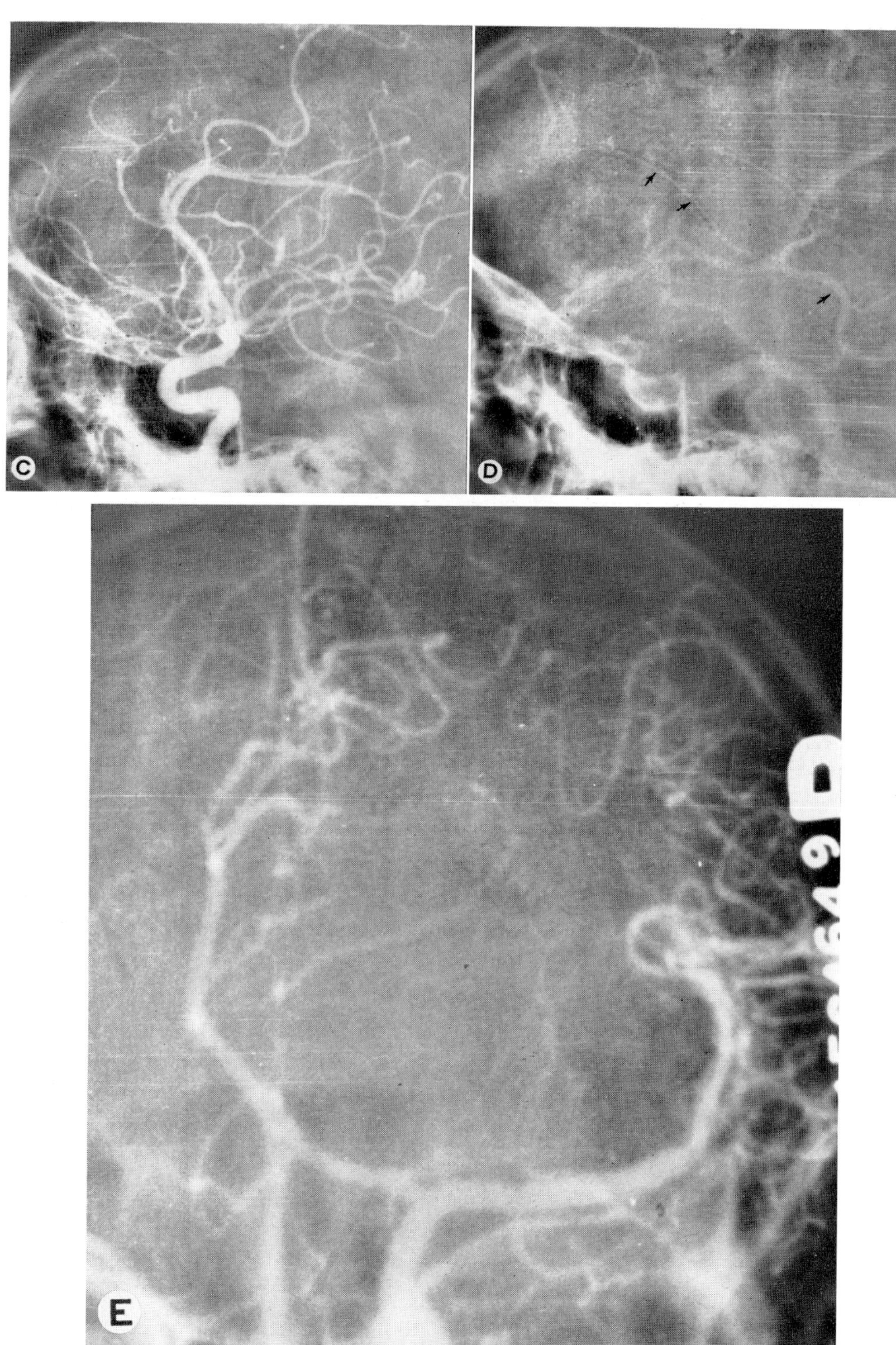

Fig. 427 (*Cont.*)

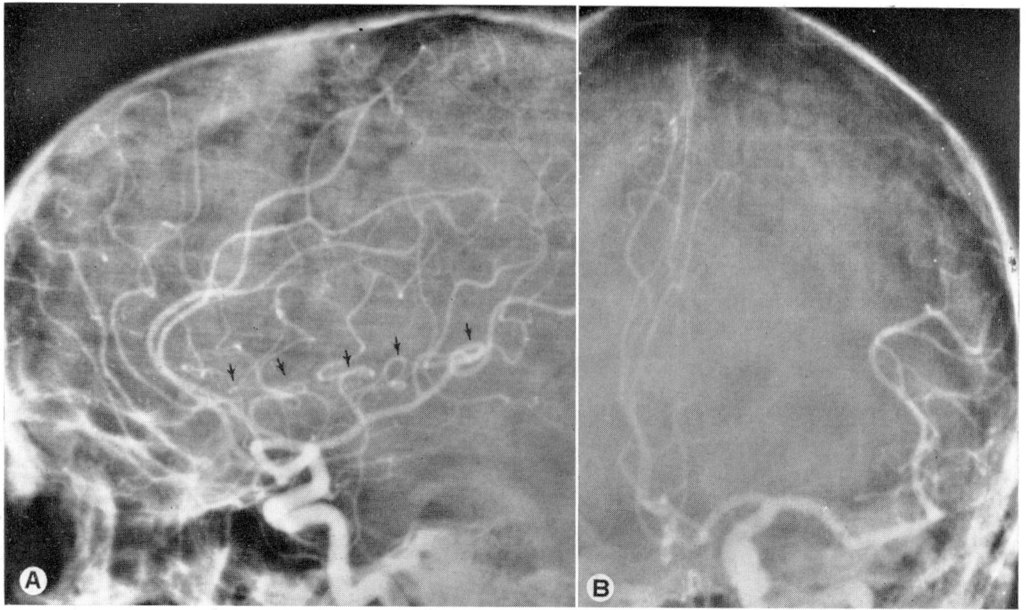

FIG. 428.—FRONTAL PARASAGITTAL TUMOR

In the lateral projection (A), there is slight flattening of the upper portion of the pericallosal artery, but the displacement is not so definite that an unequivocal statement can be made. The appearance is essentially normal in the arterial phase as far as the anterior cerebral branches are concerned. However, there is a uniform downward displacement of the anterior portion of the Sylvian triangle (*arrows*) and crinkling of the frontal opercular branches. The frontal projection (B) shows a relatively rounded shift of the anterior cerebral vessels which suggests a frontal location of the mass. There is flattening of the bifurcation of the carotid siphon forming a T-shaped configuration.

Midfrontal masses. Tumors of this location may also be referred to as lateral frontal or frontal convexity masses. As before, the group also contains intracerebral and extracerebral tumors. They are represented by those tumors, which, being situated anterior or near to the coronal suture, do not fit into the previously described groups. These tumors ordinarily present the general angiographic signs of frontal masses described above. They may extend backward or produce edema which then causes them to simulate the next group, the frontoparietal (supra-Sylvian) tumors.

Supra-Sylvian Tumors

The lesions of this group include the posterior frontal, frontoparietal, and parietal masses. They may be situated (1) on the convexity (low, mid, or high), (2) in the parasagittal region, and (3) in the midline.

General manifestations. The masses usually produce a midline shift of the anterior cerebral vessels. The shift does not have a "rounded" configuration characteristic of anterior frontal lesions. Instead it may be "square," or it may be more marked distally, depending on the exact location of the mass. The supraclinoid portion of the internal carotid artery is displaced downward (closing of the siphon). The ascending branches of the middle cerebral artery often exhibit stretching and bowing with or without loss of undulations. The loss of undulations is often accompanied by *spreading* of these arteries. The internal cerebral vein may be displaced across the midline and, with the high convexity and parasagittal lesions, it is depressed. In more posteriorly situated tumors, the vein is shifted across the midline to a greater degree than the anterior cerebral artery.

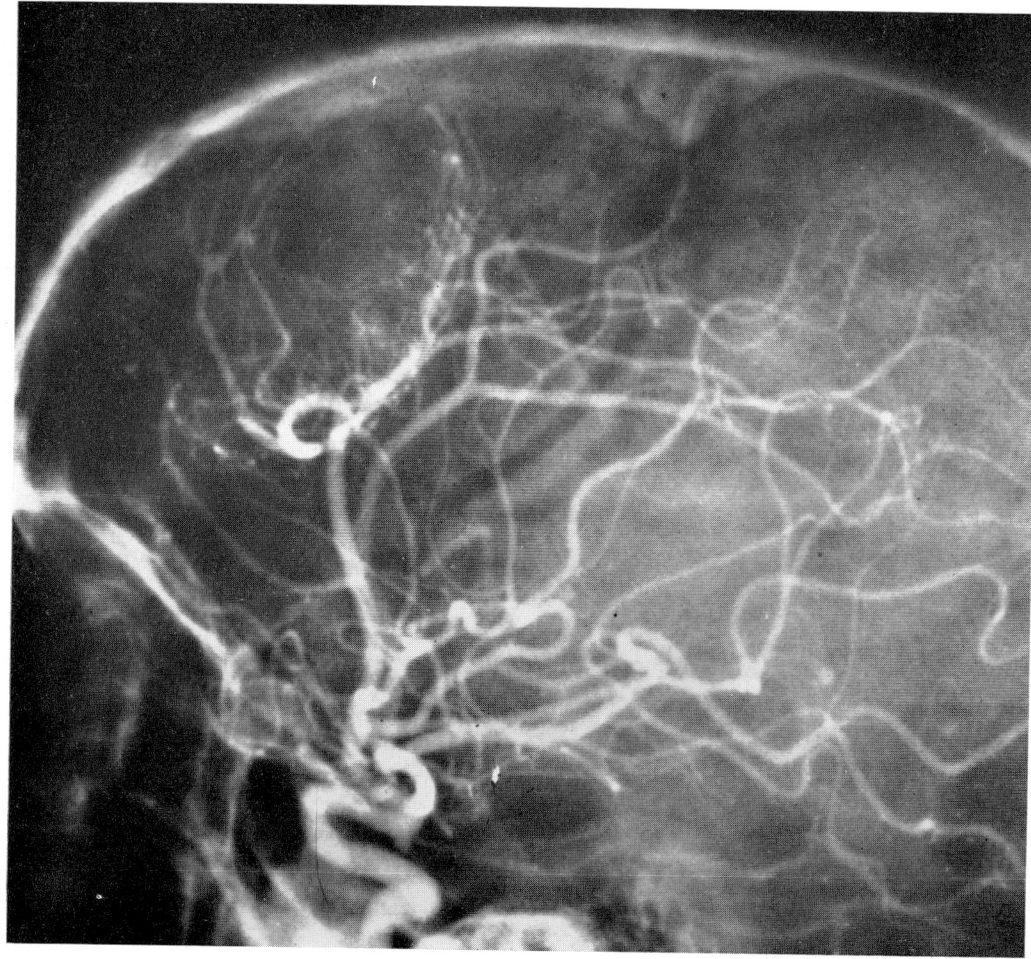

FIG. 429.—MIDLINE FRONTAL MENINGIOMA ARISING FROM THE FALX

In spite of the fact that this tumor arose from the falx, there is very little distortion of the branches of the callosomarginal artery and only a slight blunting of the curvature of the pericallosal artery. The position of the tumor is clearly shown by the abnormal vascularity. Other signs of frontal lobe tumor are present.

Convexity masses. The more anterior masses are frontoparietal (anterior supra-Sylvian) and the more posterior ones are parietal (posterior supra-Sylvian). These two groups are distinctly separable. Attention is called to the fact that radiographic projection in the lateral view causes the mid-portion of the convexity to project near the top of the skull (fig. 432).

Frontoparietal convexity masses have the characteristic features listed below.

1. *Spreading* of the opercular arteries is usually accompanied by loss of undulations. It indicates that the sulci in this region have been spread apart by tumor infiltration or by edema (figs. 433, 419, and 420).

2. Depression of the upper boundary of the Sylvian triangle is common. As mentioned under "Anatomy," and explained in Figure 375, in normal cases the upper margin of the Sylvian triangle is fairly regular in configuration when it is clearly visible. Although in normal cases, one vessel may sometimes be lower or higher in position than the one anterior or posterior to it, it is uncommon to see two or more adjacent

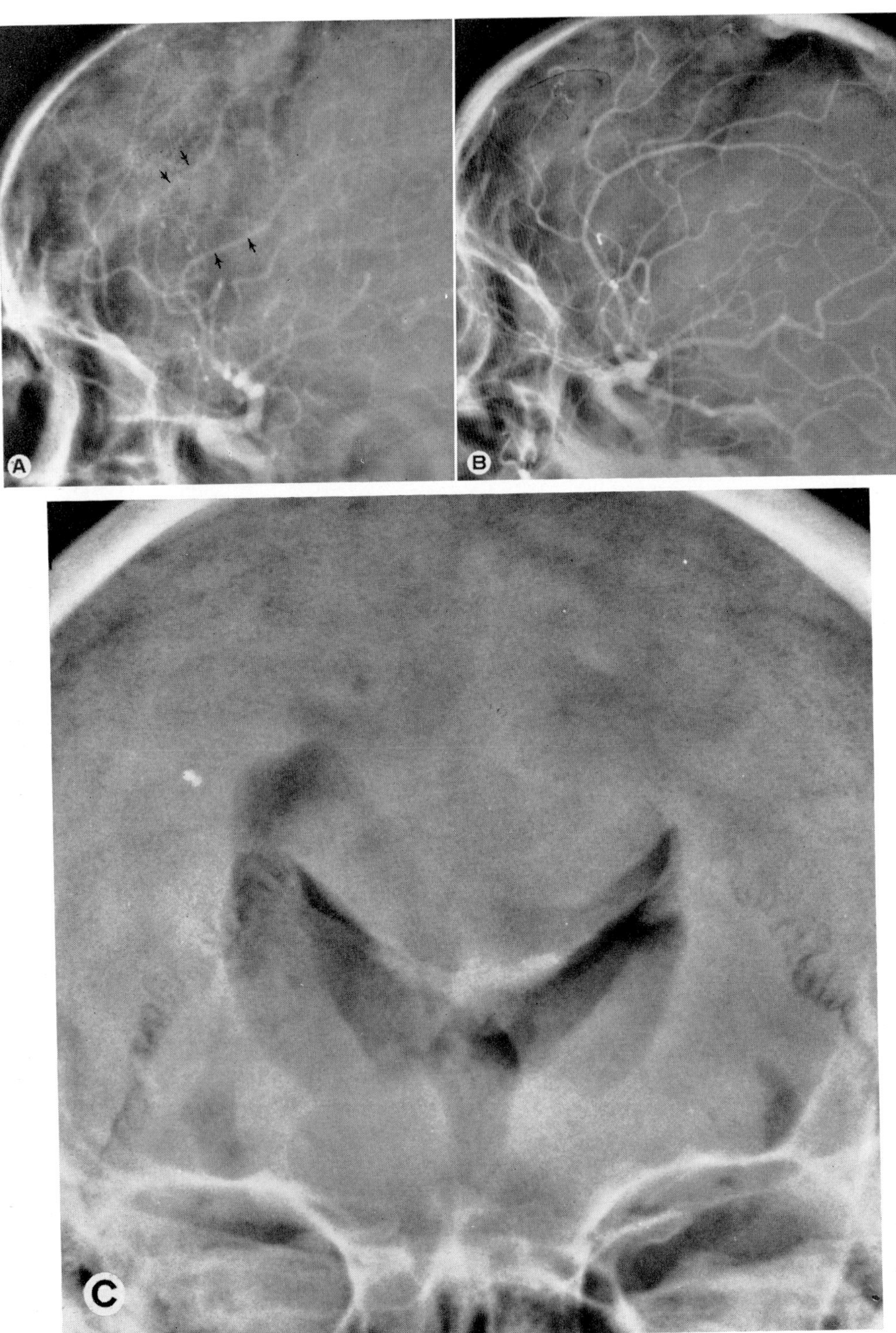

Fig. 430

(*Revised 1963*)

arteries vary in this way. The convexity tumors tend to bow downward the upper margin of the Sylvian triangle, particularly those lesions involving primarily the operculum (figs. 419B, 420, and 433C).

3. Depression of the proximal portion of the major branches of the middle cerebral artery, as seen in the lateral view, is commonly present, depending on the size of the mass (fig. 420).

4. Medial displacement of the more anteriorly situated opercular arteries often occurs before they turn around the lower margin of the operculum (fig. 434). This is more apparent when it can be compared with the opposite normal side.

5. If the tumor is accompanied by edema extending backward into the parietal region or if it is large enough, there may be depression of the angiographic Sylvian point (fig. 435); otherwise the frontoparietal masses are situated in front of this point and do not displace it downward significantly.

6. There is usually displacement of the internal cerebral vein across the midline and, in addition, it may be displaced downward with the high convexity tumors. The thalamostriate vein is displaced medially or medially and downward. The basilar vein is displaced medially and downward.

Parietal convexity masses characteristically displace the angiographic Sylvian point downward. Downward displacement may be recognized by measurement on the frontal film, as explained under "Anatomy" (p. 1.517). If this point measures more than 1.0 cm. below the center of the distance from the midline convexity inner table to the upper margin of the orbit or petrous pyramid (whichever is lower), it may be considered as displaced downward (fig. 410). Sometimes downward displacement may be easily ascertained by comparing it with the opposite normal side and an anteroposterior view with compression of the opposite side often is helpful (fig. 436). The downward displacement of the angiographic Sylvian point causes the artery marking its position to ascend obliquely upward and outward if the center of the tumor is some distance under the surface or if it is in the high convexity or parasagittal region (figs. 436 and 412). If the tumor is more superficial, it may cause the angiographic Sylvian point and the emerging branches to be equally displaced downward (fig. 435).

Medial displacement of the angiographic Sylvian point is common; see under "Anatomy" for normal measurements. The latter indicates either that the tumor is superficial or that it is causing edema of the operculum (fig. 436). If the tumor extends even deeper, the Sylvian vessels may be displaced laterally, toward the inner table of the skull (fig. 437).

There may be stretching and bowing of the branches of the middle cerebral artery in the region of the tumor (fig. 435). Spreading of the arteries, which also often is present, is difficult to ascertain in this region due to the great variability in the configuration of these vessels in normal subjects.

The posterior cerebral artery and its branches are usually displaced down and medially by posterior supra-Sylvian tumors (fig. 438).

The internal cerebral vein is almost always displaced across the midline by parietal masses; the anterior cerebral artery is not shifted across the midline in some cases, although in the majority of cases it is shifted. However, *the vein is usually more displaced than the artery.* The posterior half of the

Fig. 430.—Midline Frontal Tumor, Intracerebral

The lateral view of the left side (A) shows depression of the pericallosal artery (*arrows*) which is separated from the callosomarginal artery (*upper arrows*). An angiogram of the opposite side (B) shows that the pericallosal artery is rounded in configuration and elevated. This indicates that on the left side, the tumor is situated in the cingulate gyrus and has separated the pericallosal from the callosomarginal artery, but it grows into the corpus callosum and elevates the right pericallosal artery. It is evident that the right and left pericallosal arteries have been split apart by the neoplasm or else, if the two arteries were together, they would probably be affected in the same manner. A pneumoencephalogram (C) shows the position of the tumor in relation to the lateral ventricles.

(Revised 1963)

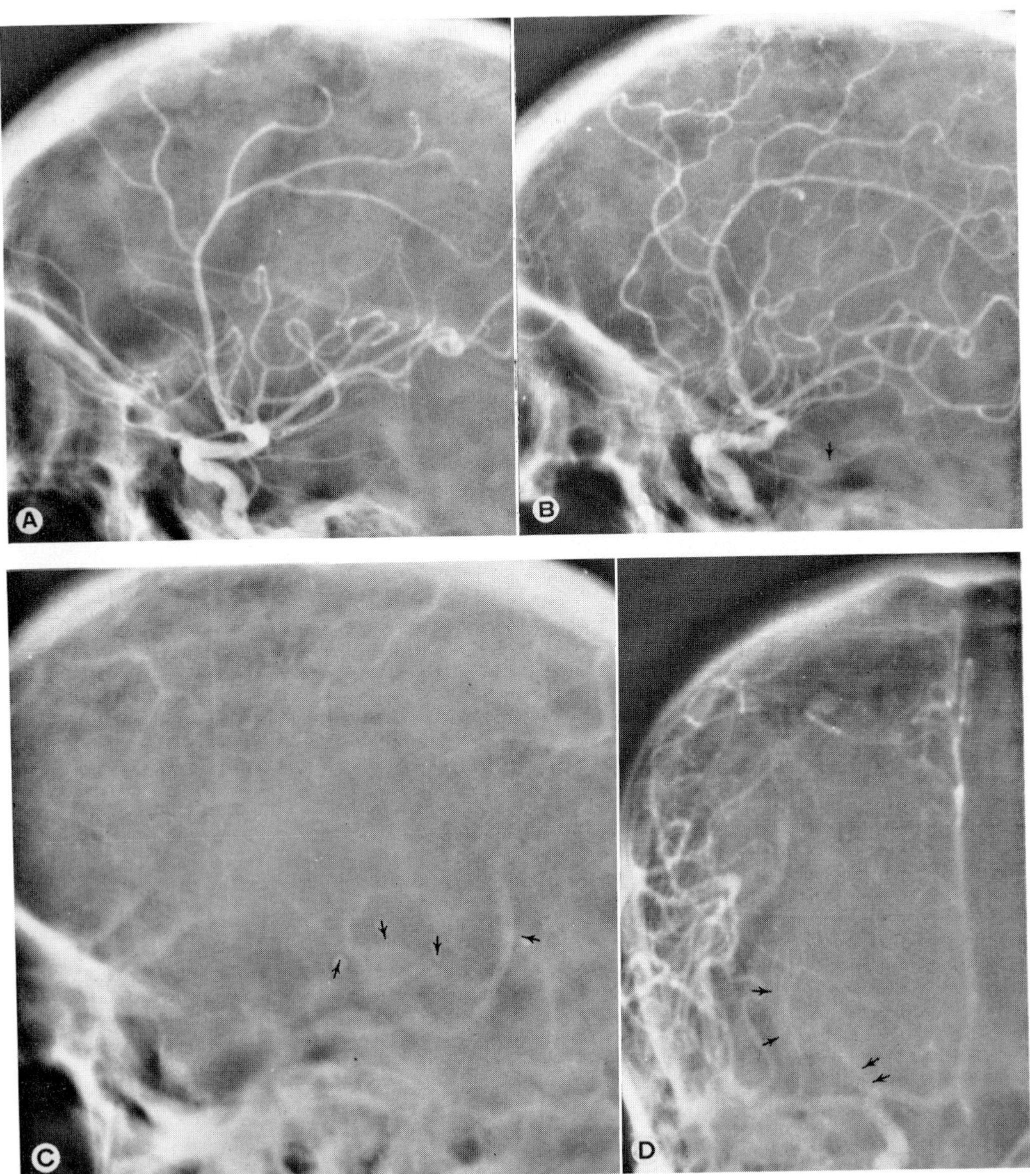

FIG. 431.—BIFRONTAL INTRACEREBRAL NEOPLASM (BUTTERFLY TUMOR)

The lateral views of both the right and the left sides ((A) and (B)) show blunting of the curve of the pericallosal artery and posterior displacement of the bifurcation of the internal carotid artery with closing of the siphon on both sides. There is downward displacement of the horizontal portion of the middle cerebral artery. The anterior chorioidal arteries are slightly stretched, and on one side the artery is displaced downward (*arrow*). The lateral view of the venous phase (C) shows marked downward and posterior displacement of the internal cerebral vein and of the venous angle as well as of the basilar vein, which indicates a high degree of transtentorial downward herniation. The vein of Galen is vertical in position (*posterior arrow*). The venous phase was similar on both sides, and only one side is shown. In the frontal projection (D) there was no evidence of midline shift of the anterior cerebral vessels, indicating that the tumor is situated in both frontal lobes, and in these cases, it always involves the corpus callosum. The tumor must have been very bulky as judged by the herniation demonstrated in (C). There

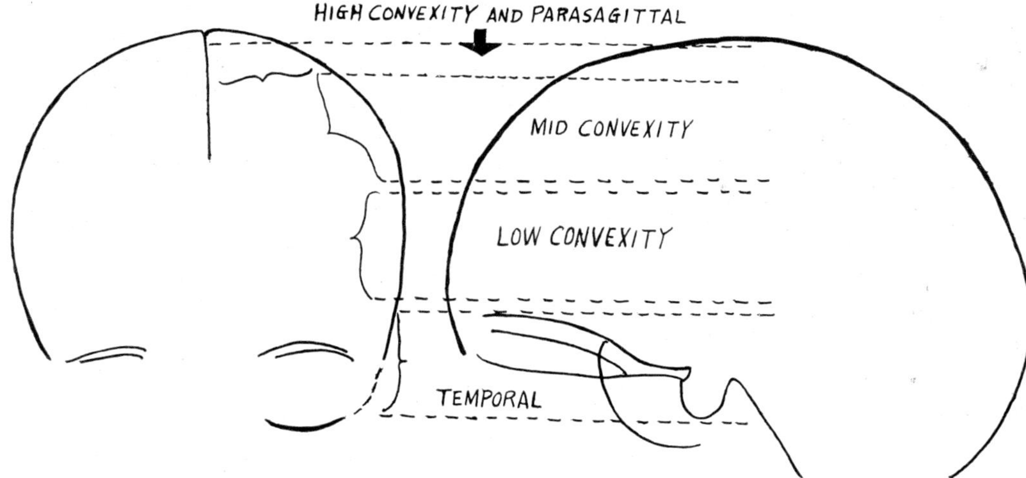

FIG. 432.—EFFECT OF PROJECTION ON THE APPARENT POSITION OF A TUMOR IN THE LATERAL VIEW IN RELATION TO THE CORONAL SECTION OF THE SKULL

The midconvexity of the skull actually projects very high in the lateral view, and it is not uncommon to call a tumor parasagittal in location because in the lateral view it projects very high. This emphasizes the importance of considering the curvature of the skull at all times when planning surgical flaps.

curve of the internal cerebral vein may be flattened; sometimes the entire curve of the vein is flat. The degree of flattening is dependent on the position of the tumor. The higher the tumor is in the convexity of the brain, the greater the chances of producing significant flattening of the vein. Parietal parasagittal tumors produce the greatest degree of flattening, as might be expected, but this again is related to the size of the mass. Invasion of the corpus callosum is frequent in parietal gliomas, and this also produces flattening of the internal cerebral vein (fig. 437).

The thalamostriate vein may be unchanged in position. If the internal cerebral vein is flattened, the venous angle between the thalamostriate and the internal cerebral vein, as seen in the lateral view, is widened (fig. 437). The basilar vein is displaced downward and medially to a degree dependent on the size of the mass and accompanying edema.

Parasagittal masses. The diagnosis of parasagittal tumors by angiography may be difficult. The difficulties are mostly related to the anatomy of the region. In the first place, the normal pericallosal artery often presents a downward curve or depression in its course which is an anatomic variant (fig. 366). Second, the branches of the middle cerebral artery become progressively attenuated as they ascend to this region and do not have a reliable, relatively constant configuration. Third, the branches of the pericallosal and callosomarginal arteries are of sufficient size, but they are situated on the inner surface of the hemisphere, against the falx, and cannot be displaced significantly by small tumors. Another factor is the absence of any vascular structure posteriorly, 2 to 3 cm. lateral to the midline where the center of the tumor is often located. (More anteriorly, the thalamostriate vein serves this purpose.) On the other hand, the roof of the lateral ventricle is in a very favorable

---

is enlargement of the lenticulostriate arteries which are also stretched (*arrows*) and have lost their usual slightly irregular curves. The anterior chorioidal artery is displaced laterally and its normal curve has changed. The appearance indicates an associated central transtentorial herniation which is seen in midline tumors and large masses within the 3d ventricle. In these cases, the medial portions of the temporal lobes are pushed laterally.

(Revised 1963)

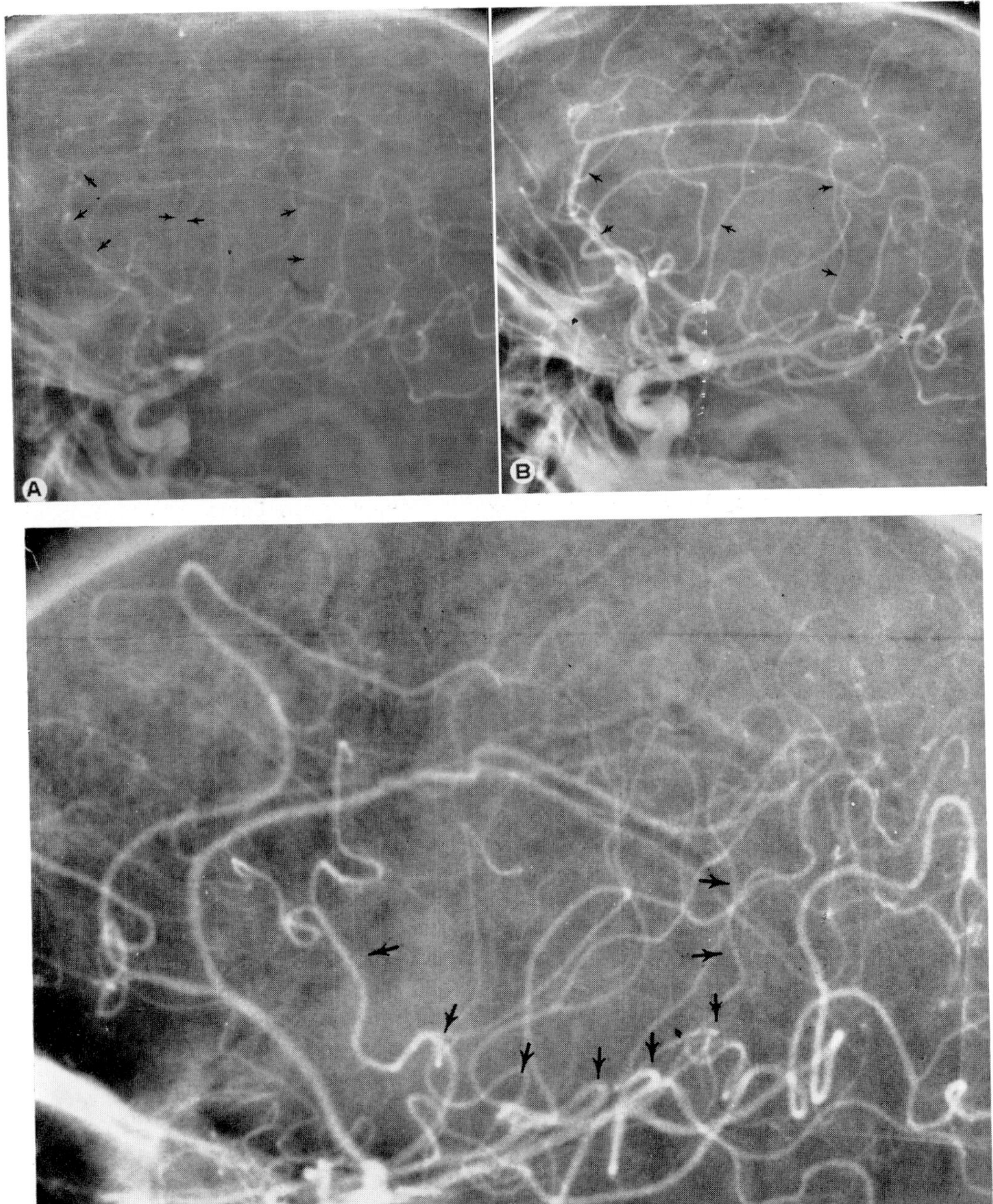

Fig. 433.—Anterior Supra-Sylvian (Frontoparietal) Intracerebral Tumor

The lateral view of the initial examination (A) shows that there is spreading of the branches of the middle cerebral arteries over the frontoparietal operculum. The Sylvian triangle is not significantly deformed but there is spreading with some virtually straight arteries (*arrows*) presumably in or near the

(*Revised 1963*)

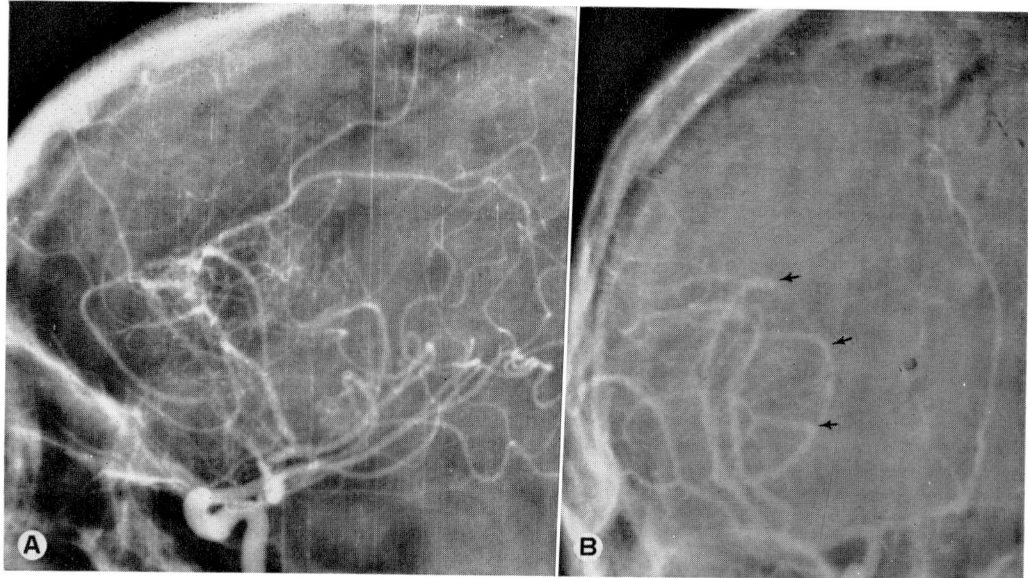

Fig. 434.—Posterior Frontal Opercular Tumor (Anterior Supra-Sylvian)

There is disruption of the anterior aspect of the Sylvian triangle as seen in the lateral view (A). There is downward displacement and bowing of the anterior portion of the branches of the middle cerebral artery. The frontal projection (B) shows medial displacement of the opercular branches of the middle cerebral artery without disturbing the more posterior branches which describe their normal curve around the insula. The angiographic Sylvian point is in normal position (*upper arrow*).

position to reflect local pressure and generally shows deformity on pneumography at an earlier stage of tumor development than it does on arteriography. This is not to say that parasagittal tumors cannot be diagnosed by angiography; on the contrary the majority can be diagnosed, and a good number of them may present abnormal vascularity, even though they do not produce characteristic vascular displacements (fig. 524). Angiography is often helpful in determining the type of tumor, whether intra- or extracerebral, and in this respect it may be superior to pneumography. Several angiographic changes may be observed.

1. Depression of the pericallosal artery, both its presence and degree, depends upon the position and the size of the tumor. If the tumor is over the convexity, it may only produce a midline shift without depression, and a small tumor will usually produce no appreciable depression.

2. Localized lateral shift of the pericallosal artery is always posterior, or at least

center of the disturbance, and bowing of branches in front and in back of the straight ones, presumably at the periphery of the mass lesion (*arrows*). Because of the absence of midline shift (the anteroposterior views are not shown here), the diagnosis of a mass lesion was not considered as sufficiently secure. Reexamination was performed five months later and at that time, there was no significant change in the appearance of the vessels in the lateral view (B). Exactly the same stretched vessels were seen, and bowing of the vessels anterior and posterior to it was again noted. The Sylvian triangle was now slightly flattened and irregular when compared with (A). In the frontal projection (not shown here) there was now a moderate shift of the anterior cerebral vessels and of the internal cerebral vein which was not present previously.

(C) represents an anterior supra-Sylvian mass in another case, which is causing bowing of the upper boundaries of the Sylvian triangle (*arrows*). The Sylvian triangle is also too low in its vertical dimension anteriorly. There is evidence of spreading, of straightening, and of bowing, without complete loss of undulations, of two arteries, one in front and one behind the center of the disturbance (*horizontal arrows*).

(*Revised 1963*)

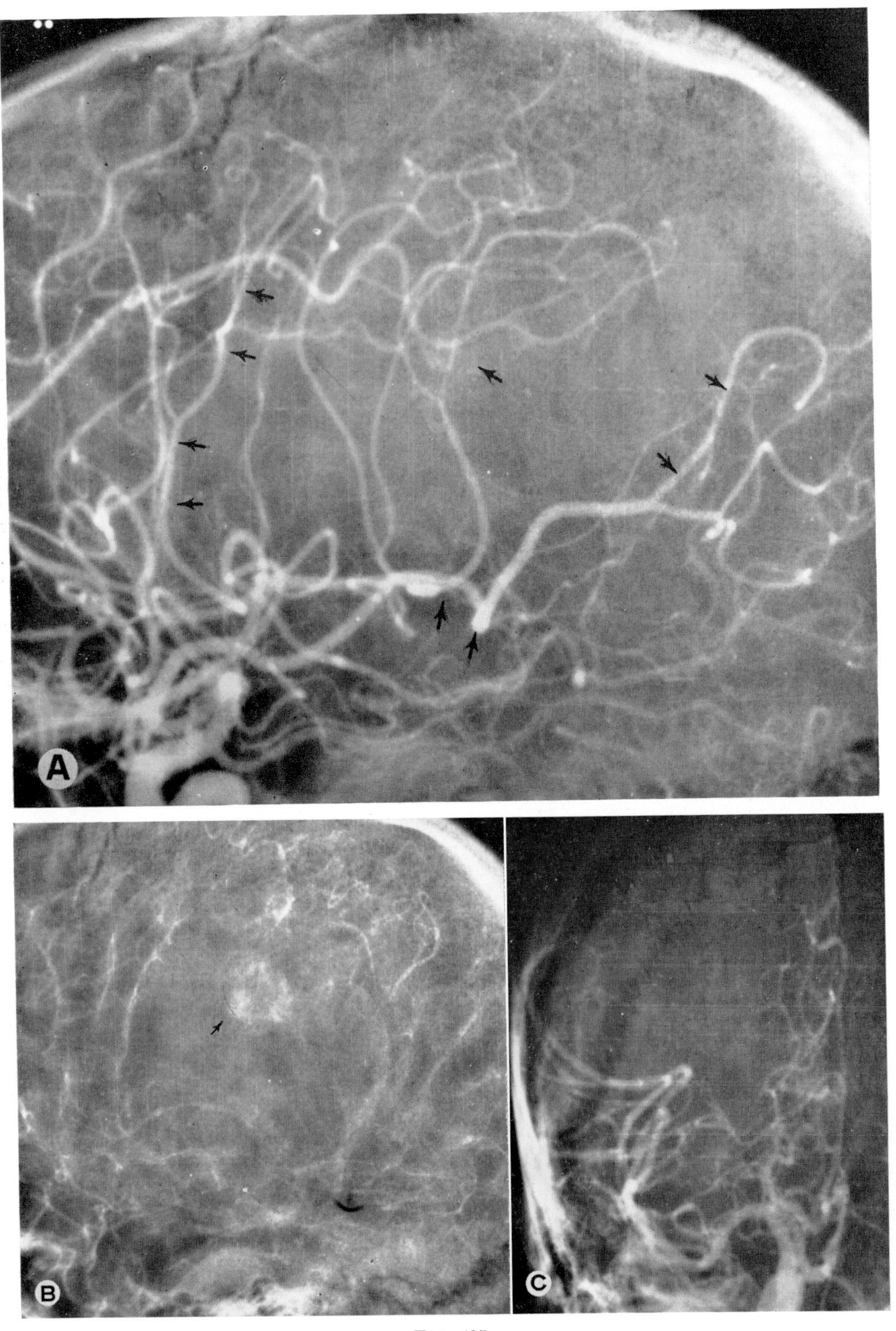

FIG. 435

(Revised 1963)

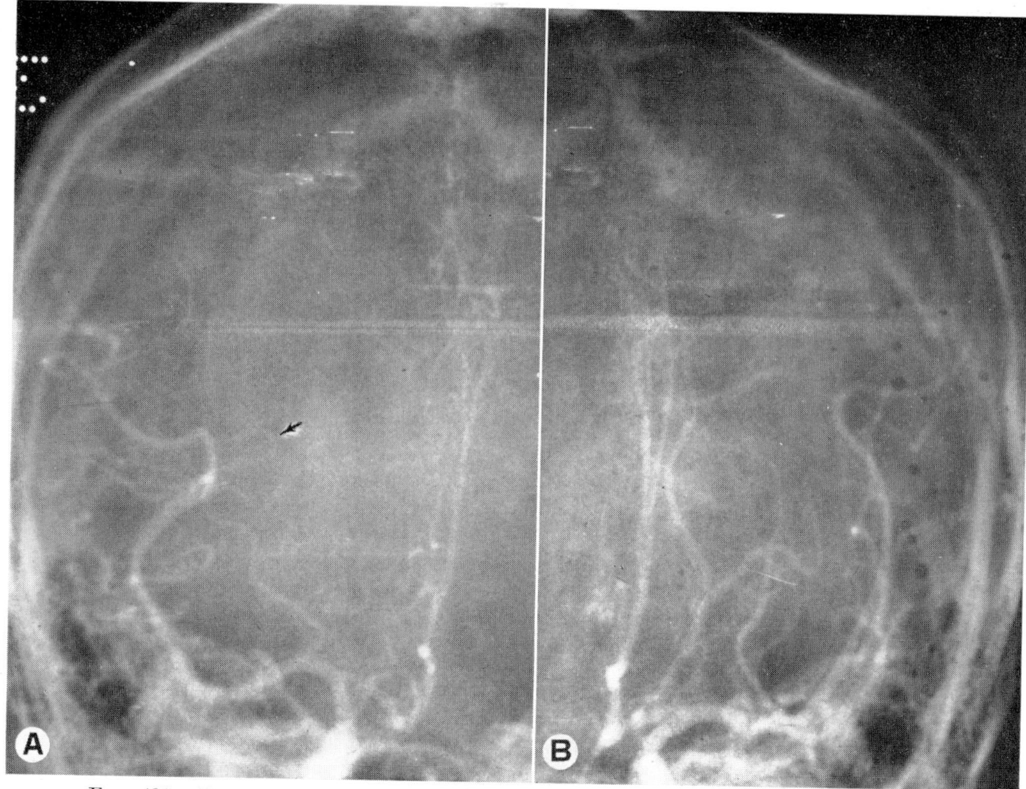

FIG. 436.—DOWNWARD DISPLACEMENT OF THE ANGIOGRAPHIC SYLVIAN POINT DUE TO A PARIETAL TUMOR

On the side of the tumor there is downward displacement of the Sylvian point (*arrow*), which is also displaced medially. From its depressed position, the branches emerge from the Sylvian fissure obliquely upward and outward; the vessels are directed upward much more so than on the opposite (normal) side (B). There is only distal, subfalcial shift because the tumor was situated in the upper half of the hemisphere.

more pronounced posteriorly; that is, it involves the upper or distal portion of the anterior cerebral artery as seen in the anteroposterior view (fig. 439). Sometimes, this midline shift is very inconspicuous; the pericallosal artery is seen to cross the midline and return almost immediately to the side of the mass, making a short horizontal "V"

FIG. 435.—SUPRA-SYLVIAN (ANTERIOR PARIETAL) CYSTIC ASTROCYTOMA

The center of the tumor is situated at the frontoparietal junction or a little behind it. In the lateral arteriogram (A), there is stretching and spreading of the vessels in the frontoparietal operculum. The vessels near the center of the tumor, the nodular center of which is outlined by "capillary blush," are relatively straight, whereas on the anterior aspect of the tumor, bowing of a vessel at a fairly wide distance from the center is present (*anterior arrows*). On the posterior aspect, it is always more difficult to detect with certainty the posterior margin of the disturbance because of the irregular distribution of the vessels in this region. However, the posterior arrows also indicate a loss of undulations of the main branch of the middle cerebral artery with bowing, and this probably indicates the posterior margin of the mass. Bowing, however, in this area, is often present in normal cases. There is downward displacement of the Sylvian point (*lower arrows*) and of the posterior portion of the Sylvian triangle. The intermediate phase (B) shows the exact size of the mass represented by the area of relative avascularity. The frontal projection (C) shows a straight downward displacement of the angiographic Sylvian point and emerging middle cerebral branches. This points to a superficial position of the center of the tumor. Compare with Fig. 436A. The astrocytoma nodule persisted into the end of the venous phase and was homogeneous.

(Revised 1963)

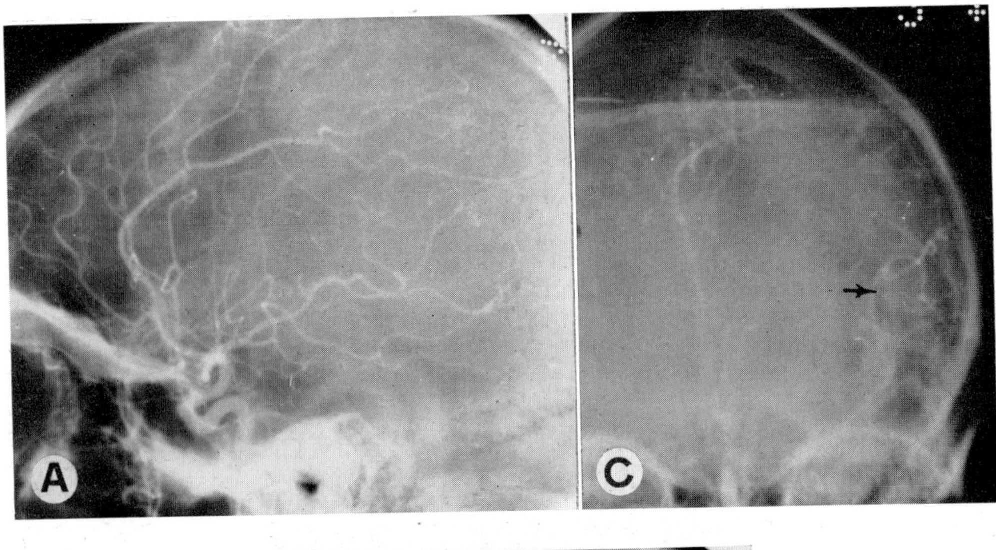

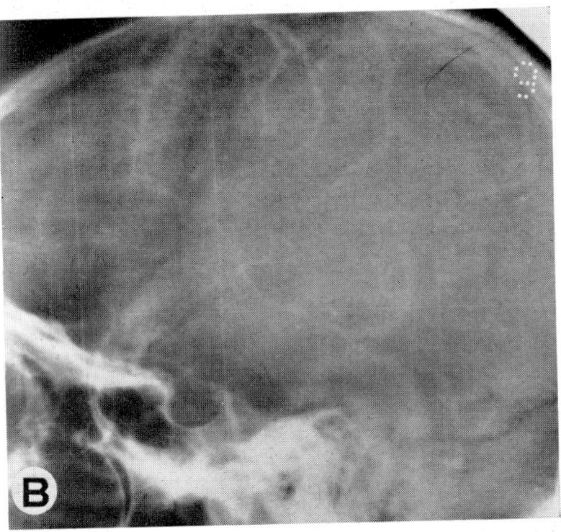

Fig. 437.—Parietal Tumor (Posterior Supra-Sylvian)

The lateral view (A) shows no obvious abnormalities except for the elevation of the pericallosal artery. There is actually spreading of the vessels in the parietal region, but this is difficult to ascertain, as explained in the text. The venous phase (B) shows marked depression of the internal cerebral vein, which causes apparent widening of the venous angle. The frontal projection (C) shows that there is displacement of the anterior cerebral vessels across the midline in its distal portion, which indicates that the tumor is situated in the upper half of the hemisphere. The Sylvian point is displaced laterally (*arrow*). The lateral displacement of the Sylvian point indicates that there is deep extension of this tumor, and the marked flattening of the internal cerebral vein with elevation of the pericallosal artery most probably indicates that the tumor has extended into the corpus callosum.

that must be looked for carefully (fig. 440). At other times these tumors cause a pronounced shift with complete herniation of the cingulate gyrus (fig. 412). See under "Cerebral Herniations" for greater detail.

3. Spreading and distortion of the upper portion of the middle cerebral artery branches, as mentioned above, is often difficult to discern because the arterial branches taper as they ascend. Sometimes the vessels may be stretched and generally deranged in their relationship with one another (figs. 437 and 438), but at others, no appreciable abnormality of these vessels can be detected.

(Revised 1963)

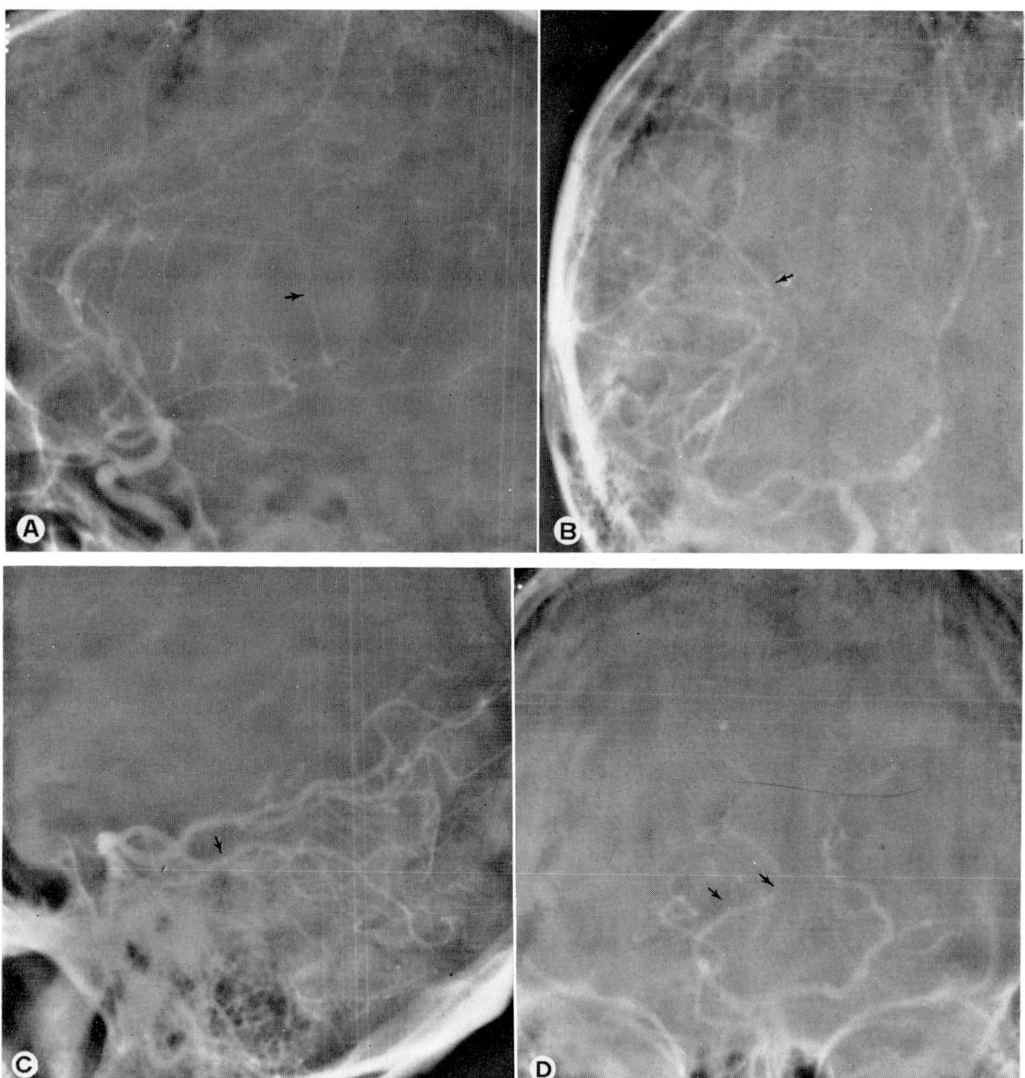

FIG. 438.—SUPRA-SYLVIAN TUMOR CAUSING DEPRESSION AND MEDIAL DISPLACEMENT OF THE POSTERIOR CEREBRAL ARTERY

The lateral view (A) shows stretching and spreading of the branches of the middle cerebral artery. The straightened vessel at the arrow probably is at or near the center of the tumor. The frontal projection (B) shows a downward and medial displacement of the Sylvian point *(arrow)*. The distal (upper) portion of the anterior cerebral artery is displaced more than the proximal portion, which probably indicates extension to the upper portion of the hemisphere. A vertebral angiogram shows, in the lateral view (C), downward displacement of the posterior cerebral artery on the side of the tumor *(arrow)*. The downward displacement involves chiefly the posterior portion. In the frontal projection (D) there is medial displacement of the posterior cerebral artery in the posterior half of its curve around the midbrain *(arrows)*. This could be produced by a posterior herniation. The tumor was an extensive primary reticulum cell sarcoma; some pathologists classify the tumor as a microglioma.

4. Depression of the angiographic Sylvian point is an important sign of parietal parasagittal masses. It is present whenever the tumor has grown to appreciable size, or when there is sufficient edema of the adjacent brain even with small tumors (fig. 439).

5. Depression of the internal cerebral vein is characteristic of parasagittal tumors

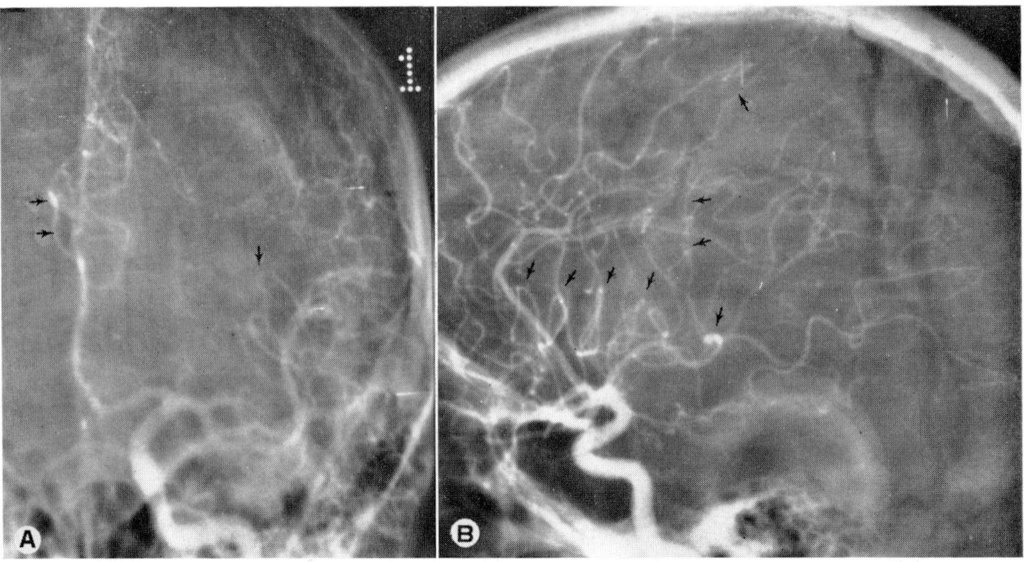

Fig. 439.—Parietal Parasagittal Meningioma

The frontal film shows a typical shift involving only the distal portion of the anterior cerebral artery (*arrows*). There is marked downward displacement of the angiographic Sylvian point. The lateral view (B) shows a slight bowing without loss of undulation of branches of both the anterior and the middle cerebral artery on the anterior aspect of the mass (*arrows*). The pericallosal artery, on the other hand, does not show any significant depression or deformity or, at least, a depression that may be unequivocally called pathological. The angiographic Sylvian point (*lower arrow*) is depressed, but the anterior portion of the Sylvian triangle is in normal position (*arrows*).

of perceivable size. The flattening may be more pronounced anteriorly or posteriorly, depending on the location of the center of the mass, or the entire vein may be depressed and its curvature flattened. The thalamostriate vein may be depressed in the more anteriorly located masses, termed closing of venous angle (figs. 442 and 524), but it may remain in normal position if the mass is more posterior. Parasagittal meningiomas may be attached to the bone adjacent to the midline, or they may arise from the junction of the falx and the superior longitudinal sinus with the meninges of the convexity of the calvaria. These meningiomas may, and often do, invade the wall of the superior longitudinal sinus and produce first a narrowing of the lumen of the sinus and, later, complete obstruction. In these cases the venous flow can be seen on the serialogram to be reversed; that is, it is caudad in direction in the frontal veins to reach the anastomotic venous systems on the surface of the brain in order to bypass the area of obstruction. Sometimes the blood will simply drain by way of the middle cerebral veins. At other times it enters the vein of Trolard and thence the superior longitudinal sinus, if the obstruction is in front of this vein. Sometimes the superior longitudinal sinus may be displaced downward without being obstructed. At other times the sinus is obstructed and can also be seen to be displaced downward by the meningioma (fig. 441).

In order to visualize the superior longitudinal sinus to better advantage on the angiogram, simultaneous frontal and lateral views are made with compression of the opposite carotid artery in the neck. At the same time a greater quantity of contrast substance (12 cc.) may be used. The anteroposterior projection is altered by rotating the head slightly to the side opposite the injection (10 to 15 degrees). This opens the curve of the superior longitudinal sinus and does not affect the quality of the frontal projection as

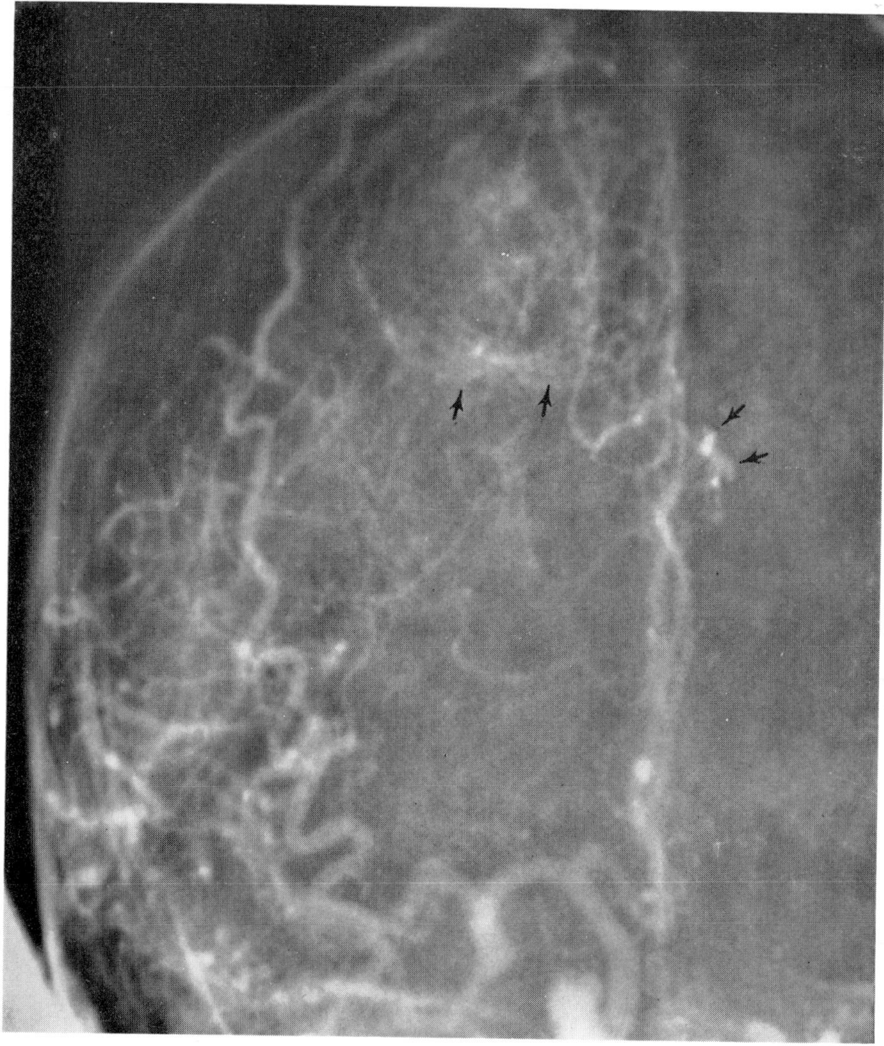

Fig. 440.—Parietal Parasagittal Tumor (Meningioma) Causing Only Slight Distal Shift
The anterior cerebral vessels are in the midline all the way through except for the small V-shaped shift under the falx (*arrows*). The position of the tumor in the parasagittal region, partly outlined by abnormal vascularity, can be seen (*arrows*). There is Pantopaque in the subarachnoid space from myelography performed prior to admission.

made for this particular purpose. A sinogram performed by injecting contrast substance into the anterior portion of the superior longitudinal sinus through a burr hole made in the frontal region is usually not necessary, although the radiographic contrast by this method is superior to that obtained by carotid angiography. We have not found it necessary to perform a sinogram to determine patency of the superior longitudinal sinus during the last few years.

(Revised 1963)

Midline supra-Sylvian masses. As in the case of midline anterior frontal masses, the supra-Sylvian tumors may arise from the falx or they may be intracerebral lesions. Meningiomas may arise from the lateral surface of the falx, in which case they displace the branches of the anterior cerebral

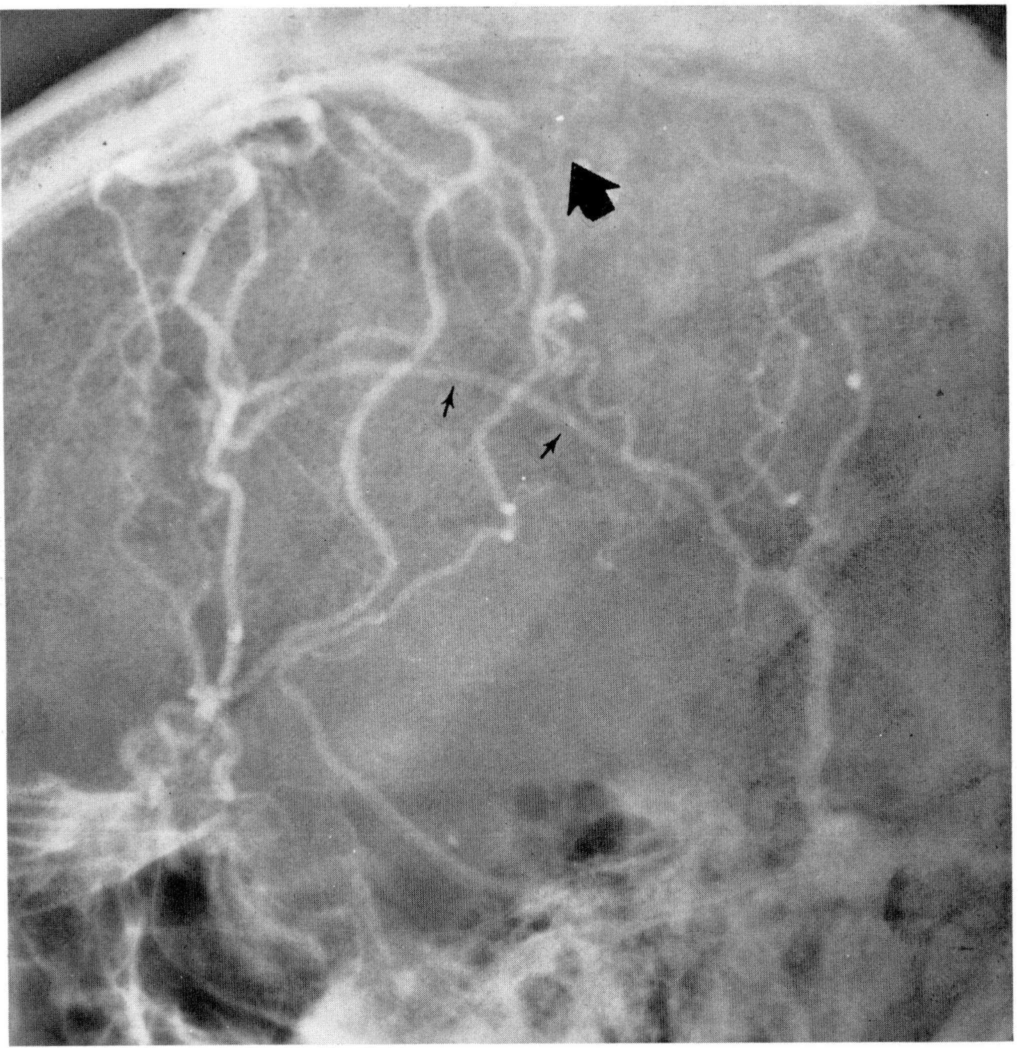

Fig. 441.—Supra-Sylvian Parasagittal Meningioma Producing a Block of Superior Longitudinal Sinus

A large meningioma was present in the parasagittal region which obstructed the superior longitudinal sinus and displaced it downward (*arrow*). The sinogram disclosed reversal of the venous flow which is draining toward the sphenoparietal sinus and to the lateral sinus via the anastomotic veins. The midline veins drain into the inferior longitudinal sinus (*arrows*) and the straight sinus. The obstructed segment is bypassed, and a parietal vein is seen to fill and drain again into the superior longitudinal sinus. With the passage of time, the anastomotic pathways develop, and it is possible surgically to remove the obstructed segment without any ontoward reactions, chiefly retrograde venous thromboses. On the other hand, before the sinus is completely obstructed, it is hazardous to perform surgical removal of the sinus.

artery in an arc away from the midline as seen in the frontal view (fig. 442). The arc described by the vessel does not necessarily indicate the size of the tumor; the vessel may be at or near one pole of the tumor, or the x-ray beam may not be perpendicular to the plane of the vessels (figs. 442 and 443). Bowing of the vessel in this manner is characteristic of falx meningiomas. If the tumor arises from the edge of the falx, it may grow

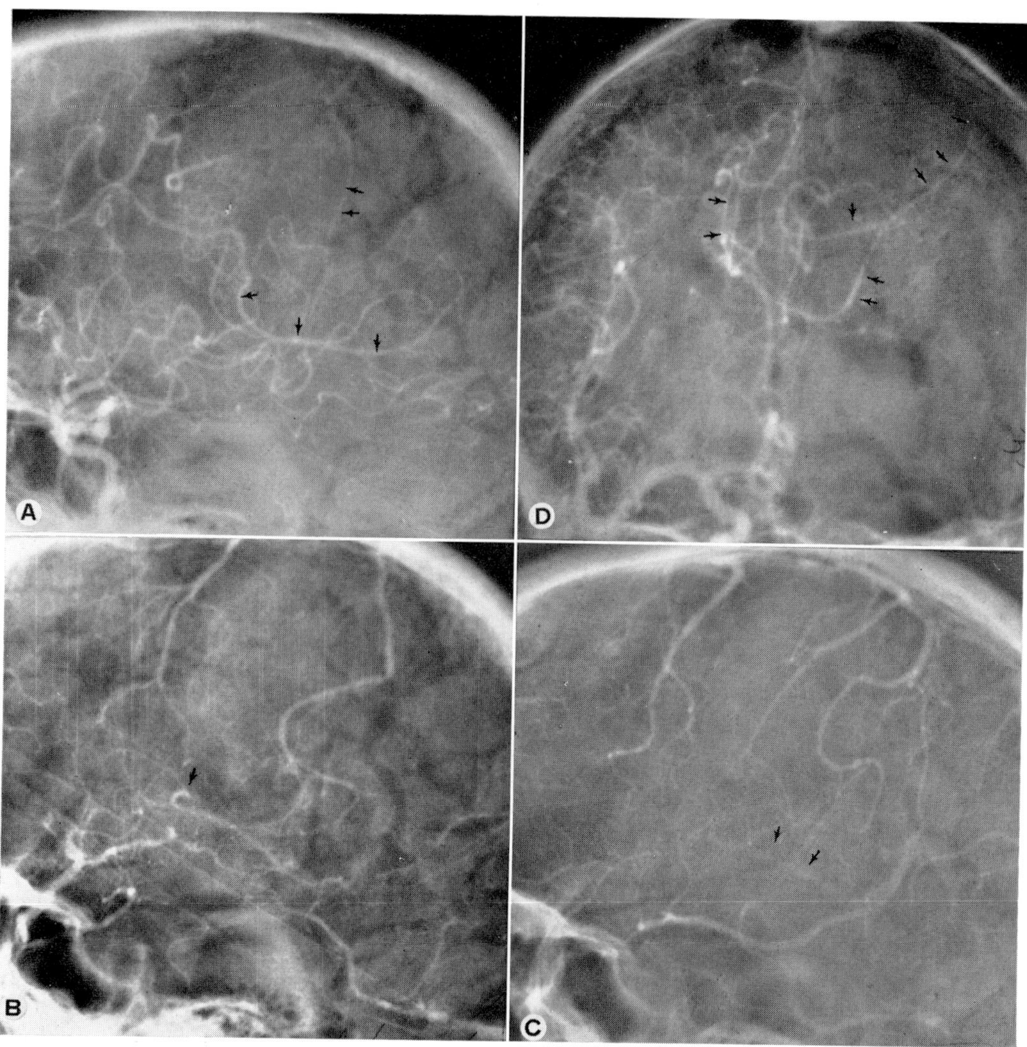

FIG. 442.—MIDLINE SUPRA-SYLVIAN TUMOR (FALX MENINGIOMA)

The lateral view (A) shows downward displacement of the posterior portion of the pericallosal artery (*arrows*). There is a meningeal arterial branch which becomes larger as it goes distally (*double arrow*). In the venous phase (B) there is flattening of the internal cerebral vein and closing of the venous angle due to downward displacement of the thalamostriate vein (*arrow*). The venous phase on the opposite side (C) reveals flattening of the internal cerebral vein, but there is relative widening of the venous angle because the thalamostriate vein is not depressed. The frontal projection film of the opposite side (D) demonstrates to better advantage, because of bilateral anterior cerebral artery filling, the lateral displacement of the callosomarginal artery branches which is pathognomonic of a midline mass. The rounded displacement of one of the arteries (*upper arrows*) is probably at or near the widest circumference of the tumor, and this is a reliable sign of midline (falx) meningioma. On the other hand, another artery (*lower arrows*) is not displaced as far laterally and does not describe a rounded curve. On the basis of this vessel, which is not situated near the greatest circumference of the tumor, an unequivocal diagnosis of midline rounded mass cannot be made since intracerebral tumors can produce a similar finding, provided that the vessel is situated deep in the cingulate sulcus. There is also some displacement away from the midline on the opposite side of the tumor (the side of the angiogram), indicating that the tumor mass is wrapped around the lower aspect of the falx and has a component on the other side.

(*Revised 1963*)

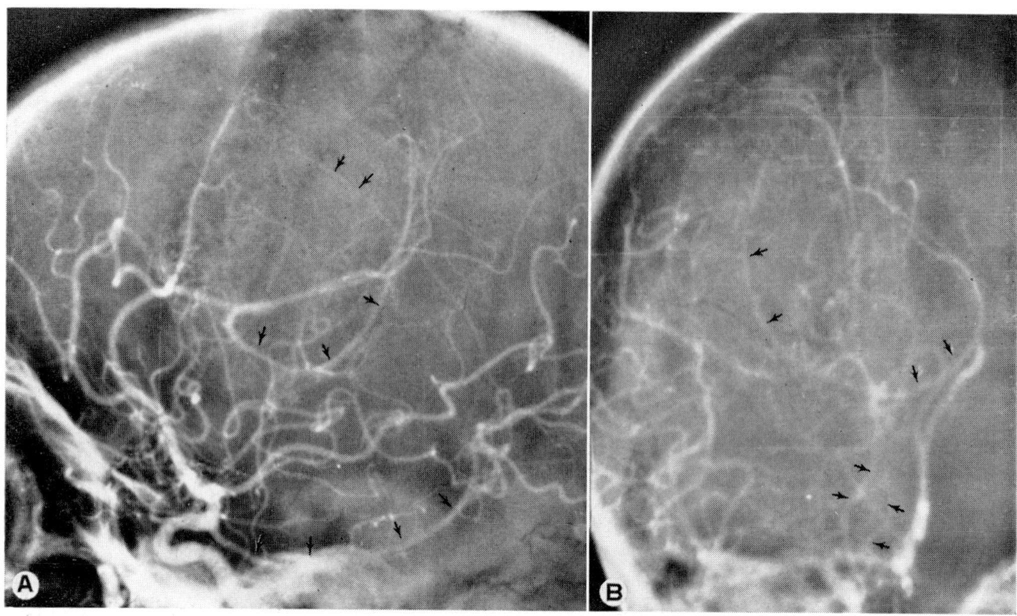

FIG. 443.—LARGE MIDLINE (FALX) MENINGIOMA IN THE SUPRA-SYLVIAN REGION

The lateral projection (A) shows a stretching and spreading of the branches of the pericallosal and callosomarginal arteries. There is depression of the pericallosal artery with one branch being markedly displaced downward (*arrows*). The same branch is seen to describe a semicircle in the frontal projection. A straight arterial branch (*upper arrows*) represents, most probably, a meningeal branch running along the edge of the falx which supplies the meningioma. An extreme degree of downward displacement of the posterior communicating and posterior cerebral arteries is seen indicating a complete downward herniation (*lower arrows*) with the typical step at the tentorial edge. The anteroposterior view (B) shows marked distal shift. The same artery that describes an arc in the lateral projection is seen in the frontal projection (*arrows*), which is typical of meningioma arising from the falx. The posterior cerebral artery is displaced medially, thus confirming the presence of complete downward herniation suspected from the lateral view (*lower arrows*). The anterior chorioidal is also medially displaced (*lower medial arrows*). The case emphasizes the importance of caution in performing pneumoencephalography in patients with supratentorial tumors. An unsuspected complete herniation was present in this case which would have possibly resulted in severe complications if a pneumoencephalogram performed without extreme care were carried out.

more to one side or the other, or it may be almost centered on the midline. These tumors produce early and pronounced downward displacement and bowing of the pericallosal artery (fig. 443), as well as outward displacement of the branches of the callosomarginal artery.

Subdural hematomas localized in this re-

FIG. 444.—PARASAGITTAL INTRACEREBRAL TUMORS SHARPLY CIRCUMSCRIBED

(A) There is a posterior frontal midline tumor which is sharply circumscribed by two branches of the callosomarginal artery (*arrows*). This is an unusual appearance for an intracerebral tumor, and an erroneous pre-operative diagnosis of meningioma was made in this case. Actually, the tumor was intracerebral, involving the region of the brain between these two vessels which were displaced concentrically because they were situated deep within sulci. There was exact correlation between the separated vessels and the gross specimen at autopsy in this instance. A certain degree of edema of the adjacent area is present, as evidenced by the slight downward displacement of branches of the Sylvian triangle and the slow filling of the opercular branches in the area outlined by the arrows. The delayed filling of local arteries is usually an indication of a neoplasm in the immediate neighborhood. No neoplasm was encountered in this region at autopsy. The photograph of the specimen taken at autopsy (B) shows the localized nature of the tumor, which was a glioblastoma, and the edema of the adjacent white matter.

(Revised 1963)

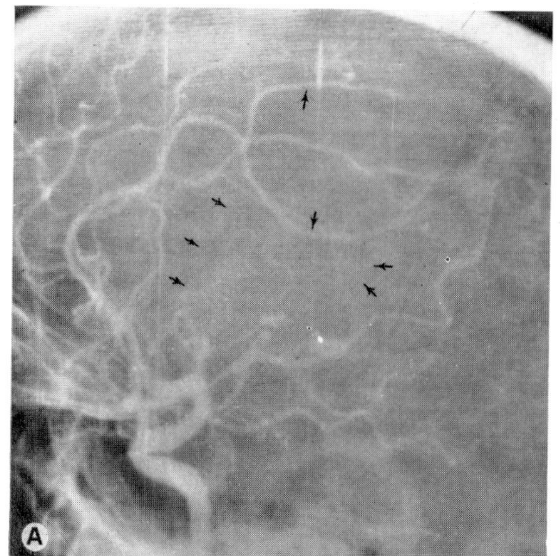

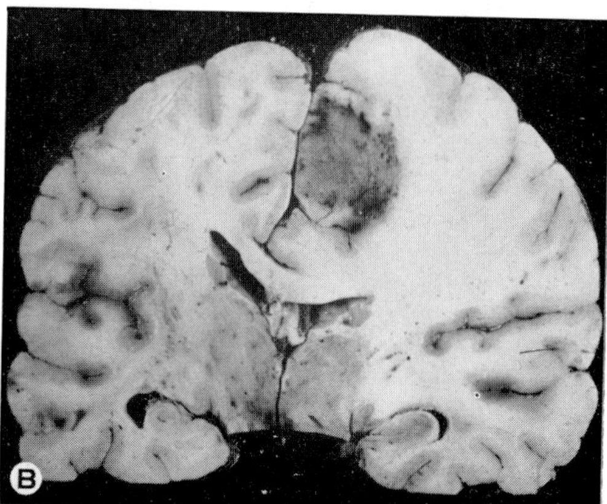

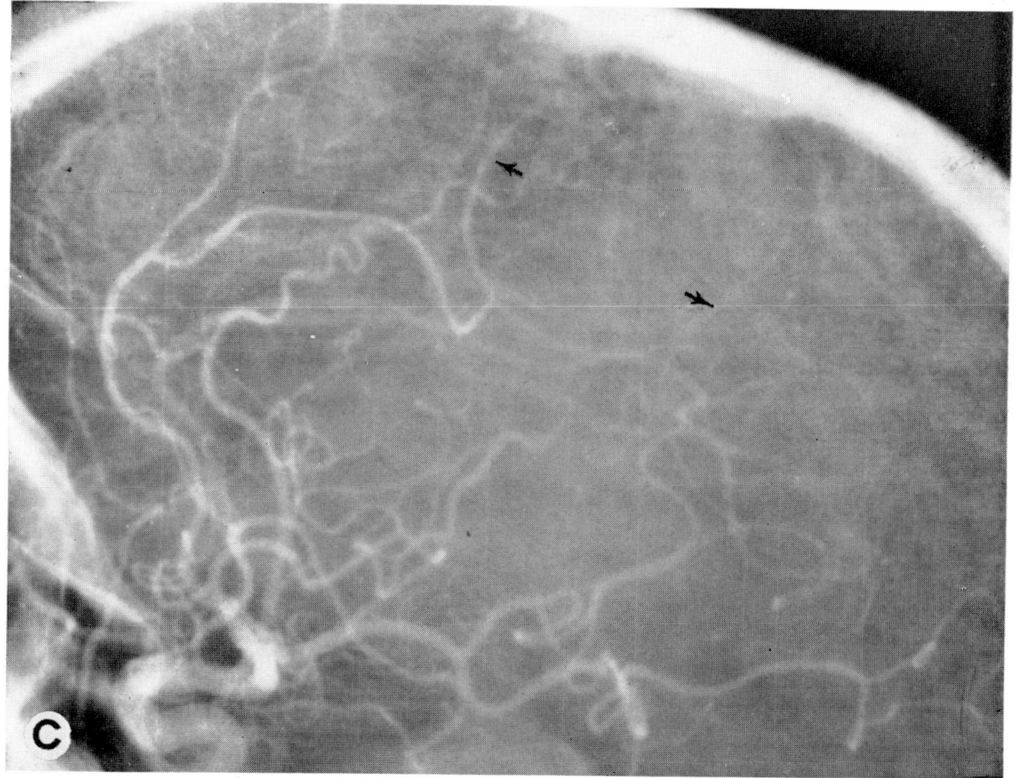

FIG. 444 (*Cont.*).—(C) WELL-CIRCUMSCRIBED FALX MENINGIOMA PRODUCING SHARP DISPLACEMENT OF THE MIDDLE AND POSTERIOR INTERNAL FRONTAL BRANCHES OF THE CALLOSOMARGINAL ARTERY (*arrows*)

This appearance should be compared with that noted in (A) because it would be difficult to differentiate this picture from the previous one. In fact, the diagnosis of meningioma must be made as the first choice in cases where such an appearance is observed.

(*Revised 1963*)

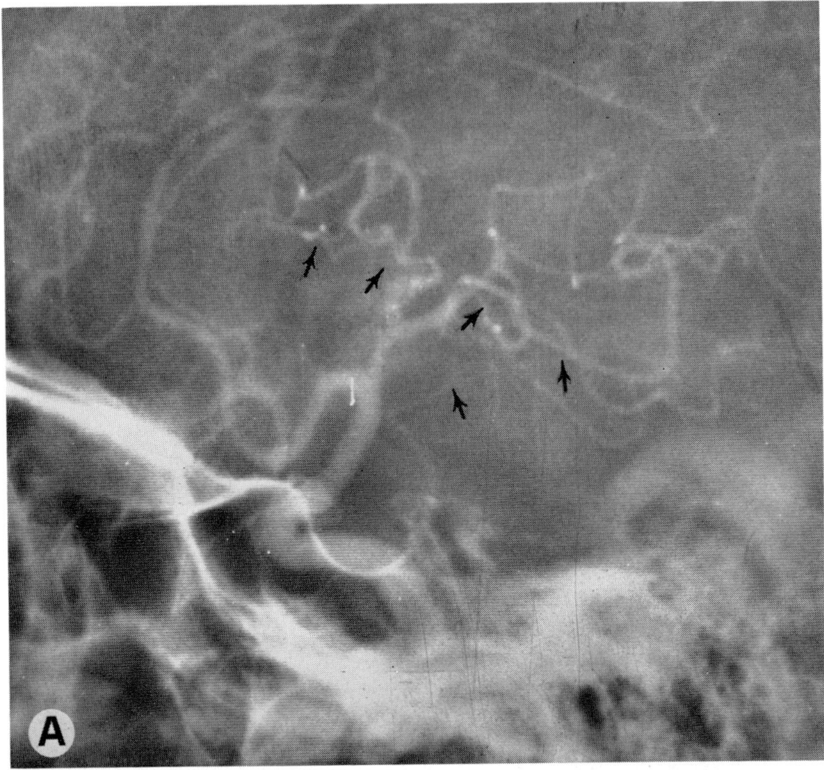

FIG. 445.—ANTERIOR TEMPORAL TUMOR (EPIDERMOID)

The lateral view (A) shows upward displacement of the anterior branches of the middle cerebral artery (*arrows*) which is causing complete disruption of the Sylvian triangle. There is marked elevation of the supraclinoid portion of the internal carotid artery with elevation of the bifurcation of this artery. The anterior chorioidal artery (*lower arrows*) is elevated and stretched. The frontal projection (B) discloses marked elevation of the horizontal portion of the middle cerebral artery, and medial displacement and stretching of the supraclinoid portion of the internal carotid artery with elevation of the bifurcation. There is only a slight shift of the anterior cerebral artery across the midline, with the proximal portion displaced to a greater extent. The anterior chorioidal artery is seen to describe a wide semicircle, and it is actually beyond the midline (*arrows*). This artery demarcates the medial extent of the tumor which was rather large. The midline shift is slight because the tumor was growing very slowly. It might be mentioned that all of the branches of the middle cerebral artery are elevated because the entire temporal lobe was elevated by the tumor situated under it.

gion are rare but may occur. As might be expected, they are situated between the falx and the inner surface of the hemisphere and therefore produce separation of the anterior cerebral artery branches and displacement from the midline. When associated with hematoma of the convexity, they may be overlooked at operation unless preoperative angiography has been preformed and the full extent of the lesion thus recognized (fig. 611). (See "Head Injuries and Their Complications.")

The intracerebral midline masses usually involve the cingulate gyrus which becomes wider, thus causing separation, stretching, and sometimes bowing of the pericallosal and the callosomarginal arteries (fig. 444). The vessels, particularly those that are deep in a sulcus, may be displaced away from the midline, due to edema of the adjacent gyrus, but not in a characteristic manner such as seen in falx meningiomas. It might be mentioned here that separation of the pericallosal and callosomarginal arteries does not

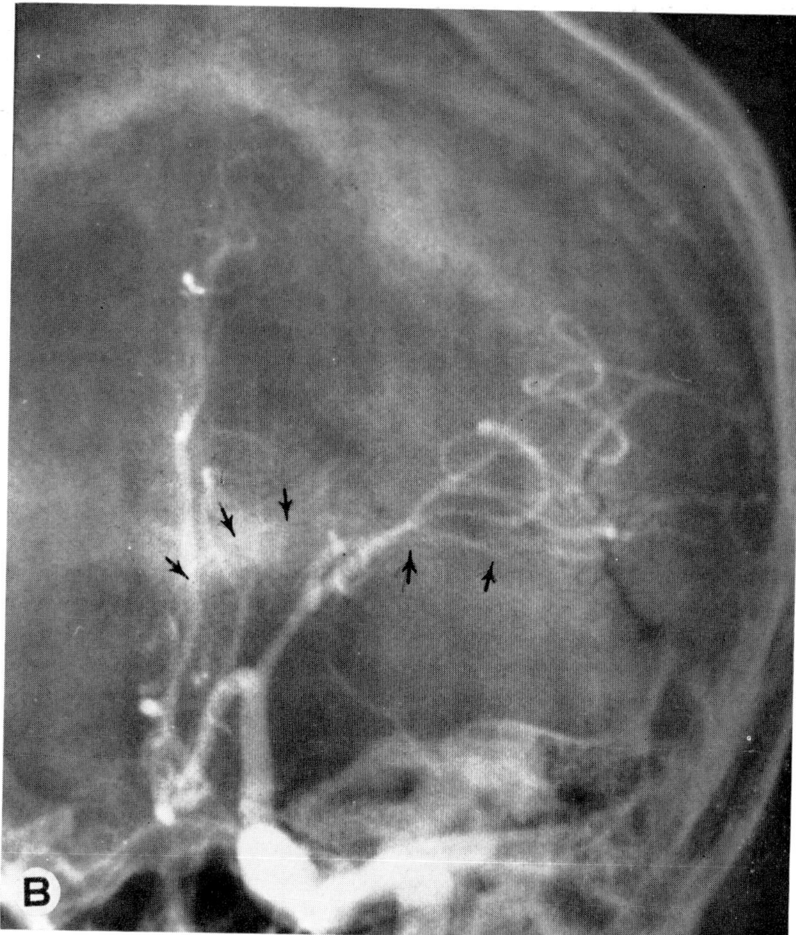

Fig. 445B

always mean tumor invading the cingulate gyrus; edema may also cause this to happen in some cases. In each instance, all of the findings should be noted first and their relative importance weighed before arriving at a definite conclusion. The internal cerebral and thalamostriate veins may be affected in a manner similar to the parasagittal masses.

Infra-Sylvian Tumors

Temporal tumors are among the best located for study by cerebral angiography. It is only infrequently that even a small infiltrating temporal tumor should go undetected by angiography.

In this group belong the temporal lobe intracerebral masses (neoplasm, hematoma, and abscess), and the temporal extracerebral masses, usually meningiomas arising from the sphenoid ridge or the floor of the middle fossa and temporal subdural hematomas. Sometimes a pituitary adenoma extends subtemporally, and a chordoma can grow mostly toward one side. Epidermoid tumors in the middle fossa are rare, but do occur; the same applies to 5th nerve neurinomas. In addition, "dumbbell" or "saddle" tumors centered at the tentorial incisura are partly infratentorial and partly subtemporal. These tumors are most commonly meningiomas attached (1) to the medial portion of the floor of the middle fossa, (2) to the tip of the petrous pyramid, and (3) to adjacent portions of the dorsum sellae and clivus. Evi-

(*Revised 1963*)

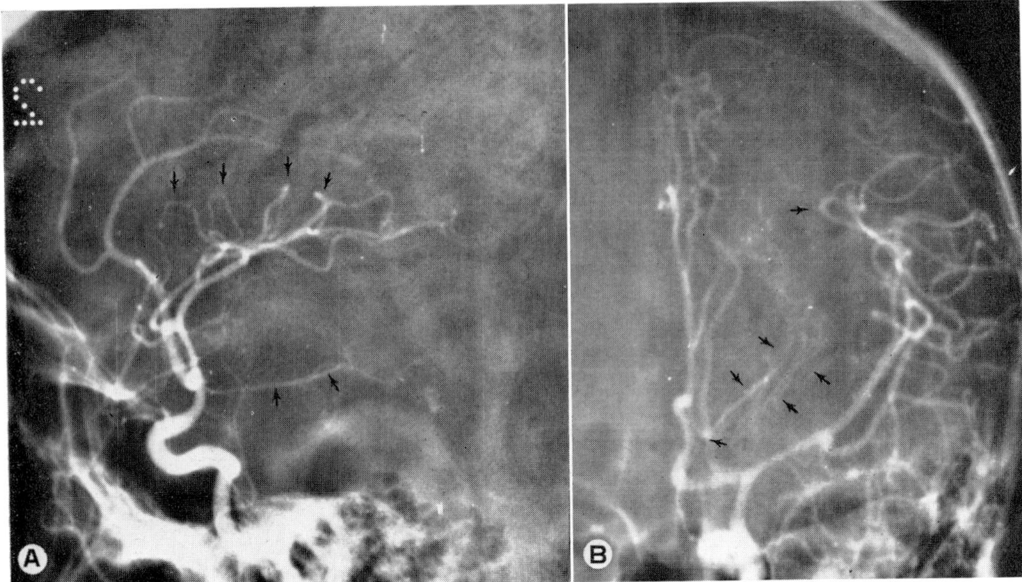

FIG. 446.—TEMPORAL TUMOR OCCUPYING THE ANTERIOR TWO-THIRDS OF THE TEMPORAL LOBE
The lateral view (A) shows marked elevation of the middle cerebral artery and its branches. The Sylvian triangle is markedly elevated (*arrows*). The supraclinoid portion of the carotid siphon is slightly elevated and displaced forward. The anterior chorioidal artery is enlarged (*arrows*). The frontal projection (B) shows elevation of the horizontal portion of the middle cerebral artery and slight elevation of the angiographic Sylvian point (*upper arrow*). There is medial displacement of the lenticulostriate arteries and of the anterior chorioidal artery (*arrows*). There is only a slight degree of midline shift involving the distal and proximal portion of the middle cerebral artery with the central portion of the vessel returning to the midline.

dence of isolated or multiple areas of attachment may be found. Trigeminal nerve neurinomas and some chordomas also may be included in this group of "saddle" tumors.

Temporal masses produce vascular displacement patterns that are dependent upon their site of origin within the middle fossa as well as their location and size. Therefore, it is advantageous to subdivide them, from the point of view of diagnosis, according to the portion of the temporal area in which they arise. They may be (1) anterior temporal (those involving the anterior half of the temporal lobe), (2) posterior temporal (masses located here tend to blend with the retro-Sylvian group), (3) deep temporal (medial), or may be (4) infiltrating neoplasms, or (5) extracerebral masses.

General manifestations. The common features of infra-Sylvian tumors may be listed as shown below.

1. The most characteristic and, statistically, the most common finding in temporal tumors is elevation of the middle cerebral artery and its branches (figs. 445–454).

2. The middle cerebral branches may be displaced medially, away from the inner table (figs. 448 and 450).

3. The supraclinoid portion of the internal carotid artery is displaced medially and its bifurcation often is elevated (figs. 445 and 453). "Opening of the siphon" is a term used to describe elevation of the supraclinoid portion of the internal carotid artery, but this appearance is not identical with that of intrasellar tumors which produce "true" opening of the siphon (fig. 485).

4. The anterior chorioidal artery usually is displaced medially and may also be displaced upward or downward (figs. 446, 448, and 453).

5. The basilar vein is displaced medially.

6. There is usually a midline shift of the internal cerebral vein and anterior cerebral

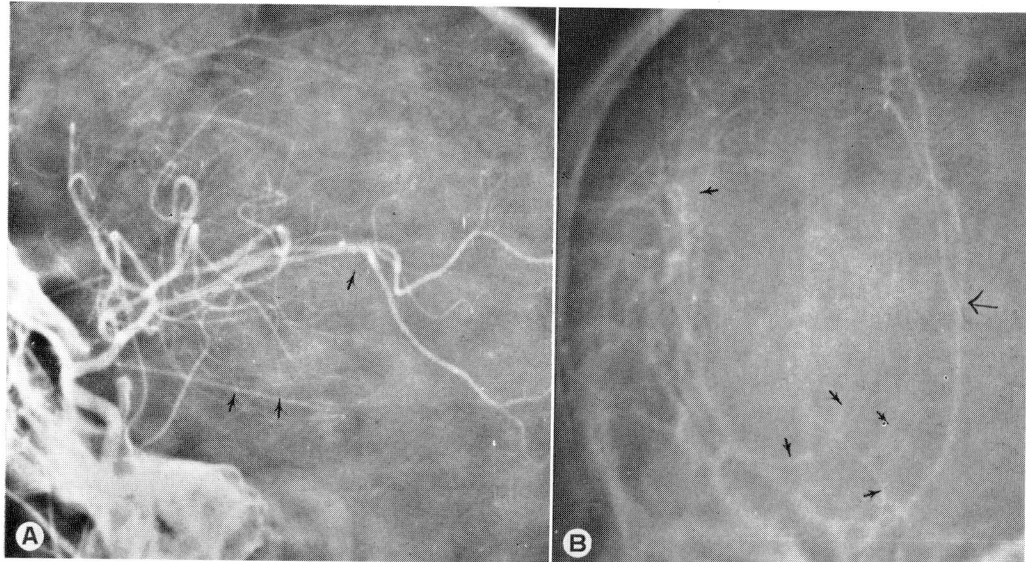

FIG. 447.—POSTERIOR TEMPORAL TUMOR CAUSING EDEMA OF THE ANTERIOR PORTION OF THE TEMPORAL LOBE

The lateral view (A) shows that the maximum displacement is posterior, under the angiographic Sylvian point (*arrow*). The posterior portion of the Sylvian triangle is slightly more elevated than the anterior portion. The anterior chorioidal is markedly stretched and also enlarged. The frontal projection (B) discloses a moderate degree of elevation of the horizontal portion of the middle cerebral artery which is felt to be due to edema of this portion of the lobe. There is medial displacement and rounding of the anterior chorioidal artery due to associated uncal herniation (*arrow*). The lenticulostriate branches are markedly stretched and displaced medially (*upper arrows*). This is probably a sign of deep extension of the tumor. The deep extension is further confirmed by the fact that there is lateral displacement of the angiographic Sylvian point, which is also elevated (*arrow*).

artery. This shift of the artery may involve more the proximal than the distal portion in some cases (figs. 445 and 448).

These various findings may be altered by the presence of hippocampal herniation and by deep extension of the tumor; some will be present in one case and not in others.

The following discussion refers to the location of the maximum deformity, which usually indicates the center of the mass. Edema of the adjacent brain may modify the picture to a certain extent, but based on proper evaluation of all the findings, it should be possible to state whether the mass is anterior, posterior or deep, as well as intracerebral or extracerebral.

Anterior temporal masses. Anterior lesions are characterized by the fact that they elevate the horizontal portion of the middle cerebral artery because the center, or at least part, of the tumor is actually located under this portion of the artery (fig. 445). There is usually elevation of the proximal or anterior portion of the middle cerebral artery branches. The anterior chorioidal artery usually is displaced medially and may also be pushed upward. Its arc usually is distorted as seen in the frontal projection; it most often becomes wider (but sometimes narrower) than usual. As mentioned under "Cerebral Herniations," the medial displacement of this artery indicates that there is at least some degree of hypocampal herniation, or the tumor itself is straddling the edge of the incisural opening. The anterior chorioidal artery frequently is stretched and straightened and often enlarged (fig. 446).

The anterior portion of the Sylvian triangle is elevated. The basilar vein may be displaced medially or medially and upward, in its anteroinferior portion.

Posterior temporal masses. In these

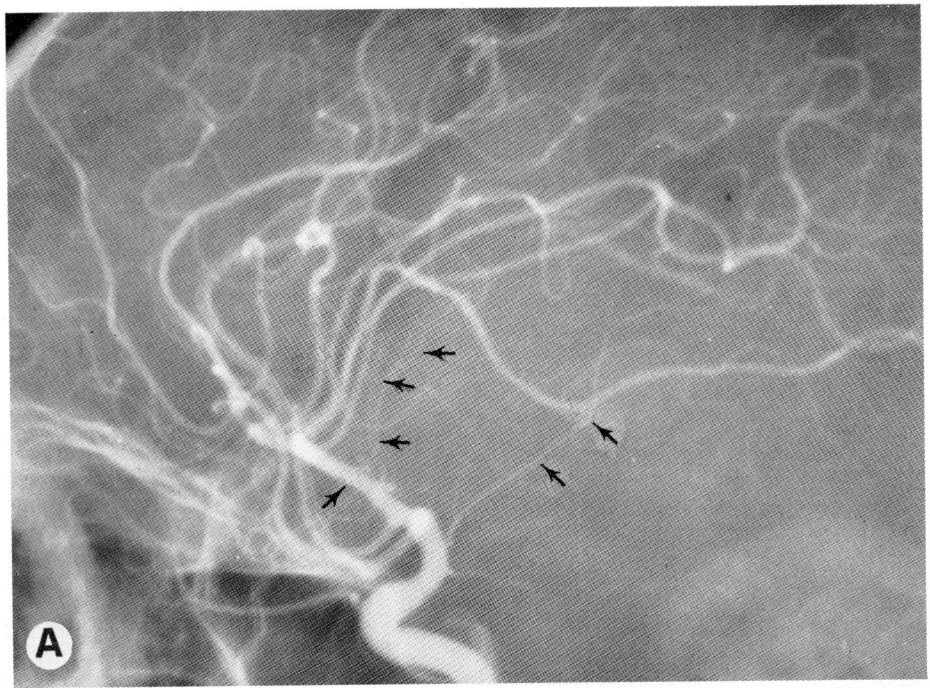

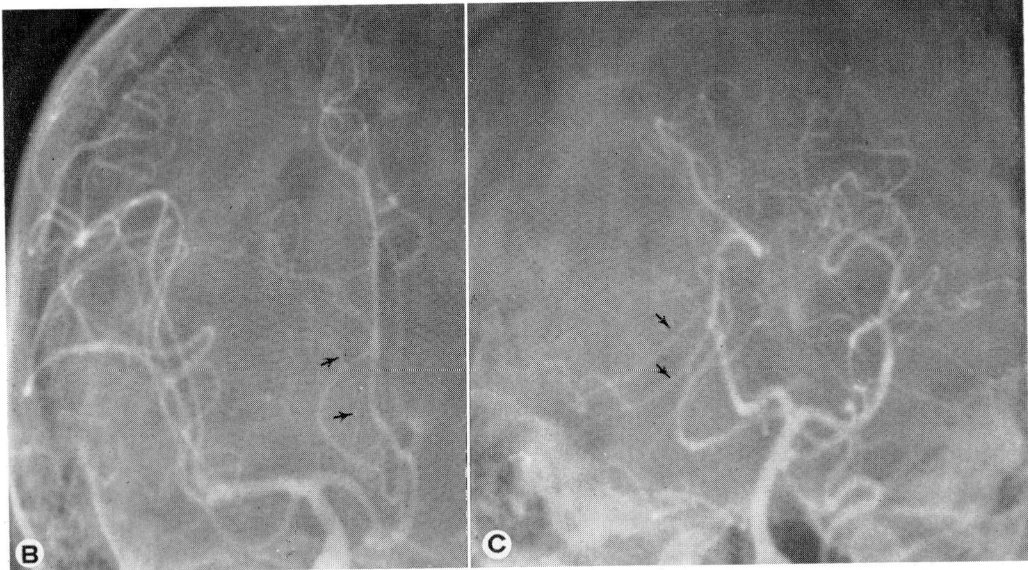

FIG. 448.—TEMPORAL INTRACEREBRAL TUMOR OCCUPYING THE ENTIRE TEMPORAL LOBE

The lateral view (A) shows moderate forward displacement and elevation of the horizontal portion of the middle cerebral artery (*anterior arrow*), as well as marked elevation of the branches of the middle cerebral arteries posteriorly. The anterior chorioidal artery is elevated, stretched, and enlarged (*arrows*). The lenticulostriate arteries are also displaced forward (*forward arrows*). At least two branches of the middle cerebral artery are seen to drape over the area occupied by the tumor, indicating the intracerebral position of the mass. The frontal projection (B) discloses a marked degree of medial displacement and bowing of the anterior chorioidal artery (*arrows*) which extends to the most posterior portion of the artery. Because the center of the tumor is more posterior, the supraclinoid portion of the carotid siphon is essentially normal in position. There is medial displacement of the branches of the middle cerebral artery away from the inner table of the skull, which is an indication of involvement of the temporal operculum. A vertebral angiogram (C) disclosed the presence of involvement of the posterior temporal branches of the posterior cerebral artery which are distorted (*arrows*). There is flattening of the curve of the posterior cerebral artery around the midbrain as compared to the other side. The distortion of the posterior temporal arteries indicates that the tumor has extended posteriorly to a considerable ex-

(*Revised 1963*)

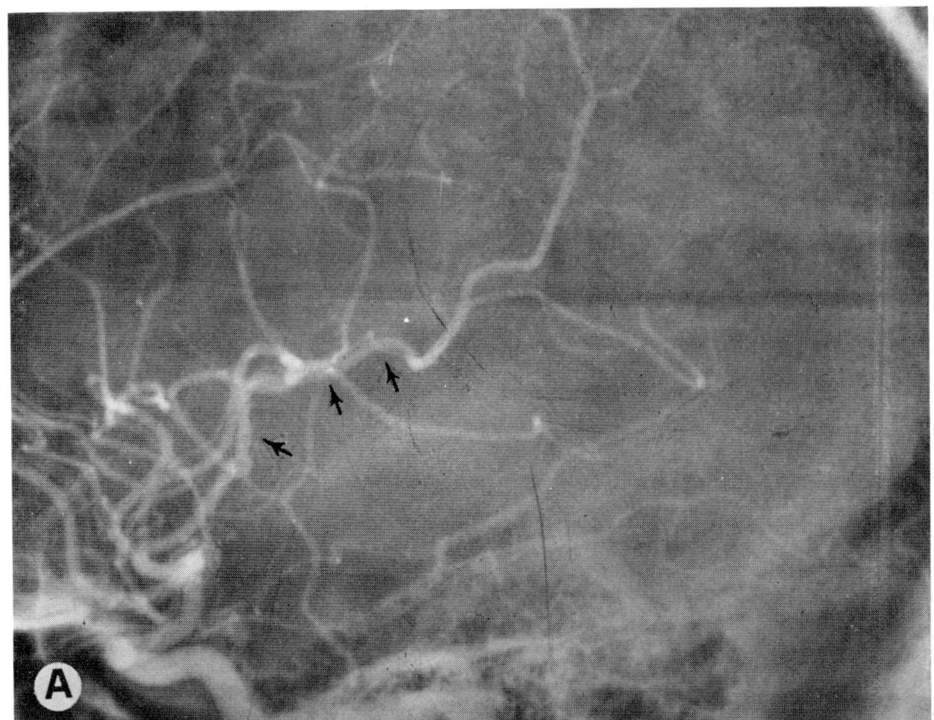

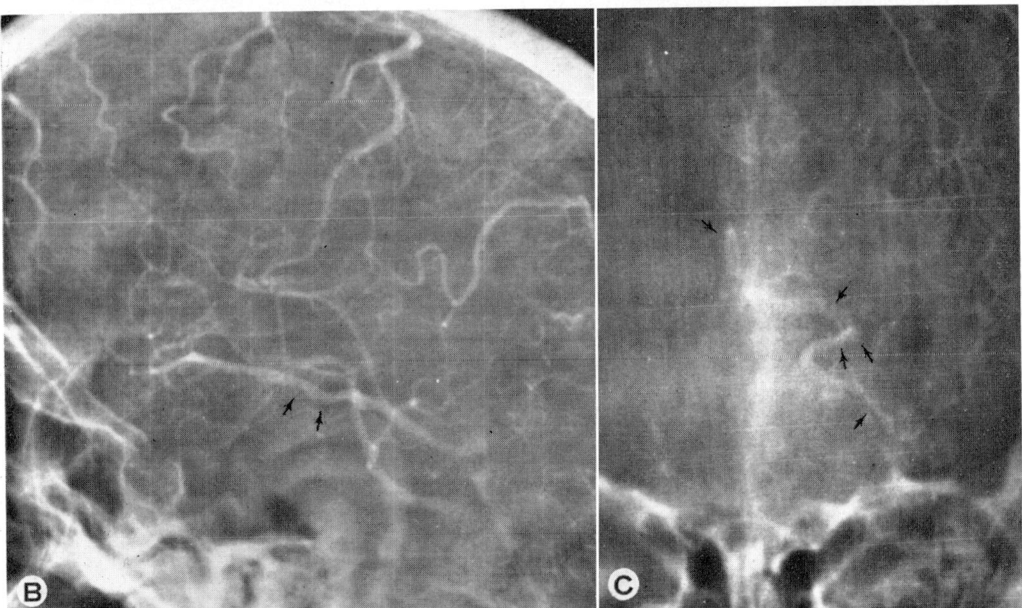

FIG. 449.—POSTERIOR TEMPORAL TUMOR

The lateral view (A) shows elevation of the posterior portion of the Sylvian triangle. The lateral view in the venous phase (B) shows elevation of the basilar vein (*arrows*). The frontal projection in the venous phase (C) confirms the elevation of the basilar vein which is also displaced medially to a significant degree (*arrows*). The *lower arrow* points at the deep middle cerebral vein which drains into the basilar vein. The *arrow* on the opposite side points at the displaced internal cerebral vein.

---

tent, or it is possible that the deformity could be produced by diffuse swelling. The lack of a large shift, however, which involves chiefly the proximal portion of the artery, would indicate that there is not very much cerebral edema, and we are probably dealing with a relatively slowly growing mass. The tumor was an extensive astrocytoma. (Courtesy of Dr. Franklin Reed and Dr. Faith Walsh, Morristown, N. J.)

(*Revised 1963*)

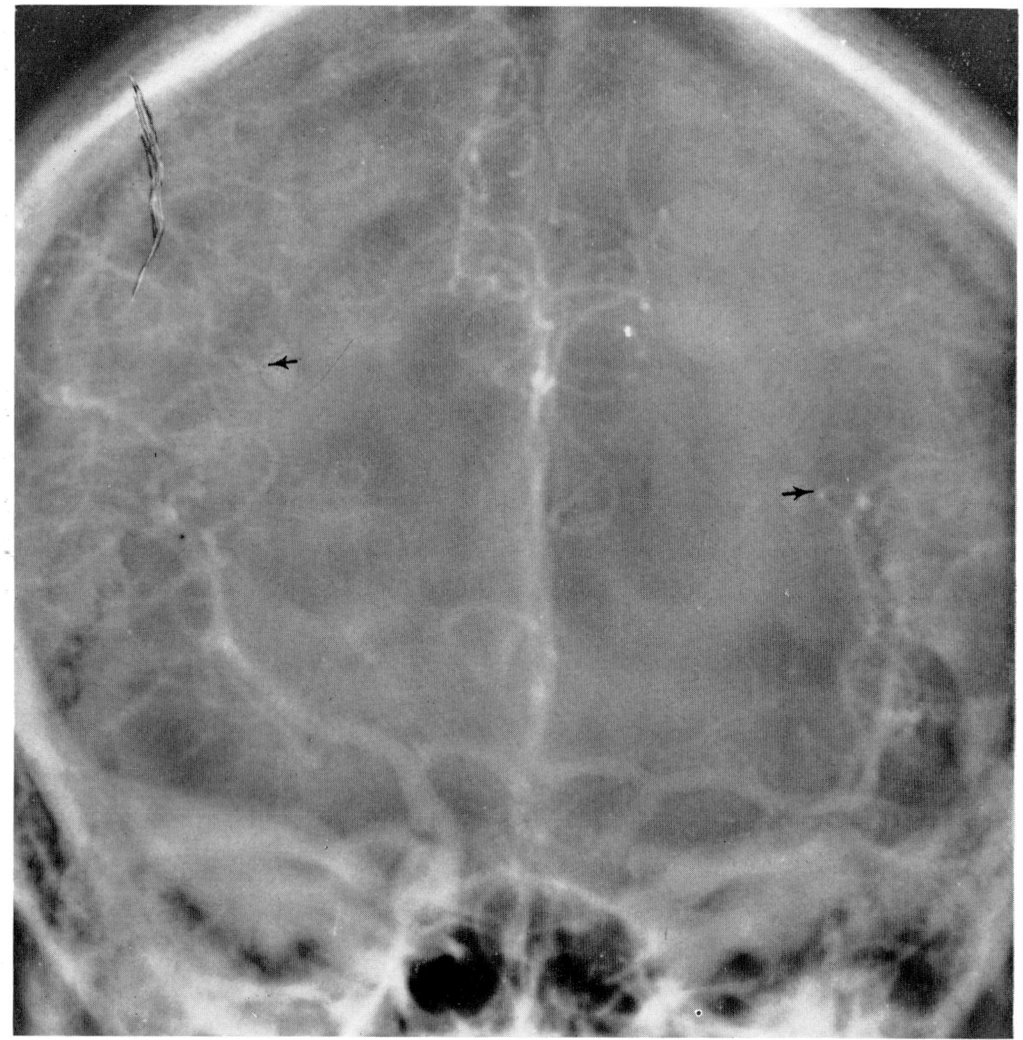

FIG. 450.—TEMPORAL LOBE TUMOR WITH BILATERAL FILLING OBTAINED BY APPLYING COMPRESSION TO THE OPPOSITE SIDE

The bilateral filling emphasizes the difference in the configuration of the middle cerebral branches. There is rounding of the knee of the middle cerebral artery which is often an early sign of temporal tumors. There is elevation of the angiographic Sylvian point (*arrow*) in comparison with the opposite, normal side. There is medial displacement of the branches of the middle cerebral artery and of the insular surface in a diffuse manner.

cases there is frank elevation of the middle cerebral artery branches as seen in the lateral view. In the frontal projection, there may be only slight elevation of the horizontal portion of the artery, which is produced by a certain amount of brain edema (fig. 447). Sometimes the tumor occupies the entire temporal lobe if it is very large (holotemporal tumor) (fig. 448). The midtemporal tumors tend to produce findings similar to those of the anterior temporal masses as regards displacement of the carotid siphon and anterior chorioidal artery. If a posterior tumor is very large or if it is accompanied by extensive edema, it will also produce signs of an inferior retro-Sylvian mass.

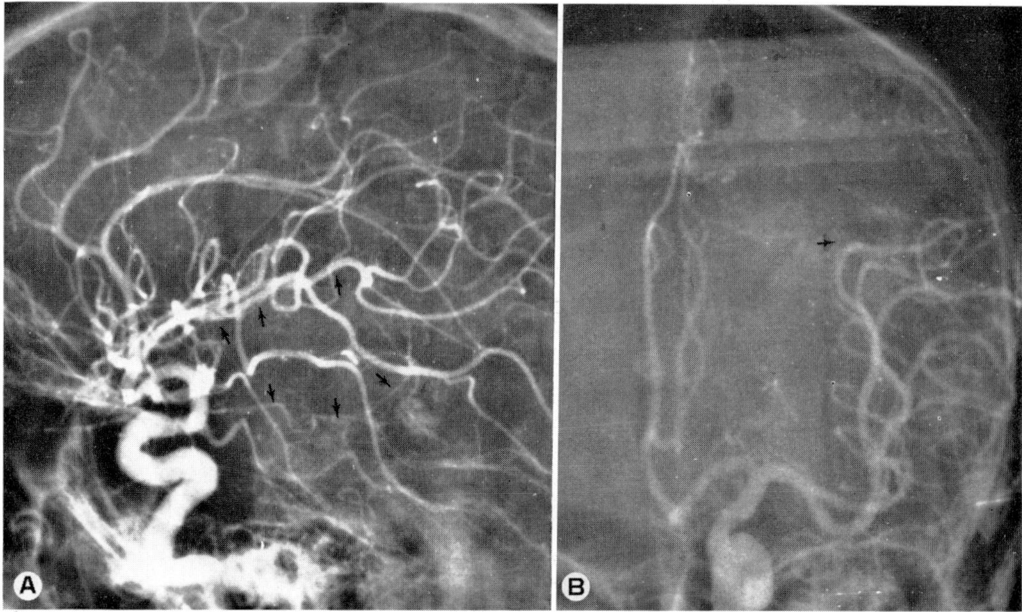

FIG. 451.—INTRACEREBRAL TEMPORAL TUMOR

The lateral view (A) shows general elevation of the branches of the middle cerebral artery and the lower aspect of the Sylvian triangle *(upper arrows)*. There is draping of the branches of the middle cerebral artery, which, being on the surface of the brain, go downward and backward over the outer surface of the temporal lobe. There is enlargement of the anterior chorioidal artery which can be traced backward around the atrium *(lower arrows)*. The frontal projection (B) shows that there is no elevation of the horizontal portion of the middle cerebral artery, which indicates that there is no tumor or edema in the anterior portion of the temporal lobe. There is slight medial displacement of all of the branches over the insula. The angiographic Sylvian point is only slightly elevated.

The angiographic Sylvian point is elevated in these cases (figs. 447, 448, and 450). Such elevation is a characteristic finding of posterior temporal masses. Medial displacement of the same point as well as of the branches over the insula may be present.

The basilar vein is displaced medially and upward (fig. 449), or downward (fig. 452). The latter finding may indicate deep extension. The internal cerebral vein usually shows a greater midline shift than the anterior cerebral artery.

The appearance of the anterior chorioidal artery is not crucial in the diagnosis of posterior temporal masses. Its behavior depends on the size of the tumor and on the presence or absence of hippocampal herniation. The anterior chorioidal artery often is enlarged. The posterior communicating and posterior cerebral arteries are not significantly affected by temporal tumors except in extracerebral lesions (see below), and when there is hippocampal herniation (see under "Cerebral Herniations").

(Revised 1963)

Deep temporal masses. Tumors may arise deep in the temporal lobe or may extend deeply from a more superficial location. The group considered here comprises only those that are primarily deep in position. These tumors produce less elevation of the branches of the middle cerebral artery, but usually some degree of elevation is present. The anterior chorioidal artery is deformed early as its curve is made wider, and later, when the mass is large enough, it will be displaced medially (fig. 451). The basilar vein may be sharply and selectively angled or kinked (fig. 452). The latter deformity is not usually produced in more superficially placed tumors which extend medially.

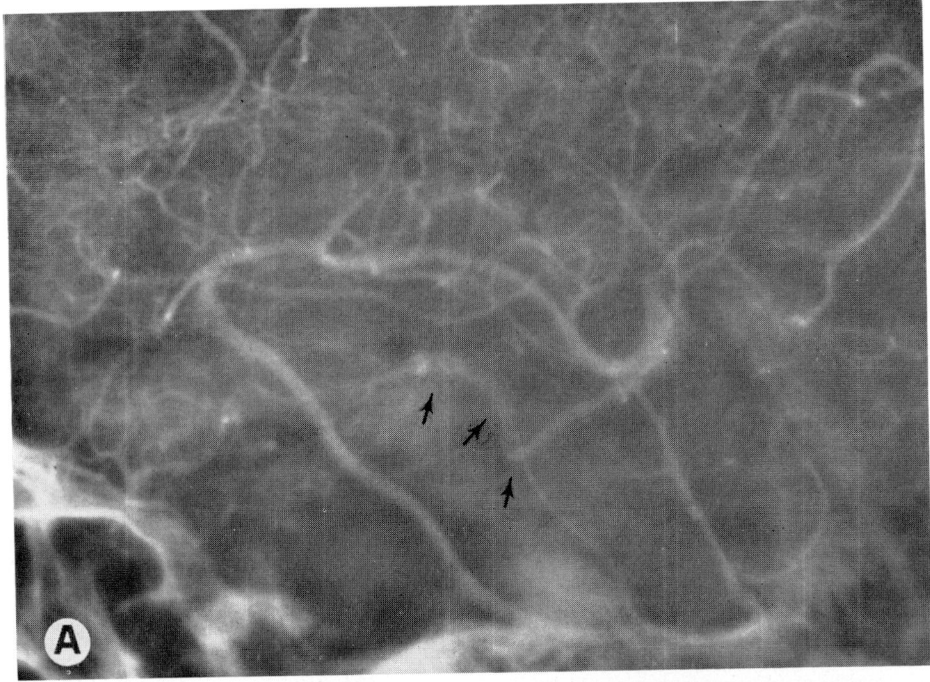

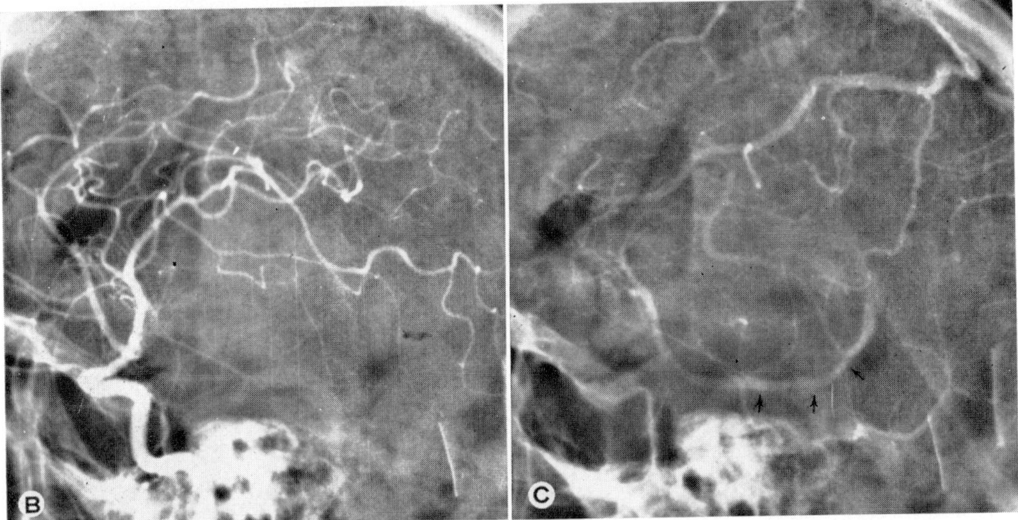

FIG. 452.—DEEP TEMPORAL LOBE TUMOR

The lateral view in the arterial phase, not shown here, shows only slight elevation of the middle cerebral vessels. The most conspicuous finding was the marked elevation and buckling of the basilar vein (A) which indicated the deep location of this intracerebral tumor. Surgical intervention disclosed an astrocytoma situated in the medial portion of the temporal lobe, anteriorly. (B) represents a lateral view of another case with a large midtemporal lobe tumor causing extremely marked elevation of the branches of the middle cerebral artery and of the angiographic Sylvian point. The venous phase (C) revealed marked downward displacement of the basilar vein (*arrows*). The junction of the basilar vein and the internal cerebral vein is also displaced downward and slightly backward, making the vein of Galen closer to vertical in position. In the frontal projection (not shown), the basilar vein was markedly displaced medially. If the basilar vein is widely separated from the internal cerebral vein, deep extension of the tumor is probably present. Compare with Fig. 470.

(*Revised 1963*)

Infiltrating neoplasms. Deep, infiltrating temporal tumors may be difficult to diagnose by angiography or in fact by any method, until they acquire a certain size. Unless they are shown by angiography or pneumography, the neurosurgeon also may overlook them because of their deep location. Only on histological section of tissue removed at operation can a diagnosis be made in some cases. Later, when the tumors become more bulky it is possible to visualize them. Some tumors of this region are accompanied by a localized cerebral atrophy until they become large. See page 410 for further details.

Temporal intracerebral tumors do not usually cross the Sylvian fissure. However, some glioblastomas and an occasional astrocytoma may grow through the Sylvian fissure into the frontal lobe. In the latter cases, the angiographic appearance would be modified and may be difficult to interpret. Signs of a temporal as well as of a frontal mass may be present on the angiogram. Posterior temporal intracerebral tumors often infiltrate deeply into the basal ganglia region as part of their customary growth.

Extracerebral masses. Tumors of the temporal fossa represent an important group. As mentioned above, the majority are meningiomas arising most commonly from the sphenoid ridge, but they may arise also from the floor of the middle fossa or the lateral or medial walls. Some may be dumbbell or saddle meningiomas, partly in the middle fossa and partly in the posterior fossa. An occasional 5th nerve neurinoma or epidermoid is found in this location, and chordomas may extend laterally. Subdural hematomas may be localized to the temporal fossa.

All of these tumors lift the temporal lobe and with it the middle cerebral vessels. The sphenoid ridge meningiomas behave as anterior temporal tumors and produce some of the most beautiful examples of upward displacement of the horizontal portion of the middle cerebral artery and medial displacement of the supraclinoid portion of the carotid siphon with elevation of the bifurcation. The transverse portion of the middle cerebral artery often describes a rounded curve (fig. 453C).

Extracerebral tumors situated on the floor of the middle fossa produce marked elevation of the anterior chorioidal artery, particularly if they are more medially placed (fig. 453). In addition, they will produce the usual signs of a temporal mass. Sometimes the anterior chorioidal artery is elevated almost to the exclusion of other signs (fig. 454).

In general, extracerebral masses produce *upward displacement of all of the branches* of the middle cerebral artery because they lift the temporal lobe. On the other hand, intracerebral temporal tumors lift the branches within and above the Sylvian fissure, but those on the surface of the temporal lobe still descend on the outer surface of the enlarged lobe. This phenomenon may be referred to as the "draping sign" because the temporal arterial branches drape over the tumor (fig. 451). Draping can be seen in extracerebral tumors arising from the medial aspect of the floor of the middle fossa because they lift selectively the medial portion of the temporal lobe. However, they also elevate sharply the anterior chorioidal artery as explained above (fig. 453). In interpreting the draping sign, it should be kept in mind that if the tumor is anterior temporal in location, even though extracerebral, the temporal vessels descend over the temporal lobe behind the tumor suggesting an intracerebral location (fig. 445). Some temporal intracerebral tumors situated deeply and involving the medial inferior portion of the temporal lobe may elevate the anterior chorioidal artery (fig. 455).

Retro-Sylvian Tumors

General manifestations. The term retro-Sylvian is applied to all masses that are situated behind the Sylvian point. In this area, the temporal and parietal lobes come together and behind this region is the occipital lobe. If a lesion is situated directly in back of the Sylvian point, it may be called a retro-Sylvian mass. If the lesion is situated in the upper portion more than in the lower, it is referred to as *superior retro-Sylvian*. If the lesion is situated more toward the temporal lobe, the term *inferior retro-Sylvian* is used. It is common for a posterior temporal lobe tumor to extend backward into this general area, and reference here is made rather to the group of lesions which appear to

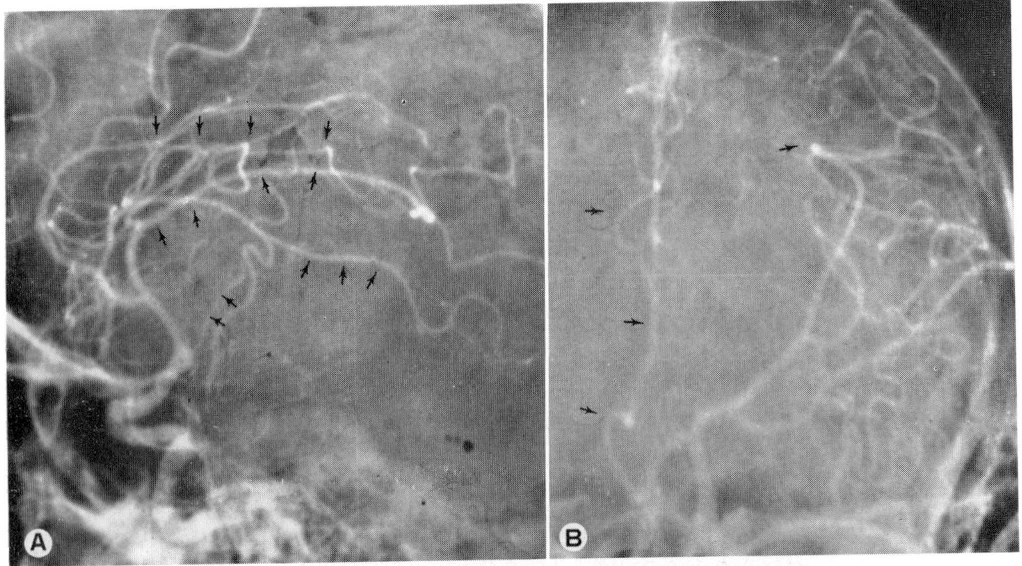

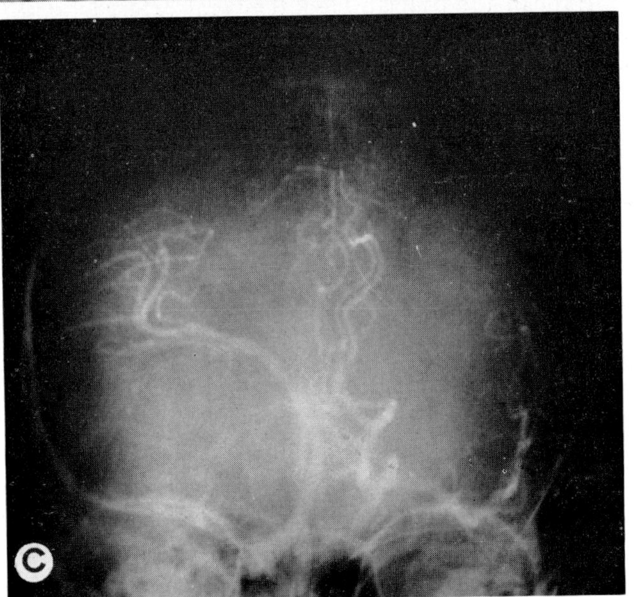

FIG. 453.—MIDDLE FOSSA MENINGIOMA

The lateral view (A) shows a marked degree of elevation of the middle cerebral artery and its branches. The Sylvian triangle is extremely high in position (*arrows*). The anterior chorioidal artery is markedly elevated, almost vertical in position (*two lower arrows*). One branch of the middle cerebral artery (*posterior three arrows*) seems to drape over the tumor even though it is a meningioma. The reason is that the tumor is very deeply placed in the middle fossa, and, in fact, it could not be removed surgically; thus some of the lateral aspect of the temporal lobe was not lifted off the floor of the middle fossa. The frontal projection (B) reveals the marked degree of elevation of the middle cerebral vessels and the extremely high position of the angiographic Sylvian point (*arrow*). The supraclinoid portion of the siphon is displaced medially, and the bifurcation is high. The shift of the anterior cerebral artery is more pronounced on its proximal (*inferior portion*) and to a lesser degree in its distal segments, but the central portion (*midline arrow*) is practically in the midline. (C) shows an anteroposterior view in another case with typical rounded configuration of middle cerebral artery displacement in a patient with sphenoid ridge meningioma.

(Revised 1963)

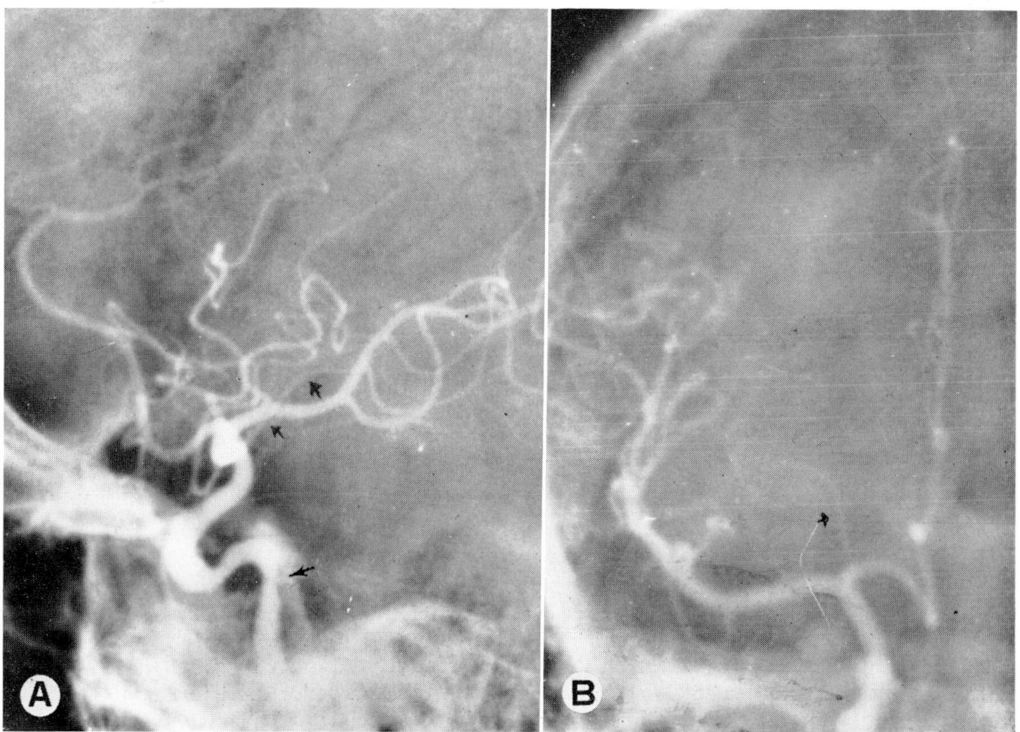

FIG. 454.—DEEPLY PLACED MIDDLE FOSSA MENINGIOMA

The lateral view (A) shows marked elevation of the anterior chorioidal artery (*arrows*). There is only slight elevation of the anterior portion of the middle cerebral group. The frontal projection (B) shows no evidence of midline shift. The anterior chorioidal artery is slightly laterally displaced, and its curvature is abnormal. This indicates that the meningioma has grown on the lateral aspect of the sella turcica, thus producing lateral displacement of the uncus of the temporal lobe. The lower arrow in (A) points at the narrowing of the intracavernous portion of the internal carotid artery due to invasion of the wall of the cavernous sinus.

arise in the retro-Sylvian region and from there extend either toward the parietal or toward the temporal lobe.

The majority of the retro-Sylvian lesions are intracerebral tumors, and when in the dominant hemisphere, they almost always produce aphasia and sometimes, also, a hemianopia. Some retro-Sylvian masses are meningiomas arising from the occipital bone, the tentorium or the falx in the posterior parietal region and displacing the brain forward.

Angiographically, the most important finding is *forward displacement of the angiographic Sylvian point.* The angiographic Sylvian point is difficult to locate exactly in the lateral projection. However, a fairly good approximation can be made of its position by following the upper margin of the Sylvian triangle. The point where the last middle cerebral branches are seen to emerge from the depths of the Sylvian fissure onto the surface of the brain usually indicates the position of the angiographic Sylvian point. A forward displacement of the Sylvian point results in a telescopic, or closed accordion, deformity of the branches of the middle cerebral artery which is rather typical when it is present (fig. 458). If the lesion extends toward the temporal lobe, the posterior portion of the middle cerebral branches are displaced upward; this is the most common configuration. If the tumor extends toward the parietal lobe, the branches are displaced downward.

In frontal projection, the angiographic

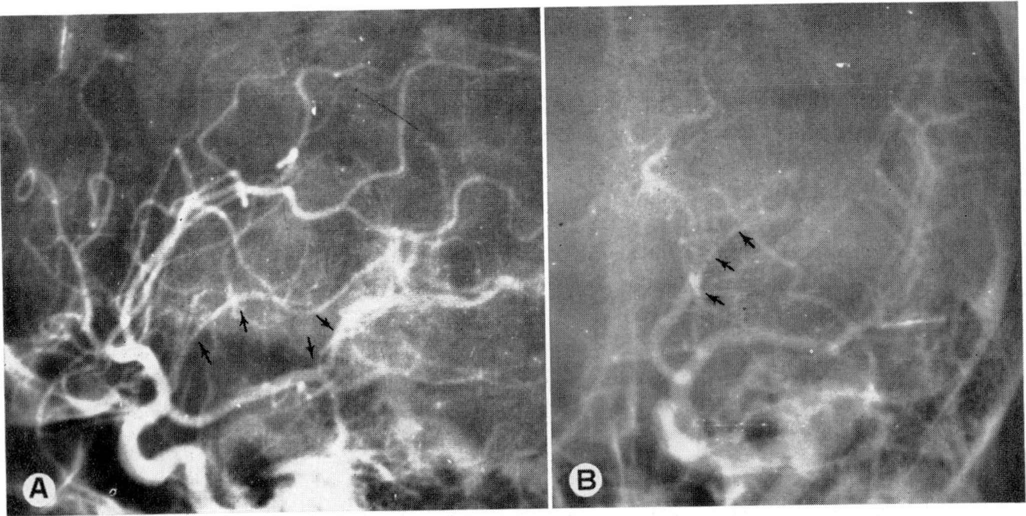

Fig. 455.—Temporal Lobe Tumor, Intracerebral, Producing Elevation of the Anterior Chorioidal Artery

The lateral view (A) shows elevation of the branches of the middle cerebral artery typical of mid- and posterior temporal tumors. The anterior chorioidal artery is elevated and enlarged (*arrows*). The posterior cerebral artery is depressed and makes a step over the edge of the tentorium (*arrows*) which probably indicates some degree of transtentorial herniation. The frontal projection (B) discloses an increase in the curvature and slight medial displacement of the anterior chorioidal artery (*arrows*). The broad curve of the anterior chorioidal artery is probably associated with infiltration of the medial portion of the temporal lobe by tumor and with the downward herniation. The horizontal portion of the middle cerebral artery is not elevated because the tumor was posterior to it.

Sylvian point is displaced downward because forward displacement of this point is equivalent to downward displacement. Therefore, even if the angiographic Sylvian point is not displaced downward, as seen in the lateral view, still when visualized in the frontal projection, it lies well below the center of the reference line described under "Anatomy." Of course, when the angiographic Sylvian point is seen to be displaced downward in the frontal projection, the lateral projection will demonstrate whether or not the deformity of the vessel is above the Sylvian point, that is, in the parietal region, and is displacing the point downward. If the tumor is retro-Sylvian, the area of the Sylvian point would be displaced foward. Use of the sella turcica as a reference point to determine forward displacement is helpful because the angiographic Sylvian point normally is well behind and above the dorsum sellae, usually directly above the density of the petrous pyramid.

Another important angiographic sign of retro-Sylvian tumors is that they displace the brain forward, thus causing bowing of the middle cerebral arterial branches as they ascend in the cerebral sulci, describing a curve concave backward. This curvilinear distribution of the vessels can extend for a considerable distance forward and may be seen better in the late arterial or early intermediate phase than in the early arterial phase (fig. 456). Sometimes the venous phase also shows the same configuration of the surface veins (fig. 457). This appearance of the vessels is referred to by us as "onion peeling" because as the gyri of the brain are bent for a distance in front of the tumor, it is somewhat reminiscent of the successive layers of an onion.

Superior retro-Sylvian masses. In general, retro-Sylvian tumors tend to produce a greater displacement of the internal cerebral vein than of the anterior cerebral artery and its branches, but the degree of

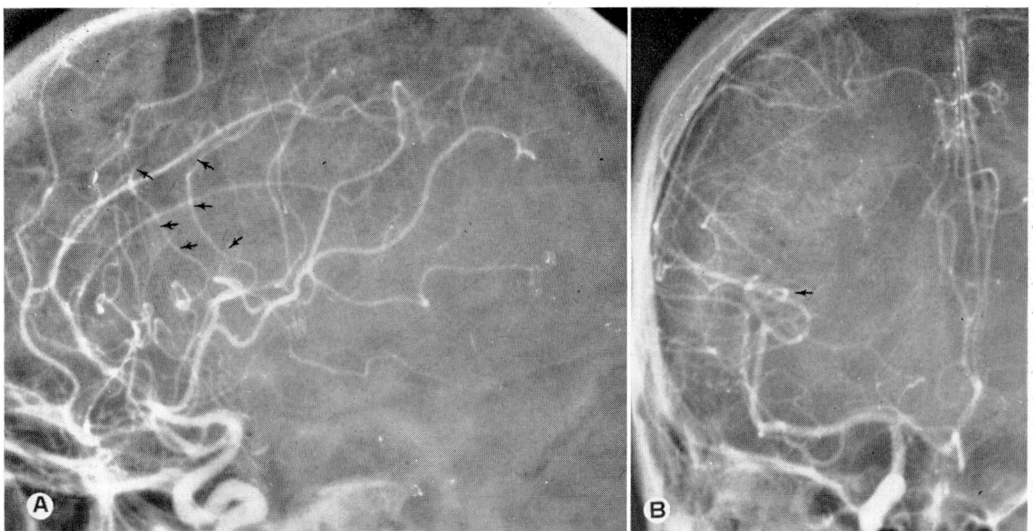

Fig. 456.—Retro-Sylvian Mass

The lateral projection (A) shows separation, loss of undulations, and spreading of the branches of the middle cerebral artery in the region behind the Sylvian triangle. The region of the Sylvian point is displaced forward. There is bowing of the branches of the middle cerebral artery dorsally, extending forward as far as the coronal suture (*arrows*), due to the telescopic effect on the brain of these posteriorly placed tumors. The frontal projection (B) shows marked downward displacement of the angiographic Sylvian point (*arrow*) which is due to forward displacement of this point. As explained in the text, forward displacement of the angiographic Sylvian point is equivalent to downward displacement such as is produced by supra-Sylvian masses.

displacement is, to a certain extent, as in the case of tumors located elsewhere in the brain, dependent on the degree of edema present. If the tumor is high, the posterior slope of the internal cerebral vein is flattened (fig. 457) and, if the tumor is low, the internal cerebral vein may be normal in position or it may be elevated, particularly if there is deep extension of the tumor. The basilar vein is usually displaced medially, not only because of the tumor itself, but because there is often an associated posterior herniation through the incisura of the tentorium which would, in itself, displace the basilar vein and the posterior cerebral arteries medially.

In the retro-Sylvian group belong certain meningiomas arising, as mentioned above, from the occipital bone or from the posterior parietal region and also meningiomas arising from the tentorium and the posterior aspect of the falx. The ones arising from the tentorium are inferior retro-Sylvian masses whereas the ones arising from the posterior aspect of the falx are midline retro-Sylvian masses. The latter may displace the vessels away from the midline in a manner similar to that seen in parasagittal or midline meningiomas more anteriorly situated in the falx.

Posterior retro-Sylvian masses. *Occipital lobe tumors* will produce deformity of the branches of the posterior cerebral artery. The calcarine branch may be displaced upward. The parieto-occipital branch may be separated from the posterior temporal branch (fig. 459). The separation of the parieto-occipital branch and the posterior temporal branch is also evident in the frontal projection. If the tumor is large enough, it will produce the forward telescoping of the Sylvian vessels which is seen in any retro-Sylvian mass.

Inferior retro-Sylvian masses. The extracerebral tumors attached to the tentorium elevate all of the branches of the

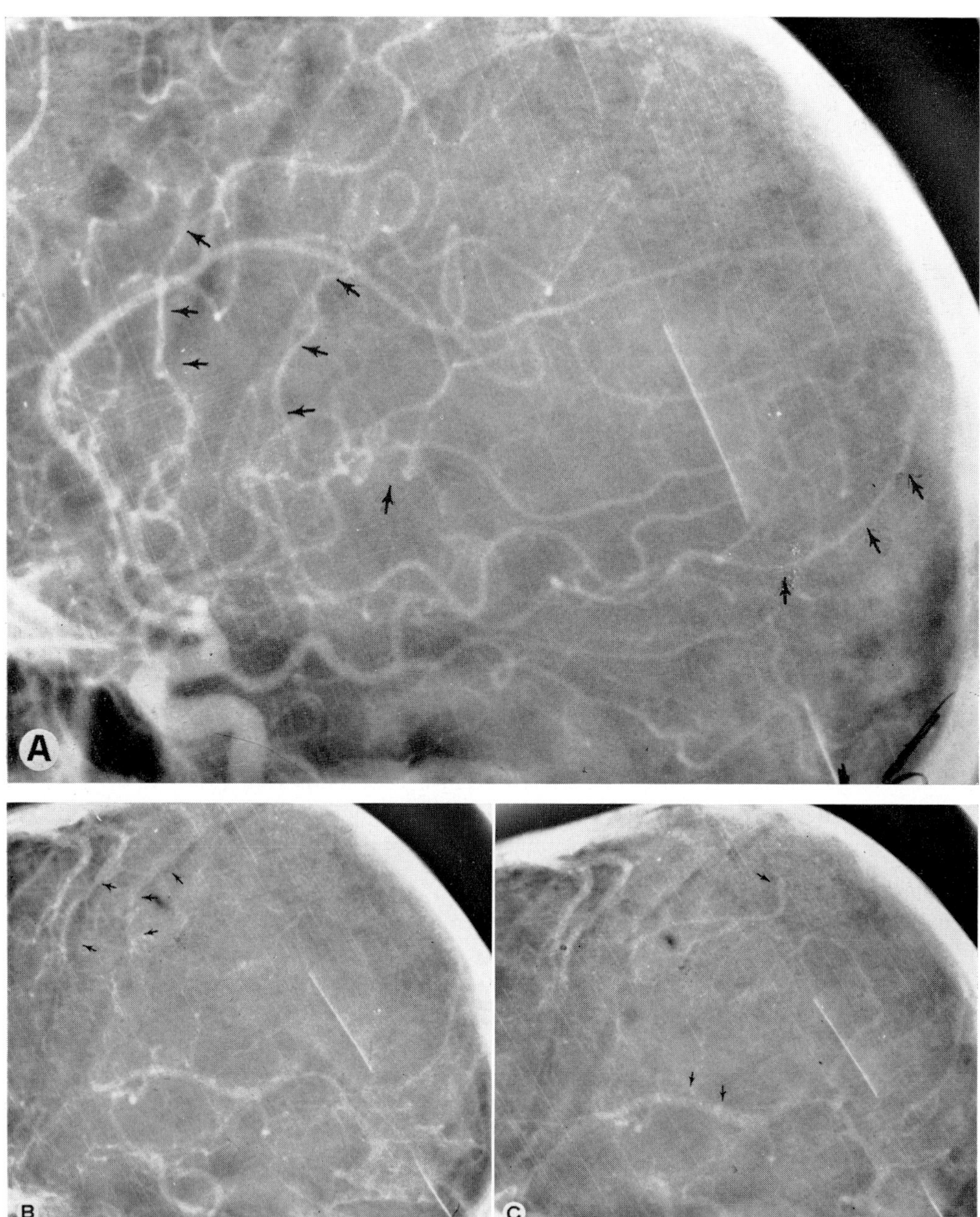

Fig. 457.—Superior Retro-Sylvian Mass (Parasagittal Meningioma)

The lateral view (A) shows disruption of the vessels in the retro-Sylvian region extending over the parietal area outlined by the arrows. There is bowing of the parieto-occipital branch of the posterior cerebral artery (*arrows*) and only a slight general bowing without loss of undulations in the ascending branches of the middle cerebral artery extending fairly far forward (*forward arrows*). The area of the angiographic Sylvian point is displaced forward (*arrow*). In the early venous phase (B) there is an area with delayed venous filling. The bowing of the surface veins in the area anterior to the tumor is evident (*arrows*). A later film made in the venous phase (C) shows that the surface veins over the region of the tumor could not quite reach the superior longitudinal sinus and stop at a certain distance from the top of the skull (*arrow*). This was related to the presence of obstruction of the superior longitudinal sinus which caused reversal of the venous flow in this region. There is moderate downward displacement and flattening of the curve of the internal cerebral vein.

(*Revised 1963*)

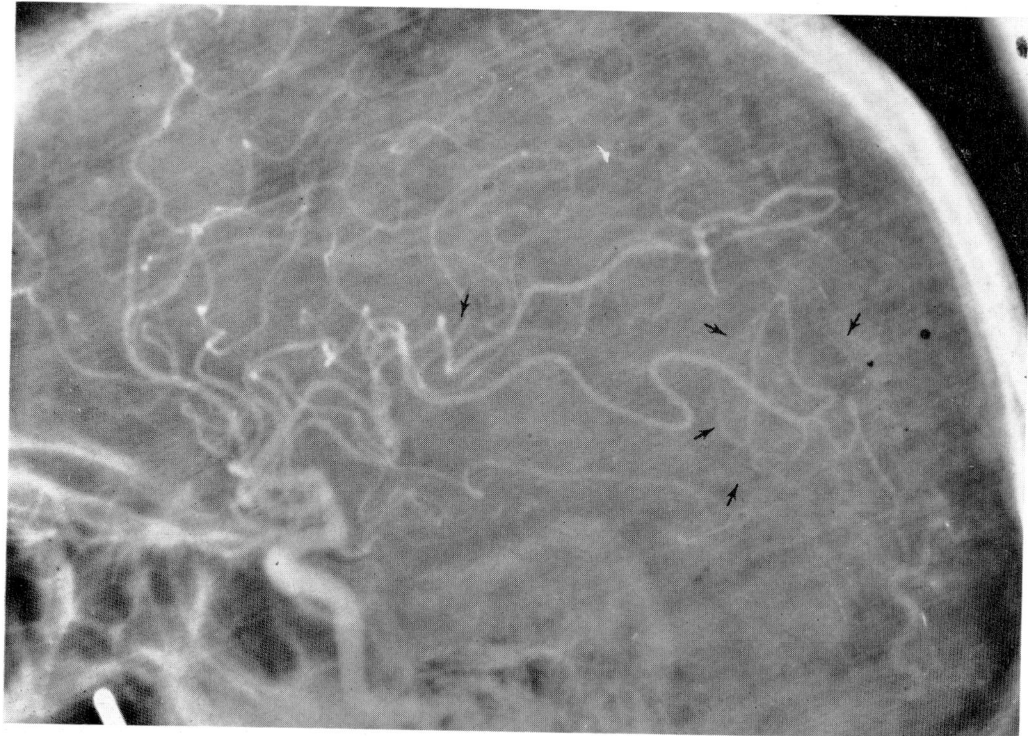

Fig. 458.—Retro-Sylvian Tumor Producing Telescoping of the Middle Cerebral Branches
The region of the angiographic Sylvian point is displaced forward (*arrow*); it is almost straight above the dorsum sellae. There is stretching of the posterior branches of the middle cerebral artery and beginning abnormal vascularity in the area outlined by the *posterior arrows*. A later phase demonstrated abnormal vascularity extending forward and not further than the *three posterior arrows*.

middle and posterior cerebral arteries if the tumor is broad enough extending beneath the medial portion of the inferior surface of the temporo-occipital region. If a tentorial meningioma is occupying more the lateral aspect, it will elevate the branches of the middle cerebral artery and displace the posterior cerebral vessels medially. On the other hand, if the meningioma is arising from the most medial portion of the tentorial surface, it will produce upward displacement of the posterior cerebral vessels. Of course, the findings involving the posterior cerebral artery and its branches are most apparent when there is good filling of the posterior cerebral artery through the carotid system or on vertebral angiography.

While some tentorial meningiomas may be grouped with the posterior temporal masses, others arising further posteriorly should be included with the inferior retro-Sylvian masses. The inferior retro-Sylvian tentorial meningiomas produce telescoping and upward displacement of the angiographic Sylvian point as seen in the lateral view, while the more anteriorly situated ones produce only elevation of the Sylvian point without forward displacement (fig. 460).

Some tentorial meningiomas are supplied by a branch of the internal carotid artery, which is an enlarged branch that normally supplies the wall of the cavernous sinus and tentorium. This artery was first described by Bernasconi and Cassinari (1957) and can be seen to best advantage in arteriograms where only the internal carotid artery is injected (fig. 460). The presence of such a vessel usually is an indication that the tumor is a tentorial meningioma. Meningiomas arising in the parasagittal region may ob-

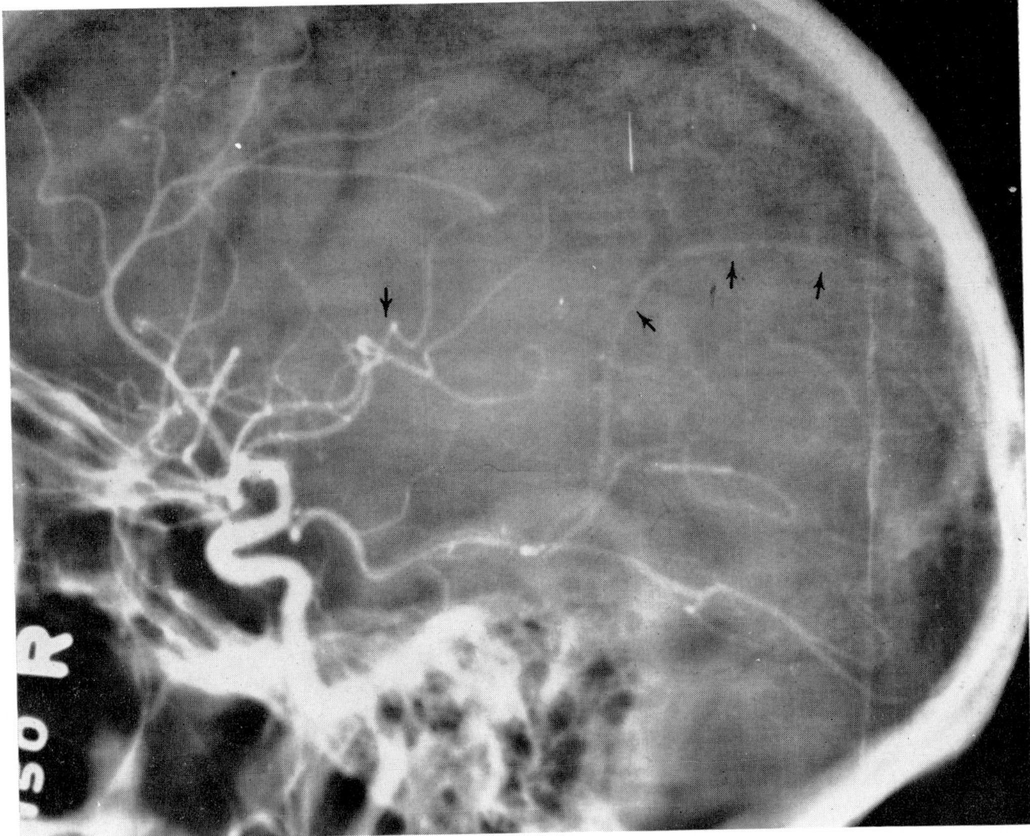

FIG. 459.—RETRO-SYLVIAN MASS IN THE OCCIPITAL LOBE

There is stretching and spreading of the branches of the posterior cerebral artery which filled adequately in this carotid angiogram. There is marked separation of the parieto-occipital branch and the posterior temporal branch of the posterior cerebral artery with marked elevation and bowing of the parieto-occipital branch (*arrows*). The area of the angiographic Sylvian point is displaced forward (*anterior arrow*).

struct the superior longitudinal sinus and produce a reversal of venous flow around the obstructed area (fig. 457). For details, see "Supra-Sylvian Tumors: Parasagittal Masses." Tentorial meningiomas arising from the free edge of the tentorium and other lesions around the tentorium are described separately under "Incisural Tumors."

Intra-Sylvian Tumors

As the name indicates, the group comprises neoplasms that occur between the lips of the Sylvian fissure. The tumors are relatively rare and usually are meningiomas. The authors have seen at least one case of an astrocytoma arising deep within the temporal operculum, or from the lateral aspect of the insula, which grew outward apart from the surrounding brain cortex of the Sylvian fissure and produced findings somewhat similar to those encountered in intra-Sylvian meningiomas (fig. 462).

Characteristically, such masses produce very sharp displacement and stretching of the branches of the middle cerebral artery. Some of the branches will rise above and some will be situated below the tumor, thus producing a rather characteristic splitting of the branches of the middle cerebral artery (fig. 461). If the tumor bulges out of the Sylvian fissure, it may displace the middle cerebral branches away from the inner table

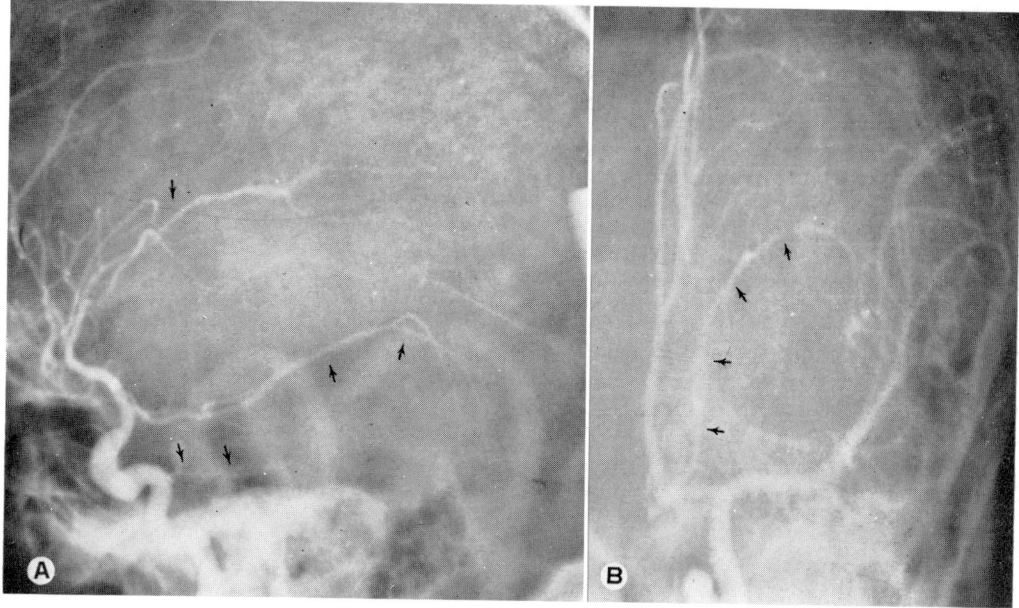

FIG. 460.—LARGE TENTORIAL MENINGIOMA (INFERIOR RETRO-SYLVIAN TUMOR)

The lateral view (A) shows marked forward displacement of the area of the angiographic Sylvian point. This area is so distorted, however, that it is difficult to determine without stereoscopic films just where the vessels are emerging. There is marked elevation of the posterior branches of the middle cerebral artery behind the area of the angiographic Sylvian point. There is elevation and bowing of the posterior temporal branch of the posterior cerebral artery. The parieto-occipital branch apparently was not filled at the time that this film was made. The frontal projection (B) discloses a marked degree of medial displacement of the posterior cerebral artery and its posterior temporal branch (*arrows*). It was felt that this finding confirmed the possibility of a tentorial meningioma. In addition, the lateral film demonstrates a tentorial vessel arising from the internal carotid artery (*lower arrows*) which is usually only see in meningiomas. (Courtesy of Dr. S. Unger and Dr. Erich Krueger, Bronx Veterans Administration Hospital, N. Y.)

of the skull. If the tumor tends to grow more toward the midline, some of the branches of the middle cerebral artery are displaced toward the inner table. The most outstanding feature is the splitting of the branches with sharp stretching and bowing as described above. Intra-Sylvian meningiomas, not attached to the inner table of the skull, are relatively rare.

Latero-Sylvian Tumors

Masses situated lateral to the Sylvian region may be either neoplasms or hematomas. Meningiomas arise from the inner table of the skull in the pterional region or from the temporoparietal convexity. As the name indicates, lateral Sylvian masses are situated mostly in relation to the mid and lower convexity of the brain; if they were situated along the high convexity or the parasagittal region, they would belong in the category of supra-Sylvian masses.

Characteristically, such lateral masses produce a medial displacement of the branches of the middle cerebral artery and of the angiographic Sylvian point. The displacement is usually typical in appearance and easy to evaluate except in thin subdural hematomas where the degree of displacement may be only slightly above the normal range of 43 mm. for the Sylvian point and 30 mm. for the branches over the outer surface of the island of Reil. Because these masses are extracerebral in location, they simply displace the middle cerebral artery branches inward and not upward or downward.

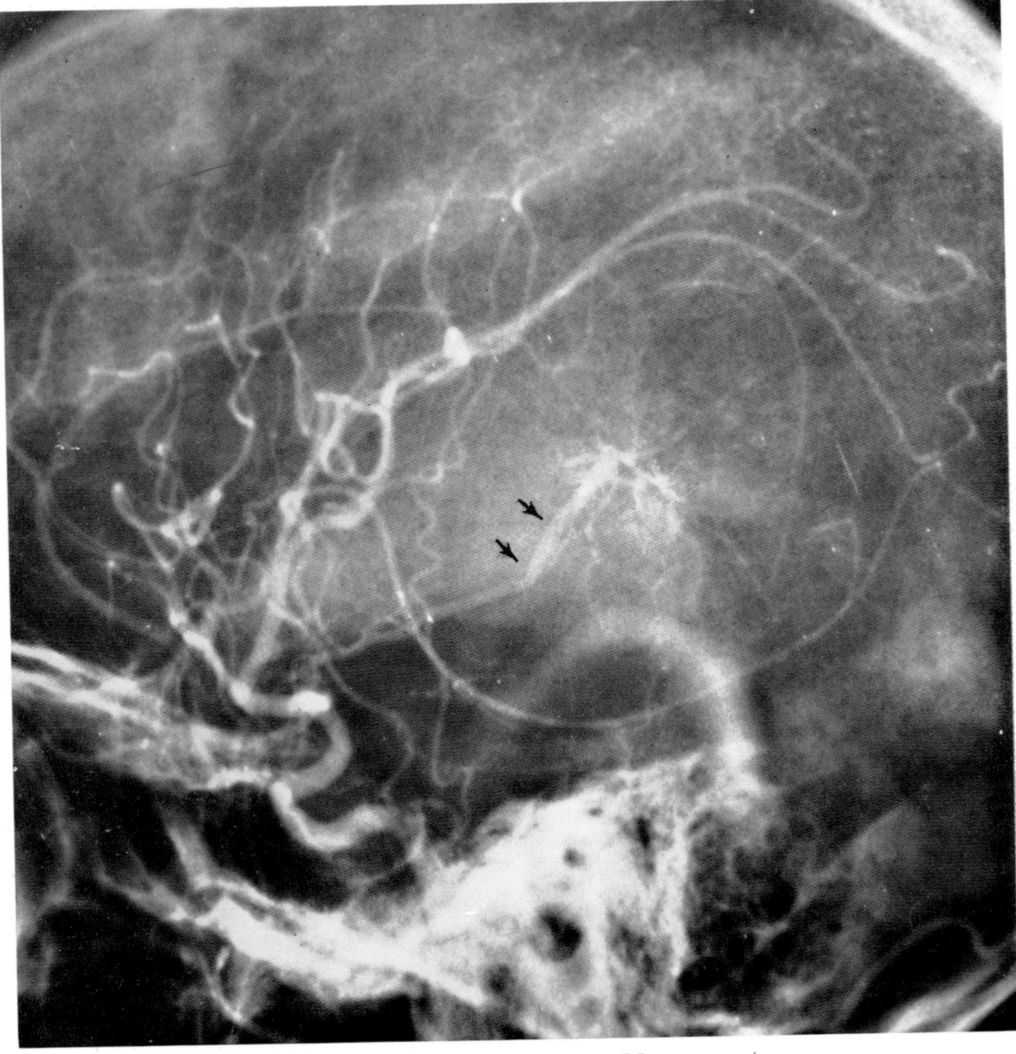

FIG. 461.—INTRA-SYLVIAN TUMOR (MENINGIOMA)

There is splitting of the branches of the middle cerebral artery, some of which go up and some go down, outlining the meningioma. A meningeal vessel is seen to feed this meningioma (*arrows*).

If the tumor is slightly more anterior, in front of the angiographic Sylvian point near the pterional region, it displaces mainly the branches related to the island of Reil (fig. 463). If the tumor is more posteriorly situated, it produces a more localized displacement which clearly involves the angiographic Sylvian point and vessels adjacent to it (fig. 464). A more complete discussion of subdural hematomas will be found in the discussion of "Head Injuries and Their Complications."

Centro-Sylvian Tumors

General manifestations. The group comprises thalamic and deep posterior frontal masses and in several respects is related to groups 8 and 9 of this classification (miscellaneous deep tumors, intraventricular tumors, corpus callosum tumors, and hydrocephalus). Discussion, therefore, will overlap because the diagnosis of these conditions depends to a considerable extent on the behavior of the deep veins of the brain.

Thalamic masses. Under the deep tu-

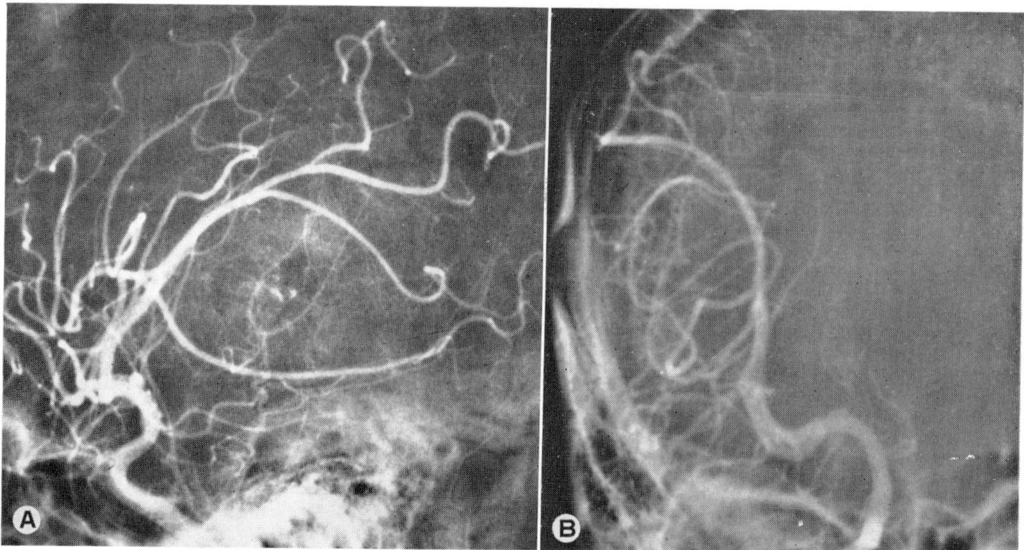

FIG. 462.—INTRA-SYLVIAN ASTROCYTOMA SIMULATING INTRA-SYLVIAN MENINGIOMA

The lateral view (A) shows an apparence quite similar to that noted in the preceding figure. The frontal projection (B) shows medial displacement of the middle cerebral branches with flattening of the insular curve.

mors we will describe masses of the thalamic and the posterior deep frontal locations which are often difficult to distinguish even on air studies. It is obvious that some thalamic tumors extend forward to invade the posterior frontal area, and vice versa. The tumors are adjacent to the 3d ventricle and, therefore, situated, at least partly inferolateral to the internal cerebral vein. The thalamus is situated partly beneath the floor of the lateral ventricle and above the vein (fig. 465). It will be remembered that the thalamostriate vein lies in the sulcus between the caudate nucleus and the thalamus along the wall of the lateral ventricle. Therefore, thalamic tumors may be expected to produce an upward displacement of the thalamostriate vein which causes what has been described by Ecker and Riemenschneider (1955) as "opening of the venous angle." The internal cerebral vein usually is displaced upward and its curvature would become more rounded and the arc deeper. The elevation involves more frequently the posterior half of the vein (Potts and Taveras), as shown in Figure 466. In the frontal projection there is almost always displacement of the internal cerebral vein toward the healthy side and there is upward and medial displacement of the thalamostriate vein (figs. 466 and 467).

The arterial phase also is important in the diagnosis of deep tumors. As seen in the *frontal projection*, the angiographic Sylvian point is displaced laterally, toward the inner table. This produces a vertical or straight configuration to the middle cerebral branches as they ascend, instead of the usual curved configuration (fig. 468). Straightening is not specific for thalamic and deep tumors, however, and may be seen in the presence of extreme ventricular dilatation. The lenticulostriate arteries are displaced outward and downward; more so in the anterior thalamic or posterior deep frontal masses (fig. 468).

In the lateral projection, the arterial phase may be normal or, in many instances, there will be some degree of *upward displacement* of the branches of the middle cerebral artery. The mechanism responsible for the upward displacement of the middle cerebral branches is not well understood. It is possible that there may be an actual rotation of the insula in which its inferior

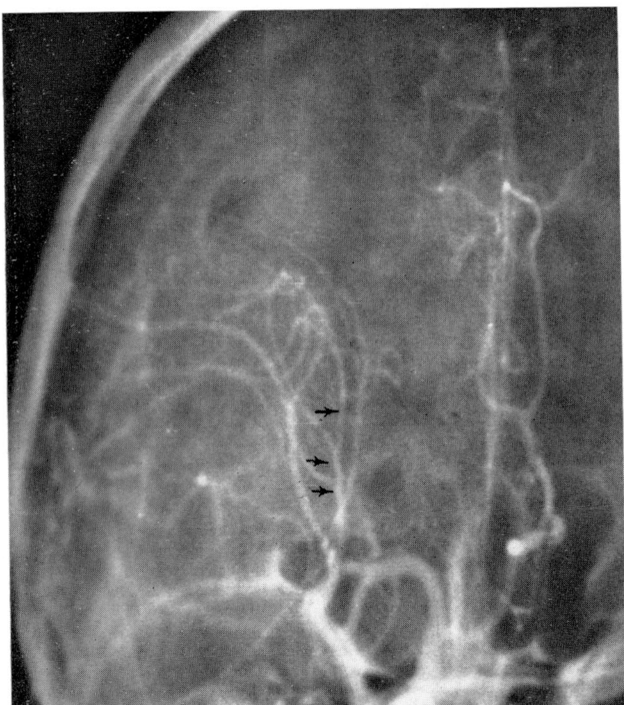

Fig. 463.—Latero-Sylvian Tumor (Pterional Meningioma)

There is medial displacement of the insular vessels and reversal of the usually convex curve of the insula (*arrows*).

portion is displaced outward and upward; the insula will then carry with it the branches of the middle cerebral artery. Another possibility is that there is tumor extension downward to involve the midbrain, which then bulges laterally to displace and rotate the lower portion of the insula and temporal lobes. The temporal lobe itself may be invaded by tumor. The pericallosal artery may be elevated in very large lesions and thereby may produce an increased rounding of its posterior portion.

The anterior chorioidal artery is usually enlarged and sometimes can be traced around the posterior portion of the thalamus. As might be expected, the vessel shows an increase in the radius of its curvature (fig. 469). The anterior chorioidal may be displaced downward in its proximal portion and straightened. If the posterior communicating and posterior cerebral arteries are visible, they may be displaced downward. The lateral posterior chorioidal arteries show an enlargement of their curvature. Usually, however, vertebral angiography is not carried out in cases of suspected thalamic tumors, but sometimes they fill from the internal carotid artery (fig. 469). The medial posterior chorioidal arteries are not specifically displaced.

The basilar vein of Rosenthal may be displaced downward, and if the tumor extends into the upper portion of the brain stem, it also will be displaced laterally. It should be pointed out that some thalamic tumors may produce atypical venous manifestations in the angiogram. Sometimes a very large thalamic tumor fails to produce elevation of the internal cerebral vein, and some tumors may produce depression of this vein if they involve chiefly the upper portion of the thalamus. In one case, the internal cerebral vein was markedly elevated on one side and yet the angiogram of the healthy side showed no evidence of elevation of the internal cerebral vein in spite of the fact that these two structures are so very close to each other in the midline.

Thalamic tumors characteristically do not produce displacement of the anterior cerebral artery across the midline, but the internal

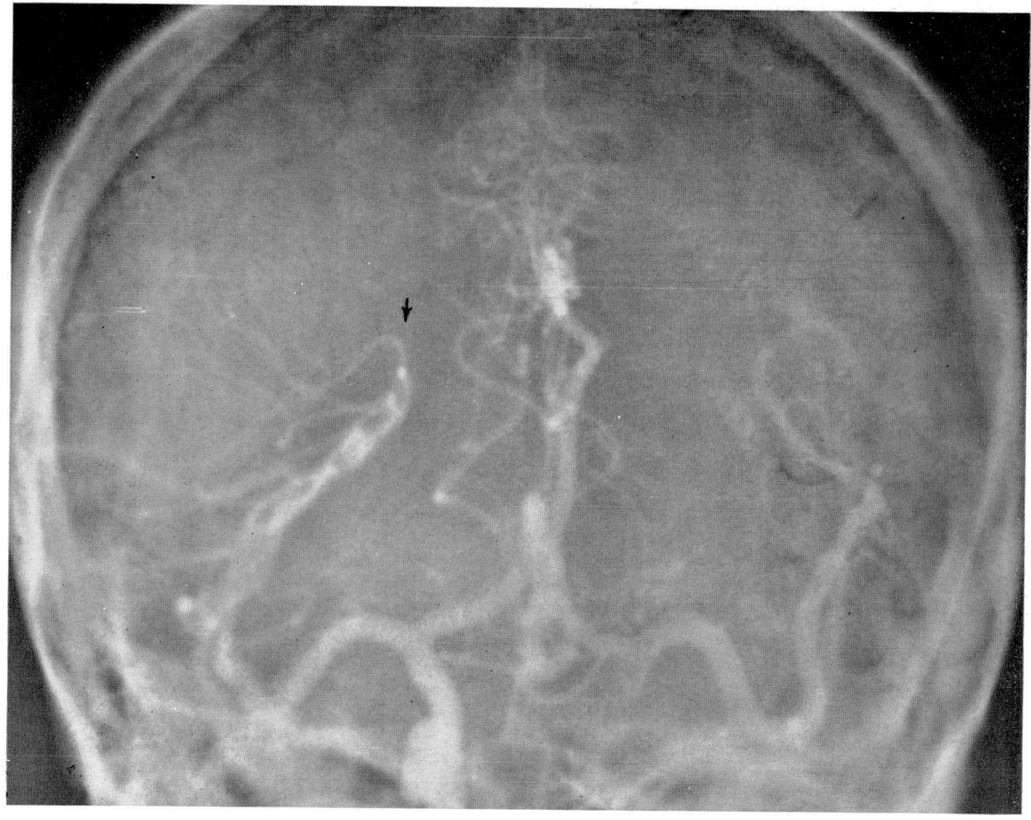

FIG. 464.—LATERO-SYLVIAN TUMOR (MENINGIOMA)
The film was made with compression of the opposite side and shows the extreme medial displacement of the angiographic Sylvian point (*arrow*) in contrast to the one of the opposite side.

cerebral vein is almost always shifted (figs. 467 and 468).

The thalamus may be secondarily invaded by a tumor situated in the parietal or posterior temporal regions, and some of the signs that such tumors produce may be modified by their deep extension (figs. 470 and 471). Primary thalamic tumors, on the other hand, may be associated with extension outside of the thalamus or they may produce downward transtentorial herniation which may modify to a certain extent their typical appearance. A very large thalamic tumor can produce downward displacement of the bifurcation of the basilar artery and the proximal portion of the posterior cerebral artery, particularly if there is downward herniation. Extension of the tumor to involve the midbrain also causes increase in the width of the curvature of the posterior cerebral artery (fig. 472). Deep posterior frontal tumors produce an increase in the height of the anterior portion of the Sylvian triangle.

Ventricular Dilatation

When the ventricles become dilated, they elevate the corpus callosum and, if the temporal horn is sufficiently enlarged, the Sylvian fissure will be high. The elevation of the corpus callosum produces an upward displacement and rounding of the curve of the pericallosal artery. However, the ventricles must be moderately to markedly enlarged before ventricular dilatation can be appreciated by an increased curvature of the pericallosal artery. Because of the normal anatomical variation of the configuration

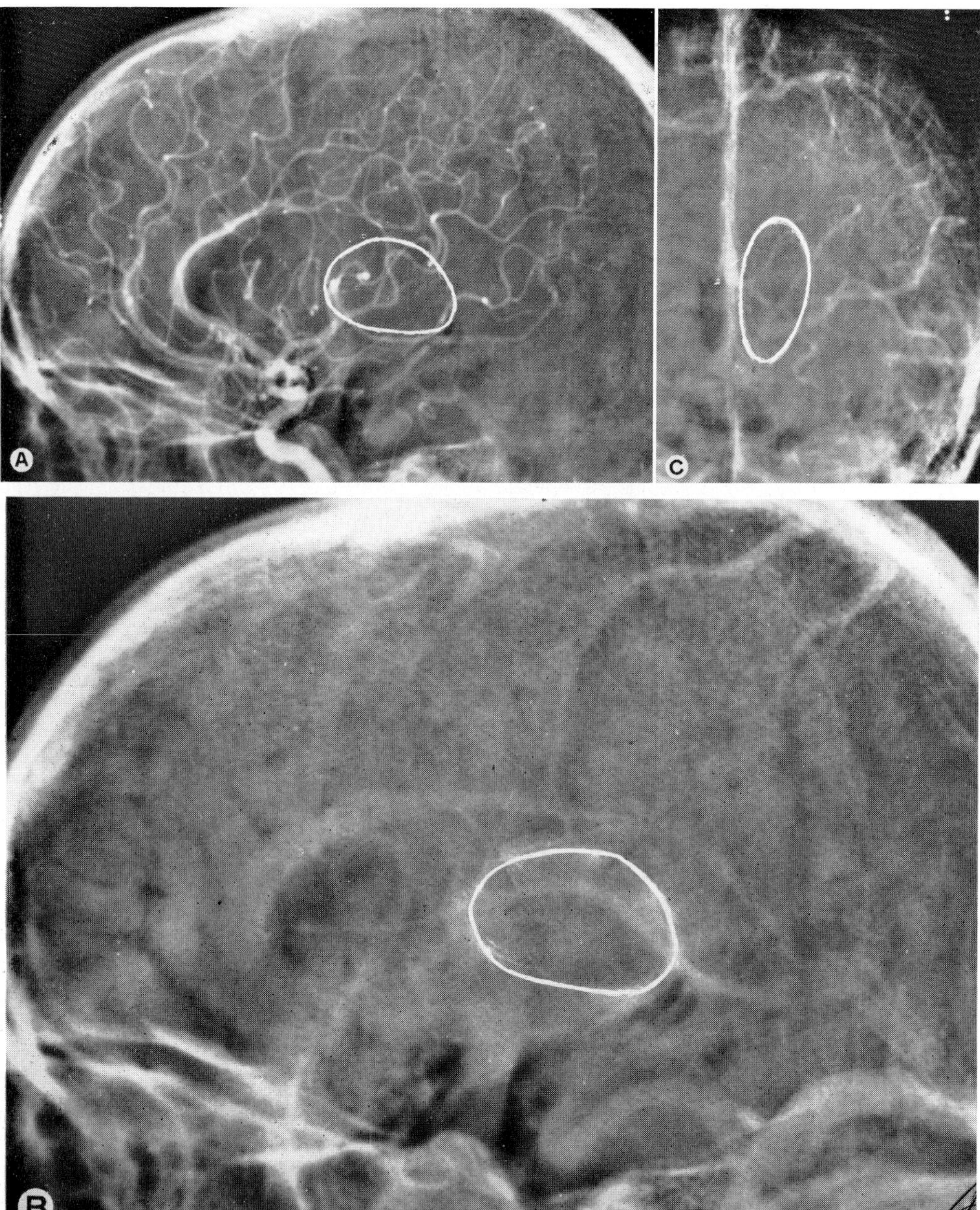

FIG. 465.—THE APPROXIMATE POSITION OF THE THALAMUS IN RELATION TO THE VESSELS, IN THE LATERAL ANGIOGRAM ARTERIAL PHASE (A); IN THE VENOUS PHASE (B); AND IN THE FRONTAL PROJECTION VENOUS PHASE (C)

The thalamus lies approximately one-third above the level of the internal cerebral vein and two-thirds below this vein, as indicated in (B).

---

of the arterial branches attached to it. The posterior communicating and cerebral arteries are displaced (*arrows*). The lateral view in the venous phase (B) discloses elevation of the internal cerebral vein which involves chiefly the posterior aspect of this vein (*arrows*). There is also a separation of the internal cerebral and basilar veins. In this respect, the picture is not dissimilar to what is seen in pinealomas. However, there is elevation of the thalamostriate vein (*arrow*) which causes "opening of the venous angle." This does not occur in pinealomas or posterior third ventricle tumors. The frontal projection in the venous phase (C) demonstrates the elevation and medial displacement of the thalamostriate vein (*arrows*) and the displacement of the internal cerebral vein across the midline (*arrow*). The latter is almost a constant finding in thalamic tumors.

(Revised 1963)

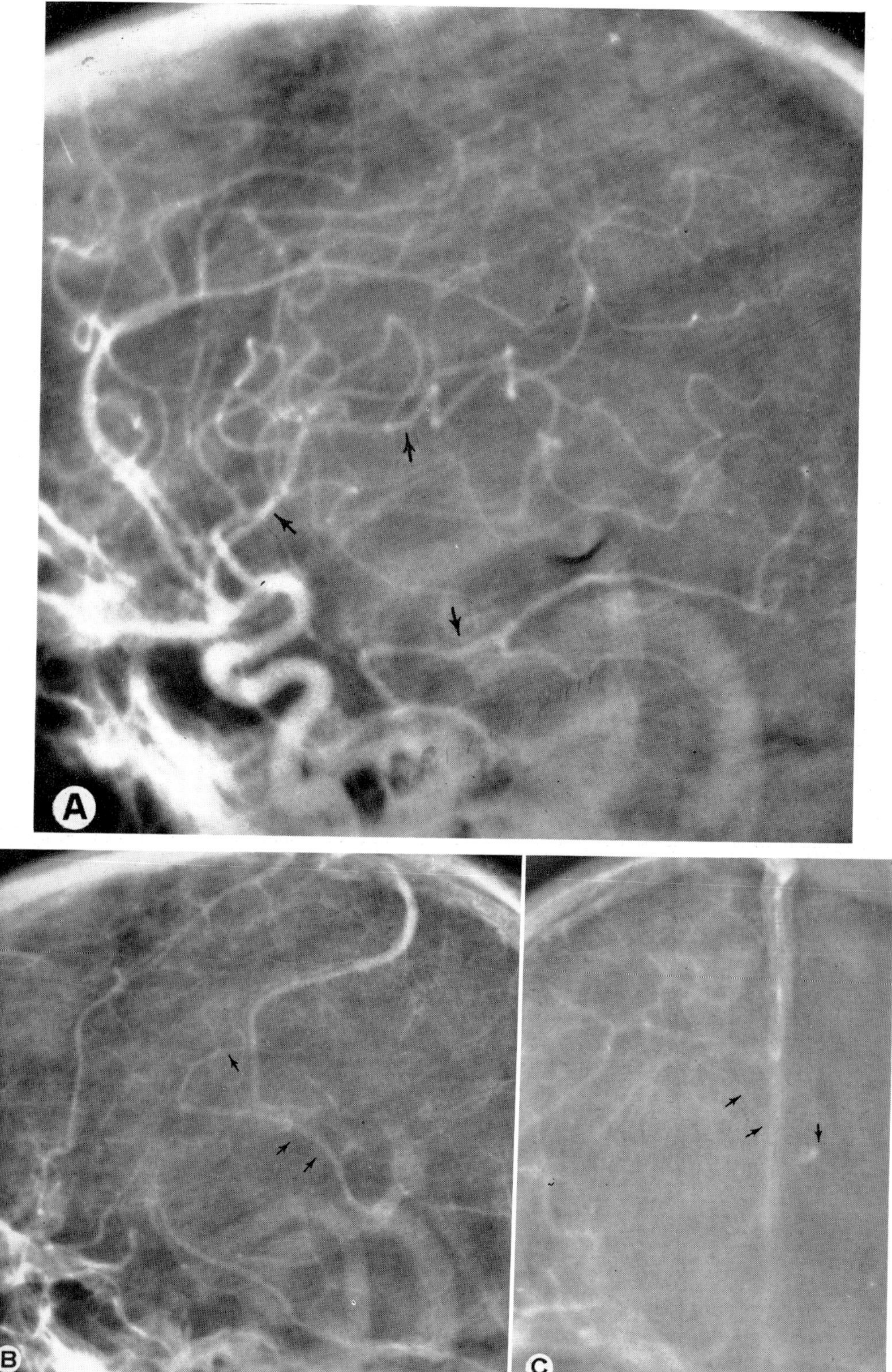

FIG. 466.—THALAMIC TUMOR

The lateral view in the arterial phase (A) shows moderate elevation of the branches of the middle cerebral artery, which is somewhat suggestive of a temporal lobe intracerebral tumor. This is felt to be due to rotation of the insula by lifting of the lower portion of this structure which results in elevation

(Revised 1963)

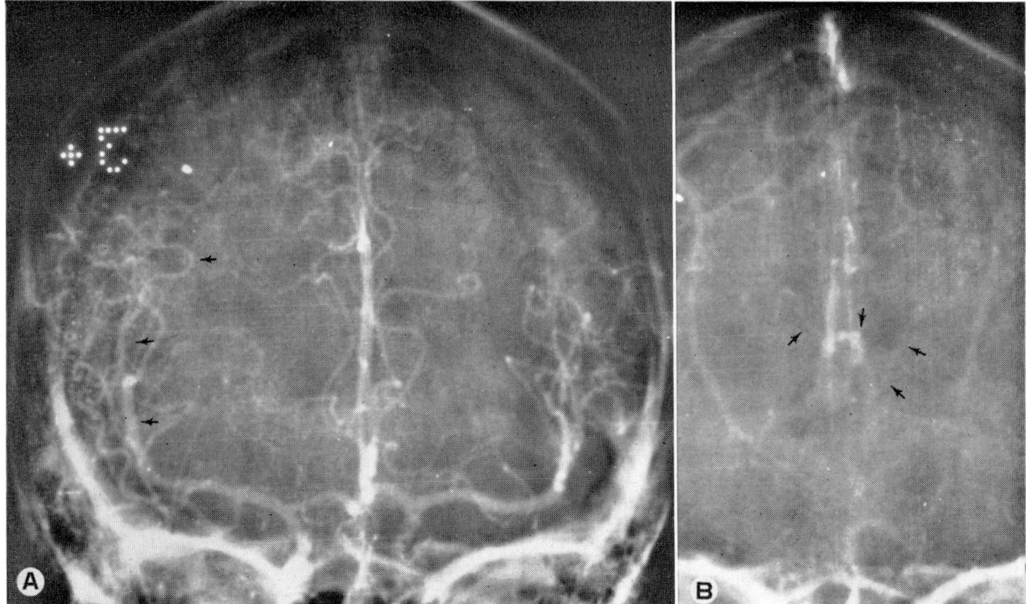

FIG. 467.—THALAMIC TUMOR

Bilateral filling obtained with compression of the opposite side at the time of the injection demonstrates in the arterial phase (A) that there is no evidence of midline shift of the anterior cerebral arteries. There is a discrepancy, however, in the space between the anterior and middle cerebral arteries when the right side is compared with the left. The branches over the insula on the left side have been displaced laterally, although the angiographic Sylvian point still seems to be normal in position (*arrow*). In the venous phase (B) the discrepancy in the position of the thalamostriate veins is noticeable. There is upward displacement of the vein on the reader's left side (*arrow*). Slight shift of the internal cerebral vein to the right is also noted (*vertical arrow*). The contralateral thalamostriate vein is also filled (*two arrows*).

of the ventricles, some patients show definite rounding of the pericallosal curve when the ventricles are not too large whereas, in others, the ventricles can become extremely large with a relatively normal pericallosal curve.

Attention should be called here to an anatomic variant which may be confused with ventricular dilatation. Not uncommonly, both pericallosal arteries fill from one side, but on the side opposite the injection only the callosomarginal artery fills, which normally describes a wider curve than the pericallosal artery (fig. 364). In such cases, a false impression of ventricular dilatation on the anomalous side is gained.

Another sign of ventricular dilatation in the arterial phase is elevation of the branches of the middle cerebral artery. The elevation is straight and does not suggest the usual rounded configuration seen with temporal tumors (fig. 479). In frontal projection, the Sylvian point may not be elevated. In the same projection, however, the arterial phase may show lateral displacement of the angiographic Sylvian point if the ventricles are extremely enlarged. The greater the degree of ventricular enlargement, the greater the lateral displacement of the angiographic Sylvian point and of the vessels over the island of Reil (fig. 473).

In our hands, the most reliable index of ventricular dilatation has been found in the frontal projection in the venous phase. The thalamostriate vein, which is situated along the floor of the lateral ventricle, is displaced laterally and its curvature is increased. The greater the degree of ventricular dilatation, the wider this curve is apt to be (fig. 474).

(Revised 1963)

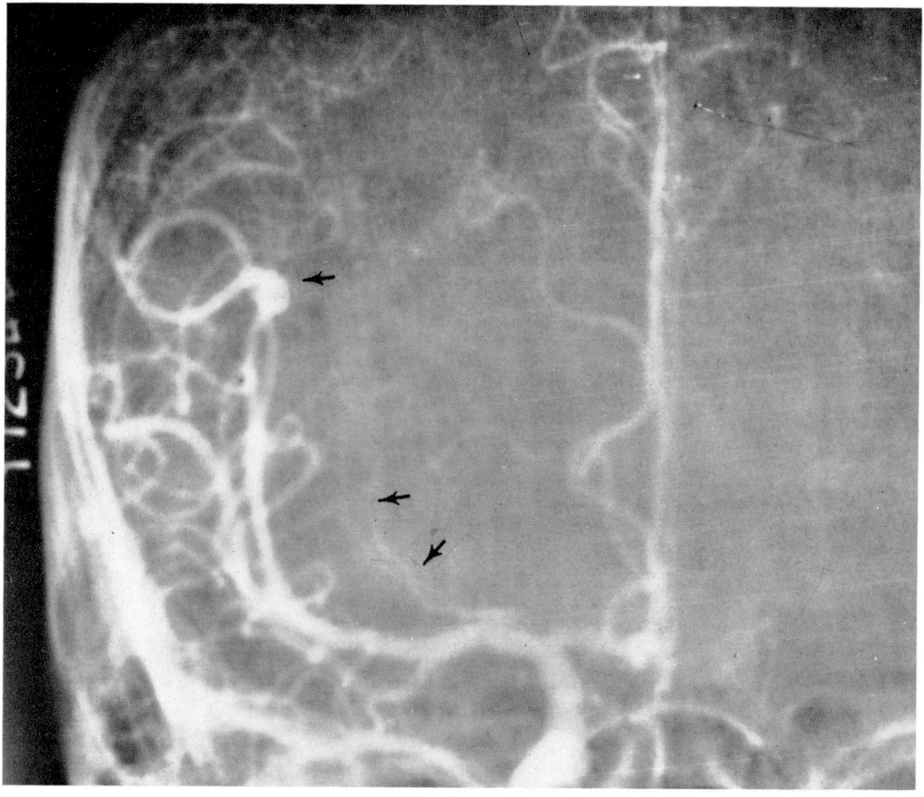

FIG. 468.—THALAMIC TUMOR

There is no evidence of shift of the anterior cerebral vessels. There is a straight upward course to the branches of the middle cerebral artery over the insula with lateral displacement of the angiographic Sylvian point (*arrow*). There is also downward displacement and bowing of the lenticulostriate arteries (*arrows*).

The venous phase in the lateral projection may show that the internal cerebral vein is relatively normal in position when all the ventricles are equally enlarged. Enlargement of the lateral ventricles tends to displace the internal cerebral vein downward, but proportionate enlargement of the third ventricle produces upward bulging of its roof and, therefore, the vein may remain in normal position or, perhaps, its curvature is slightly flatter than normal. As was described under "Anatomy," the veins that are tributaries of the thalamostriate vein and internal cerebral veins, including the septal veins, become visible as they reach the ventricular wall. Therefore, the point at which the veins become visible is usually the upper margin of the ventricular wall. The vessels are clearly seen in a high percentage of cases, and if the ventricles are enlarged, the visible section of the veins is longer (fig. 478).

When there is extreme ventricular enlargement, as in congenital internal hydrocephalus or aqueduct stenosis occurring in childhood, there is, in addition to the findings described above in the arterial phase, considerable stretching and loss of the normal undulations of the arteries of the brain. This can reach a marked degree and, in some cases, it may be associated with narrowing of the vessels that are stretched and straight (fig. 473).

The lenticulostriate arteries are usually displaced laterally and downward in cases of extreme ventricular dilatation. In this re-

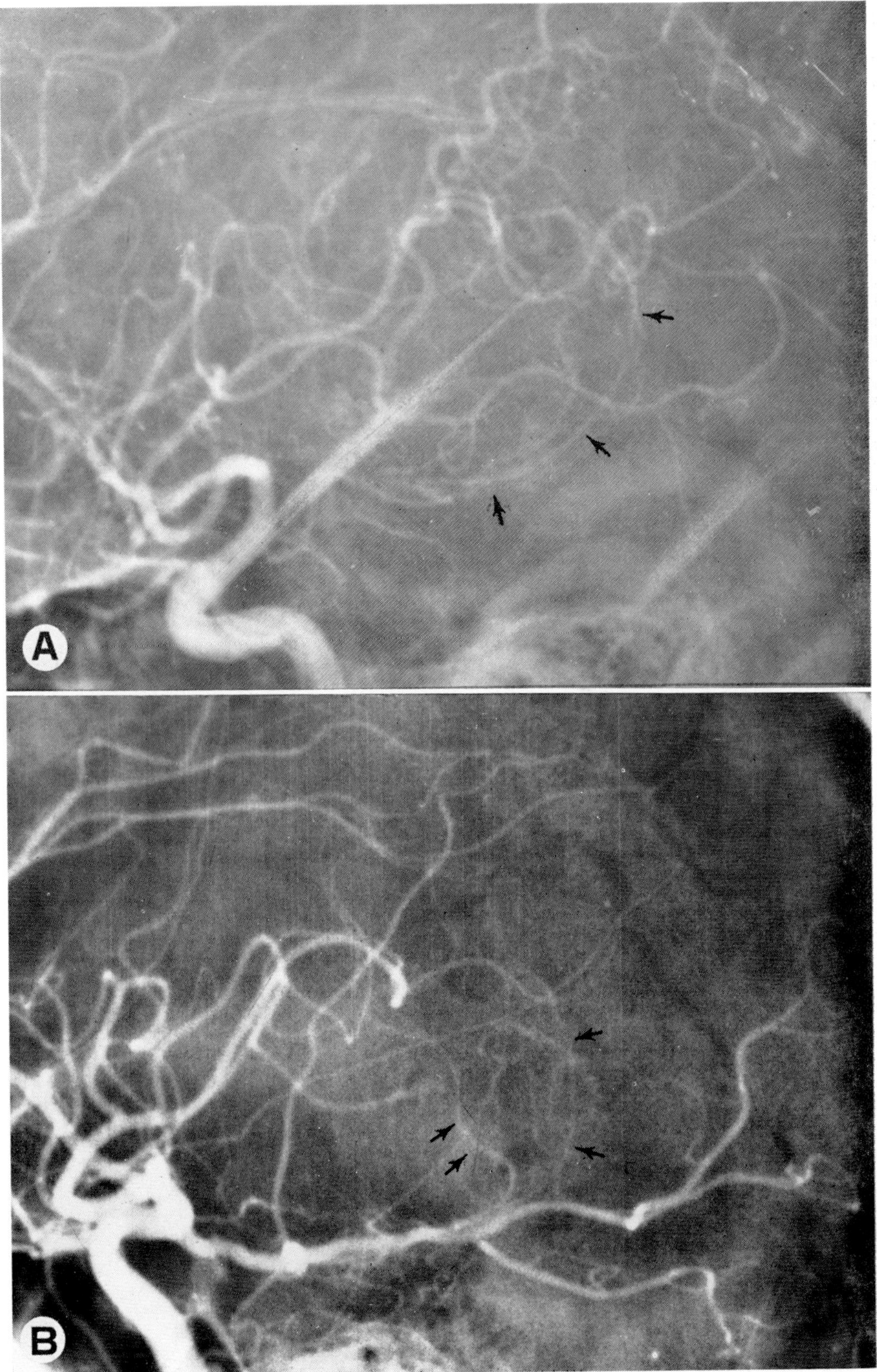

FIG. 469.—THALAMIC TUMOR

(A) The anterior chorioidal artery is enlarged and shows downward displacement of its posterior portion. The curvature in its posterior portion shows an increase in its radius due to the thalamic mass.

(Revised 1963)

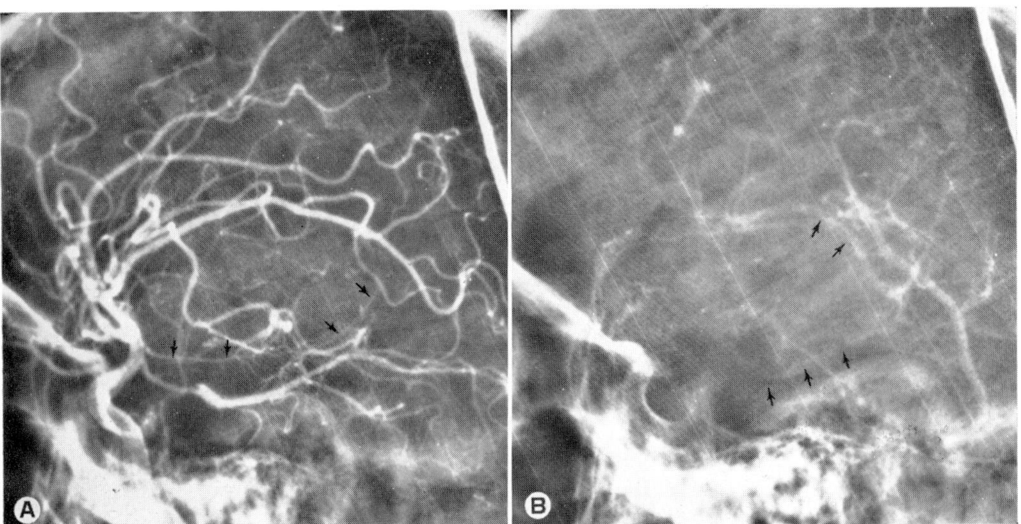

Fig. 470.—Temporal Lobe Tumor with Thalamic Extension

The lateral view in the arterial phase shows typical features of a temporal lobe tumor with elevation of the middle cerebral vessels. There is depression of the posterior communicating and posterior cerebral arteries as well as the anterior chorioidal artery (*arrows*). In addition, the lateral posterior chorioidal artery filled because of the good posterior cerebral filling, and this shows an increase in the width of its curvature (*arrows*). The lateral view in the venous phase (B) shows some elevation of the internal cerebral vein and depression of the basilar vein (*arrows*). The findings indicate that the posterior temporal tumor extends into the thalamus.

spect the appearance is similar to that of posterior deep frontal and anterior thalamic tumors, which may also produce lateral and downward displacement and stretching of these vessels (fig. 468).

Dilatation of the lateral ventricles without enlargement of the third ventricle, such as may be seen in tumors involving the foramen of Monro, causes the internal cerebral vein to be flattened; its curve may disappear completely and it is usually displaced downward. Such flattening indicates a collapse of the third ventricle with the roof of the third ventricle being displaced downward by the enlarged lateral ventricle (figs. 477 and 478). Specific lesions that produce the deformity are tumors that arise from the septum pellucidum to obstruct the foramen of Monro, and colloid cysts of the third ventricle, which have the same effect (Potts and Taveras, 1963).

On the other hand, if the third ventricle is enlarged because it contains a tumor or cyst, then the lateral ventricles are dilated and the third ventricle may be relatively larger than the lateral ventricles. An upward displacement and increased curvature of the internal cerebral vein then results. Third-ventricle gliomas, and sometimes large suprasellar tumors that project upward, elevate the roof of the third ventricle, having the same effect. Pinealomas produce a slightly different deformity, but they do also fall into this category. As mentioned above, if the block is in the aqueduct of Sylvius or below, the enlargement of the lateral ventricles and of the third ventricle is uniform and the internal cerebral vein probably

---

There is also elevation of the middle cerebral branches as was also noted in Fig. 465. In (B) an angiogram of another case, there is downward displacement of the posterior cerebral artery. The lateral posterior chorioidal artery is filled and shows widening of its curvature (*arrows*). The medial posterior chorioidal artery is not displaced (*double arrows*). There is elevation of the middle cerebral branches.

(Revised 1963)

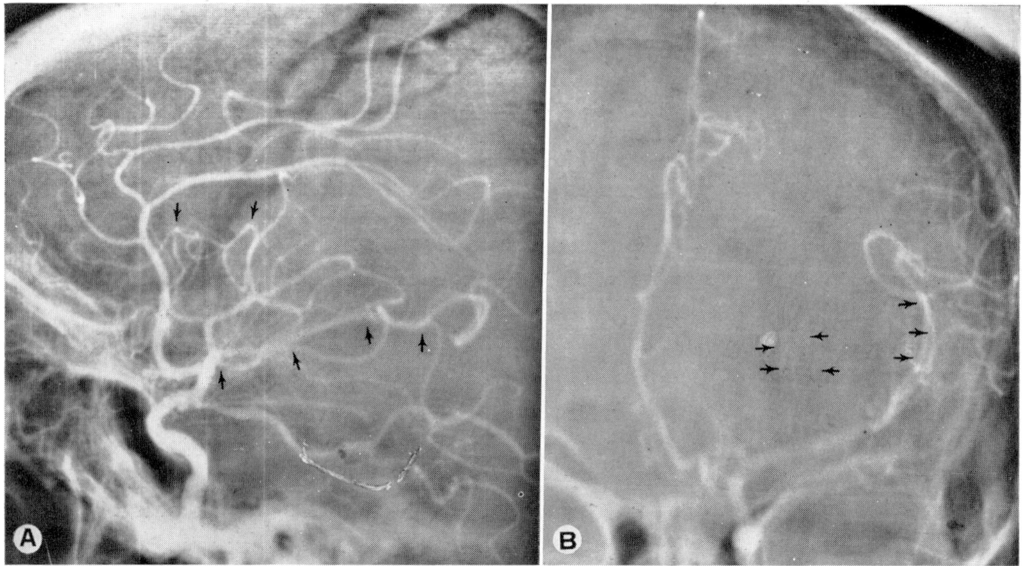

Fig. 471.—True Frontotemporal Tumor

The lateral view in the arterial phase (A) shows elevation and distortion of the inferior and posterior aspect of the Sylvian triangle (*arrows*). At the same time, there is an increase in the vertical diameter of the anterior portion of the Sylvian triangle with distortion of the vessels (*arrows*). Many fine, straight vessels can be seen in the general area of the Sylvian triangle. The frontal projection (B) shows shift of the anterior cerebral artery, slight elevation of the horizontal portion of the middle cerebral artery with rounding of the knee of the middle cerebral artery. However, there is lateral displacement of the vessels over the outer surface of the island of Reil (*arrows*). The latter cannot be explained on the basis of a temporal lobe tumor which usually produces the reverse and cannot be explained on the basis of involvement of the frontal operculum; there must be a tumor medial to the vessels to produce this finding. In addition, there is stretching of the lenticulostriate arteries which are straight up and down and do not have their usual S-shaped curve (*arrows*). At autopsy there was an oligodendroglioma which had infiltrated across the Sylvian fissure to involve both the temporal and the frontal lobes deeply. Increase in the vertical width of the Sylvian triangle is a feature of deep posterior frontal tumors.

will remain in normal position or be slightly flattened.

Porencephalic dilatation of certain portions of the ventricles may cause a displacement of vessels somewhat similar to that caused by tumors. This is particularly true in cases that involve the temporal horn and the atrium of the lateral ventricles. Sometimes the displacement caused by porencephaly can be extremely marked, such as is shown in Figure 615. The most reliable finding is the absence of midline shift of the anterior cerebral artery or of displacement of the internal cerebral vein toward the opposite side in cases of porencephaly. Moreover, in porencephaly, sometimes the shift may be toward the atrophic side due to cerebral hemiatrophy of the entire corresponding hemisphere.

In diffuse cerebral atrophy the ventricles do not usually become as large as in cases of obstructive hydrocephalus and for this reason the characteristic angiographic signs of ventricular dilatation are not seen. Because the ventricles dilate through loss of substance of the hemispheres, there is usually no appreciable elevation of the corpus callosum and no upward displacement of the anterior cerebral artery. When marked cerebral atrophy is present there is often an increase in the cerebrospinal fluid cushion over the surfaces of the hemispheres, thereby increasing the distance between the pial vessels and the inner table of the skull. It is therefore possible, in severe cases, to diagnose the presence of diffuse cortical atrophy by the fact that the vessels on the surface of the brain are separated by several

(*Revised 1963*)

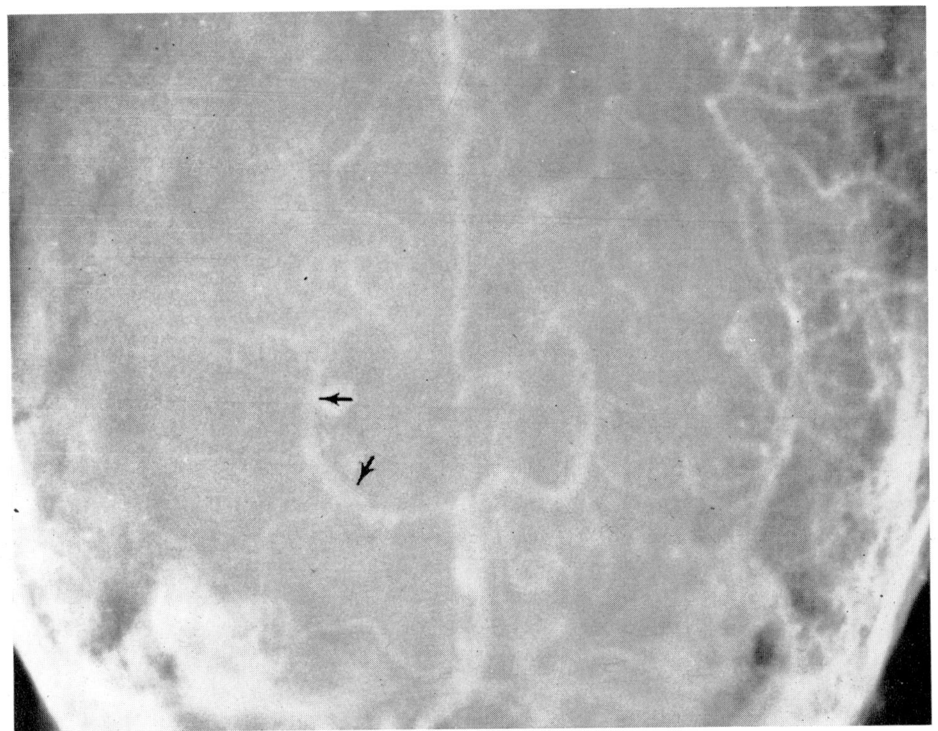

FIG. 472.—THALAMIC TUMOR WITH EXTENSION INTO THE MIDBRAIN

The child had a left thalamic tumor extending downward and producing stretching and increase in the width of the curvature of the posterior cerebral artery on the tumor side as compared with that on the opposite side (*arrows*). The lesion was demonstrated by a right retrograde brachial angiogram so as to visualize the carotid and vertebral systems simultaneously.

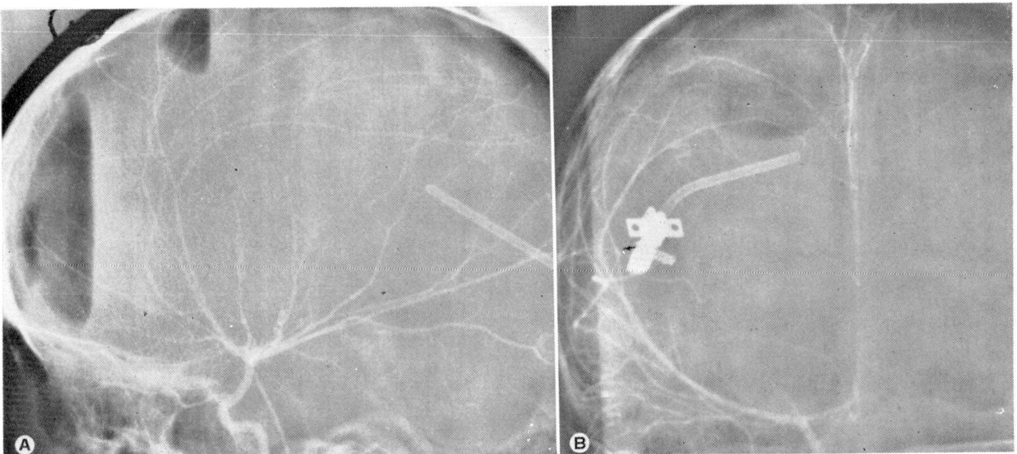

FIG. 473.—MARKED VENTRICULAR DILATATION

The lateral view (A) shows the extreme degree of stretching and loss of undulations resulting from the marked ventricular dilatation; the pericallosal artery shows increase in rounding, and there is a straight appearance to the middle cerebral vessels as they extend backward and upward. The frontal projection (B) demonstrates the lack of midline shift and the marked lateral displacement of the angiographic Sylvian point (*arrow*). The venous phase was not recorded in the serialogram, even though a span of 9 seconds was covered during the examination. The obstructive hydrocephalus was secondary to a tumor of the posterior third of the third ventricle in a 2-year-old child.

(Revised 1963)

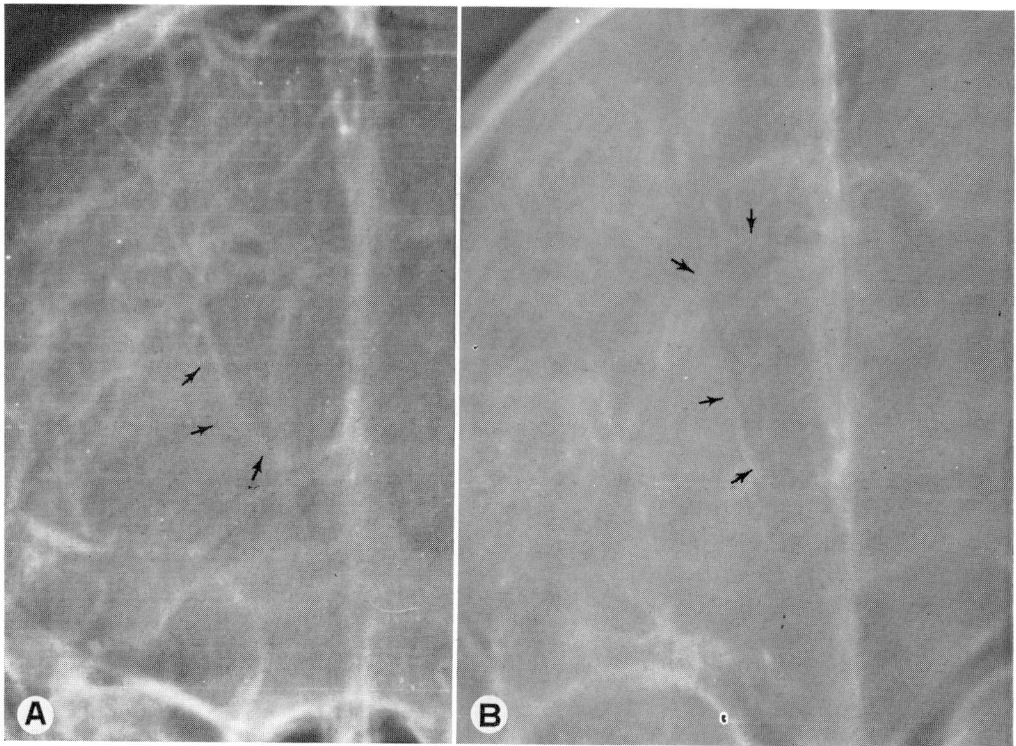

FIG. 474.—VENTRICULAR DILATATION, MODERATE

The anteroposterior film in the venous phase (A) demonstrates the increase in the width of the curve of the thalamostriate vein (*arrows*). The larger the ventricular enlargement is, the wider is the curve of the thalamostriate vein. In (B), an anteroposterior film of another case taken in an intermediate phase while there was some arterial and some venous filling, shows the radiolucent, avascular shadow of the ventricle completely outlined against the opacified background of the brain. This appearance is sometimes seen in the intermediate phase when there is some degree of ventricular dilatation. The thalamostriate vein is already filled and contributes to the enhancement of the ventricular shadow. A more constant demonstration of the ventricles can be obtained by laminagraphy in the anteroposterior projection made in the venous phase.

millimeters from the inner table of the skull. In these instances the vessels maintain the outwardly convex configuration of the cerebral surface and are not flattened or locally depressed as with subdural hematoma.

Miscellaneous Deep Tumors

The majority of lesions in this group arise within the ventricles or from the corpus callosum. The intraventricular tumors may be divided into two groups, those that involve the lateral ventricles and those that involve the third ventricle.

Lateral intraventricular masses. The tumors that occur in the lateral ventricles are usually intraventricular meningiomas, ependymomas, chorioid plexus papillomas, and mixed gliomas (usually oligodendrogliomas and astrocytomas). Tumors that arise from the septum pellucidum are usually mixed gliomas; in our series a few have been ganglioneuromas and gangliogliomas. Intraventricular epidermoids can occur either in the midline or in the lateral ventricles. Generally, intraventricular tumors are best diagnosed by pneumography. However, it is common to see such cases first examined by angiography because of the practice prevalent in many centers of studying any clinically suspected supra-tentorial lesion by angiography first, with pneumography as

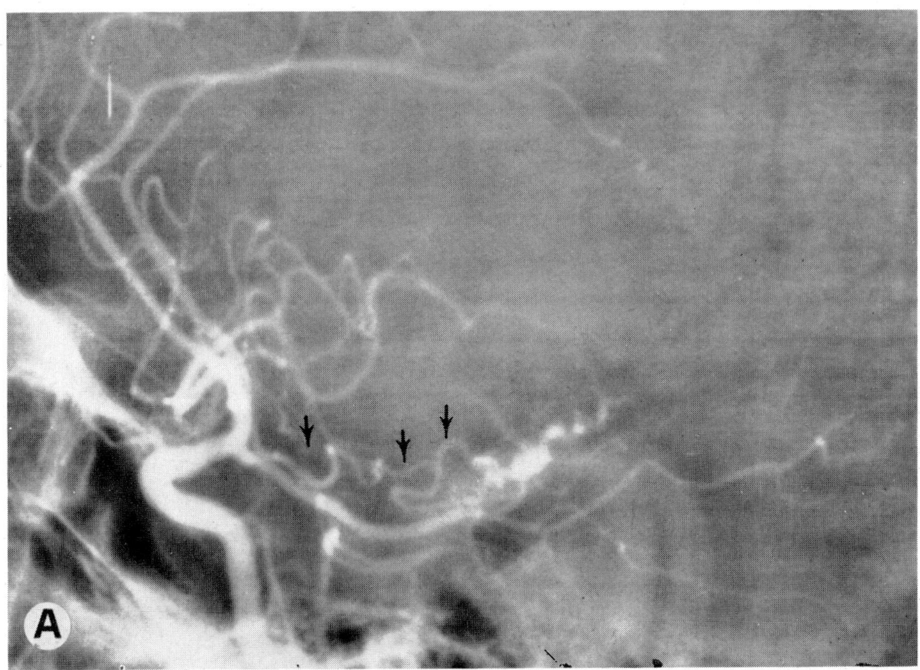

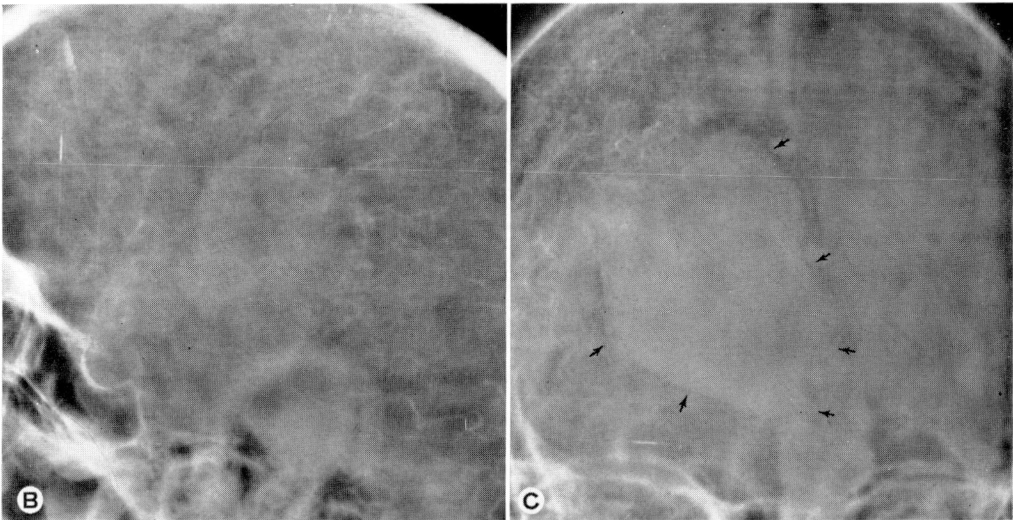

FIG. 475.—INTRAVENTRICULAR MENINGIOMA WITH ABNORMAL BLOOD SUPPLY

In the arterial phase (A) there is enlargement and considerable tortuosity of the anterior chorioidal artery (*arrows*). There is evidently enlargement of the posterior chorioidal arteries arising from the posterior cerebral artery as well (*posterior arrow*). The film made at 3.5 seconds (B) shows a homogeneous, almost perfectly round, radiopacity in the center of the skull having an appearance consistent with the cloud of a meningioma. The frontal film (C) made at the same time (3.5 seconds), shows the position of the homogeneous cloud just off the midline and partly beyond the midline. The position of the collection of contrast material would place the tumor most likely within the ventricles, and therefore a diagnosis of intraventricular meningioma was justified in this case preoperatively.

(Revised 1963)

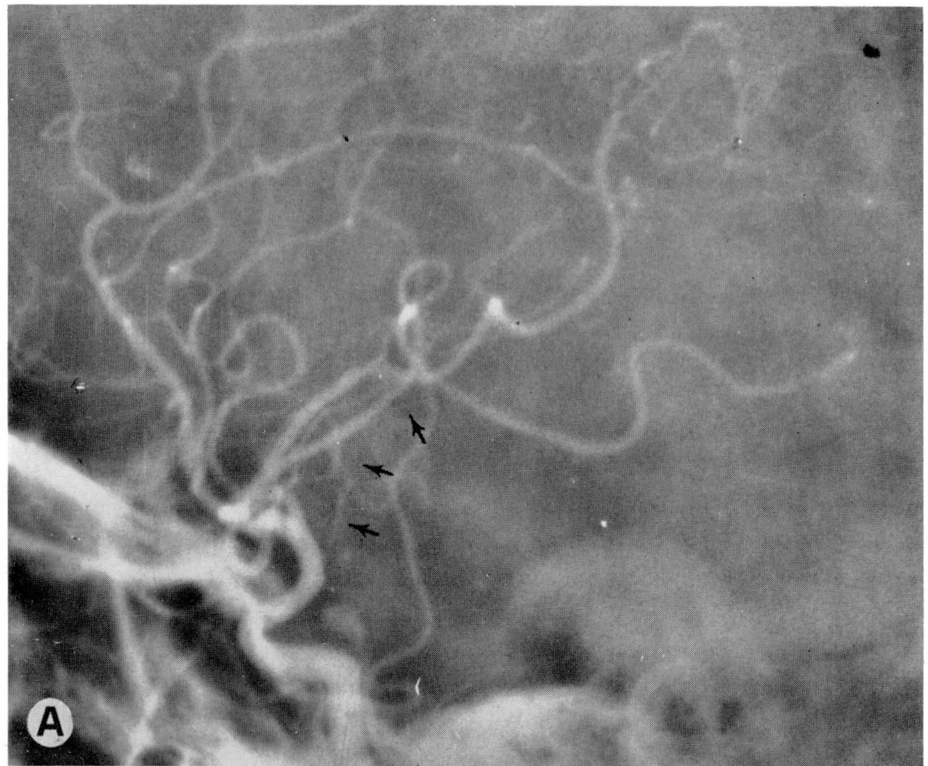

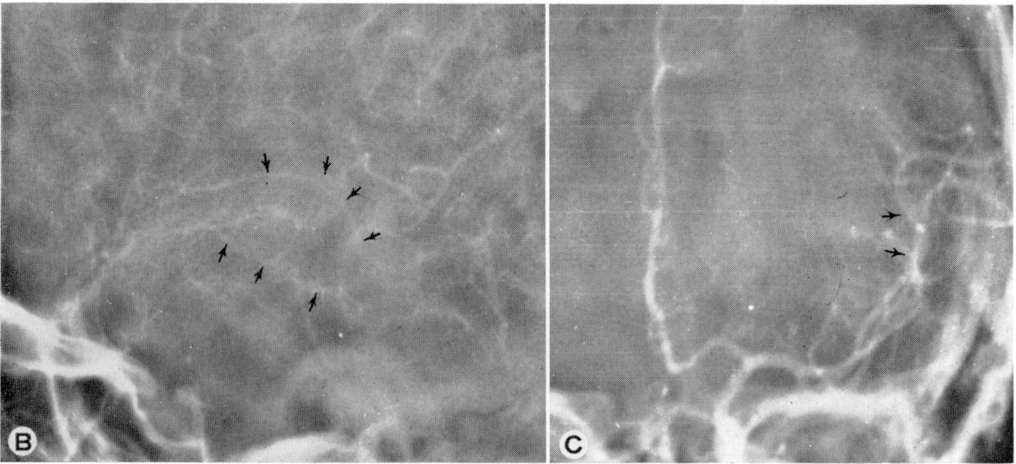

FIG. 476.—INTRAVENTRICULAR CHOLESTEATOMA OF THE TEMPORAL HORN

The lateral view in the arterial phase (A) shows moderate elevation of the branches of the middle cerebral artery chiefly involving the anterior portion. The siphon shows a forward displacement of the bifurcation. The anterior chorioid artery (*arrows*) is markedly elevated. The lateral view in the venous phase (B) shows marked elevation of the anterior portion of the basilar vein which only filled momentarily in the serialogram (*arrows*). In addition, there is rounding and elevation of the curve of the internal cerebral vein (*upper arrows*). The frontal projection (C) reveals minimum shift of the anterior cerebral artery. There is lateral displacement of the middle cerebral branches over the insula, with the resultant increase in the width of the space between the middle and anterior cerebral arteries. Unfor-

(Revised 1963)

the second diagnostic procedure. When these tumors are studied first by pneumography, an angiogram is unnecessary (see "Intraventricular Tumors" under "Intracranial Pneumography").

The chorioid plexus papillomas arise more frequently in the atrial portions of the ventricles than elsewhere. The same applies to intraventricular meningiomas which arise from the walls of the chorioid plexus. Unless these intraventricular tumors present abnormal vascularity, they probably will not be localized by angiography. Usually only ventricular dilatation is demonstrated without any specific findings. When these tumors are vascular, an abnormal blood supply may be present through the chorioidal arteries. In the case of intraventricular meningiomas, the anterior chorioidal or the posterior chorioidal arteries may be markedly enlarged (fig. 475). In some instances a true tumor cloud, typical of meningiomas, can be seen. Chorioid plexus papillomas also are extremely vascular, and the same applies to mixed gliomas which, in our experience, have been rather richly vascularized. Large veins draining the tumor by way of the thalamostriate and internal cerebral vessels may be seen. By visualizing the position of the abnormal vascular pattern in the lateral and frontal projections, it is possible to diagnose a mass deep in location. A diagnosis of cholesteatoma or epidermoid of the lateral ventricles cannot be made by angiography because these tumors are avascular. The intraventricular location of the mass can be suspected when they are in the temporal lobe (fig. 476). On the other hand, diagnosis by pneumography is relatively easy because these tumors do have a rather characteristic configuration (see under "Intraventricular Tumors" in the section on "Intracranial Pneumography").

Tumors that arise from the septum pellucidum often produce blockage at the foramen of Monro and there is an associated collapse of the third ventricle. The diagnosis can be suspected, at least, even in the absence of abnormal vascularity in these cases. The septal veins may be enlarged and deformed. Lateral ventricular obstruction and the collapse of the third ventricle causes a marked degree of flattening of the internal cerebral vein. The thalamostriate vein may be enlarged even in the absence of visible abnormal vessels because it usually drains the neoplasm; it also may be distorted (fig. 477).

Juxtavtenricular tumors, which secondarily invade the lateral ventricles and which have an abnormal vascularity, may be confused angiographically with intraventricular tumors. In both frontal and lateral projections, such tumors lie in the general location of the lateral ventricles. This confusion, however, may occur even at pneumography.

Third ventricular masses. The intraventricular tumors of the third ventricle may be divided into three types: those of the anterior portion, typically the colloid cysts; those of the posterior portion, typically pinealomas; and those which involve the entire third ventricle. The latter may arise from the wall of the third ventricle or in the suprasellar region, secondarily obliterating the lumen of the third ventricle almost completely. Colloid cysts of the anterior superior third ventricle produce marked dilatation of the lateral ventricles and collapse of the third ventricle by virtue of the fact that they block the foramen of Monro.

---

tunately, the anterior chorioidal artery could not be identified definitely in the frontal projection. An analysis was made in the following manner. The marked elevation of the anterior chorioidal artery and of the basilar vein indicated the presence of a deeply placed tumor capable of producing this marked upward displacement. However, in the frontal projection the tumor appeared to be medial to the insula because there was lateral displacement of the insular branches and there was also elevation of the internal cerebral vein. In the frontal venogram (not shown here), there was a slight elevation of the thalamostriate vein. A thalamic tumor was not considered as a possibility because of the marked elevation of the chorioidal artery and the basilar vein. Therefore, an intraventricular tumor within the temporal horn was considered most likely because it was felt that a subtemporal lesion, similar to that shown in Fig. 454, should not produce lateral displacement of the middle cerebral branches.

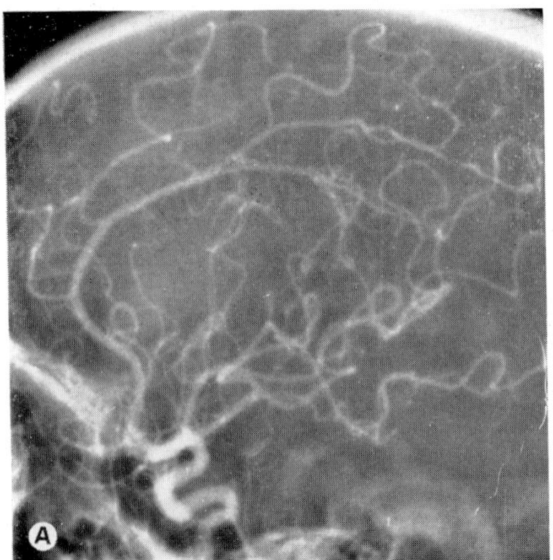

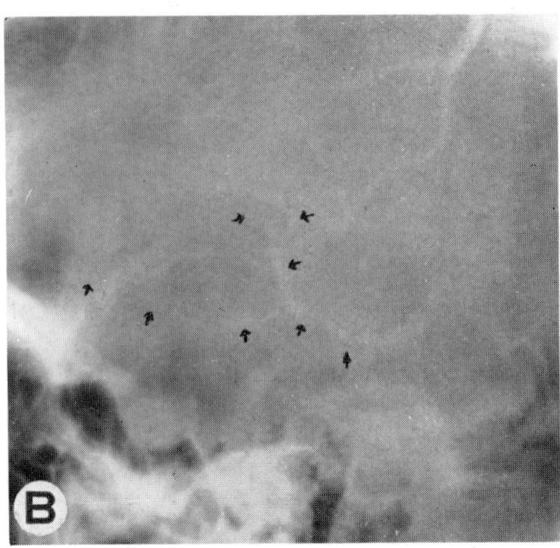

FIG. 477.—LARGE TUMOR OF THE SEPTUM PELLUCIDUM

The lateral projection in the arterial phase shows typical signs of ventricular dilatation with rounding of the pericallosal artery and straight general elevation of the inferior boundary of the Sylvian triangle. The lateral view in the venous phase (B) reveals a markedly low position of the internal cerebral vein which, nevertheless, has preserved its curvature (*arrows*). There is an enlarged thalamostriate vein which also receives large tributaries (*arrows*). The septal vein can be seen for a certain distance due to the ventricular dilatation and is low in position. The findings were considered to be those of marked ventricular dilatation associated with depression without deformity of the internal cerebral vein which was interpreted as due to collapse of the 3d ventricle; that is, the tumor was above the 3d ventricle and was blocking the foramen of Monro. The enlarged veins indicated an abnormal drainage by this route. The angiogram of the opposite side also revealed depression of the internal cerebral vein. There was no midline shift.

In this respect they resemble the septum pellucidum tumors. With colloid cysts, however, the internal cerebral vein is flattened in its posterior portion, but in its anterior portion it describes a sharp curve concave downward which is not present in the tumors situated within the anterior portion of the lateral ventricles. Presumably the extra anterior curve of the vein develops owing to pressure from the cyst below (fig. 478). Such a typical appearance has been seen in several instances of colloid cyst.

Tumors of the posterior portion of the third ventricle usually are diagnosed as pinealomas, but some of these are ordinary gliomas, perhaps even one-third of such lesions (Cummins, Taveras, and Schlesinger, 1960). Tumors of the pineal region usually produce separation of the posterior portions of the internal cerebral and basilar veins owing to elevation of the internal cerebral vein in its posterior segment. Typically, the roof of the third ventricle is displaced upward by the tumor and the internal cerebral veins are displaced upward symmetrically (fig. 479). On the other hand, the internal cerebral vein may not be displaced by a small pineal tumor, and it is possible for relatively large pineal tumors not to displace the vein to an extent that can be recognized as abnormal in the angiogram. Sometimes only a small depression on the inferior aspect of the vein is shown (fig. 480). If the tumor is large, however, the vein is usually truly displaced and it tends to form an angle with the vein of Galen instead of the usual normal S-shaped configuration (Löfgren, 1958). The internal cerebral vein was displaced in 12 of the 21 cases described by Löfgren.

In patients in whom the posterior cerebral artery fills well at carotid angiography and ordinarily at vertebral angiography, it is possible to see backward displacement and an increase in the curvature of the posterior

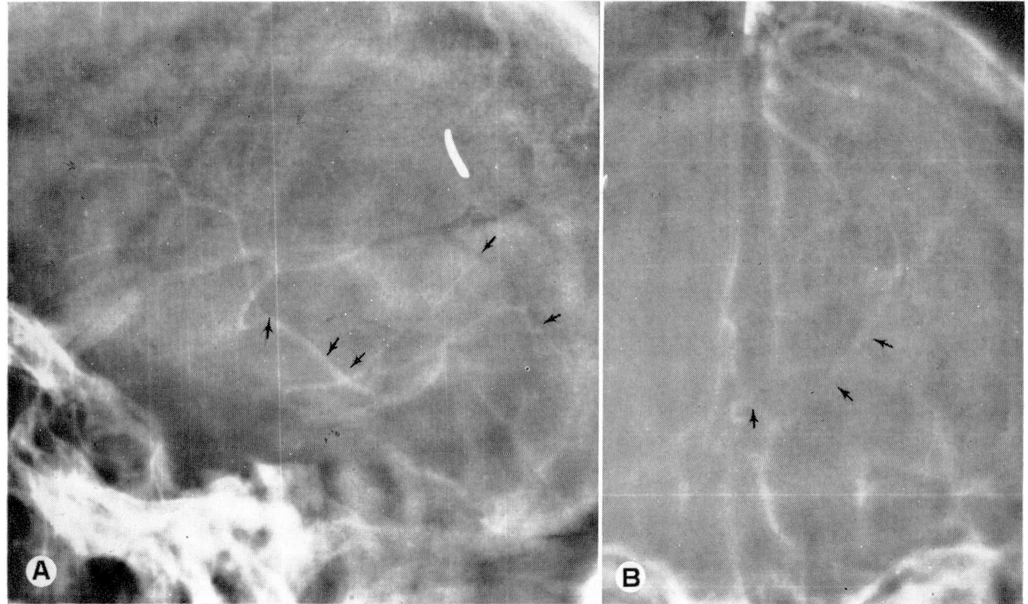

FIG. 478.—COLLOID CYST OF THE THIRD VENTRICLE

The carotid angiogram showed general signs of ventricular dilatation as seen in the arterial phase. The lateral venogram (A) shows a downward displacement of the internal cerebral vein which, on its anterior aspect, makes a curve concave downward (*arrow*). This appearance can be produced by a tumor in the anterior portion of the 3d ventricle which blocks the foramen of Monro and causes collapse of the posterior portion of the 3d ventricle. The frontal projection (B) demonstrates a curve concave downward, formed by the thalamostriate vein (*arrow*). The thalamostriate vein demonstrates the extreme degree of ventricular dilatation which is present. In fact, in the lateral projection, it is possible to visualize the actual size of the ventricles which are outlined by the most peripheral portion of the deep veins outlined in the lateral venogram (*arrows*).

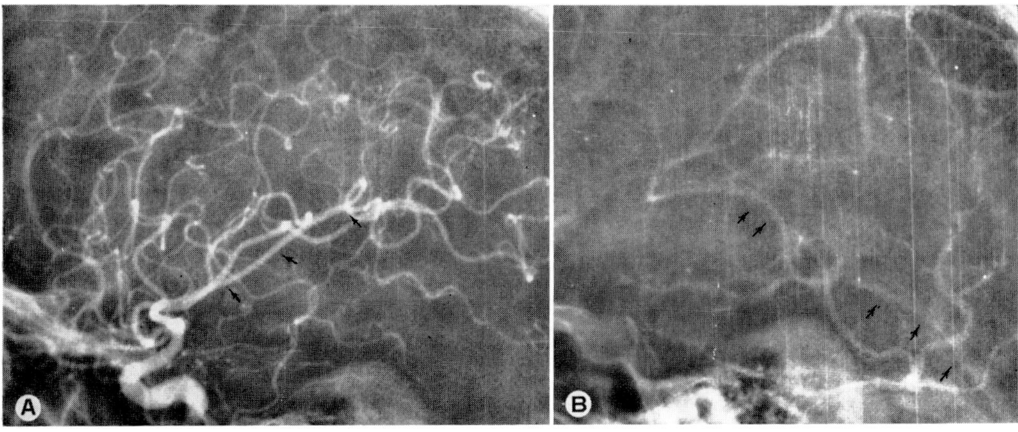

FIG. 479.—TUMOR OF THE POSTERIOR THIRD OF THE THIRD VENTRICLE (PROBABLY PINEALOMA)

The lateral view in the arterial phase (A) shows no significant elevation of the pericallosal artery, but there is moderate elevation of the lower boundary of the Sylvian triangle (*arrows*). The elevation of the middle cerebral branches is straight and uniform due to the dilatation of the temporal horn. The lateral venogram (B) discloses elevation of the posterior portion of the internal cerebral vein (*arrows*) without any deformity of the basilar vein. A ventriculogram (not shown here) disclosed a small posterior 3d ventricle tumor which, on superimposition of the air study films with the lateral venogram, corresponded to the elevation of the internal cerebral vein. The straight sinus is curved in this instance (*posterior arrows*).

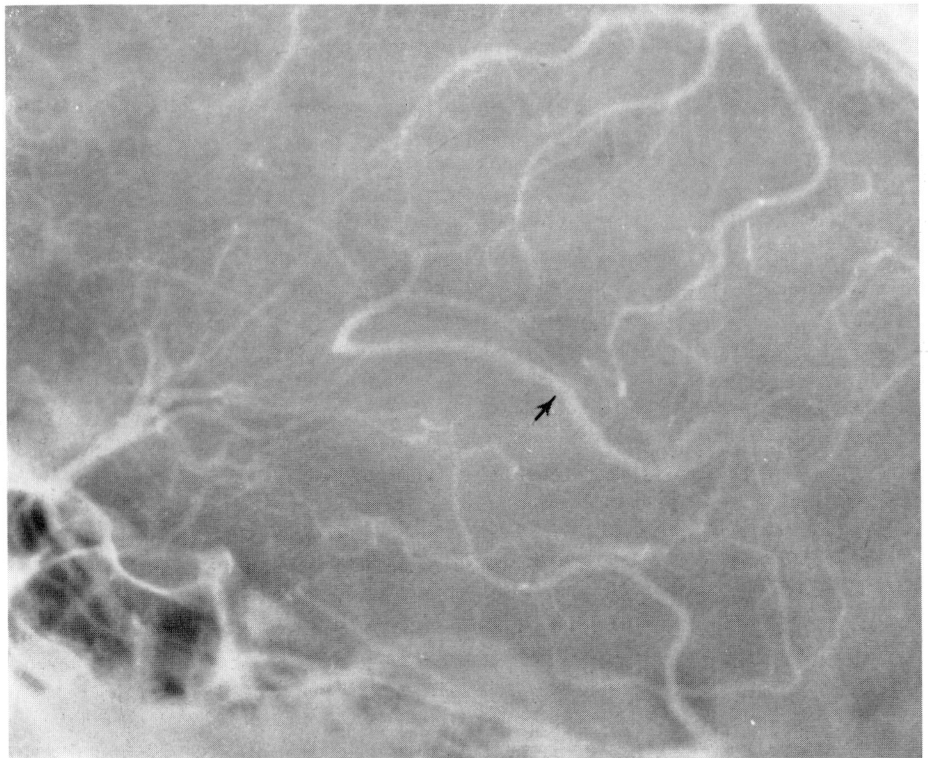

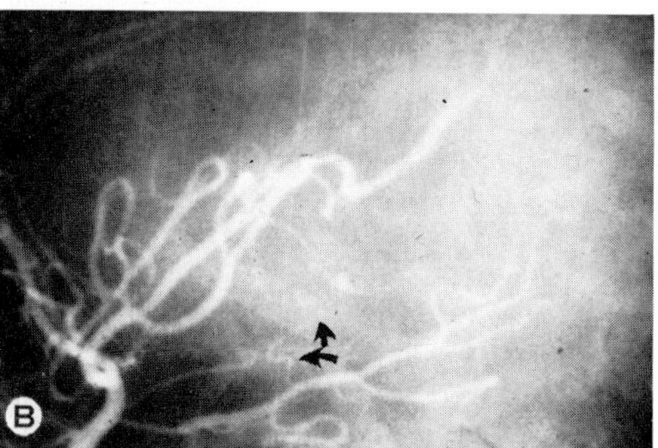

FIG. 480.—SMALL TUMOR OF THE POSTERIOR PORTION OF THE THIRD VENTRICLE

The lateral venogram shows only a very slight localized elevation of the internal cerebral vein (*arrow*). A ventriculogram performed later revealed a tumor in that location. The appearance noted here, however, is sometimes seen in normal cases. In another case of pinealoma the medial posterior chorioidal artery was displaced forward as shown by the *arrows* in (B). The posterior portion of the internal cerebral vein was slightly elevated as shown in (C). The *arrow* points to the calcification seen on the plain films. A ventriculogram (D) demonstrates the typical tumor encroachment on the posterior portion of the third ventricle. The calcification is seen to be approximately in the center of the tumor mass.

chorioidal branches in the presence of pinealoma. It is the medial posterior chorioidal arteries that can be expected to be displaced earliest in these cases (Galloway and Greitz, 1960). The internal cerebral vein, however, remains the most important structure in the diagnosis of pinealoma by angiography. In one of our cases the medial

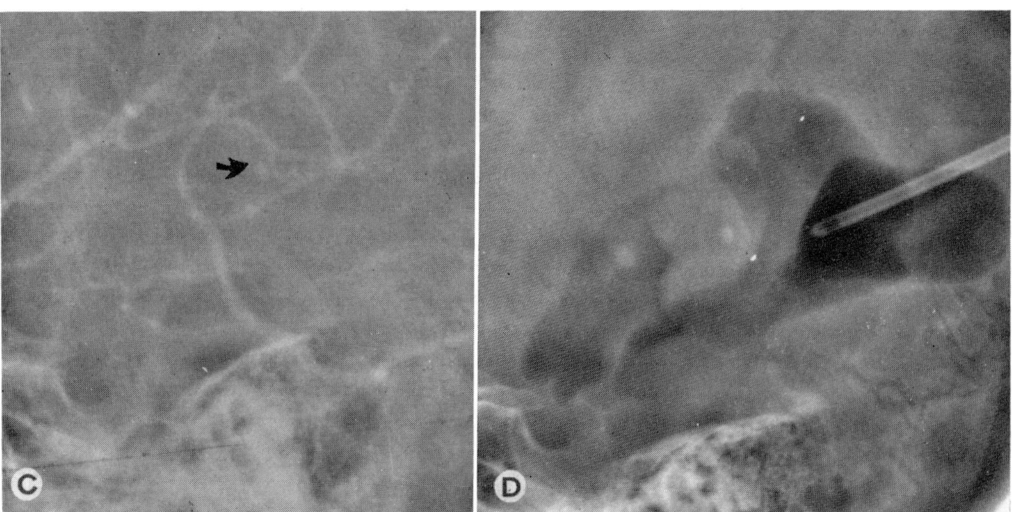

FIG. 480. C–D

posterior chorioidal artery was displaced downward and forward but the posterior portion of the internal cerebral vein and vein of Galen were displaced upward (fig. 480 B, C, and D).

Tumors that involve the entire third ventricle produce an increase in size of this ventricle through invasion and elevation of its roof. The internal cerebral veins are elevated in these cases, as well as in the presence of suprasellar tumors which extend upward sufficiently to cause elevation of the roof of the third ventricle (fig. 481). The internal cerebral veins usually are not displaced from the midline, and this differentiates the intraventricular from the thalamic and other hemispheric tumors with deep extension. The latter may cause elevation of the internal cerebral vein but may also produce a shift of the veins to the opposite (normal) side. The lateral ventricles usually are markedly enlarged, and other signs of ventricular dilatation will be present in the angiogram. For this reason the thalamostriate vein shows widening of its curvature whereas in thalamic tumor, it is displaced medially and upward. Large third ventricle tumors also may bulge inferiorly and produce a downward displacement and kinking of the basilar artery near its bifurcation, similar to that which may be seen in some severe cases of bilateral transtentorial herniation (fig. 482).

Corpus callosum tumors. It is often difficult to localize a tumor to the corpus callosum on the basis of the angiogram. Cerebral pneumography on the contrary usually permits accurate diagnosis of these tumors. The chief angiographic characteristics of these masses are elevation of the pericallosal artery with depression of the internal cerebral vein, which may or may not remain in the midline (fig. 483). Because corpus callosum tumors are often malignant, abnormal vessels are frequently seen on the angiogram.

Suprasellar and Parasellar Tumors

Lesions of the parasellar region may be intradural or extradural in location. The extradural masses are chiefly the carcinomas of the sphenoid sinuses and nasopharynx which extend upward, and the chordomas. An occasional rare lesion was found in our material, a meningocele through the foramen ovale. Meningiomas can sometimes extend extradurally and involve the sphenoid sinus as well as the nasopharyngeal tissues. Certain pituitary adenomas also are extradural. The latter lesions may extend laterally, pushing aside the dural walls of the cavernous sinus and undermining this struc-

(Revised 1963)

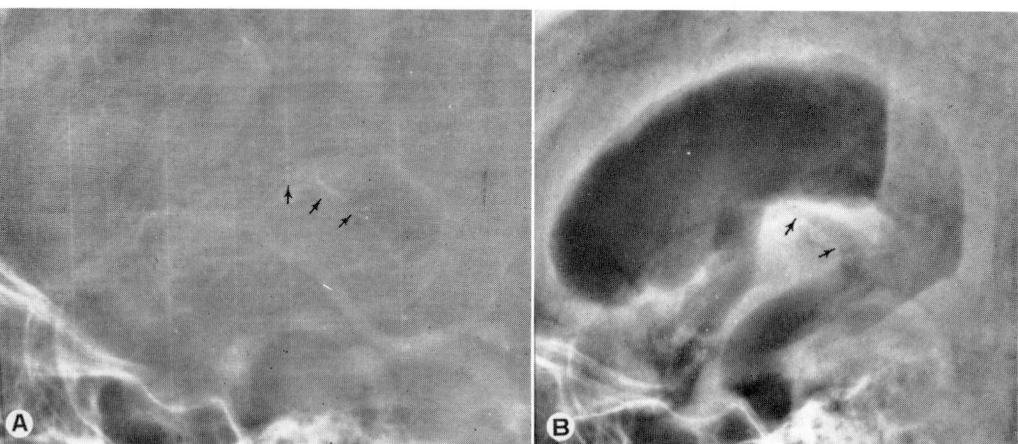

FIG. 481.—LARGE THIRD VENTRICLE TUMOR

The lateral venogram shows elevation of the internal cerebral vein (*arrows*). Signs of ventricular dilatation were present in the arterial phase and in the frontal venographic film. A ventriculogram (B) demonstrates the 3d ventricle tumor, which was causing elevation of the roof of the 3d ventricle.

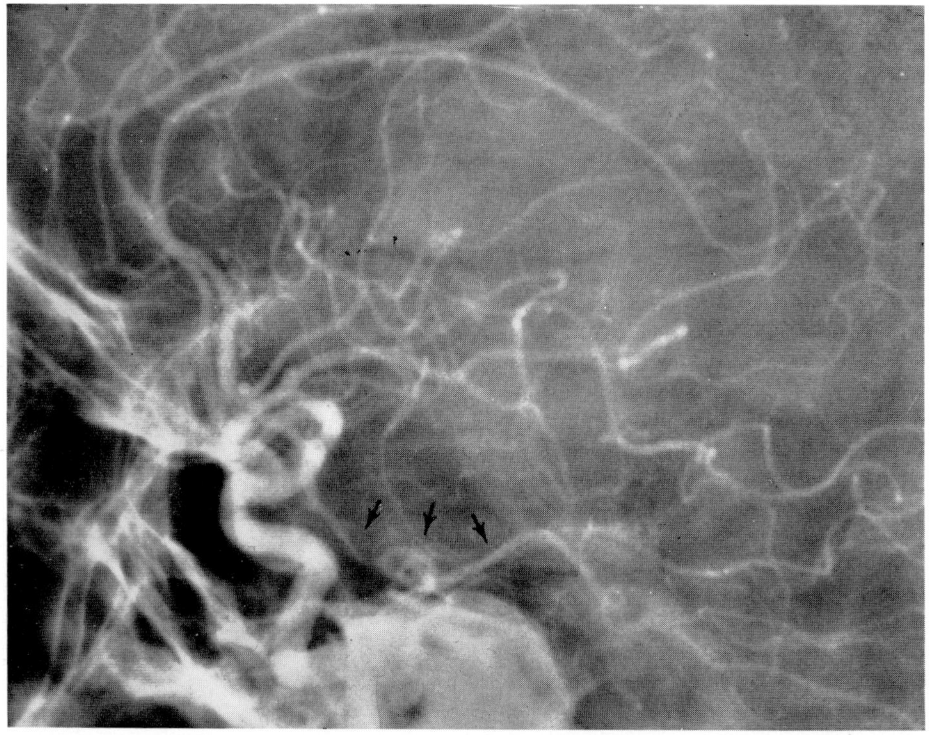

FIG. 482.—LARGE THIRD VENTRICLE TUMOR (INTRAVENTRICULAR CRANIOPHARYNGIOMA)

There was a large 3d ventricle tumor which produced marked downward displacement of the posterior communicating artery and the anterior portion of the posterior cerebral artery (*arrows*). In addition, there was a slight regurgitation into the basilar artery which discloses downward displacement of this artery as well.

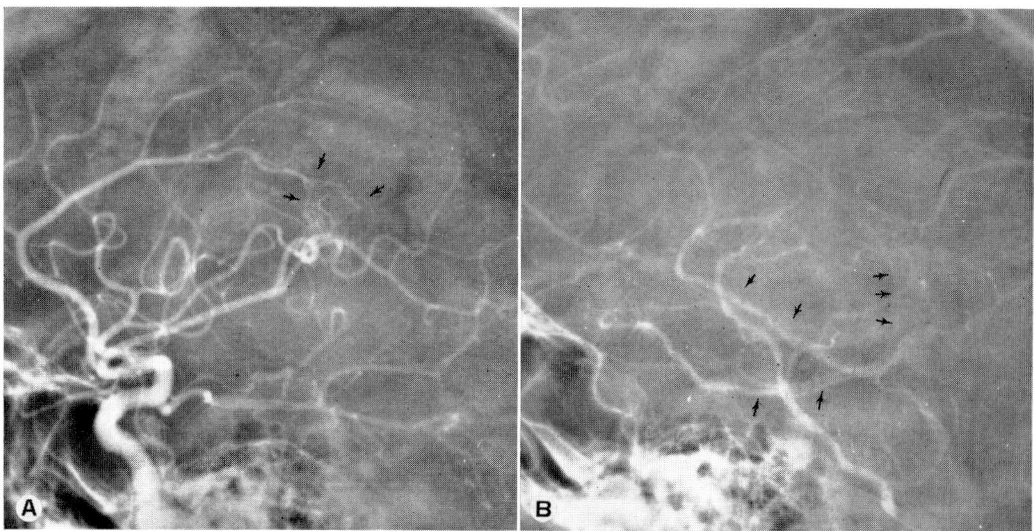

FIG. 483.—TUMOR OF THE CORPUS CALLOSUM

The lateral view in the arterial phase (A) reveals elevation of the pericallosal artery with a slight rounding. The pericallosal artery in its posterior portion shows a few abnormal vessels (*arrows*). The lateral venogram (B) shows marked flattening of the internal cerebral vein (*arrows*). The basilar vein is also depressed. On the contrary, the thalamostriate vein remained in normal position, which tends to differentiate this appearance from that noted in a parasagittal tumor, which would tend to displace the thalamostriate downward. The vein of the splenium is displaced backward (*three arrows*).

ture and its arterial contents, even extruding into the temporal fossa. Other adenomas extend inferiorly into the sphenoid sinus and nasopharynx, remaining confined beneath the diaphragma sellae.

Intradural masses. The *intradural tumors* are by far the more common and important lesions of the group. They may be pituitary adenomas, craniopharyngiomas, meningiomas, epidermoid tumors, and optic gliomas. The intradural tumors may be partially intrasellar in location and partially suprasellar. Such suprasellar masses occur owing to upward extension through the diaphragma sellae of a primarily intrasellar tumor, which is often the case with pituitary adenomas and most craniopharyngiomas, and they also may be entirely suprasellar in location without any intrasellar component, such as is the situation with meningiomas, the optic gliomas, and epidermoid tumors. Saccular aneurysms are suprasellar masses and may produce vascular displacements similar to those caused by other lesions, but it is rare for saccular aneurysms to be large enough to cause vascular displacement and not be filled with contrast substance, making the diagnosis obvious. Saccular aneurysms are discussed under "Subarachnoid Hemorrhage."

Angiographically and pathologically, intradural parasellar masses should be divided into straight suprasellar, anterior suprasellar, and posterior suprasellar lesions (fig. 484). Such a classification is advantageous because each location produces relatively well defined displacement of the vessels in this region (Chase and Taveras, 1961). The most frequent tumor in the area is a pituitary adenoma. Because these tumors are primarily intrasellar, they produce a rather characteristic displacement of the internal carotid artery siphon. The intracavernous portion of the carotid siphon is usually displaced laterally along its mid and posterior aspects. The displacement is best shown in the frontal projection (fig. 485). Displacement also may be demonstrated in mentovertical views, but such special views are unnecessary in most instances. As seen in

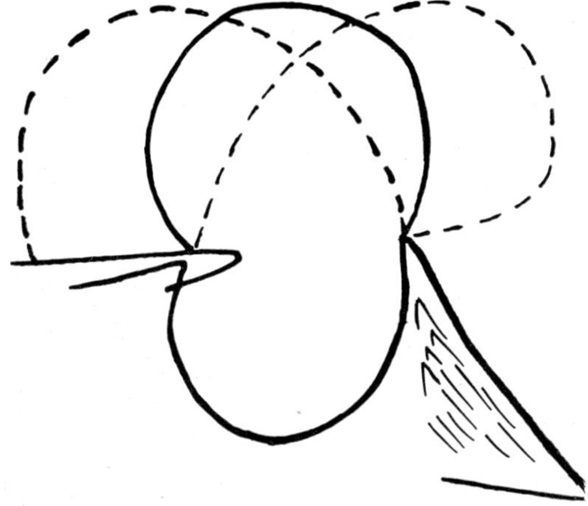

Fig. 484.—The Classification of Suprasellar Tumors in Relation to the Sella Turcica

Angiographically and pathologically it is advantageous to divide the suprasellar masses or the suprasellar extension of intrasellar masses into anterior suprasellar, straight suprasellar, and posterior suprasellar. Each one of these suprasellar locations would produce characteristic angiographic findings. A large tumor can occupy any two of the areas or all of the areas outlined in this diagram

the lateral view, the intracavernous portion of the internal carotid artery remains in its normal position, but it is common for it to appear elevated in relation to the floor of the sella turcica because the floor has been displaced downward by the enlarging tumor.

Upward displacement of the supraclinoid portion of the siphon (*opening of the siphon*) is common with pituitary adenoma. Suprasellar mass lesions arising outside of the sella turcica may or may not cause opening of the carotid siphon. Lateral displacement of the supraclinoid portion, as seen in frontal projection, is fairly common as well as elevation of the bifurcation of the internal carotid artery (fig. 485).

Upward and forward displacement of the horizontal portion of the anterior cerebral artery usually is seen in the frontal projection. If there is a straight upward displacement, this can be demonstrated in films made in any frontal view. If there is more forward than straight upward displacement, a film made in the orbital projection (see "Radiographic Technique") demonstrates the displacement and bowing of the anterior cerebral vessels to best advantage. It might be mentioned here that apparent upward displacement of the horizontal portion of the anterior cerebral artery is sometimes a normal finding, particularly in younger adults and in children (fig. 365).

More reliable evidence of significance is elevation of the proximal portion of the anterior cerebral artery with a reversal of the normal downward convex curve of the initial segment of the anterior cerebral artery as seen in the lateral projection (figs. 485 and 487). However, this appearance may also be normal. A small suprasellar extension of a pituitary adenoma or a primary suprasellar tumor may be present and not displace the anterior cerebral vessels in any direction. Sometimes even relatively sizable tumors may not displace the vessel if the masses extend backward. Craniopharyngiomas, even large ones, can grow superiorly without producing significant angiographic signs of a suprasellar tumor due to the fact that they may extend out of the sella by means of a thin stalk which mushrooms above (fig. 486).

Because of the lateral displacement of the carotid siphon in its supraclinoid portion, it is obvious that the origin of the anterior chorioidal artery and of the posterior communicating artery will be displaced outward along with the internal carotid artery. The anterior chorioidal artery and the anterior portion of the basilar vein usually are not displaced upward unless there is lateral extension of the tumor (see below).

Some suprasellar masses may extend upward to a considerable extent, which produces blockage of the foramen of Monro and elevation of the internal cerebral vein. This type of lesion is difficult to differentiate from primarily intraventricular tumors in the third ventricle, but the latter tumors

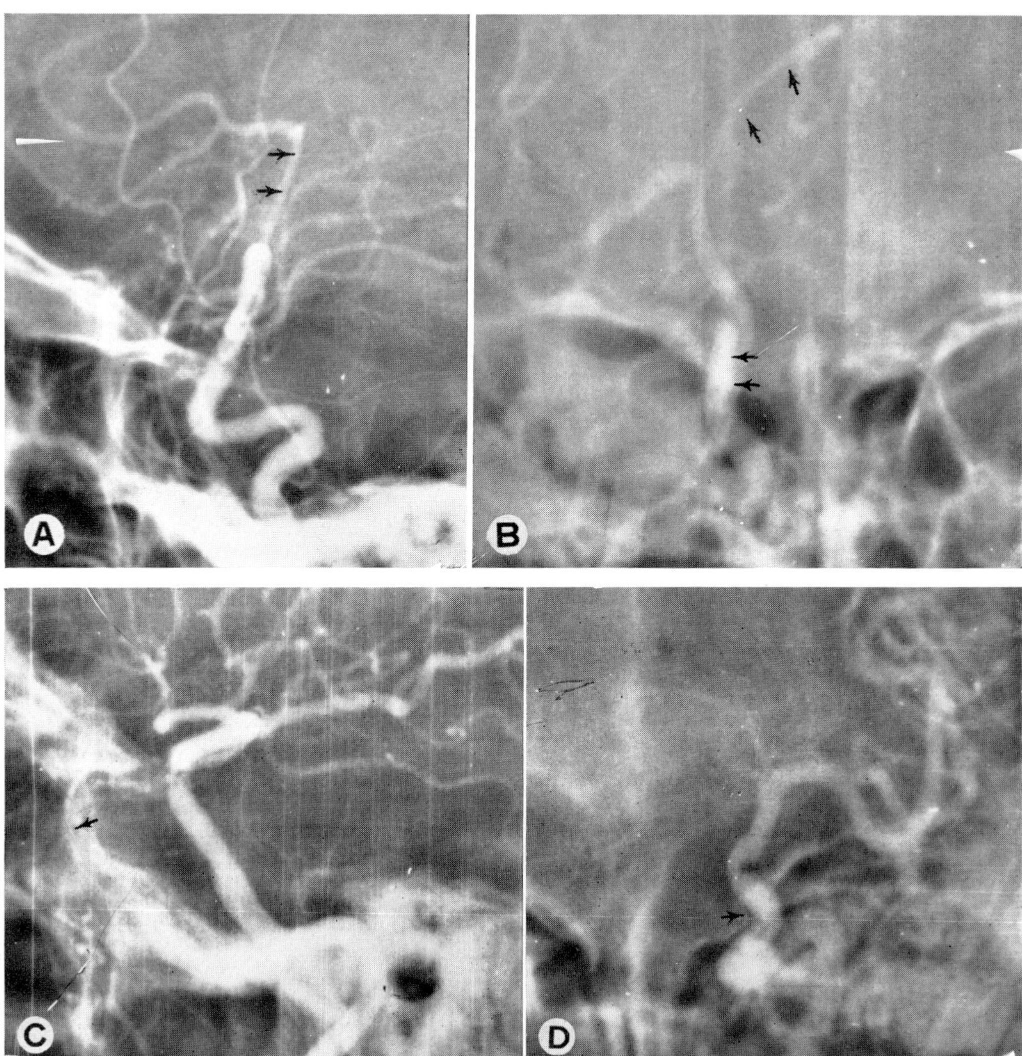

FIG. 485.—PITUITARY ADENOMA WITH SUPRASELLAR EXTENSION

The lateral view in the arterial phase (A) shows that the carotid siphon has remained in essentially normal position although the sella turcica floor is markedly depressed and the sella is destroyed. There is upward and forward displacement of the carotid siphon (opening of the siphon). There is marked straight upward displacement of the horizontal portion of the anterior cerebral artery (*arrows*) and of the adjacent portion of this artery. The frontal projection (B) shows lateral displacement of the intracavernous portion of the internal carotid artery (*arrows*). There is lateral displacement of the supraclinoid portion of the internal carotid artery with elevation of its bifurcation. The anterior cerebral artery (*arrows*) is also markedly elevated.

(C) and (D) represent lateral and frontal angiograms of another patient with an extensive pituitary adenoma. In this case, the intracavernous portion of the artery was straightened, probably due to a slight degree of lateral extension under the cavernous sinus. The floor of the sella is markedly displaced forward and indicated with an arrow in the lateral view. The frontal film of that case (D) reveals lateral displacement of the intracavernous portion (*arrow*). Because of the elevation of the bifurcation of the internal carotid artery, the middle cerebral artery must go outward and downward but probably is not elevated. Compare with Fig. 490.

(*Revised 1963*)

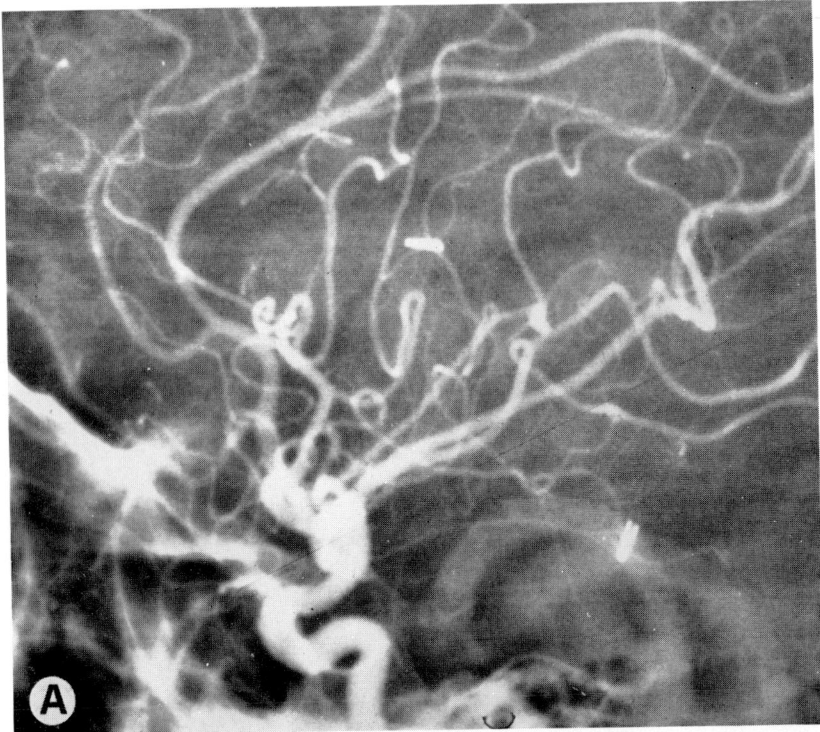

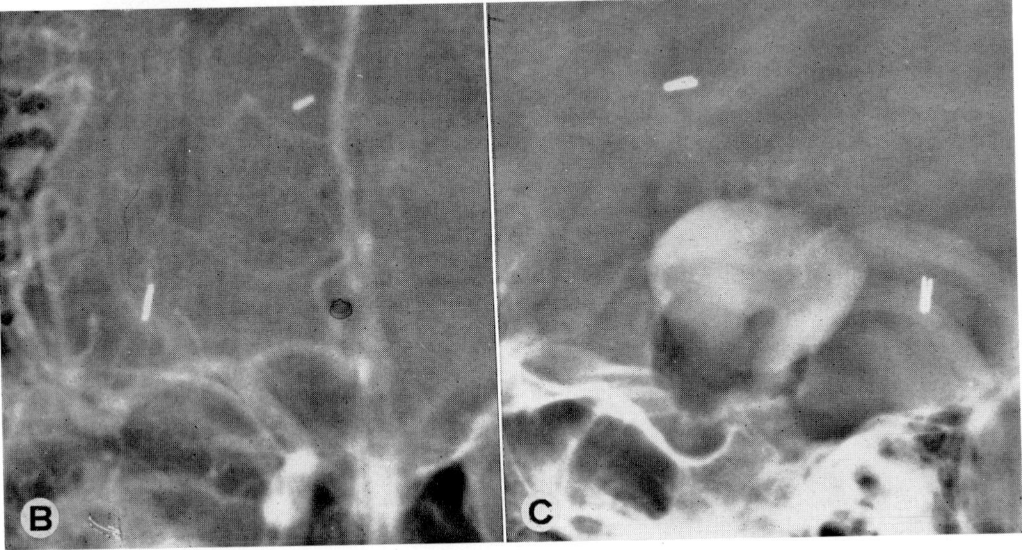

FIG. 486.—CRANIOPHARYNGIOMA, LARGE, PRODUCING ESSENTIALLY NO FINDINGS ON THE ANGIOGRAM

The lateral view in the arterial phase (A) reveals an essentially normal angiogram except for rounding of the pericallosal vessels which indicated ventricular dilatation. The frontal projection (B) revealed essentially no abnormal findings. The anterior chorioidal artery is not well shown on this film, but its curve is only slightly decreased. A lateral film of the skull made after the injection of opaque material into the cyst (C) shows the superior retrosellar position of the cyst. Intrasellar calcifications are seen, indicating that the tumor extends into the sella turcica. It is evident that the tumor mushroomed above the sella and passed through the medial suprasellar region on a thin stalk, thus avoiding the vessels.

(*Revised 1963*)

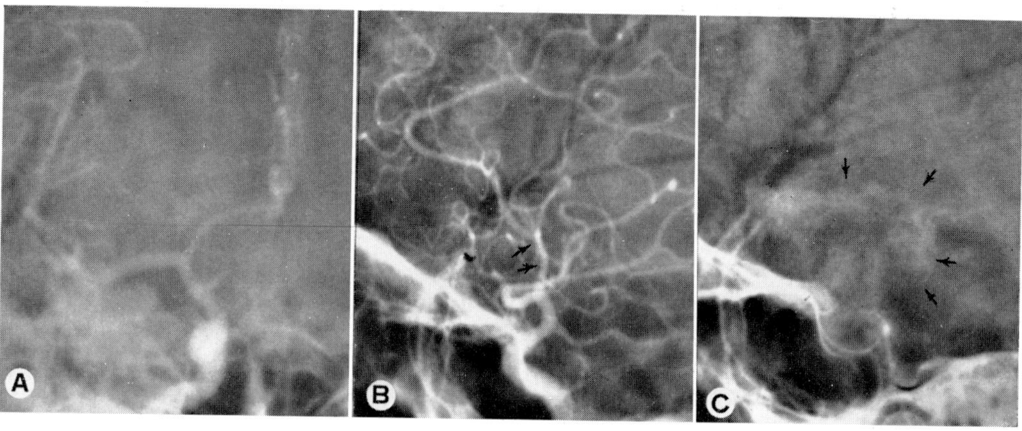

Fig. 487.—Suprasellar Meningioma

The frontal projection (A) shows marked elevation and rounding of the horizontal portion of the anterior cerebral artery and lateral displacement of the carotid siphon. The lateral view in the arterial phase (B) confirms the elevation of the proximal portion of the anterior cerebral artery (*arrows*) and the elevation of the bifurcation of the carotid siphon which is also in a forward position in relation to the sella turcica. The posterior communicating and posterior cerebral arteries are normal in position (compare with Fig. 488). The lateral venogram (C), reveals an opacity situated directly above the sella turcica and representing the meningioma. The disclosure of an occasional tumor cloud is one good reason for performing cerebral angiography in suprasellar tumors.

usually do not produce evidence of optic chiasmal compression.

The *anterior suprasellar tumors* usually are meningiomas attached to the tuberculum sellae or to the planum sphenoidale. Some may arise from the region of an anterior clinoid process or from the meninges around the optic nerves. Characteristically they produce sharp elevation and backward displacement of the anterior cerebral artery and may produce *closing of the siphon* owing to downward and backward displacement of the supraclinoid portion of the internal carotid artery. The group is related to the subfrontal masses which are situated slightly further forward.

Optic gliomas vary somewhat in their angiographic presentation, depending on their point of origin along the optic tract and the location of the bulk of the mass. Such tumors even may be entirely within the orbital cavity. When the tumor arises intracranially from one of the optic nerves or extends forward from the chiasm, the transverse portion of the anterior cerebral artery will be elevated and the internal carotid artery displaced downward and backward, as with suprasellar meningioma. Chiasm masses presenting directly in the suprasellar area produce lateral displacement of the internal carotid arteries and of the proximal portions of the posterior communicating and the anterior chorioidal vessels. Some tumors grow primarily upward and compress the hypothalamus, even extending to obstruct the foramen of Monro. Large optic chiasm gliomas not only elevate and straighten the anterior cerebral artery, but also elevate the internal cerebral vein and exhibit the usual features of lateral ventricular dilatation.

The *posterior suprasellar masses* characteristically produce lateral displacement of the anterior chorioidal artery and of the posterior communicating artery (fig. 488). In addition, they produce elevation and forward displacement of the bifurcation of the internal carotid artery. The tumors may be pituitary adenomas, growing more in a dorsal direction, epidermoid cysts, and chordomas.

Pituitary adenomas may extend laterally beneath the temporal lobes. Likewise meningiomas may grow laterally along the medial portion of the sphenoid ridge and the floor of the middle fossa (fig. 490).

(*Revised 1963*)

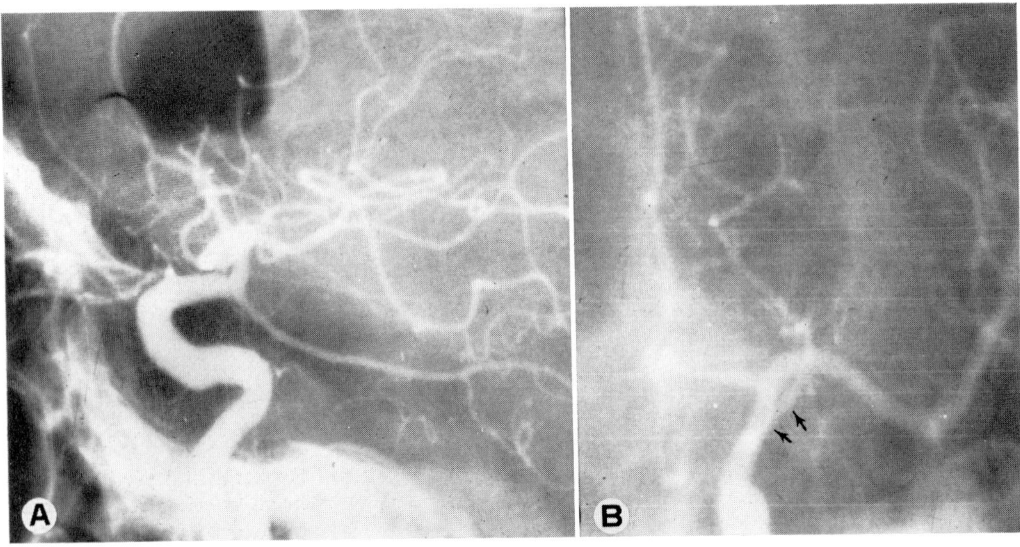

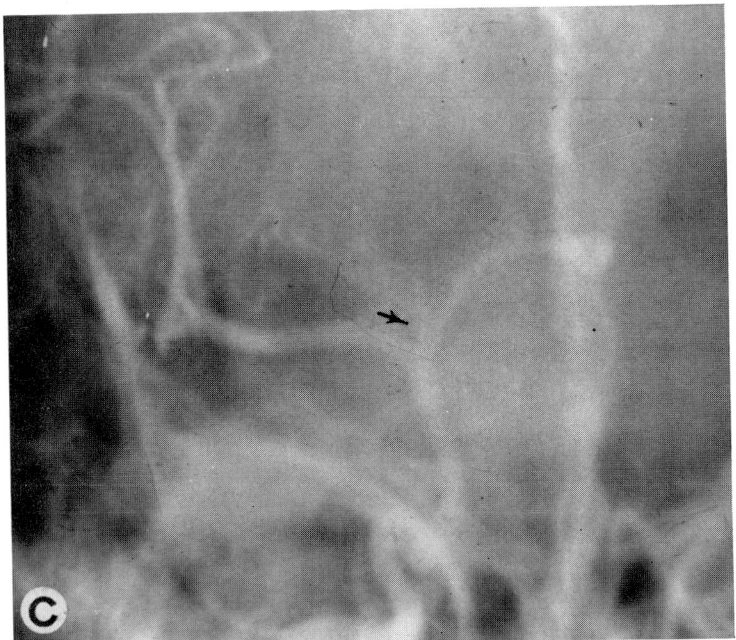

FIG. 488.—RETROSELLAR EXTENSION OF PITUITARY ADENOMA

The lateral view in the arterial phase (A) reveals a slight forward displacement of the bifurcation of the internal carotid artery without significant elevation of the proximal portion of the anterior cerebral artery. The posterior communicating and anterior chorioidal arteries are not significantly displaced. In the frontal projection (B) there is a marked degree of lateral displacement of the posterior communicating artery which normally should project medial to the carotid siphon (*arrows*).

(C) shows an anteroposterior angiogram of another patient that demonstrates lateral displacement of the anterior chorioidal artery due to a posterior suprasellar extension of a pituitary adenoma. Note also lateral displacement of the intracavernous portion of the internal carotid artery.

(*Revised 1963*)

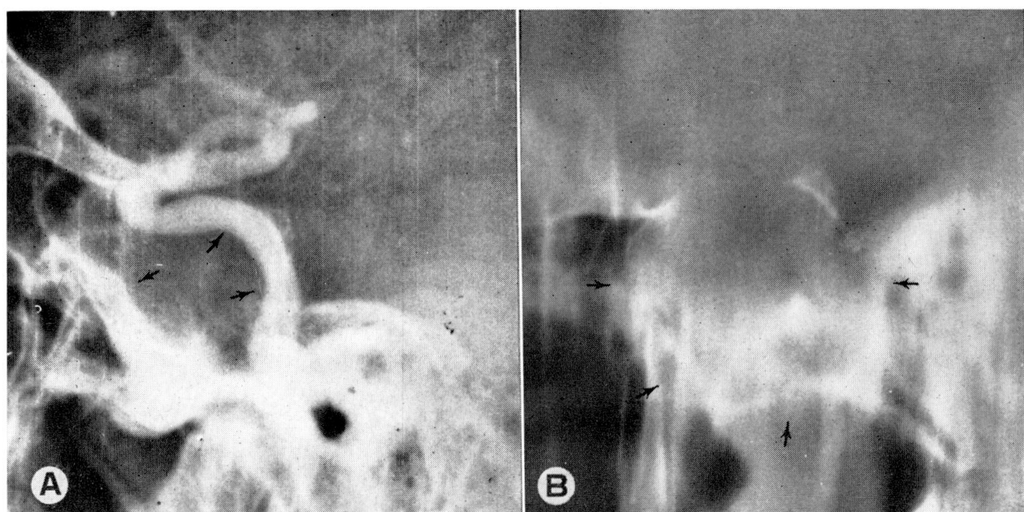

FIG. 489.—LARGE PITUITARY ADENOMA WITH LATERAL EXTRADURAL EXTENSION
The lateral view (A) reveals considerable elevation of the intracavernous portion of the internal carotid artery. The destroyed sella is seen to extend much further anteriorly (*arrows*). A laminagram of the sella turcica (B) discloses the extent of sellar enlargement only on one side; the other side of the sella was normal in size. The patient had clinical signs of partial 3d and 6th nerve involvement but no evidence of chiasmal compression.

When pituitary adenomas extend laterally, they may project beneath the intracavernous portion of the internal carotid artery to produce elevation of this portion of the vessel (fig. 489). In addition, there may be elevation of the horizontal portion of the middle cerebral artery (fig. 490), which should be distinguished from elevation of the origin of the artery. The latter occurs whenever the bifurcation of the internal carotid artery is pushed upward. The difference is clear when Figure 485 is compared with Figure 490. Such cases also show elevation of the basilar vein and of the anterior chorioidal artery (fig. 490).

Some craniopharyngiomas produce very few findings at angiography, even though they are quite large. This is apparently possible because a craniopharyngioma may originate within the pituitary fossa, but extend by means of a thin stalk through the diaphragma sellae and mushroom well above the sella turcica, thus avoiding some of the arterial branches in the suprasellar region (fig. 486). Moreover, some craniopharyngiomas may originate in the hypothalamus or even may be entirely intraventricular (fig. 482).

Extradural masses. *Epidural parasellar tumors* are characterized by the fact that they displace and deform the intracavernous portion of the internal carotid artery, which may move upward, medially, or laterally. In our experience at the Neurological Institute, the most numerous groups have been the pituitary adenomas, with meningiomas and nasopharyngeal carcinomas somewhat less frequent (Chase and Taveras, 1963). Some extradural lesions are chordomas and metastatic tumors. We also have encountered cases of osteochrondroma, osteogenic sarcoma, and fibrous dysplasia in this region. Fifth nerve neurinomas may be partly extradural. Mucoceles of the sphenoid sinus extending upward extradurally may be expected to produce lateral and upward displacement of the intracavernous portion of the carotid artery. If the extradural tumor is large enough, the middle cerebral artery will be elevated due to lifting of the temporal lobe. The most characteristic finding as previously mentioned, however,

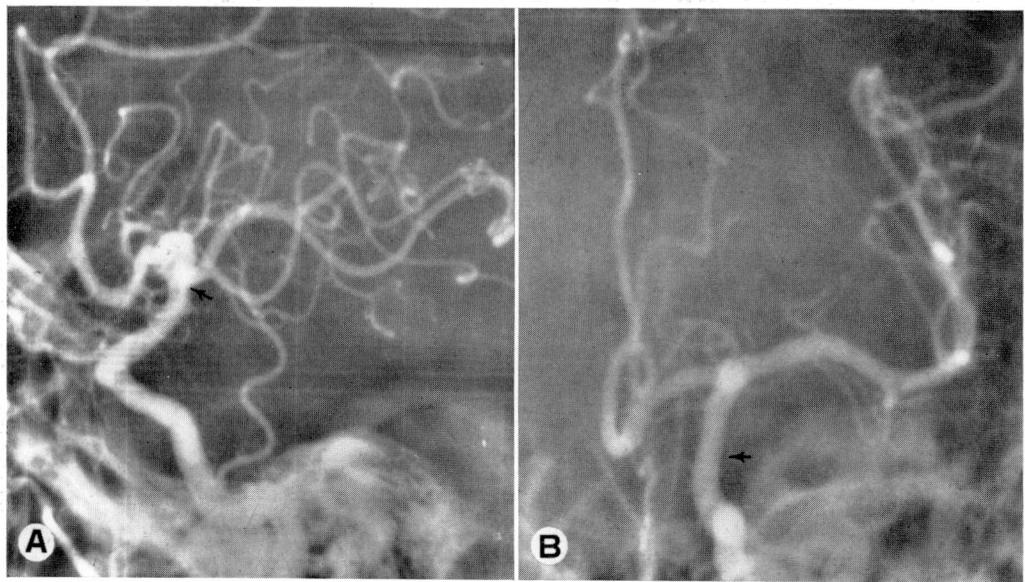

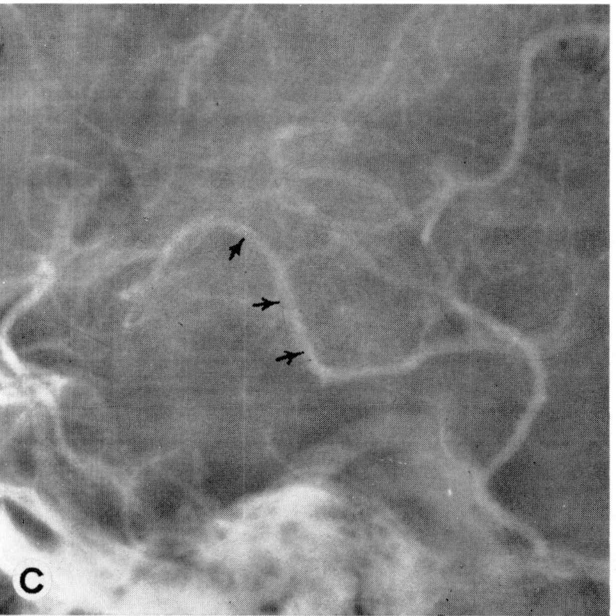

FIG. 490.—LATERAL EXTENSION OF PITUITARY ADENOMA

The lateral projection (A) demonstrates the typical opening of the siphon with elevation of the supracavernous portion. However, the intracavernous portion is in normal position. There is elevation of the horizontal portion of the middle cerebral artery and of the anterior portion of the middle cerebral group (*arrow*). The frontal projection (B) reveals medial displacement of the supraclinoid portion of the carotid siphon (*arrow*) and elevation of the horizontal portion of the middle cerebral artery. The lateral view in the venous phase (C) shows a sharp upward displacement of the basilar vein (*arrows*). This confirms the subtemporal extension of this pituitary adenoma.

(*Revised 1963*)

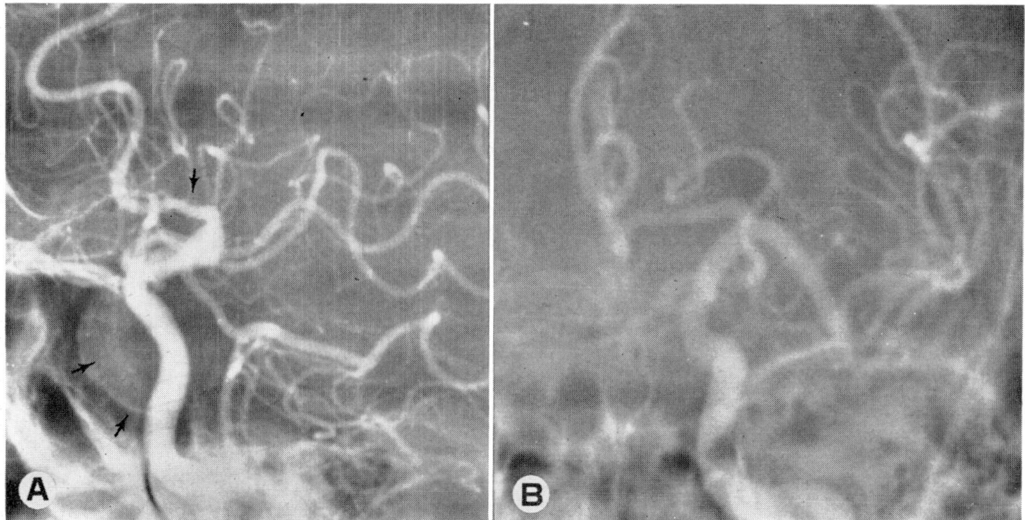

FIG. 491.—APPARENT LATERAL EXTENSION OF PITUITARY ADENOMA

The lateral projection (A) shows a relatively high position to the intracavernous portion of the carotid siphon due to marked depression of the floor of the enlarged sella turcica. There is elevation of the carotid bifurcation and of the proximal portion of the anterior cerebral artery (*arrow*). The frontal projection (B) reveals slight lateral displacement of the carotid siphon and elevation of the bifurcation of this artery which causes the middle cerebral artery to pass downward and lateralward, but this does not indicate lateral extension.

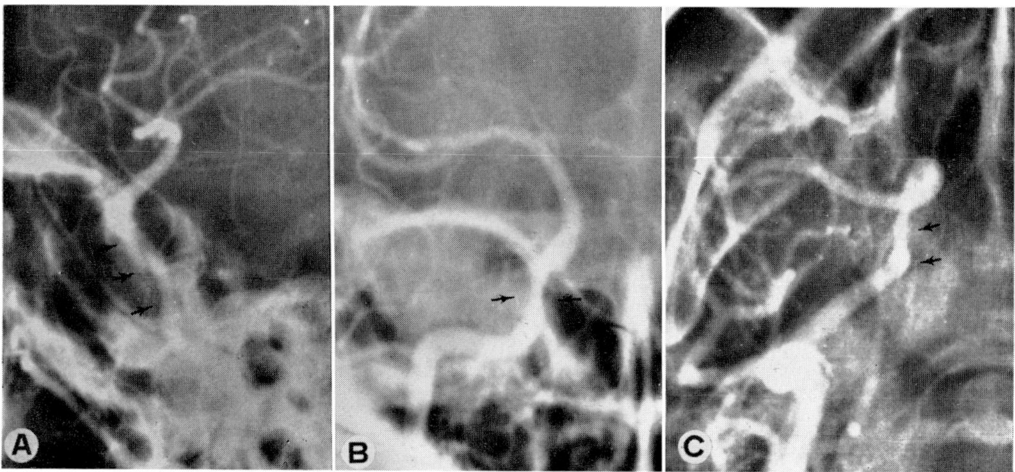

FIG. 492.—MENINGIOMA WITH EXTRADURAL EXTENSION

The lateral view (A) shows irregularity and constriction of the internal carotid siphon in its intracavernous portion localized to an area about 2 cm. in length (*arrows*). No evidence of arteriosclerosis is seen elsewhere. The frontal projection (B) demonstrates the area of narrowing in this plane, and the base view (C) reveals lateral displacement as well as irregularity of the intracavernous segment.

is displacement and sometimes deformity of the intracavernous portion of the carotid artery. Elevation of this portion of the artery implies elevation of the cavernous sinus (fig. 489). This should not be confused with relative elevation secondary to depression of the floor of the sella (fig. 491). Medial displacement of the intracavernous or pre-

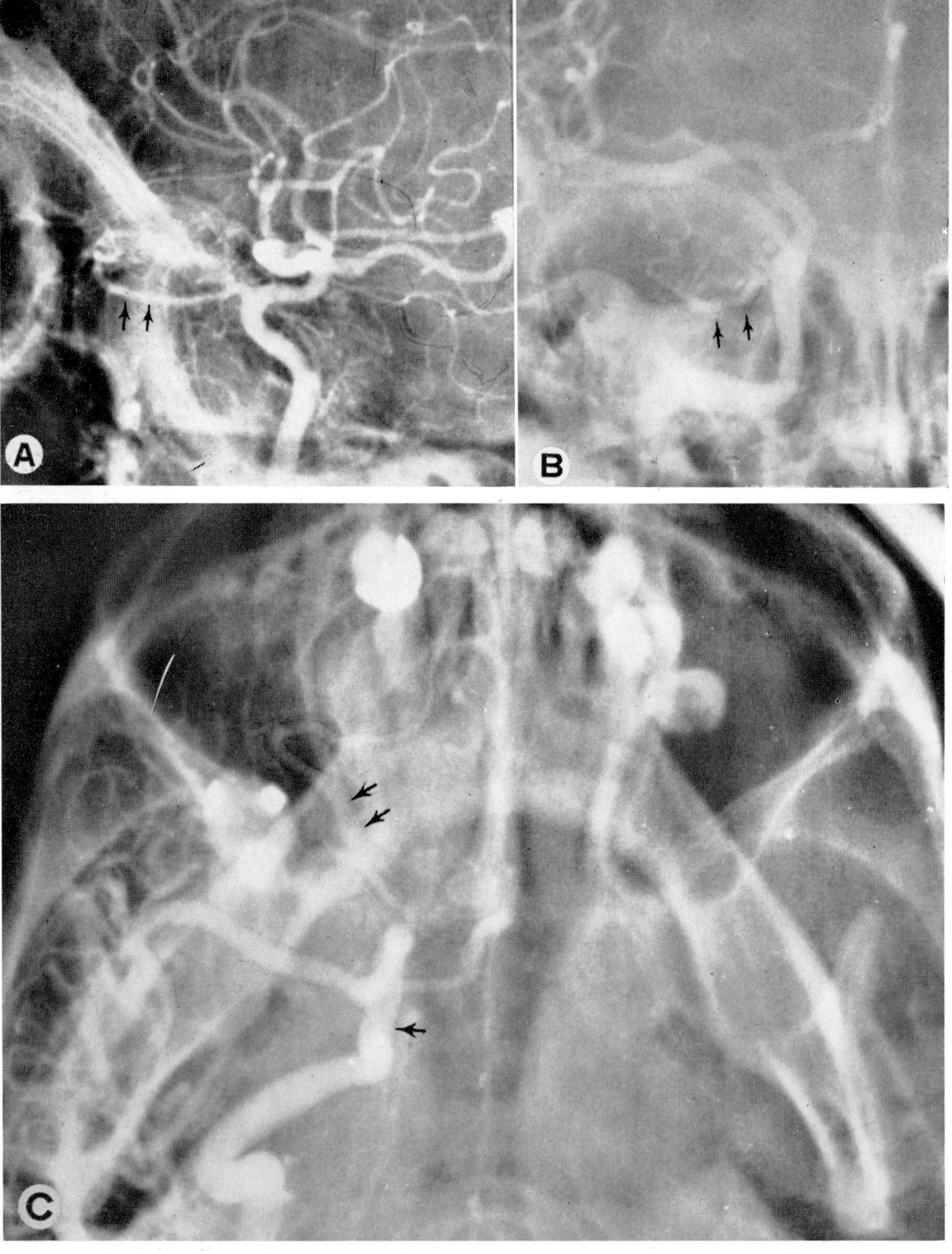

FIG. 493.—PERISELLAR MENINGIOMA INVOLVING THE ORBITAL ROOF

The tumor invaded the sphenoid sinus and the ethmoid sinuses and produced bone destruction in this region. The lateral view (A) shows no significant deformity of the carotid siphon which is only slightly displaced upward in its intracavernous portion. The ophthalmic artery is displaced downward (*arrows*). In the frontal projection (B) it is difficult to appreciate the downward displacement of the ophthalmic artery (*arrows*). The base view (C) shows lateral displacement of the ophthalmic artery (*arrows*). The posterior portion of the intracavernous segment is slightly displaced laterally (*arrows*).

(*Revised 1963*)

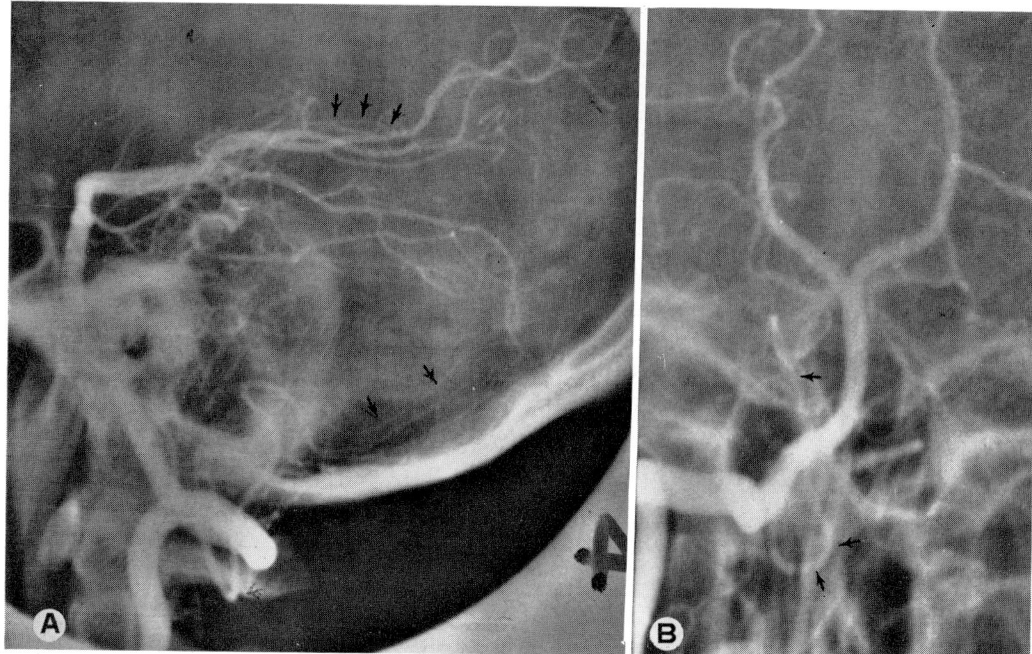

FIG. 494.—CEREBELLAR TUMOR CAUSING CEREBELLAR TONSILLAR HERNIATION

The lateral view (A) shows the basilar artery to be displaced forward against the clivus; only in its upper 1.5 cm. does it separate from the clivus. The caudal curve of the posterior inferior cerebellar artery goes down below the lower margin of C1 (*arrow*). At least one of the superior cerebellar arteries is seen to bulge upward above the medial branch of the posterior cerebral artery (*arrows*), which indicates upward transtentorial bulging. In the frontal projection (B) the caudal curve of the posterior inferior cerebellar artery is again visualized (*arrows*). The posterior inferior cerebellar artery is displaced to the right (*upper arrow*), which places the tumor on the left side.

cavernous portion is evidence of extradural mass. Involvement of the precavernous or intracavernous segment of the artery as evidenced by irregularity, narrowing, or even occlusion is direct evidence of extradural extension (fig. 492). Meningiomas that invade the bone and extend downward into the sphenoid sinus or nasopharynx may produce constriction as well as displacement of the intracavernous and even of the intrapetrosal portion of the internal carotid artery. Extension into the orbital roof causes displacement of the ophthalmic artery (fig. 493). The bone changes seen on plain films of the skull in each of the conditions described above usually are helpful in arriving at the correct preoperative diagnosis.

Infratentorial Tumors

The indications for angiography in the diagnosis of infratentorial masses are fairly well defined. It is the opinion of the authors that cerebellar tumors, with the exception of some lesions such as hemangioblastomas, which may exhibit abnormal circulation, should be diagnosed by pneumography. The same applies to brain stem tumors and cerebellopontine angle tumors. The indications for vertebral angiography to diagnose space-occupying lesions in the posterior fossa are: (1) to differentiate an intrapontine mass from a prepontine lesion, particularly to exclude an aneurysm of the basilar artery as the basis for a mass which produces posterior displacement of the aqueduct and floor of the fourth ventricle; (2) in cases of suspected cerebellopontine angle tumor when pneumography is inconclusive; (3) in the study of incisural masses when air studies need supplementation, particularly if aneurysm is suspected; (4) whenever a posterior fossa lesion is suspected clinically

(*Revised 1963*)

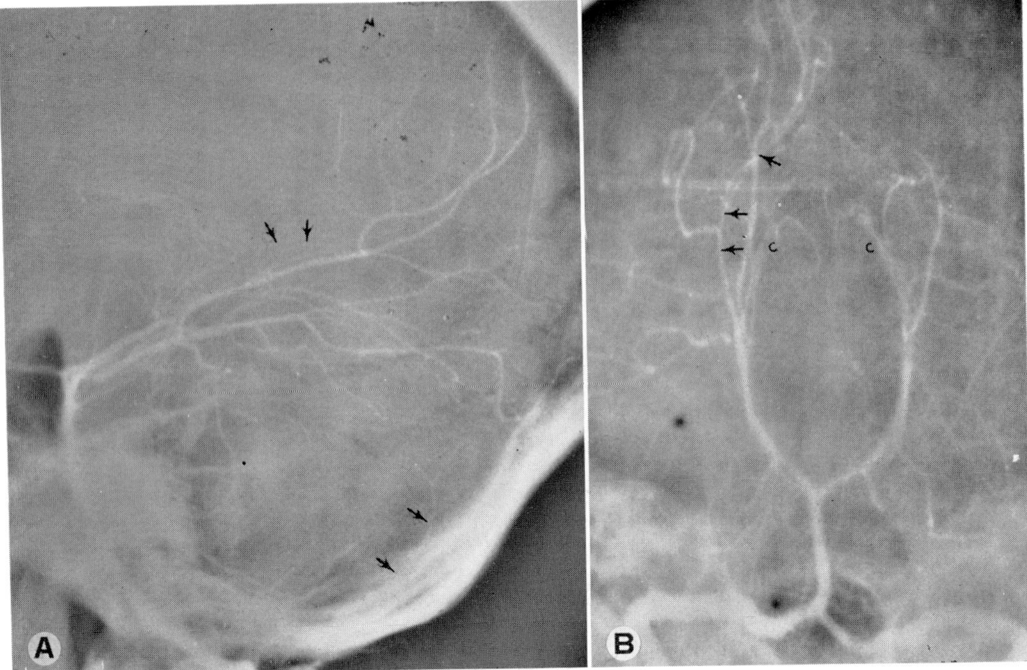

FIG. 495.—CYSTIC CEREBELLAR TUMOR IN A TEN-YEAR-OLD CHILD

The lateral projection (A) reveals forward displacement of the basilar artery which is pressed against the clivus. Although the trunk of the posterior inferior cerebellar arteries cannot be visualized clearly, they probably arise from the basilar artery in this instance. There is stretching of the vermis branch of the posterior inferior cerebellar artery (*arrows*), and there is stretching of both the posterior cerebral and superior cerebellar arteries in their proximal portions, forming a straight line upward and backward. However, this patient has a relatively low bifurcation of the basilar artery, and the stretched appearance is exaggerated by this anatomical variant. The superior cerebellar artery branches are displaced upward on one side to a greater degree than on the other side (*arrows*). On the side marked by the arrows, they project beyond the branch of the posterior cerebral artery which is itself probably elevated. There is stretching of the parieto-occipital branches of the posterior cerebral artery probably due to ventricular dilatation. The frontal projection (B) reveals lateral bulging of the posterior cerebral artery on the reader's left side, probably due to a fairly large transtentorial herniation (*arrows*). The medial posterior chorioidal arteries are seen on both sides and marked by the letter (c).

of being either a hemangioblastoma or an arteriovenous malformation; and (5) when it is suspected that a lesion may be a meningioma, particularly in the case of a mass arising from the tentorium which may require a special surgical approach. Aside from the indications listed, the authors believe that vertebral angiography is indicated only infrequently.

Generally, tumors of the cerebellum or of the brain stem produce forward displacement of the basilar artery, which is pressed against the posterior aspect of the clivus and dorsum sellae (fig. 494). This is a nonspecific finding. The posterior inferior cerebellar artery may be displaced downward beyond the foramen magnum and may reach the level of the second cervical vertebra in cases where there

cerebellar artery (*arrows*). There is also evidence of tonsillar herniation; the caudal curve of the inferior cerebellar artery goes beyond the lower margin of the posterior arch of the atlas (*arrow*). The frontal projection (B) does not reveal any significant abnormalities except for the displacement of the posterior inferior cerebellar artery (*arrows*), which is better shown in a film made later after the basilar artery had emptied (C). The posterior inferior cerebellar artery was actually displaced across the midline to the opposite side.

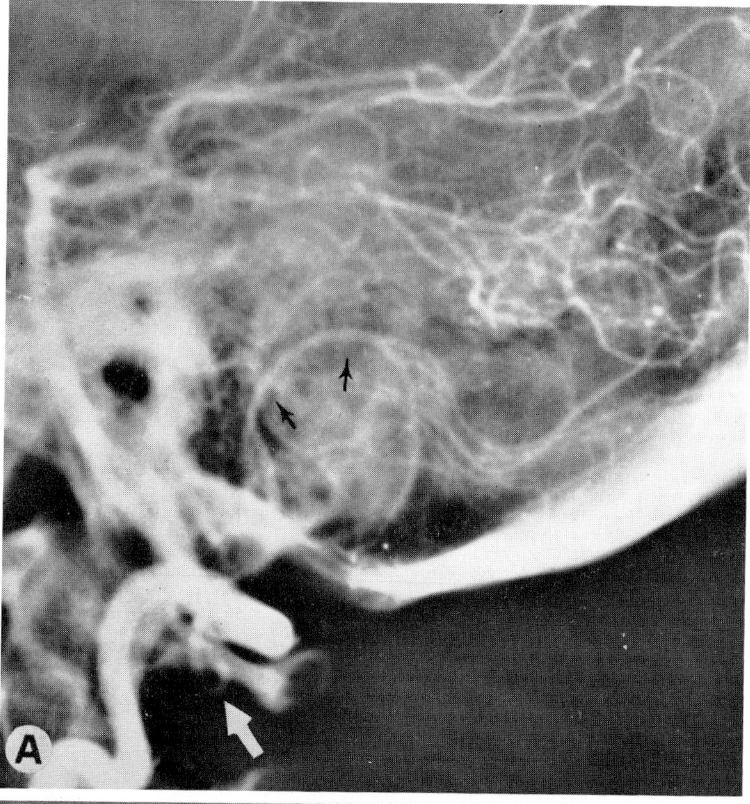

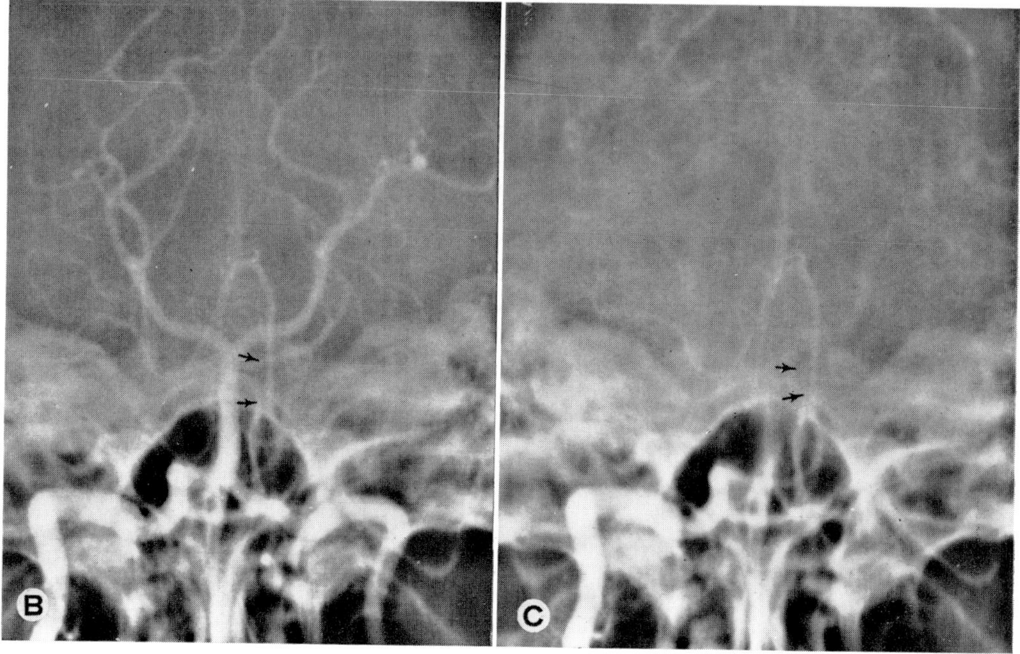

FIG. 496.—LOW CEREBELLAR TUMOR, METASTATIC

The lateral view (A) disclosed diffuse forward displacement of the basilar artery which is an almost constant finding in cerebellar tumors. There is a marked elevation and rounding of the posterior inferior

(Revised 1963)

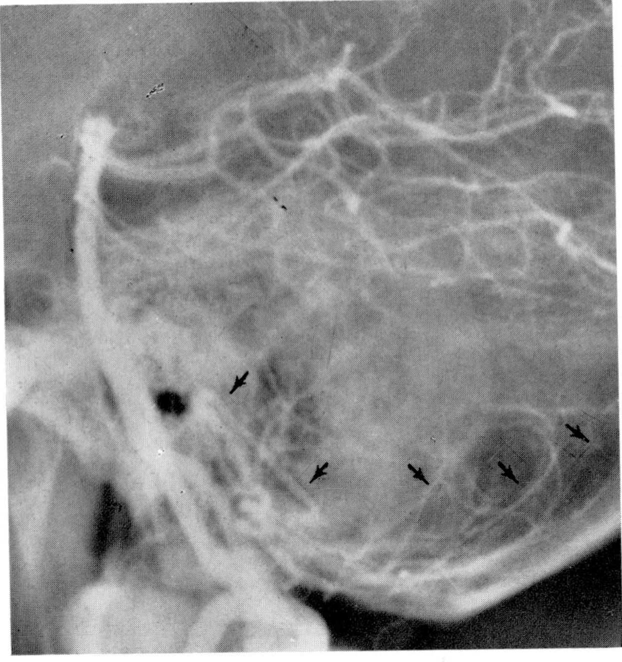

Fig. 497.—Vermis Tumor of the Cerebellum

There is marked forward displacement and stretching of the cephalic curve of the posterior inferior cerebellar artery (*arrows*). Some abnormal branches can be seen between the two arrows. In addition, there is stretching of the branches of the posterior inferior cerebellar artery (*posterior arrows*) which also show an increase in their number, probably due to abnormal vessels. Two metastatic nodules were encountered in this patient in the lower half of the cerebellum and invading the 4th ventricle wall, causing the forward displacement of the posterior inferior ceribellar artery. (Courtesy of Dr. Solomon Unger and Dr. Erik Krueger, Bronx Veterans Administration Hospital, New York.)

is herniation of the cerebellar tonsils (fig. 494). The posterior cerebral arteries may be stretched and displaced upward from their usual position, but this finding also is nonspecific (fig. 495). The superior cerebellar vessels are often seen to project higher than the posterior cerebral artery after passing around the brain stem. This is due to transtentorial bulging or upward herniation of the cerebellum (figs. 494 and 495).

In spite of the fact that the cerebellar arteries are not in the most favorable anatomical position to permit diagnosis of cerebellar tumor, it is possible in a fairly high percentage of cases to arrive at a diagnosis by angiography. Although it is not considered to be the procedure of choice, it does have the advantage of not requiring immediate surgical intervention such as is the case with ventriculography. Two other cases of cerebellar tumors are shown in Figures 496 and 497. The vermis branch of the posterior inferior cerebellar artery is useful because it is usually in the midline and is displaced by unilateral cerebellar masses.

More specific signs of posterior fossa tumors are encountered in connection with masses of the clivus and of the cerebellopontine angle. With tumors arising from the clivus, usually *meningiomas* or *chordomas*, there is posterior displacement of the basilar artery which is characteristic of a prepontine mass (fig. 498). Not all prepontine tumors produce posterior displacement of the basilar artery; in one instance a congenital epidermoid cyst lay between the basilar artery, which was in front of the tumor, and the pons, which was posterior to it. The air study in this instance was superior to the angiogram because the former disclosed dorsal displacement of the pons and marked enlargement of the prepontine cistern. If a tumor is anterolaterally placed, the basilar artery is displaced posteriorly and to the opposite side (figs. 498 and 499). If the tumor is midline in location, the basilar artery will be displaced straight posteriorly and form a concave curve around the posterior aspect of the mass (fig. 498).

A tumor of the *cerebellopontine angle* produces elevation of the corresponding superior cerebellar artery as it passes around the anterolateral aspect of the upper brain stem (fig. 499). This is seen both in the lateral and in the frontal projections. Abnormal

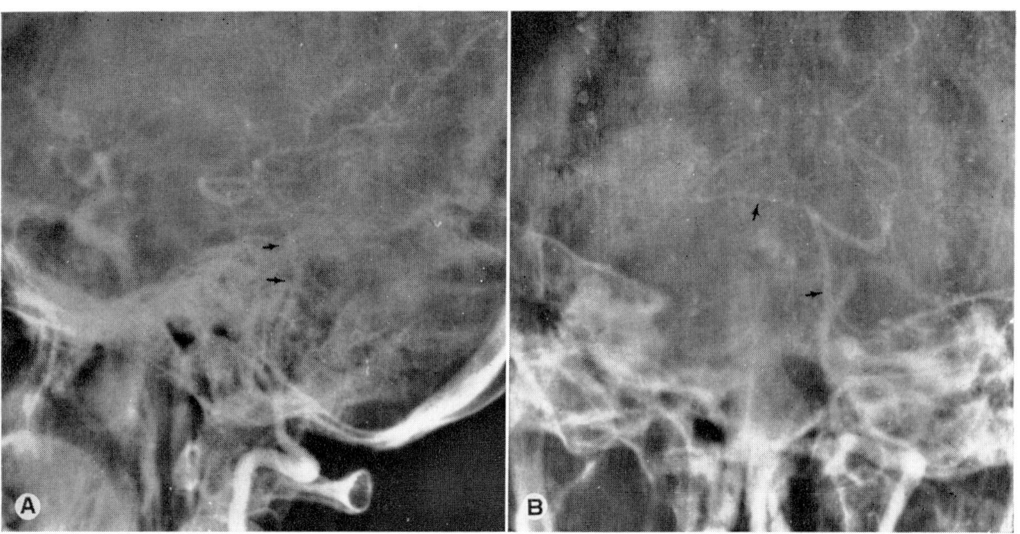

FIG. 498.—CHORDOMA OF THE CLIVUS

The lateral view (A) discloses marked posterior displacement of the basilar artery (*arrows*) which extends up to the bifurcation of this artery. The frontal projection (B) shows that there is also lateral displacement of the basilar artery as well as marked elevation of the posterior cerebral artery on the right side. The latter indicates the upward extension of the mass.

vessels may sometimes be present in neurinomas of the 8th nerve, as pointed out by Olsson (1953). Lesions situated in the midline at the incisura produce posterior displacement of the basilar artery, while anterolateral incisural masses produce upward and dorsal displacement of the proximal portion of the posterior cerebral artery (fig. 501). The hemangioblastomas of the cerebellum, meningiomas of the tentorium, and angiomatous malformations present certain vascular features that are described under "Diagnosis of Intracranial Masses by Abnormal Circulation."

Incisural Tumors

Lesions of the free tentorial edge often belong partly to the supratentorial group and partly to the infratentorial category. It appears appropriate, therefore, to have delayed consideration of incisural tumors until after both supratentorial and infratentorial lesions have been described. Pneumography usually is employed to localize these lesions most accurately. Angiography of the carotid system and, if necessary, of the vertebral system is indicated after pneumography, if an aneurysm is suspected or to complete a study in order to make preoperative localization more precise (fig. 500).

Angiography is very helpful in the study of incisural tumors situated anteriorly in the midline which displace the basilar artery backward. Anterolateral lesions displace the posterior cerebral artery upward and backward and sometimes produce downward displacement of the superior cerebellar artery (fig. 501). Some masses of the region are large aneurysms which fill directly at angiography (fig. 502). The procedure is also very useful in the case of posterior midline masses which produce separation, or "splitting," of the two posterior cerebral arteries in the portions beyond the turn around the brain stem. In addition, midline posterior incisural masses arising from the tentorium may produce forward and downward displacement of the vein of Galen and of the posterior portion of the internal cerebral vein, if their supratentorial extension is great. Such displacements differentiate incisural from posterior third ventricle tumors,

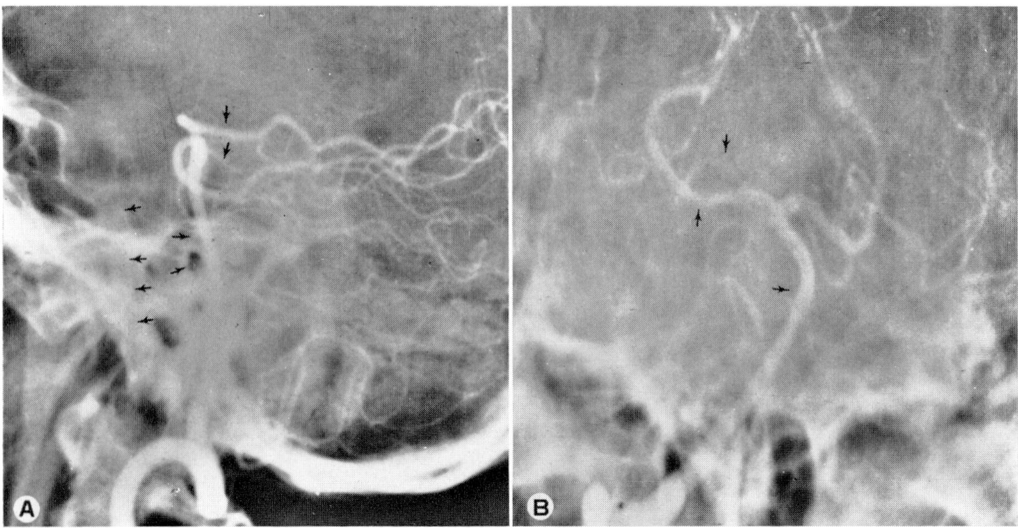

Fig. 499.—Cerebellopontine Angle Meningioma

The lateral projection (A) reveals moderate posterior displacement of the basilar artery (*arrows*). The *anterior arrows* outline the clivus. The posterior cerebral artery and superior cerebellar arteries on one side are elevated (*upper arrows*). In the frontal projection (B) there is displacement of the basilar artery to the opposite side and the elevation of the posterior cerebral and superior cerebellar arteries on one side becomes more pronounced. The superior cerebellar artery is more elevated (*upper arrow*) than the posterior cerebral artery.

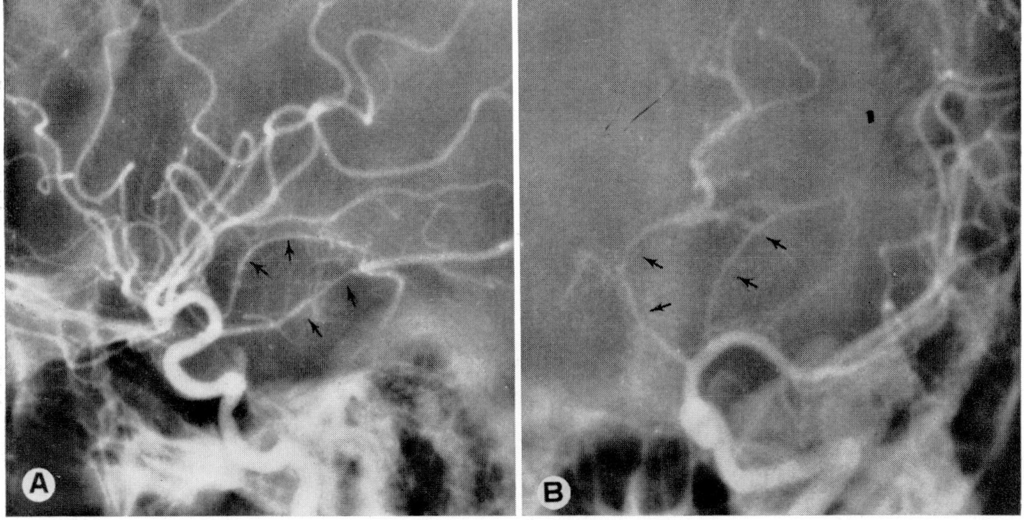

Fig. 500.—Incisural Tumor Demonstrated by Carotid Angiography (Cholesteatoma)

The lateral view (A) demonstrates elevation and enlargement of the anterior chorioidal artery (*arrows*). The posterior communicating artery is well shown, and the anterior portion of the posterior cerebral artery is thin due to stretching (*lower arrows*). The frontal projection (B) demonstrates an increase in the width of the curve of the anterior chorioidal artery (*arrows*). There is marked medial displacement of the posterior communicating artery and backward and upward displacement of the posterior cerebral artery (*arrows*). It was felt that these findings indicated the presence of an incisural mass, anterolateral in location, and vertebral angiography was deemed unnecessary. (Courtesy of Dr. Thomas Mason and Dr. G. Hines, Schenectady, New York.)

(*Revised 1963*)

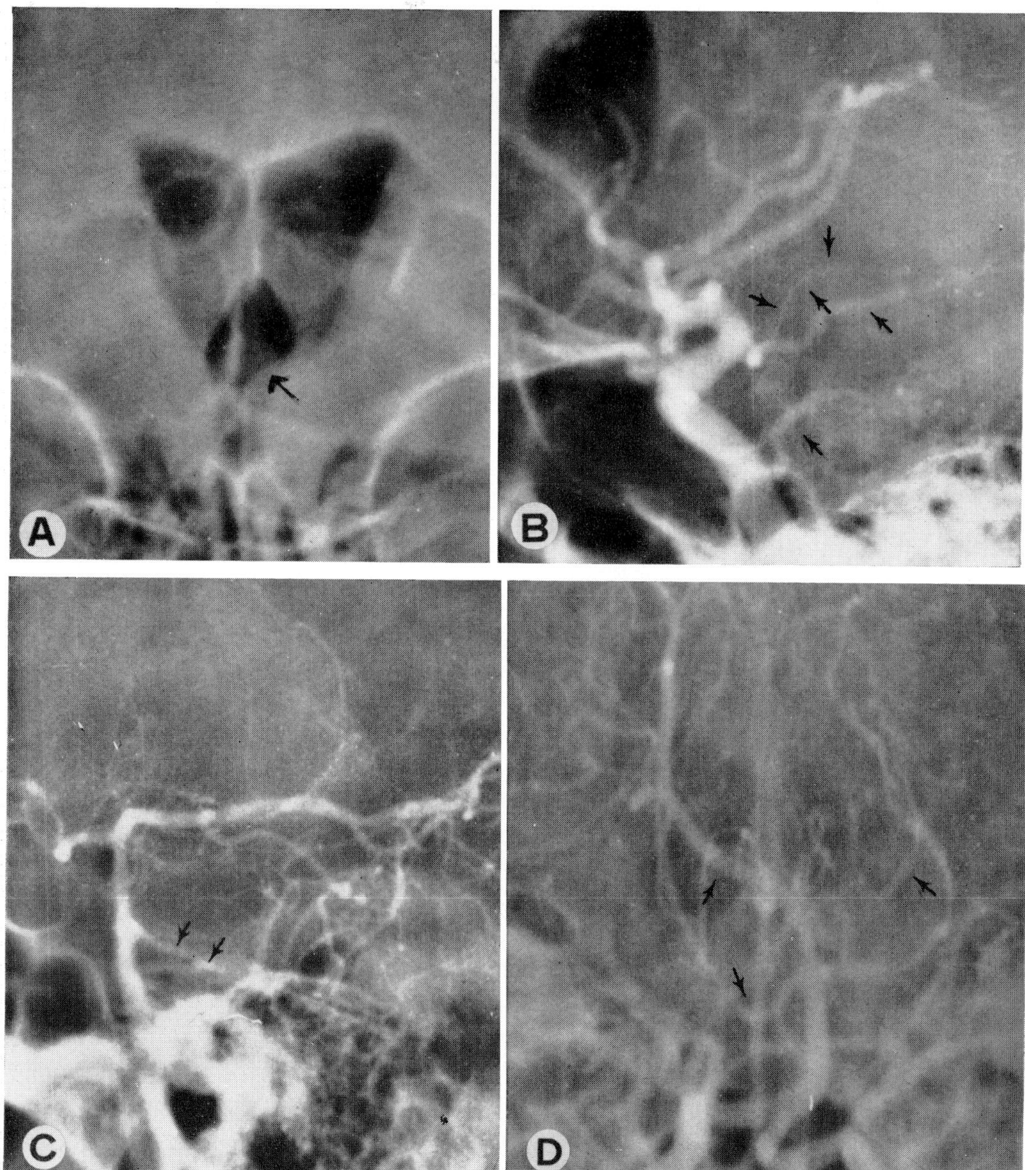

Fig. 501.—Incisural Tumor (Meningioma Arising from the Tentorial Edge)

The patient had had a previous air study (A) which was inconclusive but demonstrated the usual indentation on the posteroinferior aspect of the 3d ventricle (*arrow*). A carotid angiogram (B) demonstrates elevation of the anterior chorioidal artery and of the posterior cerebral artery (*arrows*). There was also filling of a tentorial meningeal branch arising from the internal carotid artery (*lower arrow*). A vertebral angiogram was then performed which demonstrated, in the lateral view (C), an elevation of the only posterior cerebral artery that filled.

There was depression of the superior cerebellar artery (*arrows*). The frontal projection (D) demonstrates elevation of the posterior cerebral artery and depression of the superior cerebellar artery (*arrows*). The basilar artery was slightly displaced to the opposite side. The posterior cerebral artery on the contralateral side only filled slightly (*arrow*), and its curvature can be compared with that of the abnormal side.

(*Revised 1963*)

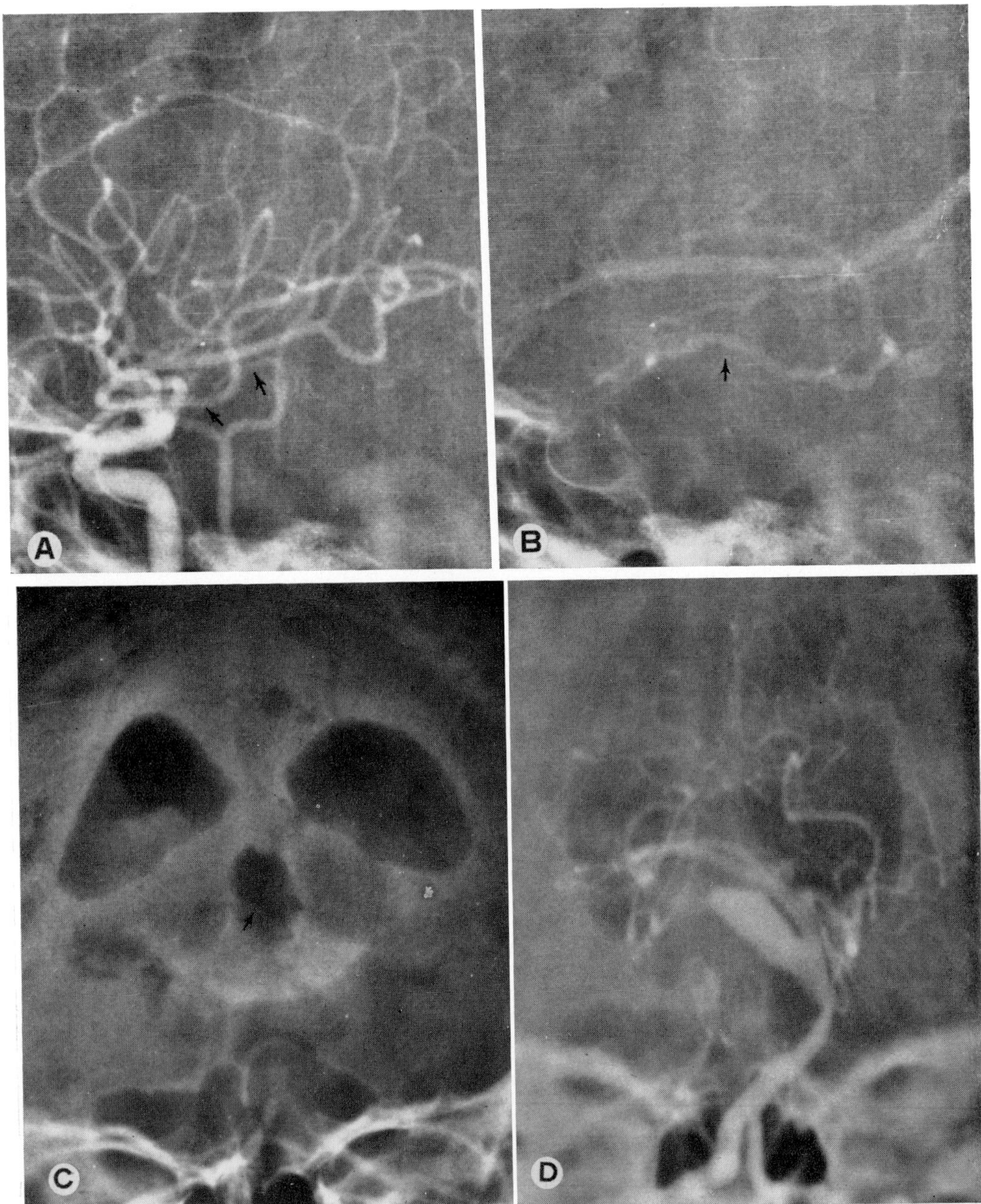

FIG. 502.—INCISURAL MASS (PARTLY THROMBOSED BASILAR ARTERY ANEURYSM)

A carotid angiogram was performed first and the lateral projection (A) revealed upward displacement of the anterior chorioidal artery (*arrows*). The arteriogram was otherwise normal. In the venous phase (B) the basilar vein was elevated (*arrow*). A pneumoencephalogram was then performed (C) which showed the typical posterolateral indentation on the third ventricle (*arrow*). Because the possibility of aneurysm was suspected, it was decided to perform a vertebral angiogram (D) which demonstrated a marked degree of lateral displacement of the basilar artery and elevation of the posterior cerebral as well as of the superior cerebellar arteries. An aneurysm filled, and it was felt that the remainder of the mass probably represented a large, partly thrombosed aneurysm.

(Revised 1963)

and these angiographic findings may be important since the two can produce a similar appearance at pneumography (Taveras, 1960). The incisural masses are described in more detail in the section on "Intracranial Pneumography."

DIAGNOSIS OF INTRACRANIAL MASSES BY ABNORMAL CIRCULATION

Intracranial masses, particularly certain neoplasms, contain a vascular supply that is rich enough to be demonstrated angiographically. The percentage of tumors that present abnormal vascularity will depend to a certain extent on the technical quality of the examination. If serialograms of excellent grade are obtained in every case in frontal and lateral projections, a large number of cases will exhibit abnormal vessels in the arterial or in the venous phase, or in both. By careful examination of the character of the abnormal vessels, it is possible, in a very high percentage of cases, to predict the histologic type of tumor present; the most important differentiation is between a meningioma and a malignant glioma or metastatic tumor. It cannot be overemphasized that in order to maintain a high degree of accuracy of histologic diagnosis by angiography, it is essential to have complete serialographic examinations and, in some instances, to do separate angiograms of the external and of the internal carotid arteries.

In general terms the findings that may be observed at cerebral angiography when abnormal circulation develops in connection with an intracranial mass are: (1) enlargement of pre-existing afferent arteries (most conspicuous when an artery which is enlarged is compared with adjacent vessels); (2) the appearance of new arterial channels, plainly visible irregular thin vessels which represent either new vessels or sometimes enlarged old vessels; these may be straight and smooth or they may have a "beaded" appearance; (3) "capillary blush," "tumor cloud," or "stain" (a general increase in density produced presumably by the opacification of many dilated tiny vessels); and (4) the appearance of new or enlarged veins (seen in the tumor area, at the periphery of the tumor or distal to the lesion draining into the surface veins or into the deep veins).

From the standpoint of pathologic physiology, tumors that present abnormal vascularity may be divided into two main groups, (1) those that have an increase in the speed of circulation through the tumor and (2) those that do not have an increase in the speed of circulation through the lesion. Such a classification is useful because neoplasms accompanied by a local increase in the speed of circulation are usually malignant tumors with very few exceptions. The chief exceptions are occasional cases of angioblastic meningioma or hemangioblastoma. In the description to follow, the tumors that do not increase the speed of circulation will be described first.

Abnormal Circulation Pattern with Normal Circulatory Rate

Meningiomas. Tumors of the meningioma group are usually very vascular and often produce enlargement of the arteries which supply them. The most characteristic vascular finding of meningioma is a contribution to the blood supply of the neoplasm by branches of the external carotid artery. Whenever it is possible to show that the external carotid artery shares in the blood supply of an intracranial tumor, the likelihood that it is a meningioma is extremely high. On the other hand, cranial tumors that invade the meninges may have an evident blood supply in the angiogram from a branch of the external carotid artery, but bone destruction usually is also evident. Metastatic tumors which invade bone or the meninges and, rarely, even glioblastoma multiforme may result in such a finding.

With meningioma, the artery which most often becomes enlarged is the middle meningeal or its branches and the other meningeal arteries. Only after a meningioma has invoked a reaction of the outer periosteum of the skull will the superficial temporal or some other branch of the external carotid artery participate in the tumor blood supply.

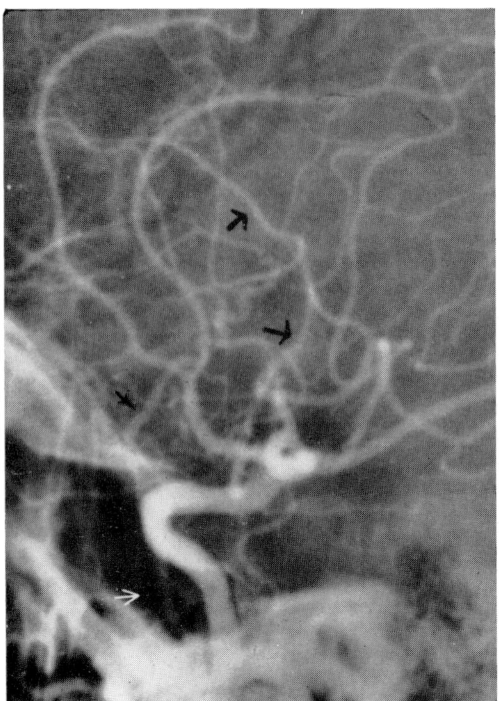

Fig. 503.—Tortuous Middle Meningeal Artery Which Is Slightly Enlarged in Patient with Meningioma in the Lateral Subfrontal Region

The tortuosity is accompanied by enlargement of the middle meningeal artery which can be traced as it crosses the air-containing shadow of the sphenoid sinus (*lower arrow*). The two upper arrows point at an elevated posteriorly displaced anterior opercular branch of the middle cerebral artery. This is the same case as that shown in Fig. 425.

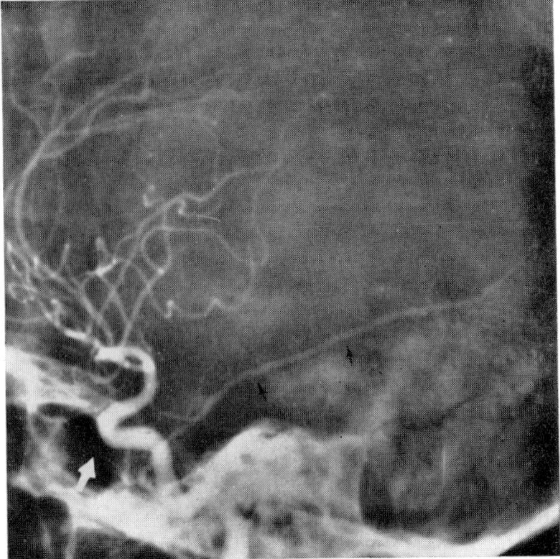

Fig. 504.—Earlier Filling and Larger Size of Feeding Branch of Middle Meningeal Artery in Meningioma

This patient had a tentorial meningioma which was supplied by the large posterior branch of the middle meningeal artery (*arrows*). On the other hand, the main branch, which is usually more conspicuous, is not filled as yet and is quite thin (*lower arrow*).

In attempting to determine whether the external carotid artery is indeed involved in the supply of a tumor, it is essential to pay careful attention to the relative size of the branches of the middle meningeal artery in particular and to try to determine whether small branches enter the tumor area from the artery in question.

Several routine steps may be helpful to determine whether a branch of the external carotid artery is or is not supplying a tumor. First, the size of the trunk of the middle meningeal artery should be scrutinized. If there is an increased blood flow through the middle meningeal trunk, which is necessary to supply a tumor, the artery usually becomes tortuous in its initial portion before it bifurcates (fig. 503). The presence of tortuosity per se is not necessarily an indication of an increased blood flow through this artery, since some patients have a tortuous initial portion of the middle-meningeal artery without having a neoplasm. Second, the relative size of the various branches of the middle meningeal artery should be noted since a branch involved in the supply of a tumor will fill slightly earlier and be larger than the other branches (fig. 504). Third, while a branch may not appear to be enlarged at its origin from the middle meningeal trunk, if the artery is followed to its periphery, it will be noted that instead of getting smaller, it will actually get larger as it approaches the region of the neoplasm (figs. 442 and 505). Such a finding is an important sign of blood supply of a tumor and is believed to be due to a reversal of blood flow in the many arterioles which anastomose within the bone. Similarly, other arterioles proceeding either from an ad-

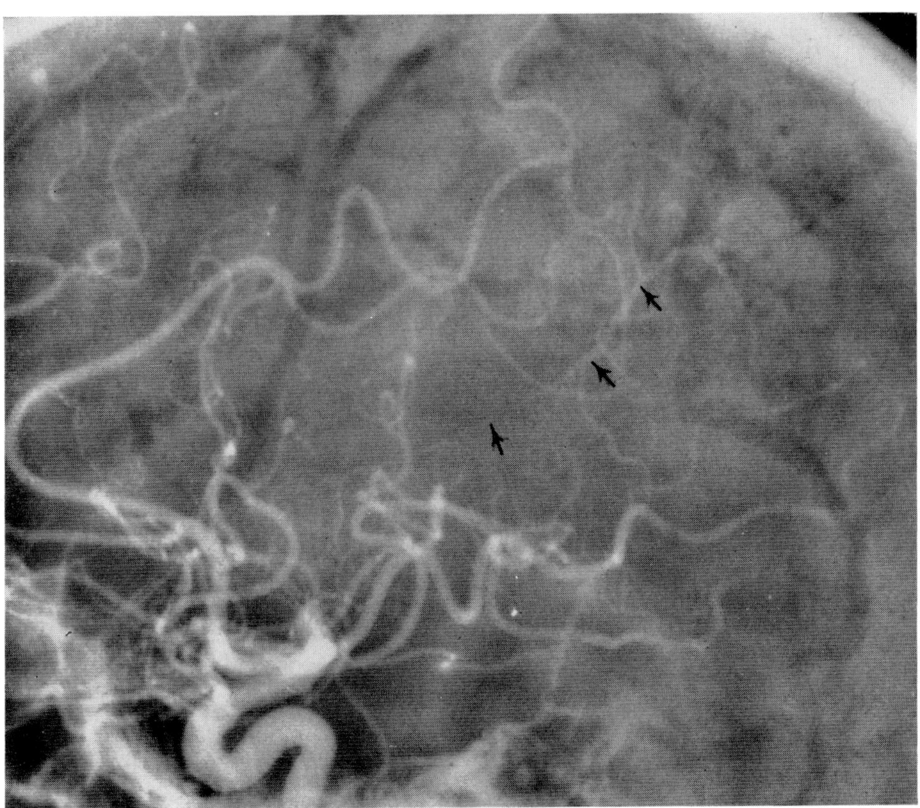

FIG. 505.—INCREASE IN THE SIZE OF A MIDDLE MENINGEAL CHANNEL IN ITS PERIPHERAL PORTION DUE TO MENINGIOMA

A branch of the middle meningeal artery gets considerably larger and seems to branch out into large branches after it goes further peripherally (*arrows*).

jacent branch of the middle meningeal or from accessory meningeal branches or superficial temporal arteries involved in the blood supply of the bone, may join the vessel feeding the tumor. By virtue of this reversal of flow, more blood is drawn into the final segment of the artery to increase the blood supply of the neoplasm. Finally, one should look carefully for multiple branches arising from any vessel in question, especially near its termination. Such branches may be very inconspicuous, as is shown in Figure 505, or they may be extremely prominent, as is shown in Figure 506. When *external carotid angiography* alone is performed, the abnormal vessels are easier to visualize than when there is superimposition of branches of the internal carotid artery. The term sunburst appearance has been applied to this very distinctive finding by angiography which is characteristic of meningiomas. It is believed that the sunburst appearance is due to a radial distribution of the small arterial branches which seem to spring from a central point. This focal point has been called by us the hilus of the meningioma, and probably represents the original site from which the blood supply was drawn at the beginning of the growth of the tumor (figs. 506 and 507).

The majority of meningiomas which occur over the cranial vault are supplied by branches of the middle meningeal artery and, as explained above, sometimes by the superficial temporal artery. Some meningiomas situated in the frontal fossa may be supplied by meningeal branches which normally feed the bone in this region and which

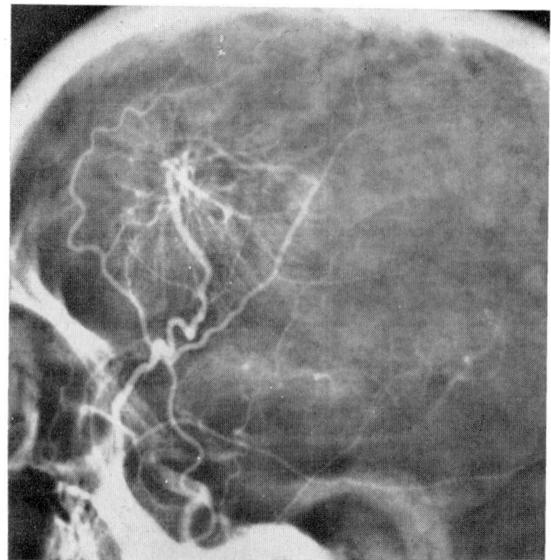

FIG. 506.—SUNBURST APPEARANCE IN MENINGIOMA SUPPLIED BY THE MIDDLE MENINGEAL ARTERY

It is evident that the anterior branch of the middle meningeal artery is quite large and tortuous whereas the posterior branch is small. This external carotid angiogram is advantageous to demonstrate the appearance of the radiating vessels springing from the hilus of the meningioma in a radial fashion.

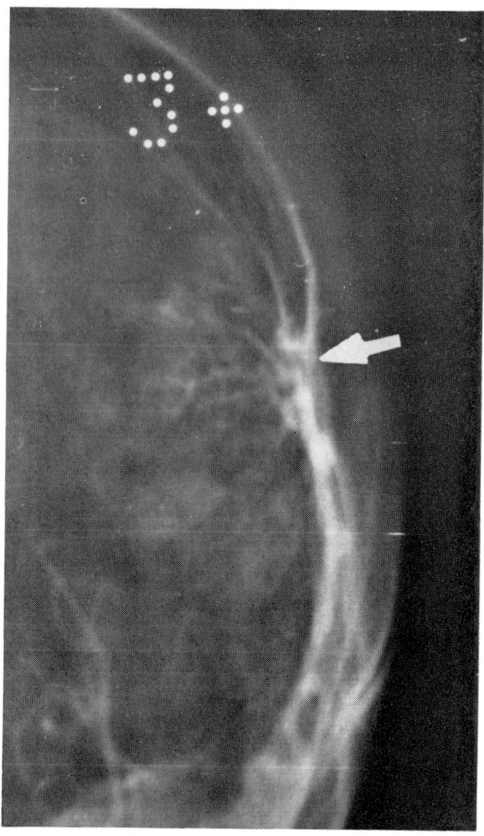

FIG. 507.—DEMONSTRATION OF THE RADIAL DISTRIBUTION OF THE VESSELS IN MENINGIOMA SUPPLIED BY THE MENINGEAL ARTERIES

The vessels appear to start from a point (*arrow*) which may be termed the hilus of the meningioma and from there radiate in all directions as shown in Fig. 506 in the lateral projection.

anastomose with branches of the ophthalmic artery. Since the blood supply through the internal carotid artery is swifter, eventually a significant proportion or most of the tumor blood supply may be by way of the ophthalmic artery, and this vessel becomes enlarged. In such cases it is possible to demonstrate angiographically branches arising from the superior aspect of the ophthalmic artery and extending upward to the roof of the orbit (figs. 508 and 509). Falx meningiomas arising higher up may receive their blood supply partly through the ophthalmic artery. The anterior meningeal artery (arising from the anterior ethmoidal branch of the ophthalmic) may become enlarged and can be followed along the inner table of the skull in the frontal region (fig. 510). While frontal midline meningiomas and subfrontal (olfactory groove) meningiomas usually receive their blood supply through the ophthalmic artery, tuberculum sella meningiomas do not appear to do so (Lombardi *et al.*, 1960; DiChiro, 1961). Falx meningiomas arising in the posterior frontal region may still receive their blood supply partly by way of the anterior meningeal branch (fig. 511).

Another example of blood supply through the internal carotid artery by way of its meningeal anastomotic branches is found in some tentorial meningiomas. The case illustrated in Figure 512 demonstrates a small branch arising from the posterior aspect of the internal carotid artery and extending backward to supply a meningioma. The tumor also received branches from the external carotid system and thus a common carotid angiogram demonstrated a rich

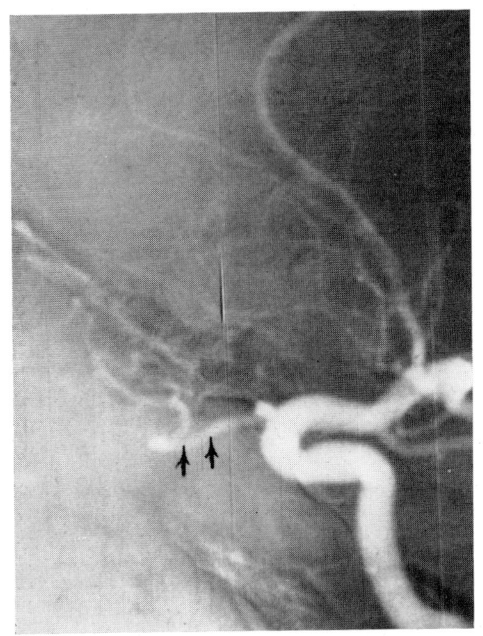

Fig. 508.—Branching of the Ophthalmic Artery Supplying Small Subfrontal Meningioma Demonstrated by the Subtraction Method

The ophthalmic artery (*arrows*) is seen to give off branches which go cephalad to supply an area of abnormal bone in the planum sphenoidale region. The bone is completely blotted out by the photographic procedure used, and only the vessels stand out.

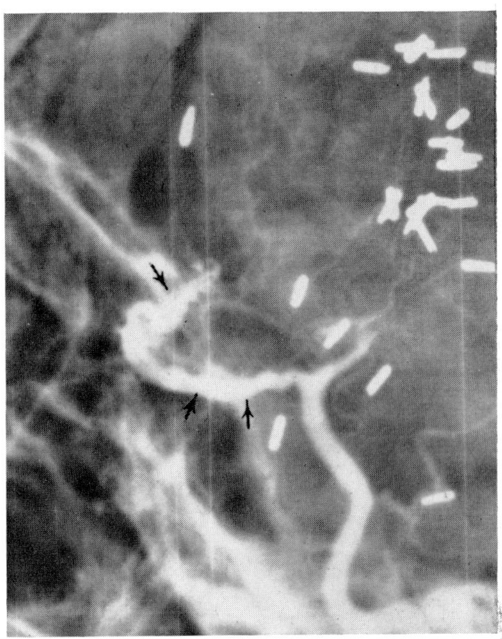

Fig. 509.—Recurrent Sphenoid Ridge Meningioma Supplied by a Huge Ophthalmic Artery

Following surgical ligation of the middle meningeal artery at the time of the first operation, the supply then took place by way of the ophthalmic artery and its anastomoses with the meningeal arteries (*arrows*).

blood supply with a large "capillary blush" not shown when only the internal carotid artery was injected. (See also Figures 460 and 501.) Meningiomas in the posterior fossa also may be supplied by accessory meningeal arteries, which are branches of the external carotid system entering the skull by way of the condyloid foramen and through the foramen lacerum.

Occasionally, branches of the middle meningeal and superficial temporal arteries overlie the area of a neoplasm, but this does not mean necessarily that they are supplying the lesion (fig. 513). The rules explained above, especially progressive vascular enlargement, should be followed in trying to evaluate the significance of vessels in or about a tumor area.

An occasional branch of the external carotid artery, most often the superficial temporal artery, may appear to enlarge on the late films of a serialogram. It is necessary, however, to differentiate between actual enlargement of a vascular segment and apparent enlargement which may be seen because of *laminar flow*. Since the main stream of contrast substance is through the center of the artery, and the periphery of the vessel becomes opacified after the center, the later of two films may show an arterial diameter which appears to be larger than at the earlier time. Such an appearance usually can be differentiated in the angiogram from true enlargement.

Not all meningiomas are supplied principally by the external carotid artery and its branches. In fact, a significant number are supplied by both the external and the internal carotid arteries, and a small percentage are supplied exclusively by intracranial branches of the internal carotid

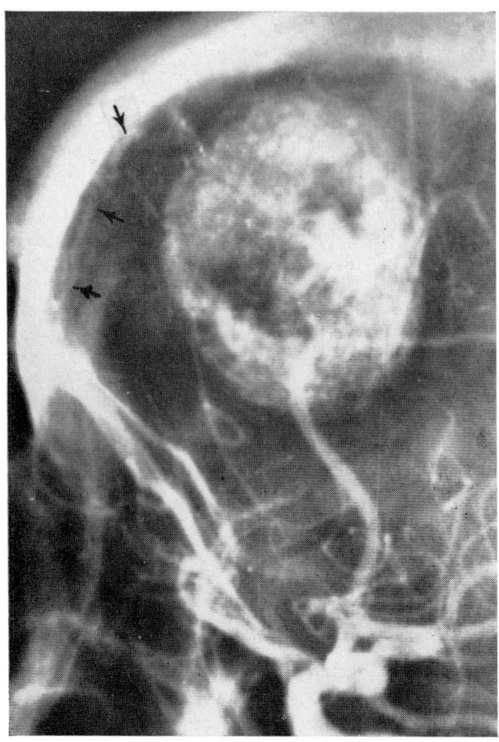

Fig. 510.—Anterior Meningeal Branch of the Ophthalmic Artery Supplying Frontal Falx Meningioma

The artery can be followed just beneath the inner table of the skull in the frontal bone (*arrows*).

artery. An example of exclusive supply by the internal carotid artery is found in the case of intraventricular meningioma, a tumor which usually is fed by the chorioidal arteries (fig. 475).

While vessel or vessels that actually supply a meningioma often can be seen in the angiogram, sometimes these cannot be visualized and only a large area of abnormal density can be discerned. Previously the intrinsic vascularity of a tumor has been referred to as the "tumor cloud," "stain," or "capillary blush." A homogeneous tumor cloud in which there is a fairly even distribution of the contrast material throughout the tumor is characteristic of meningiomas. In addition, persistence of the tumor cloud for a considerable period of time throughout the serialogram is of great importance in the diagnosis of meningioma. The stain actually still may be visible even on the last film taken 8 or 9 seconds after the beginning of the injection.

The intrinsic vascular outline of meningiomas usually is sharply circumscribed and yet irregular in lobular configuration. This characteristic is in contradistinction to some gliomas (usually mixed oligodendrogliomas and astrocytomas), which may present a homogeneous cloud but are not sharply circumscribed (fig. 514).

Meningiomas usually fail to exhibit prominent draining veins. With some meningiomas a few thin veins may be seen at the periphery of the tumor. An occasional case of angioblastic meningioma may present numerous large veins with an increase in the speed of circulation through the tumor that produces early venous filling similar to that seen with malignant tumors (fig. 515). Such lesions, however, which present draining veins, may exhibit all other characteristics of meningiomas. In these cases, the draining vessels are usually superficial cerebral veins, although sometimes deep veins drain into the vein of Galen, as in the case illustrated by Figure 515. Such veins indicate that there is invasion of brain tissue by the meningioma or, at least, that "tumor" vessels have appeared which bridge the space to the surface of the brain. Intraventricular tumors, of necessity, must drain by way of the tributaries of the thalamostriate vein and the internal cerebral veins.

In trying to evaluate the importance of the above described characteristics of the abnormal circulation of meningiomas, the most significant features are considered to be (1) a blood supply from the external carotid system, (2) a homogeneous but sharply circumscribed cloud, and (3) the persistence of the contrast substance within the tumor. Often no blood supply can be traced from the external carotid artery into the meningioma, and a diagnosis must be based on other observations. Of the latter two findings, persistence of the tumor cloud appears to be slightly more reliable than homogeneity alone (fig. 516).

(*Revised 1963*)

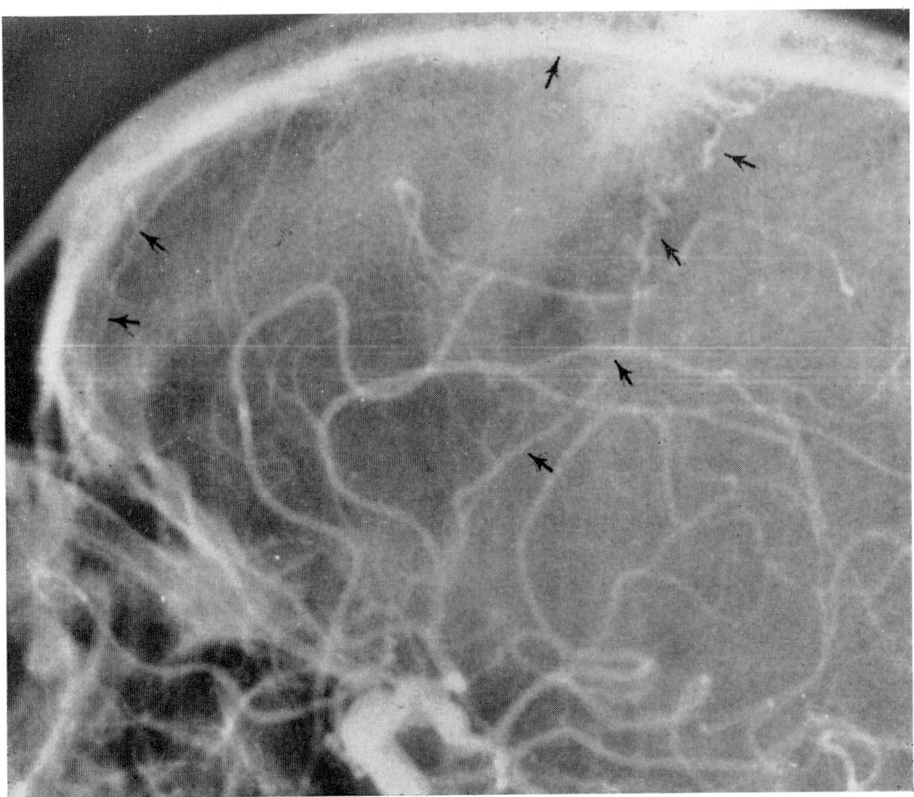

FIG. 511.—POSTERIOR FRONTAL FALX MENINGIOMA RECEIVING BLOOD SUPPLY THROUGH OPHTHALMIC ARTERY

The anterior meningeal branch of the ophthalmic artery can be followed along the inner table of the skull (*arrows*) to join the middle meningeal artery (*posterior arrows*) in supplying the meningioma. The presence of these meningeal channels made the diagnosis certain, even though the vascular displacements were not typical.

Because of pressure on superficial cerebral veins, slowing of the circulation through the area of a meningioma may be seen in the absence of abnormal vascularity. The surface veins in the tumor area fill later than those elsewhere in the brain, owing to local slowing of the circulation (fig. 457). The finding is nonspecific and may be seen in cases of intracerebral tumor as well (Leeds and Taveras, 1963).

Abnormal Circulation Pattern with Increased Circulatory Rate

The chief characteristic of tumors of this category is that blood is shunted through them, with the result that veins fill more rapidly in the region of the tumor than they do in the remainder of the brain. The increase in the speed of circulation through the tumors is presumably due to the presence of many new or enlarged arterioles with incomplete walls, usually referred to as "sinusoids." Such vessels actually represent small arteriovenous communications. Usually many draining veins are visible but sometimes only one or two venous channels can be visualized clearly. The veins that fill are, in the majority of instances, on the surface of the brain, either the outer or the medial surface of a hemisphere. Deep veins can be

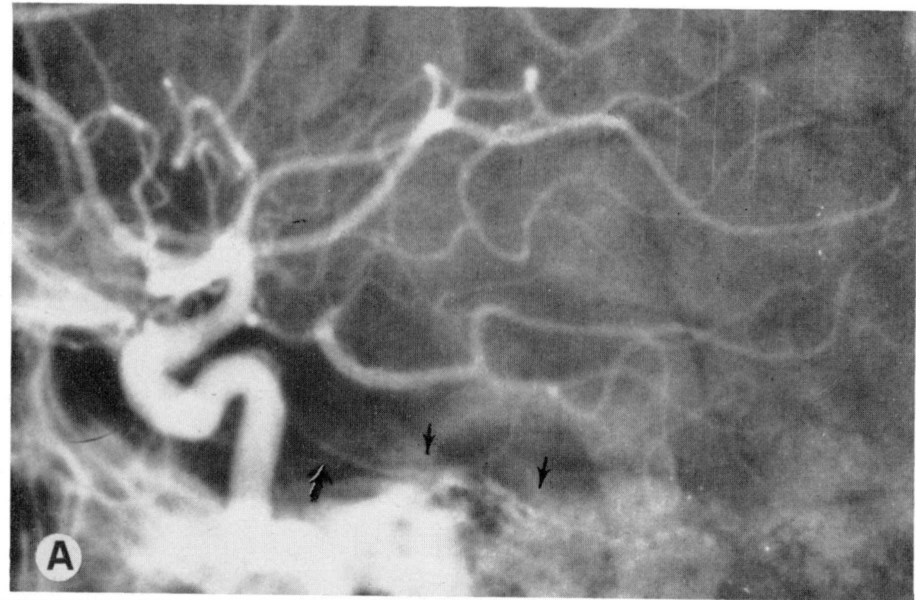

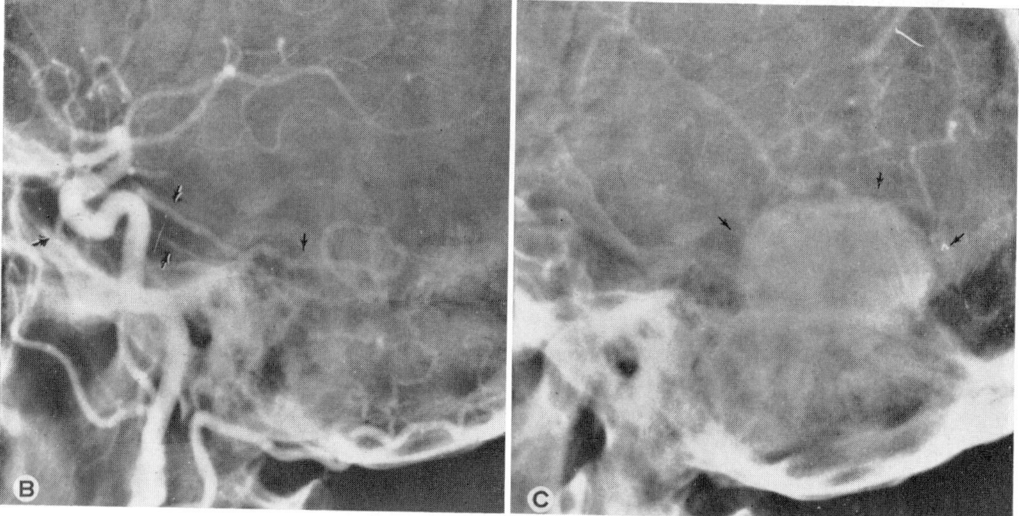

FIG. 512.—TENTORIAL MENINGIOMA SUPPLIED BY MENINGEAL BRANCH OF INTERNAL CAROTID ARTERY

The internal carotid angiogram (A) demonstrated a meningeal branch of the internal carotid artery (*arrows*), but no other abnormalities were noted. It was then decided to perform a common carotid angiogram. The lateral view on this angiogram (B) revealed a large middle meningeal artery which gave off large branches to supply the tentorial meningioma (*arrows*). The serialographic film (C) made at 6 seconds revealed the presence of a large tumor stain which was homogeneous and persisted, typical of meningioma. The occipital artery also seemed to supply the lesion.

visualized which indicate that the tumor has originated in or has invaded the depths of the brain. The drainage of such a tumor is by way of the branches of the internal cerebral vein.

Malignant gliomas. Tumors of the glioblastoma multiforme group often present many irregular looking, or beaded vessels. Such vessels are not seen exclusively in glioblastomas but a similar appearance may

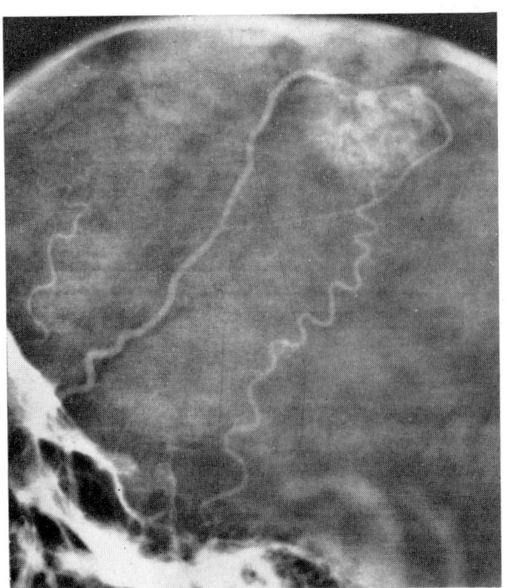

FIG. 513.—EXTERNAL CAROTID ANGIOGRAM IN PARASAGITTAL MENINGIOMA

The middle meningeal artery divides into two branches, both of which are seen to enter the meningioma to supply it. The tumor area was homogeneous from the start, and the radial distribution of vessels was not visible in this instance at any stage during the serialogram. A branch of the superficial temporal artery is seen to pass over the tumor, but on later serials was seen to go beyond the tumor and to diminish in diameter progressively. It is common to find external carotid branches overlying the area of the tumor, and unless certain criteria are met, it should not be considered that the overlying external carotid vessel is involved in the blood supply.

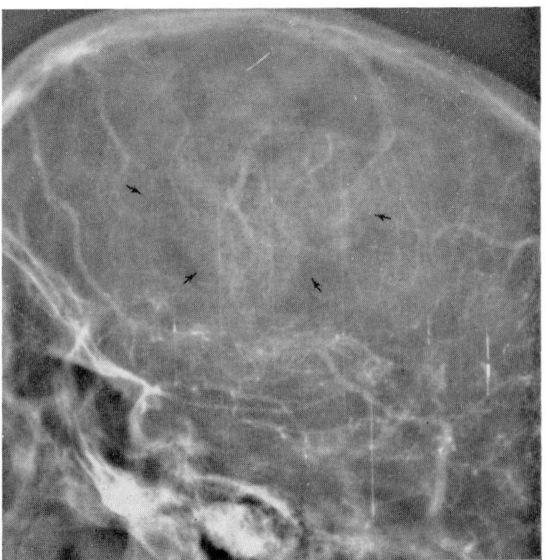

FIG. 514.—HOMOGENEOUS MODERATELY PERSISTENT CLOUD IN MIXED GLIOMA (OLIGODENDROGLIOMA AND ASTROCYTOMA)

There is a homogeneous collection of contrast material which is somewhat irregular in configuration (*arrows*). The capillary blush is not sharply circumscribed and seems to blend with the remainder of the brain. The latter differentiates it from meningiomas which are usually well demarcated. The cloud persisted (this film was made at 6 seconds) but reveals cerebral veins overlying the tumor, which is unusual in meningioma.

be seen also in some meningiomas (fig. 516). They are presumed to represent immature vessels with incomplete walls and "sinusoid" formation. The abnormal vessels of glioblastomas tend to be predominately situated, or at least are more numerous, in the periphery of the mass (Lima, 1950), presumably due to central necrosis which glioblastomas often present, and only the growing border shows a rich vascularity (fig. 517).

The abnormal vascularity of glioblastomas tends to disappear fairly rapidly (Tönnis and Schiefer, 1959). In following the progress of the contrast substance in serialograms, it will be noted that toward the end of the examination no abnormal vessels may be visible in glioblastoma, contrary to the situation with meningioma (fig. 518).

Drainage by deep veins is, with few exceptions, an indication of a malignant intracerebral growth (fig. 519). The rapidity with which abnormal vascularity can develop is demonstrated in Figure 520.

Enlargement of feeding vessels is common in glioblastomas (fig. 521). Vascular thrombosis, endothelial proliferation, and collagenous thickening of the walls of larger vessels also occur (fig. 522). One case of glioblastoma was seen in which the meningeal branches of the internal carotid were enlarged similar to what is found in tentorial meningiomas (fig. 523).

Occasionally, no abnormal vascularity is seen within a glioblastoma, and only early filling of draining veins is visible in the angiogram. It is very important, therefore,

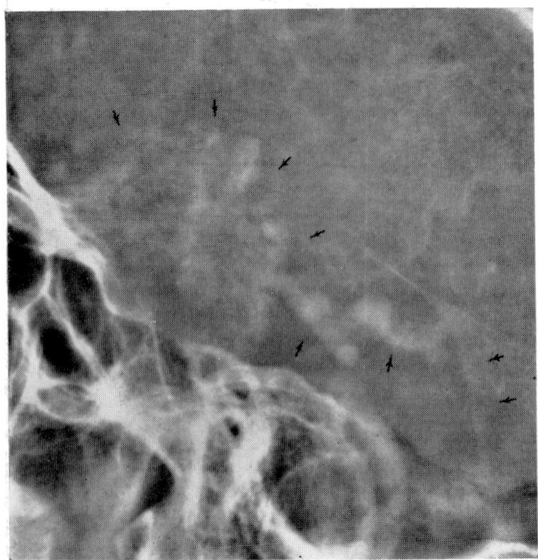

FIG. 515.—ANGIOBLASTIC MENINGIOMA WITH INCREASED SPEED OF CIRCULATION AND DRAINAGE BY WAY OF DEEP CEREBRAL VEINS

The tumor cloud was well circumscribed (*arrows*) and at one stage during the serialogram, it was homogeneous. At this stage (3.5 seconds) there is irregularity within the area of increased density due to very large draining veins. The tumor was seen to drain by way of the basilar vein, which was extremely tortuous and enlarged, into the straight sinus. Such drainage would indicate invasion of the brain.

to look for early venous opacification which may be the best clue, not only to the presence of tumor, but also to the nature of the neoplasm (fig. 524).

Metastatic tumors. Secondary neoplastic deposits exhibit an abnormal vascularity very similar to that of glioblastoma. It has been stated by Ethelberg and Vaernet (1953) that one finding that helps one to differentiate metastatic tumors from glioblastomas is that a single artery feeds the metastatic lesion, which is not usually the case with glioblastoma. The authors, however, have seen glioblastomas supplied by one vessel which becomes enlarged, in the same manner as a metastatic growth (fig. 521). Presumably, the significance of a single enlarged artery in a metastatic tumor is that the original neoplastic cellular embolus occurred by way of this particular vessel (fig. 525).

Regarding early venous filling, there is no appreciable difference from glioblastoma. The immature beaded vessels also are seen in metastatic tumors, and such masses exhibit central areas of necrosis in the same manner as do glioblastomas.

The only reliable angiographic evidence of metastatic tumor is multiplicity. Multiple lesions are almost always of metastatic origin, although cases of multiple glioblastomas are known to occur rarely (figs. 526 and 527). When metastatic brain tumor is accompanied by invasion of the meninges and the skull, the branches of the middle meningeal artery may participate in the blood supply and angiographic differentiation with meningioma may be difficult. However, the plain films are usually diagnostic of a destructive bone lesion.

Metastatic tumors sometimes present a homogeneous type of cloud, although accompanied by an increase in the speed of circulation. One impressive example of such circulation was seen in a case of metastatic brain tumor from the thyroid. Metastatic deposits from the kidneys also may tend to have a slightly more homogeneous distribution of abnormal vascularity than tumors originating in the lungs or in the breast. Generally, however, secondary tumors are usually not confused with meningiomas because of early venous filling with the former lesions.

Attention should be paid to early draining veins which may drain some metastatic nodules, whereas a tumor stain may be seen in other nodules (fig. 528).

Other cerebral tumors. Four cases of mixed tumor (oligodendroglioma and astrocytoma) have been seen presenting a relatively homogeneous tumor cloud which, although not sharply circumscribed or lobulated, tended to persist, as occurs with meningioma (fig. 514). Draining veins could be seen in the area of the tumor in some cases. A few mixed intraventricular gliomas have been seen which presented an increased vascularity and rapid venous drainage by way of branches of the thalamostriate vein. These can usually be identified as intraventricular because of their location

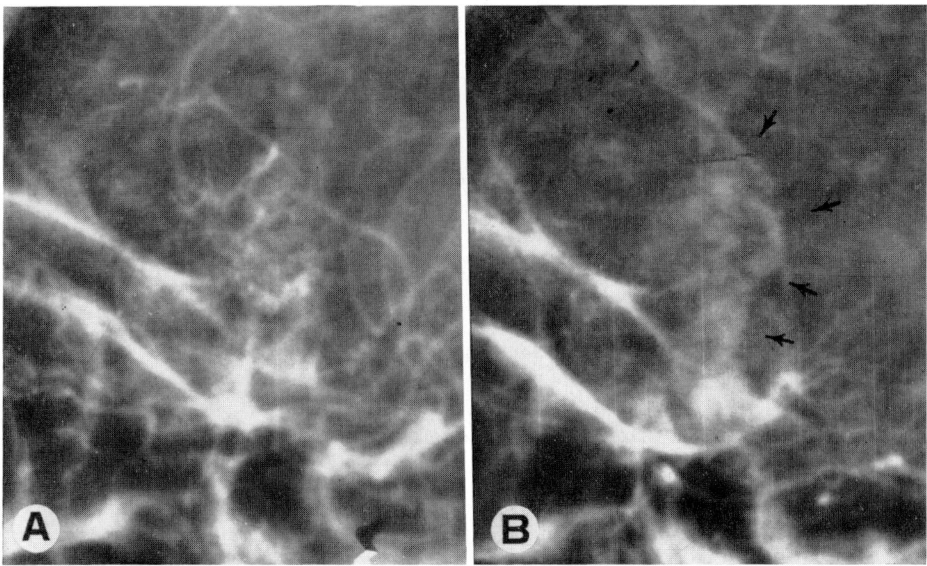

Fig. 516.—Subfrontal Meningioma Showing Beaded Vessels

The film made in the arterial phase (A) shows many beaded vessels in the area of the tumor. The appearance was considered as atypical for meningioma. However, the film made at 5.5 to 6.0 seconds (B) shows a persistent, fairly homogeneous cloud (*arrows*) and the diagnosis of meningioma was felt most likely, which proved to be the case.

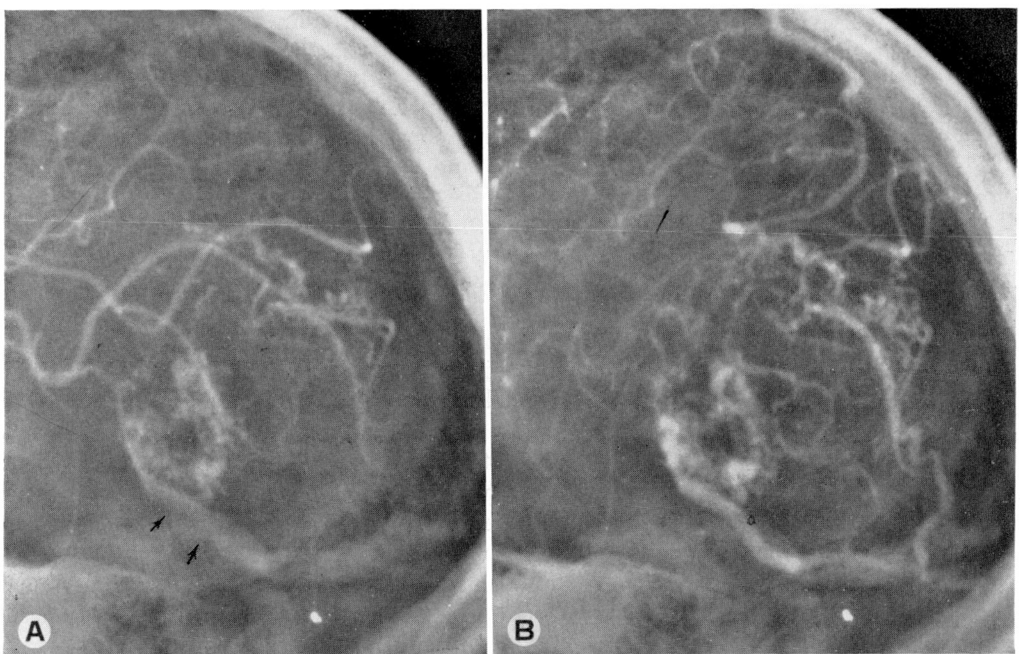

Fig. 517.—Glioblastoma Multiforme Showing Peripheral Distribution of Vascularity Probably Due to Central Necrosis

The film in the early arterial phase shows a distribution of abnormal beaded vessels around the periphery of a lesion which does not show any significant vascularity in the central portion. Already a vein (*arrows*) is draining into the lateral sinus. A film made 1.0 second later (B) shows considerable venous drainage in the region of the tumor, while in the remainder of the brain the circulatory phase is still in the late arterial phase. This is due to shunting of blood through the malignant tumor.

(Revised 1963)

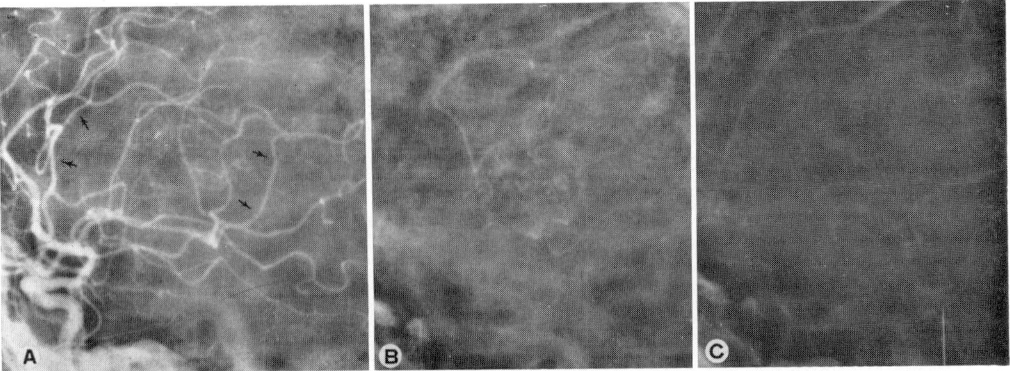

FIG. 518.—GLIOBLASTOMA SHOWING DISAPPEARANCE OF TUMOR STAIN IN 5.5 SECONDS

The film made in the arterial phase (A) shows a capillary blush in the supra-Sylvian opercular region. The arteries in the region of the tumor are somewhat straight, and one artery in front and another in back of the lesion show concentric bowing (*arrows*) which delimits the area of edema accompanying the neoplasm which is rather sharply circumscribed, as shown in (B), a film made at 2 seconds after the beginning of the injection. Already early venous drainage can be seen, whereas the remainder of the brain is in the intermediate phase. A film made at 5.5 seconds (C) shows complete disappearance of the abnormal vascularity and of the veins draining the tumor, whereas the brain is now at the peak of the venous phase.

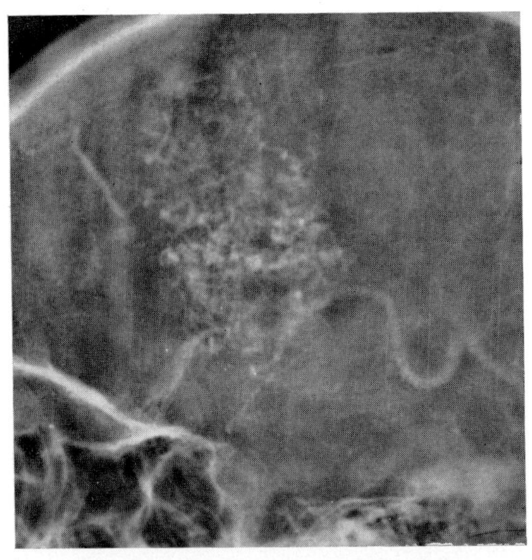

FIG. 519.—TYPICAL APPEARANCE OF A MALIGNANT INTRACEREBRAL TUMOR (GLIOBLASTOMA MULTIFORME)

The film demonstrates the irregularity of the vascular components of the tumor with conglomerations of contrast substance representing the sinusoids which are actual areas of arteriovenous communications within the malignant tumor. Early venous drainage is seen in the frontal region and particularly by way of the internal cerebral vein, which is conspicuously outlined. Drainage by way of deep veins is almost always an indication of malignancy.

close to the midline in the frontal projection, and in the lateral projection situated in the region where the ventricles are placed. One case which was diagnosed histologically as lymphosarcoma of the frontal lobe of the brain has been seen which presented a relatively homogeneous cloud and a perfectly rounded and sharply circumscribed configuration (fig. 529).

Astrocytomas usually show no angiographically demonstrable tumor vascularity; rarely a well differentiated astrocytoma is encountered with a visible capillary blush (fig. 435).

In the presence of extremely vascular tumors, particularly the malignant ones which exhibit early and extensive venous filling, the question is sometimes raised whether they are a vascular arteriovenous malformation rather than a neoplasm. It usually is easy to differentiate between the two because the arteriovenous malformations are fed by very large arteries and are drained by extremely large veins and the circulation time through an arteriovenous malformation is much faster than through a neoplasm. In addition, neoplasms usually are accompanied by other signs of an intracranial mass, such as displacement of vessels

(*Revised 1963*)

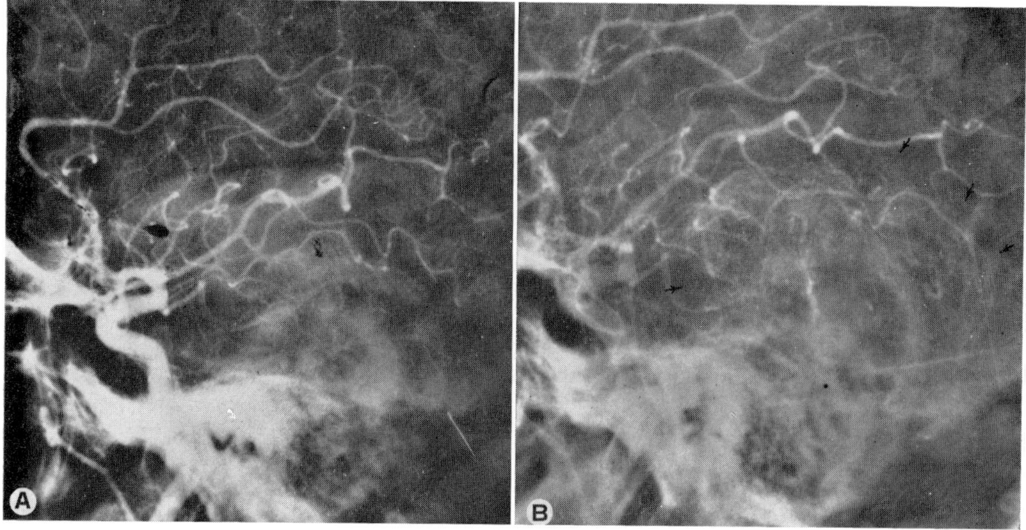

FIG. 520.—RAPID DEVELOPMENT OF NEOPLASTIC VESSELS IN GLIOBLASTOMA

The film shown in (A) demonstrates minimum abnormalities of the temporal region and no abnormal vessels were demonstrated in the serialogram. In fact, the arteriogram was called essentially normal at that time. Eight weeks later (B) repeat angiography demonstrated a large area of abnormal vascularity and vascular displacement indicating the rapid growth of the tumor and the formation of neoplastic vessels.

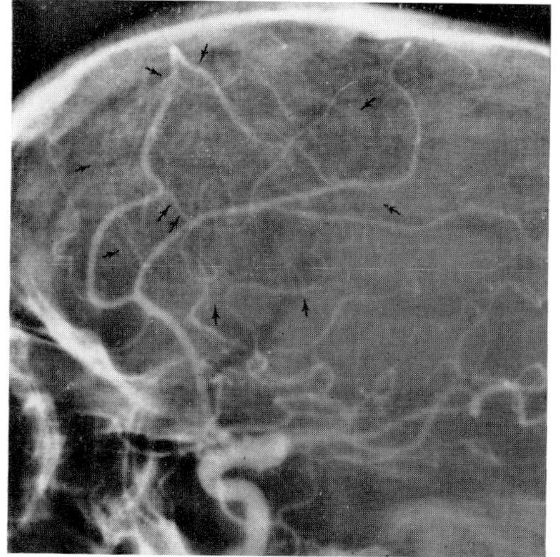

FIG. 521.—ENLARGEMENT OF A BRANCH OF THE CALLOSOMARGINAL ARTERY SUPPLYING A GLIOBLASTOMA

There is enlargement of the internal frontal branch which is supplying this parasagittal glioblastoma (*upper arrows*). Note that the middle internal frontal branch, which springs from the same artery (the callosomarginal artery) is small (*two arrows*), whereas the one supplying the tumor is much larger. Many fine straight vessels which are slightly irregular in contour are seen occupying a fairly broad area outlined by the circumscribing *arrows*.

(Revised 1963)

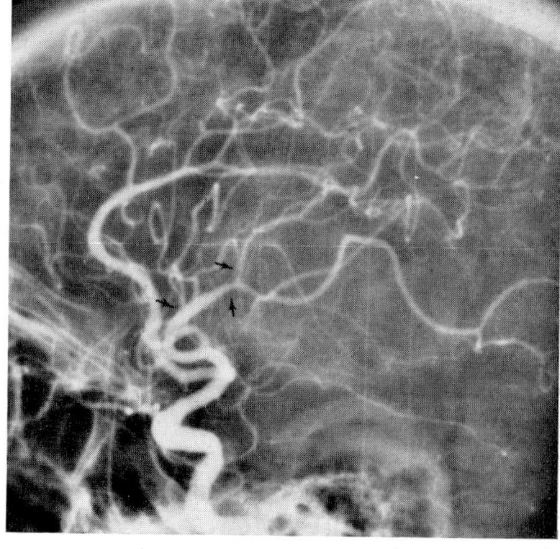

FIG. 522.—TEMPORAL GLIOBLASTOMA PRODUCING ENLARGEMENT, NARROWING, AND IRREGULARITY OF THE VESSELS

There is irregular elevation of the middle cerebral branches. The branches of the middle cerebral artery reveal considerable irregularity and variation in the width of the lumen (*arrows*) which, in glioblastomas, may be associated with collagenous thickening of the vessel wall and possibly, actual invasion.

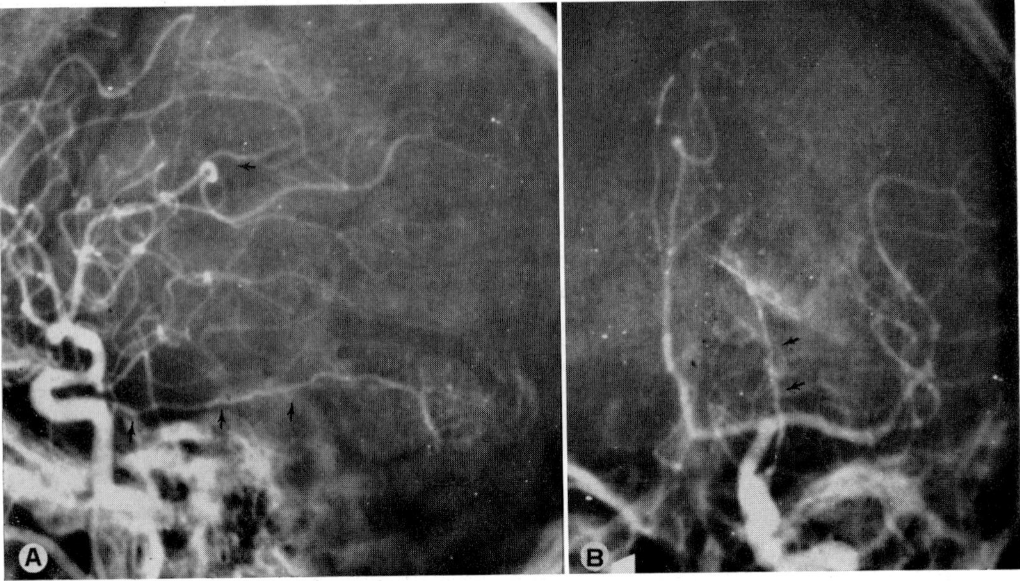

FIG. 523.—GLIOBLASTOMA SHOWING ENLARGEMENT OF TENTORIAL BRANCH OF INTERNAL CAROTID ARTERY

The lateral view (A) demonstrates an inferior retro-Sylvian mass which is producing upward and forward displacement of the angiographic Sylvian point (*arrow*). There is a very large meningeal branch arising from the intracavernous portion of the internal carotid artery (*arrows*) which is seen to give off branches in its posterior portion. The frontal projection (B) confirms the position of this artery which is following the edge of the tentorium (*arrows*). A diagnosis of tentorial meningioma was made, but surgical intervention demonstrated anaplastic glioma which was growing through the subarachnoid space and invading the tentorium. The latter invasion probably explains the blood supply by this branch of the internal carotid artery. This appearance is extremely unusual. (Courtesy of Dr. Norman Chase, New York.)

or midline shift. Only occasionally, when an arteriovenous malformation has recently bled and produced an intracerebral hematoma is a relatively atypical configuration produced which may be confused with a tumor.

Brain abscess rarely has sufficient vascularity to show clearly on the angiogram. Some cases, however, do present a halo of increased density due to vascular congestion around the mass.

Abnormal Circulation Pattern of Posterior Fossa Tumors

Meningiomas of the posterior fossa present the same characteristics by angiography as were described above. A tentorial meningioma may be supplied by branches of the external carotid artery through accessory meningeal arteries. It also may be supplied by way of branches of the internal carotid artery which supply the meninges and the tentorium. As previously mentioned, these

---

of the tumor, but this does not indicate a vascular supply by the meningeal artery. In fact, this is an intracerebral tumor of the malignant type. The film made in the intermediate phase (B) shows early filling of posterior frontal veins (*arrows*) with no other veins visible in the remainder of the brain. There was no visible capillary blush, the apparent increase in density in the area was seen on the plain films. The film made at 3.5 seconds (C), the full venous phase, shows the filling of the remaining cerebral veins. The thalamostriate vein is depressed and the venous angle is closed (*arrows*) which is a feature of parasagittal tumors. The curve of the internal cerebral vein, on the other hand, is normal.

(Revised 1963)

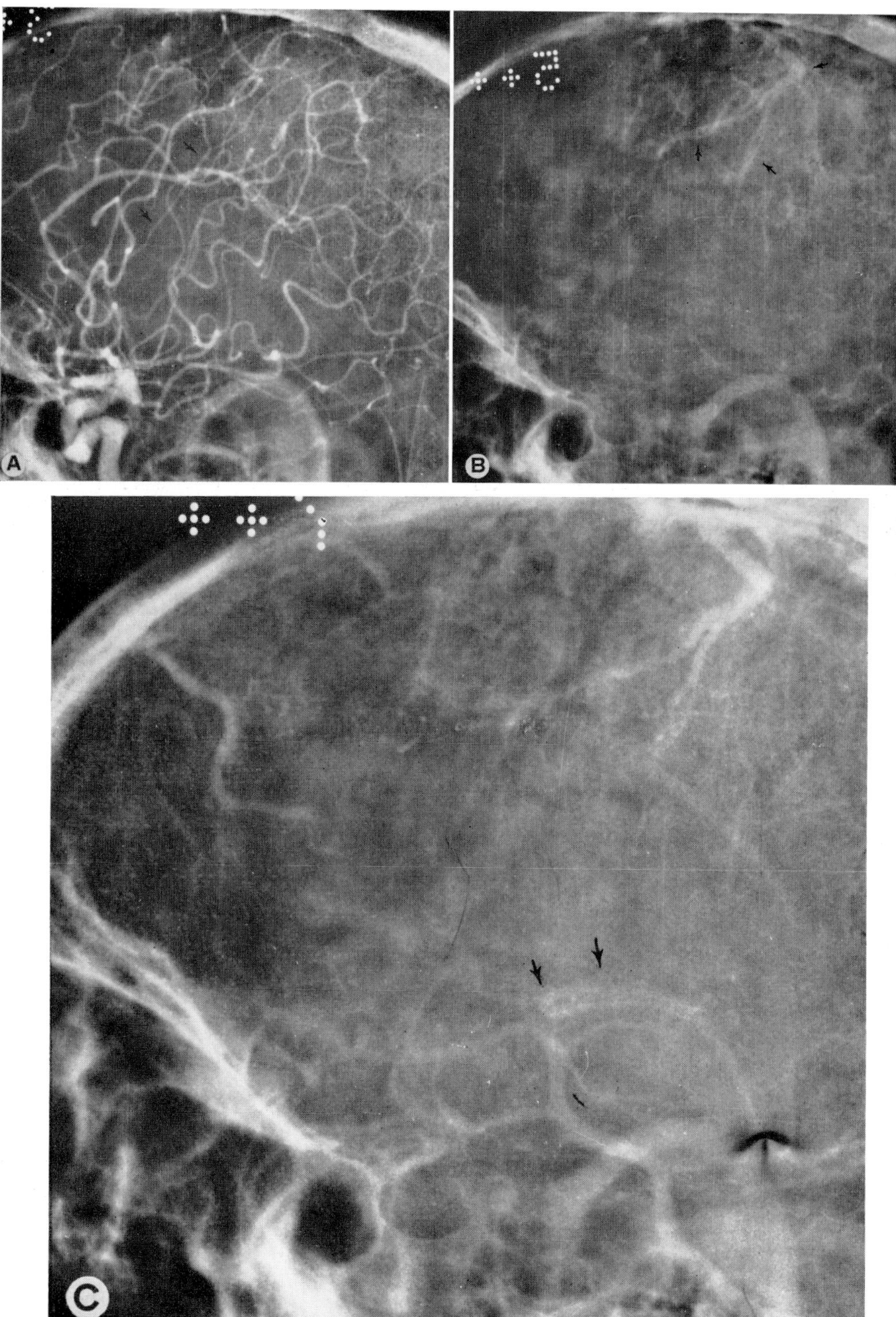

Fig. 524.—Parasagittal Tumor Showing Early Drainage of Vein and No Definite Findings in the Arterial Phase

The arterial phase (A) does not reveal any definite abnormalities. The pericallosal artery shows slight rounding which is not necessarily abnormal. There may be slight depression of the Sylvian triangle, but this is questionable. A middle meningeal branch (*arrow*) is seen to ascend toward the area.

(Revised 1963)

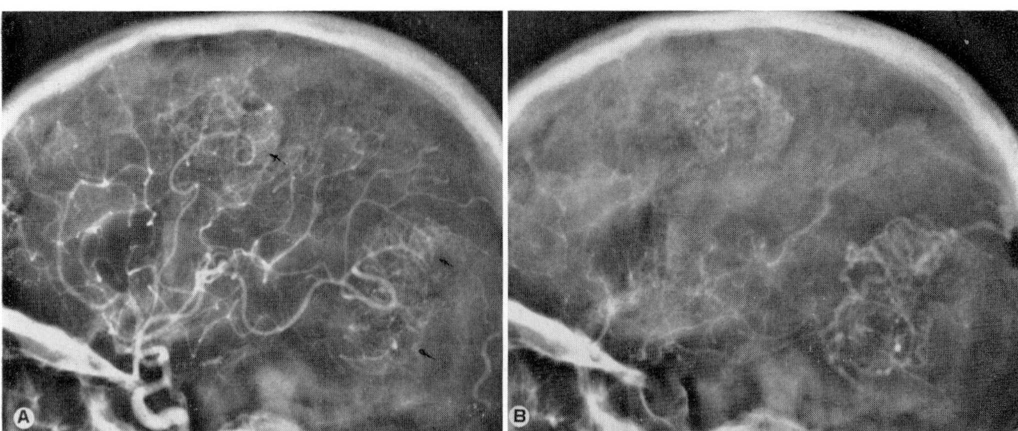

FIG. 525.—MULTIPLE NODULES FROM METASTATIC MELANOMA

(A) Three nodules are seen (*arrows*) which are supplied by single slightly enlarged arteries. In the film made at 2.5 seconds in the intermediate phase (B), there was rapid and extensive venous drainage from these metastatic nodules similar to that seen in glioblastomas.

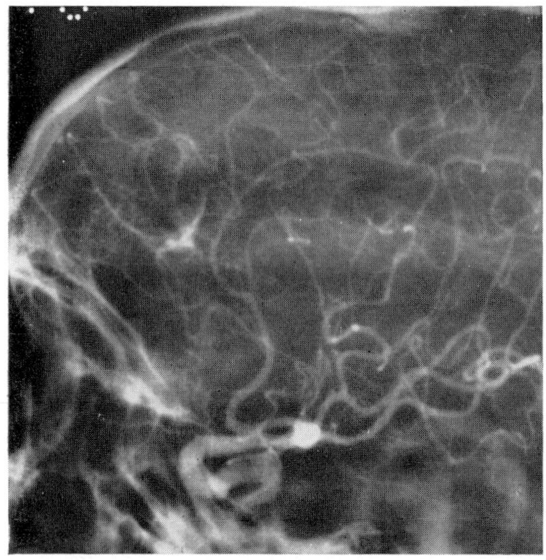

FIG. 526.—MULTIPLE GLIOBLASTOMAS

Four separate tumors were found, the largest in the left frontal area. Another frontal tumor was found on the right side, and in addition, a temporal tumor was found on this side. Even in retrospect, only one tumor could be diagnosed with certainty, the left frontal mass. The case emphasizes the difficulty of diagnosing multiple intracranial masses. Fig. 526 shows the left side; Fig. 527 shows the right side.

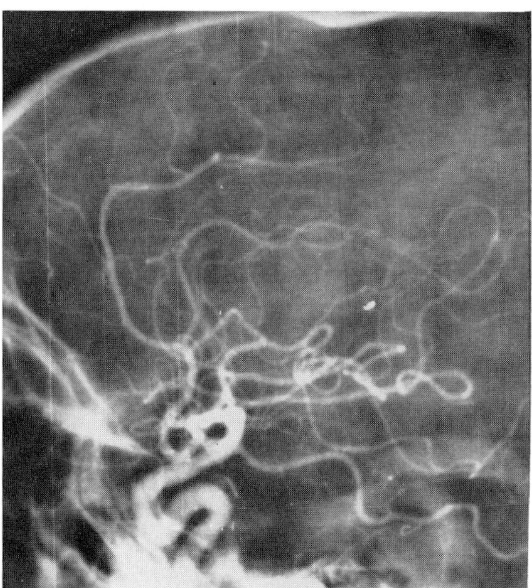

FIG. 527.—MULTIPLE GLIOBLASTOMAS

Same case as Fig. 526; right side.

branches probably originate in the intracavernous portion of the internal carotid artery and are almost never visualized angiographically unless they become enlarged (fig. 512). Branches of the vertebral and basilar artery also may participate in the blood supply of posterior fossa meningiomas.

The most striking lesion angiographically of the posterior fossa is the *cerebellar hemangioblastoma*. These tumors are usually extremely vascular. They may consist of a simple mural nodule in the wall of a large cyst. In some instances the central portion of the mass is a cyst surrounded partially or completely by a vascular tumor. In still

(*Revised 1963*)

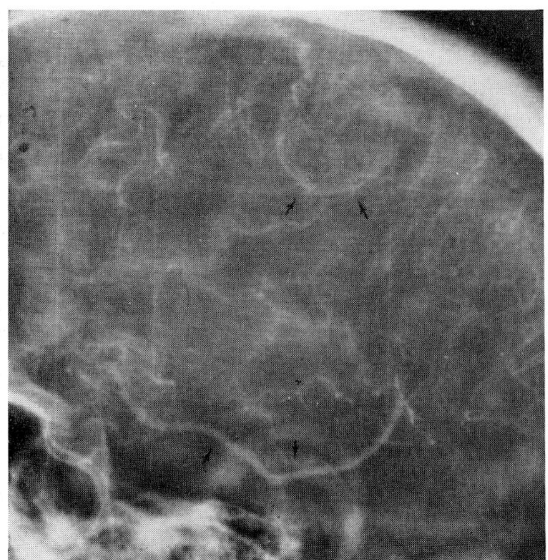

FIG. 528.—TWO METASTATIC NODULES OUTLINED BY CEREBRAL ANGIOGRAPHY

One is seen in the parietoparasagittal region (*arrows*); the other one is detected by the early draining tumor into the basilar vein (*arrows*). Even if no tumor nodule is visible, the early draining vein would detect the metastatic deposit.

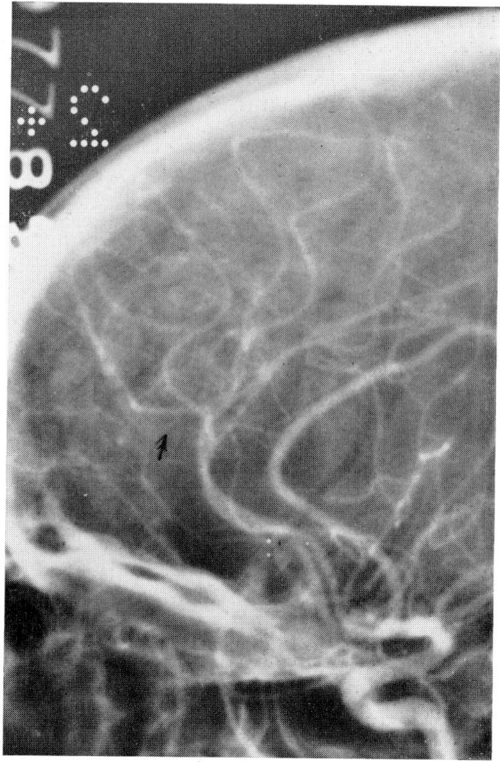

FIG. 529.—LYMPHOSARCOMA OF THE FRONTAL LOBE

There is a sharply circumscribed, perfectly round tumor nodule in the frontal region (*arrow*) which did not persist. The tumor was called primary lymphosarcoma of the brain or microglioma. Other lymphosarcomas that have been seen have not had abnormal vascularity (Fig. 438).

other cases the tumor is solid without any cystic component. Angiographically, three different types of vascular patterns have been seen: (1) a mural nodule with a cyst, within which the nodule is usually well shown by its vascular bed and one or more draining veins may be seen originating from the nodule (fig. 530); (2) a circular or coronal arrangement of abnormal vessels surrounding a clear cystic space; and (3) a large mass with many abnormal vessels throughout and distinct draining veins (fig. 531).

Also in the cerebellar area, *metastatic tumors* may produce findings similar to corresponding secondary lesions of the supratentorial region. In one instance, a small rounded vascular shadow produced by a metastatic tumor was mistaken for the nodule of a hemangioblastoma.

Glomus jugulare tumors are richly vascularized. They act somewhat like arteriovenous malformations with early filling of large veins and there is also usually an enlargement of the feeding vessels. The tumors are supplied by branches of the external carotid artery since they are extradural in location; a tumor cloud is usually shown. The tumors may grow and destroy along the petrous pyramid which, because of its position, can simulate an extradural mass, especially after a common carotid artery injection, although the tumor is localized to the bone. The lesion is shown to best advantage in subaxial projection following injection of the external carotid artery (fig. 532). An intracranial mass sometimes can be shown by pneumography (fig. 532E). The subtraction method, as advocated by Ziedses des Plantes (1935), can be used to bring out the tumor vascularity which is usually obscured, sometimes completely, by the bone of the base of the skull.

These tumors are also known by the name of chemodectoma and non-chromaffin para-

(*Revised 1963*)

ganglioma. They arise in chemoreceptor tissue situated in the region of the jugular fossa around the superior ganglion of the vagus nerve (jugular body). Other sites of occurrence are around the auricular branch of the vagus nerve and tympanic branch of the glossopharyngeal nerve. In addition, chemoreceptor tissue can be found along the cervical portion of the vagus nerve (glomus intravagale) where tumors of this type can occasionally be found (Berk, 1961).

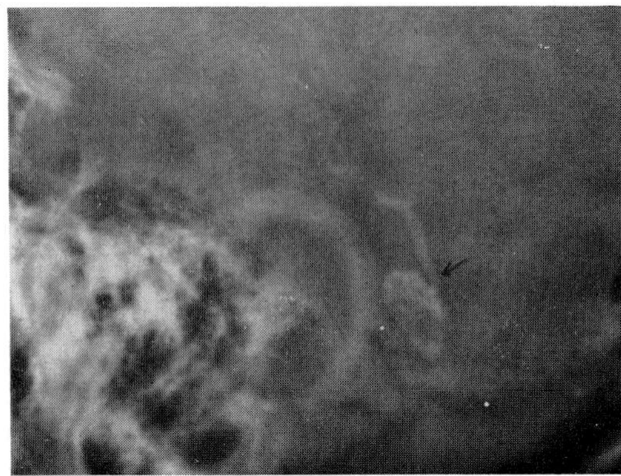

Fig. 530.—Hemangioblastoma of the Cerebellum, Cystic, with a Nodule Outlined by Vertebral Angiography

The small, homogeneous, nodule reveals an early draining vein. The cystic component did not show any abnormal vascularity.

Abnormal Circulation Pattern of Other Lesions

Several cases of sarcomatous metaplasia in Paget's disease have been observed. Some patients present an increase in the size of the branches of the middle meningeal and superficial temporal arteries, even in the absence of sarcomatous change owing to the marked vascularity of bone involved by Paget's disease. In the cases that have shown sarcomatous changes there have been seen, in addition, "lakes" of contrast substance probably in dilated venous channels associated with a slowing of circulation through the area (fig. 533). One patient with a destructive lesion of the base of the skull, which was diagnosed histologically as possibly fibrous dysplasia at one time and osteogenic sarcoma at another, had a cere-

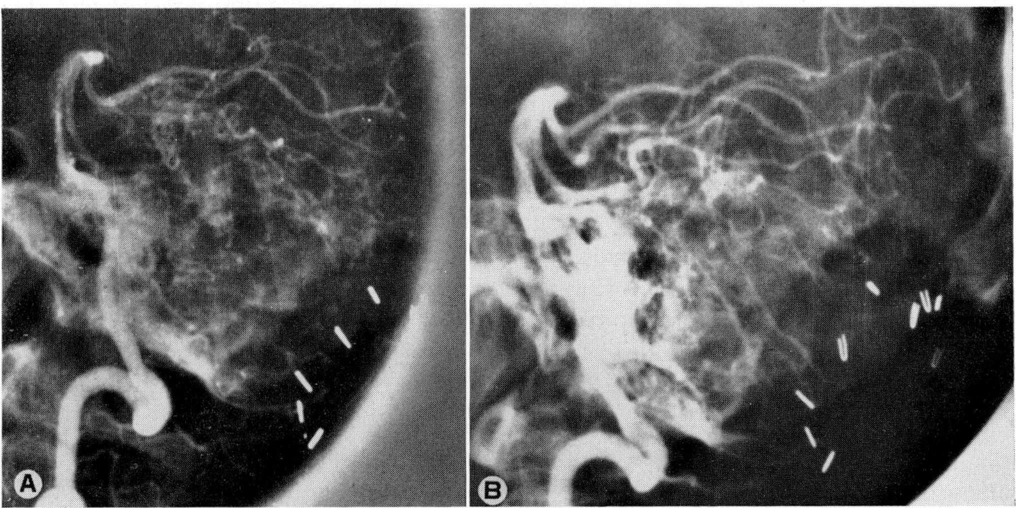

Fig. 531.—Recurrent Hemangioblastoma with Abnormal Vascularity

(A) There are numerous small convoluted vessels situated high in the cerebellum which are distributed mostly around a semicircular area. The anterior position of some of the abnormal vessels indicates that the vessels may be in the cerebellar peduncles or possibly invading the brain stem. Following treatment with iridium seeds, the patient had another recurrence of symptoms 14 months later. Repeat angiography at that time (B) revealed decrease in the vascularity, but now the vessels are more stretched, indicating the presence of a large cyst. Some abnormal veins were still present in the venous phase, however. The cyst was drained.

(Revised 1963)

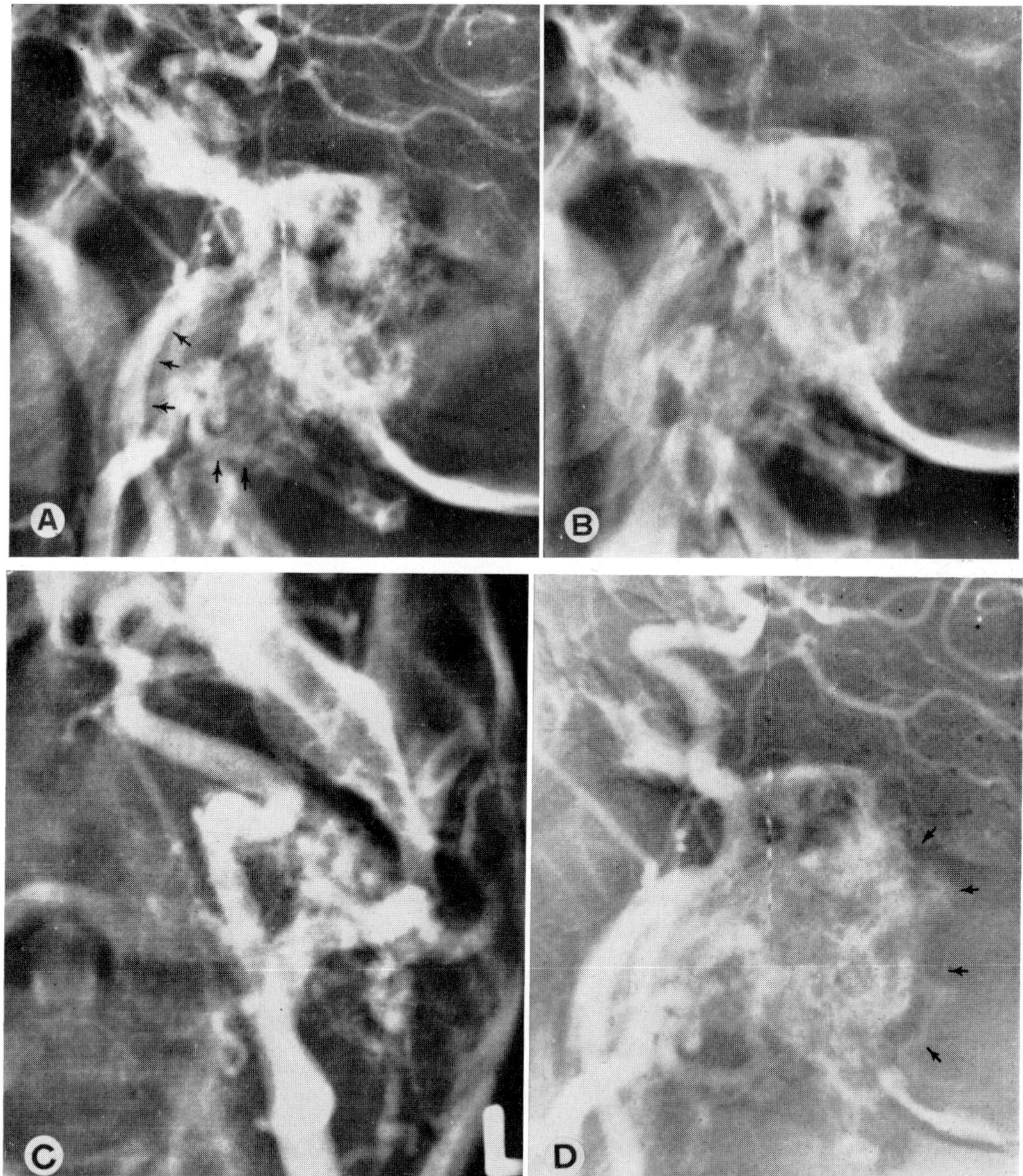

Fig. 532.—Glomus Jugulare Tumor with Abnormal Vascularity

The common carotid angiogram revealed in the lateral view taken in the arterial phase (A) the presence of large external carotid branches (*arrows*). In addition, there is forward displacement of the cervical portion of the internal carotid artery which describes an arc (*arrows*). This, however, can be seen in normal cases.

In the intermediate phase (B) there is a fairly homogeneous collection of contrast material (*arrows*), and one vein is already draining in the deep cervical group. The frontal projection was not very helpful because of overlying shadows. However, a subaxial projection demonstrated the vascularity supplied by the external carotid in the arterial phase (C). These tumors drain by way of the jugular vein even though the intracranial venous drainage on the side of the tumor may be obstructed at the jugular foramen by the neoplasm. The subtraction film (D) demonstrates a larger area of vascularity than is apparent in (A) because here it is confused with mastoid shadows. (E) Pneumoencephalogram on another patient with glomus jugulare tumor demonstrated intracranial extension of the mass (*arrows*). There is medial displacement of the cerebellar tonsil and actual enlargement of the cerebellopontine cistern. The vallecula (v) has remained in the midline. (*Fig. 532-E on next page.*)

(*Revised 1963*)

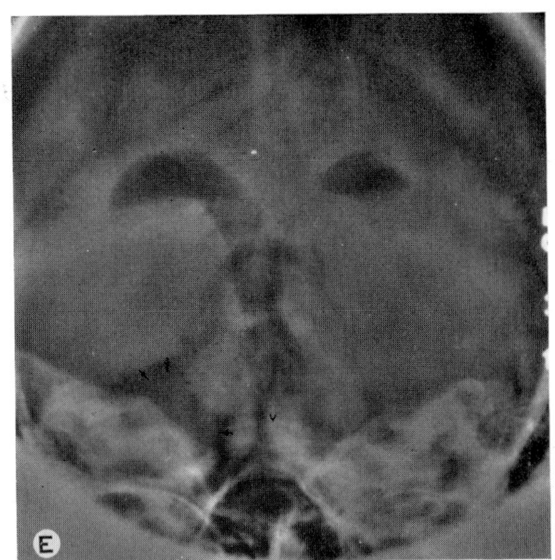

Fig. 532E

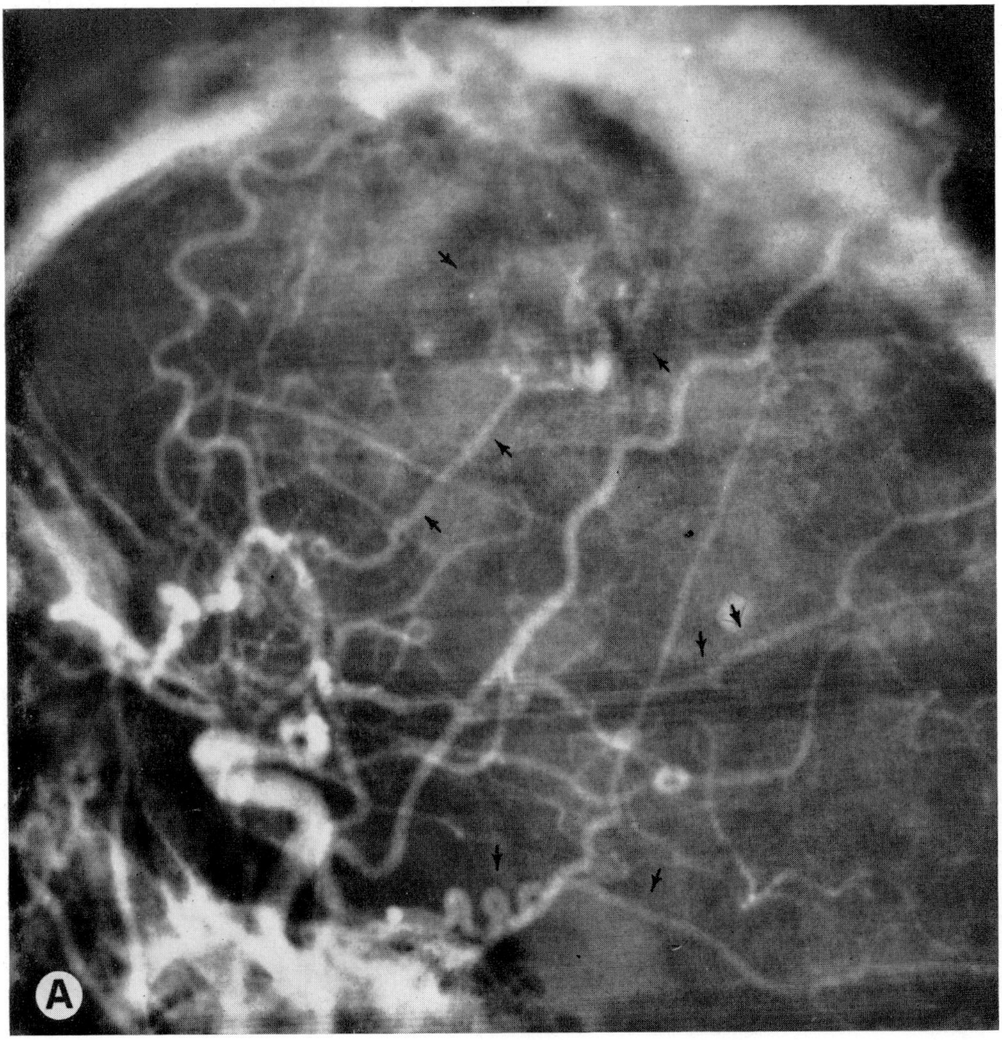

Fig. 533A

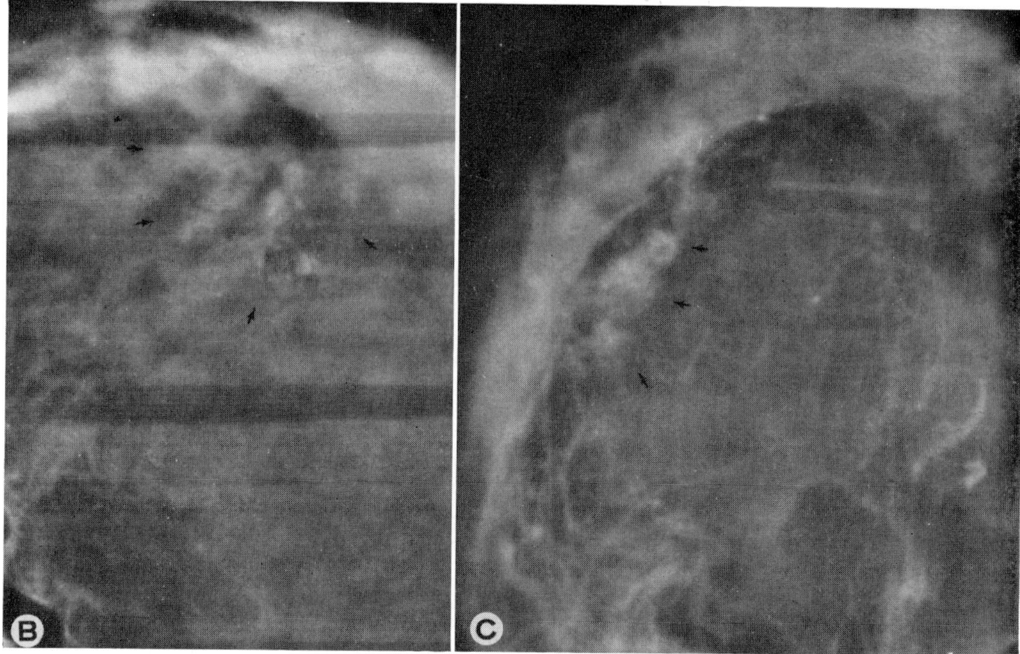

Fig. 533.—Paget's Disease with Sarcomatous Degeneration

The film in the arterial phase (A) shows marked enlargement and tortuosity of the branches of the middle meningeal artery and prominence of the superficial temporal vessels as well (*arrows*). The posterior branch of the middle meningeal artery and other meningeal arteries not in the area of the neoplasm are also enlarged (*posterior arrows*). The anterior branch leads to an area of abnormal vascularity underneath the markedly dense bone in the region of the coronal suture. A film made at 3.5 seconds (B) reveals pooling of contrast substance in the parasagittal region due to intracranial extension of tumor. There was lengthening of the circulation time in the brain due to increased intracranial pressure, and no venous channels are visible in the brain as yet. The frontal projection (C) shows the area of abnormal vascularity beneath the bone (*arrows*).

bral angiogram which demonstrated abnormal vascularity with some venous lakes not dissimilar to those occurring in Paget's disease with sarcomatous changes.

Several patients with malignant nasopharyngeal tumors invading the base of the skull have been examined by angiography. Vascular displacement has been seen in these cases, usually involving the carotid siphon (Chase and Taveras, 1963). No abnormal vascularity has been observed, but faintly opacified vessels could be easily overlooked because of overlying bone.

Carotid body tumors usually show abnormal vascularity. The vessels are numerous and irregular, and a nonhomogeneous tumor cloud is seen in typical cases. The findings are unmistakable because of the characteristic location of the tumors at the bifurcation of the common carotid artery.

Vascular Diseases of the Brain and Extracerebral Vessels

One of the chief advantages of cerebral angiography is that it allows the diagnosis of diseases affecting the blood vessels of the brain. The subject constitutes an extensive segment of angiography and comprises the following subjects: (1) cerebral arterial

(Revised 1963)

spasm, (2) occlusive and stenotic vascular disease of the intracranial and extracranial vessels, and (3) subarachnoid hemorrhage. The last heading includes saccular aneurysms, arteriovenous malformations and arteriovenous fistulas, and other causes of subarachnoid hemorrhage.

ARTERIAL SPASM

By spasm of the arteries, as demonstrated by cerebral angiography, is meant a narrowing of the lumen of an artery which cannot be explained on the basis of atherosclerosis, extrinsic pressure, or other structural change. The narrowing may be localized, involving a short segment of a vessel, or it may be diffuse, extending throughout one vessel and involving also other vessels. It may, in addition, be segmental and involve several segments of more than one vessel.

It is not uncommon to see evidence of spasm of the internal carotid artery in the neck near or above the site of injection. Decker (1956) reported several cases of this type of spasm and demonstrated its disappearance on follow-up examination. It is possible that adequate local anesthetic infiltration of the internal carotid artery in the neck prior to the insertion of the needle would diminish the irritability of the vessel wall. In our experience, spasm, that is, narrowing of the cervical portion of the internal carotid artery attributable to a muscular

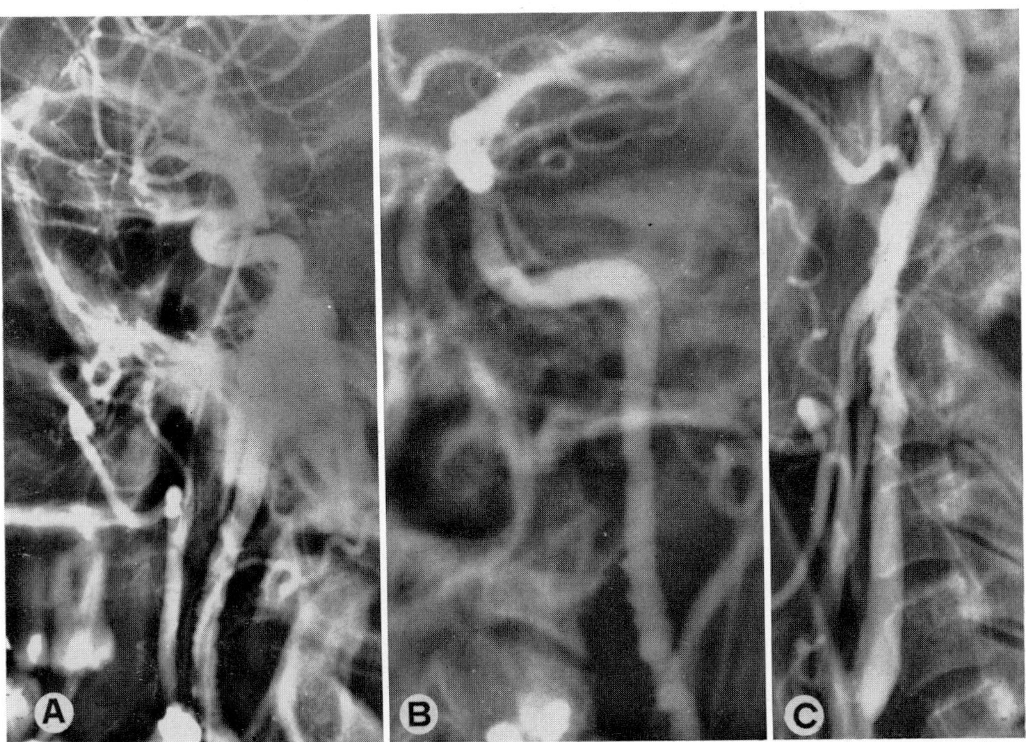

Fig. 534.—Irregular Appearance of Cervical Internal Carotid Artery Bilaterally Probably Due to Congenital Defect in the Media

(A) right side. (B) left side. The patient had multiple intracranial aneurysms. Following intracranial surgical ligation of one of the aneurysms (the one that was thought to be bleeding) repeat angiography (C) two months after the original angiogram, showed no change in the appearance of the irregular portion of the internal carotid artery, which indicates that the appearance was not temporary. (Courtesy of Dr. F. C. Boykin, Shreveport, Louisiana.)

(Revised 1963)

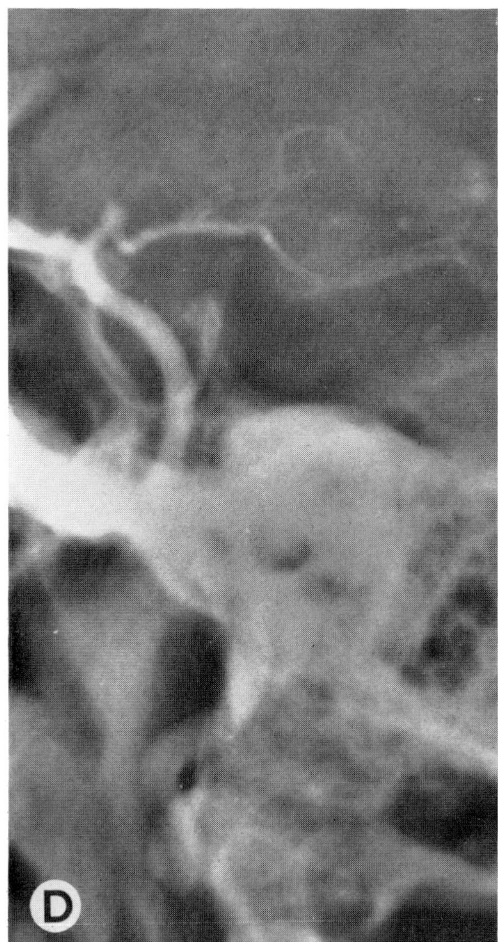

FIG. 534(*Cont.*)—(D) OCCLUSION OF INTERNAL CAROTID ARTERY ABOVE THE POSTERIOR COMMUNICATING ARTERY SHOWING A SLOW FLOW AND NARROWING OF CERVICAL AND INTRACRANIAL PORTION OF INTERNAL CAROTID ARTERY DUE TO DIMINISHED FLOW

contraction of the vessel, is rare. Even in patients having general anesthesia, a local infiltration of the neck with procaine is recommended to prevent spasm.

A curious phenomenon which was attributed by Theander (1960) to "stationary arterial waves," possibly as a result of intermittent or discontinuous injection of the contrast substance, has been seen by the authors on a few occasions. The "waves" consist of very short constrictions followed by areas of dilatation between the constrictions, extending for a distance of several centimeters along the vessel. Similar appearances have been attributed by Wickbom and Bartley (1957) to spasm. In one case the change was bilateral and symmetrical and it was thought that it might be a congenital malformation in a patient with multiple aneurysms. It is probable that in these cases there is defective formation of the arterial wall (fig. 534).

When occlusion of the supraclinoid portion of the internal carotid artery occurs, spastic contraction of the cervical portion of this artery ensues. The narrowing is due to the fact that there is not sufficient flow through the ophthalmic and the posterior communicating arteries (if the occlusion is above these vessels) to maintain the lumen of the carotid artery at its preocclusion diameter. If the posterior circulation is maintained by way of the vertebral system, very little flow takes place through the internal carotid artery, which then undergoes a diffuse and marked reduction in caliber (figs. 534D and 535). Extension of thrombus downward as far as the bifurcation of the common carotid artery may occur later.

The most frequent cause of spasm of the intracranial vessels is bleeding of an intracranial aneurysm. In these cases, the narrowing may be localized to the supraclinoid portion of the internal carotid artery or it may involve this artery and also the anterior and middle cerebral branches (fig. 536). The narrowing of the internal carotid artery in such cases extends to the level of the anterior clinoid process but usually does not involve the intracavernous or the cervical portions. Sometimes the siphon contracts in such a way as to produce two areas of narrowing; one above the anterior clinoid process and the other one at the bifurcation, with a less narrow portion in the segment between these two constrictions. The phenomenon also may be observed along the anterior and middle cerebral arteries (fig. 537). An explanation may be an irregular distribution of contractile elements in the vessel wall.

Spasm localized to the area of a bleeding aneurysm may be an important sign in determining which aneurysm is in fact bleed-

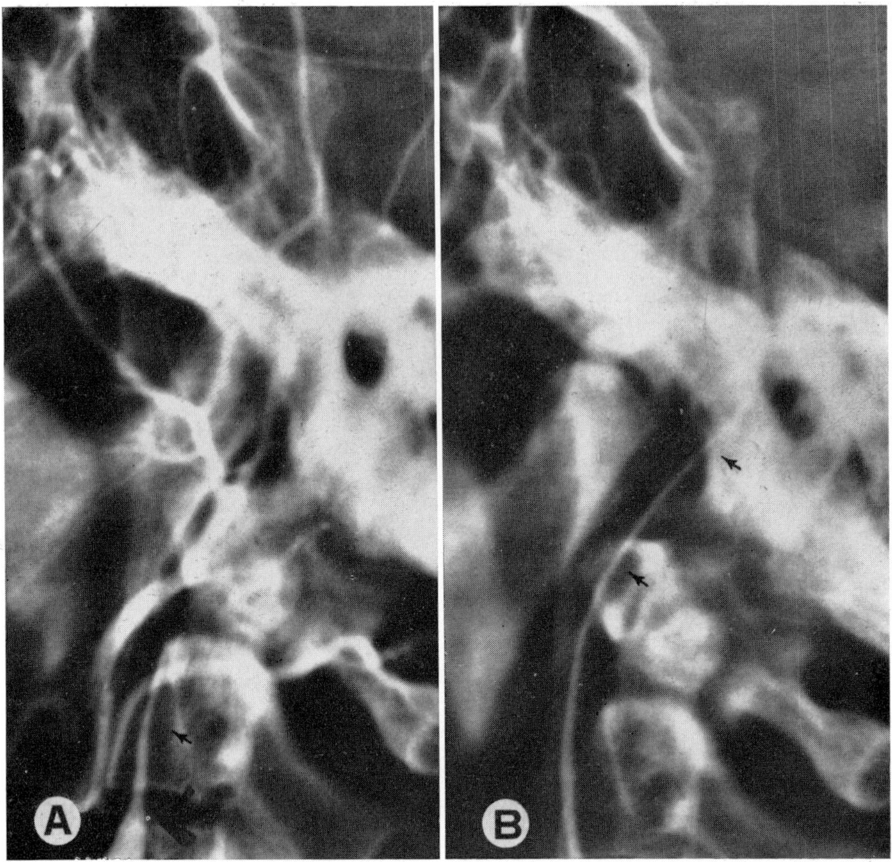

FIG. 535.—THROMBOSIS OF INTERNAL CAROTID ARTERY IN THE REGION OF THE CAROTID SIPHON; SECONDARY CONTRACTION OF CERVICAL INTERNAL CAROTID ARTERY DUE TO ABSENT FLOW

The lateral view made at 1 second (A) shows the origin of the internal carotid artery and extension of the contrast substance for about 4 cm. above the bifurcation (*arrows*). A film made at 4.5 seconds (B) shows that the contrast substance has slowly penetrated to the intracranial portion of the artery (*arrows*). Eventually, the thrombosis may extend down to the bifurcation.

ing in cases where there are multiple lesions. Narrowing of the arteries is present more frequently in the first days following the rupture of an aneurysm and tends to disappear in a few weeks. In the 100 cases reviewed by Fletcher, Taveras, and Pool (1959), there was a marked difference in incidence of spasm when examinations performed in the first 3 weeks after bleeding were compared with those performed after 3 weeks. In the same series it was found that patients in the older age group (above 55 years of age) usually showed no narrowing of the vessels, even in angiograms performed within a few days of the bleeding episode. It was concluded that there was a probable relationship between the arteriosclerosis of the vessels in these patients and the lack of contractility of the vessel wall as a result of it, which prevented spasm from occurring.

The various causes of the narrowing of the vessels are not clear. It is probable that irritation by the blood around the ruptured aneurysm and the ruptured aneurysm itself, as a mechanical factor, may cause narrowing to occur. Surgeons know that at the operating table it is possible to cause a vessel to contract visibly by tapping its walls. An-

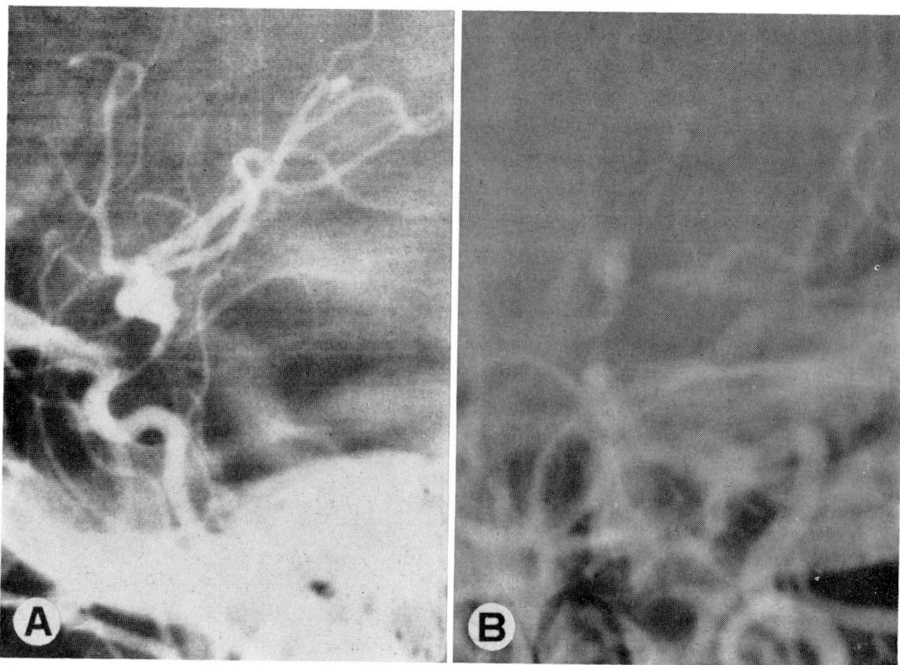

Fig. 536.—Internal Carotid Aneurysm in an 8-year-old Girl with Marked Spasm
(A) Lateral projection. (B) Frontal projection.

other possible factor is the meningeal reaction caused by the presence of blood in the cerebrospinal fluid. In one instance, shown in Figure 537, there was segmental spasm of various vessels in a child who did not have a bleeding aneurysm but who, instead, had bleeding into the ventricles or into the subarachnoid space as a result of injury to a vessel that occurred unintentionally when a tube was placed for a short-circuiting procedure to control hydrocephalus. Narrowing of the vessels of the same type as that described above has been seen in cases of infectious meningitis (fig. 538).

Diffuse narrowing of the distal branches of the anterior and middle cerebral arteries is difficult to ascertain. It definitely is observed in patients with hydrocephalus where there is stretching of the vessels, and it undoubtedly occurs under other circumstances. The authors have seen one case of brain abscess in which the initial examination, during the acute stage of cerebritis, revealed the vessels to be diffusely narrowed; repeat angiography 10 days later after the abscess had become localized showed that the vessels were much larger. It was thought that spasm was present originally. In another instance, diffuse carcinomatosis of the meninges was accompanied by diffuse narrowing of all of the vessels. The facts are difficult to assess, however, because one cannot be sure that technical factors related to the force of the injection, such as the location of the needle (that is, common carotid as against internal carotid artery) and injection time do not play a role to influence the caliber of the vessels.

The low incidence of arterial narrowing as demonstrated angiographically in the older group of patients reported by Fletcher, and co-authors (1959) would appear to indicate that cerebral vasospasm may not be an important factor in the production of the stroke syndrome.

One criticism of attaching pathologic significance to arterial spasm, as demonstrated angiographically, is that a foreign substance is introduced into the vessels and that this in itself may cause sufficient me-

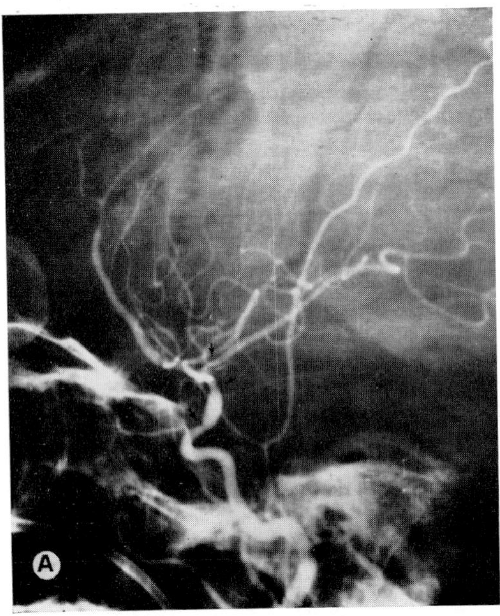

FIG. 537.—(A) DIFFUSE SPASM OF SEGMENTAL DISTRIBUTION IN THE INTERNAL CAROTID, ANTERIOR CEREBRAL, AND MIDDLE CEREBRAL ARTERIES IN PATIENT WITH SUBARACHNOID HEMORRHAGE

Areas of narrowing are seen in these arteries in a child who had intraventricular hemorrhage for a period of a few weeks due to vascular injury while trying to perform a ventriculopleural shunt.

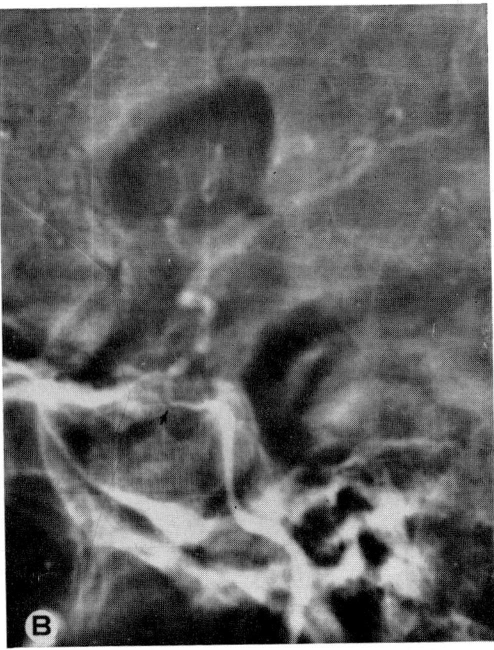

FIG. 537 (*Cont.*)—(B) DIFFUSE NARROWING OF INTERNAL CAROTID ARTERY IN EIGHT-YEAR-OLD CHILD, PROBABLY DUE TO ARTERITIS

This child had developed excruciating localized headache and diminished vision leading to blindness over a short period of time. He developed a third nerve paresis, and the pupil was constricted. Diffuse narrowing of the internal carotid artery particularly, extending from its entrance into the epidural space to the supraclinoid portion, is present (*arrows*). The middle cerebral branches are of normal caliber. The ophthalmic artery was extremely thin (*arrow*). A pneumoencephalogram, which was normal, had been performed immediately prior to the angiogram.

chanical or chemical irritation to provoke a contraction. The question also may be asked whether the arterial narrowing demonstrated angiographically is a *persistent constriction* of the vessel or whether it represents *hyperirritability* of the vessel which, upon the injection of contrast substance, undergoes a temporary contraction. It is difficult to answer this question. The absence of spasm 3 to 4 weeks after a bleeding episode, such as is shown in the case in Figure 538, could be explained by hyperirritability of the vessel which was present originally but disappeared.

The authors have had occasion to perform several injections of different substances in some patients during angiography in whom arterial spasm was demonstrated, including the use of Thorotrast, without change in the narrowing. Thorotrast is considered to be essentially nonirritating to the endothelium of the vessels at the time of injection and is thought not to incite contraction. The observations of Raynor and Ross (1960) in cats suggest that a state of hyperirritability of vessels can exist owing to previous manipulation. The investigators mechanically irritated vessels by stroking and found that a second stroking followed by Hypaque (50 per cent) injection was followed by prolonged contraction. In one cat, spontaneous hemorrhage occurred after Hypaque injection (attributed by them to a hypersensitive state), and in this instance the vessel remained contracted for the entire period of observation, at least 20 minutes.

As stated above, we have had occasion

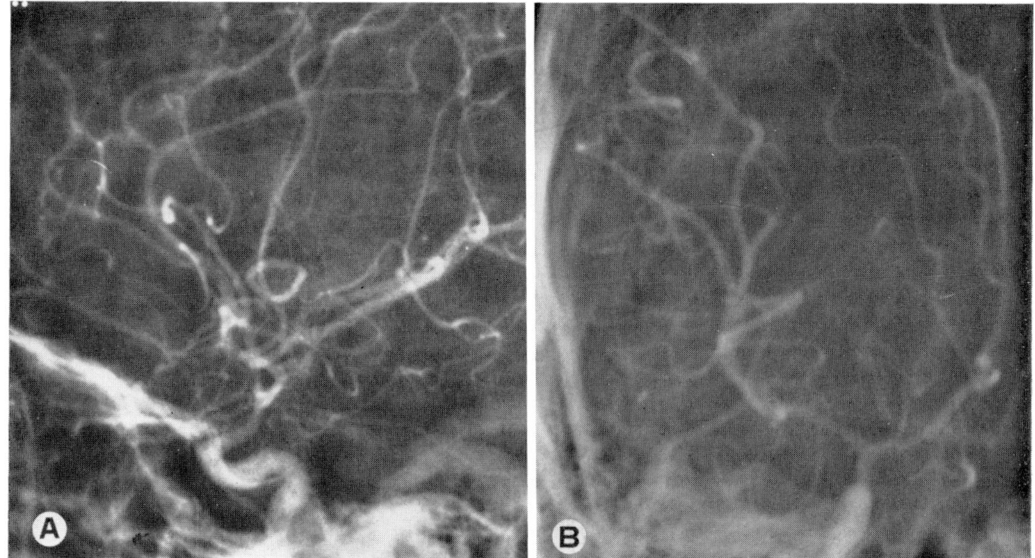

Fig. 538.—Spasm of the Supraclinoid Portion of the Internal Carotid Artery and Adjacent Segments of the Artery in Patient with Subdural Empyema and Frontal Lobe Abscess

The lateral view (A) demonstrates the marked narrowing of the internal carotid artery and the adjacent portions of anterior and middle cerebral arteries similar to that seen in aneurysms. The frontal projection (B) shows evidence of a subdural collection which displaces the vessels away from the inner table of the skull. A midline shift is also noted. Spasm, or at least a state of hyperirritability of the vessel wall, which causes a contraction at the time of the injection of the contrast material, exists in the presence of subarachnoid bleeding as well as infection, or trauma.

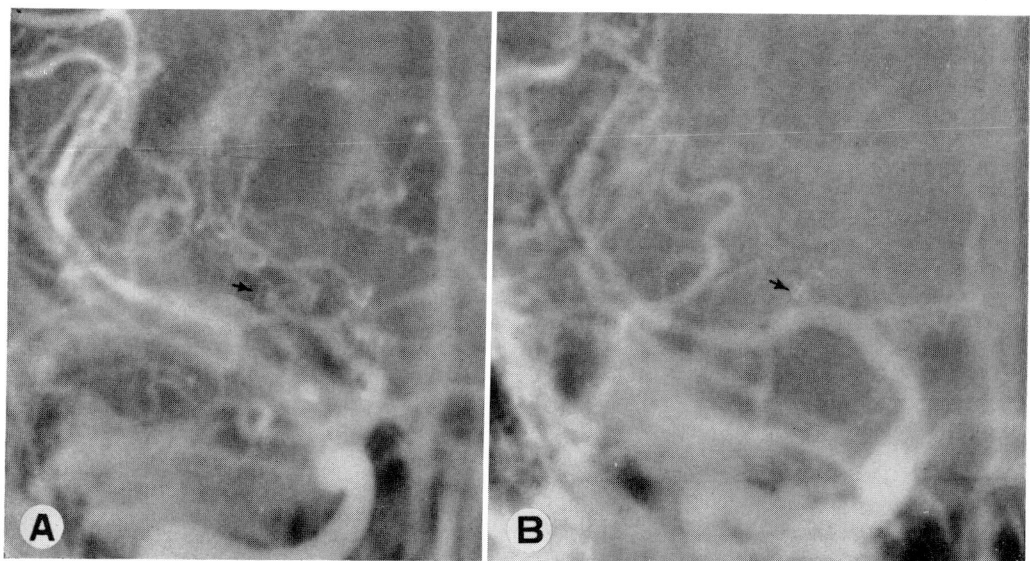

Fig. 539.—Spasm of Middle Cerebral Artery in Patient with Bleeding Aneurysm Arising from Middle Cerebral Artery at Origin of Lenticulostriate Artery

The original angiogram (A) reveals spasm in the horizontal portion of the middle cerebral artery. A small out-pouching (*arrow*) indicates the presence of a small aneurysm at this point. Re-examination ten days later (B) discloses the disappearance of the spasm previously noted and the aneurysmal sac has now become larger. The sac was successfully clipped surgically.

(Revised 1963)

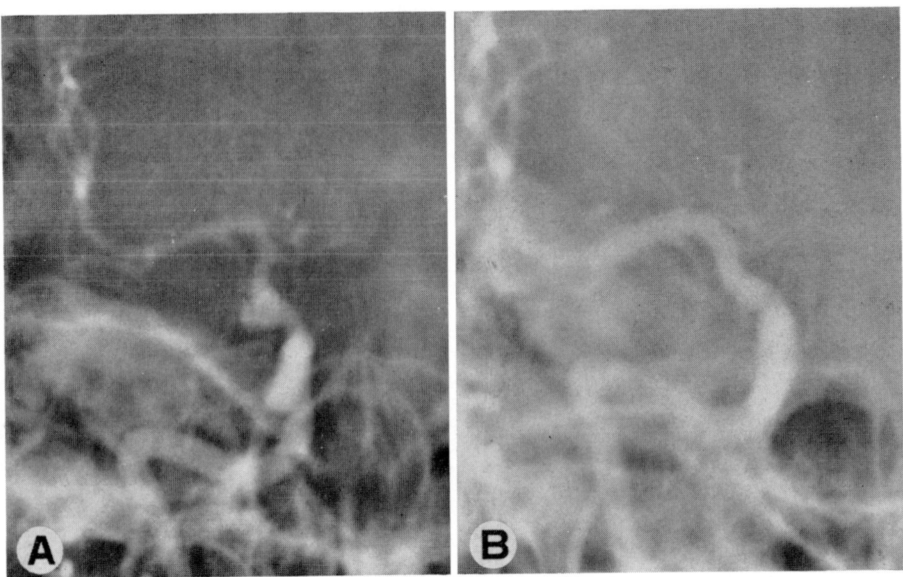

FIG. 540.—BLEEDING ANEURYSM OF THE POSTERIOR COMMUNICATING ARTERY SHOWING SPASM OF ALL THE INTERNAL CAROTID AND MIDDLE CEREBRAL VESSELS DISAPPEARING THREE MONTHS LATER

The initial angiogram (A) shows considerable diffuse spasm. The subsequent angiogram (B) performed three months later showed disappearance of the spasm. The aneurysm has become thrombosed at east partially.

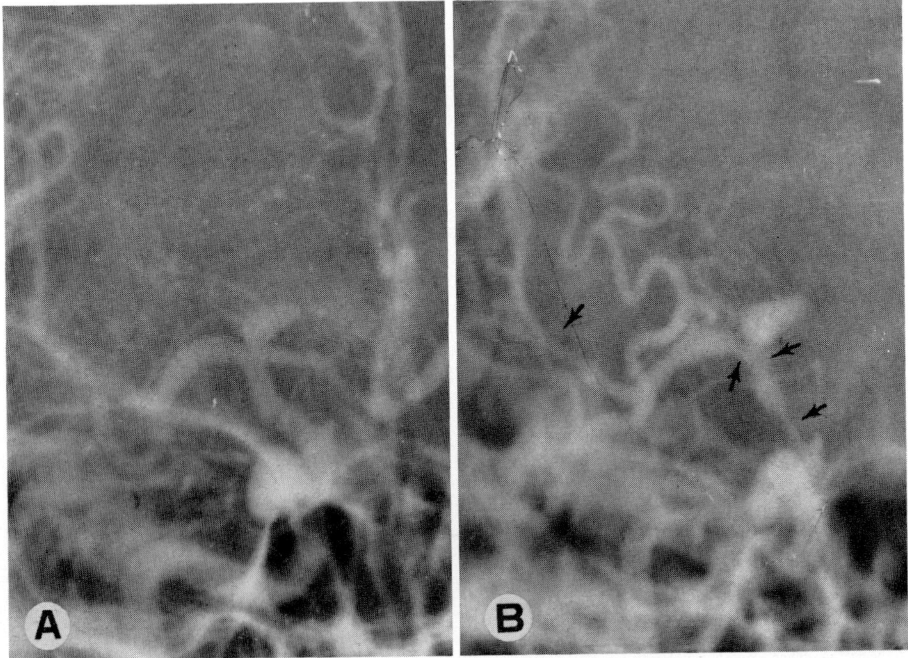

FIG. 541.—ANEURYSM OF THE BIFURCATION OF THE INTERNAL CAROTID ARTERY SHOWING NO SPASM IN THE ORIGINAL EXAMINATION AND SPASM DEMONSTRATED TWO WEEKS LATER FOLLOWING ANOTHER BLEEDING EPISODE

(A) original angiogram. (B) angiogram performed two weeks later showing marked segmental spasm (*arrows*) of the internal carotid and middle cerebral arteries. The aneurysm is very slightly larger by measurement.

to see the narrowing of a vessel disappear over a period of several days or months when a repeat angiogram was carried out (figs. 539 and 540). The reverse also has been seen. An angiogram performed on a patient with an aneurysm showed no narrowing initially but a second angiogram following an acute episode suggesting bleeding, revealed a marked degree of spasm (fig. 541).

Inflammatory processes of the vessels (*arteritis*) may be a cause of diffuse arterial narrowing. In children several cases have been seen for which no other explanation is found (fig. 537B).

OCCLUSIVE AND STENOTIC LESIONS

Clinical and Pathologic Considerations

The "stroke" syndrome may be produced by a variety of conditions involving the vessels of the brain. Among these may be listed: (1) stenotic and occlusive lesions of the extracranial and intracranial arteries (thrombosis and embolism); (2) intracranial hemorrhage due to rupture of an artery, an aneurysm, or an arteriovenous malformation; (3) systemic hypotension; (4) venous and dural sinus thrombosis; (5) conditions of undetermined origin.

The stenotic and occlusive lesions of the extracranial and intracranial vessels may be due to localized atheromatous changes in such portions of the arteries, usually at the sites of bifurcation, or they may be part of a more generalized degenerative process with more pronounced changes in certain focal areas. They also may develop as the result of an inflammatory process of the vessel. In these cases arteritis is associated with a known inflammatory disease, such as syphilis or septic embolism of pyogenic or tuberculous origin. Cerebral arteritis may be part of certain diseases of undetermined origin, such as lupus erythematosus and polyarteritis nodosa; or it may be a solitary arteritic process of unknown etiology.

A large number of lesions responsible for the stroke syndrome are demonstrable by cerebral angiography. The majority of cases can be diagnosed clinically and the indication of angiography for diagnosis of cerebrovascular accidents should be reserved for those cases that offer diagnostic difficulties. The latter are common, however, and a sizable proportion of patients even with extracranial occlusive or stenotic disease of the arteries present with a clinical syndrome which simulates a cerebral neoplasm. In recent years, cerebral angiography has been used much more frequently to determine the site of obstruction of the vessel with a view to possible surgical correction of the obstructive process.

Clinically the stroke syndrome can be divided into several stages or types. First, that of *intermittent ischemic attacks*, which may be produced by stenotic or occlusive lesions of the extracranial vessels and also by disease of the intracranial vessels. The attacks also may be associated with some other conditions, such as heart block. This is the stage at which the diagnosis preferably should be made because the obstruction lends itself to removal of the cause, in many instances leading to complete recovery. Between the attacks of circulatory insufficiency the patients may be entirely normal. The symptoms may involve the carotid or the vertebral basilar circulation. No evident permanent damage to the brain may result from such attacks.

The second stage or *intermittent progressive type* indicates that the patient did not quite recover from an ischemic attack and days or sometimes weeks later another attack occurs from which the patient recovers even less. At any time the patient may have a third or fourth attack or more attacks which eventually will leave him hemiplegic. *Advancing stroke* constitutes type three. The term may be applied to a clinical evolution in which the patient's condition, following the first partial involvement of his functions, continues to deteriorate over a period of hours or within a day or two. The condition is similar to the intermittent progressive type mentioned above but differs from it in that the increase in functional deficit takes place more rapidly.

(*Revised 1963*)

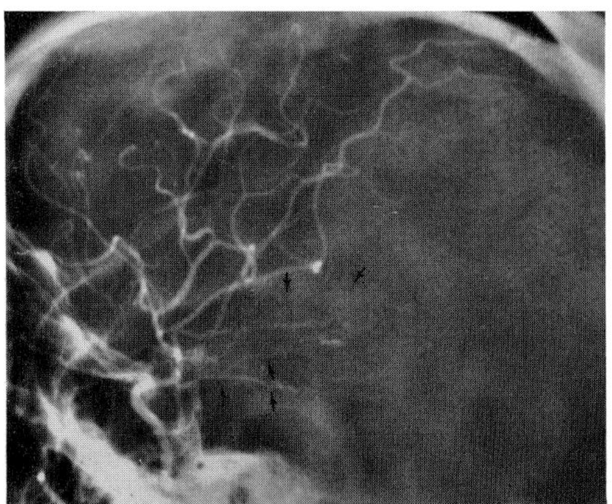

FIG. 542.—PROGRESSIVE THROMBOSIS OF THE CEREBRAL VESSELS

An initial angiogram demonstrated thrombosis of several branches of the middle cerebral artery with dilatation of the small perforating branches in the region of the lenticulostriate group and thalamic area (*arrows*). The patient recovered partially from the first stroke only to undergo another stroke six months later, at which time angiography (not shown here) demonstrated thrombosis of the internal carotid artery at the bifurcation of the common carotid.

The final type is the *completed stroke.* Siekert (1960) defined the completed stroke as a state in which the neurologic deficit is stable and persistent over a period of hours or days. If the patient is completely disabled, it is easy to determine that a completed stroke exists. On the other hand, the stroke process may reach termination when only partial, or even minimum, deficit has occurred. Undoubtedly, some of these patients belong in what Gurdjian and coauthors (1960) have called "intermittent progressive stroke," since a patient who has partial neurologic involvement may later have another attack with advancement toward greater disability, as in the case shown in Figure 542.

On examination of the brain the pathologist usually finds evidence of a cerebral infarct. This may be a white or a hemorrhagic infarct or it may be mixed in type. Either a pale or a hemorrhagic infarct may be due to embolism or to thrombosis, and the conditions leading to the development of a hemorrhagic as against a pale or white infarct are not well understood. Cerebral hemorrhage may be associated with a disturbance of the blood-clotting mechanism, it may be associated with the rupture of an aneurysm or an arteriovenous malformation, it may be secondary to the rupture of an artery in the course of hypertensive cardiovascular disease or it may be of undetermined cause.

The *indications* for angiography in the diagnosis of cerebral vascular disease are varied. First, angiography is helpful when there is doubt clinically whether the patient has a stroke syndrome or an intracranial mass. Some neoplasms, particularly metastatic tumors and some glioblastomas, may produce a sudden occurrence of neurologic findings very suggestive of vascular occlusion. Spontaneous intracerebral hematomas often produce clinical findings similar to those produced by vascular occlusion, and angiography can show the presence of a mass for which surgical removal may be indicated. Second, angiography should be performed when a stroke is associated with bloody cerebrospinal fluid, because in these patients the lesion may be a saccular aneurysm or an arteriovenous malformation. The third and most important indication for angiographic examination of patients with the cerebrovascular stroke syndrome in recent times is the possibility of surgical correction of the obstructing lesion if it is in one of the extracranial vessels.

The matter of surgical treatment of an obstructing lesion in a major cerebral vessel in the neck deserves particular consideration. In the first place, occlusive and stenotic lesions of the internal carotid and vertebral arteries, and even of the common carotid and subclavian arteries, occur commonly without producing symptoms; that is, they occur in patients who have no old or recent history of a cerebrovascular accident. Martin, Sayre, and Whisnant (1960), after a study of 100 embalmed cadavers over 55 years of age, reported an 11 per cent incidence of complete occlusion of at least one major artery, either the internal carotid, the common carotid, or the vertebral artery. In 3 patients there was occlusion of two major extracranial arteries. A few of these patients had a history of neurologic disease in the past, but the material was an unselected, consecutive series. Fisher, in 1954, found a 9.5 per cent incidence of occlusion or severe stenosis of the cervical carotid arteries in a large necropsy series. A startling finding in the series of Martin and co-authors (1960) was that, in addition to the 11 per cent incidence of complete occlusion, there was a 29 per cent incidence of partial occlusions in which one or more of the four major vessels was at least 50 per cent reduced in caliber. Thus, an over-all incidence of 40 per cent of occlusive and severely stenotic lesions was demonstrated.

Because the incidence reported by these authors was so high, one of us decided to perform arteriographic studies on cadavers under conditions that simulated those existing *in vivo*. The injections were made employing a contrast substance of moderate viscosity which did not pass readily through the capillaries. It was possible, therefore, to distend the major vessels to a degree similar to that encountered in the living subject. A pressure ranging between 120 and 200 mm. of mercury was used during the injection. A total number of 130 cadavers was injected and the findings were as follows. Of 121 patients without neurologic symptoms prior to death, there was a 22 per cent incidence of stenotic lesions greater than 50 per cent that involved the carotid or vertebral systems, and sometimes both systems (7 cases). The patients who had a neurologic history (9 cases) prior but not necessarily related to death all had stenotic lesions involving both the extracranial and intracranial vessels. Only 6 cases of complete occlusion were found of which one was thought to be preagonal (Stein *et al.*). The lower incidence (4 per cent) of complete occlusion (as against 11 per cent as found by Martin *et al.*) is more in keeping with our daily experience in cerebral angiography. That is, we rarely encounter carotid occlusions in performing vertebral angiograms in older patients without related clinical manifestations.

As can be seen, the incidence of partial or complete obstruction is lower than that described in the pathologic specimens but is still moderately high. How, then, is it possible to decide, regarding a patient who presents with a stroke syndrome and who has occlusion or stenosis of a cervical vessel, whether symptoms are due to occlusive intracranial or extracranial arterial disease. The problem is further complicated by the fact that an obstructing lesion in the neck may promote or provoke the production of an occlusion in an intracranial vessel. In a certain patient, for example, it may happen that both intracranial and extracranial segments of one carotid artery system contain stenotic lesions, and the cervical obstruction becomes complete. The lowering of pressure resulting from the cervical occlusion would tend to provoke completion of the occlusion in the intracranial artery. This is illustrated by the case in Figure 543, a patient with an intracranial aneurysm. Following the application of a clamp to the internal carotid artery in the neck, the patient became hemiplegic. The clamp was released promptly but the neurologic deficit did not change. An angiogram was then performed which showed complete occlusion of the middle cerebral artery. It is quite possible that the lowering of the blood pressure subsequent to application of the clamp produced a slowing of circulation time through the middle cerebral territory which lead to the deposition of thrombus and subsequent occlusion. Indeed, multiple lesions of the intracranial and extracranial vessels probably are the rule rather than the exception.

The case shown in Figure 544 is even more complicated because, in addition to an extremely stenotic lesion in the neck, the patient had a partial thrombosis of the middle cerebral artery and an intracranial neoplasm in the frontal region. A pneumoencephalogram was performed since the history suggested more the evolution of a neoplasm with gradually progressive development rather than the intermittently progressive development characteristic of vascular insufficiency. Because of the problem of multiplicity of lesions, all of the extracranial vessels as well as the intracranial vessels should be visualized to assure complete diagnosis. It is imperative that all of the extracranial vessels be visualized in cases that are not clear-cut

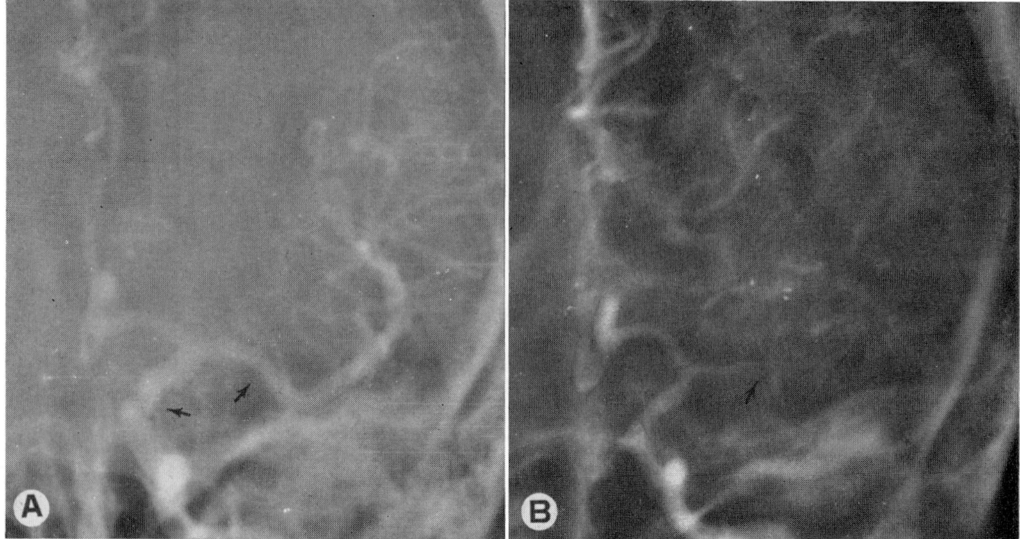

FIG. 543.—MIDDLE CEREBRAL THROMBOSIS OCCURRING AFTER APPLICATION OF SELVERSTONE CLAMP IN THE INTERNAL CAROTID ARTERY

The original anteroposterior angiogram (A) shows a normal cerebral angiogram except for a density behind the carotid siphon which represented a posterior communicating aneurysm. There is only a slight irregularity of the horizontal portion of the middle cerebral artery (*arrows*). A Selverstone clamp was applied in the internal carotid artery as the treatment for the intracranial aneurysm. The patient developed a hemiplegia after complete closure of the clamp for four hours. The clamp was released within five minutes but the hemiplegia persisted. Repeat angiography was carried out at that time (B), and it revealed a complete occlusion of the middle cerebral artery just beyond the anterior temporal branch (*arrow*). There was collateral circulation on the surface of the brain by way of the anterior cerebral vessels.

clinically, prior to surgical intervention. In addition, the intracranial circulation must be studied by means of serialograms. Individual films do not suffice.

Methods of Examination

In visualizing angiographically both carotid and both vertebral arteries in their cervical portions, it is important to choose a procedure that will be accompanied by as little morbidity as possible. Ideally, retrograde femoral catheterization should be the procedure of choice because via a remote route, it is possible to visualize the cervical portions of these arteries without producing any local mechanical trauma. Unfortunately, many patients with arteriosclerotic cerebral disease also have generalized arteriosclerosis with a particularly high incidence of occlusive and stenotic lesions in the lower abdominal aorta and iliac arteries. Therefore, attempted retrograde femoral catheterization is often unsuccessful because the catheter cannot be passed through the iliac arteries and lower aorta. In addition, there is danger of dislodging an atherosclerotic plaque by manipulation of the catheter, thus producing femoral arterial occlusion and ischemia of the lower extremity. At least one such case has been seen at our institutions and the authors know of several other occurrences elsewhere.

Retrograde brachial arteriography, with or without a catheter, is a reasonably satisfactory procedure but may cause circulatory difficulties in the upper extremity. Such a complication is particularly undesirable in view of the fact that for unilateral injection, the right arm is the better side to use in performing this type of examination. Bilateral retrograde brachial injections may be necessary to visualize the right common

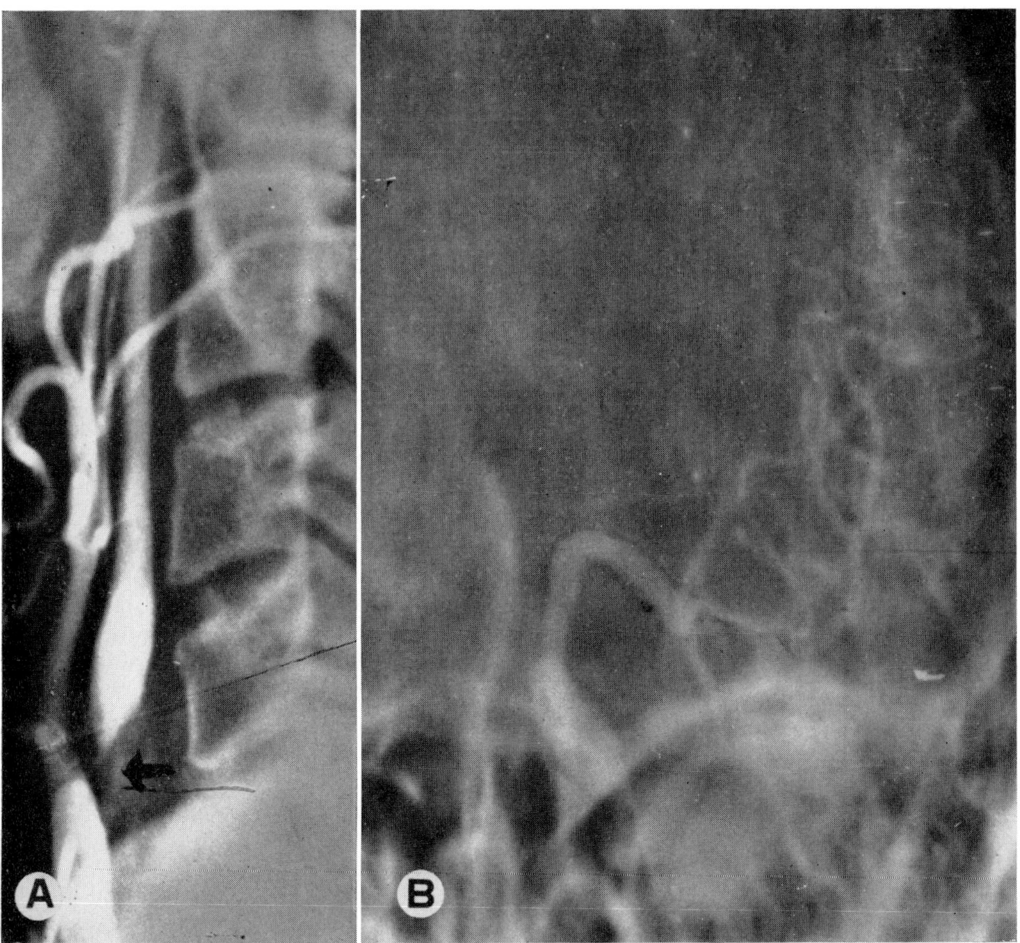

Fig. 544.—Partial Thrombosis of Internal Carotid Artery, Middle Cerebral Artery, and Frontal Lobe Tumor in Same Patient

The common carotid angiogram (A) demonstrates a very high degree of stenosis of the origin of the internal carotid artery in the neck. A simultaneous anteroposterior view was also made of the head (B) which demonstrated occlusion of some of the branches of the middle cerebral artery at the trifurcation of this artery (*arrow*). There was no filling of the anterior cerebral artery. Because the patient's clinical history was more compatible with that of tumor with a gradual progression of symptoms, pneumoencephalography was then performed which revealed a frontal mass, and surgical intervention disclosed a frontal glioma. The case emphasizes the fact that multiple lesions are common.

carotid and right vertebral arteries via the innominate and the left vertebral artery via the left subclavian artery. Because the left common carotid artery arises directly from the aorta, it usually is not visualized by the retrograde brachial route. A direct puncture of the left common carotid artery with the needle pointing downward may be required in addition to the other injections. Unless the stream of contrast material is directed downward toward the aorta, a relatively blind segment of the proximal portion of the common carotid artery is present. The internal carotid may be compressed at the time of the injection to force the contrast material caudad.

Another method is that of bilaterial puncture of the subclavian arteries which produces the same results as retrograde brachial arteriography. Here again, a left common

(*Revised 1963*)

carotid arteriogram must follow. It is unfortunate that this method, as well as the previous one, requires a puncture of the left carotid which is usually on the side of the dominant hemisphere.

The procedures outlined above ordinarily produce poor visualization of the intracranial vessels, thus making evaluation of individual cerebral branches of the internal carotid artery and of the basilar artery more difficult. At the present time there is no single clinical procedure completely adequate to visualize the intracranial and extracranial portions of the vertebral and carotid systems, including the main vascular orifices. A choice must be made between good intracranial *or* extracranial visualization and a compromise of excellence of demonstration of both cervical and cranial regions. When the latter is necessary, attention usually is focused on the neck but at the same time some information concerning the cerebral vascular status is needed. Under these circumstances stereoscopic lateral views are recommended in place of the serial films because with bilateral filling, particularly as obtained with retrograde femoral catheterization and intra-aortic injections, there is considerable superimposition of the intracranial vessels. The stereoscopic views may be obtained with a single injection if special apparatus is available. We prefer to obtain simultaneous anteroposterior and stereoscopic serial lateral views as pioneered by Chamberlain and Stauffer (1951) in these cases. In some instances, it is advantageous to take an additional anteroposterior projection with the chin well extended, in order that the cervical portions of the arteries may be followed to the base of the skull without being obscured by the mandible. Another way of visualizing all of the cervical vessels is by direct puncture of both common carotid and of both vertebral arteries. This, of course, is too traumatic for endorsement, and there is a high percentage of failure of visualization of both vertebral arteries.

An *increased morbidity* as a result of angiography is observed in patients with cerebrovascular disease. The reported incidence of *permanent complications* (that is, deterioration of the patient's clinical condition following the angiogram, after which the symptoms persist or improve only to remain at a level less favorable than before the angiogram) varies from almost none to as high as 9 per cent (Baker, 1960). In our own material, in the first 60 patients with thrombosis of the internal carotid artery in the neck, two developed permanent hemiplegia, an incidence of 3.3 per cent. In these cases, a direct puncture of the common carotid artery was performed. In the cases reported by Crawford *et al.* (1959) and by DeBakey, Crawford, and Fields (1961), there was a 15 to 20 per cent incidence of pneumothorax following bilateral percutaneous subclavian injections. Two patients in their series died and two were made worse but improved after operation, which followed immediately.

The use of intravenous angiography has not met with success in the study of cerebrovascular disease because of the poor concentration of the contrast substance in the cerebral vessels. The neck vessels are seen only faintly. It is to be hoped that further refinements in contrast media and techniques may permit better visualization of the extracranial portions of the vessels by the intravenous method. Such a method would be most desirable to study cerebrovascular disease, because morbidity should be very low, but it is doubtful whether it can ever provide adequate visualization of the intracranial circulation. It might be possible to combine a direct percutaneous common carotid injection on the side of the patient's symptoms with an intravenous arteriogram to visualize the extracranial portions of all the remaining vessels.

Other methods of approach based on modifications of the patient's blood pressure and intrathoracic pressure during brachial artery injection deserve investigation.

Radiologic Diagnosis

Extracranial arteries. Occlusion of the internal carotid artery at its origin, that is, at the bifurcation of the common carotid artery, is the most frequently encountered lesion. The diagnosis is usually simple by angiography. Technical artifacts, however, chiefly the intramural injection of contrast substance, can simulate thrombosis. The differentiation of intramural injection from thrombosis can be derived objectively. First, there is absence of branches of any of the vessels, most evident by the absence of filling of the external carotid and its branches. Second, there may be a partly intramural and partly intraluminal injection so that some branches of the external carotid artery fill. In these cases, it is often possible to see the radiolucent line which represents the displaced arterial wall around the intramural collection of contrast substance (fig. 343). Third, there is a relatively greater density of contrast substance with an intramural collection than when the injection is made within the lumen of the artery, because in the latter case the contrast substance is diluted by the bloodstream, whereas when the injection is intramural, the contrast substance is not diluted (fig. 343B). Finally, there is residual contrast substance remaining in the artery at the end of the serialogram. Delayed films made several minutes later may not show any residual contrast substance in the arterial wall unless Thorotrast is being used.

Another common site of obstruction by thrombosis is in the distal internal carotid artery, usually in the region of its bifurcation intracranially. It is uncommon to find occlusion of the internal carotid artery between these two areas with patent proximal and distal ends of the vessel. On the other hand, propagation of a thrombus starting at the siphon and progressing proximally, or, vice versa, starting at the bifurcation and progressing distally, is common. The distal portion of the internal carotid artery tends to remain open when occlusion of the proximal portion has occurred under certain circumstances. Taveras *et al.* (1954) have shown that by retrograde flow through the ophthalmic artery, the distal internal carotid artery remains patent in patients with surgical occlusion of the internal carotid artery in the neck. This may be recanalization.

Under more natural circumstances, in which spontaneous thrombosis of the proximal portion of the internal carotid artery takes place, the thrombus tends to propagate fairly rapidly, often within a few hours. The lumen of the internal carotid artery as far as the origin of the ophthalmic or posterior communicating branches may be obliterated. The reason for the propagation of thrombus in this manner is probably due to the fact that no flow of blood takes place in this portion of the artery. A reversal of flow occurs in the supraclinoid portion of the internal carotid artery down to the ophthalmic artery, owing to pressure from the opposite side. The thrombus tends to stop below the ophthalmic, although this is not always so. The rapid propagation of a thrombus to the nearest branch is an important reason for prompt surgical intervention in the cases where an amenable occlusion of the proximal portion of the internal carotid artery is demonstrated.

Thrombosis of the common carotid artery is less common. It may occur just proximal to its bifurcation so that external carotid as well as the internal carotid artery are occluded. Obstruction also may develop at its origin from the innominate artery on the right side and from the aorta on the left side. Of the 409 cases of completed stroke reported by Gurdjian *et al.* (1961) and studied by angiography, there were only two instances of occlusion of the common carotid artery, indicating its relative rarity. In the same series, there were 68 cases of internal carotid occlusion, 5 of which were bilateral, and 27 cases of occlusion and stenosis of the vertebral basilar system. Occlusion of the vertebral artery occurs most commonly at its origin. Both vertebral arteries should be opacified in patients who show evidence of basilar artery insufficiency.

The possibility of involvement of major arteries *proximal* to the common carotid and vertebral arteries should be kept in mind. Of 149 cases of stenotic and occlusive lesions reported by Crawford *et al.* (1959), the internal carotid artery was involved in 93, the common carotid artery in 12, the innominate artery in 14, the subclavian artery in 21, and the vertebral artery in 9 cases. Moreover, in the cases reported by the same authors, the lesions involving the common carotid, the innominate, and the subclavian arteries were segmental in nature and restoration of circulation in many instances

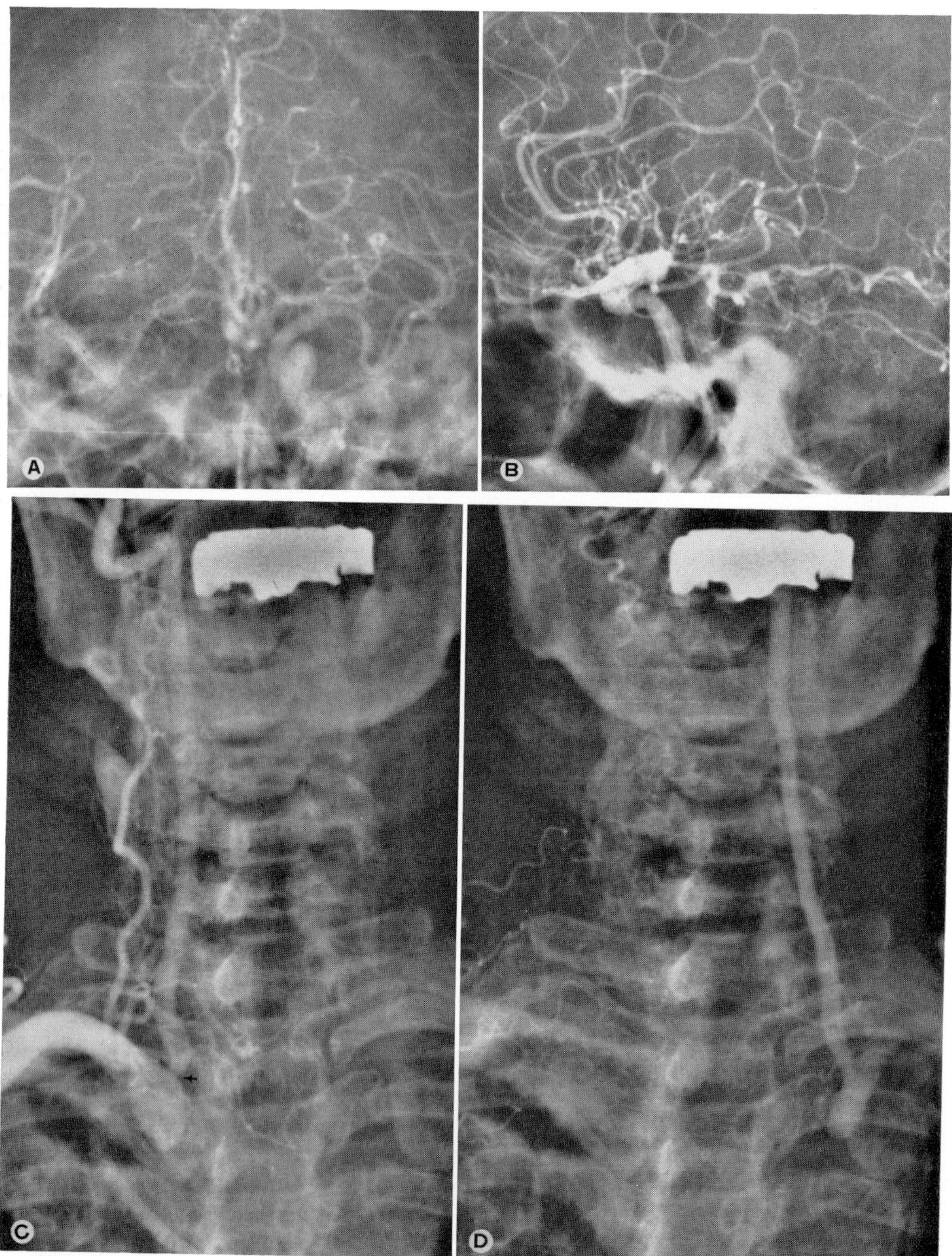

FIG. 545.—MULTIPLE OCCLUSIVE DISEASE OF EXTRACRANIAL VESSELS—"SUBCLAVIAN STEAL"
Left carotid angiogram was first performed which showed (A) in the frontal projection, bilateral filling of the anterior and middle cerebral arteries. In the lateral projection there was noted also filling of both posterior cerebral arteries and some regurgitation into the superior cerebellar arteries (B). A right retrograde brachial angiogram was then performed which revealed thrombosis of the common carotid artery on the right side which did not fill. In the frontal projection (C), there was narrowing at

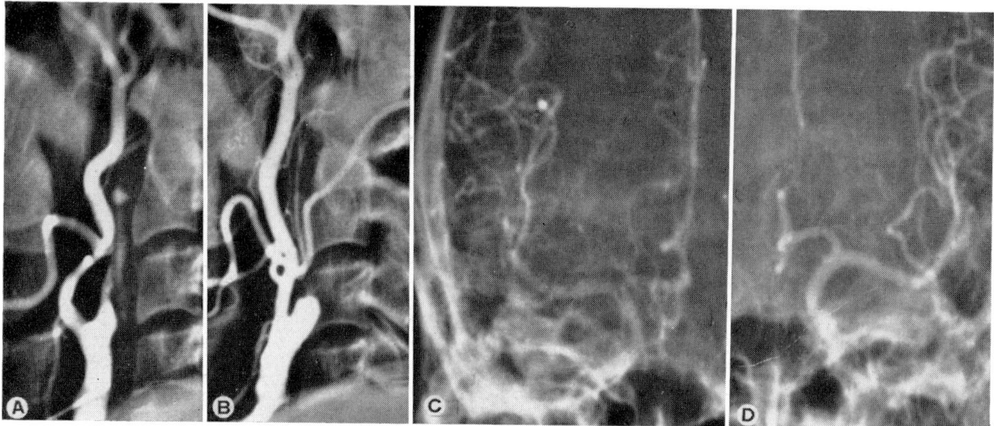

Fig. 546.—Bilateral Occlusion of the Internal Carotid Artery Near Its Origin

(A) and (B) demonstrate the occlusion of the internal carotid artery at its origin on each side. The anteroposterior serialograms on each side (C) and (D) disclose rather adequate filling of the internal carotid artery and both the middle and anterior cerebral arteries from each side by way of the ophthalmic arteries. This is unusual because the ophthalmic arteries very rarely supply both the anterior and middle cerebral arteries; only the middle cerebral artery is usually supplied. It is probable that in this case, there is some degree of hypotension in the region of the vertebral basilar system and thus the entire carotid supply is by way of the ophthalmic arteries.

was possible by surgical means. In the same series, 83 of the 93 cases involving the internal carotid artery were considered as segmental. As mentioned earlier, occlusive disease of the extracranial vessels may involve more than one vessel (fig. 545 and 546).

Obstructive lesions of a *stenotic* type involving the extracranial vessels are common. A lesion may be seen on either the frontal or the lateral angiogram, and the other projection may not reveal the narrowing. For this reason frontal and lateral views are necessary to diagnose arterial narrowing with certainty. If the stenosis is due to a lesion involving the periphery of the vessel, a concentric narrowing is produced which may be shown on either the frontal or the lateral projection. On the other hand, if, as is commonly the case, the narrowing is produced by a plaque situated only on one side of the vessel, it may be obscured in one projection. The outline of the lumen in the stenotic segment is usually irregular as seen in profile by angiography because the surface of the lumen in this region is rough. The beginning of a stenotic segment is usually fairly abrupt and can be traced to its beginning and end in the arterial lumen as a sharply defined point. Contrariwise, if the narrowing is due to spasm it is usually of greater length and begins smoothly and gradually at both ends; the lumen of the vessel is seen to decrease progressively in size and then to widen again.

Care should be taken to examine carefully the origin of the *vertebral arteries* because there is usually a slight curve at this point which may obscure a stenotic lesion (fig. 547). Narrowing of a vertebral

the origin of the right vertebral artery (*arrow*); otherwise the caliber was normal. A film made at 3 seconds (D) revealed that the left vertebral artery had now become filled and that there was retrograde flow to fill the left subclavian artery which evidently was occluded. It is obvious that the blood supply to the left arm was chiefly by way of retrograde flow from the right vertebral through the left vertebral artery. The bilateral filling of both posterior cerebral and superior cerebellar arteries from the carotid systems is often due to hypotension in the region of the basilar artery system. However, this is not always so, and many cases have come to our attention in which brachial angiography, performed after this observation, revealed normal filling by way of the vertebral artery.

(Revised 1963)

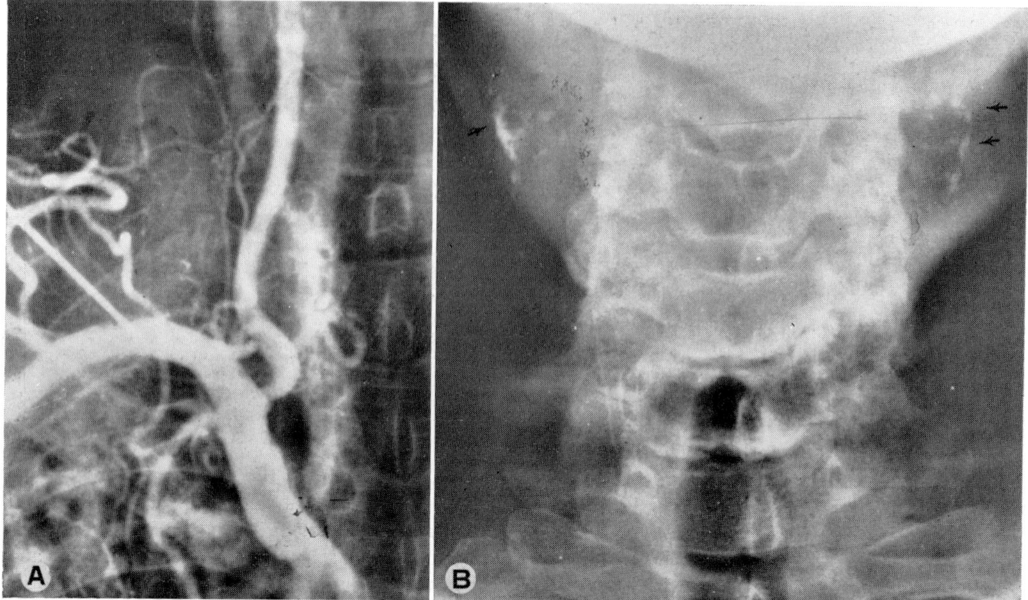

Fig. 547.—Narrowing of the Origin of the Vertebral Artery on the Right Side Partly Obscured

(A) There is narrowing of the vertebral artery at its origin followed by a slight poststenotic widening of this artery. In addition, there is an arteriosclerotic plaque on the superior wall of the subclavian artery just proximal to the origin of the vertebral artery. If the origin of the vertebral arteries is to be seen without any superimposition of the subclavian artery, it is often necessary to angle the tube caudad about 10°. (B) Bilateral calcification in the region of the bifurcation of the common carotid arteries (*arrows*). The presence of calcification is not necessarily associated with occlusive disease. (C) Arteriosclerotic narrowing (in another patient) of internal carotid artery, and occlusion of external carotid. (D) Postoperative angiogram following endarterectomy shows that both the internal and the external carotid artery are patent. On the opposite side (E), the patient had occlusion of internal carotid artery with collateral circulation by way of the ophthalmic artery.

artery may be produced within the vertebral canal by osteophytes arising from the vertebral column. Occasionally, there is an extreme degree of osteophytosis originating in the articular facettes which causes the vertebral artery to be quite irregular in its course. It has been stated that this may be a significant cause of obstruction, particularly upon turning the head, and that it may explain the occurrence of "dizzy spells" in older individuals with motion of the head and neck, but the general significance is hard to evaluate.

Calcification in the intracavernous portion of the internal carotid arteries is common in older individuals. Calcification in the supraclinoid portion is less common. It is also common to observe calcification in the cervical portion of the artery usually at the site of bifurcation of the common carotid artery (fig. 547B). Like any other arterial calcification, these calcific deposits indicate degenerative changes but are not necessarily related to the presence of vascular occlusions.

How often cerebrovascular insufficiency results from an occlusive or stenotic lesion in the vessels of the neck is not known. It has been stated that over 30 per cent of patients with the stroke syndrome have symptoms owing to occlusion of the extracranial vessels (Crawford *et al.*, 1959). Others have estimated it to be lower, approximately 20 per cent (Fields *et al.*, 1958).

Of the 600 patients with an admission diagnosis of cerebrovascular disease re-

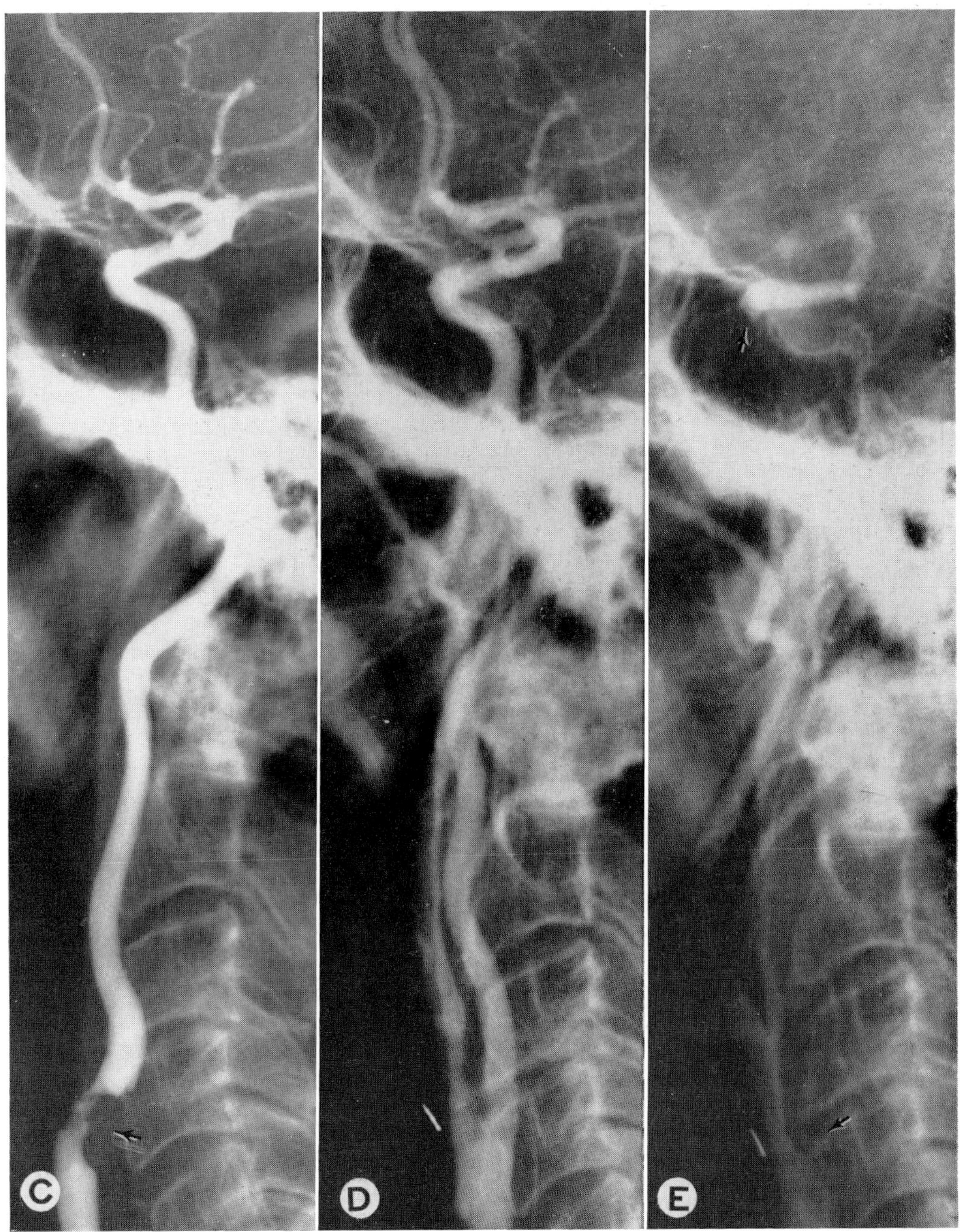

Fig. 547. C–E

ported by Gurdjian and co-authors (1961), there was an incidence of approximately 30 per cent of occlusive abnormality in the larger vessels in the neck and thorax. This is not to say, however, that the presence of an occlusive abnormality in these vessels indicates that it is the actual cause of the stroke. In addition there was a 10 per cent

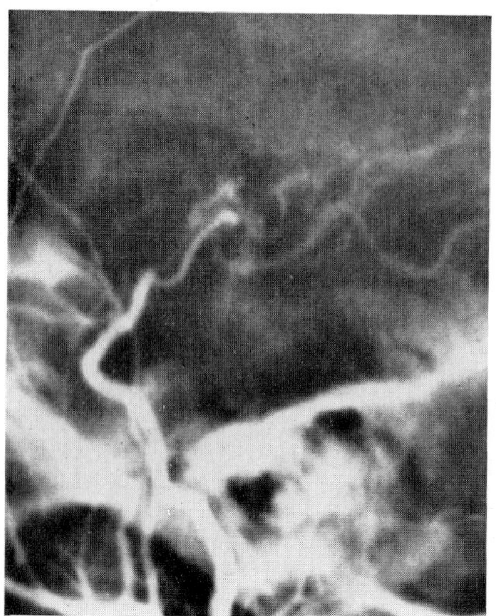

Fig. 548.—Occlusion of Internal Carotid Artery in an Infant 3 Years of Age

There is an obstruction of the internal carotid artery just above the origin of the posterior communicating artery. The artery below this point is diffusely narrowed due to decreased flow through it similar to that of Figs. 534D and 535.

incidence of mass lesions (subdural hematomas or neoplasms). Of the obstructive lesions in the internal carotid artery, 90 were classified as partial occlusions (30 of these were bilateral) and 60 showed complete internal carotid occlusion (6 of these were bilateral). In the entire group, only 25 cases of middle cerebral artery occlusion were seen, which appears to be an abnormally low incidence in this group of cases, but the patients were not studied by serialograms in every instance.

Tortuosity and kinking are seen often in patients with arteriosclerosis. Occasionally they are seen also in young subjects without arteriosclerosis. Elongation of a vessel with tortuosity and kinking is most probably not clinically significant unless it is associated with partial occlusion.

Major cerebral arteries. Consideration of obstructive intracranial vascular disease may be divided into three portions: (1) stenotic and occlusive lesions of the major cerebral vessels (internal carotid, anterior and middle cerebral arteries, and basilar and posterior cerebral arteries); (2) diseases of the branches of the major cerebral vessels; and (3) the behavior of the small vessels of the brain and of certain collateral channels.

Occlusion of the intracranial portion of the *internal carotid artery* is not as common as is obstruction of the cervical portion. It usually occurs just above the origin of the posterior communicating artery (figs. 534 and 548). Arteriosclerotic narrowing with irregular plaques in the walls of the artery are common in this region. Spastic narrowing is also common but usually is seen with bleeding aneurysms, as described under "Arterial Spasm."

Occlusion of the *middle cerebral artery* most often occurs in its horizontal portion, either immediately distal to its origin or at the site of the first branching. Commonly, the first large branch of the middle cerebral artery, usually the orbitofrontal or anterior temporal branch, is well filled (fig. 549). In children, occlusion of the middle cerebral artery is more frequent than obstruction of the internal carotid, in our experience. When the middle cerebral artery is thrombosed, there is usually very good visualization of the anterior and of the posterior cerebral arteries on the same side. Collateral circulation by way of the so-called meningeal arterial anastomoses is established by way of direct end-to-end anastomoses between the anterior and the middle cerebral arteries and sometimes from the posterior cerebral artery. In the cases where there is a stenotic lesion of the anterior cerebral artery coexisting with thrombosis of the middle cerebral artery, the principal collateral circulation would be established by way of the posterior circulation (fig. 564).

Thrombosis of the *anterior cerebral artery* may occur in its proximal or distal portions. Care should be taken not to diagnose thrombosis of the proximal portion of the anterior cerebral artery merely on the basis of a lack of filling from one side, since hypoplasia of the horizontal portion of the anterior cerebral artery is so common. For further evaluation, angiography on the opposite side should be carried out, compressing the carotid on the side where filling of the anterior cerebral artery was not obtained. If the

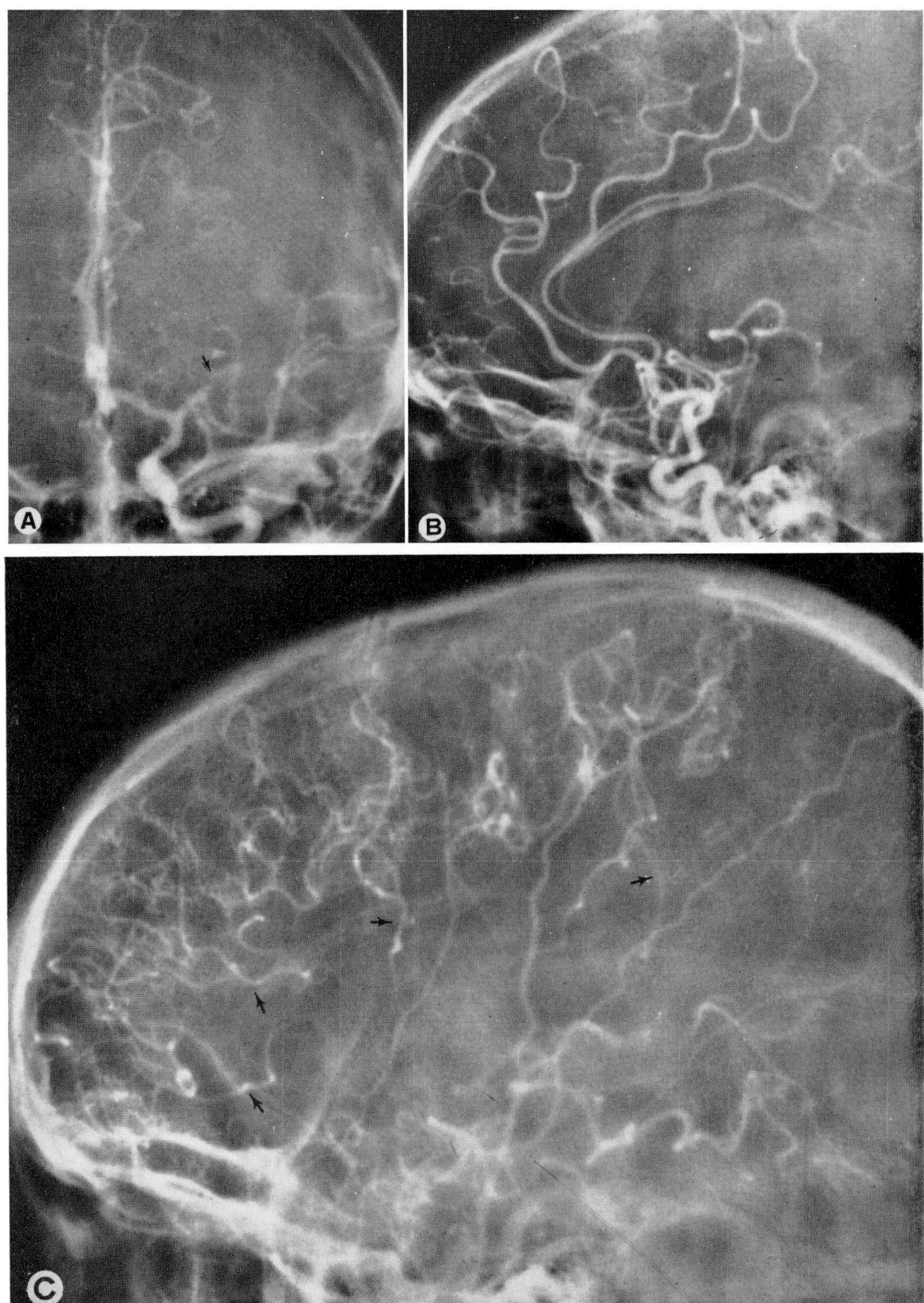

FIG. 549.—THROMBOSIS OF THE MIDDLE CEREBRAL ARTERY IN AN 8-YEAR-OLD CHILD

The frontal film (A) discloses the obstruction of the trunk of the middle cerebral artery just distal to the bifurcation of this artery (*arrow*). The lateral view made in the early arterial phase (B) demonstrates the good filling of the anterior cerebral vessels which later in the serial (C) is seen to fill in retrograde manner the branches of the middle cerebral artery (*arrows*).

(*Revised 1963*)

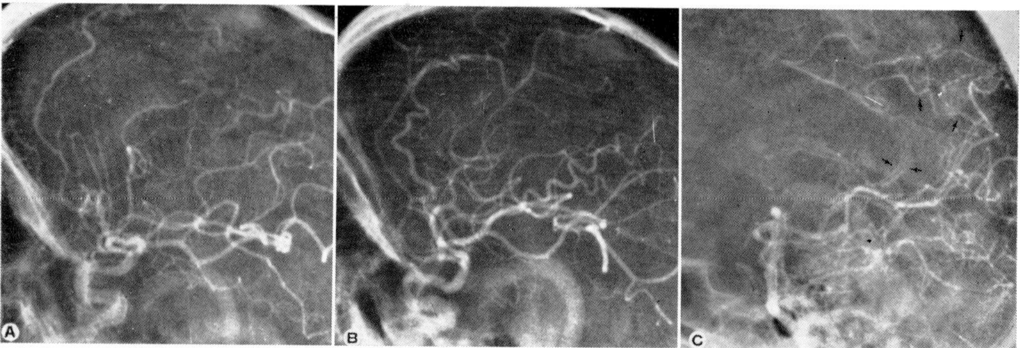

FIG. 550.—BILATERAL OCCLUSION OF THE PERICALLOSAL ARTERIES WITH COLLATERAL CIRCULATION FROM THE VERTEBRAL ARTERIES

The right and left angiograms (A) and (B) revealed nonfilling of both pericallosal arteries. The callosomarginal arteries and at least the anterior and middle internal frontal branches of these arteries are filled. A vertebral angiogram (C) revealed retrograde flow by way of anastomoses between the parieto-occipital branches of the posterior cerebral arteries and the branches of the pericallosal artery (*arrows*). There is also filling of the arteries of the splenium or posterior pericallosal arteries which anastomose with the terminal branch of the pericallosal artery (*lower arrows*).

artery is only mildly hypoplastic, the segment usually will fill from the opposite side when compression is used. If the horizontal segment is markedly hypoplastic, it may not fill even though it is not completely atretic. Only a small percentage of such patients actually have a true occlusion of this portion of the anterior cerebral artery. It has been reported by Riggs (1937) from an anatomical study of 1647 specimens of the circle of Willis obtained at autopsy that no instance of an absent horizontal portion of the anterior cerebral artery was encountered, even in this large group. On the other hand, Webster and co-authors (1960) believed that occlusion of the proximal portion of the anterior cerebral artery may be fairly common. This position, however, is open to question since conclusions were drawn from angiographic material without the benefit of serialographic studies and routine ipsilateral neck compression when the contralateral side was being injected.

Occlusion of the distal portion of an anterior cerebral artery is easier to demonstrate angiographically than obstruction of the proximal portion. In cases of anterior cerebral thrombosis, collateral circulation is often seen over the medial surface of the brain from branches of the posterior cerebral artery (fig. 550). Occasionally anastomotic channels over the superior surface of the hemisphere may be seen extending from the middle cerebral artery arborization.

Thrombosis of the *basilar artery* and the intracranial portion of the *vertebral arteries* occurs not infrequently. Marked atherosclerotic changes are common in the basilar artery. The artery becomes elongated, tortuous, and irregular in contour, showing some areas of narrowing and some areas of dilatation of the lumen. As the artery becomes elongated, it may project upward higher than usual, sometimes making an indentation on the inferior aspect of the third ventricle (fig. 388). Care should be taken in diagnosing stenosis of the basilar artery; it is very common to see laminar flow in the basilar artery when only one vertebral artery is injected since the nonopacified blood from the opposite vertebral tends to confine the contrast substance to one side of the vessel. Therefore, the arterial lumen may appear narrow when it actually is normal in caliber (fig. 406).

Another finding often encountered in vertebral angiography performed by direct puncture is true narrowing of the basilar artery due to contraction of the arterial wall, a reaction to local lowering of the blood pressure. Such local hypotension occurs when the needle in the vertebral artery causes some extravasation of blood or contrast substance at the injection site, thus producing obstruction to blood flow. In these cases the contrast substance is seen to remain in the basilar and in the vertebral arteries for a relatively long period of time. Only faint or no opacification of the branches of the basilar artery can be seen on the films, falsely suggesting an occlusion of the artery. In some instances the posterior inferior cerebellar artery is well visualized, which also should not be interpreted as evidence that distal occlusion of the basilar artery is present. As mentioned under "Anatomy" and "Physiology," a good vertebral injection usually produces some regurgitation of the contrast substance into the opposite vertebral artery. A diagnosis of thrombosis of the basilar artery probably should not be made unless some regurgitation takes place into the opposite vertebral artery. Thrombosis of the basilar artery usually occurs just proximal to the bifurcation of the artery into its main branches. The lesion may develop above the junction of the two vertebral arteries but at the site of this confluence, obstruction is less frequently encountered. In these cases, carotid angiography usually shows filling of both posterior cerebral and both superior cerebellar arteries and such collateral flow through the circle of Willis tends to confirm the presence of thrombosis of the basilar artery.

Isolated thrombosis of a *superior cerebellar artery* or *posterior cerebral artery* occurs, but the authors have seen such obstructions only rarely. Thrombosis of branches of a posterior cerebral artery are encountered more often.

Thrombosis of the *posterior inferior cerebellar artery* is a well recognized clinical entity. The diagnosis of obstruction of the artery by angiography, however, is tenuous because there are normal anatomical variants which include absence of this artery. It is possible, moreover, that thrombosis of this artery is an accompaniment of occlusion of the vertebral artery from which it arises, in which case no filling of the vertebral trunk in this region is obtained.

Divided cerebral arteries. The diagnosis of thrombosis of the principal branches of the middle, anterior, and posterior cerebral arteries can be made, provided serial films are taken routinely during angiography. If routine serial films are not made, it is possible to confuse the lack of filling of a given branch with an anatomical variant or even a small tumor. Adequate films usually demonstrate the presence of collateral flow into the area normally supplied by the obstructed vessel. In the case of thrombosis of a middle cerebral branch, collateral flow most often comes from the anterior cerebral arterial branches and retrograde filling of the obstructed territory usually can be traced on serial films (fig. 551). In the case of anterior cerebral branch occlusions, the middle cerebral subdivisions, which anastomose directly with those of the anterior cerebral artery, may be the source of collateral supply. In our experience, however, the posterior cerebral artery is a more common source of collateral supply for the anterior cerebral area (fig. 550). In one instance of thrombosis of the posterior temporal branch of a posterior cerebral artery, retrograde filling took place by way of anastomoses with branches of the parieto-occipital division of the posterior cerebral and with the middle cerebral arteries (fig. 552). When the occluded branches do not fill by collateral flow, propagation of thrombus into these branches may have occurred.

When the branches of the cerebral arteries remain occluded for a period of time such as may be produced by propagation of thrombus from the original site of occlusion, there is no way in which blood can get to the area supplied by these vessels inasmuch as the perforating branches arising from them will also be occluded. Eventually the thrombus may disappear and be completely reabsorbed, but the damage to the territory of this vessel will persist and a cerebral infarction will probably occur. After the thrombus is dissolved, filling of the previously obstructed portions of the vessels may then take place by retrograde flow from a territory of an adjacent nonobstructed vessel. However, the damage to the perforating vessels has already taken place and capillary block will probably persist in the infarcted area.

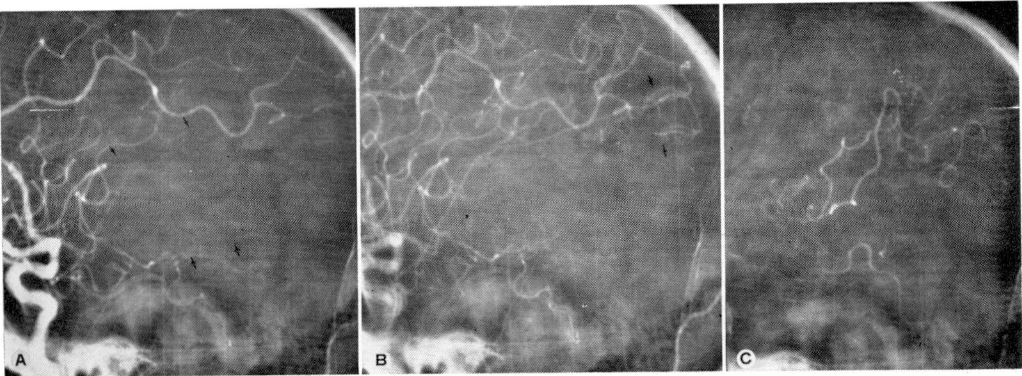

FIG. 551.—THROMBOSIS OF BRANCHES OF MIDDLE CEREBRAL ARTERY SIMULATING TUMOR

The film made at one second (A) shows an avascular area in the anterior retro-Sylvian area. A film made at 1.5 seconds (B) discloses a persistence of the avascular area with some fine vessels in this region. A film made at 2.5 seconds (C) now discloses retrograde filling of branches of the middle cerebral artery from the anterior cerebral artery which fill the avascular area. In (B) it is already possible to see the prominent branches of the anterior cerebral artery which have turned downward after reaching the upper margin of the hemisphere (*arrows*).

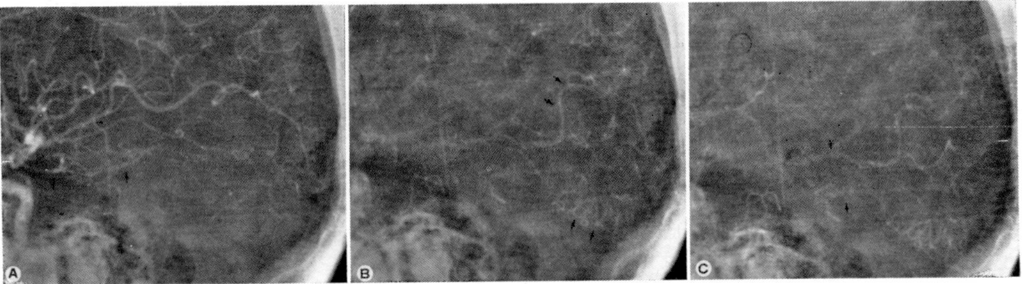

FIG. 552.—OCCLUSION OF BRANCHES OF THE POSTERIOR CEREBRAL ARTERY

A film made at one second (A) shows partial filling of the posterior cerebral artery by way of the posterior communicating artery. As progress of the contrast substance was followed in the serialogram it was noted, at 2.0 seconds (B) that the arterial phase was finished in the remainder of the brain, but in the occipital area there was now retrograde flow into the parieto-occipital branches and many fine branches are also seen in the region of the undersurface of the occipital lobe (*arrows*). The film made at 2.5 seconds (C) shows filling of the posterior temporal branch as well as more proximal filling of the parieto-occipital branch of the posterior cerebral artery (*arrows*). If a serial had not been made in this case, it would have been concluded that the posterior cerebral artery showed simply partial filling, which is common in carotid angiography.

There will be a persistence of the contrast material in the vessels filled by collateral flow. The persistence of the contrast substance, which we have come to call "stasis in the collaterals" is evidently the result of block of the perforating branches arising from those cerebral arteries which are visible by angiography. The diagnosis of cerebral infarction can, therefore, be suggested under these circumstances (fig. 564). Generalized stasis in collateral channels has also been seen in cases of occlusion of the trunk of the middle cerebral artery with infarction of almost the entire hemisphere. These patients usually die (Taveras, 1961).

Single branch occlusions of the cerebral arteries, particularly branches of the middle cerebral artery, may also be diagnosed accurately by angiography. The diagnosis is based on the demonstration of retrograde flow into the area of the occluded vessel in the later phases of the serialogram. Local

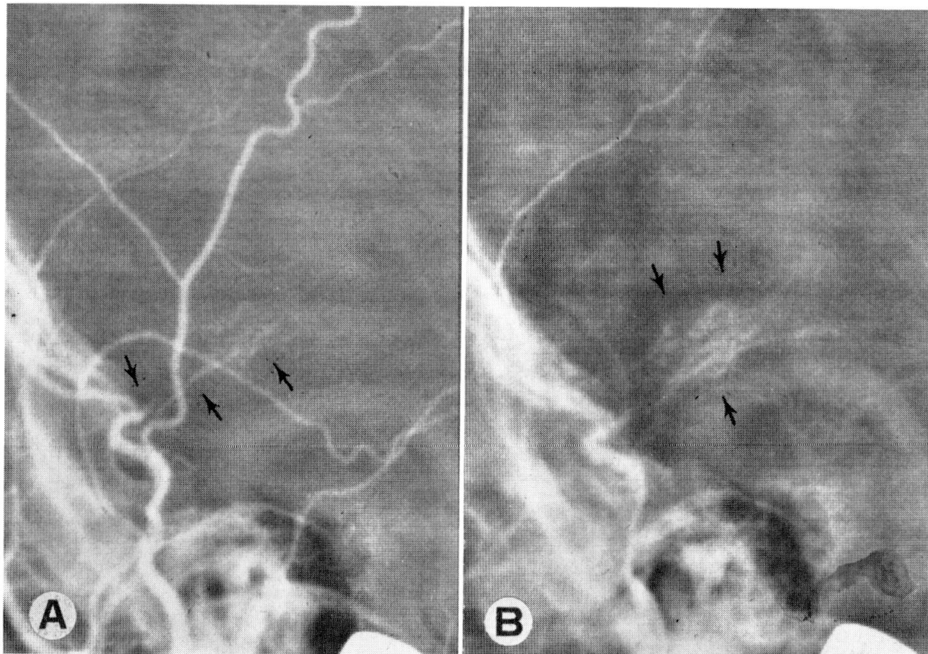

FIG. 553.—THROMBOSIS OF THE INTERNAL CAROTID ARTERY IN 20-MONTH-OLD INFANT ABOVE THE ANTERIOR CHORIOIDAL ARTERY

The film made at 2.5 seconds (A) reveals the dilated trunk of the anterior chorioidal artery with a capillary blush around it (*arrows*). The film made at 4.5 seconds (B) discloses a wider area of staining. This is probably due to hypoxic vasodilatation of the arterioles, branches of the anterior chorioidal artery, but it may also be an attempt to establish collateral circulation at the capillary level. The child had developed an infantile hemiplegia.

stasis may be demonstrated in the distal 1 or 2 cm. of the occluded vessel, and it may take several seconds for the segment beyond the occlusion to fill in a retrograde manner from an adjacent territory (fig. 552). This type of diagnosis requires careful scrutiny of the areas in question because the arteries which fill by retrograde flow may be confused with veins. Care should be taken not to confuse retrograde flow and filling of a given vessel with the usual late emptying which takes place in the parieto-occipital region. The latter phenomenon is caused by the longer length of these arteries and also by the fact that the last amount of contrast material left at the end of the injection, by gravity, tends to fill the posterior arteries, the contrast material being heavier than the blood.

Minor cerebral arteries and collateral circulation. It has been demonstrated by anatomic dissections that there are direct end-to-end anastomoses between branches of the anterior, middle, and posterior cerebral arteries on the surface of the brain. This fact is repeatedly demonstrated angiographically. Whether anastomoses exist between such small "end" arteries as the lenticulostriate, anterior chorioidal, and other perforating branches of the cerebral vessels has not been shown. It is likely that anastomoses for these vessels exist by way of the capillary bed, but the anastomotic pathways are insufficient to carry the circulation from one territory to another. On cerebral angiograms in cases of thrombosis, it is common to see dilatation of many small perforating branches of the cerebral arteries which are not usually visualized on normal cerebral angiograms. It is not known whether, in the acute stage, the dilatation is the result of hypoxia with relative stasis within the

(*Revised 1963*)

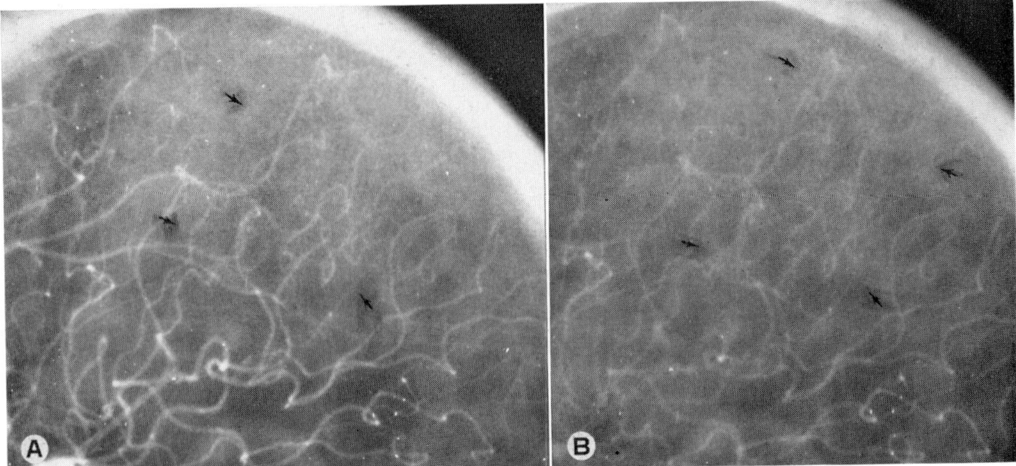

FIG. 554.—THROMBOSIS OF DISTAL BRANCHES OF MIDDLE CEREBRAL ARTERY IN PARIETAL REGION WITH ARTERIOLAR VASODILATATION

The film made in the midarterial phase (A) reveals many dilated thin vessels surrounding a group of arteries in the parietal region (*arrows*), but no individually obstructed vessels can be seen. In the intermediate phase (B) there is an isolated area of increased vascularity which was felt to be most likely a neoplasm. However, pneumoencephalography was performed following the angiogram, and it revealed only ventricular dilatation and some cortical atrophy.

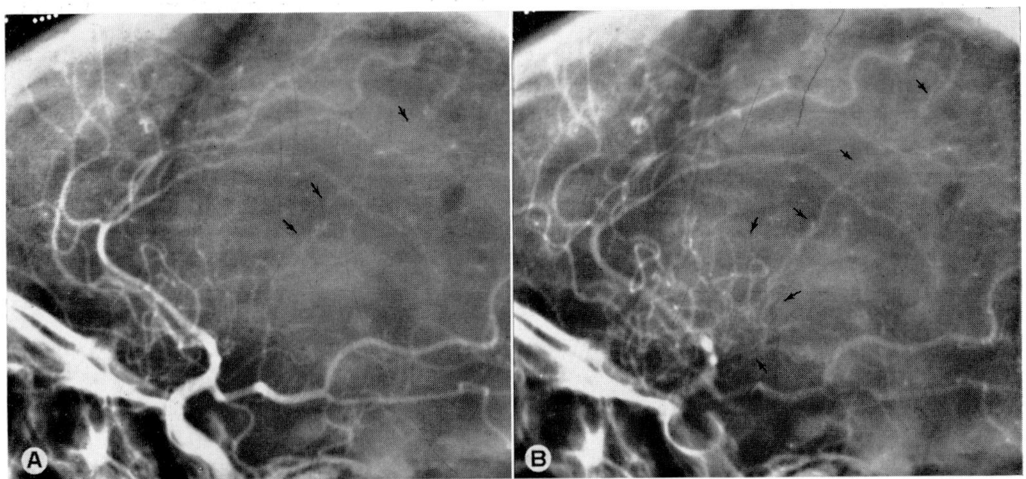

FIG. 555.—THROMBOSIS OF THE MIDDLE CEREBRAL ARTERY WITH SMALL VESSEL ENLARGEMENT

In the midarterial phase (A) there is filling and dilatation of lenticulostriate branches and one anterior opercular branch. A single channel is seen to cross the brain going from the parasagittal region to the middle cerebral territory (*arrows*). In the later phases, one or two others could be traced. It is curious that the branch outlined by the arrows is apparently not on the surface of the brain but represents a deep perforating branch. Film taken 0.5 second later (B) shows rich vascularity in the region of the lenticulostriate branches which became more prominent later in the serialogram (not shown). Yet the surface branches of the middle cerebral artery in the posterior frontal and parietal regions never filled, except for the periphery of the hemisphere. Probably all of these branches have become occluded.

(Revised 1963)

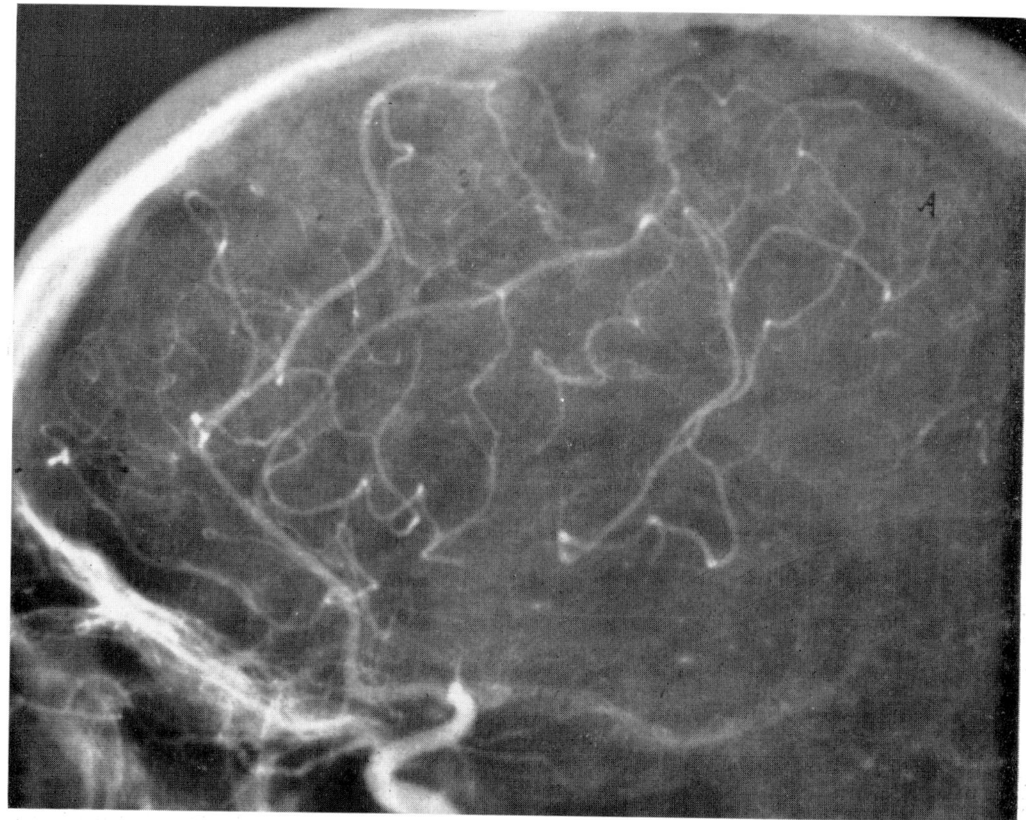

Fig. 556.—Thrombosis of the Middle Cerebral Artery with Surface Collateral Circulation from the Anterior to the Middle Cerebral Vessels

There is excellent retrograde flow by way of the anterior cerebral branches which filled practically all of the middle cerebral artery branches. The last one is marked with the letter (A). The more posterior ones are filled by way of the posterior cerebral artery. In this case there is practically no small vessel dilatation although there are some visible lenticulostriate branches. These become easier to visualize when there is middle cerebral thrombosis because of the lack of overlying middle cerebral branches. It is obvious that in this case the middle cerebral branches remained patent following occlusion of this artery, whereas in the case shown in the preceding figure, there must have been occlusion of the major branches of the middle cerebral artery and thus they could not be filled by retrograde flow.

vessels, or whether they are dilated to serve as a means of collateral flow. The case shown in Figure 553, in which a thrombosis of the internal carotid artery occurred just above the level of the origin of the anterior chorioidal artery, illustrates extreme dilatation of the branches of the anterior chorioidal artery that produces a relatively wide area of staining in the angiogram. The evidence of increased vascularity remained on the serialogram for several seconds, and it is likely that there was stasis here within the arterioles. The enlargement of numerous small perforating branches is sometimes so pronounced that it suggests the presence of a tumor, such as was mistakenly thought to exist in the case illustrated in Figure 554. Whether or not small vessels will become dilated and be visible in the angiogram probably depends on the status of arteries distal to the site of obstruction. That is, if a thrombus propagates within the branches of the obstructed main vessel, the perforating branches arising proximal to the obstruc-

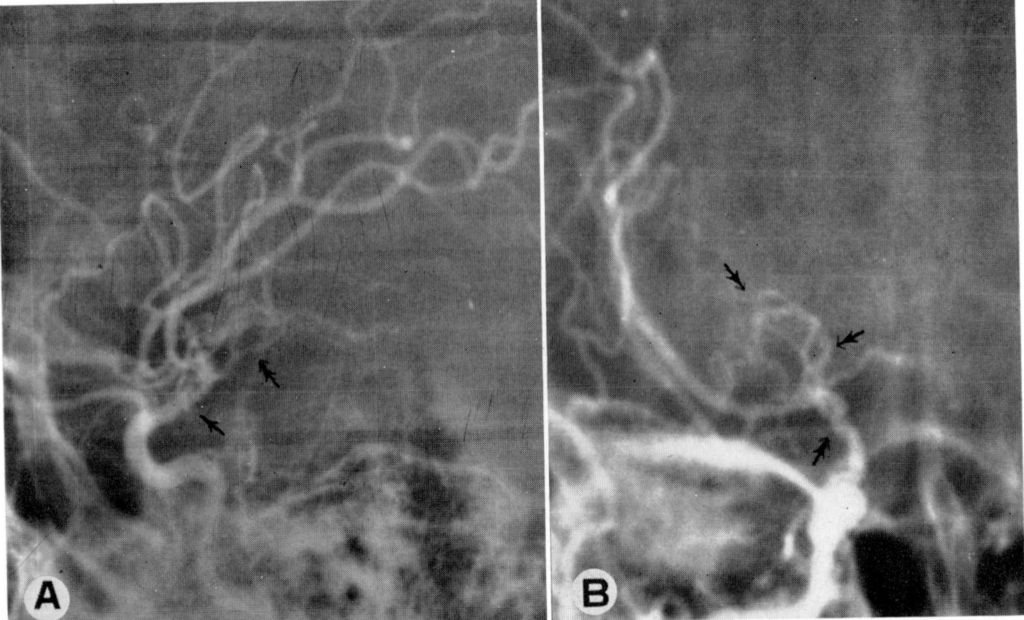

Fig. 557.—Old Thrombosis of Internal Carotid Artery with Recanalization and Collateral Circulation from the Internal to the Middle Cerebral Artery by Way of Perforating Branches

The lateral projection (A) demonstrates poor filling of the middle cerebral branches and considerable irregularity and narrowing of the supraclinoid portion of the carotid siphon. The *two-headed arrow* points to what is felt to be a dilated anterior chorioidal artery. The frontal projection (B) reveals irregularity of the carotid artery (*lower arrow*) which is felt to be due to recanalization of a previously thrombosed vessel. The extremely enlarged anterior chorioidal artery is seen to anastomose with lenticulostriate arteries (*upper arrows*) and to bypass the old area of obstruction. The proximal portion of the middle cerebral artery is extremely thin. It is felt that recanalization took place, and perhaps this anastomotic pathway is no longer needed. Hemiplegia had occurred in this 14-year-old girl 7 years before and the onset was sudden. Unfortunately, no angiogram was available at the time of the original injury, which was felt to be most likely an occlusion of the supraclinoid portion of the internal carotid artery, probably above the anterior chorioidal origin. Although this is an atypical appearance for the anterior chorioidal artery, it must be remembered that this vessel does not always arise at the same place (see anatomy of the anterior chorioidal artery).

tion probably will become dilated and may succeed in supplying at least a part of the ischemic area. On the other hand, if the arteries beyond the point of obstruction remain patent, blood supply can be effected by retrograde flow from anastomoses on the surface of the brain. The case illustrated in Figure 555 shows a combination of filling of only a few branches of the middle cerebral artery by way of surface anastomoses following thrombosis of the main stem of this artery, but there is considerable small vessel enlargement seen in the region of the trunk of the middle cerebral artery. It is probable that thrombus had extended into some of the branches of the middle cerebral artery and therefore retrograde flow was not possible in most of them. On the other hand the case illustrated in Figure 556 shows no small vessel enlargement and only collateral flow by way of the surface anastomoses with the anterior cerebral artery. In the case illustrated in Figure 557 it is thought that anastomoses between the anterior chorioidal and the lenticulostriate arteries permitted the bypassing of an obstruction of the internal carotid artery proximal to its bifurcation. Unfortunately, in this case no angiogram

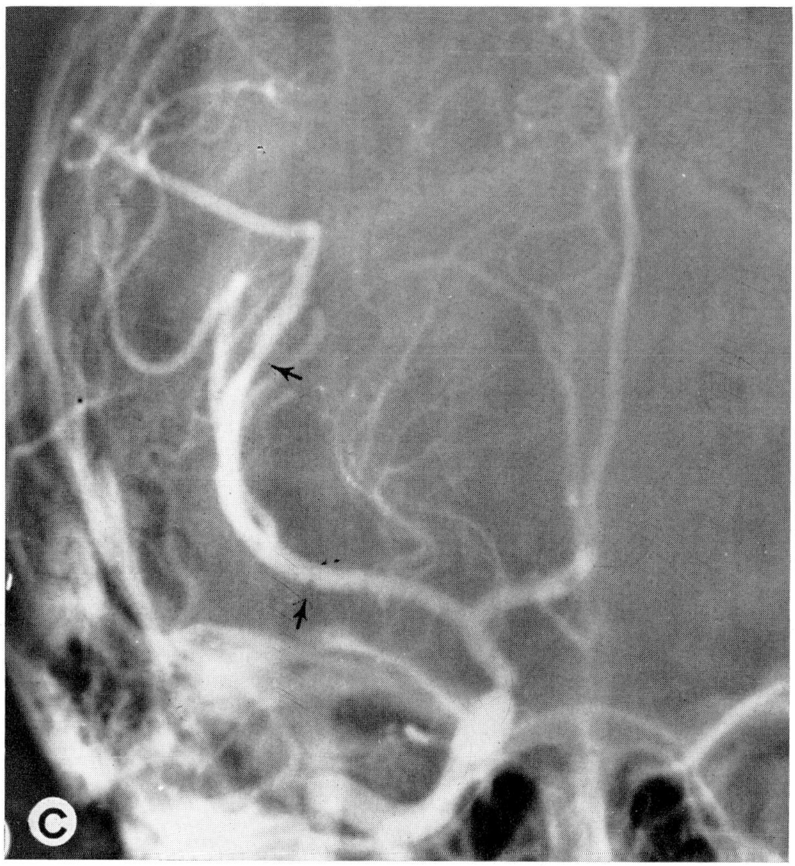

FIG. 557 (cont.).—OLD MIDDLE CEREBRAL THROMBOSIS IN 11-YEAR-OLD CHILD, WITH PROMINENT ANTERIOR CHORIOIDAL AND LENTICULOSTRIATE ARTERIES

There is irregularity of the horizontal portion of the middle cerebral artery extending into the distal branches as well (*arrows*), and there is also a marked diminution in the number of branches in the middle cerebral territory; only three branches can be seen. This indicates an old thrombosis of the middle cerebral artery with possible recanalization of only some of the branches. The lenticulostriate arteries and the anterior chorioidal arteries have evidently become dilated, possibly to supply adjacent areas by way of capillary connections.

made soon after the infantile hemiplegia had occurred was available which might have provided a valuable comparison.

Sometimes the presence of small dilated perforating branches of the cerebral vessels adjacent to an area of thrombosis is helpful in differentiating a neoplasm from an edematous area secondary to occlusion of vessels. We may refer to these, in the acute stage, as "anoxic vessels" (fig. 554). Later, these vessels remain dilated and tend to surround each one of the larger arteries or groups of arteries with a "corona" of fine vessels (figs. 554 and 560). In early stages of vascular occlusion there usually is cerebral edema which may be localized, and in some cases it may be sufficiently pronounced to suggest a tumor (Wood and Farmer, 1957). Midline shift may be present and sometimes it is very marked, as in the case illustrated in Figure 558. It probably takes about 2 weeks for edema to disappear, provided that no subsequent vascular occlusion occurs such as takes place in the intermittent progressive type of stroke syndrome.

Discussion of *collateral circulation* may

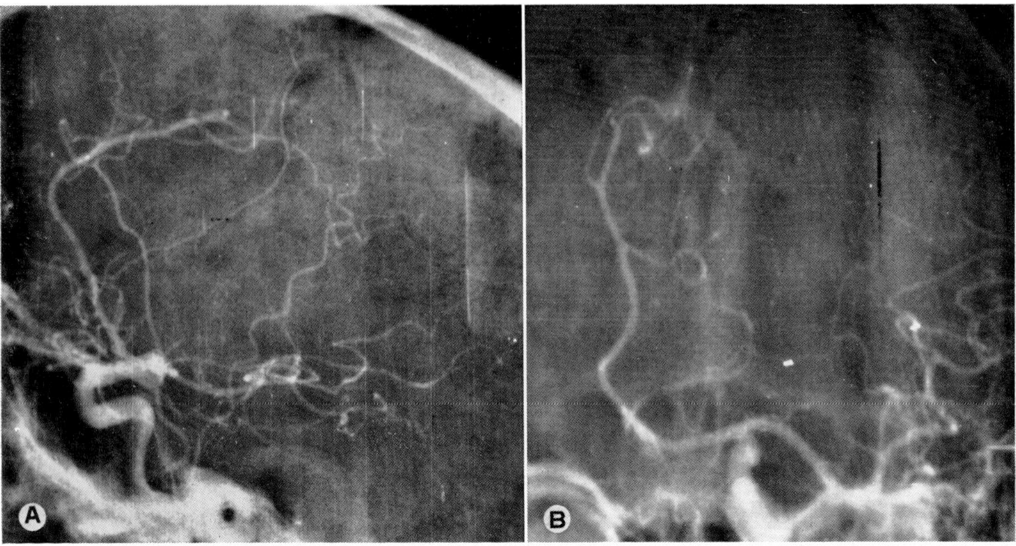

FIG. 558.—PARTIAL MIDDLE CEREBRAL THROMBOSIS IN THE ACUTE STAGE WITH MARKED CEREBRAL EDEMA

The lateral view (A) shows filling of some anterior opercular branches and some posterior branches of the middle cerebral artery, but there is a paucity of vessels in the supra-Sylvian region. This was thought to be due to thrombosis of branches of the middle cerebral artery rather than to spreading from an intracerebral mass. The frontal projection (B) revealed a marked degree of shift of the anterior cerebral vessels. The clinical history and findings were in agreement with the diagnosis of thrombosis.

be divided into circulation from the external carotid to the internal carotid system and circulation from branches of the internal carotid or basilar artery to other branches.

Circulation from the external carotid arteries to the intracranial vessels may take place by way of the ophthalmic artery, the most common route. Branches of the ophthalmic artery anastomose with those of the superficial temporal, external maxillary, and internal maxillary arteries as well as with branches of the middle meningeal artery. Since the ophthalmic is a sizable branch of the internal carotid system, reverse circulation can be established fairly easily. It probably requires some time, however, for significant collateral circulation to be established by way of the ophthalmic artery. Just how long a time this takes cannot be stated, but it may be as long as a few weeks before there is voluminous flow. For this reason there does not seem to be any relationship between the presence of collateral circulation through the ophthalmic artery and the degree of recovery from a stroke following occlusion of the internal carotid artery in the neck (Bossi and Pisani, 1955). The reversal of circulation through the ophthalmic artery does not become established unless the obstruction is proximal to the ophthalmic artery and the carotid siphon remains patent.

The second most important source of collateral supply from the extracranial to the intracranial circulation is that resulting from anastomoses between the branches of the external carotid and the muscular branches of the vertebral artery. This is sometimes a very efficient way for collateral flow to be established, as shown in the case in Figure 559.

Other sources of collateral supply from the extracranial to the intracranial vessels occur only uncommonly. In our first observed case, direct anastomosis between a branch of the middle meningeal artery and a division of the middle cerebral artery, occurring directly through the subdural space, resulted in good filling of many of the branches of the middle cerebral artery following intracranial liga-

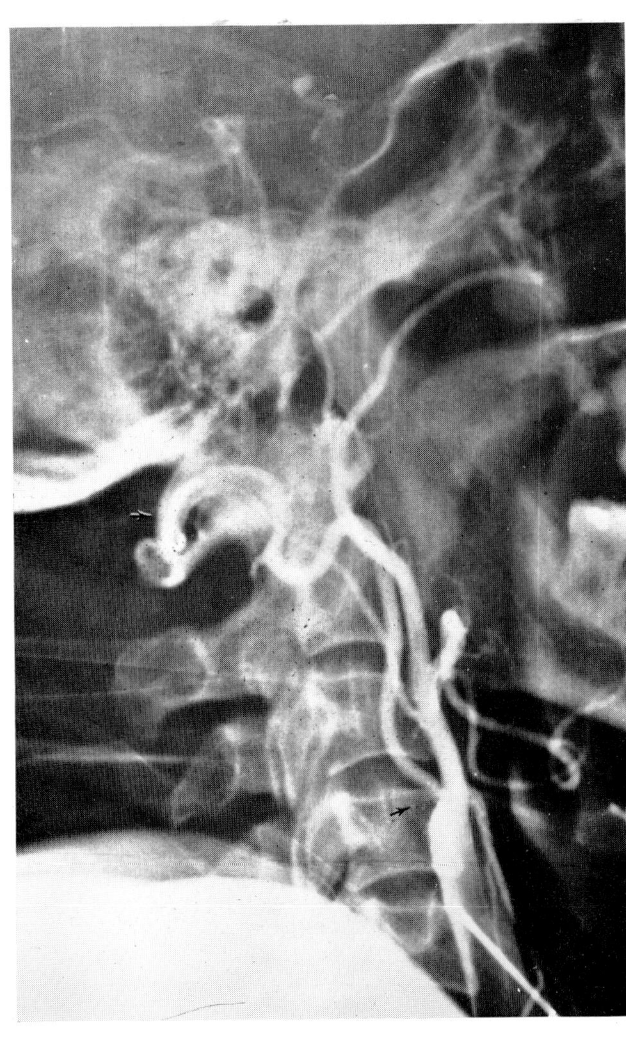

Fig. 559.—Thrombosis of the Internal Carotid Artery and of the Vertebral Artery with Collateral Circulation from the External Carotid to the Vertebral Artery

The injection was made in the common carotid artery, and the internal carotid artery is not visualized (*arrow*). There is a large artery that goes from a point just beyond the origin of the external carotid artery backward and upward and fills the vertebral artery directly. Later films showed fairly adequate vertebrobasilar filling. We believe this is a communication between the external carotid and the vertebrobasilar system by way of the occipital artery and not a persistent hypoglossal artery, because it does not arise from the internal carotid artery.

tion of the internal carotid artery (Mount and Taveras, 1957). Other cases have been seen with more extensive communications following old thromboses (fig. 561). Enlargement of middle meningeal channels is visible on plain films (fig. 562). While the *retia mirabilia* are functional in some animals, such as the cat, the anastomoses in man are clinically important only in the presence of long standing occlusion of the internal carotid system.

Of great physiologic and clinical significance are the direct end-to-end anastomoses between the branches of the anterior, middle, and posterior cerebral arteries. The channels are physiologically available for bidirectional flow at all times and are naturally utilized readily to support general circulation whenever there is a lowering of arterial pressure on one side which demands a reversal of the usual direction of flow. In a manner similar to that operating in the circle of Willis, the flow of blood can be reversed very rapidly in these small arteries following occlusion of a major vessel by an embolus or a thrombus.

Since many of the branches of the anterior and middle as well as the posterior cerebral arteries anastomose with one another directly, the flow of blood must stop at some point in these vessels. The anterior cerebral artery flow is upward and backward along

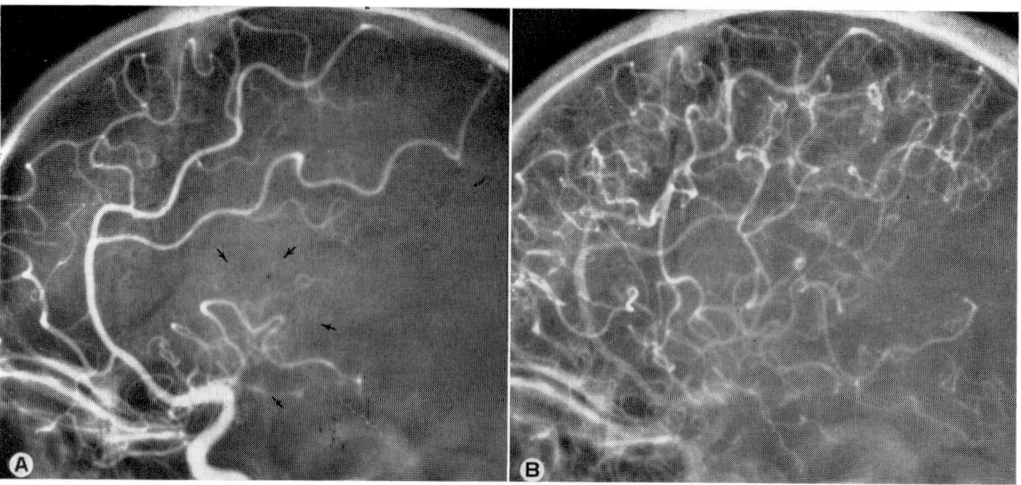

Fig. 560.—Thrombosis of the Middle Cerebral Artery with Collateral Circulation from the Anterior to the Middle Cerebral Artery and "Anoxic" Dilated Arterioles

The first film (A) discloses complete thrombosis of the middle cerebral artery with excellent filling of the anterior cerebral vessels. There is enlargement of the lenticulostriate group of arteries (*arrows*). A later film made at 2 seconds (B) reveals excellent collateral flow from the anterior to the middle cerebral vessels. There is also an extra added density around all of the vessels which is due to dilated arterioles. A film made at 3 seconds (C) reveals further prominence of the halo of increased density and fine vessels around each one of the larger collateral channels, which is more prominent when there is a group of vessels together and may suggest the presence of a tumor stain. The basilar vein was filled at this time, and in fact, in the previous film taken 0.5 second earlier, it was already filled. This represents an instance of more rapid shunting of blood through the deep structures, such as that noted in Fig. 563. A later film taken at 4 seconds (D) shows even more accumulation of fine vessels. This patient also exhibited local stasis in the collaterals; that is, a film made at 5.5 to 6.0 seconds still showed that the venous phase was nearing its end, but the lower portion of some of the middle cerebral branches filled by collateral flow were still visible (*lower arrows*). In spite of this, the patient made a fairly good recovery from his hemiplegia.

the medial surface of the hemisphere to the parasagittal margin of the brain and thence lateralward and downward as the branch vessels curve outward onto the lateral hemispheric surface for a short distance. In the middle cerebral branches, the flow of blood is upward to reach the superior portion of the hemisphere. Usually, the middle cerebral branches can be followed at angiography only to a point 2 to 3 cm. below the upper edge of the hemisphere. Beyond this point they ordinarily are not visible. This is clearly shown in cases where there is no contrast filling of one anterior cerebral artery, but in which flow is normal as a result of both arteries filling from one side. At such a junction point, the pressures in the anastomotic vessels between the anterior and middle cerebral arteries become equalized, and no flow results except toward the perforating branches which supply the brain. If, however, the pressure is lowered in either the middle or the anterior cerebral system, retrograde flow into the territory of the hypotensive vessel will occur and can be seen with contrast substance on serial films (figs. 551 and 556). As mentioned above, retrograde flow can be established only if there is no propagation of thrombus distally from the site of obstruction, since extension will cause obliteration of the arterial branches (fig. 555).

The arterial circulation time as well as the arteriovenous circulation time are increased in patients with thrombosis. It is our impression that proportionately, the arterial circulation time is increased more than the arteriovenous circulation time. The

(Revised 1963)

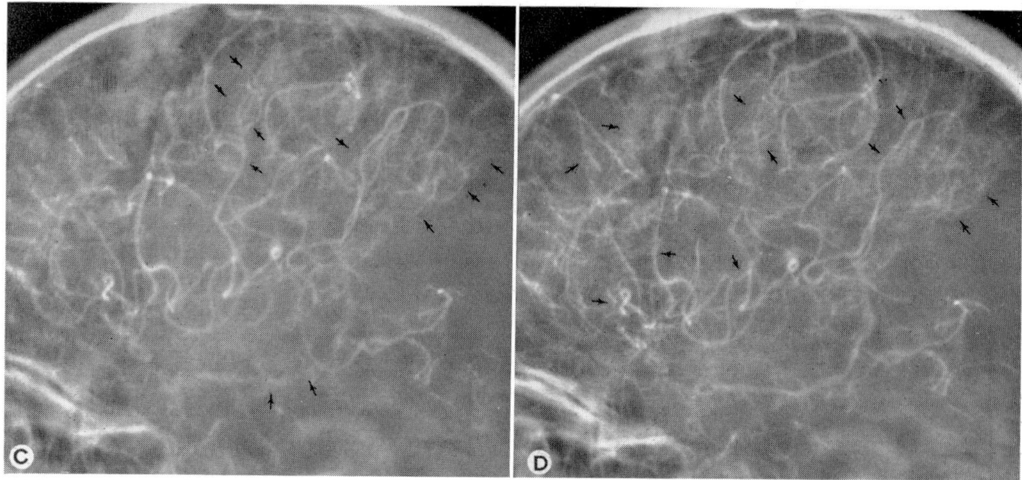

FIG. 560. C-D

collateral circulation time, measured as the time from appearance to disappearance of collateral channels, may last from 2 to 6 seconds. Over 4 seconds, however, is considered as excessively slow.

Usually the contrast substance is still visible in collateral channels when it has disappeared from other arterial branches (fig. 551). Some patients present what is considered to be definite stasis of the contrast substance in the collateral channels and, in some cases, narrowing of the collateral vessels also is observed. Stasis suggests the possibility of propagation of the thrombus for some distance along branches of the main artery. Stasis also may develop owing to partial thrombosis within distal branches or to parenchymal changes in the brain resulting in capillary block, either of which may impede normal flow.

The phenomenon of *generalized stasis* in collateral channels has been observed in four patients with middle cerebral artery thrombosis, in their 3d and 4th decade of life, all of whom died, usually within several hours or a few days (fig. 563). Generalized stasis in the collateral channels is thought, therefore, to indicate a bad prognosis. On the other hand, *local stasis* in collateral channels has not necessarily been associated with poor prognosis. In the case shown in Figure 564, the patient had a fairly good recovery in the three to four weeks after the angiogram.

(Revised 1963)

It is quite likely that local stasis is associated with damage to the perforating branches supplying the brain, with consequent diminished flow, and indicates the presence of an area of cerebral infarction.

A number of miscellaneous observations concerning small vessels and collateral channels should be mentioned. The increased circulation time in collateral channels may be related to some extent to a local change in the vessels, which allows only a reduced speed of flow, and also to the length of the vessel observed. Since blood flow may be expressed in centimeters per second, a column of contrast substance which must travel a greater distance to reach its final arborization will be visible in more frames of the serialogram (fig. 551). When stasis within the collateral channels is present, the vessels may appear narrower than normal. It is considered probable that a diffuse decrease in caliber of the collateral channels is not due to spasm but to simple contraction that results from diminished pressure and flow.

Obstruction of the arterioles or the capillaries, such as may be produced by multiple tiny emboli, causes only a lengthening of the arterial circulation time. Several such instances have been observed, in one of which diffuse tumor embolization occurred in a patient with carcinoma of the lung. Two other patients had multiple emboli as

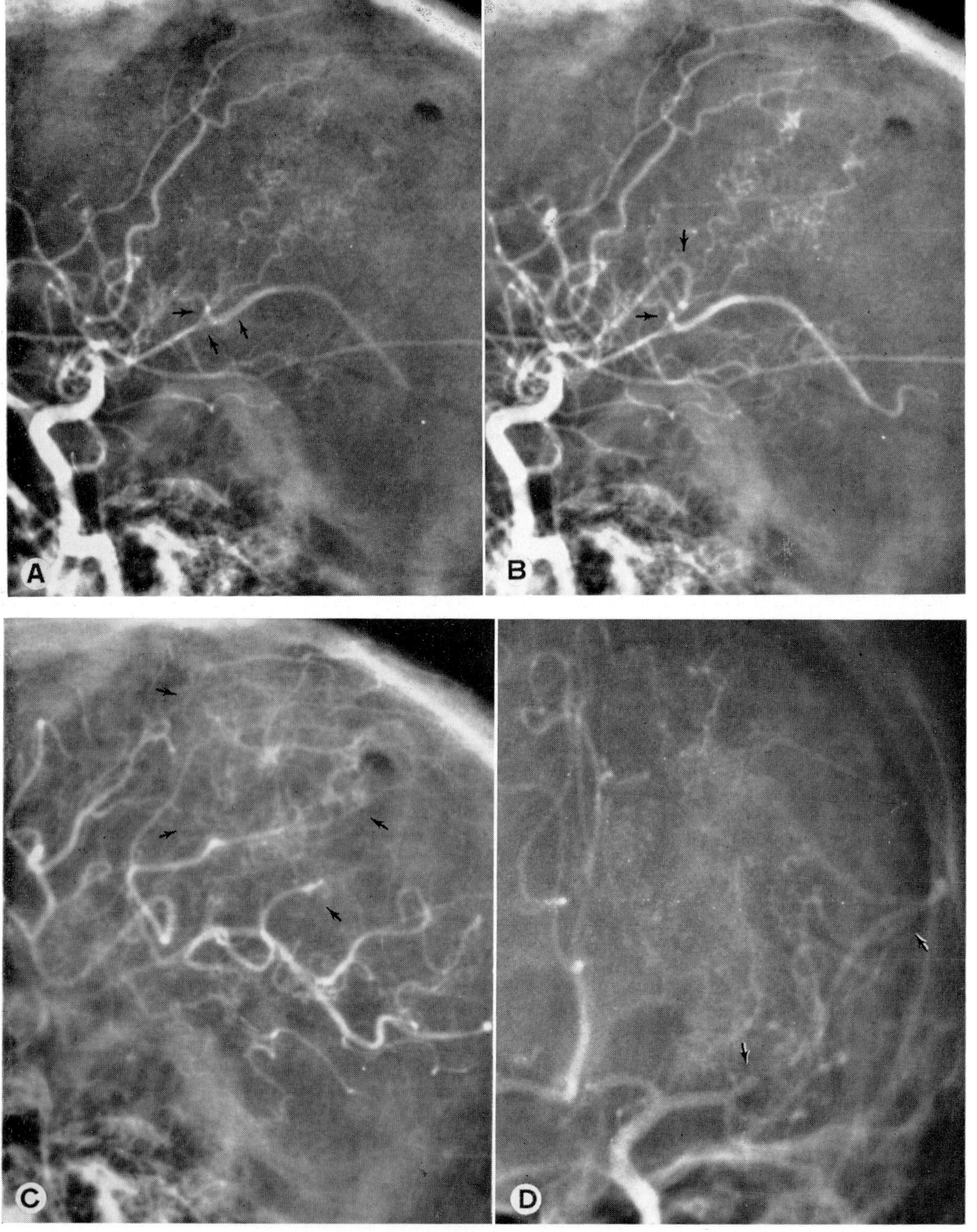

FIG. 561.—CIRCULATION FROM THE EXTERNAL TO THE INTERNAL CAROTID ARTERY THROUGH THE *RETE MIRABILE* MECHANISM

The first film (A) demonstrates direct connection between a branch of an enlarged middle meningeal artery with an important branch of the middle cerebral artery (*arrows*). From this point it is possible to trace on the next film (B) flow proximal to this vessel which indicates that this was indeed the point of connection between the external and the internal circulation. Other connections could also be seen but not as clearly as the one shown here. There are numerous fine vessels particularly involving the deep circulation. In fact, similar to the case shown in Fig. 560, there is a "corona" of fine vessels around each one of the larger vessels representing dilated arterioles. This has become more obvious in (C) where the appearance is quite prominent (*arrows*). The patient had had a severe stroke with a hemiplegia a year and a half previously. The hemiplegia improved and at the time of readmission to the hospital, he was brought in because of mental deterioration, loss of memory, and a general downhill course. Subdural hematoma was the suspected clinical diagnosis at that time. The anteroposterior projection (D) shows the interruption of the middle cerebral artery (*arrow*) with retrograde filling distally.

(*Revised 1963*)

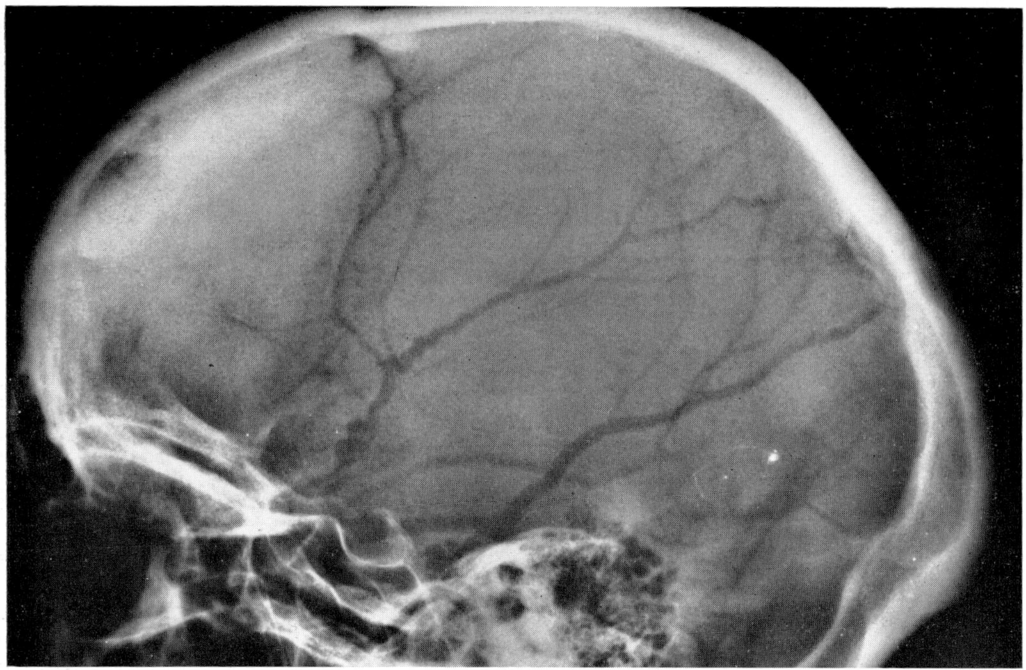

FIG. 562.—ENLARGED CHANNELS OF THE MENINGEAL VESSELS IN A PATIENT WITH OLD THROMBOSIS OF BOTH INTERNAL CAROTID ARTERIES AND COLLATERAL CIRCULATION FROM THE EXTERNAL TO THE INTERNAL CAROTID ARTERY THROUGH THE *RETIA MIRABILIA*

a result of the injection of improperly suspended Thorotrast which apparently had flocculated. The presence of anomalies of the arteries of the brain may tend to modify the clinical course in some cases (fig. 565).

It may be worth noting that in view of the difficulty of visualizing all of the vessels of the brain well, an obstruction in the cervical portion of the internal carotid artery may be accompanied by an intracranial occlusion without angiographic evidence of obstruction of any of the branches of the intracranial vessels when, indeed, the latter might be the direct cause of the patient's symptoms at the time of the diagnostic examination.

Cerebral veins and dural sinuses. Thrombosis of the dural sinuses is a well known cause of atypical stroke syndrome. As a result of obstruction of the sinus, there is a back pressure of blood in the cerebral veins which leads to hypoxia of brain tissue and even to hemorrhage. Sinus thrombosis may be the result of inflammation, usually following an infection of the mastoid or paranasal sinuses, or it may be associated with dehydration and cachexia, particularly in children. Venous thrombosis also may be seen in the postpartum period and in some cases may be associated with hemic disorders, such as polycythemia and sickle cell disease. Retrograde thrombosis of cerebral veins starting at the sinuses is not uncommon. In the case of thrombosis of the lateral sinuses, only intracranial hypertension may result. Extrinsic pressure on the sinus may produce the same effect (fig. 566). Slow occlusion of the superior longitudinal sinus by meningiomas may not lead to retrograde venous thromboses because it occurs slowly. Sinus occlusion may also result from direct invasion of the sinus by an adjacent malignant bone lesion; *e.g.* from neuroblastomas (fig. 567).

Carotid angiography may be used to demonstrate an obstruction of the dural sinuses, particularly if an increased amount of contrast material is used and compression

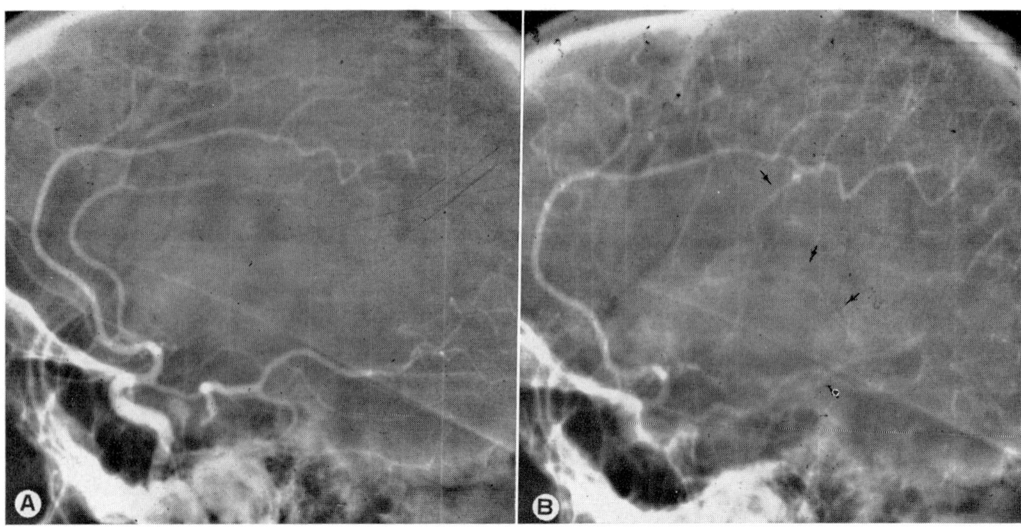

FIG. 563.—MIDDLE CEREBRAL THROMBOSIS SHOWING STASIS IN COLLATERAL CHANNELS FROM ANTERIOR AND POSTERIOR CEREBRAL ARTERIES TO MIDDLE CEREBRAL TERRITORY

The film made in the arterial phase (A) shows typical middle cerebral thrombosis with good anterior and posterior cerebral artery filling. A film made at 1.5 seconds after the injection (B) shows that the patient moved slightly during the exposure, but it demonstrates some further filling of the branches of the anterior cerebral artery with beginning filling in the territory of the middle cerebral artery (*arrow*). It is also noted that the basilar and the internal cerebral veins are well shown (*arrows*), indicating a rapid shunting of contrast substance through deep vessels to the deep veins. A film made at 3.0 seconds (C) shows further filling of the deep veins without any significant filling of the superficial veins as yet. There is visualization of only the branches of the middle cerebral artery which have filled by collateral flow from the anterior and posterior cerebral arteries. These look narrow and remained filled for the entire period of the examination, 7 seconds. It was felt that this represented cerebral shunting through deep vessels and generalized stasis within the collateral channels. The patient, a 30-year-old woman, died within several days.

of the side opposite the injection is carried out. Occlusion of the sinuses also may be demonstrated by means of a sinogram. Meningiomas invading and obstructing the superior longitudinal sinus may cause retrograde venous thrombosis, and this complication may modify the clinical picture of tumor in some cases. Trauma also is an important cause of obstruction of the dural sinuses.

SUBARACHNOID HEMORRHAGE

Arterial Saccular Aneurysms

General considerations. An aneurysm is an abnormal dilatation of an artery. It may be saccular, arising at a site of vascular bifurcation, or it may be a fusiform dilatation, involving a lengthy segment of a vessel. The latter type is seen uncommonly, affecting the intracranial vessels except for the basilar artery.

It is thought that the majority of intracranial aneurysms represent a congenital anomaly, presumably a congenital weakness of the vessel wall permitting localized bulging to occur. This contention is supported by the fact that the tunica media is absent in the region of saccular aneurysms and the internal elastic lamina is frayed or completely absent. There is considerable discussion in the literature, however, about whether only the weakness of the wall is present originally, with subsequent development of the aneurysmal sac, or whether the

(Revised 1963)

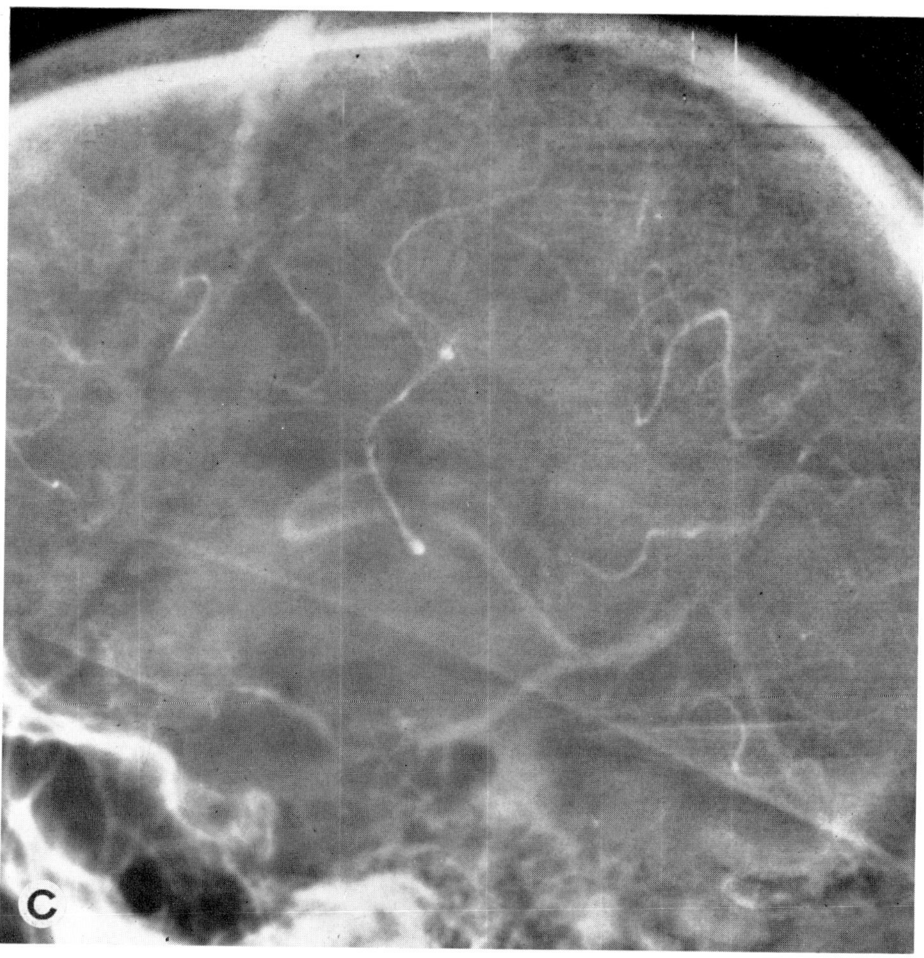

Fig. 563C

aneurysmal sac is actually present from birth. The factors responsible for such a localized weakness of the arterial wall are, of course, not known. The congenital theory is disputed by many, since there are multiple areas of relative weakness in the walls of intracranial vessels, and a higher incidence of aneurysms would, therefore, be expected than is actually found. The available statistics on the occurrence of intracranial aneurysms in children, however, indicate a low incidence. Children rarely suffer a subarachnoid hemorrhage. This could be due to infrequent rupture of aneurysms in children caused by short duration of disease and low blood pressure. Riggs and Rupp (1943) found 131 aneurysms in 1437 necropsy examinations of the circle of Willis, an incidence of 9 per cent. All were located in relation to arterial branchings. They found no aneurysms in the 102 specimens from children under 10 years of age. No cases of intracranial aneurysms in children were found in the 3000 brains of children from the Presbyterian Hospital (Housepian and Pool, 1958).

The congenital theory of the origin of intracrianial aneurysms is further strengthened by the embryological studies of Padget (1944) on the cerebral circulation. Many arterial channels that are seen in the fetus in the earlier stages of development later disappear. It is presumed that at the sites where these "experimental vessels" arose, a rela-

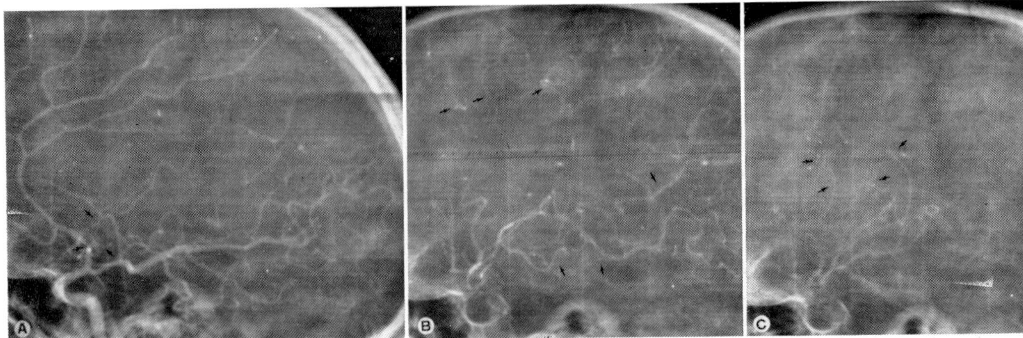

Fig. 564.—Middle Cerebral Thrombosis with Collateral Circulation and Local Stasis in Collateral Channels due to Cerebral Infarction

The film made in the middle of the arterial phase (A) reveals beginning collateral flow from the posterior and some from the anterior cerebral territory. It is noted, however, that the proximal portion of the anterior cerebral artery presents an extreme degree of local narrowing (*arrow*). Enlargement of lenticulostriate branches apparently originating from the internal carotid siphon is also noted (*arrows*). A film made one second later (B) shows now adequate collateral flow, mostly from the posterior cerebral artery with the anterior cerebral vessels supplying only the upper portion of the hemisphere (*arrows*). A film made at 5 seconds (C) shows collateral channels in the posterior frontal region which have not disappeared, whereas other collateral channels have disappeared (*arrows*). The venous phase is seen in the remainder of the brain. A film made 2 and 3 seconds later revealed the same degree of stasis in the area outlined by the arrows. This patient had a moderate degree of recovery following the initial severe hemiplegia.

tive weakness of the wall remains which may later become the site of a saccular aneurysm.

In support of the congenital origin of intracranial aneurysms is the fact that anomalies of the circle of Willis are commonly associated with intracranial aneurysms. Anomalies outside of the brain, such as polycystic kidneys (Sahs, 1950), and coarctation of the aorta (Baker and Shelden, 1936) are often present.

Other types of aneurysm are: (1) arteriosclerotic (probably a common cause); (2) mycotic (caused by emboli of—or containing—pathogenic organisms); (3) traumatic (extremely rare); and (4) luetic (probably a very rare occurrence, although it was previously thought to be frequent).

Saccular aneurysms are more frequent in women than in men. In Dandy's series (1944) of 91 patients, 50 were in women and 41 in men. In the series at the Neurological Institute, the incidence was 99 in women and 50 in men. Hamby (1952) reported 61 in women and 47 in men in his 108 cases.

The incidence of aneurysms in the general population may be in the range of 0.5 to 1.0 per cent. This is suggested by the data of Courville (1950), who reported 96 aneurysms in 30,000 autopsies, of which the brain was examined in 55 per cent; Mitchell and Angrist (1943) found 42 aneurysms in 36 cadavers from a total of 3080 routine consecutive autopsies.

According to Dandy, intracranial aneurysms are usually found in patients between 20 and 70 years of age, each decade containing about an equal number of aneurysms. Under the age of 20, and over the age of 70, they are much less common. They are quite rare in patients under 10 years of age; only four cases have been seen at the Neurological Institute in the last 14 years. Of 149 aneurysms seen at the Neurological Institute between 1957 and 1960, 108 (72 per cent) occurred in patients between the ages of 30 and 60, and 11 occurred in patients between ages 20 and 30 (fig. 568). Of a total of 313 consecutive cases of subarachnoid hemorrhage seen at the Neurological Institute there were: 177 aneurysms, 11 tumors, 28 arteriovenous malformations, 21 intracere-

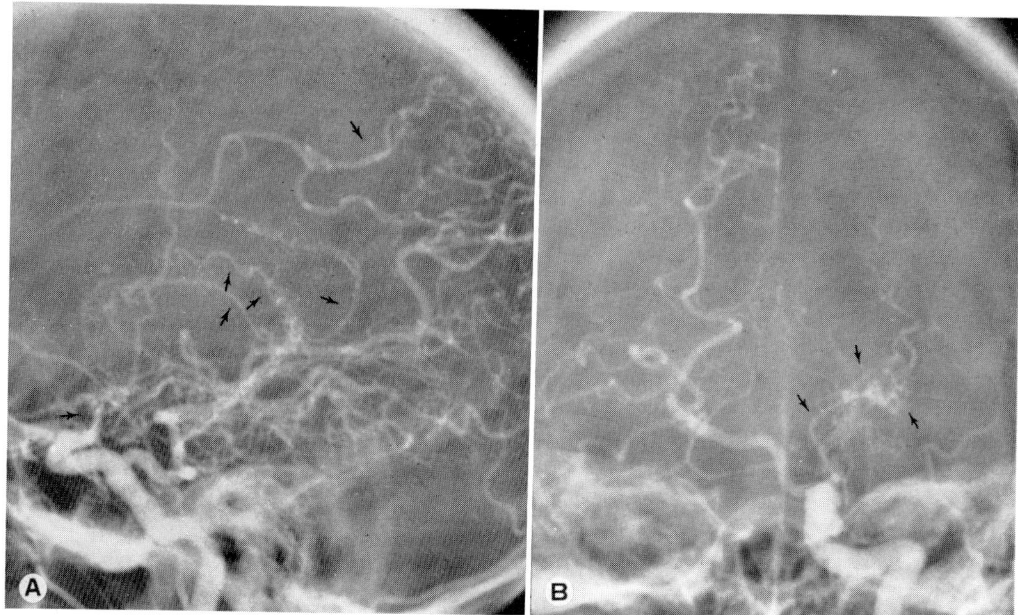

FIG. 565.—THROMBOSIS OF INTERNAL CAROTID ARTERY IN PATIENT WITH PERSISTENT PRIMITIVE TRIGEMINAL ARTERY

Thrombosis of the left internal carotid artery just above the posterior communicating is shown (*arrow*); the persistent primitive trigeminal artery resulted in filling of the distal portion of the basilar system (A). The right posterior cerebral artery is large and there is striking prominence of many small branches. The medial posterior chorioidal artery (*arrow*) is large and evidently serves as a collateral channel; the lateral posterior chorioidal arteries (*two arrows*) are dilated and tortuous. A conspicuous posterior pericallosal artery (*posterior arrow*) apparently supplies the territory of the pericallosal branch of the anterior cerebral artery; the latter vessel also fills by anastomoses with collateral channels (*upper arrow*), some of which are supplied by the parieto-occipital branch of the posterior cerebral artery. In the frontal projection (B) many small superior cerebellar branches supply the territory of the thrombosed posterior cerebral artery (*arrows*), whereas the prominent anastomotic channels are on the right. Subsequently, a right carotid angiogram was performed which disclosed that a thrombosis of the right carotid siphon also was present. The clinical findings were those of basilar artery insufficiency. (Courtesy of Dr. Faith Walsh and Dr. Franklin Reed, Morristown, New Jersey.)

bral hemorrhages (6.7 per cent), and 76 cases (24 per cent) where no lesion was demonstrated.

Aneurysms are usually situated in the region of the circle of Willis but may be seen proximal or distal to the circle. The majority are on the carotid side of the circle of Willis (approximately 80 per cent). However, the exact statistical incidence varies in the different series reported. McDonald and Korb (1939) reported 83 per cent incidence in the carotid system and 17 per cent in the vertebral system. Martland (1939) reported 71 per cent in the carotid system and 29 per cent in the vertebral system in a group of 54 patients who died of spontaneous subarachnoid hemorrhage.

(Revised 1963)

As mentioned above, aneurysms are usually situated at the sites of vascular bifurcation. When they occur at a site where no branch appears to arise, this may have been the site of origin of a branch present during embryologic development which later disappeared.

Aneurysms of the *internal carotid artery* are most commonly located at the origin of the posterior communicating artery. Less commonly, they occur on the anterior aspect of the carotid siphon at, or near, the origin

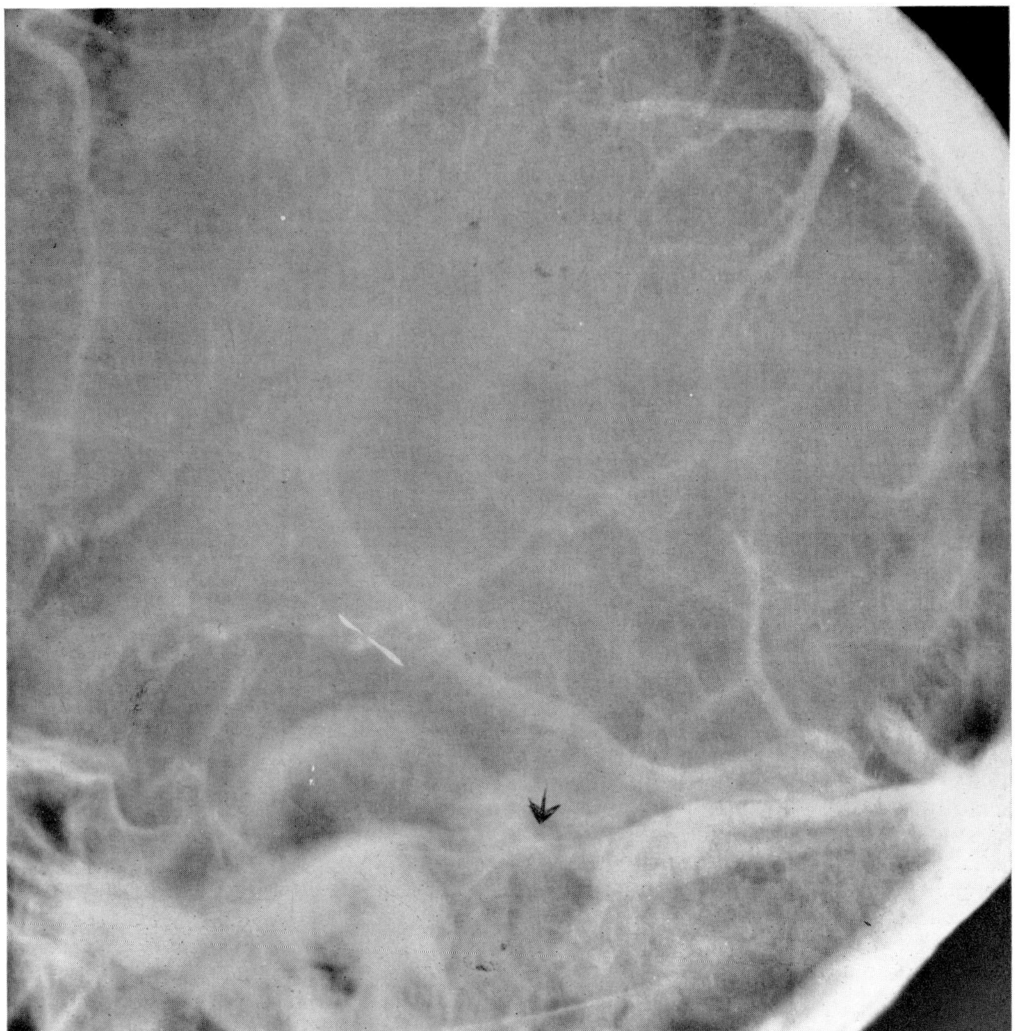

FIG. 566.—OBSTRUCTION OF LATERAL SINUS DUE TO EXTREME PRESSURE FROM MASTOID ABSCESS

The arrow points at the radiolucency in the anterior aspect of the lateral sinus in this seven-year-old child who had developed acute intracranial hypertension following an attack of acute mastoiditis. Surgical intervention revealed a suppurative mastoid and pressure on the sinus, but no sinus thrombosis appeared to be present. An appearance suggestive of obstruction such as is seen in this case may be encountered in normal patients at times.

of the ophthalmic artery; more distally, they are found at the bifurcation of the internal carotid artery.

Along the *anterior cerebral artery*, the most frequent site of aneurysm is at the junction with, or directly from, the anterior communicating artery. Sometimes they occur slightly more proximal, but angiographically they cannot be differentiated from an anterior communicating aneurysm. More distally, aneurysms of the anterior cerebral artery may arise from the pericallosal artery at any of the sites of branching (fig. 569). In the latter cases, it is not infrequent to find a common trunk to the anterior cerebral artery where the two sides join for a distance of 1 or 2 cm. and then divide higher up. Aneurysms of the distal arterial branches

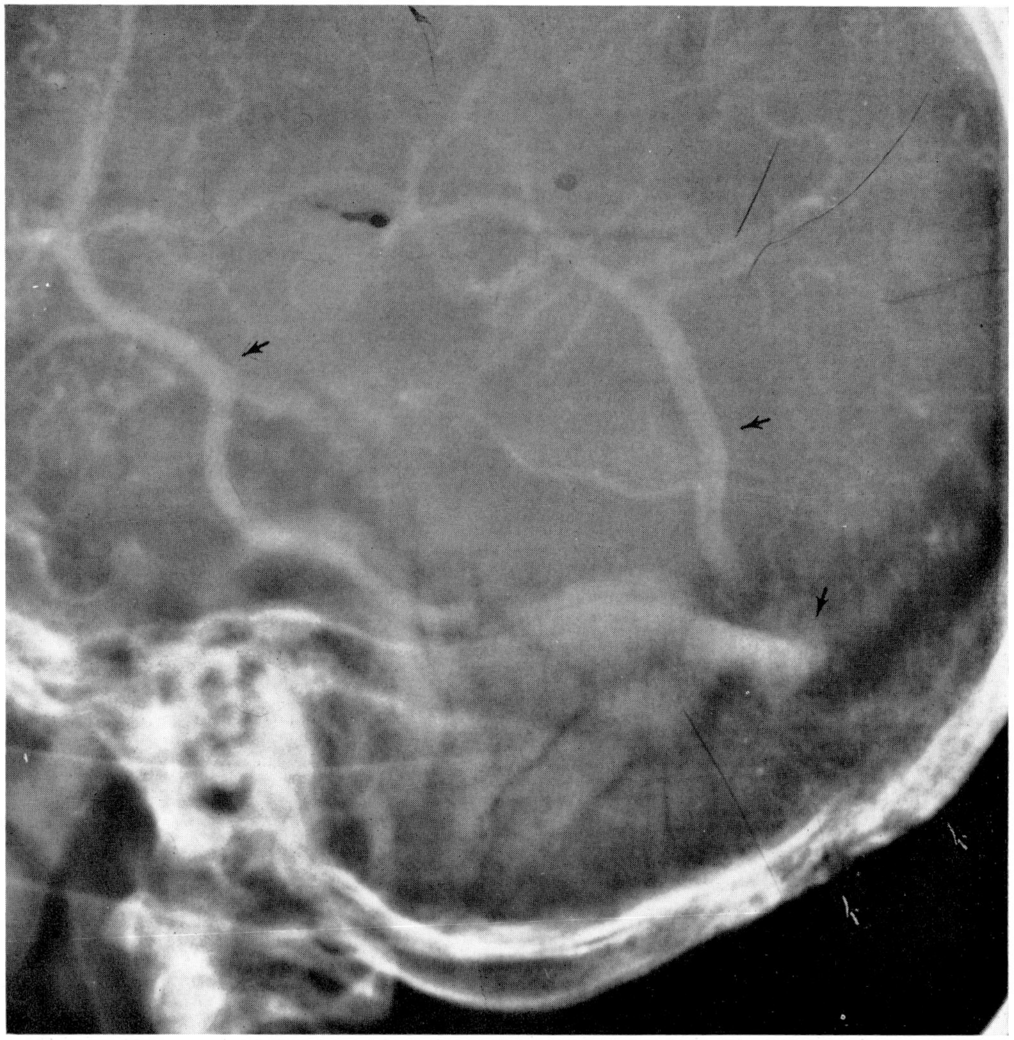

FIG. 567.—OBSTRUCTION AT THE TORCULAR HEROPHILI DUE TO INVASION BY METASTATIC NEUROBLASTOMA

There is irregularity in the occipital bone (*arrows*) indicating the site of metastasis. The posterior portion of the superior longitudinal sinus is not opacified because the contrast material is being shunted by way of the surface venous anastomoses to the lateral sinus. Two large veins (*arrows*) are seen to drain into the lateral sinus; one of them might be called the vein of Labbé. The child had developed marked increased intracranial pressure, and the angiogram was performed in order to visualize any intracerebral metastases; instead, the intracranial hypertension was secondary to venous obstruction.

are probably more truly congenital, in view of associated anomalies often found, such as a common anterior cerebral trunk (Potts, 1960). We have found two cases of aneurysms in children under 10 years of age in this location.

Middle cerebral artery aneurysms are most frequently situated at the site of the first bifurcation (fig. 578). Less frequently, they occur distally. Aneurysms arising from the trunk of the middle cerebral artery near its origin are difficult to differentiate from those which arise from the internal carotid bifurcation. Rarely do aneurysms arise at

(Revised 1963)

TABLE VI

Sex Incidence	
Male	50
Female	99
Total	149

Age Incidence	
0–10 years	1 (0.67%)
11–20 years	4 (2.7%)
21–30 years	11 (7.4%)
31–40 years	27 (18.1%)
41–50 years	44 (29.5%)
51–60 years	44 (29.5%)
61–70 years	16 (10.7%)
71+	2 (1.34%)
Total	149

Location	Number of Cases
Internal carotid	68
Anterior communicating	41
Middle cerebral	25
Anterior cerebral	9
Basilar and vertebral	5
Posterior cerebral	1
Total	149

FIG. 568.—INCIDENCE AND LOCATION OF ANEURYSMS IN 149 CASES SEEN AT THE NEUROLOGICAL INSTITUTE

the origin of the lenticulostriate arteries (fig. 539).

The *posterior communicating artery* is only infrequently the site of an aneurysm, except for those arising at its junction with the internal carotid artery; these are considered internal carotid aneurysms.

Along the posterior circulation, aneurysms may arise at the basilar artery bifurcation or below, from its trunk. The posterior cerebral arteries may give origin to aneurysms which usually are situated distally, at the site of the first major branching. Vertebral artery aneurysms may arise at the origin of the posterior inferior cerebellar artery, or higher, just before the two vertebrals join (fig. 570).

Multiple aneurysms of the intracranial vessels are fairly common. In Dandy's 108 cases, there was an incidence of 15 per cent. In Riggs and Rupp's material, the incidence was 21 per cent. At the Neurological Institute, the incidence was 24 per cent of 149 cases. We have seen as many as five aneurysms, demonstrated by angiography, on one carotid tree (fig. 571). Two patients of the 149 had saccular aneurysms and arteriovenous malformations. When an aneurysm involving the intracavernous portion of the internal carotid artery is found, the possibility of bilateral aneurysms becomes a strong consideration because such lesions are often symmetrical (fig. 572). The same applies to middle cerebral aneurysms.

Rupture of aneurysms. When an intracranial aneurysm ruptures, it may do so suddenly and completely. Blood escapes from its lumen, leading to what is termed clinically "spontaneous subarachnoid hemorrage." The blood may pass only into the subarachnoid space, or it may pass partly into the brain substance and partly into the subarachnoid space. The blood may, on occasion, be entirely within the cerebral substance, forming an intracerebral hematoma. Some aneurysms, upon rupturing, tear the arachnoid and an accumulation of blood may be found in the *subdural space* as well as in the subarachnoid space. Aneurysms of the anterior communicating and middle cerebral arteries are often associated with an intracerebral hematoma.

An aneurysm may rupture with extravasation of blood through the intima but not beyond the wall of the vessel; at other times a local thinning and bulging of the wall may occur without intramural hemorrhage. In these cases, the size of the aneurysmal sac increases rapidly and the patient may complain of headache, or there may be involvement of the cranial nerves which are adjacent to the aneurysm (fig. 573C).

Cerebral angiograms carried out as soon as the patient is brought into the hospital usually show the aneurysm, and only rarely has the contrast material been seen to spurt out of the ruptured sac. This was seen in one case during the second injection of contrast substance when it was not present on the first injection (fig. 573). In this particular instance, it is possible that angiography may

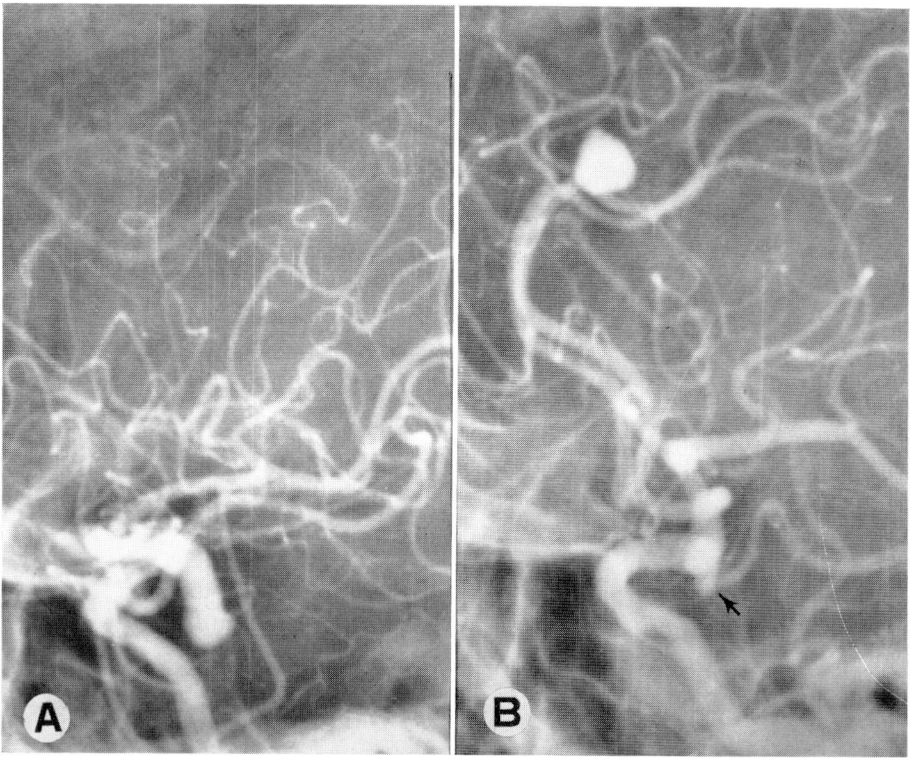

Fig. 569.—Multiple Aneurysms

On the right side (A) there is an elongated aneurysm of the internal carotid artery at the junction with the posterior communicating artery. On the left side (B) an aneurysm of the distal anterior cerebral artery is disclosed; it exhibits a punctum but there is no evidence of a local mass. A junctional dilation or infundibulum at the left posterior communicating artery also is present (*arrow*). Spasm of significant degree is not present on either side.

have contributed to the second rupture of the aneurysmal sac. For the most part, however, cerebral angiography does not appear to cause significant deterioration of the patient's condition when carried out at almost any stage of the clinical course.

It is very common to see arterial spasm in the region of a ruptured aneurysm. It is common, also, for all of the major vessels on the side of the lesion to be involved by spasm with poor filling of minor branches. Spasm may be seen affecting the carotid systems bilaterally, and the basilar branches as well when diffuse spasm is present; however, it often is most severe in the neighborhood of the bleeding lesion. In occasional cases spasm may be seen only contralateral to a ruptured aneurysm. The authors have found severe, localized spasm to be one useful feature in deciding which aneurysm has bled, when more than one aneurysm is present (see below).

A bleeding aneurysm often has an irregular contour in the angiogram (figs. 573 and 574). One or more pointed or rounded projections at the periphery of the lesion frequently are seen. Similar puncta, however, may be observed along the margin of aneurysms that give no evidence of having ruptured, even when examined by histopathologic methods. Contrast media within the lumen of an aneurysm that recently has bled ordinarily does not outline the point of rupture because of a coagulum at this site.

In cases where intracerebral bleeding has occurred and a localized hematoma has been formed, the usual signs of a mass may be encountered in the angiogram (fig. 575). Aneurysms of the anterior cerebral-anterior

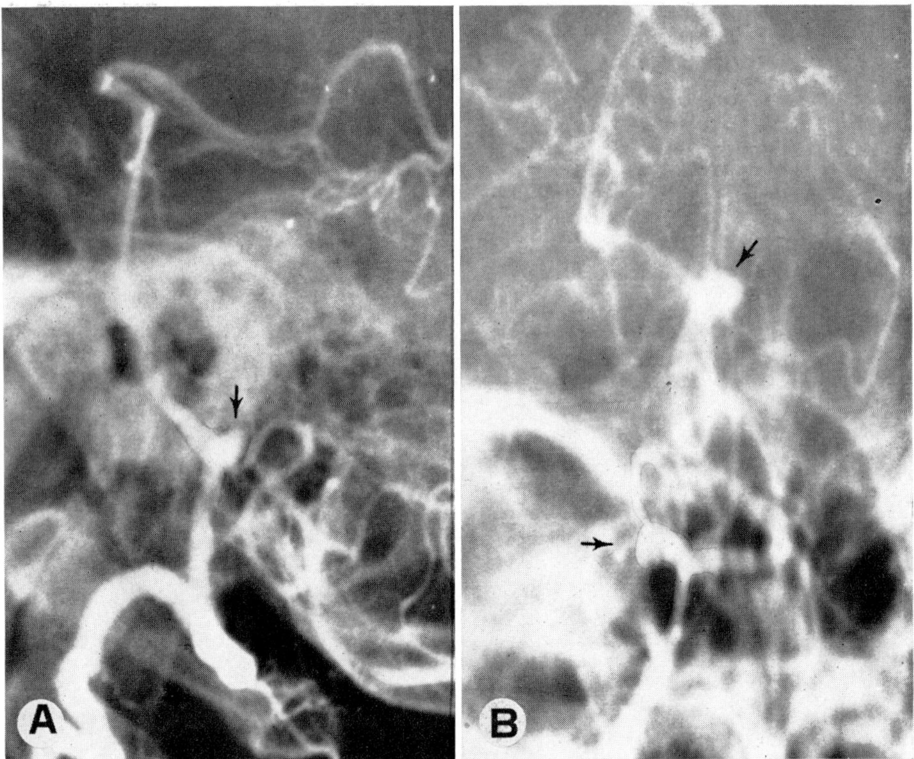

FIG. 570.—ANEURYSM ARISING FROM THE VERTEBRAL ARTERY AT THE ORIGIN OF THE POSTERIOR INFERIOR CEREBELLAR ARTERY

An aneurysm at the posterior inferior cerebellar artery points backward (*arrow*) in the lateral view (A). There appears to be narrowing of the lumen of the right vertebral artery proximal and distal to the lesion, with limited filling of the basilar artery and its branches. The frontal film (B) discloses a tortuous basilar artery with a rounded shadow suggesting an aneurysm at the bifurcation (*upper arrow*) but now shown on lateral view; superimposed is the medial branch of the posterior inferior cerebellar artery (see Fig. 385). The proximal aneurysm points lateralward, being projected through the petrous tip (*lower arrow*).

communicating artery junction rupture, not uncommonly, into the medial portion of the contralateral frontal lobe. Lesions of the medial cerebral surface elsewhere, not adjacent to the falx, may adhere to the opposite hemisphere and rupture contralateral to their origin.

Arterial narrowing indicative of spasm is seen predominantly in the first three weeks after bleeding of ruptured intracranial aneurysms. Thereafter, the incidence of spastic narrowing decreases (Fletcher, Taveras, and Pool, 1959). Spasm is much less common in the age groups over 50 years. Fletcher *et al.* considered this absence as possibly a manifestation of arteriosclerosis.

In considering further the problem of rupture in patients with *multiple* cerebral aneurysms, it frequently is not clear from the clinical standpoint which of two or more aneurysms has bled when a subarachnoid hemorrhage occurs. Desirable surgical treatment may be withheld or inappropriate treatment may be instituted. By studying a large group of patients who had multiple aneurysms demonstrated in life by angiography and who eventually had necropsy examination of the various cerebral aneurysms, it has been possible to develop radiologic criteria that serve to identify the ruptured lesion in a very high percentage of cases (Wood, 1963). In many patients the rupture of an aneurysm is followed by the development of a subarachnoid, an intra-

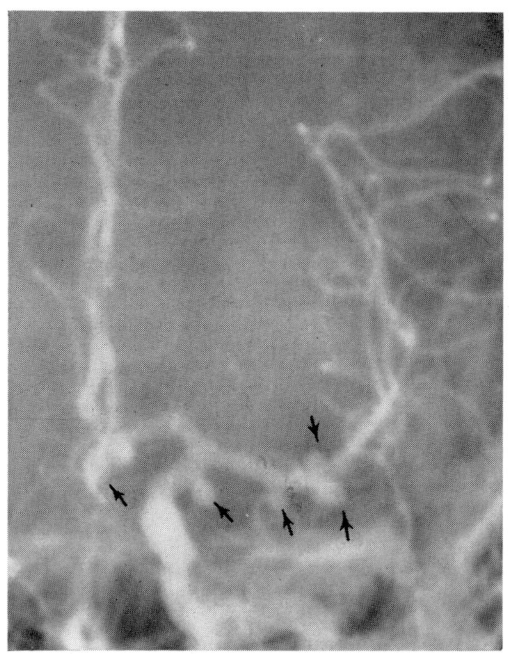

FIG. 571.—MULTIPLE ANEURYSMS DEMONSTRATED BY CAROTID ANGIOGRAPHY

Five aneurysms are visible in this patient on a single side, one in the anterior communicating, one at the posterior communicating, and three arising from the middle cerebral artery (*arrows*).

cerebral, or a subdural hematoma, or an edematous infarct may form; major or minor angiographic displacements signifying a mass may be found in these cases. In approximately 80 per cent of patients with multiple aneurysms, the offending lesion is indicated by angiographic evidence of a major mass or of a minor mass plus localized spasm of moderate to marked severity. In three-fourths of the remaining 20 per cent of cases features of the aneurysms, which include their size, configuration, and opacification patterns, will be helpful in diagnosis. In the vast majority of patients (85 to 90 per cent), as shown by Wood (1963), the following rule applies: the *larger* of two aneurysms, or the *largest* of more than two aneurysms, is the lesion that ruptures.

Radiographic technique. The first question to be answered is when to perform an angiogram on a patient who is brought into the hospital with a clinical diagnosis of ruptured intracranial aneurysm. Until approximately six years ago, angiography was not performed at the Neurological Institute until the patient had become relatively stable clinically. An effort was made, however, to perform an angiogram within the first 10 days following the episode of bleeding. Aneurysms tend to rupture a second time in a fairly high percentage of cases if left alone during the first three weeks following the initial bleeding episode. With widespread acceptance of prompt intracranial surgical treatment whenever applicable, angiography is now performed soon after admission of the patient to the hospital. Some modifications of this general policy have been necessary when unusual situations arise. Angiography is performed as soon as feasible in spite of the fact that some patients in poor clinical condition or who show evidence by angiography of marked diffuse spasm, are not operated upon immediately after the diagnosis is made. It is considered advantageous to have a correct diagnosis as soon as possible, in case the treatment policy has to be altered. It also has been found that angiography does not jeopardize the patient's condition, particularly if it is performed by an experienced operator.

The examination usually is performed under local anesthesia. Careful infiltration of the artery in the neck should be performed, perhaps with even more care than in patients who have not bled. The technique used is identical to the routine previously described, as far as the introduction of the needle and the amount of contrast material injected is concerned.

Frontal and lateral serialograms are exposed simultaneously during the injection, and the anteroposterior view is taken in the standard angiographic projection (12 degrees caudad from the orbitomeatal line).

The films are viewed immediately, and additional injections are made if necessary. An oblique view with the use of a 25- to 35-degree rotation to the side *opposite* that being injected is taken almost routinely. The oblique films serve to visualize in another plane aneurysms shown on the preliminary films, as well as to "uncoil" the vessels, in case another aneurysm may be

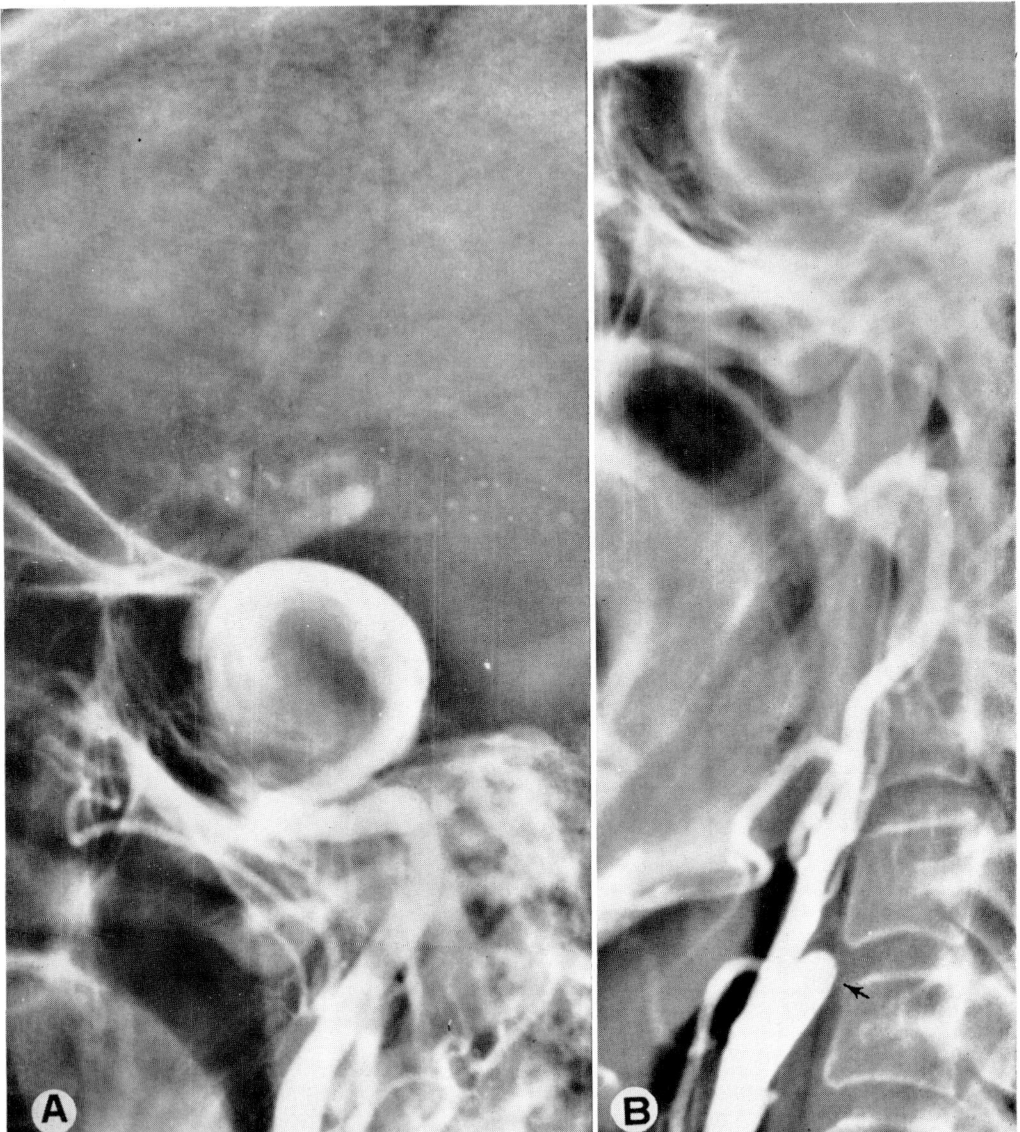

FIG. 572.—BILATERAL INTRACAVERNOUS ANEURYSMS OF THE INTERNAL CAROTID ARTERY IN A 52-YEAR-OLD WOMAN

The right-sided angiogram (A) shows an aneurysm arising from the intracavernous portion of the artery with eddying. The left-sided angiogram (B) shows thrombosis of the internal carotid artery in the neck (*arrow*). The sella turcica was considerably enlarged and rounded in configuration on both sides. It is thought that an aneurysm on the left side became thrombosed, and the thrombosis extended proximally in the internal carotid artery. The patient had a long history of difficulties; at age 25 she had had eye muscle operations and 2 years prior to admission she had ptosis of the left lid, which slowly improved. Her vision was 20–30 for the left eye, but she could only count fingers with the right eye. The patient had a blood pressure of 210/130.

hidden owing to tortuosity. The contralateral oblique view is essential for anterior communicating artery aneurysms (figs. 576 and 577). It is our practice to take a simultaneous oblique view in the anteroposterior and in the lateral projection by rotating the patient 25 degrees. In this manner, an oblique anteroposterior film is made and an off-lateral film obtained with only one injection.

Sometimes it is necessary to rotate the patient to the same side as that being injected. This is particularly important for aneurysms in the region of the posterior communicating artery which, in the frontal projection, are seen to project posteriorly and medially. In these cases, an oblique view made rotating the head toward the opposite side actually obscures the origin of the aneurysm further.

Orbital views are useful to study the horizontal portion and genu of the middle cerebral artery, as well as the bifurcation of the internal carotid artery. A small aneurysm projecting directly posteriorly from the middle cerebral artery may be obscured by the trunk of the vessel in the standard anteroposterior projection, but may be shown well in the orbital films (fig. 578).

Axial views are usually obtained for studying the vertebral basilar system. They may be very useful in demonstrating aneurysms which are obscured by the mastoid shadows and petrous pyramids in the lateral projection. Anteroposterior half axial films are sometimes made in an attempt to visualize the neck of an aneurysm to better advantage. It is, however, a standard view for vertebral angiography.

In practice, if an aneurysm is demonstrated along the carotid circulation, vertebral angiography is not performed, unless there is clinical evidence of a coexisting lesion of the posterior circulation. If no bleeding point is demonstrated on bilateral carotid angiography, a vertebral angiogram is performed. It should be emphasized that an aneurysm arising at the origin of the posterior inferior cerebellar artery may not be shown on angiography of the opposite side unless adequate regurgitation occurs proximally into the involved vertebral artery. Under certain circumstances, therefore, it may be necessary to perform bilateral vertebral angiography, in order to be absolutely certain of the absence of an aneurysm in this location. Since bilateral percutaneous puncture of the vertebral artery at the same sitting is not advisable, the other side may be visualized by way of a subclavian or a retrograde brachial angiogram.

Compression of the side on which an aneurysm is present, when the opposite carotid artery is being injected, is performed in order to determine whether or not the opposite artery is capable of filling both anterior and both middle cerebral arteries. The practice is valuable, also, to determine how much filling of the aneurysm can take place from the opposite side. Bilateral angiography is always performed in aneurysms arising from the carotid system.

Inasmuch as angiography is performed with an intent to apply the proper surgical treatment, a study of the exact relationship of the vessels to the aneurysmal wall is essential. An effort should be made to determine this point before removing the needle. Some cases require several injections before a complete study is made. It is in this type of case that simultaneous biplane angiography is extremely useful, not only by shortening the time of the examination but also by diminishing the amount of contrast material that must be injected. Ten minutes should be allowed to elapse between successive injections and, at our institution, no more than seven injections are performed under any circumstances. In the last several years, since simultaneous biplane angiographic equipment has been installed, no case has received more than four injections of 8 cc. of contrast material.

Radiologic diagnosis. The actual angiographic diagnosis of an aneurysm is extremely easy, once it has been demonstrated on films made in proper projections. Aneurysms may be overlooked if all the vessels are not carefully scrutinized in frontal and lateral projections; an error also may result when poorly visualized arteries are not studied further by making a second injection and rotating the head in the most desirable direction to uncoil a loop of the vessel. A

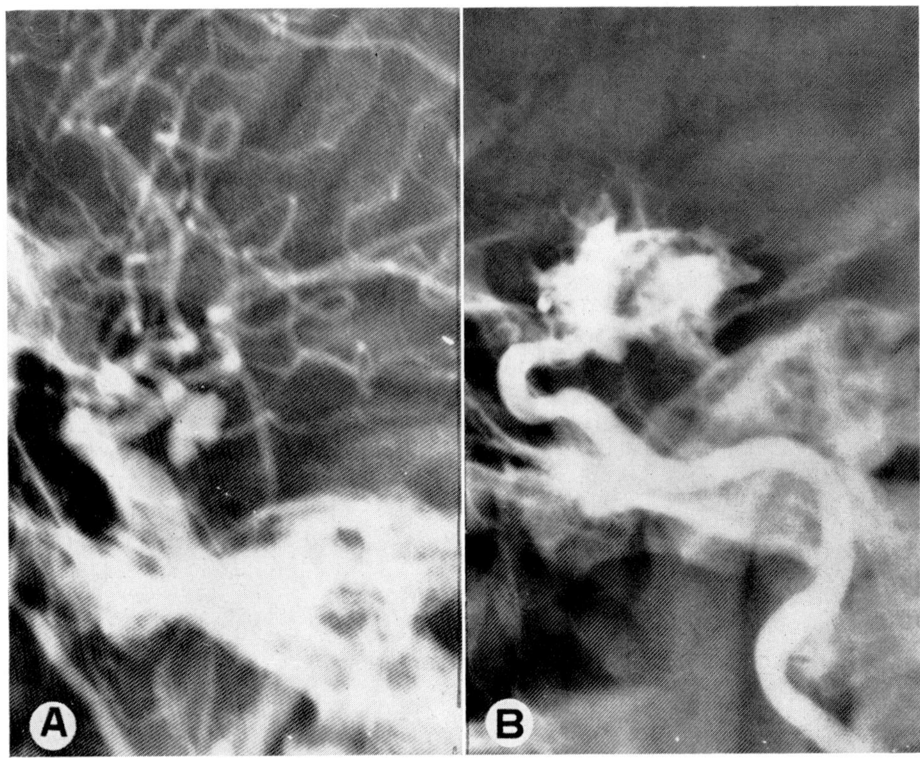

FIG. 573.—ANEURYSM SHOWING RUPTURE DURING ANGIOGRAPHY

An injection on the right side disclosed an aneurysm arising at the junction of the posterior communicating artery with the internal carotid artery. When the opposite side was opacified to complete the routine bilateral carotid examination, another aneurysm at the same location on the left was disclosed (A). A second injection then was made on the right at the same sitting (B); at that time the aneurysm was found to have ruptured and the contrast material had extravasated. The patient died 48 hours later, following intracranial clipping under hypothermia. (Courtesy of the Veterans Administration Hospital, Durham, N. C.)

In another case (C) an aneurysm was demonstrated at the bifurcation of the basilar artery. Angiography performed 3 months later because of recurrent symptoms revealed that the aneurysm had doubled in size and had become bilocular (D); enlargement during a brief interval through the development of a new loculus indicates deterioration of the wall of the sac that may be ominous (see text). Ligation of the basilar artery between the posterior cerebral arteries and the superior cerebellar arteries was performed. Postoperative angiography (E) reveals filling of only the superior cerebellar artery and no posterior cerebral artery filling. The arrow points toward an enlarged inferior cerebellar artery. Previous carotid angiography had demonstrated that the posterior cerebral arteries filled from the carotid arteries bilaterally. Postoperatively, gastrointestinal bleeding occurred, probably due to involvement of the hypothalamus. Gastrointestinal examination at that time (F) disclosed an extremely large posterior wall duodenal ulcer. The patient recovered.

common error of commission is incorrect interpretation of a vessel seen on end, which may give the impression of an aneurysm. A segment of vessel seen "end on," however, is always denser than the same vessel immediately proximal or distal. Since the lumen of the vessel is visualized containing a column of contrast substance possibly 0.5 to 1.0 cm. in length, it obviously must be denser than the vessel itself which only measures 0.2 cm. On the other hand, an aneurysm which has approximately the same diameter as the vessel from which it arises should have the same density as the parent vessel (fig. 539). In fact, the density of the aneurysmal sac on films, with few exceptions, is usually less than that of an artery of the same diameter.

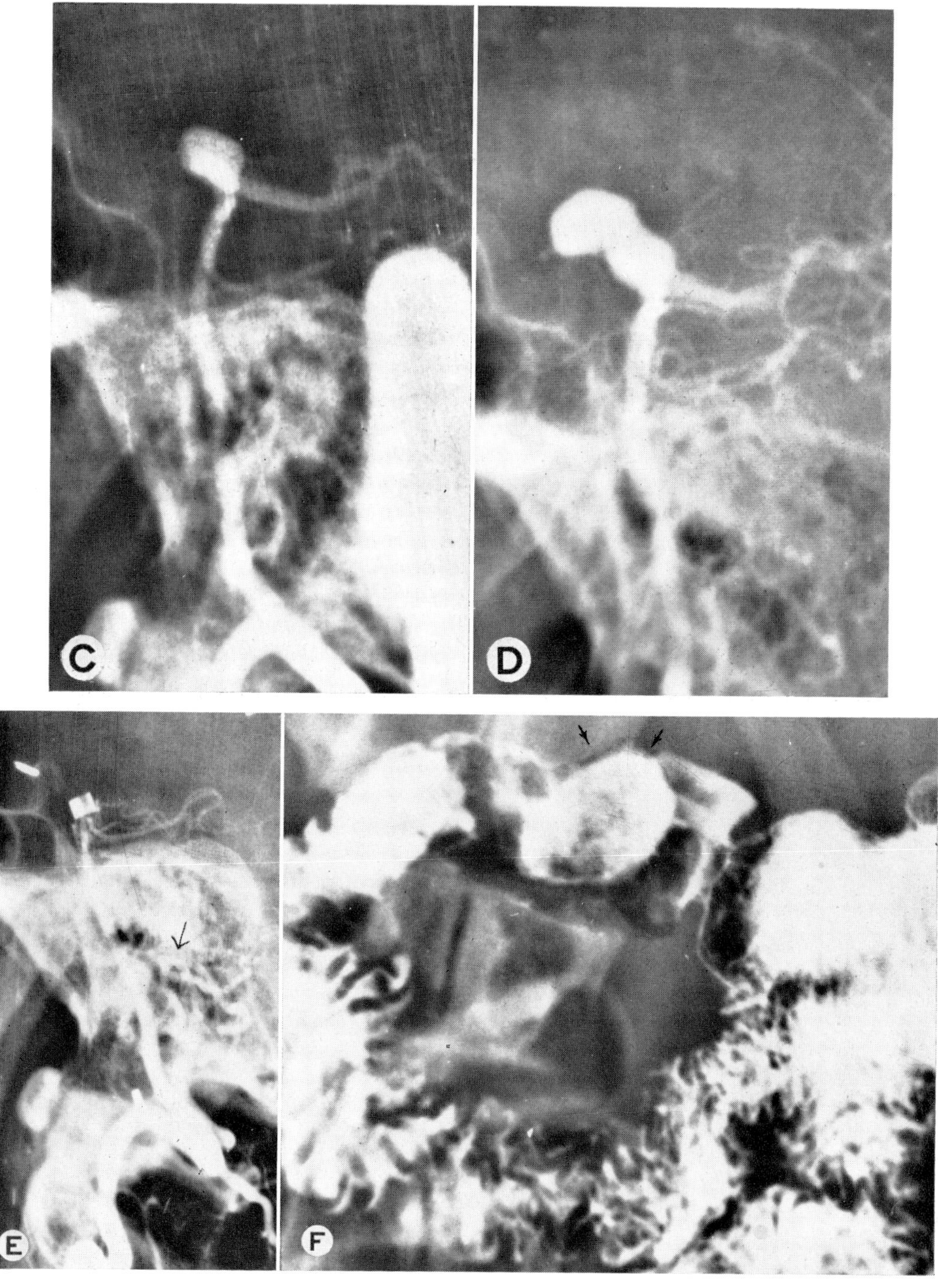

Fig. 573. C–F

Some aneurysms are not visualized on the angiogram even though complete angiography has been performed, including angiography of both carotid and both vertebral arteries. This may be due to spontaneous thrombosis within an aneurysm or to the extremely small size of an aneurysm. As one sees many cerebral angiograms, it becomes

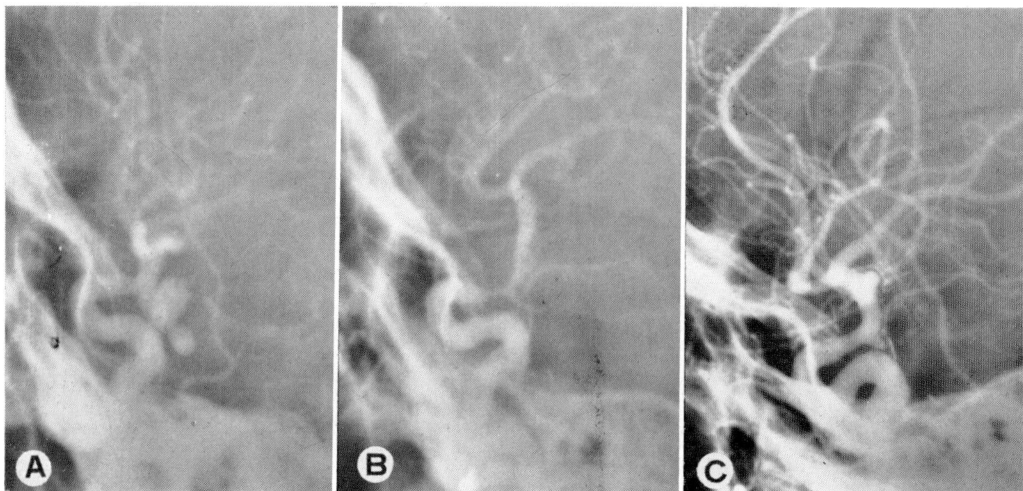

FIG. 574.—ANEURYSM OF THE POSTERIOR COMMUNICATING ARTERY WITH SPASM ON THE OPPOSITE SIDE INDICATING CORRECT SIDE OF BLEEDING

On the left side (A), the angiogram discloses a multilocular aneurysm arising from the junction of the internal carotid and the posterior communicating arteries. There is slight narrowing of the supraclinoid portion of the carotid siphon and very poor opacification of the distal internal carotid branches owing to spasm. An angiogram of this right side, performed at the same sitting, reveals segmental narrowing of the supraclinoid portion of the internal carotid artery and of several carotid branches; there is poor filling of the distal branches on the right, similar to that observed on the left. A second right carotid angiogram performed 1 week later (C) shows that the spasm has largely subsided, although areas of segmental narrowing are still evident; the peripheral branches are much better opacified than originally (B). At this time, a "junctional or infundibular dilatation" at the origin of the right posterior communicating artery was noted.

apparent that some arterial branches do not fill as well as others, particularly if the injection is made manually and the needle is placed in the common carotid artery. A stronger injection within a very short period of time, with the needle in the internal carotid artery, fills all the vessels more adequately. Under the former circumstances, it is possible to fail to fill an aneurysm that is present. It should be mentioned, however, that those patients who have had a subarachnoid hemorrhage, and in whom complete angiography fails to demonstrate the source of bleeding, have a better prognosis than patients in whom an aneurysm is found. This tends to indicate that angiography is a fairly accurate means of diagnosing aneurysms, and that when aneurysms are not shown on the angiogram, there is a good chance that they have been excluded from the circulation; this exclusion may persist.

The importance of routine serialograms is emphasized in the case shown in Figure 579. Compression films, even when adequate filling is obtained, cannot be trusted to rule out an aneurysm on the contralateral side (fig. 580).

Some aneurysms may exhibit calcification in their walls; others may produce local erosion of bone, particularly those in the intracavernous portion of the internal carotid artery. These changes have been described under "Intracranial Calcification" and "Local Bone Erosions."

Postoperative evaluation. Following ligation of the internal carotid artery for the treatment of intracranial aneurysms, certain observations of interest have been made in follow-up cerebral angiograms (Mount and Taveras, 1956). It was found very often that the clamp or tantalum band used to ligate the artery actually was not producing occlusion. Five out of six cases with a tantalum band applied, and five out of 28 cases with a Selverstone clamp applied, were found to have patency. Re-establish-

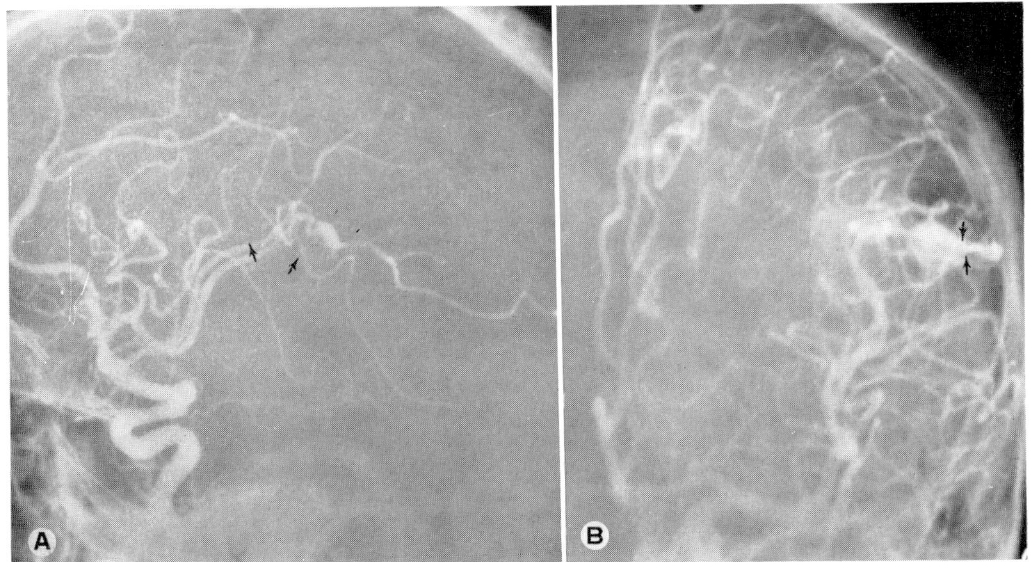

FIG. 575.—ANEURYSM OF THE MIDDLE CEREBRAL ARTERY WITH INTRACEREBRAL CLOT AND RUPTURE DEMONSTRATED BY CEREBRAL ANGIOGRAPHY

The lateral projection (A) demonstrates a partially thrombosed aneurysm (*arrows*) which only fills along one side. It evidently contains some clot because a very faint shadow of the aneurysmal wall can be seen along the opposite side (*lower arrow*). A marked degree of elevation of the middle cerebral branches with draping of the branches over the area of the mass, indicates an intracerebral tumor that is most likely a hematoma. The frontal projection (B) shows a streak of contrast substance extending toward the surface of the brain (*arrows*). This became clear in other films of the serialogram. Surgical exploration followed immediately, which demonstrated the aneurysm to be still bleeding. The patient recovered.

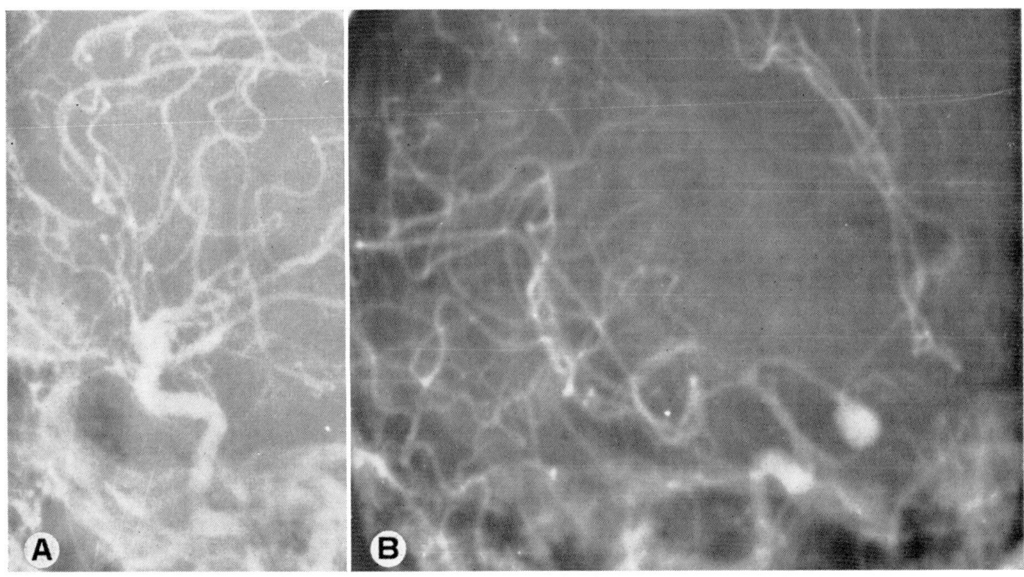

FIG. 576.—ANEURYSM OF THE ANTERIOR COMMUNICATING ARTERY BEST DEMONSTRATED IN THE OBLIQUE PROJECTION

(A) lateral view. (B) oblique view. Oblique views are necessary not only in the frontal projection but often in the lateral projection as well, in order to demonstrate the neck of the aneurysm free from overlying vessels and in order to study the exact anatomical relationship of the aneurysmal sac with the arterial branches prior to operation.

(*Revised 1963*)

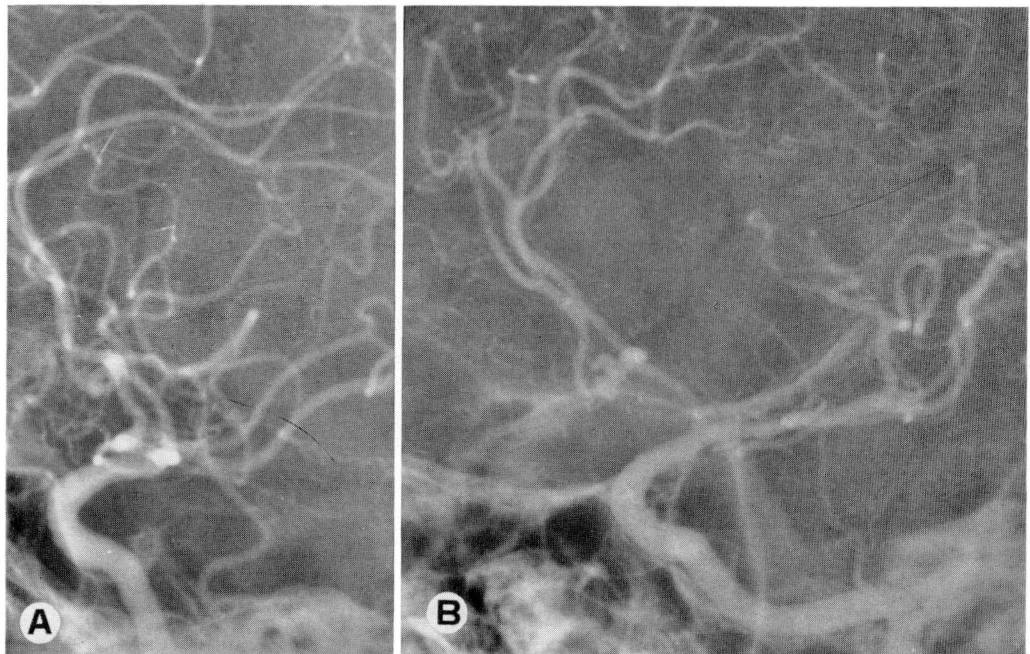

FIG. 577.—ANTERIOR COMMUNICATING ANEURYSM SHOWN ONLY IN THE OBLIQUE PROJECTION
(A) lateral projection. (B) oblique projection. Frontal projection is not shown here, but the aneurysm was not visualized.

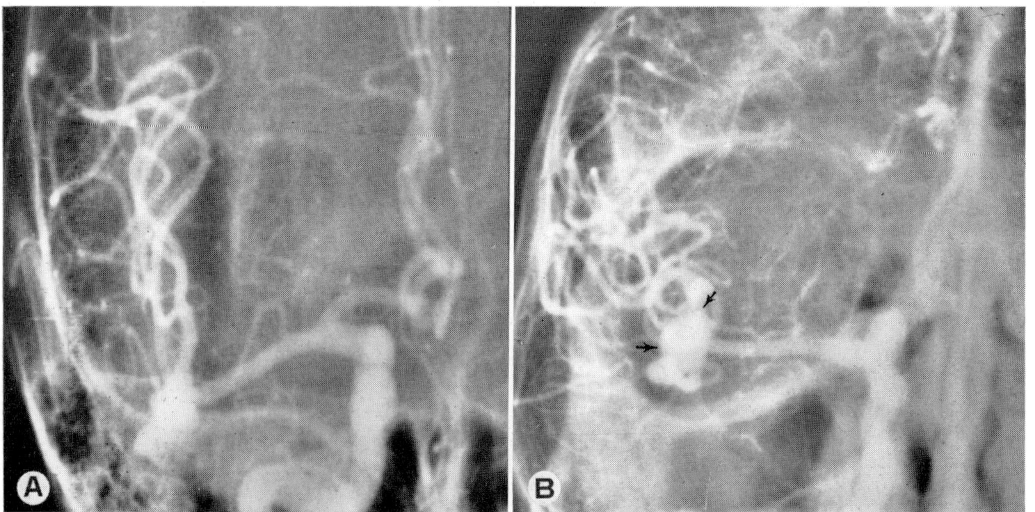

FIG. 578.—ANEURYSM OF THE MIDDLE CEREBRAL ARTERY SHOWN BEST IN THE ORBITAL VIEW
(A) standard view. (B) orbital view.

ment of flow through an area of ligation probably is due in part to the arterial wall undergoing atrophy over a period of time; the clamp that originally produced complete occlusion later produces only partial occlusion after atrophy. Another possibility is that circulation becomes re-established through enlarged *vasa vasorum*.

(Revised 1963)

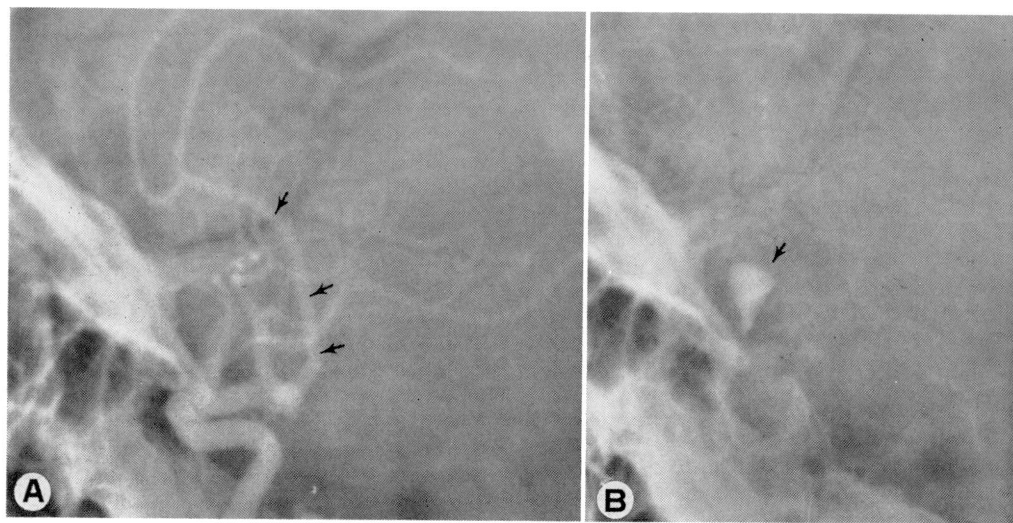

Fig. 579.—Aneurysm Arising from the Supraclinoid Portion of the Internal Carotid Artery

The arterial phase (A) did not show filling of the aneurysm. There is closing of the siphon, similar to that which is seen in a subfrontal mass, and elevation of the anterior cerebral artery (*arrows*). The aneurysm, however, did not fill at that time, but in the serialogram film made in the intermediate phase, at 3 seconds (B), the aneurysm had filled and remained filled throughout the venous phase. It is obvious that the aneurysm is partly thrombosed (it is displacing the vessels), but because of slow flow, it did not fill in the initial films. Again the importance of serial studies made routinely is emphasized.

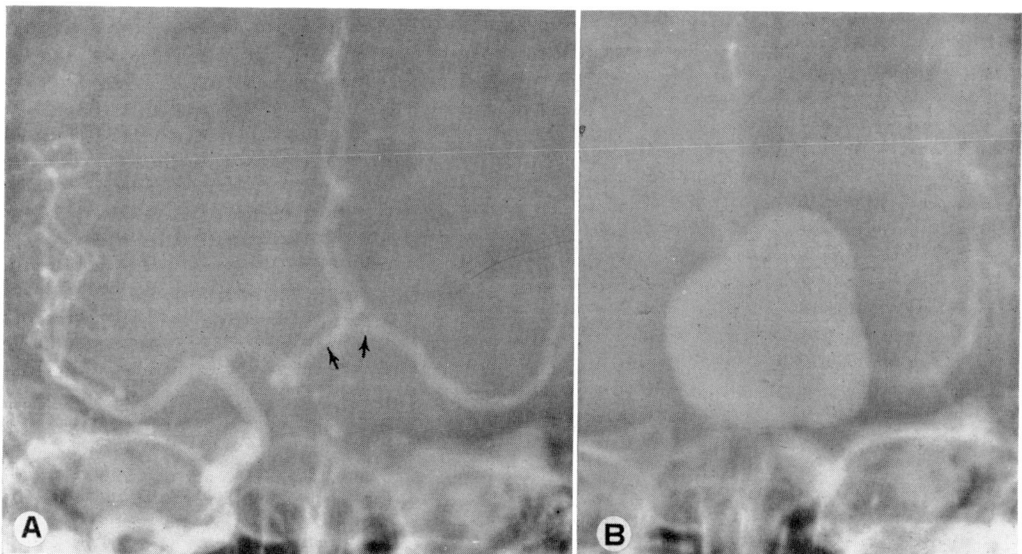

Fig. 580.—Aneurysm of the Supraclinoid Portion of the Internal Carotid Artery

The patient presented with a bitemporal hemianopia, and a pneumoencephalogram was performed first which revealed a suprasellar mass. Because of the anterior position of the mass, it was decided to do an angiogram. The right-sided angiogram was performed first and an anteroposterior film with compression of the opposite side was made which demonstrated the upward displacement of the anterior cerebral vessels in the midline. No aneurysm was seen. The left side was then injected, and this demonstrated the presence of a large aneurysm. (A) right-sided angiogram. (B) left-sided angiogram, frontal projection.

(Revised 1963)

In the cases in which the area of the previous aneurysm was visualized in the postoperative angiogram, disappearance of the aneurysmal sac was seen only with internal carotid aneurysms. The middle cerebral aneurysms did not disappear, although they usually became smaller. No anterior communicating aneurysms were included in this group of carotid ligations.

In cases in which complete postoperative studies (including vertebral angiograms) were carried out, it was noted that the anterior cerebral artery on the nonligated side usually supplied both anterior cerebral circulations; only occasionally did it also supply the middle cerebral artery on the ligated side. The vertebral-basilar system frequently was found to supply the middle cerebral territory on the ligated side; only rarely did the anterior cerebral artery fill from the basilar system. In one instance, there was retrograde filling of the branches of the anterior cerebral artery by way of anastomoses with the posterior cerebral artery. In this case, it is possible that there was an occlusion of the anterior cerebral artery which impeded filling by way of the opposite anterior cerebral; collateral circulation thus was established in a manner similar to that seen in thrombosis. The ophthalmic artery was usually visualized on the ligated side by way of anastomoses with the nonligated external carotid artery, when the clamp was applied on the internal carotid directly. In only a minority of cases was the ophthalmic artery sufficiently filled by way of the external carotid artery to outline the internal carotid artery and some of its branches.

Cases were reviewed in order to determine angiographic features which may indicate the patient's ability to tolerate ligation of the internal carotid or common carotid arteries. Several combinations of findings were encountered in the preoperative angiograms which were thought to have significance. It is known that whether or not a patient is able to tolerate ligation of the internal or the common carotid artery is dependent on the anatomy of the circle of Willis. Figure 395 indicates the configurations of the circle of Willis encountered in 1647 specimens, according to Hodes, Campoy, Riggs, and Bly (1953). As can be seen, a perfectly symmetrical circle is encountered in only about 18 per cent of the cases. The majority of specimens exhibited one or more components of the circle of Willis which were

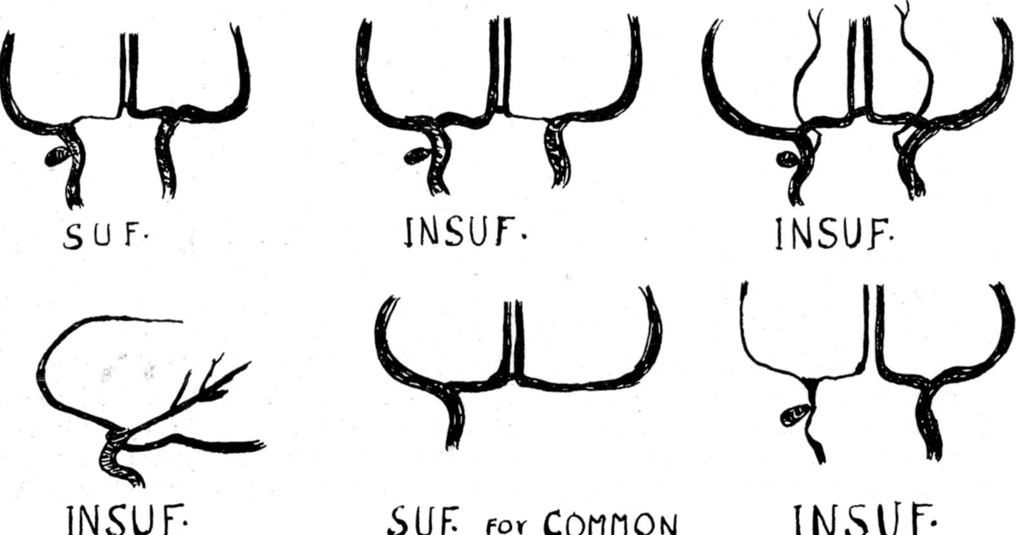

Fig. 581.—Diagram to Explain the Arteriographic Findings Which, Statistically, Were Found to Be of Significance in the Evaluation of the Collateral Circulation from Preoperative Angiograms in Patients with Intracranial Aneurysms

(Revised 1963)

hypoplastic, in relation to the other components. The pathways of collateral circulation will, therefore, depend to a significant extent on the relative caliber of the components of the circle of Willis, if the occlusion is in the cervical portion of the internal carotid artery. As indicated in the section on "Occlusion and Stenotic Lesions," the collateral circulation on the surface of the brain is more important in occlusions that are distal to the circle of Willis.

At the Neurological Institute, criteria have been found helpful as a guide to determine whether or not a patient is capable of tolerating ligation of the internal carotid or of the common carotid artery. The analysis pertains to bilateral common carotid angiography (fig. 581).

1. If, on the initial carotid angiogram, there is noted smallness of the trunk of the anterior cerebral artery on the side opposite the one to be ligated, this is evidence of insufficient collateral circulation; none of the seven patients who had a small or a nonvisualized horizontal segment of anterior cerebral artery contralaterally had sufficient collateral for immediate ligation of the internal carotid artery. Smallness of the horizontal portion of the anterior cerebral artery on the side of the aneurysm is not

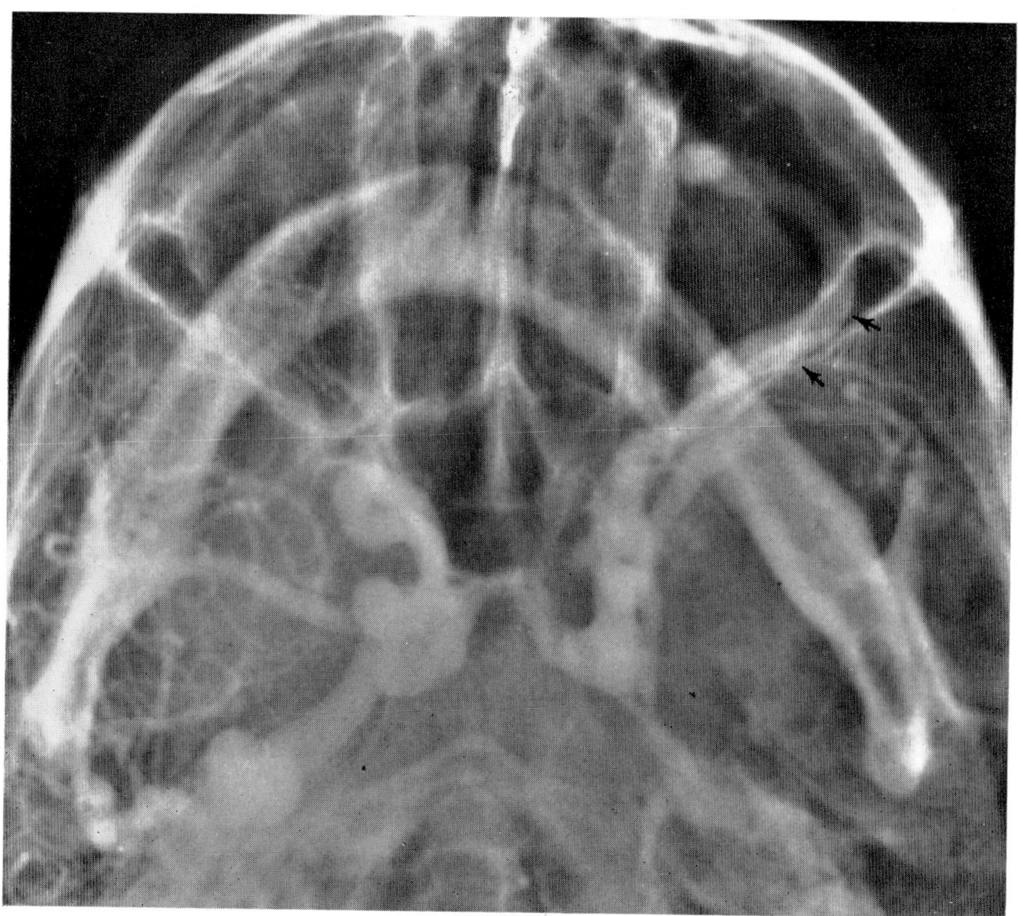

FIG. 582. CAROTID CAVERNOUS FISTULA DRAINING THROUGH THE OPPOSITE OPHTHALMIC VEINS

The patient had a left-sided proptosis, and the left-sided angiogram was normal. A right angiogram was then performed, and the base view demonstrates the filling across the coronary sinus and drainage by way of the ophthalmic veins on the side of the proptosis (*arrows*).

(Revised 1963)

necessarily an indication of insufficient collateral circulation.

2. Bilateral demonstration of the posterior cerebral arteries is an indication of deficient collateral circulation; only one patient in five tolerated ligation of the internal carotid artery. Similarly, filling of both posterior cerebral arteries, when one internal carotid artery is injected and the other is compressed, is an indication of deficient collateral circulation.

3. Bilateral filling of the anterior and the middle cerebral arteries, when the opposite side is compressed, is an indication of sufficient collateral circulation for ligation of the common carotid artery. On the other hand, it is not sufficient grounds for ligation of the internal carotid artery; 13 of 24 patients did not tolerate internal carotid ligation.

4. Diffuse spasm on the side of the lesion suggests insufficient collateral circulation for any type of ligation while the spasm lasts. It is possible that if spasm later disappears, ligation may be carried out.

Two of the 31 patients that were analyzed had insufficient collateral circulation for carotid ligation, but showed no preoperative evidence of this deficiency based on the criteria just listed. In 29, the radiologic criteria of adequacy or inadequacy of collateral circulation were substantiated by postoperative results (Mount and Taveras, 1960).

At another of our institutions it was found that anatomic variants did not play such an important role when *common carotid* artery ligation alone was employed. Pathologic specimens of a large number of patients dying of cerebral infarction following rupture of an aneurysm were reviewed; it was found that smallness or largeness of segments of the circle of Willis could not be related to the development of infarction.

Vasal size and filling, therefore, were demonstrated not to be as important in the prediction of infarction after ligation as the angiographic changes listed below.

1. The presence of a hematoma, whether subarachnoid, intracerebral, or subdural, is a very significant factor in the development of infarction, owing to ischemia produced by stretching and compression of arteries, particularly the ganglionic branches.

2. Spasm was observed in a high percentage of patients developing either spontaneous or postoperative infarction, as in the Neurological Institute series.

3. Narrowing of vessels by atheromatous plaques likewise was demonstrated more frequently in patients who subsequently suffered infarction than in those who did not.

It should be noted that clinical considerations (age, state of consciousness, blood pressure, etc.) are more important than angiographic changes in predicting adverse reactions to ligation.

Arteriovenous Lesions

Fistulae. An arteriovenous fistula is a condition resulting from direct communication between an artery and an adjacent vein. The lesions are most often the result of an injury. Intracranially, they usually involve the intracavernous portion of the internal carotid artery; the fistulae may develop owing to trauma, as in 77 per cent of the cases, reported by Locke (1924), or they may result from spontaneous rupture of an aneurysm involving the intracavernous portion of the internal carotid artery, as in 23 per cent of the cases. The cause of a traumatic arteriovenous fistula in the cavernous sinus may be a penetrating wound produced by a sharp instrument or by a metallic fragment; most often it is secondary to a fracture of the base of the skull. Arteriovenous fistulae involving the smaller intracranial vessels, or the vertebral circulation, are rare; those involving the cervical portion of the internal carotid artery are not so rare.

Clinically, the most prominent symptoms of a carotid-cavernous fistula are pulsating exophthalmos and a bruit which is very annoying to the patient. These symptoms usually begin within 24 hours of the development of the fistula, but occasionally they begin several weeks or several months later (Dandy, 1938). In addition to these symptoms, the patient may present chemosis, extraoccular palsies, and loss of vision. Sometimes bilateral pulsating exophthalmos develops as the result of the presence of an anastomosis between the two cavernous sinuses. In one of our cases, flow through the circular sinus resulted in a pulsating exophthalmos only on the side opposite the fistula (fig. 582).

The carotid-jugular fistulae in the neck are usually easy to diagnose; in addition to a bruit, there is a pulsating mass felt in the neck. Only rarely do they produce exophthalmos.

The angiographic demonstration of an arteriovenous fistula is relatively easy. The contrast substance can be seen to leave the internal carotid artery in the early arterial phase of the angiogram. Filling of the cavernous sinus and its venous communications occurs ordinarily while the contrast material is still being injected. Thus, the internal carotid artery and internal jugular vein are visualized coursing parallel in the neck. There is reversal of flow in the ophthalmic veins, which ordinarily drain into the cavernous sinus, owing to increased intracavernous pressure resulting from the carotid artery opening into the sinus. Dilated, elongated superior and inferior ophthalmic veins usually are opacified, together with their tributaries (fig. 583). In some cases, other veins and sinuses are seen to participate in the runoff of arterial flow through the fistula. In one of our cases, the original angiogram demonstrated extensive drainage by way of the ophthalmic veins. Several months following ligation of the internal carotid artery, there was clinical exacerbation of the fistula. At this time, the angiogram revealed some opacification of the superficial cerebral veins (fig. 584). The internal carotid artery fills poorly distal to the fistula; there must be a relative ischemia of the corresponding hemisphere unless the opposite carotid is able to carry the entire load. Some blood from the opposite hemisphere also may be shunted through the fistula. Injection of a greater amount of contrast substance in any case suspected of having a carotid-cavernous

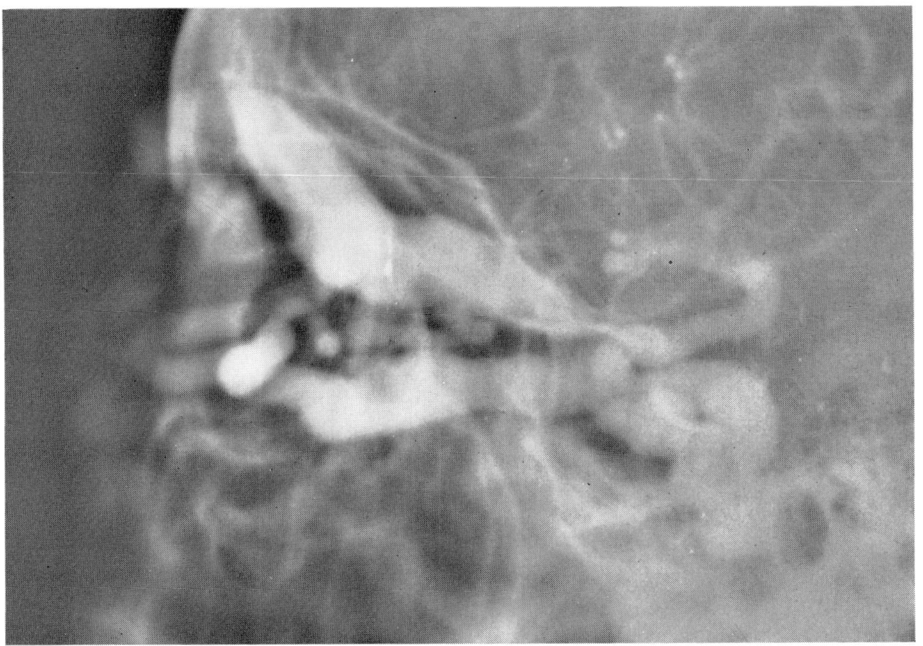

FIG. 583.—CAROTID-CAVERNOUS FISTULA WITH EXTREMELY MARKED DRAINAGE BY WAY OF THE OPHTHALMIC VEINS

There is much more contrast material leaving the cranial cavity by way of the ophthalmic veins than entering it to fill the intracranial vessels. Only the middle cerebral vessels are outlined with contrast substance. Due to hypotension on this side, both anterior cerebral arteries were filled from the opposite side.

(*Revised 1963*)

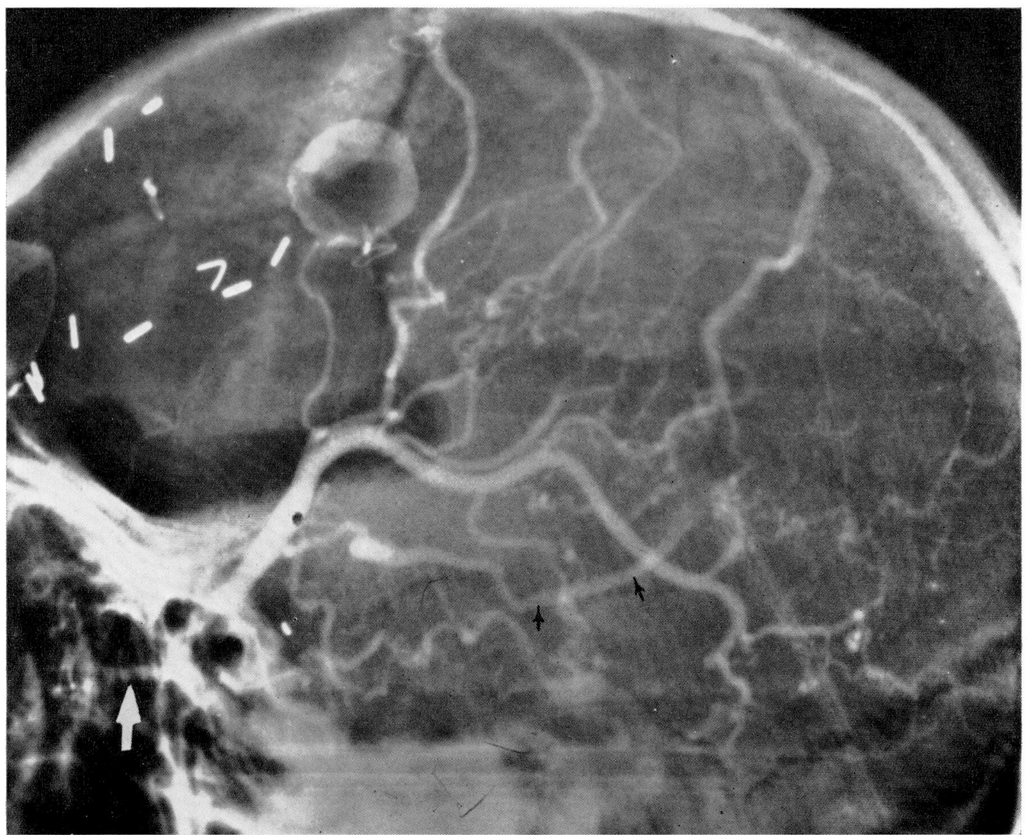

Fig. 584.—Recurrent Carotid-Cavernous Fistula

The internal carotid artery had been ligated in the neck and intracranially. Apparently, the clamp reopened in the cervical portion. At this time the flow from the internal carotid to the venous system takes place by way of the sphenoparietal sinus which then fills all of the superficial cerebral veins in a retrograde fashion. It is probable that the ophthalmic veins have now become thrombosed following their initial extremely dilated state. As a result of that, the blood is then shunted to the superficial cerebral veins and even to the deep veins (*arrows*). The anterior arrow is on one ophthalmic vein which is rather small in comparison.

fistula is advantageous since sometimes the ophthalmic veins are not well shown with the amount usually injected. The anatomic detail of the actual fistula may be best shown on rapid serialograms, particularly when the films are made at six per second during the injection and immediate post-injection arterial phases.

Full axial (basal) views may be useful in studying some carotid-cavernous fistulae to demonstrate the anastomotic channels between the two cavernous sinuses. A basal view permitted a diagnosis of the correct side of the fistula in the angiogram shown in Figure 582, while a pulsating exophthalmos clinically indicated the opposite side.

Following ligation of the internal carotid artery in the neck for the treatment of a carotid-cavernous fistula, there may be complete disappearance of the symptoms. Other cases require intracranial clipping of the internal carotid artery below the ophthalmic artery to prevent filling through the circle of Willis, and from the external carotid artery via the anastomosis of the ophthalmic artery. Even after this is done, recurrence of the fistula may occasionally take place. In one of our cases, filling probably took place by way of anastomoses between meningeal branches of the internal and the external carotid arteries in the cavernous sinus (Mount and Taveras, 1957).

Malformations. Pathologically, the malformations may be divided into (1) capillary telangiectases, (2) cavernous angiomas, and (3) venous and arteriovenous malformations (Russell and Rubinstein, 1959). The arteriovenous angiomas are by far the most common or, at least, they are the ones which can be demonstrated readily by angiography. It is possible that the lesions described as "capillary telangiectases" are overlooked in routine angiograms. If the lesion is entirely microscopic, it cannot be shown by ordinary angiography. Moreover, these lesions are more common in the pons (Russell and Rubinstein) and in this region they are extremely difficult to demonstrate with our present techniques. *Cavernous angiomas* lend themselves better to demonstration by cerebral angiography because some of them are large, measuring several centimeters in diameter; the vessels are increased in number as well as in size. The third category, that of *venous and arteriovenous angiomas*, may be subdivided into: *venous malformations*, *arteriovenous malformations*, and *capillary-venous angiomas*. The first are seen typically in the spinal cord and are similar to true varices (see under "Diseases of the Spinal Cord"). They are rare in the brain. It is possible that some, if not all, of these are actually arteriovenous anomalies in which the rate of passage of blood from the arteries to the veins is slow. Arteriovenous malformations are congenital abnormalities of the blood vessels of the brain which permit the rapid passage of blood from the arteries to the veins. The passage apparently takes place by way of anomalous, dilated capillaries. The third group, capillary-venous angiomas, are seen in Sturge-Weber disease, *i.e.*, numerous vessels are present on the surface of the brain, the majority of which are dilated capillaries or small veins.

Arteriovenous malformations may manifest themselves clinically by the production of convulsions and sometimes they may produce neurologic deficits, usually weakness of one or more extremities. At other times, they are encountered as acute clinical problems, following an intracerebral hemorrhage resulting from bleeding. The lesions are less common than arterial aneurysms. In the same period during which 149 cases of intracranial saccular aneurysm were seen, only 44 cases of arteriovenous malformation were encountered, of which two were associated with saccular aneurysms. Twenty-one of the cases were admitted because of subarachnoid hemorrhage. Bleeding from an arteriovenous malformation is more benign than the rupture of saccular aneurysms.

The venous angiomas and the arteriovenous malformations are indistinguishable pathologically, although physiologically they may be very different in the extent of the arteriovenous shunt. It is probable that the arteriovenous malformations grow over a period of time, as is the case with traumatic arteriovenous fistulae elsewhere in the body. The rate of growth is unpredictable, but some documented instances of growth have been reported (Tönnis and Schiefer, 1955; Potter, 1955; Svien, Olive and Angulo-Rivero, 1956). In the case described by Potter, angiography demonstrated the presence of a dilated venous sac which became much larger following a hemorrhagic episode. Whether growth of arteriovenous malformations takes place in this fashion—as a result of repeated rupture of some of the veins—or whether it is a continuous metaplasia cannot be stated at the moment.

Angiographically, arteriovenous malformations may be considered under several headings, as follows.

Arteriovenous malformations with extremely rapid circulation time. The classical arteriovenous malformation is one in which large draining veins are seen on the first film of the serial study, immediately after the contrast substance reaches the intracranial vessels. The draining veins appear well outlined with contrast substance and the feeding arteries are usually moderately or markedly enlarged and tortuous. What might be called the "capillary portion" of the anomaly varies in size. This area, which actually constitutes the anomaly, is usually obscured by the more spectacular appearance of the enlarged arteries and particularly

(Revised 1963)

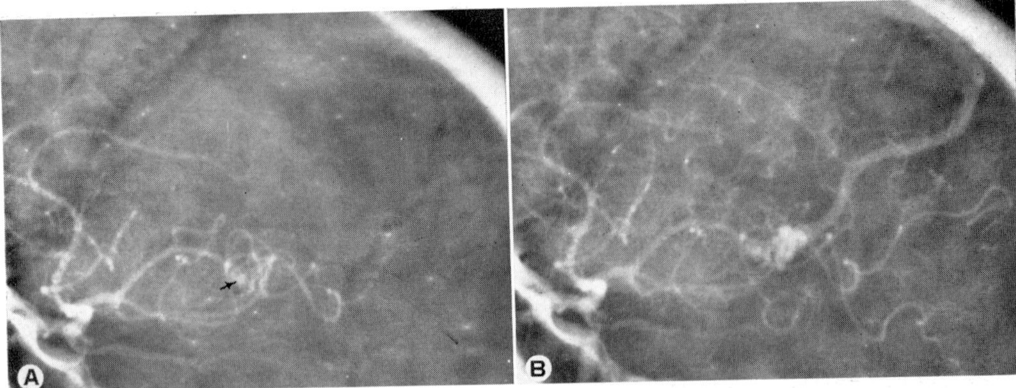

Fig. 585.—Arteriovenous Malformation without Significant Capillary Portion

The initial film (A) in the arterial phase shows possibly an enlarged arterial channel seen end-on or possibly a small conglomeration of enlarged arterioles (*arrow*). Immediately thereafter (B) filling of a vein could be seen draining into the parietal region.

by the draining tortuous venous channels on the surface of the brain. In order to visualize the true size of this capillary portion, injection of a small amount of contrast substance very rapidly, and rapid serial filming at perhaps six per second, is helpful. Sometimes, by injecting the opposite internal carotid artery, it is possible to obtain filling of the arteriovenous malformation with only a small amount of contrast substance by way of the circle of Willis. Since examination of the contralateral side must be performed routinely to determine whether or not any other lesions are present and what arterial supply is provided for the lesion, an opportunity regularly exists for capillary study of the lesion.

Some arteriovenous malformations are actually arteriovenous fistulas, in that the capillary portion of the anomaly is either completely or almost completely absent (fig. 585). In these cases, only a large vein may be seen, the origin of which cannot be determined; occasionally, an artery is seen leading directly into the dilated vein. It is not known whether such a lesion leads eventually to the formation of an arteriovenous malformation of the classical type. The arteriovenous malformations situated on the surface of the cerebral hemispheres tend to have a triangular shape, with the apex directed toward the depths of the brain (fig. 586). The disposition has something to do with the normal distribution of the vascular system of the brain; the veins usually radiate from the center to the periphery. There are actual connections between the central and the deep veins by way of very fine outward radiating veins, which extend through the brain substance (Kaplan, 1959).

Arteriovenous anomalies associated with a slight or moderate increase in the speed of circulation. This is a very important group because it is possible to overlook the lesion if an adequate serialogram has not been made (fig. 587). Sometimes only a single, relatively small, draining vein is seen. In this group should be included the "cryptic" arteriovenous malformations (Russell, 1954). They are small lesions which may bleed and produce intracerebral hematomas, and sometimes fatal hemorrhages into the ventricles. Usually such lesions are situated deeply, in or near the wall of a lateral ventricle. Niemeyer (1957) reported two such cases which were situated in the ventricular wall; they were supplied by the posterior chorioidal artery. The two patients had normal carotid angiography, but they were shown on vertebral angiography. Russell also found such lesions in the cerebellum. A few of our cases of spontaneous intracerebral hemorrhage exhibited abnormal, but ill-defined, vascularity; the cases could be considered as small arteriovenous malformations. Perhaps further improvements in technique will per-

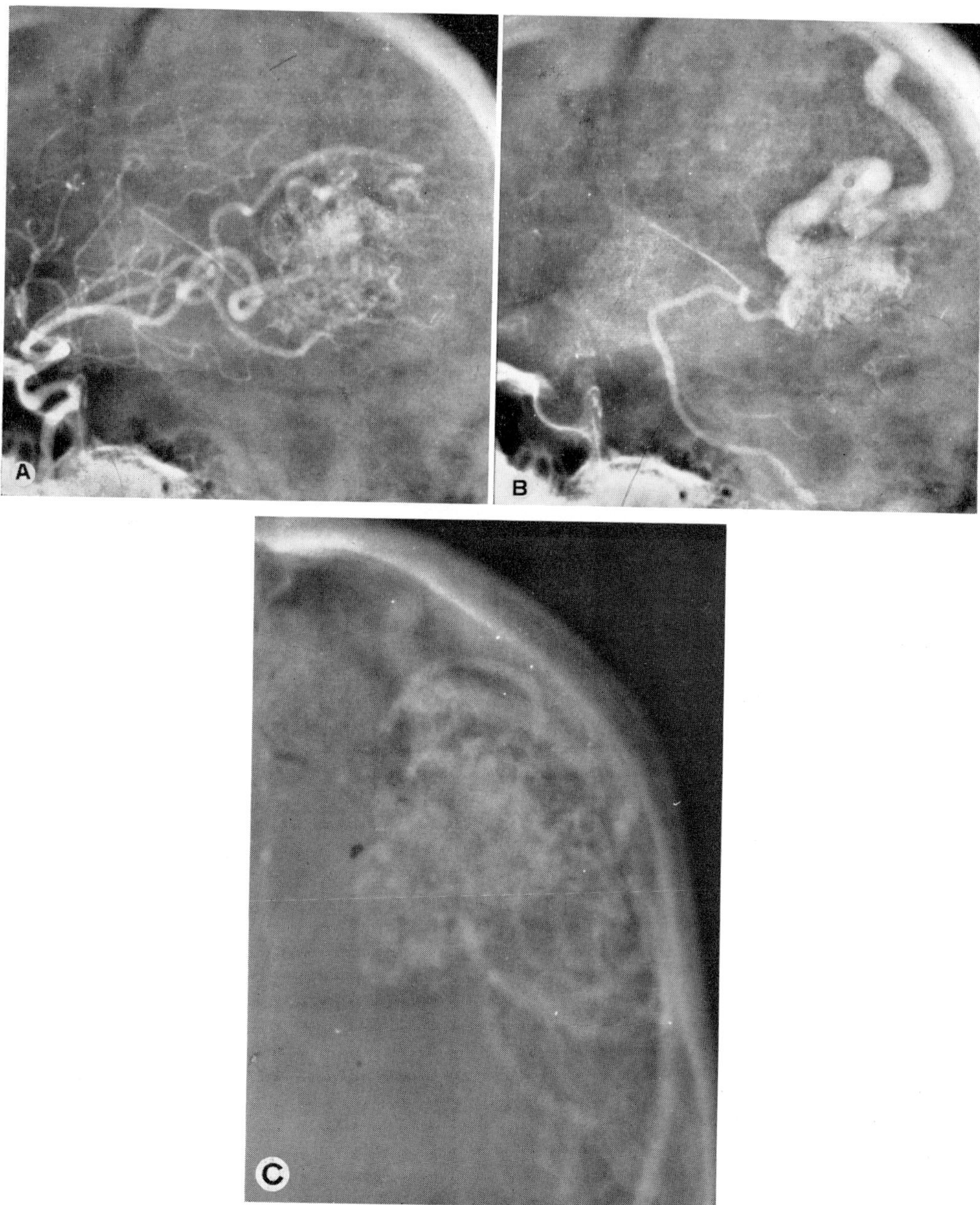

FIG. 586.—TYPICAL ARTERIOVENOUS MALFORMATION OF THE LEFT PARIETAL REGION DEMONSTRATING ITS TRIANGULAR SHAPE IN THE FRONTAL PROJECTION

(A) arterial phase. (B) venous phase. (C) anteroposterior projection.

mit the diagnosis of a greater proportion of these small lesions.

Vascular malformations without significant increase in the speed of circulation. In this group may be included (1) *Sturge-Weber disease*, (2) the so-called *venous angiomas*, and (3) the *cavernous angiomas*. Since the lesions of Sturge-Weber disease are capillary-venous angiomas, the angiogram may reveal a diffuse increase in density of the abnormal

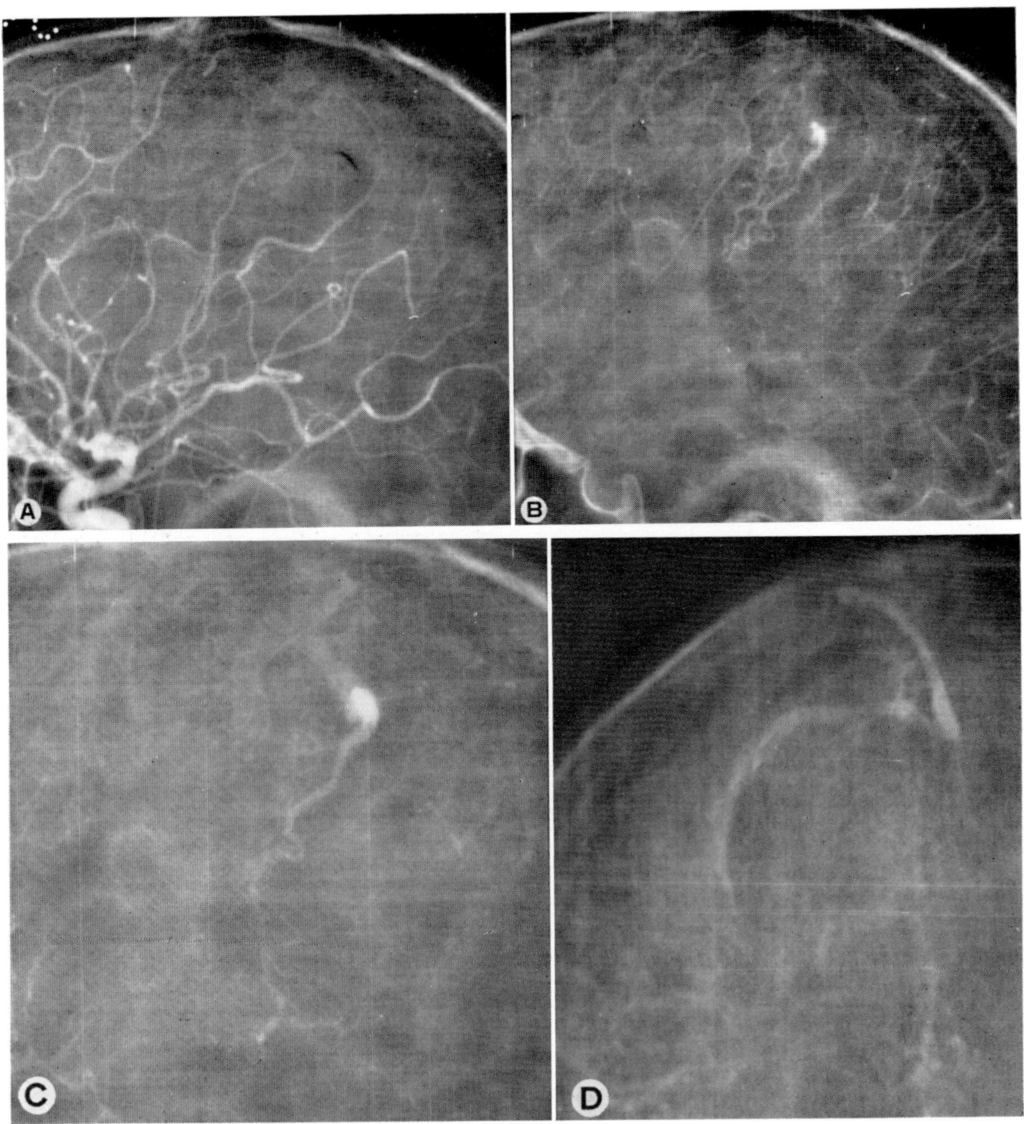

Fig. 587.—Arteriovenous Malformation without Increase in the Speed of Circulation through the Lesion

The film made toward the end of the arterial filling phase showed no filling of any abnormal vessels. A relatively avascular area is seen in the area later shown to have a vascular malformation. The film in the intermediate phase (B) reveals the abnormal vessels which in the early venous phase (C) reveals venous filling. Actually this film was made at 3 seconds after the beginning of the injection. The frontal projection (D) shows the draining vein through the substance of the brain by way of the midline superior cerebral veins. Large veins within the substance of the brain are always abnormal.

area; in some cases, large veins are seen coursing over this area of the cortex. Various types of vascular abnormalities have been seen in patients with Sturge-Weber disease (Poser and Taveras, 1957); thrombosis of major cerebral arteries, large veins coursing in unusual directions on the surface of the brain, and subcutaneous angiomas supplied by the internal carotid system.

The authors have not had occasion to see

angiographically a true *venous angioma* which was confirmed pathologically. Clusters of veins on the surface of the brain have been seen in some cases; one case, which was surgically explored, was thought to be a normal variant by the surgeon.

Cavernous angiomas should be quite easily seen by angiography; yet, they might be confused with other normal shadows in the brain, for these lesions are only rarely recognized. Statistically, they are more frequently found in the cerebral hemispheres, particularly in the region of the Rolandic fissure (Russell, 1954). They may occur in the region of the basal ganglia or in the wall of the third ventricle, and they may calcify.

Arteriovenous malformations involving the external carotid system. The group is important because the chief symptom may be a loud bruit which is most annoying to the patient. The lesions may be very small, and when they are found in the region of the petrous pyramid, the possibility of an early glomus jugulare tumor should be suspected. Arteriovenous malformations in the territory of the external carotid artery must be differentiated from glomus jugulare tumors. The chief differential point concerns the neoplastic portion of the glomus jugulare tumor which presents a homogeneous tumor cloud, in addition to large draining veins. The true arteriovenous malformations exhibit a fleeting demonstration of the capillary portion, which will rapidly disappear and be obscured by large draining veins (fig. 588).

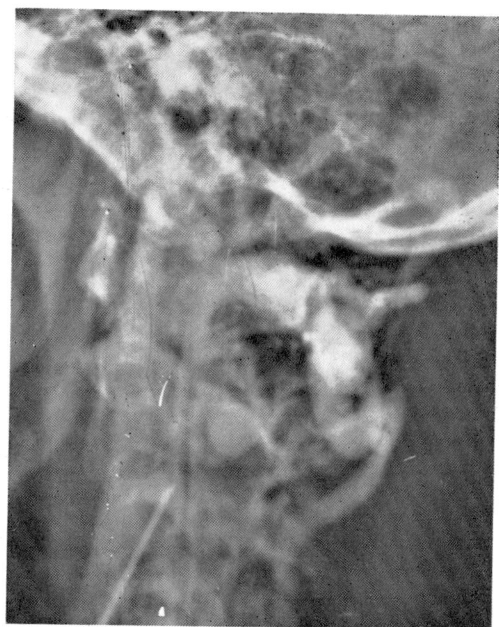

Fig. 588.—Arteriovenous Malformation in the Upper Cervical Region Supplied by Vertebral and External Carotid Arteries

Extremely large draining veins and dilated, tortuous venous channels can be seen, and there is no evidence of a homogeneous cloud such as is seen in glomus jugulare tumors. The location of this particular malformation is much more posterior than that of glomus jugulare tumors. The patient's symptoms were those of a bruit.

Postoperative angiography for arteriovenous malformations. If the arteriovenous anomaly is completely removed, the main feeding arteries, as well as the draining veins, return to normal size. Likewise, the relative ischemia of the brain on the side of the anomaly tends to disappear. If only partial removal of the malformation is accomplished, filling of some of the remaining elements will be seen; repeat angiography may show that the residual abnormality has become larger with the passage of time (Tönnis and Schiefer, 1955). Ligation of some of the arteries supplying the lesion by direct clipping will result in a decrease in size of the anomaly (fig. 589), at least temporarily. However, the arteriovenous malformation will not disappear and it probably will increase in size over a period of time, owing to enlargement of other available feeding arteries.

(Revised 1963)

Pneumoencephalography in arteriovenous malformations. If a pneumoencephalogram is carried out in patients with arteriovenous malformations, an area of atrophy with a porencephalic dilatation of the ventricle may be seen. If the lesion is more superficially located, cortical atrophy and irregularity of the air shadows of the sulci on the surface of the brain are present (fig. 234).

At other times, an arteriovenous anomaly is capable of producing pneumographic evidence of a mass lesion (fig. 590). An interesting vascular anomaly is that which has come to be called "aneurysm of the vein of Galen."

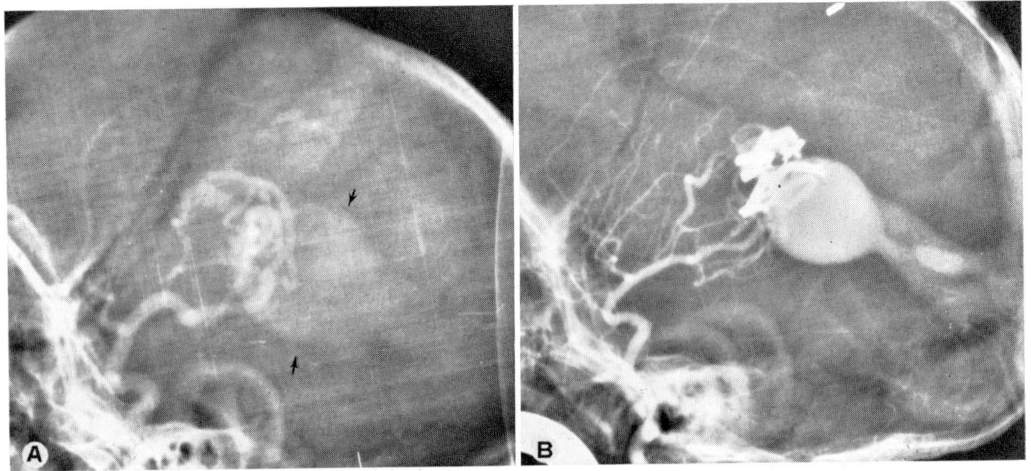

FIG. 589.—ANEURYSM OF THE VEIN OF GALEN WITH POSTOPERATIVE ANGIOGRAM

The original film (A) reveals that most of the contrast substance is going into the malformation and only a small amount is seen to fill the anterior cerebral vessels. No significant middle cerebral filling was seen anterior to the area of the aneurysm. The postoperative film (B), taken after many of the feeding vessels had been clipped, shows much improvement in the blood supply of the remaining brain, and the aneurysmal sac is considerably smaller.

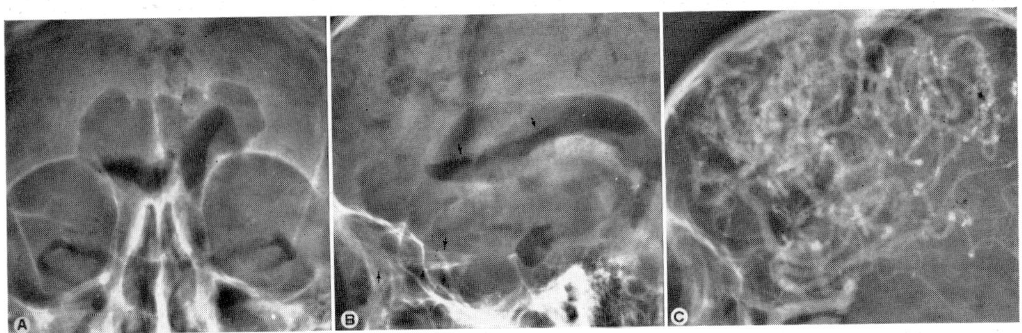

FIG. 590.—ARTERIOVENOUS MALFORMATION PRODUCING MARKED DEFORMITY OF THE VENTRICULAR SYSTEM AND ENLARGEMENT OF THE SELLA TURCICA

The pneumoencephalogram done first showed a marked deformity of the anterior portion of the lateral ventricles. (A) frontal projection. (B) lateral projection. (C) angiogram. There is also marked enlargement of the sella, clearly shown in (B). The patient had chronic, long-standing signs suggestive of increased intracranial pressure, and there was enlargement of the sella turcica and demineralization of the floor of the anterior fossa; the planum sphenoidale and the cribriform plate region are markedly demineralized (*arrows*).

FIG. 591.—ANEURYSM OF THE VEIN OF GALEN WITH OBSTRUCTIVE HYDROCEPHALUS

The lateral view (A) of the cerebral angiogram (following a ventriculogram for hydrocephalus which had demonstrated a mass in the 3d ventricle), shows the filling of the vein of Galen by way of branches of the middle cerebral artery. In Fig. 589 the filling was mostly by way of the posterior communicating and posterior cerebral arteries.

The anteroposterior projection (B) demonstrates the partially filled aneurysmal dilatation of the vein of Galen against the background of the filled ventricles. The course of the feeding middle cerebral vessels is clear on this film. The anterior cerebral artery is not filled from this side.

An angiogram of the opposite side (C) demonstrates that the middle cerebral vessels are not supplying the arteriovenous malformation, but the anterior cerebral artery is (*arrows*); the posterior communicating artery is enlarged on this side (*arrows*).

(*Revised 1963*)

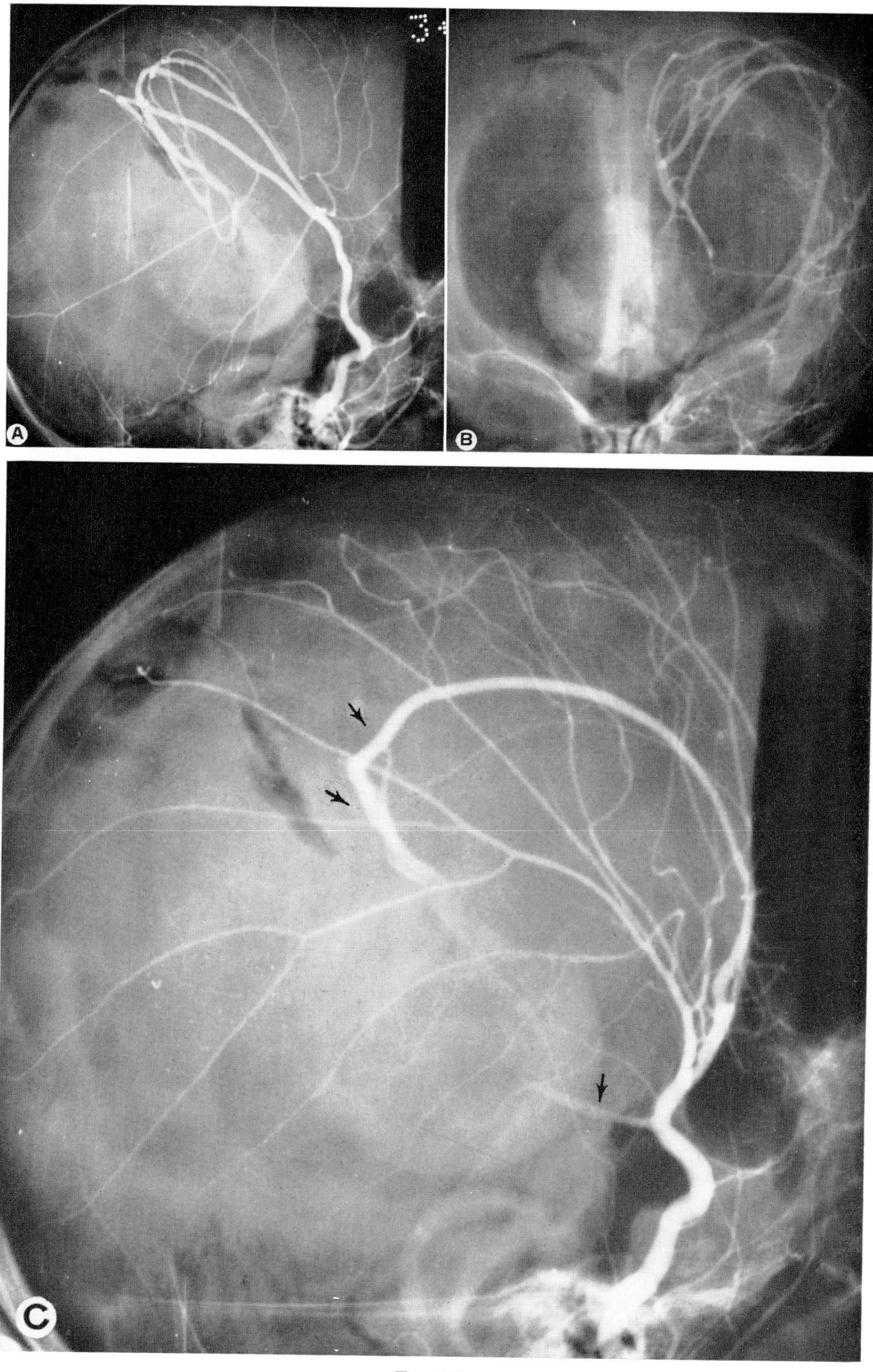

Fig. 591

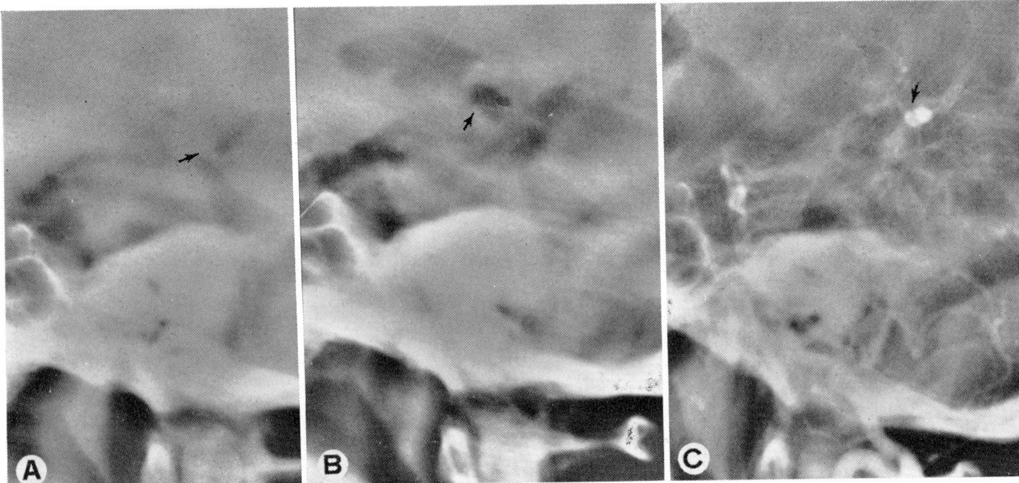

Fig. 592.—Arteriovenous Malformation Producing Partial Block of the Aqueduct

The pneumoencephalogram (A) revealed partial obstruction at the aqueduct with a slanted cut-off (*arrow*). Another film (B) showed some irregular shadows in the quadrigeminal cistern. Some air had passed beyond the partially obstructing lesion and outlined both sides of the aqueduct. The upper end is slightly dilated (*arrow*). A vertebral angiogram was performed which revealed a small vascular malformation (C) in the region of the quadrigeminal plate, and by measurement, the small vascular collection is in the area of aqueductal obstruction. The patient's initial symptoms appeared during pregnancy.

Actually this represents an arteriovenous malformation with aneurysmal dilatation of the vein of Galen. The feeding arteries can be branches of the posterior cerebral, of the anterior cerebral, and sometimes of the middle cerebral arteries. All three groups of vessels may participate in the blood supply in some cases. The lesions are discovered in infants or young children and the usual clinical diagnosis is hydrocephalus. A ventriculogram may indicate a mass in the posterior portion of the third ventricle which would, undoubtedly, lead to the diagnosis of a tumor. If angiography is not carried out, the diagnosis of hydrocephalus or of a tumor of the posterior portion of the third ventricle (fig. 591) usually will be made. A bruit is usually heard in these infants with enlargement of the head. In general any infant with an enlarging head and who has an audible bruit should undergo cerebral angiography rather than pneumographic examination as the first diagnostic procedure.

In one instance a small arteriovenous malformation encroached on the aqueduct of Sylvius and produced partial aqueductal obstruction with increased intracranial pressure (fig. 592).

Other Sources of Subarachnoid Hemorrhage

When bilateral carotid and vertebral angiography fail to demonstrate the source of subarachnoid bleeding, consideration should always be given to spinal structures. Some tumors and vascular anomalies of the spine can bleed without producing signs of an intramedullary lesion of the spinal cord. In the case shown in Figure 593 the vertebral angiogram succeeded in demonstrating an angioma of the cord, in an 18-year-old boy, fed by the anterior spinal artery.

Sequelae of Subarachnoid Hemorrhage

Aneurysms, particularly those that have ruptured, are often associated with ventricular dilatation when pneumoencephalography is performed. The hydrocephalus may be secondary to circulatory disturbances of the brain, in some cases, but in other instances,

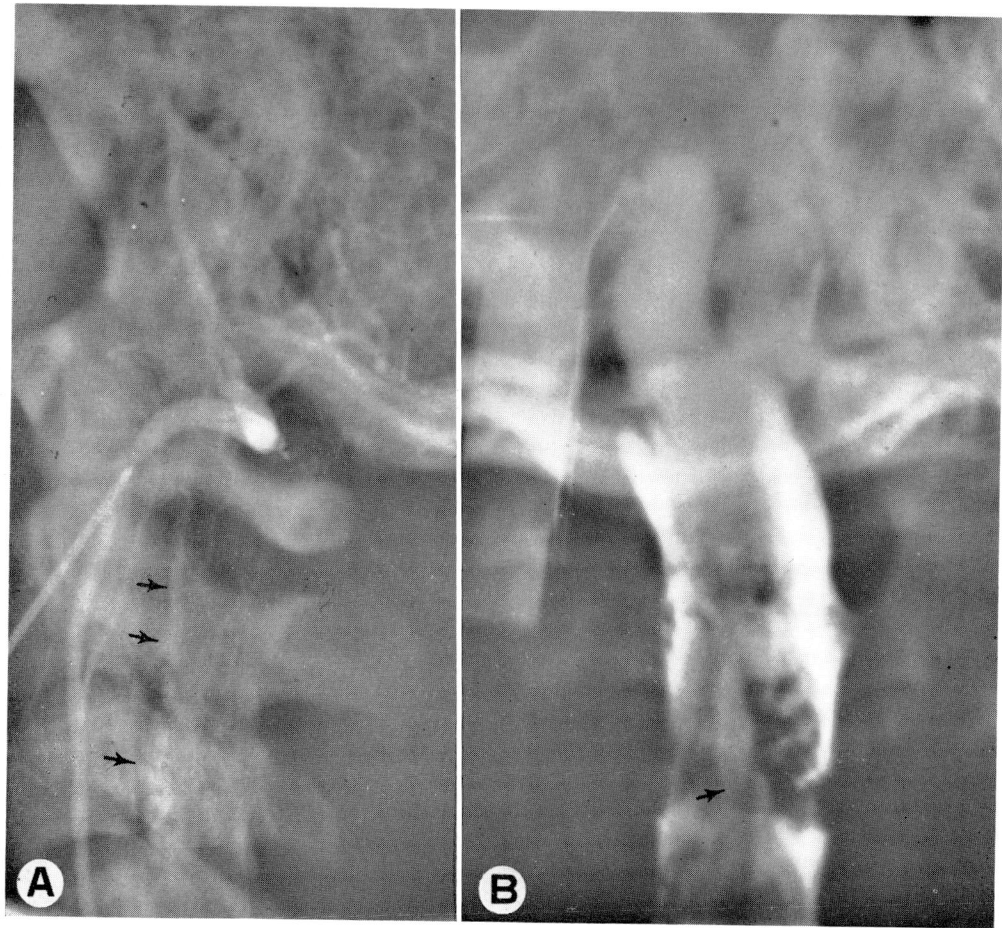

FIG. 593.—ANGIOMA OF THE CERVICAL CORD PRODUCING SUBARACHNOID HEMORRHAGE

There were no localizing signs for repeated subarachnoid hemorrhages in this 18-year-old male patient. Bilateral carotid angiography was followed by vertebral angiography which succeeded in demonstrating the presence of an abnormal collection of vessels on the anterior aspect of the spinal cord (*arrows*). The anterior spinal artery denotes the anterior margin of the cord (*arrows*), and it is seen that the lesion projects into the anterior subarachnoid space. Other arterial branches also are extending into the angioma. A Pantopaque myelogram was then performed which confirmed the presence of an anterolaterally placed mass composed of convoluted vessels in the upper cervical cord (B).

particularly when repeated subarachnoid hemorrhages have occurred, the hydrocephalus may be related to interference with the fluid absorptive mechanism. It is well known that repeated subarachnoid hemorrhage can cause experimental hydrocephalus in the dog (Dandy, 1944). When the hydrocephalus is associated with increased intracranial pressure, therefore, the possibility of performing a shunting procedure to alleviate the hydrocephalus should be considered. In other cases obstruction could be produced in the region of the incisura as a result of adhesions from hemorrhage of aneurysms in the suprasellar region (fig. 594). In one of our cases, a spino-ureteral shunt had to be performed, with satisfactory results.

Local atrophic lesions such as porencephaly may result from intracerebral hemorrhage and arterial occlusions in the region of the vascular malformations and aneurysms. These have already been mentioned in the chapter on "Intracranial Pneumography."

(*Revised 1963*)

SELECTION OF DIAGNOSTIC PROCEDURE

Even as angiography reaches the upswing of its popularity, other methods of diagnosis of intracranial disease are being developed that are complementary to this and other special procedures. Certain of these methods undoubtedly will replace angiography or pneumography in some cases. In many instances, the standard procedures probably will continue to be used, as in the diagnosis of vascular disease of the brain; it is difficult to see how any technique can substitute for angiography in providing the certainty of diagnosis and the required anatomic details concerning vascular lesions. Similarly, there is no substitute for pneumoencephalography in the evaluation of atrophic brain diseases, or ventriculography in the diagnosis of intraventricular tumors. Inasmuch as vascular lesions and degenerative diseases of the brain frequently display characteristic clinical features, problems concerning the selection of one or more diagnostic procedures revolve principally around the detection and identification of space-occupying processes.

At times, determined attempts are made on the part of radiologists, neurologists, and neurosurgeons to try to select for each individual case, depending on clinical findings, the one special neuroradiologic procedure that will result on the first trial in a definitive diagnosis. If this could be done with a high degree of success, it might be a reasonable solution. We have seen, however, cases in which angiography or pneumography was performed even without plain skull films having been made. Such an overanxious reach for a definitive diagnosis does not appear justified, even under extreme circumstances, since it not infrequently occurs that a radical approach results in an unnecessary examination.

Since there are now a variety of procedures available, not all involving radiologic methods, some orderly approach employing groups of procedures would appear desirable. It is our belief that procedures involving instrumentation, particularly the direct insertion of needles into the brain, should be avoided whenever possible. A very logical grouping of procedures has been suggested by J. W. D. Bull (yet unpublished) in which studies that are painless and, as far as is known, harmless to the patient are employed first before angiography, pneumography, and other techniques which carry with them some degree of morbidity and a definite complication rate. In accordance with this general concept, the use of the electroencephalogram and plain skull radiographs has been widely accepted for many years. Between 10 and 15 per cent of patients with a supratentorial tumor exhibit a shift of the calcified pineal gland which can be demonstrated on plain-skull radiographs; the direct diagnosis of certain intracranial lesions affecting bone, such as meningiomas, pituitary adenomas, acoustic neurinomas and a number of other conditions is well established and has been discussed elsewhere; in addition, pathologic calcification affords plain-film diagnosis in many instances. Yet, the incidence of detection of organic intracranial disease from plain radiographs remains very low.

The wide gap between the low incidence of direct demonstration of an intracranial lesion on plain films and the high accuracy of diagnosis with angiography and pneumography recently has been bridged to a significant extent by the introduction of ultrasound into neurologic diagnosis. It seems practical to determine the position of structures normally midline—chiefly the third ventricle—in relation to the midsagittal plane by ultrasonic methods in more than 90 per cent of patients (fig. 595). In addition, when a traumatic episode has resulted in a convexity hemorrhage on one side, the inner margin of such a hematoma, particularly an extradural collection, frequently may be detected, and the thickness of the hematoma may even be determined. More recently, ultrasonic techniques have been improved to allow the demonstration of enlarged lateral and third ventricles that are dilated owing either to obstruction or atrophy. The clinical diagnosis of a posterior fossa tumor or a hematoma, either spontaneous or traumatic, may be supported in this way. Future technical advances may provide a lower incidence of false negative examinations, and this would enhance the value of ultrasound as a "screening" procedure.

Scintillation scanning of the brain, with the use of isotopes of mercury or iodine, is now in widespread use. Instruments employing either a motor-driven scanning detector and multilinear recorder, or a scheme of systematic counting at specific points about the head, have been developed to a high degree of precision. Considerable experience has now been gained in many clinics concerning the value of brain-scanning techniques and, in general, a high degree of accuracy in the diagnosis of supratentorial neoplasms has been demonstrated. If an abnormal scan is found, it is so infrequently erroneous that some surgeons are now willing to carry out intracranial exploration, in certain cases, without performing another examination for confirmation. Poorly differentiated astrocytomas (glioblastomas), meningiomas, and metastatic lesions are associated with a high degree of trapping of radioactive compounds of intermediate molecular weight. The value of the method for the identification of other neoplasms and, in addition, intracranial hemorrhage and suppuration is being explored and attempts are being made to work out more refined techniques. Radioactive compounds also are being employed in the study of the cerebral circulation and for other neurophysiologic experiments.

It is conceivable that the use of ultrasonic and isotopic techniques may provide, when used in a complementary manner, a satisfactory means of "screening" patients suspected of harboring organic intracranial disease, particularly patients with mass lesions. For example, if a midline shift is found on ultrasound examination then a radioactive isotope scanogram might confirm the presence of a space-occupying supratentorial tumor, and reveal its location. The correct radiographic contrast examination to demonstrate ideally the process definitively, if required, then could be selected more satisfactorily. In patients with posterior fossa masses, the detection of a markedly enlarged third ventricle by ultrasonic techniques may serve as a guide for selecting the more informative pneumographic examination. It is obvious that a patient who is found to have a large third ventricle without a midline shift and who has markedly increased intracranial pressure on clinical examination is an ideal candidate for ventriculography; if intracranial hypertension is absent, pneumoencephalography would be preferred. In selected instances the injection of a small quantity of Pantopaque into a lateral ventricle through a parietal burr hole, without the removal of ventricular fluid, is being used when a cerebellar tumor or a midline intraventricular tumor with obstruction is suspected, in infants Pantopaque ventriculography to explore causes of hydrocephalus is easily accomplished by fontanelle puncture. Ventriculography using large quantities of air is being employed less and less and should be avoided wherever possible; occasionally, it may be necessary to fill the ventricles more completely with gas in order to diagnose an intraventricular lesion, such as a chorioid plexus papilloma.

More recently the use of measurements of skin temperature as an index of pathologic processes situated underneath has been introduced. The method allows comparison of the temperature of adjacent and contralateral areas employing very sensitive instruments that can discriminate fractions of a degree of temperature difference on the body surface. By adding a scanning device, the temperature differences can be translated into a pattern and recorded photographically as varying shades of gray (fig. 595). The resultant heat picture is copied on Polaroid film for final evaluation.

To bring out areas of increased heat, it is necessary first to lower the skin temperature. This is done by exposing the surface to be investigated in a cool room for at least 10 minutes, and moistening the surface with water so that cooling is enhanced by evaporation. Unfortunately, thermography requires clipping the hair short since hair is an effective heat insulator.

Lesions that can be detected thermographically usually are associated with increased metabolism or increased vascular supply, thereby raising the local body temperature. Preliminary trials by the authors indicate that it is possible to localize supratentorial meningiomas as well as hemispheric gliomas due to higher skin temperature on the involved side. The thermogram will not

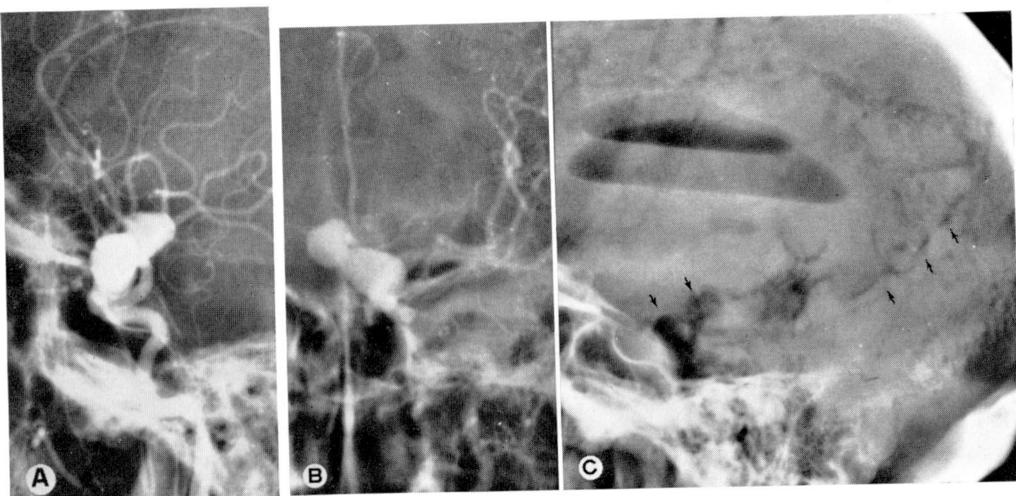

FIG. 594.—LARGE INTERNAL CAROTID ANEURYSM ARISING JUST ABOVE THE OPHTHALMIC ARTERY WITH REPEATED RUPTURE AND SUPRASELLAR ADHESIONS LEADING TO BLOCK TO THE FLOW OF CEREBROSPINAL FLUID

The frontal projection (A) and the lateral projection (B) demonstrate the irregular aneurysm which, on clinical history, had ruptured more than once. The pneumoencephalogram was performed because of developing mental symptoms (C) which demonstrated a block on the anterior aspect of the incisura (*anterior arrows*). The air was still able to pass posteriorly behind the splenium of the corpus callosum, but this route is often insufficient for the passage of all the fluid (*posterior arrows*). A moderate degree of ventricular dilatation was present. (Courtesy of Dr. George Shipman, Staten Island, New York.)

readily differentiate a benign or malignant tumor with increased heat from a local inflammatory process. Areas with decreased blood flow, however, such as result from occlusive vascular disease, may be defined thermographically as regions with a cooler temperature than the surrounding body regions.

The spine has been another region investigated with thermal apparatus, and certain lesions have shown significant heat changes from the normal. These have included spondylolithesis, an occasional neurofibroma which has produced significant compression, arteriovenous malformations and metastatic disease to the spine. The value of thermography, in comparison with other methods of examination in the diagnosis of either cerebral or spinal disease, has not yet been established.

Pneumography versus Angiography

Now that cerebral angiography has become such a popular diagnostic procedure and there is much less fear of complications than formerly, it is often necessary to decide whether angiography or pneumography should be performed. Frequently both examinations are necessary and one must decide which examination to perform first; often, however, the study that is performed first will be sufficient for diagnosis and localization of a lesion, and no further tests are required.

In certain institutions the problem is simplified by performing cerebral angiography as the first examination in any patient who shows signs of a supratentorial lesion and a pneumographic examination in any patient who presents a clinical syndrome that suggests a lesion in the posterior fossa. It is probably better to avoid oversimplifying the problem. The following criteria are suggested as a basis for selection of the procedures.

Angiography is performed as the first diagnostic procedure in cases of *subarachnoid hemorrhage*, in cases of *suspected thrombosis*, for *suprasellar lesions* (if an aneurysm is suspected) and in any patient who presents with *localizing neurologic signs* of a supratentorial mass lesion. Friedmann, Krenkel, and Tönnis recently (1962) have shown that 82 per cent of a large series of supratentorial tumors could be localized by angiography.

In general, it may be said that wherever a vascular lesion or a supratentorial lesion with localizing (sometimes lateralizing) neurologic signs is suspected, an angiogram is preferred. On the other hand, if the patient has no localizing signs, even if a supratentorial lesion is suspected, an air study is preferred in most instances because midline lesions and cases of pseudotumor cerebri are usually clarified by pneumography. There are, however, certain advantages in performing angiography, before pneumography even in these cases because ventricular dilatation is easily diagnosed by angiography. If an angiogram demonstrates no shift of the midline structures and no ventricular dilatation in a patient who has no localizing signs, it is usually safe to perform lumbar pneumoencephalography, even in the presence of papilledema. The complications from cerebral pneumography performed by the lumbar route are usually associated, in supratentorial lesions, with a shift of the midline structures which would bring the medial portion of the temporal lobe too close to the midline, or beyond the midline, allowing it to herniate through the incisura of the tentorium. On the other hand, lesions that do not produce a midline shift usually do not produce a tentorial herniation. An important exception to this general rule is bilateral subdural hematomas, but this is easily diagnosed by angiography.

A pneumographic examination is performed first in patients who have a syndrome that suggests an *infratentorial mass lesion*, in patients with suspected *atrophic lesions*, either diffuse atrophy or porencephaly, in patients suspected of having *congenital anomalies of the brain*, for *suprasellar mass lesions* (unless an aneurysm is suspected) and in patients who have no localizing signs and who may well have midline lesions. If in the latter cases there is evidence of increased intracranial pressure, one may wish to perform an angiogram first to aid in deciding whether a pneumoencephalogram or a ventriculogram should be done since, as mentioned above, pneumoencephalography is safer in patients who have no evidence of a shift of the midline structures.

Pneumoencephalography versus Ventriculography

The decision whether to perform pneumography by the lumbar route or ventriculography is often difficult to reach. Usually the final decision rests chiefly on previous training and personal experience; that is, a surgeon who becomes experienced in the use of ventriculography during his training might prefer that method. The decision, however, should be based on the type of lesion that is suspected clinically rather than on a preconceived idea of the general morbidity or complication rate of the examination. In general, a properly performed pneumoencephalogram should yield an extremely low complication rate. The morbidity rate is difficult to compare with that of ventriculography since the latter is usually followed by operation. Our own reaction to the problem is that any method that does not require the insertion of needles into the brain is preferred when it is considered safe.

Lumbar pneumoencephalography is preferred in the situations listed below.

1. Whenever patients are seen with symptoms and signs of a cerebellopontine angle lesion; in these cases, no complications have been encountered in the last ten years at the Neurological Institute, even in patients who had a high degree of papilledema. Of course, caution is always exercised in the performance of the examination. Fluid is never removed and only 10 cc. of air are injected. Further injections of air are used only after the first films have been carefully scrutinized.

2. In any case with symptoms of a brain stem tumor in the pons, in the midbrain, or in the medulla; the same care is exercised in this type of case, particularly in tumors of the lower pons and medulla. Care should be taken not to flex the head excessively, for this may cause a slight increase in the compression of the respiratory centers and the patient may develop respiratory difficulty

each time the head is flexed beyond a certain point. The use of the somersaulting chair permits the performance of the examination with the head in a slightly extended position throughout the procedure. Some of these patients with multiple cranial nerve involvement will have a prepontine lesion and, in order to differentiate between an intra-axial and an extra-axial brain stem lesion, a vertebral angiogram is recommended.

3. Lumbar pneumography is used for suprasellar tumors unless an aneurysm is suspected.

4. Patients with papilledema who have no localizing signs, and who have shown no evidence of a shift of the midline structures on the prior angiogram, may be examined by pneumoencephalography.

5. Patients who have no evidence of intracranial hypertension, but have been shown to have a hemispheric mass with very slight midline shift by prior angiography, may be safely examined.

Ventriculography is usually carried out in the situations listed below.

1. A cerebellar tumor is the most important single indication, or at least the most frequent indication, for ventriculography. It is our experience that lumbar pneumoencephalography does not usually fill the ventricles, particularly the fourth ventricle and aqueduct, in patients with cerebellar tumors owing to deformity and distortion or occlusion of the fourth ventricle. There is a certain risk of increasing the degree of cerebellar tonsillar herniation which is often present with cerebellar tumors; in addition, it is usually not possible to outline the mass; therefore, ventriculography is preferable.

2. Ventriculography is required in cases where lumbar pneumoencephalography has failed to fill the ventricles. This is commonly seen in cases of aqueduct stenosis, third ventricle tumors, and tumors or cysts in the region of the foramen of Monro and septum pellucidum.

3. Ventriculography should be used in any patient who has a high degree of papilledema with hemorrhages where angiography has not been sufficient to make an accurate diagnosis. In some cases, burr holes may be made as for ventriculography, but the needle not actually inserted into the ventricles. Lumbar pneumoencephalography is then carried out, and the burr holes are used to tap the ventricles if or when it becomes necessary. We feel that in these cases, it is preferable to attempt the ventricular puncture. If the ventricles are small and cannot be entered by the needle, it may then become necessary to do lumbar pneumoencephalography. It may be reassuring in these cases to have performed a cerebral angiogram that demonstrated no shift of the ventricular system, for under these circumstances (that is, small ventricles and no midline shift), the most frequent condition encountered is benign intracranial hypertension. The condition is also referred to as serous meningitis, pseudotumor cerebri, otitic hydrocephalus, or meningeal hydrops.

At present, there is a strong trend away from ventriculography for a cerebral hemispheric mass; angiography has replaced ventriculography to a large extent in these cases. Where a deep tumor is suspected, such as a deep posterior frontal or thalamic tumor, pneumoencephalography may be carried out if additional information is required because central tumors do not usually produce transtentorial herniations. Only in the cases presenting a significant degree of papilledema would ventriculography be performed. Urea, at half the usual dose, may be given in these cases if pneumoencephalography is to be used. If, during the performance of a pneumoencephalogram, an unsuspected supratentorial lesion is encountered in the straight posteroanterior film, the technique must be altered. If a slight shift of the normally midline third ventricle and septum pellucidum is observed (a dislocation of only 3 to 4 mm.), the examination should be terminated when 20 cc. of gas have been injected. If the shift is more than 3 to 4 mm., the examination should be discontinued immediately after the preliminary series of three scout films is made. However, the complete series of roentgenograms is taken, although no additional gas is injected. After withdrawing the needle, the patient is placed in the horizontal position, the films of this series being most advantageous in localizing supratentorial lesions. Many in-

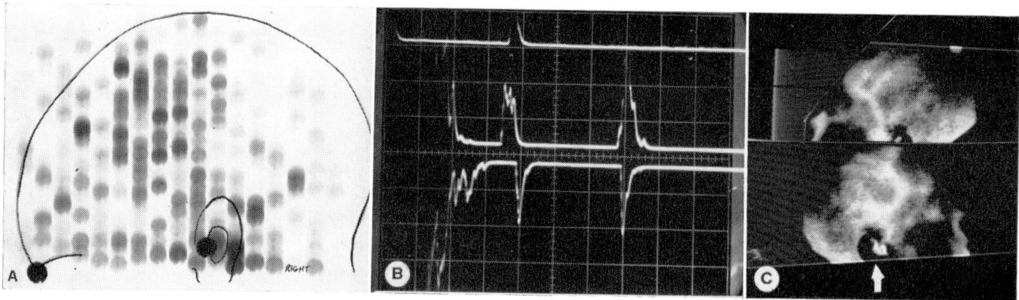

FIG. 595.—EXAMPLES OF THE NEWER TECHNIQUES

An *isotope encephalogram* (A) demonstrates an area of increased uptake of the iodinated human serum albumin at 48 hours indicating the presence of neoplasm (glioblastoma) in the frontoparietal region. An *echoencephalogram* (B) demonstrates a shift of midline structures (third ventricle) in a patient with glioma of the left cerebral hemisphere. The upper tracing is a transmission ultrasonogram which represents the width of the head from skin to skin at the upper arrow. The middle tracing depicts the echos obtained from the right side of the head. The left margin of the three pointed peak is the midline echo which normally should line up with the total distance obtained by transmission; the inner table is the peak on the right side. The lower tracing is the echo from the left side (electronically reversed) and demonstrates the off-center position of the midline echo in relation to the right. A *thermogram* of another patient with a pterional meningioma (C) demonstrates increased heat over the pterional region on the right (*lower*) side as compared to the left. The arrow points at the ear on the right side; the patient faces right for the right side and left for the left side. Increased temperature shows up as a lighter shadow in the thermogram.

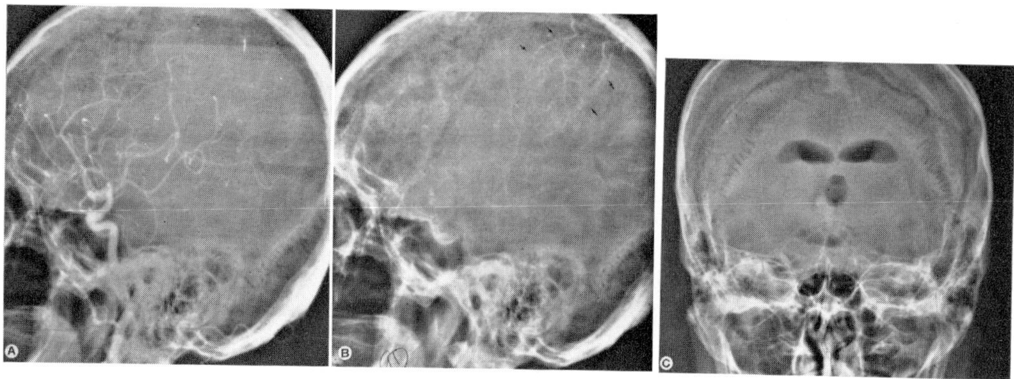

FIG. 596.—PARIETAL TUMOR DIAGNOSED BY ANGIOGRAPHY WITH NONDIAGNOSTIC PNEUMOENCEPHALOGRAPHY

In the arterial phase (A) no abnormalities are noted. In the intermediate phase (B), there is evidence of early filling of veins in the parietal region (*arrows*). No other abnormalities were noted. The venous phase was normal, and there was no evidence of a midline shift and no distortion of the deep veins. The pneumoencephalogram (C) revealed no abnormalities. A slight degree of ventricular enlargement bilaterally was present, including slight enlargement of the third ventricle. There was no evidence of flattening of the roof. The patient had an infiltrating glioblastoma which replaced brain tissue and was not accompanied by edema.

vestigators now agree that a large amount of valuable information can be obtained in numerous cases through the use of small amounts of gas if one takes care in positioning the head and moves swiftly in exposing and processing radiographs. Avoidance of unnecessary loss of time is essential when small quantities of air are used, since the gas often disappears from the areas of special interest at a rapid rate.

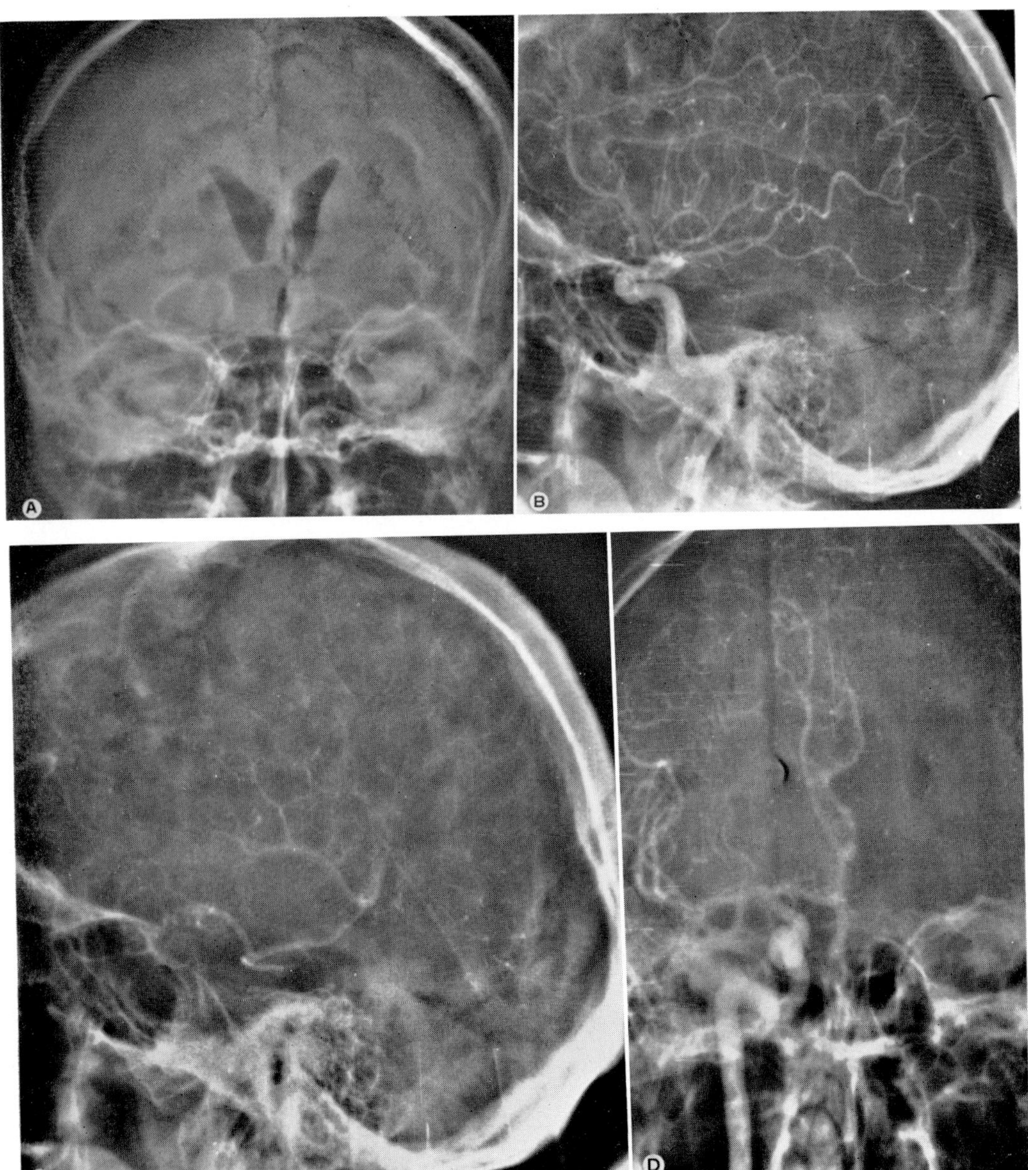

FIG. 597.—INFILTRATING TUMOR SHOWN BETTER BY PNEUMOGRAPHY THAN BY ANGIOGRAPHY

The frontal view of the pneumoencephalogram (A) demonstrates deformity of the roof of the lateral ventricle on the right side and infiltration of the septum pellucidum which is markedly widened and slightly irregular. In addition, the third ventricle is tilted, and it is obvious that the infiltration extends through the septum pellucidum and follows the right side of the brain along the thalamus. This type of infiltration cannot be demonstrated by angiography. The lateral view of the angiogram (B) shows slight flattening of the pericallosal artery, which may be a normal finding, and only minimum disruption of branches of the anterior cerebral artery in the frontal parasagittal region, which can also be a normal finding in certain cases. The venous phase demonstrates downward displacement of the internal cerebral vein and basilar veins which are generally downward with preservation of their normal contours. Slight spreading of the internal cerebral and basilar vein angle is present. Enlarged veins draining into the internal cerebral vein are also visible. These findings are consistent with a mass in the posterior frontal region which drains by the deep veins and causes a central type of transtentorial herniation. The frontal view in the arterial phase (D) demonstrates only slight shift of the anterior cerebral artery to the opposite side and slight stretching of the callosomarginal artery.

(Revised 1963)

Other Considerations

In general, one must have at his command a variety of techniques, and variations of these techniques, if he is to perform the best procedure in a given situation. It is probably best to avoid making decisions that are strictly based on habit or routine, because this often leads to the selection of an improper technique. The greatest advantage of intracranial angiography in the study of intracranial masses is that after the diagnosis is made by this means, it is not necessary to proceed at once with surgical treatment. This applies also to lesions in the posterior fossa. On the other hand, ventriculography should be followed by surgical intervention when a diagnosis is made by this method. The same may be said about lesions diagnosed by pneumoencephalography in patients who have evidence of increased intracranial pressure. However, even if there is no evidence of increased intracranial pressure, the patient should be followed carefully when a tumor has been demonstrated by pneumoencephalography, for sometimes deterioration of the clinical condition occurs several hours after the examination is performed, and surgical treatment may be required at once. Following ventriculography, it is often necessary to inject additional gas by the lumbar route to visualize better posterior fossa ventricular and cisternal areas, and this also appears to be a safe procedure, owing to removal of ventricular fluid and reduction of pressure cephalad to the lesion. It is usually desirable to tap the ventricles a second time and to remove some of the gas before performing the lumbar puncture, if aqueductal obstruction is present.

Positive contrast ventriculography is used rather infrequently by the authors. The main advantage of this technique is that it is not necessary to remove any significant amount of cerebrospinal fluid. Its use is usually restricted to obstructing lesions in the region of the aqueduct and fourth ventricle. For this type of case, "central ventriculography," as proposed by Azambuja *et al.* (1956), which requires the use of a small amount of gas, also is satisfactory; with the somersaulting chair it is possible to use a very small amount of gas for ordinary ventriculography.

The two cases shown in Figures 596 and 597 demonstrate certain of the advantages of angiography and pneumography in the evaluation of supratentorial mass lesions.

HEAD INJURIES AND THEIR COMPLICATIONS

Within a short while after the discovery of x-ray by Roentgen, the method was being used extensively in the diagnosis and treatment of traumatic disorders. A monograph by Borden (1900) describes the use of x-ray in the field during the Spanish-American War. Illustrations that deal with missile injuries of the head are included. The case of a soldier who sustained a penetrating bullet wound of the head is described; in this case, radiologic demonstration of the intracranial position of the missile affected treatment which resulted in recovery of the patient. For some time, however, the head remained one of the more difficult portions of the body to study satisfactorily by x-ray, and it was approximately 20 years after the discovery by Roentgen that skull films of good technical quality could be obtained routinely.

(Revised 1963)

Today, it is essential to have skull films of good quality not only for proper diagnosis but because of their medicolegal importance in many cases of injury. It has been our practice to attempt to obtain in traumatic cases all of the projections that are usually made in connection with the radiologic study of patients with neurologic disorders, in whom a search for an intracranial cause of the disturbance is carried out. Five films ordinarily are made, which include (1) a straight anteroposterior view, (2) an anteroposterior half axial projection, which includes the foramen magnum, (3) a straight posteroanterior projection, and (4) and (5) a lateral study of each side of the skull. This film series is considered the minimum basic examination in the case of cooperative patients for study of the cranial skull; it is not intended to comprise a completely satisfactory examination of the facial skull. In addition, any further films that may be thought to be of possible current or potential value, either on the basis of the clinical or neurologic examination or on the basis of the routine films after study by the radiologist, should be obtained. Such additional films frequently include an additional stereoscopic examination, upright films, a full axial projection in the case of suspected basal skull fracture, and other special projections.

In the case of a severely injured patient, it may be necessary in the interest of the patient's general welfare to carry out a limited study, which is understood to be only of the nature of a survey examination. In these instances, the patient usually is examined supine on a stretcher; without moving the patient from this position, it is possible to obtain the straight and inclined anteroposterior projections and lateral views made with the horizontal x-ray beam. The latter should include as much of the cervical spine as possible, because clinically occult injuries in this area may occasionally be detected by this technique. It is understood that this type of study is a compromise, calculated to be in the patient's best general interest, and that a complete routine skull examination should be carried out at a later date when the condition of the patient permits.

Fractures

The term skull fracture usually implies cranial fracture and, for the most part, is the result of direct force to the head. Fractures may be classified radiologically as (1) linear, (2) diastatic, (3) comminuted, and (4) depressed. It is very unusual to have comminution without some fragment being depressed; depression does not occur often without some degree of comminution. In addition, radiologic evidence of a compound fracture is given by (1) a line traversing one of the air sinuses of the skull, (2) intracranial foreign material, and (3) an obvious soft tissue defect in connection with a fracture line. Bursting fractures may occur as a result of injury by a high velocity missile; some investigators have emphasized the importance of contrecoup fractures with this and other types of trauma (Gurdjian, Webster, and Lissner, 1950).

It is important to try to determine whether a skull fracture is old or recent. Recurrent head trauma may occur in a patient who has had a previous bony injury but in whom the bony skull itself has escaped recurrent damage. It is very important also to differentiate normally occurring linear shadows and normal cranial variations from new and old traumatic changes.

NORMAL FINDINGS SIMULATING FRACTURE

Sutures and Accessory Ossicles

A number of specific normal findings, which may be misinterpreted as a fracture, occur with sufficient frequency to deserve special mention. Even normal sutures may resemble fractures on occasion. Sutures often are composed of two types of lines. The suture of the outer table usually has the characteristic serrated or zigzag appearance commonly associated with these structures. Inspection of the inside of a dried skull will readily show, however, that the portion of the suture extending along the inner table is often quite straight and without serrations at many points. The appearance in films of a straight line superimposed on a serrated shadow was called by Dyke (1941) a "double" suture line; it is seen only when the inner straight line portion of a suture is particularly distinct in skull films. It is important, however, not to interpret a double suture line as a fracture through a suture. Actually, sutural fractures look quite different and result in diastasis, as will be described subsequently.

Sutures of the posterior part of the skull may be particularly bothersome as far as the diagnosis of fracture is concerned. Even in straight frontal radiographs, one occipitomastoid suture may be conspicuous and strikingly resemble a vertical fracture. Only the knowledge of this pitfall and the detection of a similar line on the opposite side, although faint, may prevent misinterpretation. A separate small ossicle may occur in this same suture between the occipital bone and the mastoid portion of the temporal bone and can be mistaken for comminution. The small bone is referred to as Riolan's ossicle. Other sutural bones, both small and large, were described by the anatomist Worm (1634). They are most often seen along the lambdoidal suture; in this area, they may be quite large and encroach upon both the parietal and occipital bone territories.

In some instances, a large triangular bone is present just below the lambda, bounded inferiorly by a separate and well formed transverse occipital suture (mendosal suture). The mendosal suture is well marked at birth when it exists as a band of connective tissue between the upper and lower portions of the occipital squama, serving to separate the interparietal portion of the occipital squama from the lower or supraoccipital portion. At birth, the length of the fissure extending into the occipital squama as the mendosal suture varies in length from a short fissure to a complete suture, forming a separate interparietal bone in approximately 10 per cent of newborn infants. In the majority of cases, according to Caffey (1953), it persists only for several weeks after birth. A vertical fissure that extends in the midline from the posterior fontanelle into the upper occipital squama is seen so often that it has been named the superior longitudinal fissure. It has been pointed out by Caffey that the superior longitudinal fissure and the neonatal synchondroses of the occipital bone around the foramen magnum, and certain variations thereof, are not well known; sometimes they are erroneously interpreted as fracture lines. Similarly, long strips of connective tissue may extend into the parietal bones and simulate fracture. Usually the symmetry of the prominent parietal bone fissures is the strongest indication that they are developmental in origin.

An unusual deformity of the skull may occur in connection with the persistence of an independent interparietal bone at birth.

(Revised 1963)

It has again been pointed out by Caffey that the size, shape, and even the density of the interparietal bone varies greatly. In some instances, there is an overgrowth of the supraoccipital or lower portion of the occipital squama, with external bulging; at the same time, the interparietal bone may grow less and remain flat. In these instances, a steplike deformity results along the line of the mendosal suture and this irregular growth of the occipital area may persist into adult life. The deformity has been termed bathrocephaly; in the newborn, it may incorrectly suggest a recent depressed fracture, while in later life it may suggest an old, uncorrected depressed fracture. Bathrocephaly can also be produced in the reverse manner when the interparietal portion overgrows the supraoccipital segment, with an analogous deformity in the opposite direction at the site of the mendosal suture.

The bregmatic bone is a Wormian bone that is occasionally found at the junction of the sagittal and coronal sutures. An ossicle found at the pterion or sphenoparietal junction is often referred to as the epiteric bone. Other Wormian bones, too numerous to mention individually here, may be encountered and should be recognized for their true significance. Such sutural bones usually are normal variations but appear to be more frequent when the head is large; they are characteristically found with certain skeletal maldevelopments such as cleidocranial dysostosis and osteogenesis imperfecta.

Attention has been called by Caffey (1961) to the sutures normally found in the region of the foramen magnum in infancy. These sutures are involved in the normal development of the basiocciput, and while they are often quite prominent in neonatal life, they disappear early. The frequent occurrence of trauma to the posterior portion of the head in infancy and the conspicuous appearance of these sutures in the anteroposterior half axial view has, in the past, led to erroneous interpretations of fracture. Also, in the same view, a midline posterior cleft may occasionally be seen in the arch of the first cervical vertebra; this also should be recognized as developmental and not the result of injury.

The metopic suture is now well known as

an anatomic variant, significant only as a persistent frontal suture. In the developmental stage, the vertical portion of the frontal bone ossifies from two lateral centers. In the newborn, a distinct suture often can be seen still extending from the region of the anterior fontanelle or bregma straight downward to the nasion. The line usually is obliterated during early childhood, but in somewhat less than 10 per cent of normal persons, the suture may be visible to a varying extent throughout life. In the average case, closure of the metopic suture begins in the second year of life and union is completed during the third year. When fully persistent, the metopic suture resembles other cranial sutures with serrations and interdigitations. It is when the line persists only over a part of its length that confusion with frontal bone fracture is likely.

Vascular Channels

Blood vessel grooves may offer the greatest difficulty in the differentiation of normal shadows from fracture. Venous channels do not cause as much of a problem as arterial channels, on the average. Venous channels occur in the diploic space throughout the skull but are unusually prominent in the diploë of the parietal bones. Here they vary greatly in size and frequently coalesce to form "lakes," in some of which "islands" of bone are outlined. Their irregular course and their tendency to join one another are quite unlike a fracture. The middle meningeal veins may be straighter than veins elsewhere. While the diploic veins are usually most numerous in the parietal bones, vertically extending frontal diploic veins are frequently seen; similar, although usually less conspicuous, vertical occipital diploic veins may occur. The lines of diminished density usually called veins are actually diploic channels in which the veins of Breschet lie. The channels frequently are quite wide and their coalescence to form plexi is an outstanding characteristic. Some normal skulls have such a high degree of prominent venous vascularity that the term *phlebectasia* has been used to describe this condition. In some instances, anterior veins may be projected in an unusual manner onto the occipital area in straight anteroposterior or anteroposterior half axial radiographs and may be mistaken for linear fractures posteriorly.

Arterial grooves are more constant in their course and usually form straighter lines than those produced by veins. The middle meningeal arterial grooves, in lateral films lie behind the coronal suture; they branch chiefly backward, and spread upward and backward across the parietal bone. These shadows occasionally may be difficult to differentiate from fracture but their characteristic disposition and frequent branching — sometimes a trifurcation occurs — are uncharacteristic features of fracture. A posterior branch of the middle meningeal artery is demonstrated inconstantly; it is seen in the lateral films coursing upward and slightly backward, usually projected through the temporal squama just behind the sella turcica. The line is often quite sharp and without demonstrable divisions, except occasionally at its upper termination. The posterior branch of the middle meningeal artery arborizes in the usual way anatomically but in radiographs the branches are not often well seen, in contrast to the divisions of the anterior portion. Often a posterior middle meningeal vascular line is curvilinear, extending slightly backward as well as upward; in these instances, its true identity is more readily recognized. When the vessel is demonstrated only on one side, it is even more difficult to exclude the possibility of fracture. Bilateral demonstration, however, facilitates identification of the shadows as vascular channels.

In all instances, the study of stereoscopic films is extremely helpful in the differentiation of vascular channels from fractures. The venous channels, as noted above, are in the diploë and the arterial channels groove only the inner table of the skull. It can be appreciated from stereoscopic study that a doubtful line does or does not extend through both tables of the skull, which occurs in the case of a fracture. Furthermore, even on single-plane films, a comparison of a suspicious line with other known vascular channels will give a clue as to whether both tables are involved. Extension through both tables, as is the case with linear fracture, results in a darker shadow on the roentgenogram, often black, as compared with the gray shadow of a vascular groove. The very sharp, sometimes jagged, margin of a fracture line can be differentiated from the relatively smooth margin of a vascular channel, although the vascular groove may be irregular and tortuous. Difficulty in recognition of extension of a fracture line through both tables may occur when the fracture is viewed on the bias. Uncertainty in differentiating fractures from vascular channels develops most often, in our experience, when an injury occurs a number of months before the radiologic examination. In these instances, some repair may have occurred; the margins may not be as sharp nor the fracture line itself as dark as is customarily seen with a recent fracture. Further discussion of the healing of fractures is given below.

LINEAR FRACTURES

General Considerations

It has been pointed out by most writers in the field for many years that a fracture of the cranium is, of itself, not of great importance, unless there is depression, or unless there is some other direct complication, such as the fracture being compound, as occurs when an air sinus is opened. The extent of injury to the brain and other cranial contents is the consideration of real concern and of much greater importance than the bony injury. Severe force may be exerted upon the intracranial contents with extensive damage and death without the bony encasement being fractured. Contrariwise, patients who sustain fractures may exhibit no clinical evidence of brain damage or of subsequent complication. Nevertheless, the presence of a fracture is an indication and a graphic record of an injury of significant force and its current medicolegal significance cannot be discounted.

The location and type of fracture found radiographically often give a clue to the nature and severity of impact to the head; the mechanism of the production of various types of fractures has been a subject of extensive study of Gurdjian, Webster, and Lissner (1953). These investigators found that depressed fractures result from inbending with a blow of adequate velocity. If the bony skull is competent to withstand the inbending force, a rebound phenomenon occurs with outbending, which may be severe enough to produce a linear fracture. Linear skull fractures were found to occur at right angles to the maximum tensile stress, with the lines extending both toward the point of impact and in the opposite direction. The velocity of a blow determines to a considerable extent the type of fracture, assuming that the energy is adequate. High velocity blows produce more localized changes with a higher incidence of perforation and depression. Low velocity impacts of the same energy produce more widespread effects with the production of stellate fractures and depression over a sizable area (fig. 599). The shape of the object producing the blow also influences the pattern of fracture.

Linear fractures of the cranium, except for the skull base, are demonstrable radiologically in the great majority of cases. In films, a linear fracture appears as a line of diminished density varying greatly in length, but usually not exceeding 3 mm. in width, if it is simple linear in type. A recent linear fracture has sharp, well defined margins, with gradual narrowing at the distal end—often at both ends—until it tapers to a point beyond which it cannot be followed radiologically into normal-appearing bone. Fractures generally follow either a vertical or transverse course, depending upon the nature of the blow. The course, however, is not ordinarily straight linear or curvilinear; rather, there may be angular alterations in the course of a fracture line. Some fractures may be short, being only 1 cm. or slightly more in length; such fractures occur most often in thin bones, particularly near the sphenoparietal and temporal junctions, and often are overlooked. More frequently, however, fracture lines are several centimeters in length; frequently, their entire length cannot be determined, particularly in the case of vertical fractures which disappear behind dense structures of the skull base. The irregularity of the bones of the base of the skull, and the presence of areas of increased density in this region, cause many basal fractures to be undiagnosed. Technical problems involved in the demonstration of the floor of the skull *en face*, particularly in obtunded patients, or patients with injuries elsewhere, add to the difficulty of visualizing these fracture lines. The true incidence of basal skull fractures has never been established; all reports suggest that the frequency must be considerably greater than can be determined by conventional radiologic methods.

In addition to fractures of the base, fracture lines in other special locations assume particular significance. These locations include the major sutures, the main vascular channels of the skull, and the air sinuses. Occasional cases have been encountered in which pure *diastasis of the sutures* occurs

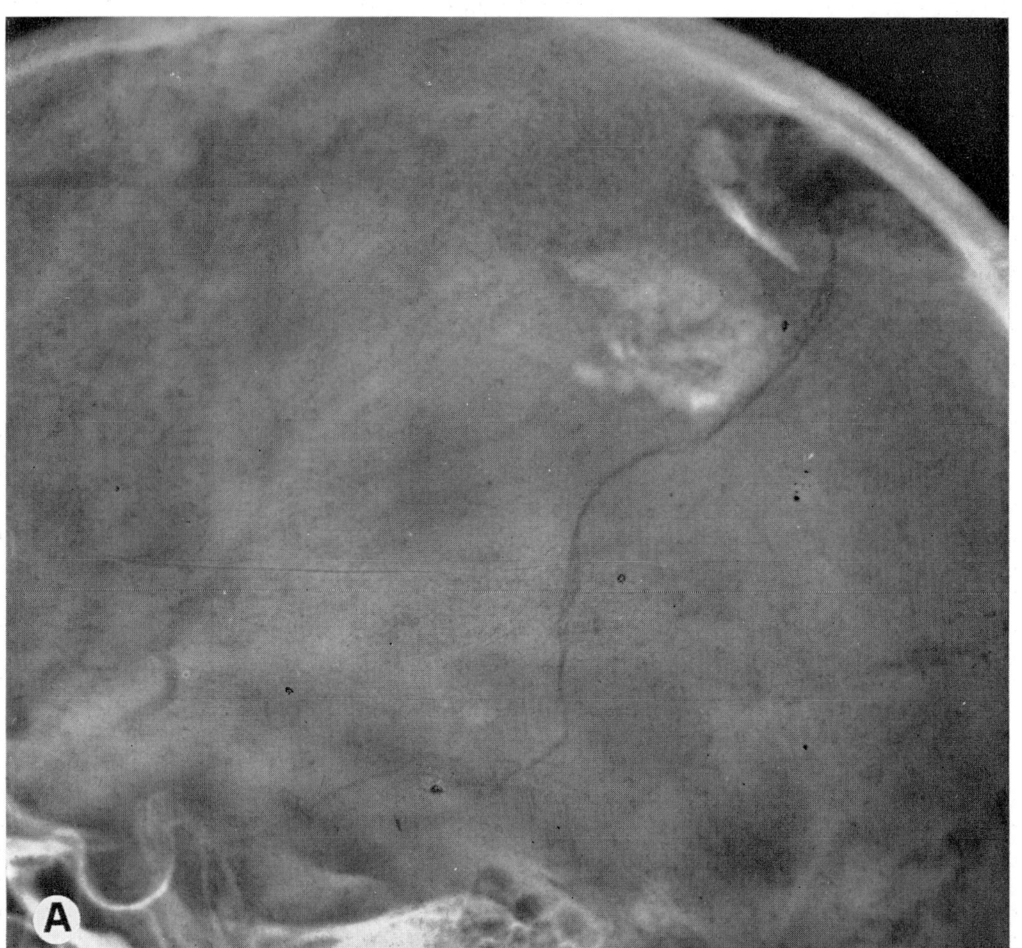

Fig. 598.—Linear and Depressed Skull Fractures

A long linear fracture is present (A), extending vertically from the midparietal region to disappear into the floor of the middle fossa. The fracture line is sharply demarcated, angular as well as curved, and exhibits a finely irregular margin at many points along its course. The sharpness of outline and density of the fracture line extending through both tables denotes the recent nature of the bony injury (see Fig. 602). A 3 cm. diameter defect is present in the parasagittal portion of the parietal bone from which bone fragments have been comminuted and impacted intracranially for a distance of 4 cm. The superior longitudinal sinus may be torn by such an injury, or it may become thrombosed, as in this case.

(Revised 1963)

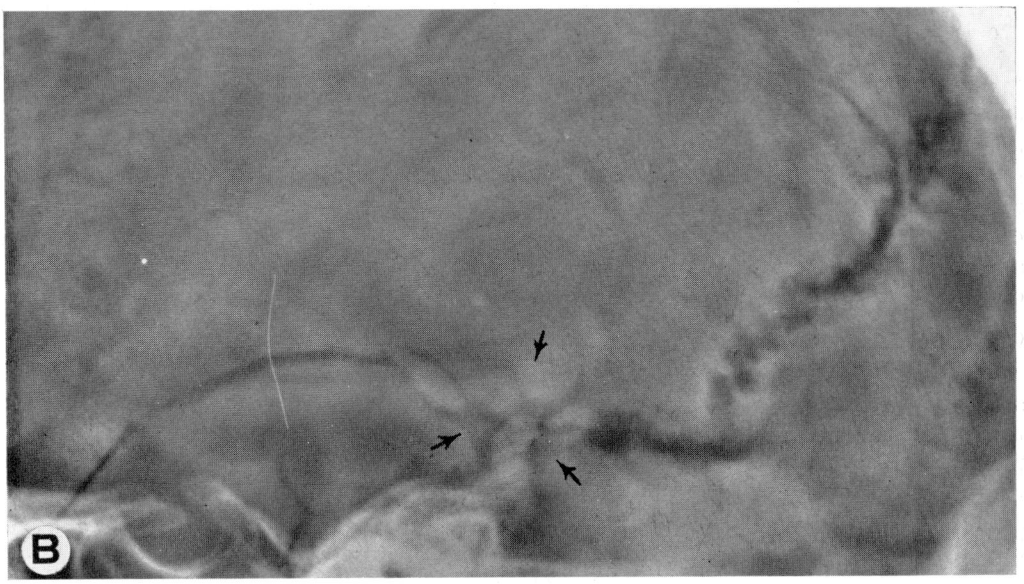

Fig. 598B

A comminuted depressed fracture is present (*arrows*) just forward of the asterion, which is in relation to the lateral sinus groove (B). Because the lateral sinus usually is bilateral, thrombosis may not produce a circulatory disturbance unless the thrombus propagates, but there may be hemorrhage from tearing of the sinus walls. Sharply defined linear fractures extend forward and downward from the comminuted depressed area. Posterior to the depressed zone, which represents the area of maximum impact at the time of injury, there is diastasis of the parietomastoid and lambdoidal sutures. When the interdigitations of a suture are separated more than 2.0 to 2.5 mm. after early life, diastasis usually is present, owing either to trauma or increased intracranial pressure.

without a demonstrable defect in any of the component bones of the vault. These occur most often in young adults owing to a headtop injury. More often, however, there is some associated crack in the bone at the beginning or termination of the point of suture widening; frequently there is a transverse line entering either the coronal or lambdoidal suture. The extent of the diastasis varies considerably, as does the length and width of the associated fracture line or lines (fig. 598).

Care must be taken to avoid interpreting a prominent suture as one involved by diastasis. The normal widths of sutures vary considerably in different individuals and at different ages. In some instances, there may be as much as 2 mm. between the interdigitating elements of the major sutures, particularly in the lambdoidal region. Firm closure of the sutures normally occurs late in life; the coronal often is not bridged until after the age of 30, and the lambdoidal usually retains a fibrous union until after the age of 60 years. Suture diastasis is not frequently seen after 30 to 35 years of age. Traumatic diastasis can be differentiated from a naturally wide suture or the widening of increased intracranial pressure by the presence of an abrupt change in the space between the interdigitations; the change usually occurs in conjunction with a fracture line.

Linear fractures that occur in close relationship to significant vascular channels of the skull, such as the middle meningeal arterial channels, may be of particular significance, since the walls of the vessels may be torn. Tearing of vascular structures may result from a force that produces a fracture either traversing or paralleling one of the vascular grooves. Linear fractures which cross either the channel of the main branch of the middle meningeal artery or its posterior branch are not infrequently associated with the development of an epidural hematoma. Similarly, linear fractures may be associated with damage to one of the main dural sinuses; more often, injury to the latter structures occurs in connection with a depressed fracture, which may result in partial occlusion and thrombosis of the sinus. A fracture line which enters the wall of one of the paranasal, or even the mastoid, sinuses may provide a communication between the sinus air spaces and the intracranial fluid spaces. Fractures in these special sites may be of particular significance as described subsequently.

Old Fractures

Skull fractures heal more slowly than similar osseous defects in other parts of the body. The time required for healing of simple linear fractures is more directly related to the patient's age than other factors. In infancy and early childhood, fracture lines frequently disappear in three to six months. In children five to twelve years of age, fractures usually heal within a year, while in adolescents, healing usually takes longer. In the adult, a linear fracture usually is clearly visible for a number of months and often for a number of years; in some instances, the site of a fracture may be recognized for the remainder of an individual's life. The average time, however, for healing of a linear fracture in the adult is two to three years (fig. 602). Healing usually occurs by the progressive laying down of bone along each side of the fracture line, with the margins becoming smooth rather than sharp and irregular. The line may become obliterated first at its tapered end, followed by one or more points of bridging along the fracture gap. The line becomes gray in the roentgenogram rather than black, and at this point may resemble closely a vascular groove. The entire line may be obliterated completely or, if still visualized in the late stages of healing, it appears clearly bridged by new bone formation.

Leptomeningeal cysts. Occasionally, particularly in children, a rent in the dura may occur in association with a linear fracture which may not be repaired in the usual manner. Rather, a small projection of arachnoid through the dural tear may occur; the pressure and pulsation of the cerebrospinal fluid in the subarachnoid space may be interposed between the two edges of dura and the two edges of bone to prevent healing. Instead, there may be erosion of bone with progressive widening of the fracture line over part, or a large portion, of its length (fig. 603). Arachnoid adhesions usually develop with an incomplete arachnoid cyst being formed, commonly referred to as a leptomeningeal cyst. The pulsation of the cyst continues to erode bone and increase the dural and bony defects; pressure atrophy of the underlying brain also may be produced. In some instances, the cranial defects may become extremely large (fig. 602). Multiloculated cysts usually are formed and produce a smoothly scalloped configuration of the eroded bone margins. The development of a wavy fracture margin with even a minimum degree of widening of the fracture line is suggestive of this type of process. If there is any question about the diagnosis, it is possible to investigate the defect by needling through the scalp and injecting a small amount of air; this will determine the extent of the cyst and its communication or lack of communication with the main subarachnoid space. While occurring infrequently, the possibility of the development of a leptomeningeal cyst makes it very important to follow, through serial roentgenograms, the healing of all skull fractures in children. It is desirable to detect the development of a leptomeningeal pocket at the earliest possible time in order to institute surgical repair before extensive adhesions and damage to the underlying brain can occur.

COMMINUTED AND DEPRESSED FRACTURES

The majority of comminuted fractures of the skull involve the cranial vault. The bones of the base are not commonly affected; occasionally, such injuries may be found in the horizontal or supraorbital portion of the frontal bone, in the ethmoid area, and in the occipital region. In some instances, comminution may be the result of a severe bursting type of fracture caused by an injury of high velocity (fig. 599). Long linear fractures often extend some distance from an area of comminution or they may occur on the opposite side of the skull. In the great majority of patients, a fracture of this type

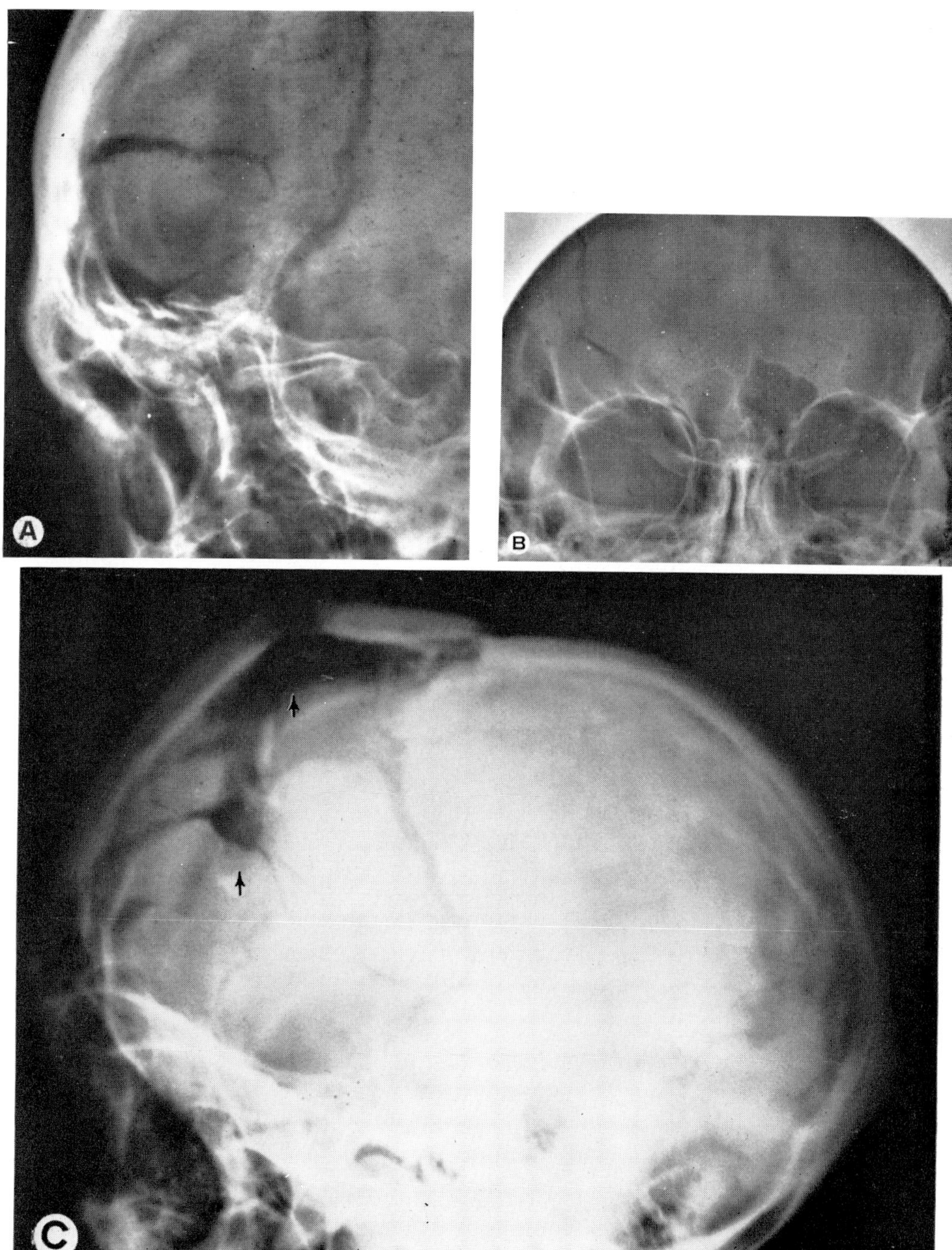

Fig. 599.—Fractures in Relation to Paranasal Sinuses

Skull fractures that involve the air sinuses of the skull, either paranasal or mastoid, are compound fractures, even though the opening to the exterior is occult. In the lateral view (A), a sharply demarcated fracture line is present which widens anteriorly. The inferior fracture limb is comminuted at its anterior extremity, with a few small bone fragments impacted intracranially from the sinus wall.

A vertical, sharply defined, angular, linear fracture is present in the right supraorbital portion of the frontal bone, which extends into the frontal sinus at its inferior extremity (B). There is clouding of the right frontal sinus and of both ethmoid areas, which contain blood and cerebrospinal fluid.

In another case, a severely comminuted fracture of bursting type has occurred. The fracture has resulted from perforation of the skull by a rifle bullet, thereby being compound extracranially. The point of entrance (*lower arrow*), because of the greater velocity of the missile, is smaller than the point of exit (*upper arrow*), where a greater bursting effect is evident.

(Revised 1963)

results from a blow of considerable energy; usually there is intracranial depression of one or more of the comminuted fragments. In such cases there may be marked impaction and brain penetration, particularly when the injury results from a missile wound (fig. 598). It is rather unusual to have a pure comminuted fracture without some degree of depression. Healing of comminuted and comminuted depressed fractures is much slower than is the case with linear fractures, and frequently it is never complete.

Except in the case of infants, a depressed fracture requires comminution. Occasionally, a rounded or oval plaque of bone may be separated from the vault by means of a more or less circular fracture line with one edge impacted intracranially more than the opposing margin. Even here, the main central fragment usually is itself comminuted; ordinarily, linear fractures extend outward from the main central area of involvement. More often, the central area of a comminuted fracture is depressed intracranially to the greatest extent. One or several comminuted fragments may be displaced internally; often the impacted fragments are turned at right angles to their plane of origin. The depressed fragments may be of any size, from very large to a tract of minute spicules or bone dust along a foreign body tract, as in the case of missile injuries.

The degree of intracranial depression of bone fragments also varies tremendously. In the case of a missile injury, a bone fragment may be driven almost the entire length of the brain. With the ordinary civilian type of injury, however, the depression may be only very slight or, at the most, a few centimeters. There is no widespread agreement concerning the degree of depression that is significant and that requires surgical treatment. An inward displacement of a fragment only 0.5 cm. in depth is sufficient to impinge upon the brain; many investigators believe that if there is depression of this degree or greater, elevation should be carried out to avoid excessive scarring, which may cause neurologic symptoms at a later date. Others feel that the location of the injury enters into the indication for surgical elevation and that a depression in a relatively silent area, such as the frontal pole, is not as strong an indication for treatment as depression in a motor area. On the other hand, elevation of a depressed frontal fracture might be indicated for cosmetic reasons. At any rate, it is unusual for a depression of more than 0.5 cm. to remain unattended; since this is essentially the thickness of the bone in many areas and since depression in the average case is 1 to 2 cm., the majority of such injuries are surgically treated.

In radiographs, a depressed fracture appears face on as a stellate or crescentic bone defect; often one, or sometimes several, of the comminuted fragments are turned so that they appear of greater density than the general portion of the bony skull (fig. 598). In other instances, a linear fracture may appear to be present in the main; at some place along its course, instead of diminished density, there may be a linear segment of increased density, representing a point where depression of one of the elements causes the bone edges to overlap, thereby creating a double thickness of bone. The presence of depression, and the extent of intracranial impingement, may be readily appreciated in face on stereoscopic views. Tangential films, often in various oblique projections, are advisable in order to measure, in a plane at right angles to the face of the fractured bone, the extent of depression. Such films are usually best obtained after the routine skull series, including a stereoscopic study, has been examined by the radiologist. In the average case, a depression of more than 0.5 cm. along even one edge of a depressed element may be considered as a probable indication that the dura has been torn, especially if the depressed edge is sharp, irregular, or turned.

In early infancy, the bones are so thin in some areas that difficulty in diagnosing a fracture, even a depressed fracture, may be encountered unless technique is exceptionally good. In this regard, the depressed skull fractures of early life resemble the greenstick fractures that may be encountered elsewhere in the skeleton. The bone may merely bend inward, as occurs when the finger impresses a ping-pong ball. This type of injury occurs most often when the head meets the force of a blunt object, such as a smoothly rounded door knob. The limitations of radiologic study in such instances should be appreciated, and close clinical correlation carried out in all cases of head injuries during infancy.

Depressed fractures in certain areas may be of particular significance, just as are linear fractures which cross important vascular channels and fractures which open air sinuses. Headtop injuries, with intracranial depression of a fragment, in particular, provide the opportunity for damage to one of the dural sinuses of the skull. A fragment impacted into the superior longitudinal sinus (fig. 598) may either lacerate the sinus walls with resultant hemorrhage or it may form the basis for a thrombosis of the sinus. Similar impactions occur frequently along one of the lateral sinus grooves, but in this instance the development of occlusion may not be as serious an event unless there is retrograde propagation of the thrombus, since the lateral sinuses are paired structures (fig. 598). In general, such venous injuries are much less serious events than injuries to arteries.

COMPOUND FRACTURES

Compound fractures occur as a result of an external communication through the scalp, although the communication may be internal and occult. *Externally compound fractures* may result from various types of injuries but are found almost always in connection with gunshot wounds. In the case of missile injuries, the cause of the damage is usually obvious radiologically. Both penetrating and perforating wounds are produced by bullets. Patients who survive such injuries more often sustain glancing blows than direct hits, although there usually is some intracranial material of metallic density. In many instances the size of the penetrating metallic fragments is small, but there is a large amount of finely fragmented bone present. Whenever such intracranial metallic and bone fragments are observed, it can be assumed that hair, pieces of cloth headgear, and other foreign material have contaminated the wound.

Osteomyelitis

All fractures, externally compounded, carry with them the danger of local secondary osteomyelitis. Indeed, in spite of antibiotics, it is considered basic that even a simple scalp laceration deserves careful surgical attention to exclude the possibility of primary injury to galea and bone and to guard against local infection and possible secondary infection in bone and brain. As with osteomyelitis elsewhere, the changes present in the skull in radiographs may lag behind the clinical evidence of infectious disease (fig. 601). On other occasions, the skull films may give the only real clue to the presence of an infectious complication. The margins of the bone deformed by fracture or the clean-cut edges of bone about a debrided fracture become decalcified and indistinct. The pattern of the destructive change is irregular and, when first seen, it may involve a segment of bony margin that is less than 1 cm. in length and extends only a millimeter or two proximal into normal bone from the edge of the defect. Varying with the nature of the infection and other circumstances, the decalcification, and eventually the osteolytic process, may advance slowly or rapidly. Since the infection usually travels by way of the diploic veins as well as by contiguity, relatively large areas of irregularly destroyed bone may appear. In some instances, a large portion of a squamous bone of the vault may be destroyed; spread may occur across suture lines to other bones. The advancing edge of bone destruction usually is very irregular; spicules and islands of undestroyed bone may remain in large areas of osteolysis. In other instances, the destruction is quite spotty; occasionally, it may be difficult to differentiate an area of spotty osteomyelitis from

(Revised 1963)

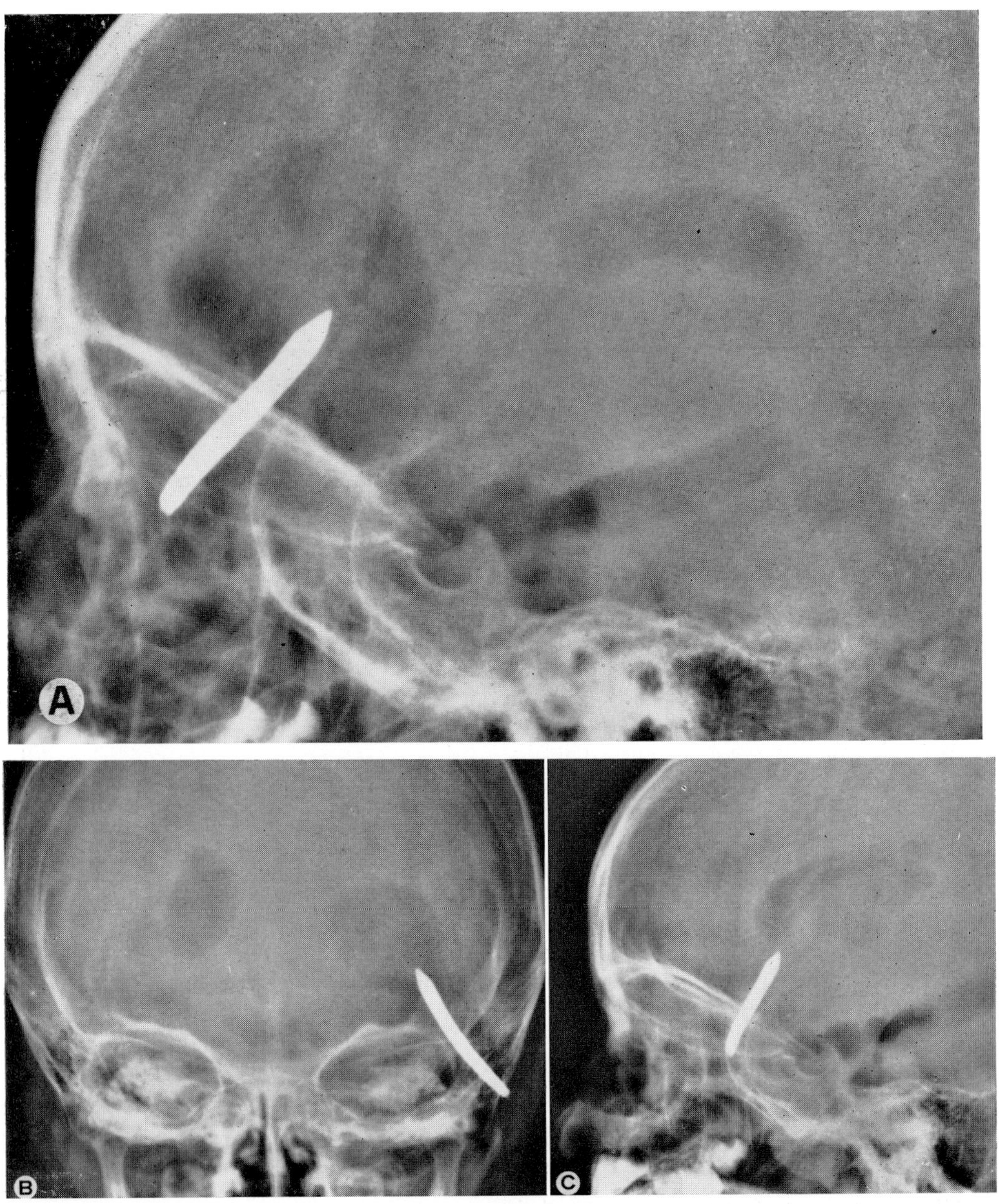

FIG. 600.—VENTRICULAR INFECTION BY GAS-FORMING ORGANISM

The child was playing in her yard while her father was cutting the lawn with a rotary power mower. The child noticed a mild stinging sensation in the region of the left temple and after a few minutes went into the house where it was thought that she had been bitten by an insect. During the next few days the patient complained of a mild headache, developed fever, and became drowsy. The films made 10 days after the injury reveal a long fragment of a nail impacted intracranially, the tip of which is surrounded by a gas collection in the left frontal lobe (A) and (B). Another lateral view (C) reveals that there is a communication from the left frontal lobe abscess to the ventricular system; the finding is similar to that frequently encountered after fractures which open the frontal or ethmoid sinuses to the intracranial cavity.

(Revised 1963)

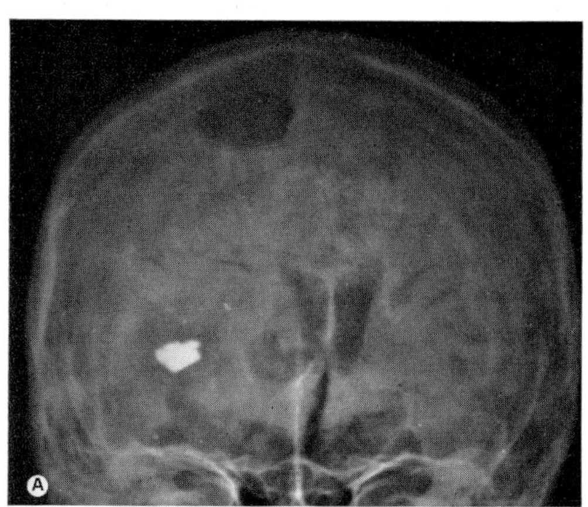

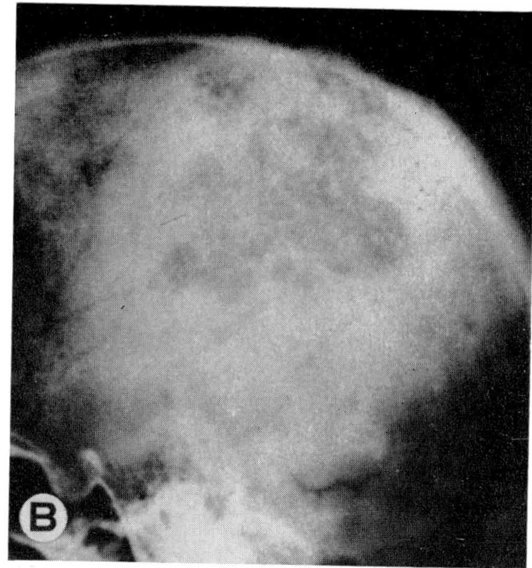

FIG. 601.—INFECTION FOLLOWING CRANIOCEREBRAL INJURY

A soldier sustained a penetrating wound of the parietal area, caused by a bursting shell fragment. Debridement of soft tissues and the bony skull was carried out and visibly damaged brain was removed. The missile tract extended deeply, and in spite of heavy antibiotic therapy, the patient developed a brain abscess about the intracranial foreign material. Following the pneumoencephalogram (A), intracranial exploration was carried out and a brain abscess evacuated.

Osteomyelitis of the skull may develop from infected scalp lacerations, even when there is no evident bony damage, and also from other causes (B). Irregular bone destruction with islands of sequestrated osseous tissue is found, often extending over a wide area. A latent period is seen in the radiologic manifestation of osteomyelitis of the skull, as in other areas. When chronic, there may be sclerosis about the margins of the osteolytic area. Osteomyelitis may be complicated by epidural and brain abscess.

an area of osteolytic metastasis from carcinoma, with coalescing secondary deposits.

In the event of prolonged chronic infection, radiologic changes of sclerosis may develop along the margins of areas that formerly exhibited destruction. Arrest of an advancing margin of decalcification, and adjacent replacement by an area of increased calcification (irregular areas of decreased density mixed among areas of sclerosis) indicates healing.

Cerebrospinal Fluid Rhinorrhea

Occult compound fractures are those linear, or sometimes comminuted, fractures that involve the walls of the air sinuses, particularly in the frontal and ethmoid regions. Many patients with injuries in these areas have associated meningeal tears and a high incidence of leakage of cerebrospinal fluid through the sinuses into the nose (fig. 599).

(Revised 1963)

Whenever such a condition exists, the pathway for bacterial contamination of the meninges and other intracranial contents exists. It is also possible for air to enter the cranial cavity through such a dural and sinus defect. While cerebrospinal fluid rhinorrhea is a common complication of injuries of the inferior frontal region, meningitis occurs much less frequently now than formerly through the benefit of antibiotics.

In radiographs, a line of diminished density often is seen traversing the inner or outer table of a sinus margin, frequently in the region of the frontal sinus. The fracture line usually can be followed into the posterior sinus plate; it is common to encounter a slight loss of apposition, displacement, or a depression of one of the fragments. Discontinuity of the posterior sinus plate, and an associated dural tear, allow fluid to enter the sinus; an air-fluid level is best demonstrated by use of the horizontal x-ray beam. In other projections, the sinus may appear diffusely, sometimes homogeneously, clouded. At times, fractures may be invisible against the complex density of the ethmoid area; a frank break in the ethmoid plate is more difficult to demonstrate than those occurring in the frontal region. Cerebrospinal fluid entering a mastoid sinus will cause opacification, but an air-fluid level rarely can be demonstrated.

There are three sites in which rhinorrhea often develops. The first is either in the frontal sinus or along the cribriform plate. The second point is in the middle fossa through the floor of the sella turcica or in the parasellar region, off the midline. If the sphenoid sinuses are large, the communication could be further lateral to the sella turcica. Another place in which cerebrospinal fluid leaks occur is the petrous pyramid and mastoid region. Defects here cause the fluid to flow into the middle ear cavity and, if the ear drum is intact, the fluid passes into the nasopharynx, from which it usually is swallowed. The sinuses on one side do not communicate with the contralateral sinuses; therefore, if cerebrospinal fluid is found in one side of the nose, this is the only side that has to be considered.

As noted above, the technique of radiographic examination in the presence of cerebrospinal fluid rhinorrhea is important. Upright Bucky films usually will disclose an air-fluid level in one or more of the sinuses. The amount of fluid varies from time to time, and more than one examination may be required for diagnosis. If the patient cannot sit, a recumbent lateral film made with the horizontal x-ray beam may suffice to demonstrate an air-fluid collection.

Occasionally, the point of cerebrospinal fluid leak is not readily demonstrated. In such cases, it may be necessary to place the patient in the position in which rhinorrhea occurs and leave him in this posture until the flow of fluid starts, at which time a film is taken immediately.

Cerebrospinal fluid rhinorrhea may occur spontaneously owing to lesions of the paranasal sinuses, as described by Cushing (1927); lesions around the sella turcica, pituitary adenomas, and small medial meningoceles also produce rhinorrhea.

Intracranial Complications

INFECTION

Aerocele

The spontaneous appearance of gas within the cranial cavity following a fracture—an aerocele, pneumatocele, or traumatic pneumocephalus—formed the basis for the first radiologic description of pneumoencephalography by Luckett (1913). An aerocele usually does not develop immediately after a compound fracture; air ordinarily appears within the cranium between ten days and three weeks after injury. Aeroceles are of three general types: the intracranial gas may be located (1) in the subarachnoid space, (2) in the brain, or (3) within the ventricles. In addition, a subdural gas collection may occasionally be found intracranially. An extracranial pneumocephalus also may develop through the dissection of gas into the subaponeurotic space of the scalp, following a break in the outer table of a cranial air cavity. The more common types of aeroceles encountered are the subarachnoid and the intracerebral gas collections. Intracerebral pneumocephalus most often occurs in one of the frontal poles of the brain; it results from the entrance of air into, or the formation of gas in, an area where a hematoma first was present following trauma (fig. 600). The hematoma and damaged brain tissue become liquified and evacuated, leaving a porencephalic area.

In roentgenograms, a gas collection, usually in the frontal lobe, may be present which in extraordinary cases measures up to 10 cm. in diameter; in most instances, it is not more than 3 to 4 cm. in size. It is of interest that the majority of intracerebral aeroceles referred to specialty hospitals have not been properly diagnosed, even with the benefit of radiologic examination. In many instances, the intracranial location of the collection of reduced air density is not appreciated; frequently, the diagnosis of a bone defect or of a benign cranial tumor has been made.

A ventricular aerocele is the end stage of an intracerebral aerocele; it usually results from communication of a frontal lobe cavity with the frontal horn of one lateral ventricle. Frequently, the ventricular system is symmetrically dilated, either a result of infection or ventricular blockage by debris. With inflammation, there is a communication of the ventricles with the subarachnoid space; in these instances, the dilatation probably is related to ependymitis with overproduction of fluid or to arachnoiditis and interference with cerebrospinal fluid absorption. Infection also may produce gliosis and obstruction in the aqueduct of Sylvius at a later time. On occasion, gas-forming organisms may be responsible for the presence of intracranial and even intraventricular gas, usually in connection with an externally compound injury (fig. 600). A naturally developing nontraumatic aerocele may be encountered rarely, as in the cases of Cushing (1927), who described several patients having orbitoethmoidal osteomas with intracranial complications. An intracerebral aerocele is, in essence, a brain abscess.

Brain Abscess

An abscess more commonly complicates a penetrating wound of the brain than any other type of craniocerebral injury. When there is radiologic evidence of intracerebral impaction of metallic and bony debris, or when a patient has a compound depressed fracture not of missile origin, then clinical and radiologic surveillance must be maintained for the possible development of a brain abscess. In such instances, a pineal shift or other evidence of an intracranial mass may be an indication of untoward developments. The usual evidences of increased intracranial pressure may not occur with a brain abscess of contamination origin. Rather, there is local evidence of pressure and bulging at the debridement site. The authors have encountered cases in which bacteria apparently remained dormant for four to five years adjacent to an impacted foreign body, only to become active after this long period of time. Cases have been reported in which a residual intracranial foreign body of metallic type has been associated with the development of frank infection 15 to 20 years after injury. More often, however, evidence of abscess develops within three to six weeks after a missile injury. Direct indication of the presence of an abscess is obtained from plain films, if movement of an impacted foreign body can be demonstrated radiologically with a change of posture, or if two examinations show that movement occurs with the passage of time (Wood, 1948). In pneumograms, evidence of a brain abscess is similar to that of other mass lesions (fig. 601). In angiograms, abnormal vascularity may denote the nature of the process present.

It is not infrequent at ventriculography for the operator to have the needle enter an abscess cavity rather than the ventricular system. On other occasions, if an abscess is suspected, needling may be carried out intentionally under antibiotic coverage. After evacuation of the suppurative contents, air often is injected to demonstrate radiologically the extent of the residual cavity and its possible extensions and loculations. Rather than air, some type of positive contrast material may be injected into the abscess, preferably one which will not be absorbed readily, such as Thorotrast or tantalum dust. Filling of the abscess with a fluid opaque material may demonstrate even better than air the cavity and its ramifications. In addition, after evacuation of the contrast material following filming, some usually will stay behind, coating the walls of the lesion. By means of this technique, reaccumulations with distention of the abscess wall may be demonstrated in serial radiographs. Likewise, continued collapse and shrinkage of the lesion with healing may be demonstrated by a progressive reduction in over-all size of the opacified abscess wall.

The development of subdural empyema is

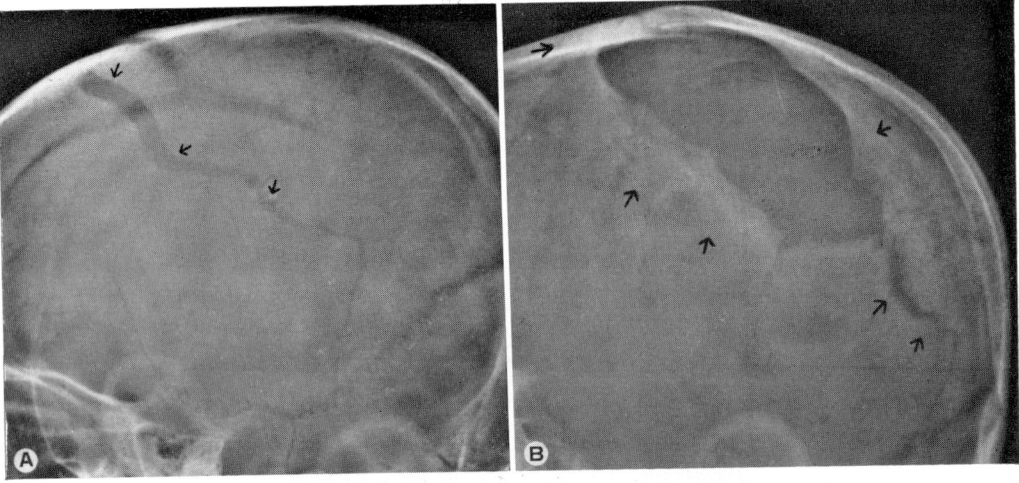

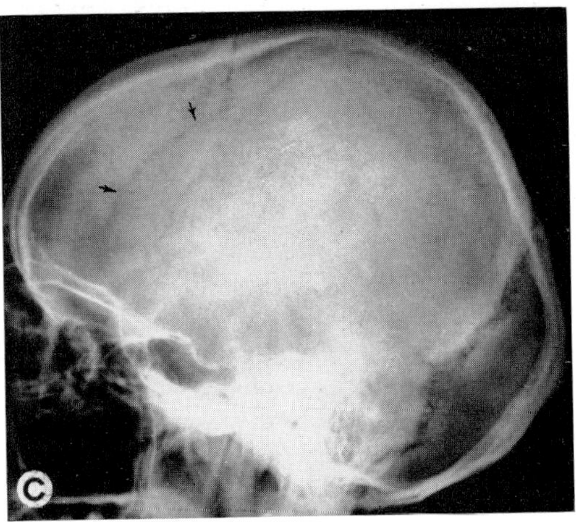

Fig. 602.—Leptomeningeal Cyst

Skull fractures in children, particularly when lengthy and wide, may be associated with tearing of the dura and the development of a leptomeningeal cyst. In the case illustrated, a severe headtop injury produced a wide fracture line (*arrows*) which extended across the midline (A). The child developed bulging of the scalp in the right parietal region which became progressively larger. A skull film made two and a half years after the injury (B) reveals that instead of healing in the normal manner, the fracture line has become much wider; the margins are scalloped in the area where marked widening has occurred (*arrows*). The most caudal extension of the fracture line on the same side also remains unhealed (*posterior arrows*). The portion of the fracture line on the opposite side of the skull appears to have healed in the usual manner.

Skull fractures which heal in the usual manner disappear gradually over a period of time (see text). A linear fracture, sustained two years before the lateral radiograph was made, has margins which are indistinct (C). The line of the fracture is not as dark as in the case of a recent injury (*arrows*); at many points the fracture line appears bridged by bony healing.

an ominous change and may be the result of natural processes as well as a compound fracture. Usually, a severe degree of brain reaction with extensive edema develops; marked dislocation of midline structures is found in pneumograms and angiograms owing to the subdural mass and the cerebral edema.

(Revised 1963)

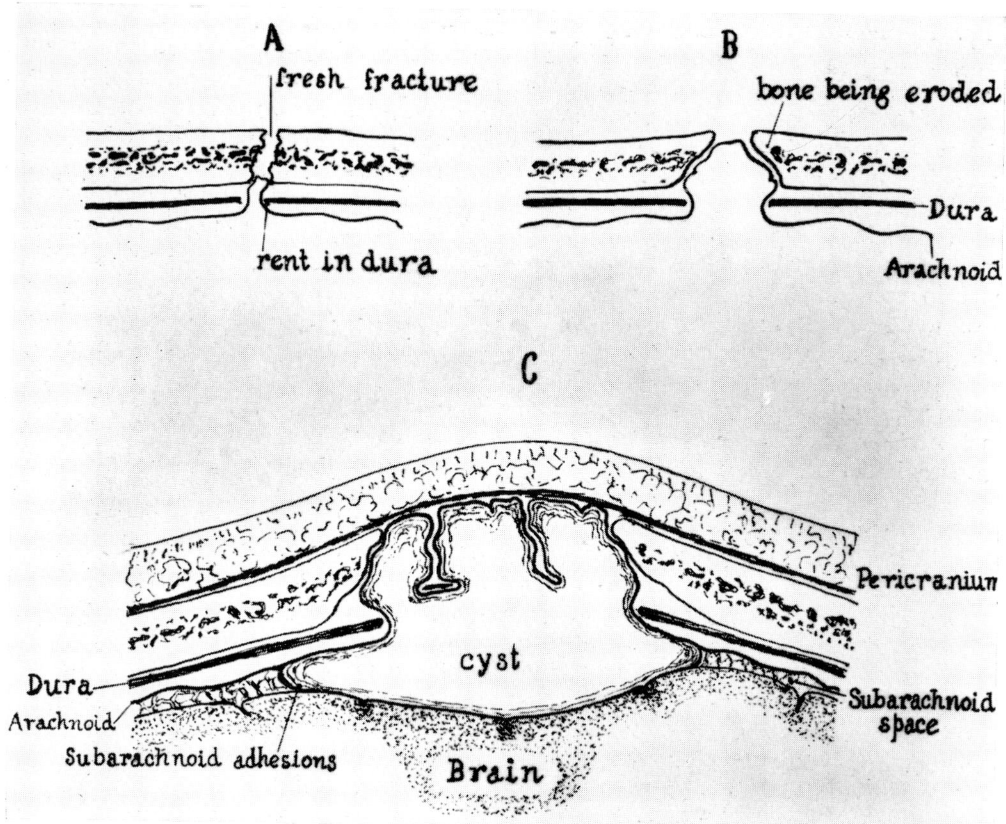

Fig. 603.—Mechanism of Progressive Changes with Leptomeningeal Cyst
The probable mechanism of production of a leptomeningeal cyst and the progressive erosion of the overlying skull is shown. The original fracture tears the dura mater, with the development of a small herniation of the arachnoid membrane through the dura (A). If soft tissue containing pulsating fluid is interposed, the bone does not heal in the usual manner, but the edges of the fracture line become smoother by erosion (B). When there is marked erosion of the bone, owing to pulsation of the cystlike collection of fluid in the partially walled-off subarachnoid space, a wide defect may be produced (C); an external prominence of the scalp usually is found, while internally there may be depression of the brain.

HEMORRHAGE

Hemorrhage and hematoma formation are an integral part of a fracture. Intracranial hematomas may occur after an apparently insignificant blow, without discernible bony skull or other damage. The majority of epicranial and epidural hematomas are of traumatic origin; others, such as subdural and intracerebral hematomas, result from trauma but also often occur spontaneously.

Cephalhematoma

Traumatic hematomas may occur in relation to the skull, the meninges, and the brain. Subperiosteal hematomas or cephalhematomas occur frequently in the newborn and they may be multiple. They occur most frequently in the parietal areas and may attain considerable size (fig. 604). Patients with such lesions are frequently referred for radiologic examination during the first few days of life in order to exclude a fracture, or a meningocele or other craniocerebral malformation. At this time, the cranial bones are found to be symmetrical but on one side enlargement of the extracranial soft tissue shadows is present over one of the bones. The increase in density may occur over the entire bone but usually is limited by the margins, where the pericranium is attached to the suture edge. In some instances, the hematoma may be several centimeters in thickness; it may produce a remarkable prominence as seen clinically and in tangential roentgenograms. Associated fracture of the underlying bone is found in approximately one-fourth of the cases.

Absorption of the cephalhematoma begins early and may be complete in as short a time as two weeks. Since the hemorrhage is beneath the periosteum, new bone formation is stimulated, as with subperiosteal hemorrhage elsewhere in the body. Often within a week, the rounded soft tissue swelling may become bounded externally by a shell of calcific density demonstrable in roentgenograms. Calcification begins in the angle between the outer table and elevated periosteum and covers the entire area of the hematoma.

After resorption of a cephalhematoma, some radiologic evidence of bony thickening may persist for months and even years. Such bony thickening, if persistent in both parietal areas, may be mistaken for rickets. In occasional cases, the space between the ossified periosteal shell and the bone persists for many years and may become filled with diploic bone. In other instances, cystlike defects remain at the subperiosteal hematoma site (cephalhematoma deformans); the changes may simulate those of an epidermoid, fibrous dysplasia, or meningioma.

Epidural Hematoma

Epidural hematomas result from hemorrhage between the inner table of the skull and the dura mater; they are found most commonly in the temporal, frontal and occipital areas. The development of such a hematoma usually is rapid, due to laceration of an arterial channel, although occasionally a large venous channel may be the source of bleeding. There is no direct evidence of the presence of an epidural hematoma; indirectly, there may be displacement of the pineal shadow or other normal calcifications The best clue on plain films is the demon

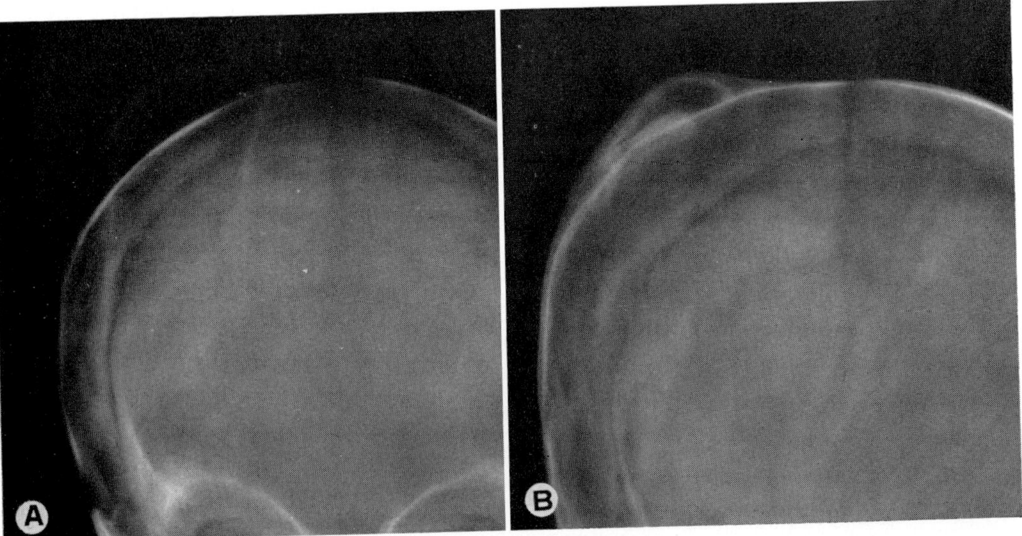

FIG. 604.—CEPHALHEMATOMA

Subperiosteal hematomas frequently are found in infancy. Calcium visible in radiographs becomes laid down along the outer (subperiosteal) margin of the hematoma at an early stage of development (A). After partial absorption, contraction, and organization, the hematoma may progressively be reduced in size, and with the passage of time, no radiologic evidence of the site of injury may be definable. In other instances, the peripheral portion of the hematoma may become more heavily calcified and ossified, and cystlike changes may be found during the intermediate stage of healing of such injuries (B).

(Revised 1963)

stration of a fracture line across or near one of the main vascular grooves of the skull, usually the middle meningeal artery or one of its branches. Recognition of a linear fracture in relation to one of these larger vasal channels may be lifesaving.

Epidural hematomas may develop at the frontal or occipital pole of the brain after trauma; the occurrence after an excessive replacement of ventricular fluid by gas for the ventriculography of hydrocephalus has been described elsewhere (see fig. 196). With hydrocephalus, such hemorrhages may be relatively silent, even though they are large. A sizable fusiform area of intracranial calcification may be the end result of such a process (fig. 157).

Whenever an epidural hematoma is suspected clinically, an angiogram is the most satisfactory method of establishing the diagnosis and, in addition, showing the exact location and extent of the collection. For hematomas in the usual parietotemporal location, frontal carotid angiograms will demonstrate the lesion to best advantage. The frontal angiogram discloses the pial vessels displaced away from the inner table of the skull a distance of 2 to 3 cm., in the average case (fig. 606). The displacement may extend from the high convexity to the inferior temporal region, but usually is more limited to the low convexity. Often the greatest thickness is near a line of fracture, if the latter is present. The avascular space of the hematoma usually has a relatively straight margin along its inner surface, resulting in a semiellipsoidal configuration. The collection may conform to the shape of the cerebral convexity, resulting in a crescentic configuration; occasionally, the hematoma is fusiform or spindle shaped, simulating a chronic subdural hematoma. Displacement of the middle meningeal arterial channels away from the inner table is characteristic of epidural hematoma; lateral views are most helpful in diagnosing the collections occurring anteriorly and posteriorly at the poles of the brain.

Subdural Hematoma

Subdural hematoma results from hemorrhage into the thin space or potential space between the dura mater and the closely applied arachnoid membrane. Trauma is considered to be the cause of subdural hemorrhage in nearly all instances, even though the injury frequently is not severe; often a history of even slight injury is difficult to obtain, particularly in infancy, in alcoholics, and in elderly individuals. Subdural hemorrhage is a frequent complication in patients with avitaminosis or a blood dyscrasia. It is now well recognized that in infancy a high incidence of hematoma occurs as a sequela of meningitis, particularly that resulting from *Hemophilus influenzae.* It has been our impression that ordinarily there is no difference between the radiologic findings in subdural hematoma following purulent meningitis or owing to trauma. In some instances, however, the postinfectious hematomas are thinner and sometimes more difficult to demonstrate satisfactorily than post-traumatic lesions. Information obtained by needling of the subdural space through the fontanelle may be equivocal or misleading in these cases if the hematoma is diffuse and thin. Bilateral subdural hematomas occur frequently in infancy, either following meningeal infection or trauma. The bleeding is most often venous in origin and usually results from tearing of the cerebral veins as they pass through the meninges; bleeding may occur from the meningeal veins and the dural sinuses. Elsewhere, the importance of careful and gentle techniques in connection with pneumoencephalography has been mentioned, particularly in instances where hydrocephalus exists. Collapse of the ventricles following replacement of fluid by gas may result in tearing of cerebral veins; we have observed not only cases in which hematomas occurred, but one instance in which a tear of a dural sinus resulted in the entrance of air into the circulatory system and death.

The pathologic anatomy and pathologic physiology of subdural hematoma have been subjects of extensive study for many years, and elaborate discussion here is not in order. It should be mentioned, however, that a subdural hematoma varies in shape with the duration of the process, and this may affect

(Revised 1963)

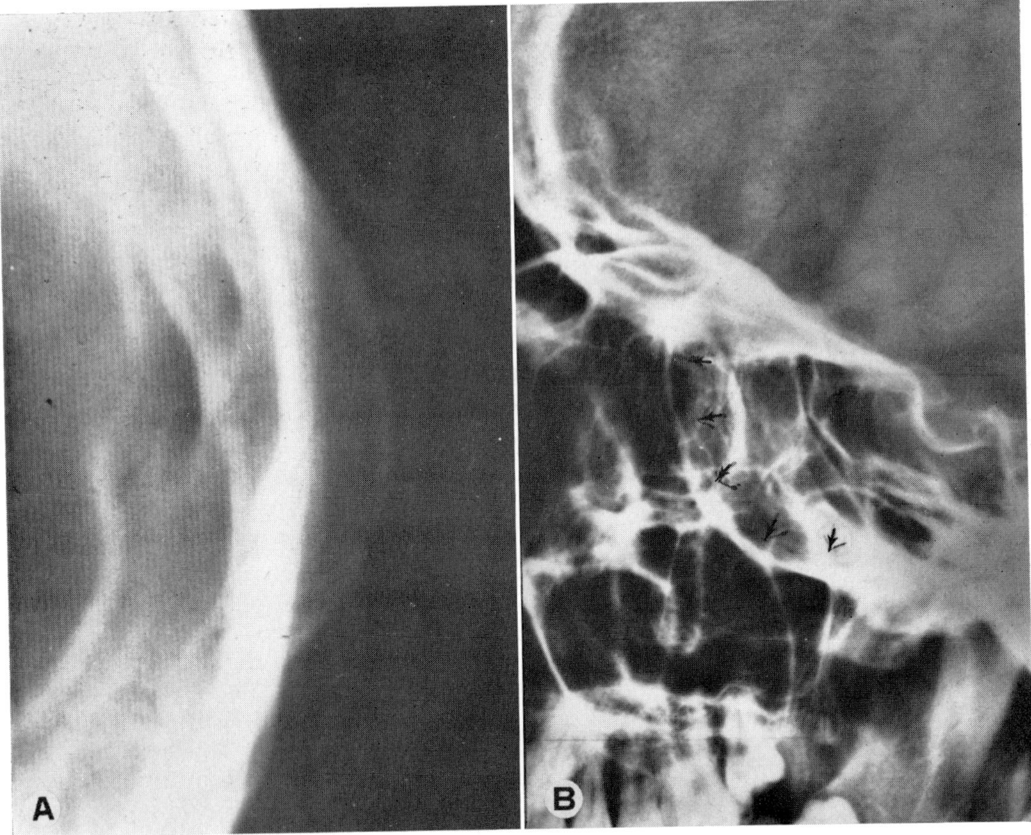

Fig. 605.—Subdural Hematoma of the Temporal Area

Cranial changes may be observed in some projections in patients who have a chronic juvenile subdural hematoma of the temporal area. In these instances, there may be outward bowing of the thin temporal bone (A). Both the inner and outer tables are convex outward, and at the dome of the prominence, the bone may be very thin. The findings are indicative of long-standing intracranial hematoma and are most frequently seen in children beyond infancy; the change is not to be confused with cephalhematoma (Fig. 604).

In other cases of subtemporal hematoma developing in early life, the sphenoid wing may be significantly affected as well as the temporal bone (B). The greater wing of the sphenoid on the involved side is bowed forward and downward (*arrows*). In frontal view (C), the greater wing is not seen tangentially and the lesser wing has a steeper slope than normal because of elevation. The picture, however, is not to be confused with neurofibromatosis, in which the posterior orbital wall and the sphenoid wing is defective in addition to being high (see Fig. 72). The angiogram (D) reveals a sizable extracerebral mass in the inferior temporal region; there is also separation of the pial vessels from the inner table of the skull laterally and superiorly. A large subdural hematoma, evidently of very long standing, was evacuated.

radiologic diagnosis. As has been pointed out by Norman (1956), the hematoma has a crescentic shape at first, following the contours of the brain surface; the fresh subdural collection is not fixed but extends as a sheath over a large area of the cerebral hemisphere. Later, the collection becomes localized and fibrous membranes develop about the hematoma, first externally and then internally. With breakdown of the blood elements, fluid is drawn into the hematoma by osmosis, producing enlargement within the membranous sac. It is thought that the abundant vascularity,

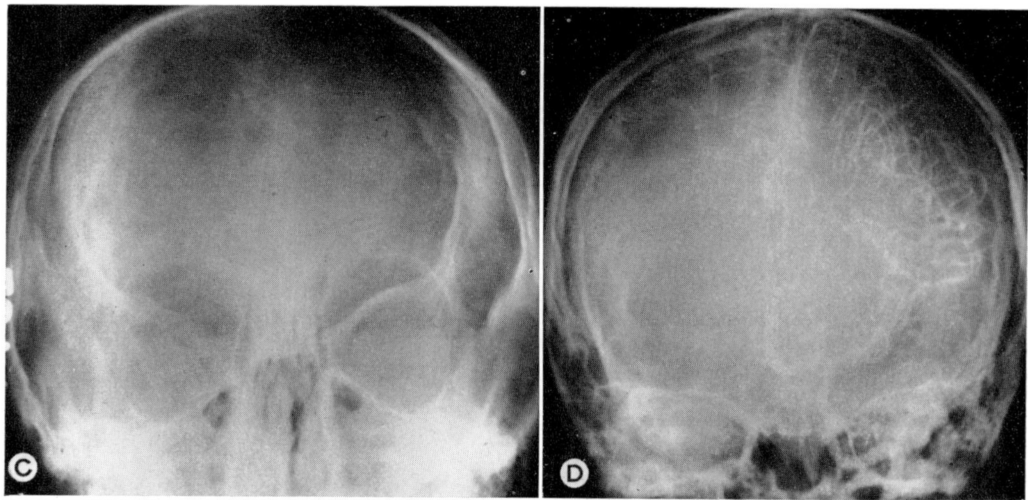

Fig. 605. C-D

developing in the membranes of some hematomas, contributes to the outflow of fluid from capillaries into the lesion. After approximately three weeks, the hematoma assumes its familiar fusiform configuration in coronal plane, having enlarged in width during this period to change from a crescentic to a semilunar and then a spindle shape. Larger hematomas which cover the entire cerebral surface do not always go through the characteristic transformation. With the passage of more time, further organization and contraction of the hematoma take place, and the characteristic fusiform or spindle shape often disappears.

Some difference exists between traumatic subdural hematoma occurring in infancy and in later life, which is of significance in roentgen diagnosis. In early life, bilateral occurrence of subdural hematoma is common, while in adults bilateral lesions occur but they are infrequent. In early life, a subdural hematoma is said often to be more fluid than in the adult; this may explain the frequent finding of uniform thickness and conformity of shape to the inner table of the skull. At one time it was thought that hematomas occurring in the middle fossa were peculiar to childhood. With the more frequent recognition of the extent of hematomas through angiography, however, it is now known that many adult lesions also have a subtemporal component. Hematomas of infancy and childhood appear to be associated more often with ventricular dilatation and underlying cortical atrophy than the lesions of later life. An infantile hematoma occurring over a large area may act as a metaventricular obstruction, thus interfering with absorption of cerebrospinal fluid. In addition, the young brain apparently may be compressed to a remarkable degree without interference with vital functions (fig. 607D); at the same time, great cortical damage may take place. The ability of the infantile head to enlarge with subdural hematoma probably contributes to the pronounced widening of the subarachnoid space which is found frequently by pneumography in lesions of long standing; the same mechanism may contribute to the hematoma being flat rather than medially convex along its inner surface.

Plain films. In plain skull radiographs, evidence of fracture is found infrequently in association with subdural hematoma. If a fracture is present, it is not uncommon for it to be located on the side opposite the hematoma. In a large series of infants with subdural hematoma, studied by Ingraham and Matson (1944), 15 per cent were found to have cranial fractures. A surprisingly frequent occurrence of multiple fractures in other parts of the body, particularly in the

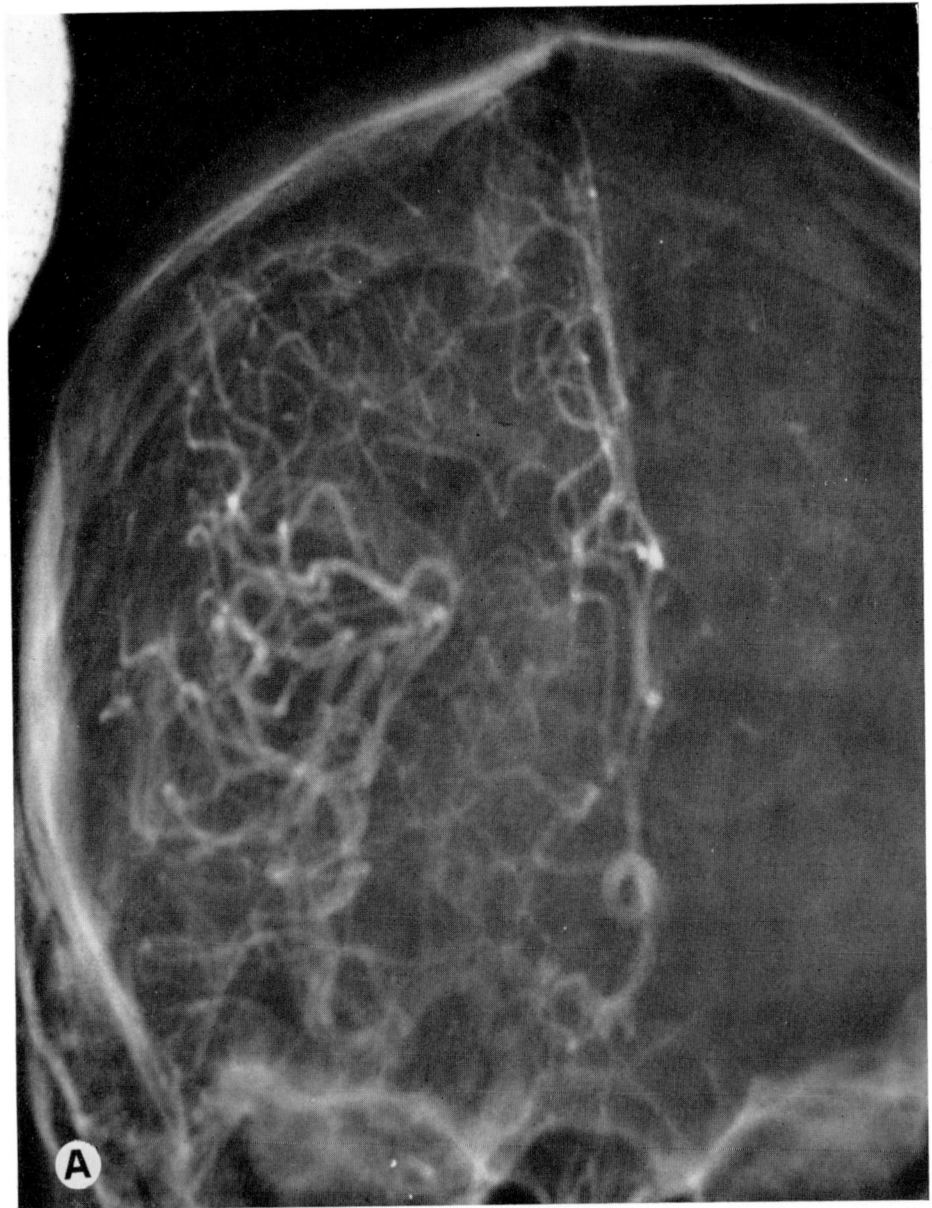

Fig. 606.—Epidural Hematoma

An adolescent boy was struck on the side of the head by a thrown baseball and rendered unconscious. After several minutes he regained consciousness, but remained dizzy and complained of severe headache. Skull films revealed a short fissure fracture of the frontotemporal region traversing the groove of the middle meningeal artery. The boy, under observation, became progressively drowsy, and the angiogram (A) reveals some branches of the middle cerebral artery displaced well away from the inner table of the skull; there is moderate contralateral displacement of the anterior cerebral artery.

In another case, a frontal epidural hematoma was found in a 15-year-old boy. The arteries are displaced away from the inner table of the skull in the frontal region (B). The venogram (C) reveals a rounded avascular area at the frontal pole of the brain extending upward (*arrows*). Venous displacement of the type shown indicates that the lesion has reached the midline. An epidural hematoma, estimated to be 150 cc. in volume, was evacuated.

(*Revised 1963*)

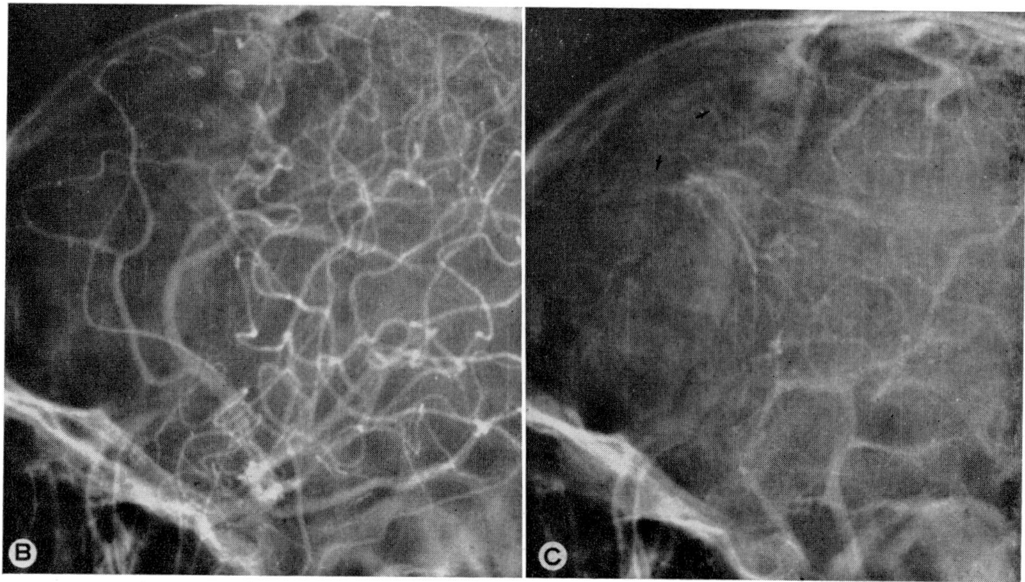

FIG. 606. B–C

long bones, was found in infants suffering from chronic subdural hematoma by Caffey (1946). A cause-and-effect relationship between subdural hematoma and the long bone fractures in infants has not been fully clarified.

Radiologic evidence of increased intracranial pressure is found in less than one-half of patients with subdural hematoma. In infancy, enlargement of the head is common, and there may be widening of the sutures and bulging of the soft tissues at the anterior fontanelle. Cranial enlargement, on the average, is not as great with subdural hematoma as with hydrocephalus, particularly of the obstructive type. Often there is more rounding of the skull in frontal projection, frequently with biparietal prominence, but without a corresponding enlargement in the sagittal plane. With megacephalus in infancy, pneumography is considered warranted, if for no other reason than to identify the cases of subdural hematoma. Some investigators (Ingraham and Matson, 1954), however, have found that many infants and children have untoward reactions following pneumography. A generalized increase in prominence of the markings does not occur as one of the evidences of increased intracranial pressure associated with subdural hematoma. Markings may be almost absent on the side of the lesion, even though the bone becomes quite thin. The inner table overlying the hematoma is often smooth, and this might be expected since the lesion is interposed between the bony skull and the brain.

Unilateral or focal pressure changes may occur with chronic subdural hematoma. These changes are more common if the hematoma forms during the first decade of life. In some instances, there is increased prominence or rounding on the side of the lesion. In other patients, with lesions of very long standing, unilateral cerebral atrophy may occur in conjunction with the hematoma and there may be an increase in the slope, or flattening, of the skull on the involved side. In other cases, there is localized bulging of one side of the skull, usually in the parietotemporal area (fig. 605). In association with the bulge, the skull is thin and the diploic space obliterated. The changes have been likened to those occurring with leptomeningeal cysts, but without fracture. Similar changes may occur with porencephalic cysts (fig. 615), and other lesions exerting focal pressure on a portion of the skull (Childe, 1953). A particular variant of such a focal change was de-

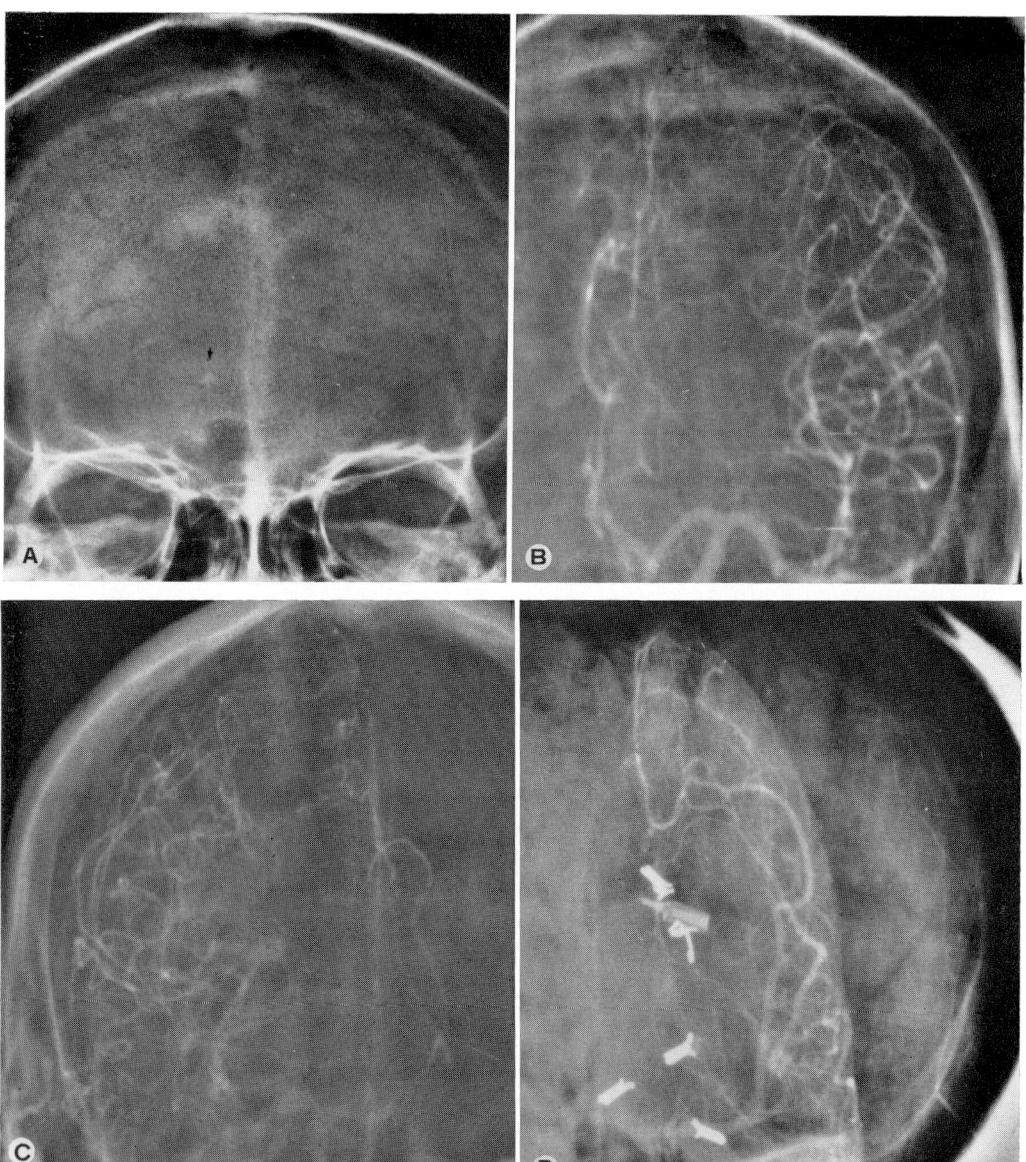

Fig. 607.—Acute Subdural Hematoma

The value of plain film examination in post-traumatic cases is illustrated by developments in the case illustrated in (A) and (B). The initial examination demonstrated a pineal which was in normal position; no fractures were identified. Because of continued headaches, the skull examination was repeated (A) and at the second examination there was moderate pineal displacement away from the midline (*arrow*). An angiogram performed at this time demonstrated a fresh subdural hematoma (B) with displacement of all of the vessels away from the inner table without loculation.

Another patient had a right carotid angiogram which reveals separation of the pial arterial vessels from the inner table of the skull a fairly uniform distance of 1.5 cm. over the cerebral convexity (C). The outline of the pial vessels maintains a normal convex curve, following the contour of the inner table of the skull. The even separation, or a crescentic separation without central fusiform enlargement, is usually associated with acute subdural hematoma (see text and compare with Fig. 609).

In a third case (D), an extremely large subdural hematoma was found following intracranial surgical treatment of an arterial aneurysm. The case illustrates the extreme degree of displacement of the brain that can occur with subdural collections.

(Revised 1963)

scribed by Davidoff and Dyke (1938) under the name "juvenile relapsing chronic subdural hematoma." These patients, who sustained injuries during the formative years of skull development, had subdural collections which were centered chiefly in the middle fossa. The most striking change consisted of deepening, widening, and lengthening of the middle fossa on one side, often with marked thinning of the contiguous bone. With lengthening of the middle fossa, the sphenoid ridge is situated further forward than its counterpart and its slope is steeper, almost vertical in some cases (fig. 605). Some elevation of the superior orbital wall may be associated. With thinning in these areas, the posterior orbital wall and often its inferior and lateral margins may be indistinct, including the outline of the superior orbital fissure. While such chronic local erosive changes are most often seen with subdural hematomas of the middle fossa, they may occasionally be seen with other lesions involving abnormalities of the dura; a congenital dural cyst was found to be the cause of the alterations in one instance observed by the authors. Sphenoid bone changes resulting from erosion are to be differentiated from those owing to neurofibromatosis (fig. 72).

After a period of time, when the hematoma is fully organized and reduced in size, there is an ipsilateral reduction in pressure, and secondary changes of unilateral cranial hypertrophy occur, similar to those in Figure 616. Such changes were an outstanding feature of the particular group of juvenile patients with subdural hematoma studied by Davidoff and Dyke (1938); they considered these changes to be a second phase of this particular disease entity (Dyke, 1941). The third phase, or "relapsing" phase, they postulated to be initiated by a second injury, usually years after the first trauma. The third phase is accompanied by clinical symptoms and signs of increased intracranial pressure. Substantiating these latter clinical observations are pneumographic changes of ventricular displacement and surgical confirmation of the middle fossa hematoma (Davidoff and Dyke, 1938).

Plain films will not disclose calcium in a subdural hematoma of average duration. Calcification and even ossification may occur in such lesions of very long standing (fig. 157). Usually, portions or segments of the inner and outer membranes of the hematoma exhibit the most prominent calcification, with irregular mottled deposits in the central part of the lesion. Two cases of such hematoma were studied in detail by Davidoff and Dyke (1938) and a third case was illustrated by Dyke in 1941. In two instances the head was large; in one of the two—probably the lesion of longer standing—there were changes of cranial thickening and hypertrophy of the air sinuses. The authors interpreted the cranial enlargement as resulting from increased pressure by the mass, and probably interference with cerebrospinal fluid circulation, at a time when the lesion was fresh. The secondary changes of cranial hypertrophy were thought to be related to later cerebral atrophy, owing to interference with cerebral blood flow by pressure on vessels. In the case of an ossified hematoma, there was a sharp slope of the cranial vault on the involved side, and the corresponding cerebral hemisphere was smaller.

Pineal displacement remains the most important plain film evidence of subdural hematoma in the average case, despite the interesting, although more unusual, plain film findings which have just been described. Except in the case of bilateral hematomas, there is readily discernible contralateral displacement of the pineal gland in almost all instances; frequently the displacement is marked. In the majority of cases, the calcified pineal body is displaced backward and frequently it is displaced downward. Upward and forward displacement do not occur.

Pneumography. Pneumographic confirmation of the presence of subdural hematoma may be obtained in a variety of ways. When there is increased intracranial pressure, ventriculography is the pneumographic procedure of choice. It is not rare for the hematoma to be encountered at the time of trephination for ventriculography. In the case of infants, direct puncture of the subdural space is usually carried out through the fontanelle prior to ventricular tap; the objective is to make a diagnosis by obtaining bloody or xanthochromic fluid from the hematoma sac itself. If the subdural hematoma is tapped directly through a burr hole or through the fontanelle, there is little purpose served by injecting air and taking radiographs, which is a practice in some institutions. Under these circumstances, rather bizarre patterns are obtained, and an accurate assessment of the extent of the lesion is difficult; the procedure usually has no significant influence as a guide to therapy. Failure to encounter a hematoma through trephination, or by means of a needle inserted through the fontanelle, cannot be accepted as valid evidence that such a lesion is absent, since the opening in the skull or the needle may not be placed at the site of the lesion. Numerous instances have been observed in which clinical reliance was placed on a negative fontanelle needle exploration, only to have a hematoma demonstrated later by means of radiologic contrast study.

If the needle is inserted deeper than usually required to tap a hematoma, it may enter a fluid space beneath the inner membrane of the lesion. The injection of air at this time may result in a pathognomonic roentgen finding. In the frontal pneumogram, the gas, which usually is collected over the midconvexity or higher, will assume a finger-shaped configuration. The shadow is medially convex, deviating away from the inner table of the skull. The soft tissue shadow between the fingerlike gas collection and the inner table of the skull represents the hematoma itself, and gives an indication of its thickness and over-all size (fig. 608). If gas fills the entire space deep to the hematoma, it will reach the inner table of the skull at the upper and lower end, demonstrating the fusiform outline of the hematoma along its entire coronal extent. The subdural gas collection beneath the hematoma usually is smooth, medially as well as laterally; the medial smoothness of the shadow results from the arachnoid being interposed between the air and brain and nonvisualization of the sulci. The lateral films are nondiagnostic. A shapeless gas collection may be observed, usually in the parietal area; a suggestion of the extent of the hematoma in sagittal plane may be gained. The typical pneumographic findings of a subdural hematoma are most readily demonstrated in the upright position.

Ordinary ventriculography provides information concerning the size and location of the mass, but does not allow definitive diagnosis. In frontal view, a shift of the midline ventricular structures away from the side of the lesion is found; often the degree of displacement is great. The septum pellucidum and upper third ventricle usually exhibit a square, or sometimes angular, shift; the type depends on the size and principal location of the hematoma. There is often some degree of ventricular dilatation, although usually it is not marked. The lateral ventricular deformity on the side of the lesion is one chiefly of flattening of the ventricular roof, owing to depression of the greater portion of the hemisphere and partial or complete herniation of the more medial structures beneath the edge of the falx. Often the entire frontal horn and ventricular

---

Fig. 608.—Chronic Subdural Hematoma

A 57-year-old man was struck by a truck and thrown to the street unconscious, two months before entering the hospital. For several weeks following injury, he complained of mental confusion and intermittent headache. The ventriculogram (A) was made after replacement of 15 cc. of ventricular fluid by gas. The right atrium and temporal horn are displaced downward and medially; the posterior portion of the ventricular body is herniated beneath the falx. A small linear collection of gas is trapped in the subdural space between a subdural hematoma and the surface of the brain (*arrows*). The cerebral surface is depressed 2 cm. beneath the inner table of the skull at the point of maximum thickness of the hematoma.

In other instances, subdural gas may follow the contour of the inner table and cerebral surface (*arrows*) to produce a configuration suggesting acute subdural hematoma (B). Unless the hematoma is chronic and contracted, however, gas usually does not collect between the hematoma and the external cerebral surface.

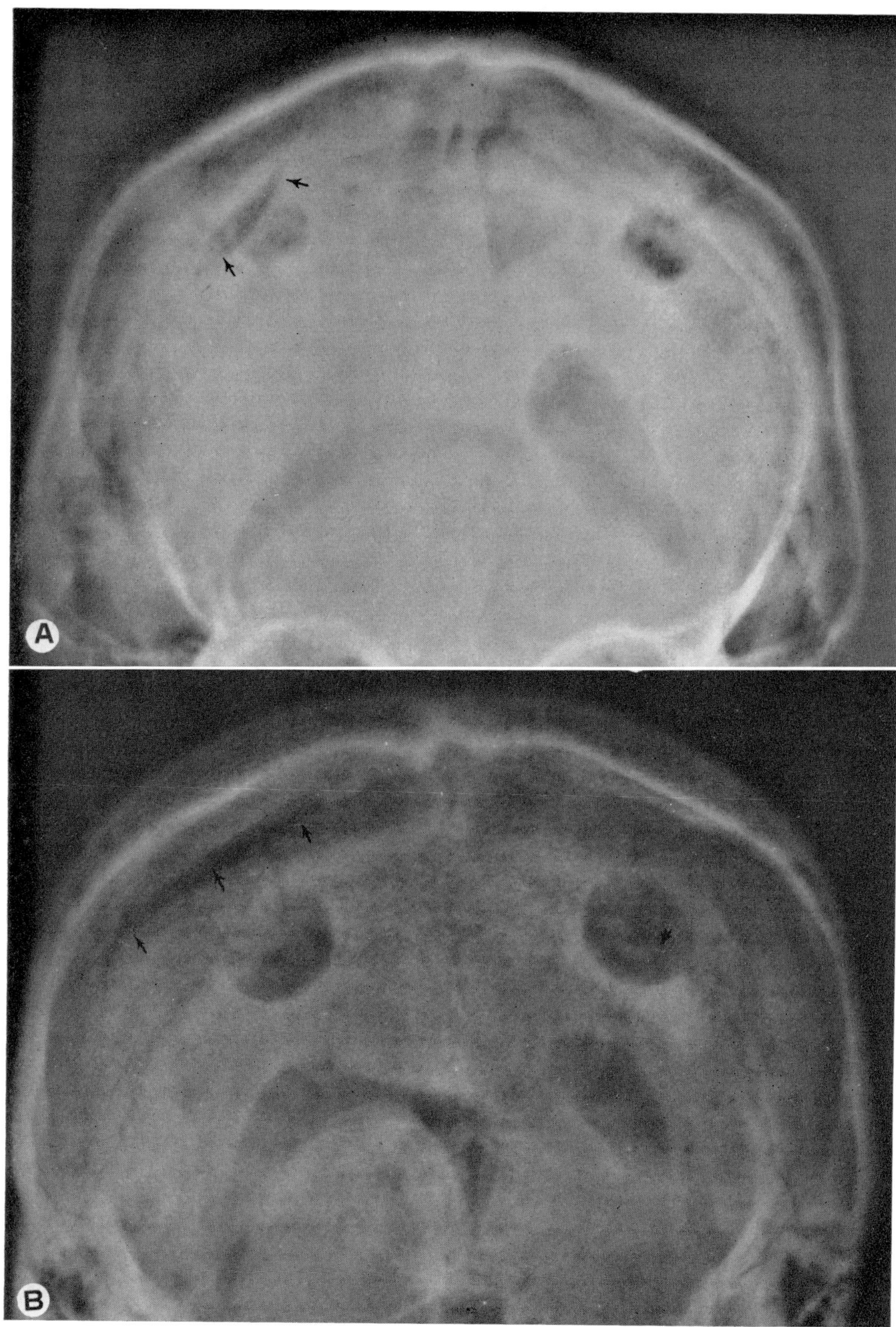

Fig. 608. A-B

body are involved in the depression, without focal change; the integrity of the ventricular lumen is protected by the great thickness of hemispheric substance, which cushions the ventricle from the direct pressure of the lesion. The length and evenness of the deformity may suggest the nature of the process, but the differentiation of subdural hematoma from other mass lesions of the frontoparietal or parietotemporal convexity by ventriculography generally is impractical. At ventriculography, there usually is not an adequate amount of gas in the subarchnoid space to visualize these pathways sufficiently to aid in diagnosis.

Pneumoencephalography may be the procedure of choice in patients with long standing lesions where retraction has occurred and increased pressure is no longer apparent. It is applicable also to those infants who are suspected of having hematoma after meningitis. In such cases, it is desirable to visualize the subarachnoid space of the convexities with regard to patency and to assess the degree of atrophy which may have taken place. Pneumoencephalography and ventriculography should be avoided if there is plain film evidence of increased intracranial pressure or a pineal shift; instead, an angiogram should be carried out. Under such circumstances, sizable unilateral lesions may be present. The displacements and deformities of the ventricular system just noted in connection with ventriculography usually are demonstrated. If there is transtentorial as well as subfalcial herniation, there is interference with ventricular filling at pneumoencephalography.

Good sulcal filling over the hemisphere usually occurs on the side opposite the lesion. On the side of the hematoma, sulcal filling may be absent entirely, or it may be seen only at the frontal and occipital poles. Full sulcal filling in the polar areas, with absence between, and with an even displacement and depression of the ventricle, suggests a surface tumor in the central area, frequently a subdural hematoma. Sulcal filling is often present along the medial aspects of the cerebral hemispheres; the markings may be displaced away from the site of the lesion, but not usually occluded by hematomas situated laterally. Occasionally, a hematoma will dissect medially and downward beside the falx; this may become an important aspect of the lesion, particularly if the lateral component is evacuated and the medial component not recognized (fig. 611). In these instances, the medial sulci do not fill, but the ventricular roof becomes more severely depressed and dislocated. Medial extension of a hematoma should be considered when the pneumographic appearance strongly resembles a parasagittal tumor. The diagnosis of medial extension is difficult, however, since in many respects the pneumographic changes of an uncomplicated convexity hematoma resemble those of a parasagittal mass. In the experience of the authors, angiography is the most successful method of diagnosis of subdural hematoma, particularly of medial extension, which will cause spreading of the anterior cerebral arteries.

In infancy, particularly in the event of bilateral subdural hematomas, there is little or no ventricular shift since the hematomas frequently are of about the same size on the two sides. The ventricular system is almost always open; a greater degree of ventricular dilatation and subarachnoid enlargement usually is seen with bilateral subdural hematomas than with a unilateral lesion. Since the ventricles frequently do not return to normal size after surgical treatment, a component of deeply seated atrophy with ventricular dilatation may be an important factor in many cases (fig. 612).

Gas over the cerebral surface in the subarachnoid space may be voluminous in the event of cerebral atrophy complicating subdural hematoma. In these instances, the outer margin of the subarachnoid gas collection is fairly smooth or only finely irregular; it outlines the inner surface of the hematoma well away from the inner table of the skull. With bilateral subdural hematoma, there is frequently a midline component of prominence; the result is that the subarachnoid gas outlines between it and the inner table of the skull a soft tissue lesion having the shape of the number 3 turned on its side, open side downward. The inner surface of the subarachnoid space is coarsely irregular in outline because the gas enters numerous wide deep sulci between shrunken hemispheric gyri. Cerebral atrophy, as a significant complication of subdural hematoma, is thought by many to be not only the result of pressure on the cortex during early stages, but also produced by an interference with cortical blood supply and nutrition. In instances where the hematoma is two or more centimeters in thickness, the lateral pneumograms will reveal a configuration resembling an inverted crescent corresponding to the shadow of the lesion. In a surprising number of instances, however, and particularly if films made in the upright position are not employed, the thickness of the hematoma cannot be appreciated satisfactorily in the lateral view.

Gas introduced at pneumoencephalography often enters the subdural space of patients with subdural hematoma, as in other cases, particularly when the patient is upright. In instances in which a hematoma is present, the finger sign described by Dyke (1936) may be outlined and is considered a diagnostic finding. It was suggested by Holt and Pearson (1936) that the presence of any subdural gas at pneumoencephalography was suggestive of subdural hematoma, in traumatic cases; Crosby and Dennis (1956), a generation later, averred that entrance of gas into the subdural space was good evidence for the presence of such a process. Most investigators, however, including the present authors, believe that air frequently enters the subdural space under normal circumstances. In some instances, undoubtedly, the gas is injected subdurally, owing to the presence of the needle bevel partially in the subarachnoid and partially in the subdural space, as occurs frequently at myelography. In more instances, perhaps, congenital communications exist between the subdural and subarachnoid spaces; in others, the introduction of gas and manipulation may produce a tear of the arachnoid which allows gas to enter subdurally.

Posterior fossa subdural hematoma occurs infrequently. In 1940, Coblentz found only four cases described in the literature and added one case of his own. Since this time, posterior fossa subdural hematoma has been described more frequently. It is unusual, however, for the diagnosis to be made preoperatively, because a history of trauma frequently is not available, and the roentgen findings are not specific. If the hemorrhage occurs during the infantile period of skull growth, there may be enlargement of the posterior fossa, such as occasionally is seen with tumors. Changes of increased intracranial pressure are found in most instances. Ventriculography, therefore, usually is performed, revealing the symmetrical lateral ventricular dilatation of internal hydrocephalus, third ventricular dilatation, and enlargement of the upper aqueduct. The aqueduct below the tentorium is either occluded or displaced forward, just as occurs in patients with tumors of the cerebellum (fig. 614). The authors have had no experience with angiography in such cases, but it is conceivable that vertebral study may be a useful procedure by demonstration of an avascular mass.

Angiography. In recent years, the use of pneumography has been largely supplanted by angiography in the diagnosis of supratentorial subdural hematoma. In typical cases, the appearance of the pial vessels in frontal view conforms to the several configurations described above concerning the shapes of hematomas at different stages of development; the vascular disposition beneath the inner membrane of a hematoma corresponds to the shape of the gas collection in the pneumogram. Thus, in the average case, the middle cerebral vessels of the midconvexity are displaced away from the inner table of the skull in the frontal angiogram, leaving a fusiform avascular clear space representing the hematoma in cross section (fig. 609). In some patients with a thin subdural collection, the displacement away from the inner table is not always conspicuous. Usually inspection of the frontal film is the most satisfactory means of detecting the vascular displacement of a hematoma; in other instances, it is possible to be more certain about medial displacement by comparing the distance of the Sylvian vessels—particularly of the angiographic Sylvian point—from the inner table on the two sides.

In single plane angiography for the possi-

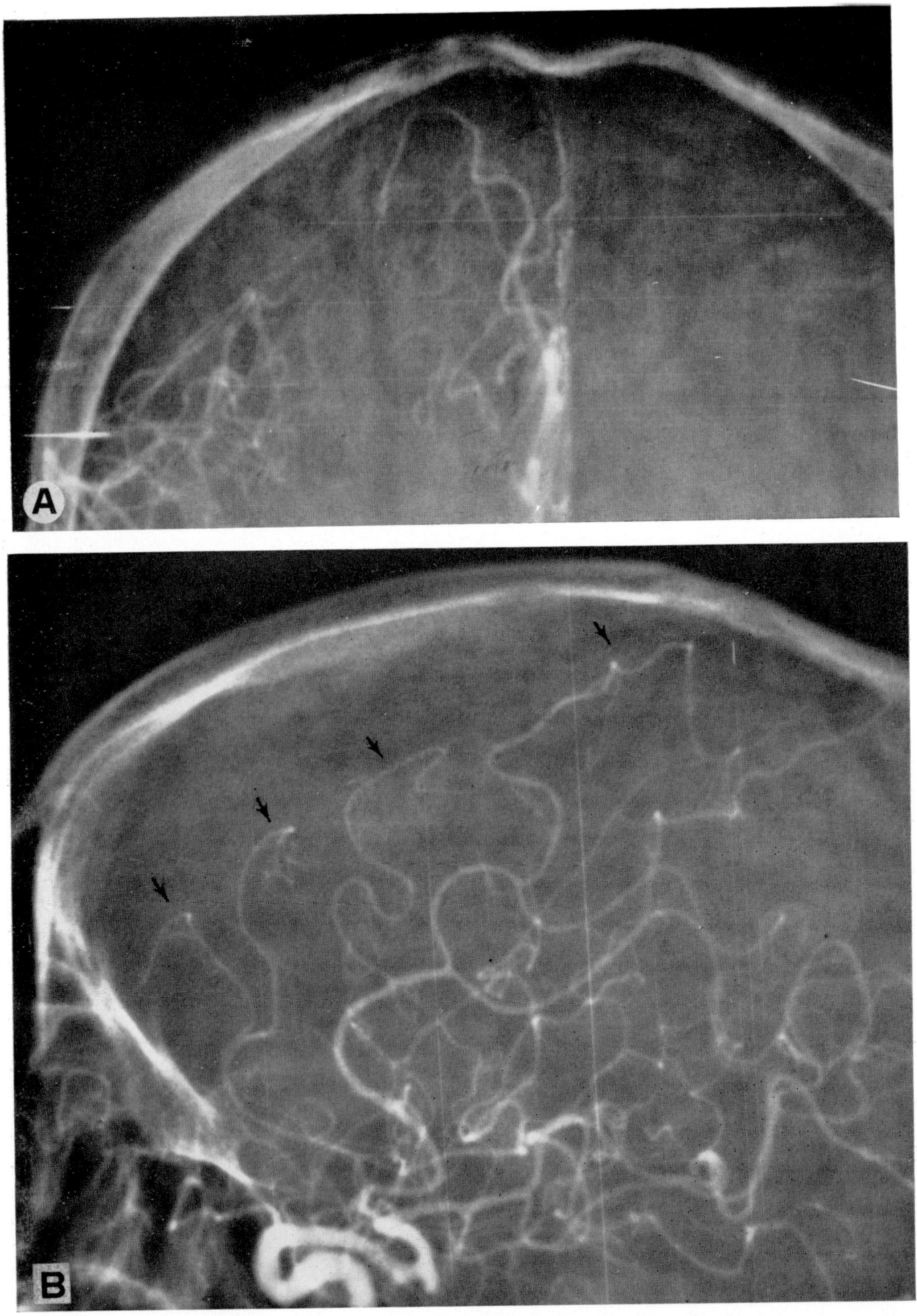

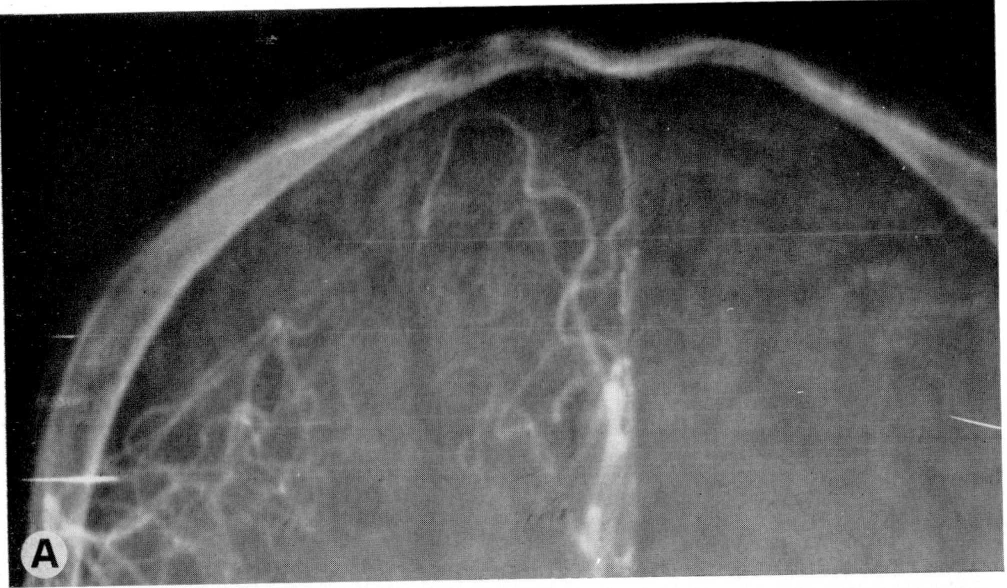

B

Fig. 609.—Subdural Hematoma only in the Frontal Region

The frontal projection (A) demonstrates medial displacement of the vessels away from the inner table of the skull over the middle cerebral convexity. A fusiform clear space (devoid of vessels) is present between the cerebral surface and the bone, characteristic of chronic subdural hematoma. In the lateral projection (B), there is marked posterior displacement of the branches of the anterior cerebral artery (*arrows*) as they pass over the periphery of the hemisphere.

(Revised 1963)

bility of subdural or epidural collections, the anteroposterior film should be made first; examination in other projections, however, should not be neglected. The anteroposterior view frequently is made with compression of the opposite side during injection in order to attempt filling of both sides with one injection; this not only allows comparison of the two sides but the diagnosis of bilateral masses, if successful. Carton (1959) recommends the taking of oblique views if the routine frontal angiogram is normal. The head is rotated slightly, both toward and away from the side being injected, in order to diagnose subdural collections in the frontal and occipital regions, which could go undetected by the routine frontal and lateral views (fig. 610).

Bilateral subdural hematomas often fail to cause any shift of the anterior cerebral vessels. Generally, the absence of shift of these vessels can be taken as an indication of the existence of bilateral subdural hematoma if a lesion is seen on the side injected (fig. 612). A minimum shift should also be regarded with suspicion when a large biconvex parietal or a subtemporal extracerebral mass is demonstrated; bilateral filling by unilateral injection, through compression, should be attempted but often fails.

It should be kept in mind that a hematoma may be localized in any part of the cranium. While the most frequent sites of occurrence are the parietal and the temporal regions, the mass is occasionally localized to the frontal region or to the occipital area (fig. 609). Both epidural and subdural hematomas localized to the frontal pole often are best shown on lateral views; in this projection, the branches of the anterior cerebral artery and the veins do not reach the inner table of the skull in the frontal region (fig. 606). In one instance of a loculated frontal subdural collection encountered, there was no filling of the anterior cerebral artery on the side of the lesion; ventriculography then revealed a frontal mass. Pneumography is required not infrequently for thorough evaluation of traumatic cases.

In the instance of the localized hema-

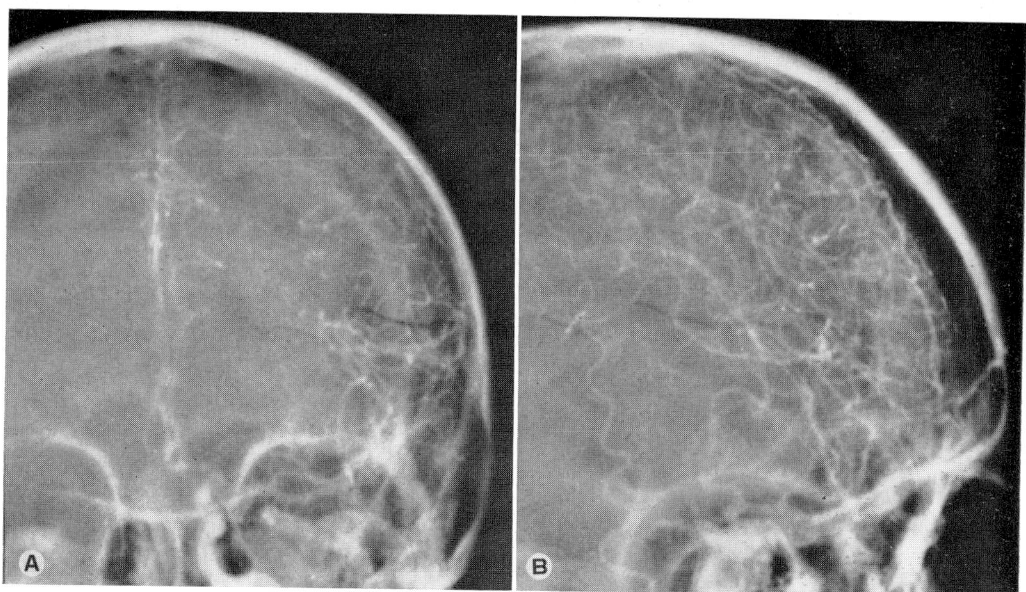

FIG. 610.—FRONTAL SUBDURAL HEMATOMA

No diagnostic change is present in the routine frontal angiogram (A), except for the presence of a linear fracture demonstrated on earlier plain skull films. An oblique projection (B), however, discloses an avascular area over the frontal convexity typical of a subdural collection. (Courtesy of Dr. Solomon Schwartz, Jewish Hospital, Brooklyn, New York.)

(Revised 1963)

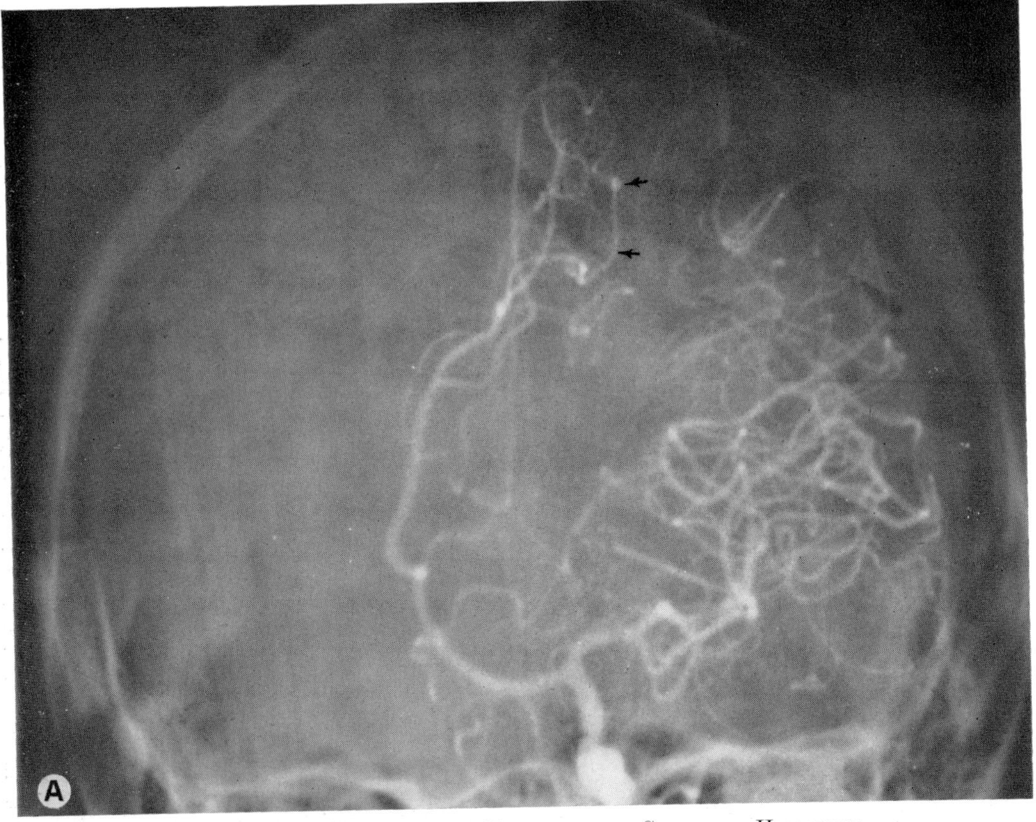

FIG. 611.—INTERHEMISPHERIC EXTENSION OF SUBDURAL HEMATOMA

The initial examination (A) reveals an extensive avascular area over the lateral cerebral surface stretching upward to the midline and spreading downward to the floor of the middle fossa. The anterior and middle cerebral arteries are markedly displaced contralaterally, except for a few distal branches of the anterior cerebral artery (*arrows*). A very large subdural hematoma was evacuated.

The patient's condition improved for a few weeks, but motor function was not fully regained. The patient's neurologic status then began to deteriorate, and because the possibility of a subdural hematoma on the opposite side was considered, a contralateral angiogram was carried out (B). Cross-filling of the anterior cerebral artery reveals displacement of the distal branches laterally, away from the midline, on the side of the original lesion. Several smaller branches are stretched. Intracranial re-exploration on the left revealed an interhemispheric hematoma, between the displaced anterior cerebral vessels (*arrows*) and the falx, which had not been evacuated at the time of the first surgical procedure. (Courtesy of Dr. Albert Heyman and Dr. Noble David, Veterans Administration Hospital, Durham, N. C.)

toma seen in older children, the so-called "relapsing juvenile chronic subdural hematoma," the loculation is usually in the temporal region. The initial hemorrhage occurs in early childhood, with the resultant development of bony changes previously described, consisting principally of elevation of the lesser wing of the sphenoid and enlargement of the middle fossa (fig. 605). Angiography is the ideal procedure to confirm the diagnosis made from plain film examination. An occasional subdural collection may be loculated in the parasagittal region, between the medial surface of the hemisphere and the falx. These collections cause a lateral displacement of the branches of the anterior cerebral artery away from the midline, spreading and stretching of the branches, and dislocation of the main portions of the vessel beneath the falx (fig. 611).

Hydroma. Subdural hydroma generally is considered to be a variant of subdural

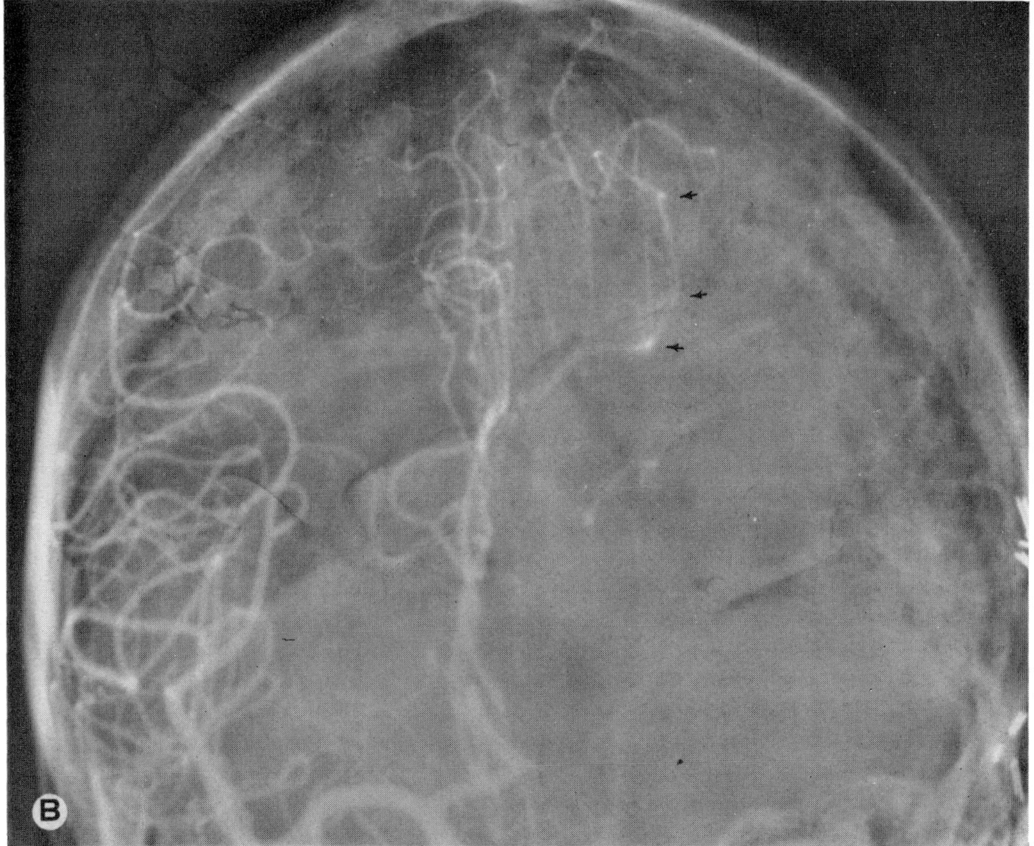

Fig. 611B

hematoma. It is thought by some that a subdural hydroma is the residual finding after resolution of a subdural hematoma. Since the chemistry of the fluid in subdural hydroma so closely resembles cerebrospinal fluid, we believe, with many others, that a subdural hydroma exists as such from the outset, always as a collection of cerebrospinal fluid without hematoma formation as an important component of the process. The mechanism suggested is an arachnoid tear—or a rent in the dura and arachnoid—which allows free entrance of cerebrospinal fluid into the subdural space. In some of the cases, the lesion is rather similar to a leptomeningeal cyst, as pointed out by Caffey (1961); an important difference is that there is no fracture of the skull associated with the subdural fluid collection.

Clinically and radiologically a subdural hydroma is usually indistinguishable from subdural hematoma. The lesions may be bilateral, or occur in the middle fossa, as is frequently the case with subdural hematoma. The plain film, pneumographic, and angiographic findings ordinarily associated with subdural hematoma are found also with hydroma. Even Dyke's "finger sign" has been described (Davidoff and Epstein, 1950). The diagnosis usually is made readily by cranial trephination. In some patients, there is a strong tendency for recurrence of these fluid collections.

Intracerebral Hematoma

Hemorrhage into the brain substance results frequently from natural causes; it also is very common for such a collection to develop owing to trauma. Hemorrhage is an integral part of penetrating wounds. Simi-

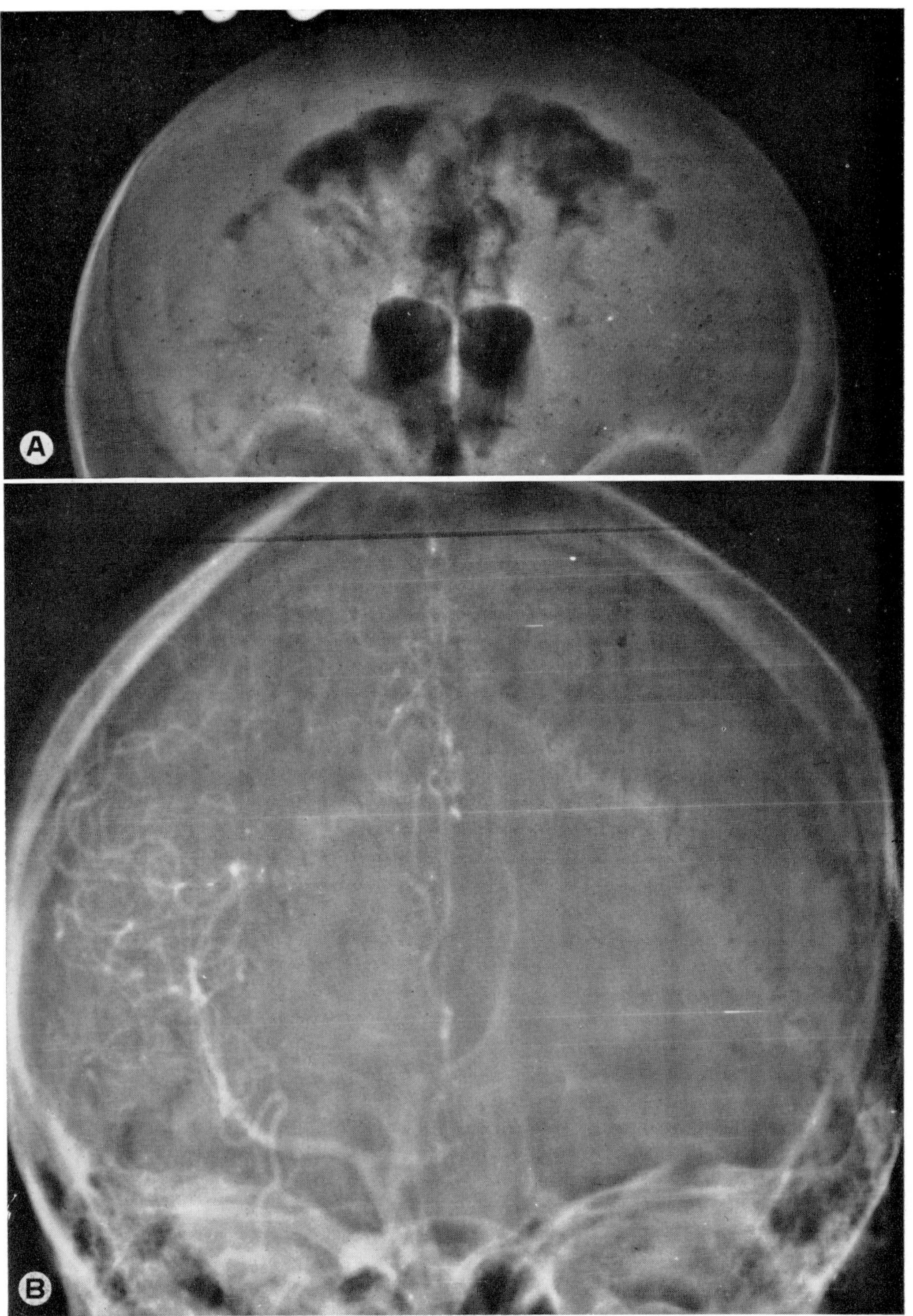

FIG. 612. A–B

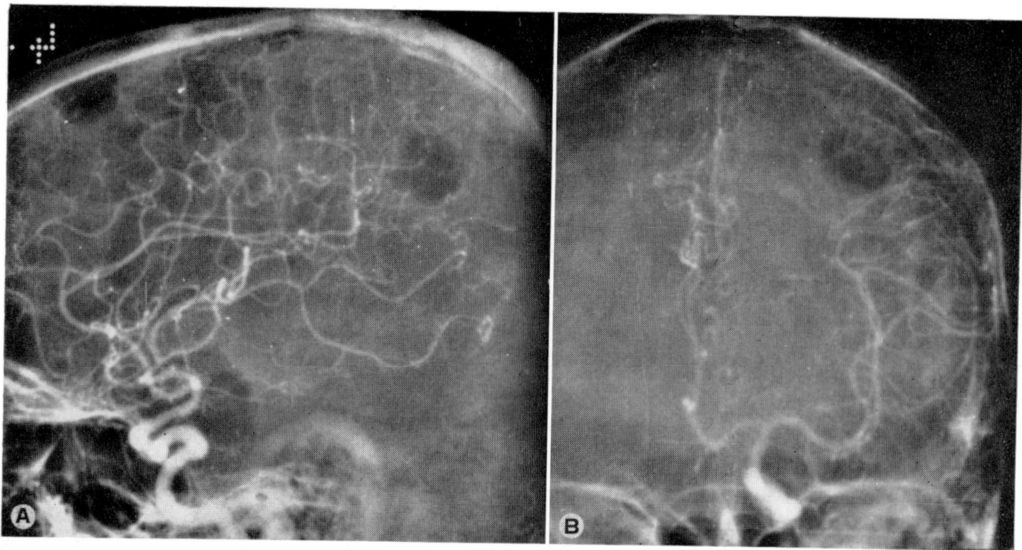

FIG. 613.—INTRACEREBRAL HEMATOMA OVERLOOKED AT TIME OF EVACUATION OF SUBDURAL HEMATOMA

The lateral view (A) demonstrates marked elevation of the middle cerebral artery with "draping" of the temporal branches. The frontal projection (B) demonstrates a moderate shift of the anterior cerebral vessels across the midline; medial displacement of the insular branches of the middle cerebral artery, due to a hematoma in the temporal operculum, is disclosed. The patient was a 57-year-old woman who had a subdural hematoma evacuated without the benefit of angiography. One week later the patient had not improved and was becoming more drowsy. Angiography at this time demonstrated no residual subdural lesion, but an intracerebral hematoma subsequently was evacuated. The case emphasizes the importance of angiography in evaluating as fully as possible the status of the patient prior to evacuation of a hematoma.

larly, bleeding of varying extent occurs with depressed fractures whether open or closed. Impaction, however, is not necessary to produce brain laceration, contusion, scattered small hemorrhages, or a massive intracerebral clot. In most instances, clinical information concerning the occurrence, type, and severity of an injury, together with neurologic examination and lumbar puncture, give the best guide to the correct diagnosis.

Except for fracture, for displacement of the pineal gland, or the finding of foreign material, there usually is no plain film evidence of the presence of the intracranial process. Ordinarily, insufficient time elapses for radiologic changes of increased pressure to develop, since the hematoma begins contraction and absorption at an early date; a possible exception is a hematoma of the cerebellum, with which pressure changes may be seen. Recovery is accompanied by

FIG. 612.—BILATERAL SUBDURAL HEMATOMAS

Bilateral hematomas are found most often in infancy, following either injury or infection. They are not rare, however, following trauma at any age. The pneumogram of a child (A) discloses a soft tissue shadow, measuring up to 2 cm. thickness, separating gas in the subarachnoid space from the inner table of the skull on each side. The subarachnoid gas outlines the inner membrane of the hematoma, and a wide subarachnoid space with prominent sulci. Widening of the subarachnoid space probably results from interference with the absorption of cerebrospinal fluid. Hematomas of long standing also undergo contraction, and there may be underlying cortical atrophy, both of which may contribute to enlargement of the subarachnoid space.

In another case (B), displacement of the middle cerebral artery upward and medially is disclosed; the avascular area also extends upward over the parietal convexity. The anterior cerebral artery, however, is not appreciably displaced. Absence of shift of the anterior cerebral artery usually indicates bilateral lesions. Large subdural hematomas were evacuated from both sides in this instance.

(Revised 1963)

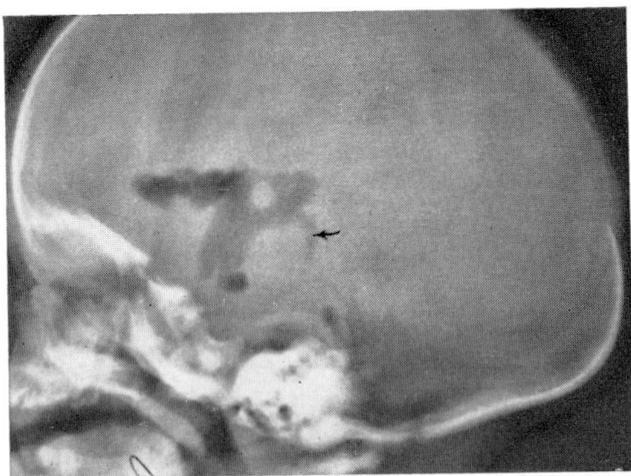

Fig. 614.—Posterior Fossa Subdural Hematoma

A hematoma may develop in the cerebellum or in the subdural space of the posterior fossa, spontaneously or owing to trauma. Ordinarily, there are no radiologic findings which are of assistance in identifying the nature of the process. In the case illustrated, in which the infant had an enlarging head, the ventriculogram revealed a mass posterior to the cerebral aqueduct. The film, made with the patient inverted, reveals ventricular dilatation and forward displacement of the aqueduct of Sylvius (*arrow*) in its subtentorial course, with obstruction of the distal iter.

absorption of the hematoma, leaving behind general or focal injuries of the brain with scarring. Fibrosis, however, usually is not a prominent feature of the healing phase of hematoma, as is the case with abscess; while calcification may occur, it is not common. An instance of a large rounded calcified mass, the end result of an intracerebral hematoma, was reported by Grantham and Smolik (1942), and recently calcific deposits in hematomas have been reported more frequently.

Pneumoencephalograms rarely are attempted early in cases of known brain injury since the added trauma of the procedure may only complicate management. In addition, ventricular filling frequently does not occur because of cerebral edema. Ventriculography, however, may be carried out to localize an intracerebral clot if evacuation is considered necessary. The findings usually correspond to those of hemispheric tumors, depending upon the location of the mass; the lesions often are polar in position. Excavation and communication with the ventricular system may occur (fig. 289). Pneumographically, it is not often possible to identify an intracerebral hematoma unless it can be shown to become smaller. Cerebellar hematomas occur much more often than appreciated in the past; they produce acute obstruction of the aqueduct of Sylvius and dilatation of the lateral and third ventricles at ventriculography, but are not distinguishable from a cerebellar neoplasm.

If an intracerebral hematoma is suspected clinically and surgical intervention is contemplated, angiography is now the procedure carried out most often for definitive preoperative diagnosis. Radiologic confirmation is considered advisable prior to intracranial exploration, because suspected subdural lesions often prove to be, instead, intracerebral hematomas. In such cases, exploration by trephination may not disclose the pathologic process. Cases have also been encountered in which a subdural collection was found and evacuated, but the patient failed to respond as well as expected to the treatment; a postoperative angiogram then disclosed a coexisting intracerebral hematoma (fig. 613).

Intracerebral hematomas tend to produce deformities similar to those caused by neoplasms, particularly in the earlier stages. Later, the edema of the surrounding brain begins to disappear and the degree of vascular displacement decreases fairly rapidly; within a period of one or two weeks, the deformity may not be recognizable in some cases. Sometimes hematomas do not produce significant midline shifts, because they tend to disrupt the brain rather than displace it, but the accompanying cerebral edema may have a dominant influence.

In cases of cerebral contusion, or when there are multiple small hemorrhages in a hemisphere, a certain degree of cerebral edema always is found causing a shift of midline structures to the opposite side. In these cases, no abnormality that would suggest an intracerebral localized mass or hematoma can be detected in the angiogram. The diagnosis of diffuse cerebral swelling is made by exclusion. The problems of radiologic diagnosis simulate, in various aspects, those presented by cerebral infarction and edema occurring without hemorrhage (fig. 287).

(Revised 1963)

ATROPHY

The causes of cerebral atrophy are legion. One of the many causes, as discussed in connection with "Hydrocephalus" under "Intracranial Pneumography," is trauma. The changes may be general, unilateral, or focal, with corresponding radiographic findings varying from diffuse atrophy to minor porencephaly; the latter may be manifested only by slight localized enlargement of a segment of the ventricular system.

Considerable attention has been given to the connection between trauma and degenerative changes; the cause and effect relationship frequently is a matter of medicolegal concern. There is no doubt that in some instances atrophy, particularly focal atrophy, is the direct result of trauma; the severity of injury and severity of degeneration, however, are difficult to correlate. It appears reasonably certain, also, that in many cases of hemicerebral atrophy the degenerative process is initiated by a traumatic event. It is not within the scope of this work to discuss the significance of atrophy as a late consequence of head injury, beyond that given in preceding sections.

An excellent study was carried out by Browder and Hollister (1945) regarding the *early* pneumographic changes that may occur as the result of head injury. The investigators found that there was often a divergence between the clinical and pneumographic findings, in that clinical improvement could occur with progressive evidence of loss of cerebral substance. Browder and Hollister were able to show that morphologic changes of ventricular dilatation can develop within 10 days of injury; the present authors have observed an instance in which a patient who sustained a war wound developed a gross porencephalic dilatation of the temporal horn within 10 days of the missile injury. For the most part, pneumography is a more satisfactory method of evaluating post-traumatic atrophy than angiography. In some instances, the shifting of vessels in association with degenerative changes may create the false impression that a mass is present (figs. 615, 616 and 617).

No attempt has been made to describe, or even list, in this section all of the radiologic manifestations of head injury. A number of conditions frequently developing as a result of trauma have not been discussed here; instead, the reader is referred to the section dealing primarily with such lesions generally, *e.g.*, carotid artery-cavernous sinus fistula following basal skull fracture. Rather than repeat much that has gone before, it was considered preferable to deal with the more commonly encountered manifestations of head injury and the direct complications. The use and interpretation of plain films, pneumograms, and angiograms have been brought together in connection with each of the conditions described. In the acute cases, and in dealing with the sequelae of trauma, the importance of careful plain-film analysis cannot be overemphasized. It is to be kept in mind, also, that a head injury may be the result, rather than the cause, of a neurologic disorder (fig. 618).

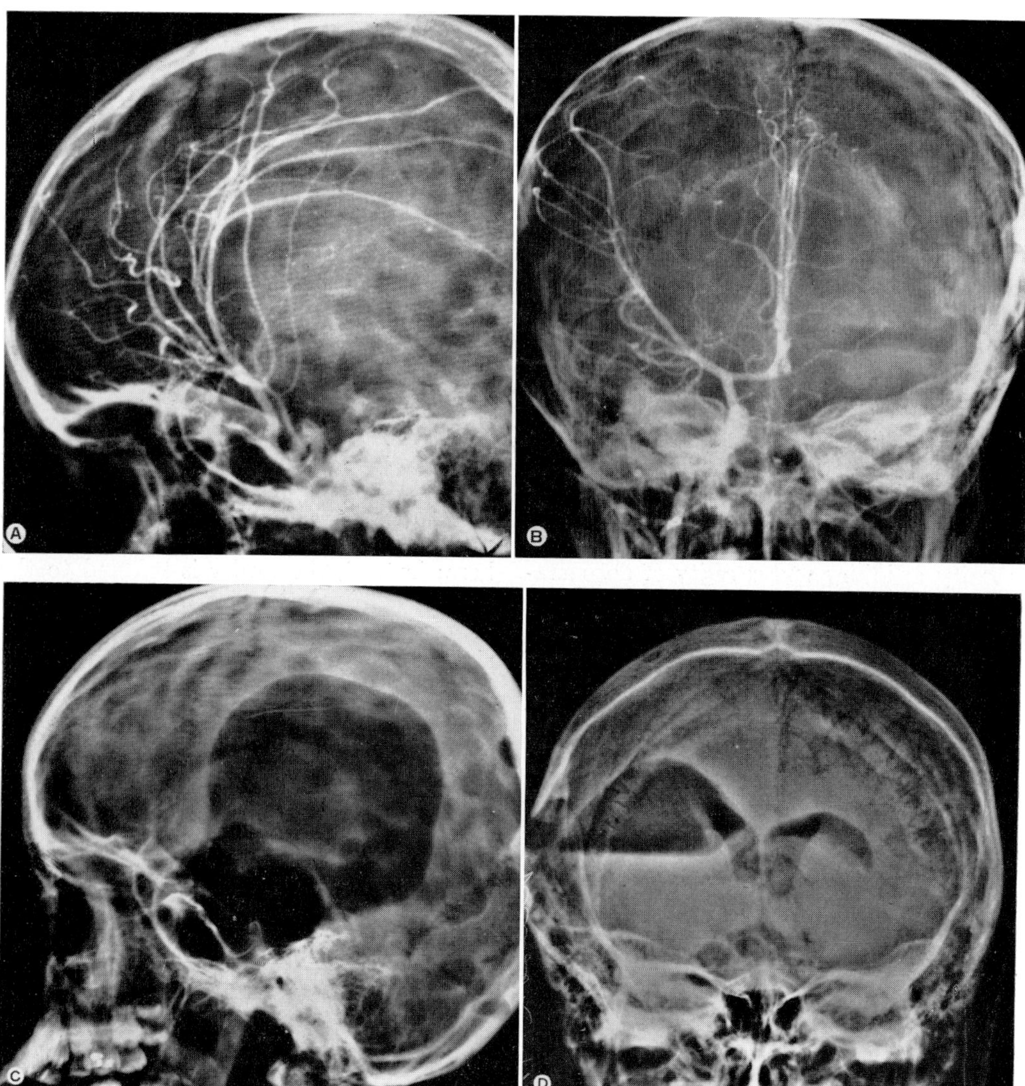

FIG. 615.—POST-TRAUMATIC FOCAL CEREBRAL ATROPHY

The findings suggest a large lesion of the temporal region. In the lateral angiogram (A), the middle cerebral vessels are markedly elevated and stretched. The frontal film, however, reveals no shift from the midline of the anterior cerebral arteries (B). The lack of midline shift suggests that either bilateral lesions are present, or that the altered position of the middle cerebral artery is not the result of a true space-occupying lesion. The ventriculogram (cystogram) discloses a large porencephalic cavity outlined by gas (C). There was no definite history of trauma, but the child was retarded and had spinal anomalies. The skull deformity may have been present since birth.

In another case (D), a parietotemporal fracture line failed to heal in the usual manner. Instead, a portion of the line of fracture became wider, suggesting a leptomeningeal cyst; thinning and outward bowing developed along the lower parietal convexity. The pneumogram reveals a large porencephalic cavity communicating freely with the atrium of the right lateral ventricle. A slight shift of the midline structures toward the area of focal cerebral atrophy is present. In this instance, the bony changes appear to be the result of erosion by pulsation of ventricular fluid in the porencephalic cavity, which extends close to the cerebral surface in the area of bony injury.

(Revised 1963)

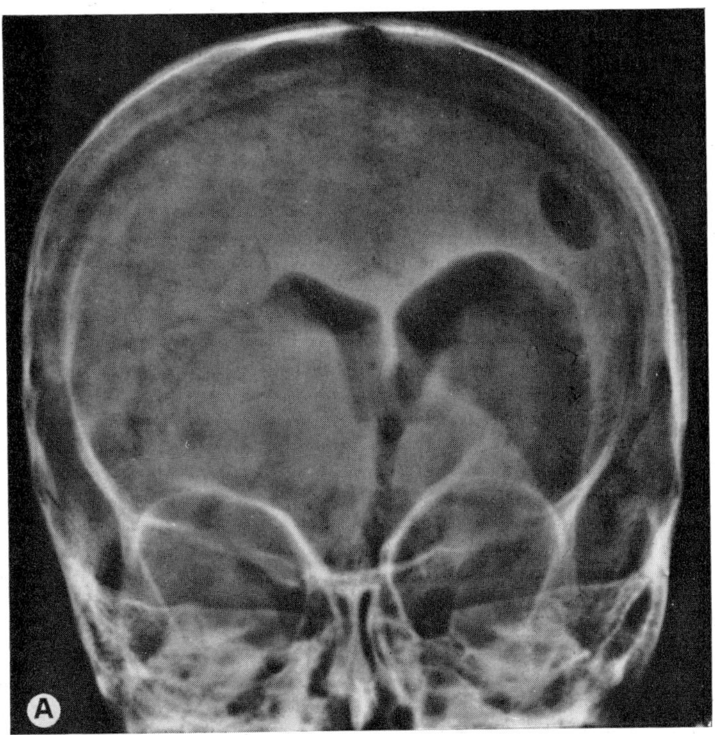

FIG. 616.—HEMICEREBRAL ATROPHY

Generalized atrophy of one cerebral hemisphere may develop owing to trauma. When pneumography is carried out a few months after injury in young persons (A), only a large ventricle may be found on the side of hemispheric degeneration. A shift of the midline structures toward the side of the atrophic lesion is shown.

Hemicerebral atrophy of long duration, which begins early in life, may result in marked unilateral ventricular dilatation and a prominent shift of midline structures toward the side of the atrophic hemisphere (B). In such instances, compensatory changes develop in the growing skull on the side of the lesion, consisting principally of thickening of the vault, high position of the bony structures of the floor of the skull, and overdevelopment of the air sinuses (see text).

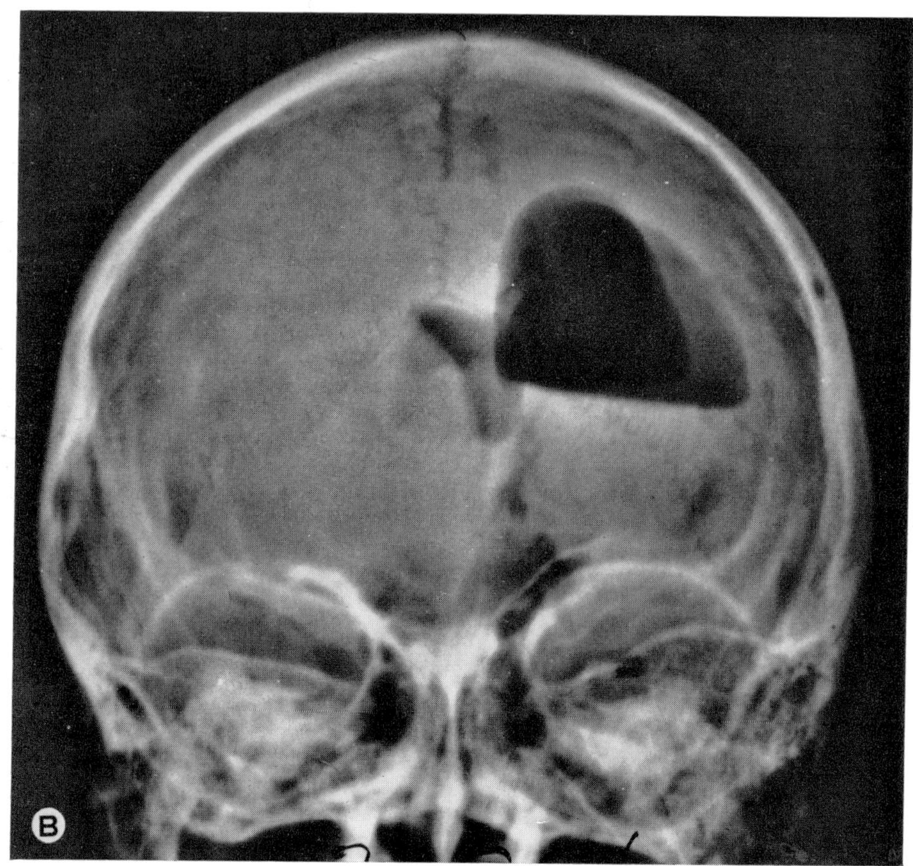

Fig. 616B

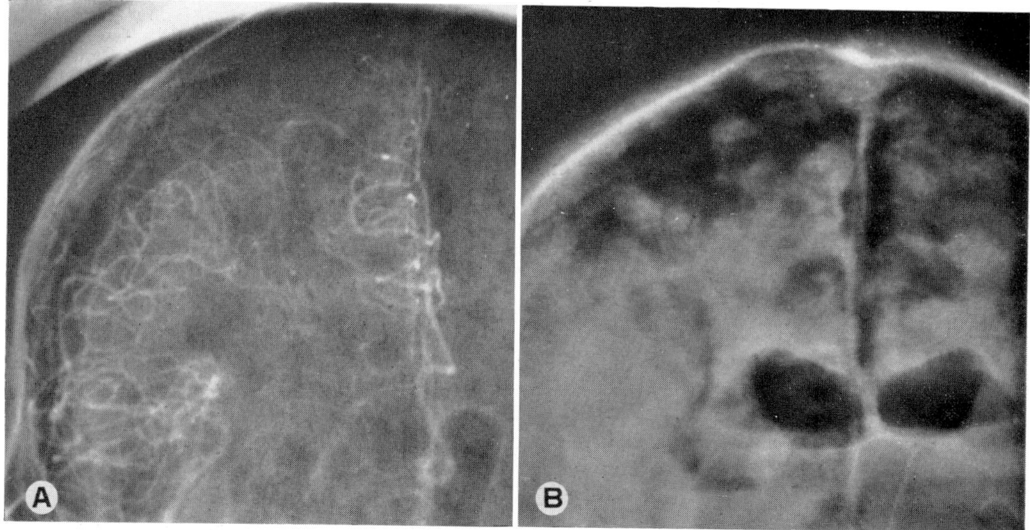

FIG. 617.—DIFFUSE CEREBRAL ATROPHY

The frontal angiogram (A) reveals the pial vessels to be projected away from the inner table of the skull 2 cm. in the parasagittal region and 1 cm. over the midportion of the cerebral convexity. A comma-shaped clear space is present which might be mistaken for the avascular zone of a subdural hematoma. There is some tortuosity of the anterior cerebral vessels but no displacement from the midline.

A pneumoencephalogram, carried out following the angiogram, reveals marked widening of the subarachnoid space over the cerebral surface bilaterally, more marked on the right (B). The sulcal gas collections are very wide and deep, and many gyri are outlined which appear shrunken and atrophic. The disproportionate cortical atrophy, as compared with the milder deep-seated change, denoted by the essentially normal appearing ventricles, is noteworthy. More often, post-traumatic atrophy results in ventricular enlargement.

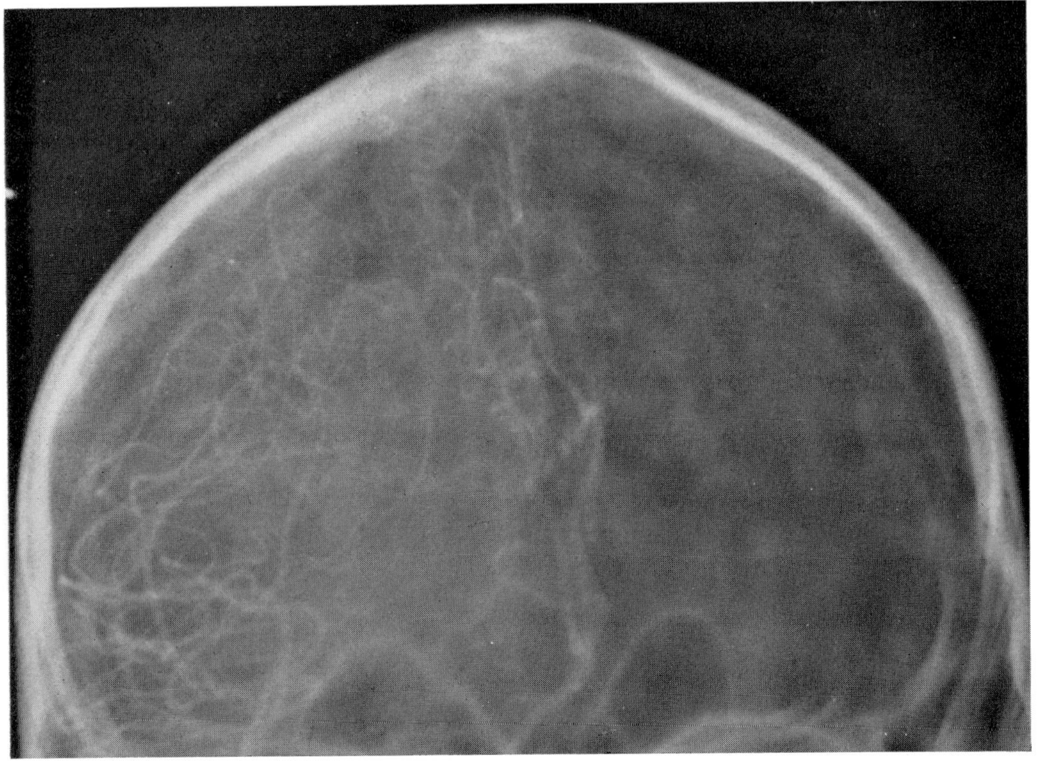

FIG. 618.—SUBDURAL EXTENSION OF A GLIOBLASTOMA MULTIFORME SIMULATING A SUBDURAL HEMATOMA

There is medial displacement of the vessels of the convexity away from the inner table of the skull, characteristic of subdural collections. Just beneath the displaced cerebral surface a number of abnormal vessels are present. The patient had an intracerebral tumor which had grown extensively outside of the brain and formed a large extracerebral plaquelike mass.

DISEASES OF THE SPINAL CORD

Anatomy

Vertebral Column

Ordinarily a vertebra can be identified by palpation of landmarks on the back, within an allowable error of one segment. Topographically, the L4–5 intervertebral space is situated at the level of the iliac crest; the 12th thoracic vertebra can be identified by palpation of the lowest ribs; the angle of the scapula ordinarily falls at the level of T7; and C7 is the highest segment to have a large and prominent spinous process. With the body flexed, individuals of average build will exhibit sessile midline prominences of the back over each vertebral spine. Identification of vertebral levels in individuals who are excessively corpulent may be extremely difficult.

A double curvature of the vertebral column in the sagittal plan is characteristic of animals that occupy the upright posture and in the absence of disease or injury, these curves are maintained throughout life. In the cervical and lumbar areas, there is a ventral convexity, while in the thoracic and sacrococcygeal areas, a dorsal convexity is presented. The cervical and lumbar curves are produced by variations in thickness of the intervertebral discs, the discs being thicker in front than behind in these regions. The intervertebral fibrocartilages are nearly of uniform thickness in the thoracic region, and the anterior concavity is dependent almost entirely on the slightly wedged shape of the vertebral bodies.

The *intervertebral discs* are composed, at their circumference, of laminae of fibrous tissue and fibrocartilage, forming the annulus fibrosus. The center of each disc is composed of a soft, pulpy, elastic substance, which bulges out when the disc is divided horizontally. The latter is called the nucleus pulposus. The nucleus pulposus is a remnant of the notochord and is particularly well developed in the lumbar region. The sizes of the intervertebral discs correspond to the sizes of the two adjacent vertebrae that they separate, except in the cervical region where they are slightly smaller in a transverse direction than the corresponding vertebral bodies. This is not strictly true, however, because there is a lateral extension of the intervertebral fibrocartilage extending into the articulation formed by the articular lip of the cervical vertebra below and the lateral aspect of the vertebra above, the so-called uncovertebral joints. Separating the intervertebral fibrocartilages from the upper and lower surfaces of the vertebral bodies is a layer of hyaline cartilage. The intervertebral discs are closely connected to the anterior and posterior longitudinal ligaments, and in the thoracic region they are joined, by means of the interarticular ligaments, to those ribs that articulate with two adjacent vertebrae.

A summation of the thicknesses of all of the intervertebral discs discloses that the fibrocartilaginous elements separating the vertebrae account for approximately one-fourth of the entire length of the vertebral column. The length of the vertebral column is greatest in the maturely developed young adult. Dehydration, loss of elasticity, and varying degrees of degeneration in the intervertebral discs occur with advancing age and result in an actual reduction in the individual's height.

The vertebral arches are joined by the ligamentum flavum which are present from the second cervical vertebrae to the sacrum. One is present on each side, commencing on either side at the base of the articular process and extending dorsally to the point where the two laminae meet to form the spinous process. There is usually a small interval present between the right and the left yellow ligaments for the passage of blood vessels and sometimes a little areolar tissue.

An adequate knowledge of the radiologic anatomy of all of the components of the vertebrae, which are often distorted by the radiologic projection and by disease, is in-

(Revised 1963)

dispensable. The reader is referred to the standard texts. However, some reference to certain anatomical structures will be made in the section on intervertebral disc disease and osteoarthritis.

Spinal Canal

The vertebral canal, in schematic cross section, has its contents arranged in a laminated manner (fig. 619). The various components, which may be considered as a series of cylinders one within another, are designated by their relationship to the meninges. The outermost tubular compartment, between the bony structures and the dura mater, is usually referred to as the *epidural or extradural space*. In this space are located spinal ligaments, connective tissue, areolar tissue, the epidural venous plexus, lymphatic channels, and supporting elements. The thickness of the epidural space varies considerably in different individuals, chiefly with the quantity of epidural fat that is present, and also in the same individual depending on the amount of blood in the epidural plexus.

Between the dura mater and the arachnoid membrane is the *subdural space*. Classically this compartment is regarded more often as a potential rather than an actual cavity. Notwithstanding the fact that the subdural space usually is very small when identified at the operating table or in the anatomy laboratory, studies in radiologic anatomy made after the injection of contrast media disclose that in some patients the subdural space is relatively wide or at least distensible. Defects, presumably developmental, may be present in the leptomeninges which allow a free passage of cerebrospinal fluid from the subarachnoid space to the subdural space, but this is debatable. Traumatic perforations of the delicate arachnoid, which are produced by piercing the meninges with a needle, frequently result in large subdural collections of cerebrospinal fluid which may

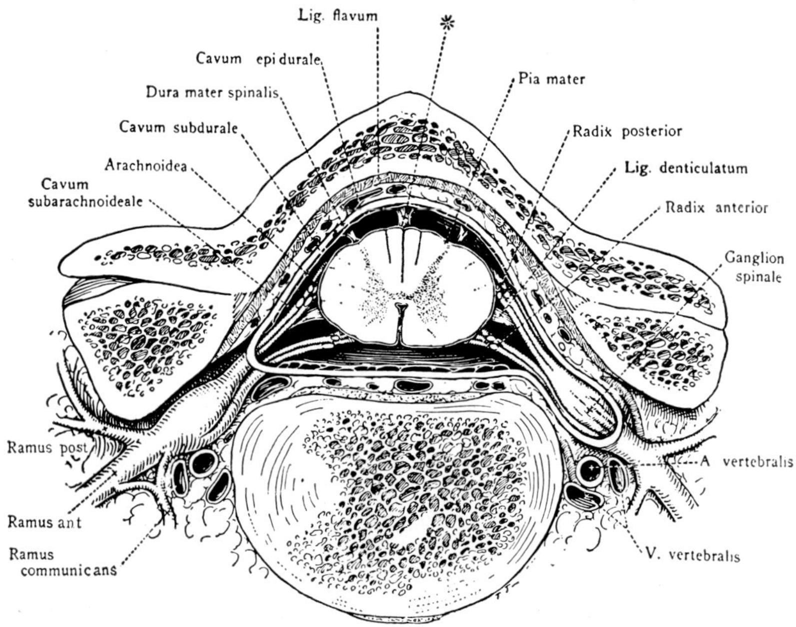

FIG. 619.—THE VERTEBRAL CANAL AND ITS CONTENTS

A transverse section at the level of C4 provides an axial view of the extradural, subdural, subarachnoid, and subpial compartments. The spinal cord, at the cervical enlargement, fills the greater portion of the vertebral canal. The relation of the spinal nerve roots and ganglia to the meningeal sheaths and the intervertebral foramina is depicted. The asterisk indicates the posterior longitudinal subarachnoid septum. (From The Manual of Surgical Anatomy, U.S. Army Medical Department, 1918.)

(Revised 1963)

persist for many days or weeks following a diagnostic lumbar puncture.

The middle meningeal layer is the *arachnoid* which, ordinarily, bounds circumferentially the compartment in which the major portion of the cerebrospinal fluid is contained. The most common anatomic variation of the arachnoid sac is in its length. At the caudal end, a tapering cul-de-sac is formed which usually terminates at the level of S2, but variations in length of as much as one vertebral segment are common. The subarachnoid space is partially divided by the *posterior longitudinal subarachnoid septum* (denoted by an asterisk (*) in Figure 619) which connects the arachnoid with the pia mater, and forms a partition, most complete in the thoracic region, along the dorsal aspect of the spinal cord. It should be mentioned that this subarachnoid septum is composed only of a few discontinuous fibers in the cervical region. It is best developed in the thoracic region but here also it is discontinuous and does not form a true septum. When the surgeon opens the dura in the thoracic region, he will often describe some "adhesions" which usually represent the dorsal subarachnoid septum. In the cervical region, it is very poorly developed.

The *dentate ligaments*, which incompletely subdivide the subarachnoid cavity into ventral and dorsal compartments, extend in the coronal plane on each side of the spinal cord. These ligaments are a series of narrow bandlike structures that extend between the pia and arachnoid and which at intervals are fixed to the dura mater. The function of the *dentate ligaments* presumably is to suspend the spinal cord in the central portion of the subarachnoid cerebrospinal fluid space. However, the spinal cord does move transversely as well as dorsally and ventrally with changes in position. This is well demonstrated in air myelography.

The *spinal pia mater* covers the entire surface of the spinal cord and is intimately adherent to it. The pia forms sheaths for the spinal nerves which are closely applied to the nerves and blend with their membranous investments.

The pia mater is a vascular membrane between and beneath the layers of which are carried the nutrient vessels of the spinal cord.

The arachnoid forms a sheath around the spinal roots as far as the point of exit from the vertebral canal. The arachnoidal sheath around the roots is sometimes quite loose and sometimes shows cystic dilatation, commonly encountered in the lumbar region (fig. 632).

The *spinal cord* forms the cylindrical core of the laminated tubular divisions of the vertebral canal. In adult life, the spinal cord extends from the margin of the foramen magnum to the level of the lower part of the body of the first lumbar segment. On the average, the spinal cord is about 45 cm. in length. The spinal cord is almost circular in shape but it is expanded transversely to an oval contour at its cervical and lumbar enlargements, which are maximum at C5 and T12 vertebral levels. The spinal cord, in the adult, tapers conically (conus medullaris) at its lower end to terminate in a filament (filum terminale) which is composed chiefly of pia mater invested by dura but which contains remnants of a few neural elements. The filum terminale is a delicate strand of tissue, measuring approximately 20 cm. in length, which extends caudad from the conus through the lumbosacral canal to attach to the first segment of the coccyx. In early fetal life, the spinal cord itself extends the entire length of the vertebral canal, but in the second and third trimesters, the vertebral column grows in length more rapidly than the spinal cord. At birth, the tip of the conus lies at the level of the third lumbar vertebra. The greater lengthening of the vertebral column in comparison to the growth of the spinal cord results in a special relationship between the spinal cord segments, the intradural arrangement of the spinal nerve roots, and the vertebrae which must be borne in mind during radiologic examination.

The *spinal cord is divided into segments* which are separated by imaginary lines drawn through the spinal cord in the transverse plane, midway between the points of origin of two adjacent nerve roots. There are 31 pairs of spinal nerves, the roots of which emerge from the vertebral canal at

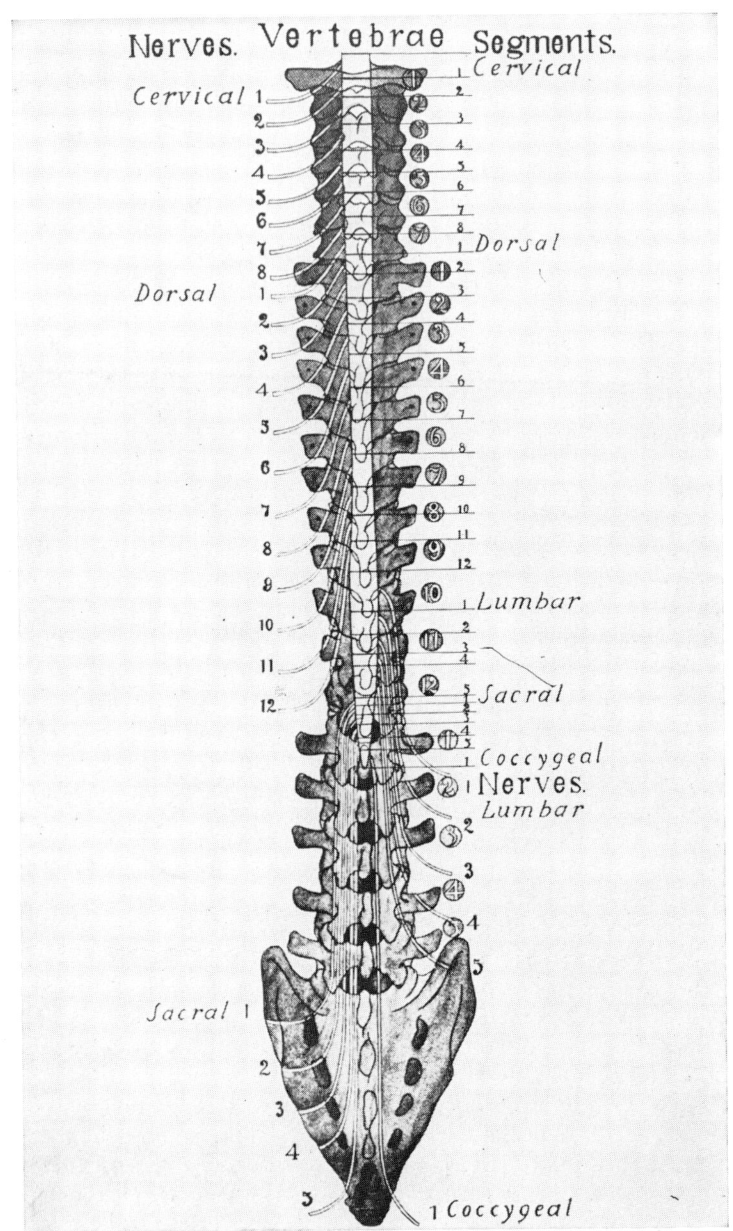

FIG. 620.—RELATION OF THE SEGMENTS OF THE SPINAL CORD AND NERVE ROOTS TO THE VERTEBRAE

The small numbers on the right are based on transverse lines which arbitrarily divide the spinal cord into imaginary segments that correspond to the level of origin of the spinal nerve roots in the cord. The encircled numerals identify the vertebrae. On the left side in the cervical, dorsal, and sacral areas and on the right side in the lumbar and coccygeal regions, the spinal nerves are numbered. (From Elsberg, C. A.: *Diagnosis and Treatment of Surgical Diseases of the Spinal Cord and its Membranes*, W. B. Saunders, 1916.)

each intervertebral level from the occipito-atlantal to the sacrococcygeal articulation. There is a marked difference between the intradural course of the nerve roots at different levels. In the cervical region the roots pass out of the dural sac at almost right angles to the cord. In the thoracic region each successive root has a slightly greater inclination caudad from the transverse plane of its origin. The lumbar and sacral nerve roots descend in almost parallel bundles to form the cauda equina surrounding the centrally located filum terminale. The fifth lumbar nerve roots emerge from the vertebral canal six vertebrae caudad to the level of their origin from the spinal cord.

The special relations of the segments of the spinal cord and the spinal nerve roots to each other and to the vertebral column are portrayed in a clearly understandable composite diagram by Elsberg (fig. 620). It is seen that the fourth cervical spinal cord segment lies approximately opposite the third cervical vertebra, and the 12th thoracic spinal cord segment lies opposite the ninth thoracic vertebra, with the result that between these levels, vertebral localization of lesions is approximately two segments higher than neurologic localization. The arrangement of the roots of the cauda equina is such that the nerve roots which originate more cephalad from the spinal cord and exit higher from the dural sac occupy the outermost position in the bundle.

The vertebral canal is thus seen to be filled by four tubular compartments separated by the three meningeal layers. The outer and innermost sections are filled with soft tissue. The two intermediate compartments are formed by membranes which are not adherent to each other. The innermost of these two compartments is the subarachnoid space, which contains the cerebrospinal fluid. The outer of these two compartments is the subdural space which ordinarily is a potential space but which can become enlarged by separating the two membranes with the formation of a subdural hygroma following spinal tap. Further discussion on subdural hygromas and subdural Pantopaque will be given below (p. 1.836).

METHODS OF EXAMINATION AND NORMAL ROENTGENOGRAPHIC APPEARANCE

Plain Film Examination

Technical considerations. The careful study of plain roentgenograms of the spine is the first step for the proper evaluation of diseases of the spinal cord. Not only the bone and joint structures of the vertebral column are important from the neurologic standpoint but also the contour and caliber of the vertebral canal and the foramina of exit of the spinal nerve roots. An attempt should be made to correlate structural abnormalities with the patient's neurologic disturbances.

Examination of the *cervical spine* should include films in frontal, lateral, and each oblique projection. The frontal film may be made with the patient supine on the radiographic table, but the erect position is preferred to avoid having to place the patient in the recumbent position and then having him sit up for the remainder of the examination. With the patient in upright position, not only is the appearance of the spine with weight-bearing depicted, but the lower cervical segments are better visualized because the shoulders are lower. In the upright position, it is much easier to take the anteroposterior or oblique projections which can be made by rotating the patient in a swivel chair or stool. In taking the oblique views, best results are obtained when the patient's body is rotated approximately 55 to 60°, and the head is turned to a true lateral position (fig. 621). In a properly taken oblique view, therefore, the sella turcica is easily visible in a true lateral position. Additional special views may occasionally yield valuable information. Ordinarily, the upper cervical vertebrae cannot be satisfactorily visualized in the frontal projection because of superimposition of the facial bones. The atlas and axis can be satisfactorily visualized in films made through the open mouth, especially when the patient is edentulous. Films made

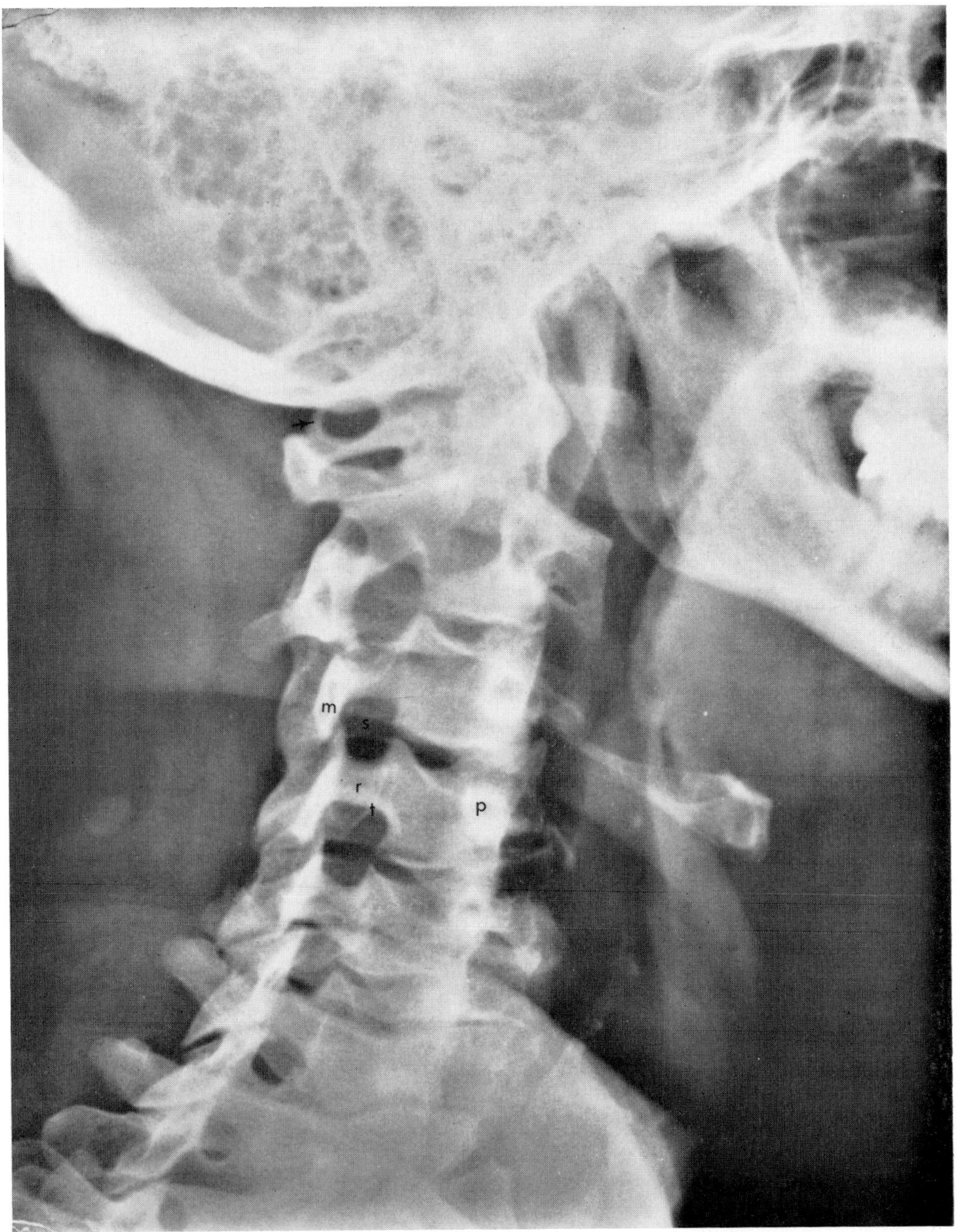

Fig. 621.—Oblique View of Cervical Spine, Normal

The film depicts the correct positioning for an oblique cervical spine film; the head is placed in a straight lateral position so that the sella turcica is visible, and the body is rotated somewhat more than 45°. The foramen at C2–3 is often larger than the others in normal cases. There is often a foramen for the passage of the vertebral artery over the posterior arch of the atlas due to calcification and ossification of the ligament (*arrow*).

The letter (m) is over the lamina on the right side in this right anterior oblique (left posterior oblique) view; (s) is over the left lamina which is seen *en face*; (p) is over the left pedicle of C4; and (r) is over the right pedicle. The letter (t) is over the anterior edge of the right transverse process, the edge of which has an arclike configuration concave upward. The apophyseal joint spaces are not usually visible in oblique views, but in lateral views.

(Revised 1963)

in subaxial projection frequently depict the odontoid process to good advantage. Laminagraphy in either coronal or sagittal plane is a satisfactory way of visualizing the upper cervical area. Lateral films of the cervical spine with the neck in flexion and extension serve as an adjunct to examination of this area. Any time that it is desired to determine whether a reduction of the lordotic curve of the cervical spine is less than normal or has disappeared altogether, films in extension in the lateral projection should be obtained. Many subjects, particularly women with relatively long necks, will tend to reverse their normal curve when they are asked to assume the erect position for filming, and this may give a false impression For this reason, it may be advisable, routinely to instruct the technicians to take the lateral cervical spine with the chin moderately elevated.

In examining the *thoracic spine,* single frontal and lateral films are usually sufficient. A film large enough to include all of the thoracic segments, and in addition the lowermost cervical and uppermost lumbar vertebrae for orientation should be used. Usually the thoracic vertebrae can be properly identified in the lateral projection by the attached ribs. In heavy-set individuals, a lead marker affixed to the skin of the back, lateral to the spine in the thoracic area, may be helpful in identifying thoracic segments in the lateral films by comparing the position of the marker in the frontal views. This should be done routinely when doing thoracic myelograms in which spot films are to be used. Stereoscopic films in frontal projection are of value when detailed examination of the component parts of certain vertebrae is desired. The highest thoracic vertebrae usually are not well visualized in the lateral view and in selected cases, oblique films or laminagrams in the sagittal plane may give the desired visualization of this area.

A routine *lumbosacral examination* includes films in frontal and lateral projection, and a film of the sacrum made with the x-ray beam angled 30° cephalad. Films in each posterior oblique projection are desirable to complete the examination. The routine views ordinarily are made with the patient recumbent on a horizontal x-ray table.

In selected cases, examination of the lumbosacral area under conditions of stress or weight-bearing may be desirable. Thus, upright frontal films with lateral bending and upright lateral films in flexion and extension give a radiographic record of the continuity and extent of movement of the vertebrae. Bending films are usually made to test the postoperative status of a spinal fusion. Cinefluorography is a promising method of evaluating preoperative mobility, as well as stability following fusion. Frequently, films made with an extension cone centered over the lumbosacral junction are necessary for clear visualization of this usually very thick area. A true lateral view of the lumbosacral area may be obtained with the patient in prone position, using a horizontal x-ray beam and a grid cassette, when satisfactory lateral views cannot be obtained by other methods. This means of examination is frequently employed in all portions of the vertebral column in the event of spinal injury where it is desirable for the patient to remain in prone or supine position until the extent of vertebral deformity has been determined.

Interpretation of plain spine roentgenograms. The examination should begin by counting the vertebrae to determine whether or not the usual number is shown. Supernumerary or infranumerary vertebrae are rare in the cervical region, although failure of segmentation in this region is a fairly frequent occurrence. An odd number of fully formed thoracic vertebrae with attached ribs is occasionally observed. Eleven thoracic vertebrae associated with six vertebrae of the lumbar type, with or without articulating transverse processes on the highest lumbar segment, is a common occurrence. Sacralization of L5 and lumbarization of S1 or a transitional vertebra is seen frequently at the lumbosacral junction. By sacralization it is usually meant that one or both transverse processes of L5 have become much thicker than normal and actually articulate with the sacrum. Bilateral sacralization is a stable condition, but unilateral sacralization is less stable. Lumbarization of the first sacral segment is present when a well formed disc space is present between S1 and S2, or when one transverse process is similar to that of the lumbar vertebrae or both. Such variations are usually designated *transitional segments.* Herniations of the intervertebral discs between the transitional segment and the sacrum is very rare or does not occur. The authors have never seen a case of herniation under these conditions at this level.

An indication of normal or abnormal mineral content of the vertebrae may be made from the apparent density of the vertebral bodies. The exact character of the various components of each vertebral segment should be determined, and specially the appearance of the pedicles of the vertebrae should be noted. A change in the normal oval contour of the pedicles or in the interpediculate distances, as shown in frontal films, may indicate the presence of an expanding lesion within the vertebral canal. The upper limits of normal separation of the pedicles in frontal view were recorded by Elsberg and Dyke (1934) and are reproduced in Table VII. The measurements can be applied to films made with the Potter-Bucky diaphragm and a target-film distance of 40 inches. Occasionally, in individuals of large stature or where there is excessive magnification of the spine in the radiograph, the interpediculate measurements may be slightly above the upper limits of normal given. The object-film distance is increased by exaggeration of the ventral cervical and lumbar curves and reduction of the dorsal thoracic curve. An abrupt change from a normal to an abnormal measurement at successive vertebral levels, however, is of great significance. In certain areas of the spine, such as the upper lumbar region, it is not uncommon to find flat pedicles in normal cases. This usually involves the first and second lumbar, and sometimes the twelfth thoracic vertebrae. Sometimes the appearance is so exaggerated that it is difficult to be sure whether this is a normal variation, and in these cases it is necessary to look at the lateral projection. In normal cases, the lateral projection will reveal a normal appearance at the posterior margin of the vertebral bodies, whereas if the erosion of the pedicles is due to expansion of the intraspinal contents, the posterior margin of the vertebral bodies will be also excavated (fig. 666).

Table VII

Upper Limit of Normal Interpediculate Measurement of Each Vertebra in Millimeters (Elsberg and Dyke).

Usual Upper Limits	Cervical	Extreme Upper Limits
cm.		*cm.*
3.0	2	3.1
3.0	3	3.2
3.2	4	3.4
3.2	5	3.3
3.2	6	3.4
3.1	7	3.3
	Thoracic	
2.7	1	3.0
2.3	2	2.5
2.2	3	2.2
2.0	4	2.0
2.0	5	2.1
2.0	6	2.1
2.0	7	2.1
2.0	8	2.2
2.2	9	2.2
2.1	10	2.3
2.3	11	2.7
2.6	12	3.0
	Lumbar	
2.8	1	3.0
2.9	2	3.2
3.0	3	3.5
3.1	4	3.5
3.3	5	3.9

The alignment of the vertebrae in both frontal and lateral projections is noteworthy. Altered alignment of the vertebrae may result from muscle spasm associated with spinal cord lesions as well as from structural deformities of the vertebrae and intervertebral discs. The articulations of the vertebral column consist of a series of slightly movable joints between the vertebral bodies and a series of mobile joints between the vertebral arches. Normally the thickness of the intervertebral disc space gradually increases from C2–3 to C6–7 and from L1–2 to L4–5. In the thoracic region, all of the intervertebral spaces are thin. The thickness of the intervertebral disc space at L5–S1 is subject to considerable normal variation and may be entirely absent with asymptomatic sacralization of L5.

The size of the intervertebral foramina can be observed in the oblique films of the cervical spine (fig. 621) and in the lateral films of the thoracic and lumbar area. It should be determined whether the intervertebral foramen is narrowed by hypertrophic spurs, by collapse of the intervertebral disc space following degenerative changes or herniation or by enlargement of portions of the vertebral bodies and vertebral arches which form the boundaries of the foramina. Localized enlargement of one foramen denotes an expanding lesion in the canal. There is variation in the appearance of the intervertebral foramina in the cervical region. The C2–3 intervertebral foramen is often large (fig. 621), and not uncommonly the C3–4 and C4–5 foramina are much larger than the lower foramina. The appearance of enlargement of a foramen, therefore, should be accompanied by a careful examination of the adjacent bony margins to determine whether or not erosion actually exists. In the oblique projections, the pedicles of the side against the film in anteroposterior oblique views are seen on end overlying the lateral aspect of the vertebral bodies and usually are rounded in configuration (fig. 621). This results from the fact that the pedicles in the cervical vertebrae are directed posteriorly and laterally from the vertebral bodies at an angle of approximately 45°, and therefore, when the patient is rotated as to take an oblique view, the corresponding pedicle would be seen on end. On the other hand, the pedicle on the opposite side will be seen in profile, forming the upper and lower margin of the intervertebral foramina that are situated immediately above and below each pedicle. Immediately lateral to the intervertebral foramina are the laminae, which in the oblique projection are seen on end, on the same side as the foramina. The lamina on the other side (the side against the film), is seen in profile and overlies not only the vertebral bodies but also part of the intervertebral foramina and pedicles (fig. 621). The lamina seen in profile will be much more clearly distinguishable in stereoscopic oblique views.

Continuing with the oblique cervical spine view, the articular pillar is seen in an oblique projection but the joint space between two articular pillars is usually not shown on the oblique views but on the lateral views. Unfortunately, in the lateral projection, the right and left joint spaces between two articular pillars (apophyseal joints) are either completely or partly superimposed and cannot be separated unless stereoscopic views are made. On an ordinary film in the lateral projection, the overlap of these joints can be avoided by rotating the patient into an off-lateral projection. If the direction of the rotation is known (the side away from the film is rotated either forward or backward), it is possible to determine which joint space is the right or the left without the need for stereoscopic lateral views.

The soft tissue shadows adjacent to the spine should be carefully examined. Small paraspinal masses are best visualized in the thoracic region where convex lateral bulges are well delineated by air-containing lung. The shadow of a tortuous aorta may make it difficult for one to be certain of the presence of a paraspinal mass on the left side of the thoracic spine. Any lateral enlargement of the retropleural space on the right side is almost surely indicative of a paraspinal mass. The prevertebral soft tissue shadow in the cervical region should always be carefully analyzed.

Myelography

Myelography refers to the visualization of the structures of the spinal canal by means of contrast agents. The simplest of contrast agents to be used is air or oxygen. In addition, radiopaque substances have been introduced, of which the first was Lipiodol, later followed by Pantopaque and by water-soluble contrast substances.

Myelography with Gases

The use of gas to visualize the spinal cord in roentgenograms was speculated on by Dandy (1919) at the time of his description of the procedure for pneumoencephalography. Gas myelography is still considered to be useful, even though radiographic demonstration of gas in the spinal canal is much more difficult than visualization of radiopaque substances (fig. 622). Fluoroscopy cannot be used and more errors in diagnosis are possible. When tomography is incorporated as a part of the filming routine, the value of gas myelography is greatly enhanced.

Air may be used, as may a number of gases, although oxygen is often employed because it is believed to be somewhat less irritating than air and it is absorbed more rapidly. Gas myelography may be carried out in several ways, as described below.

1. At pneumoencephalography, cerebrospinal fluid may be partially or completely drained. This method is satisfactory for study of the upper cervical and foramen magnum regions. It may be done immediately after a Pantopaque myelogram in order to show the dorsal and dorsolateral aspect of the foramen magnum which is not adequately demonstrated by Pantopaque in the usual manner.

2. There may be limited replacement of cerebrospinal fluid by gas with an attempt to retain the gas in the spinal subarachnoid space during the examination (Chamberlain and Young, 1939). For the lumbosacral examination, it is necessary to have the patient in such a position that the hips are higher than the shoulders at the time of the injection. Usually 30 to 50 cc. of cerebrospinal fluid are removed from the lumbar subarachnoid space and an equal quantity of gas is introduced, the exchange being carried out in fractional quantities of the total.

3. For complete myelography of the spinal canal with air it is necessary to perform a suboccipital, cisternal tap with the patient in lateral decubitus and in the Trendelenburg position. All of the cerebrospinal fluid caudad to the needle can be thus removed in fractional amounts and replaced by air. Following the complete replacement, the needle can be removed and laminagrams are made in the lateral projection which can show clearly the entire spine from the cervical to the lumbar segments. In this way, it is possible to get the anteroposterior diameter of

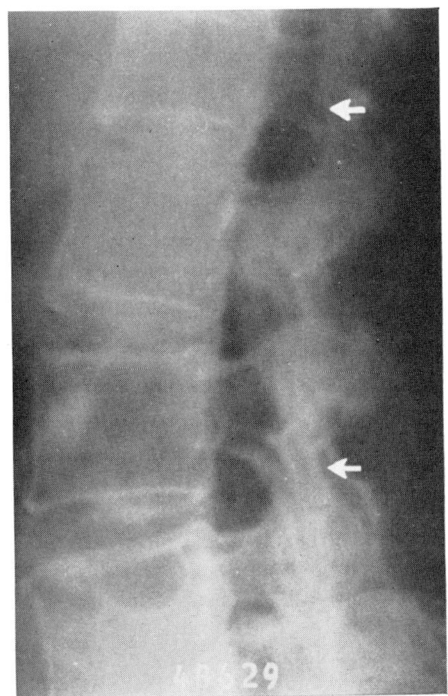

FIG. 622.—GAS MYELOGRAPHY (EXTRADURAL TUMOR, L2)

A lateral film made after the displacement of cerebrospinal fluid by oxygen discloses a smooth indentation of the dorsal aspect of the gas column extending from L1 to L3 (*arrows*). Gas provides low contrast as compared to radiopaque media because the subarachnoid space is small in caliber.

(Revised 1963)

the spinal cord in a much more satisfactory manner than by myelography with radiopaque substances which give more satisfactory visualization of the transverse diameter of the spinal cord. On the other hand, the transverse diameter cannot be satisfactorily shown by air myelography because of overlying bone shadows, although it is possible to show some of them with laminagraphy. Another difficulty in the use of laminagraphy in the frontal projection is that the curvatures of the spine throw the spinal cord out of focus at various levels. Stereoscopic posteroanterior films in the Trendelenburg position may be made of the various segments of the spine to visualize the cord in the frontal projection, and they often show it satisfactorily. The spinal cord is shown to move to the most dependent side in any given position and to follow the shortest distance when going through a curve. Thus, in the thoracic region, in the prone position the spinal cord is close to the ventral surface, whereas in the cervical region it tends to be separated from the ventral surface because of the lordotic curve here. The cord is slightly separated from the dorsal aspect of the cervical spinal canal in the prone position, but in the supine position it is against the posterior margin of the canal. In lateral decubitus position, the spinal cord tends to fall to the most dependent side. For this reason, laminagraphy is not entirely accurate in showing the same thickness of the cord throughout its extent in a lateral laminagram during air myelography. This should be taken into account when interpreting radiographs. In general, thicker laminagraphic cuts are preferable; this would tend to minimize possible errors.

Air myelography is best to diagnose atrophic lesions of the spinal cord, particularly those that are accompanied by a diminution in the anteroposterior diameter. In cases of hydromyelia, it is possible in some cases to show a thinner spinal cord in anteroposterior diameter in the cervical region when air myelography *in the sitting position* is carried out, whereas Pantopaque myelography may show a much wider cervical spinal cord. This is related to gravity. Fluoroscopy is usually not used during air myelography.

Roentgenograms are made with the patient supine, with gas in the ventral portion of the subarachnoid space against the dorsal margins of the vertebral bodies and intervertebral discs to visualize these areas in the lumbar and in the cervical regions. While it is possible to show protrusions of the intervertebral discs and various projections into the ventral surface of the spinal canal by this means, the method only is satisfactory to show the central protrusions into the canal. Lateral protrusions would go undetected unless they extend sufficiently toward the midline to indent the air column. For this reason, air myelography, although more innocuous than any other form of myelography, is not usually employed in the diagnosis of intervertebral disc disease and spondylosis, particularly in the lumbar region.

Several major indications for air myelography have been developed by the authors, and are in use at the Neurological Institute.

1. Lesions in the region of the foramen magnum may be studied. Usually Pantopaque myelography is performed first, and after the Pantopaque is removed, air is injected at the same sitting without removal of the needle. The head is placed in flexion, after the table is tilted to the desired position. Gas myelography has the advantage of showing the dorsal aspect of the cervical spinal cord and the dorsal rim of the foramen magnum; these areas are not visualized by Pantopaque myelography unless the needle is removed and the patient placed in a supine position. Supine examination may result in dissemination of the oil over the cerebellar surface, and it is mainly for this reason that air is preferred.

2. Another indication is the presence of congenital spinal anomalies in the lumbar region. These anomalies are often associated with a failure of ascent of the spinal cord which remains quite low. Therefore, in these cases, following Pantopaque myelography and removal of the oil, air is injected with the patient in the Trendelenburg position and lying on the side, and films are made in

lateral prone and posteroanterior projections stereoscopically. Laminagraphy may be used.

3. The third indication is in cases of suspected blocks within the spinal canal. In these instances, 5 cc. of gas may be injected in the semi-erect position, and the head of the air column will outline the exact site of the block. In this manner, the introduction of any potentially irritating substances is avoided. Sometimes after this is done it is found necessary to inject Pantopaque to obtain a more accurate delineation of the area, and the same applies to cases where a partial block allows the air to pass through the area of narrowing without producing a satisfactory picture.

The *gas epidurogram* is a modification of the gas myelogram (Sanford and Doub, 1941). In this procedure, the lumbar subarachnoid space is partially collapsed by the removal of 10 to 20 cc. of cerebrospinal fluid, following which large quantities of gas, usually several hundred cubic centimeters of oxygen, are injected into the epidural tissues. This method of examination, which is limited to the lumbosacral region, is only slightly more accurate for the diagnosis of herniated intervertebral disc than gas myelography and is now rarely employed. It might be said that it is also possible by this route to perform a partial retroperitoneal pneumogram because the epidural space is continuous with the retroperitoneal space.

Positive Contrast in Myelography

Myelography with Lipiodol. The use of Lipiodol to outline the spinal subarachnoid space was devised by Sicard and Forestier (1922) as an aid in the localization of spinal cord tumors. Originally, the use of radiopaque oil was restricted to injection into the cisterna magna to determine the presence or absence of a lesion which prevented its gravitation to the sacral cul-de-sac. Subsequently, larger quantities were injected into the lumbar subarachnoid space and the technique for examination with Lipiodol evolved by Hampton and Robinson (1936) is essentially the same as that now used when Pantopaque is employed as the contrast medium. Two types of Lipiodol were made, the descending Lipiodol, which gravitates in the subarachnoid space, and the ascending Lipiodol, which contains one-fourth of the quantity of iodine and is lighter than cerebrospinal fluid.

The use of Lipiodol of both types has now been largely discontinued in the United States because of the superiority of Pantopaque as a contrast substance. Pantopaque is less than 1/20 as viscous as Lipiodol, is more cohesive (that is, it does not break up in droplets as easily as Lipiodol), and is much less irritating to the meninges. The most serious sequellae of Lipiodol myelography is the latent development of chronic adhesive arachnoiditis. Iodochloral, an iodized peanut oil of American manufacture, has properties and disadvantages similar to those of Lipiodol.

Myelography with Pantopaque. Pantopaque is a mixture of ethyl esters of isomeric iodophenylundecylic acids (Strain, Plati and Warren, 1942). It has a specific gravity of 1.26 at 20° C and contains 30.5 per cent of iodine. The radiopacity compares favorably with that of other contrast media and is quite adequate for demonstration of the spinal subarachnoid space, which is encased within the bones of the vertebral column. The liquid is unctuous to the touch and common usage has designated it as an *oil* although chemically the simple esteric structure precludes its inclusion among the oleic substances of complex composition.

Injection of Pantopaque. The examination should be performed on a tilting fluoroscopic table equipped with a spot film device. It is advantageous to have a fluoroscopic table that will tilt at least 45° below the horizontal at the cephalic end. A radiographic tube on a vertical ceiling-to-floor tubestand can be used for making radiographs with a Potter-Bucky diaphragm, can be placed at the side of the table, or can be used for making radiographs with a horizontal x-ray beam on a grid-front cassette. The use of image intensifiers permits the fluoroscopist to turn off the room lights, and without accommodating, to proceed to the fluoroscopy. This facilitates the removal of Pantopaque, a procedure that usually requires that the room lights be turned on for removal and off to check the remaining Pantopaque and to place it under the needle tip.

Injection of radiopaque oil into the cisterna magna is employed rarely today because of the danger of piercing the medulla oblongata or a blood vessel of the pia mater. Cisternal puncture is reserved for those patients in whom a satisfactory lumbar puncture is technically impossible, or where there is clinical evidence of a lesion considerably higher than an obstructing lesion demonstrated at myelography by the lumbar route, so that a second spinal lesion is suspected. The most satisfactory level for insertion of the needle is the L3–4 intervertebral level in patients suspected of having a disc herniation, most frequently found at L4–5 and at L5–S1. A lower level may be used if disease is suspected in the upper lumbar, thoracic, or cervical portion of the vertebral canal. It is desirable to insert the needle at a distance from the area to be investigated since deformities of the opaque column that are of questionable significance may occur about the point of the needle.

The lumbar puncture may be made with the patient in the prone, lateral decubitus, or sitting position. Many investigators prefer the prone position because it is possible to put the tip of the needle into the center of the subarachnoid space and the patient need not be turned for fluoroscopy after the puncture is made. When the patient is sitting, a central puncture may be made more easily and the cerebrospinal fluid pressure is elevated so that the subarachnoid space is better distended with fluid for puncture. Distention of the subarachnoid space by gravity is helpful to avoid unsatisfactory puncture with resultant injection of oil outside the subarachnoid space. We prefer to perform the puncture in the sitting position.

After the skin and subcutaneous tissues have been anesthetized by infiltration with a 1 per cent solution of procaine, a 17-gauge spinal needle with short bevel is introduced into the lumbar subarachnoid space. The needle should be inserted equidistant between the two vertebral spinous processes and kept as nearly in the midline as possible. However, it is just as proper to place the needle tip slightly lateral to the midline just above the palpable lower margin of the spinous process. In this case, the needle is pushed in forward and slightly medially. When this method is used the needle should be advanced horizontally instead of with the tip pointed cephalad, as is the case when the interspinous space is used. When the operator believes that the tip of the needle is in the subarachnoid space, the stylet is removed. If there is a free flow of cerebrospinal fluid, the needle is then advanced approximately 3 mm. further to insure that the bevel of the needle tip is entirely within the subarachnoid space. In general, a relatively short beveled spinal tap needle is to be preferred for myelography. Long beveled needles should not be used.

Following the lumbar puncture the patient may lie in the lateral recumbent position on the fluoroscopic table, where manometric studies may be carried out if desired. Such examinations, however, are of academic interest only, since myelography with Pantopaque is, in itself, a more satisfactory way of determining the patency of the subarachnoid space than pressure readings. Samples of cerebrospinal fluid for laboratory examination may be obtained but usually not more than 10 cc. of fluid are removed before the Pantopaque is injected. It is our practice to perform the removal of the fluid and the injection of Pantopaque in the sitting position. If the patient is placed in the lateral decubitus position and pressure readings are then done followed by the removal of cerebrospinal fluid specimens for protein determination, etc., it is more likely that the needle tip will be dislodged from its correct position in the subarachnoid space and the Pantopaque then might be injected in the subdural space.

The quantity of Pantopaque used may vary with the requirements of the examination in each individual case. The amount to be used should be decided by the radiologist after a discussion of the clinical problem with the patient's physician and an interpretation of the plain spine roentgenograms. If it is desirable merely to locate the level of a block to cerebrospinal fluid circulation, a small quantity of contrast medium may be

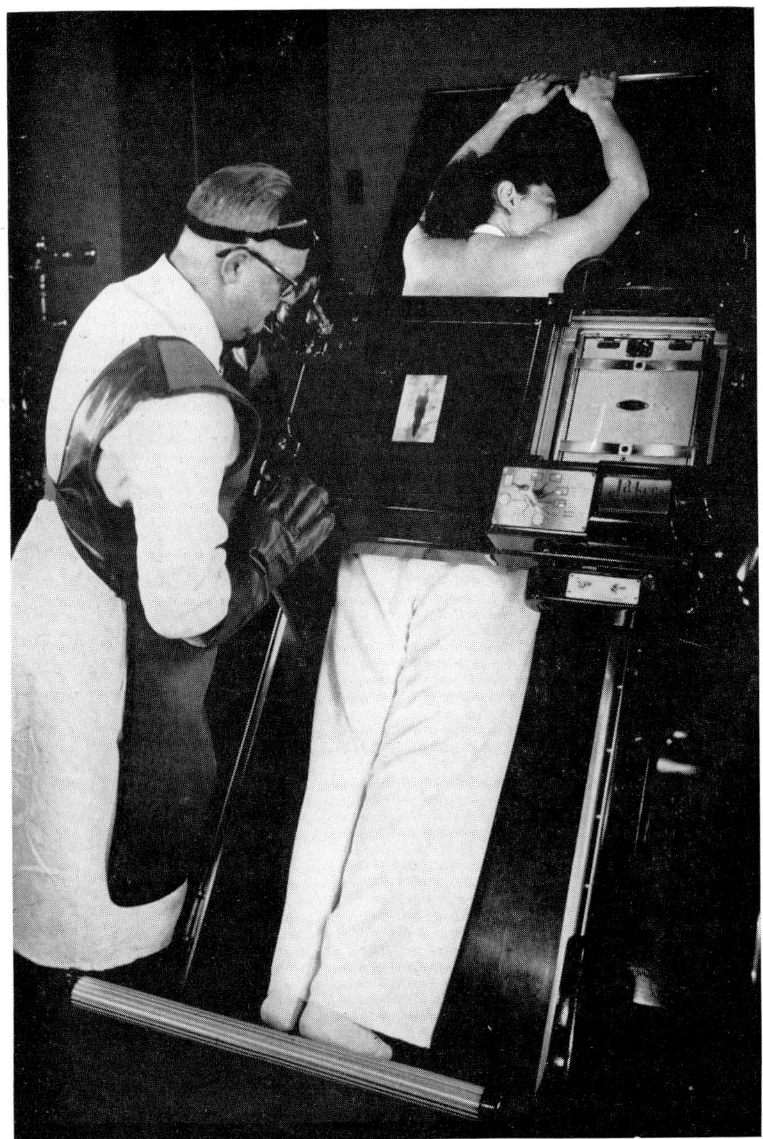

Fig. 623.—Lumbosacral Fluoroscopy

By tilting the fluoroscopic table toward the vertical position, Pantopaque gravitates to the lower end of the subarachnoid space. The lumbosacral cul-de-sac is filled with opaque oil. This is usually the preliminary step before beginning fluoroscopy for lumbar myelography.

used (2 to 3 cc.). If the thoracic or high cervical part of the subarachnoid space is to be studied, or if it is found that the vertebral canal is of large caliber at fluoroscopy, then it may be desirable to use large quantities of Pantopaque for the examination. Customarily, 6 cc. of Pantopaque are used to examine the lumbar subarachnoid space, 12 cc. for the thoracic spine, and 9 cc. for the cervical. If the patient has a large lumbar subarachnoid space, 12 or even 15 cc. of Pantopaque may be necessary in these cases to examine adequately the lumbar sac. We feel that the use of small quantities of Pantopaque (3 cc.) to examine the lumbar subarachnoid space for disc disease often makes

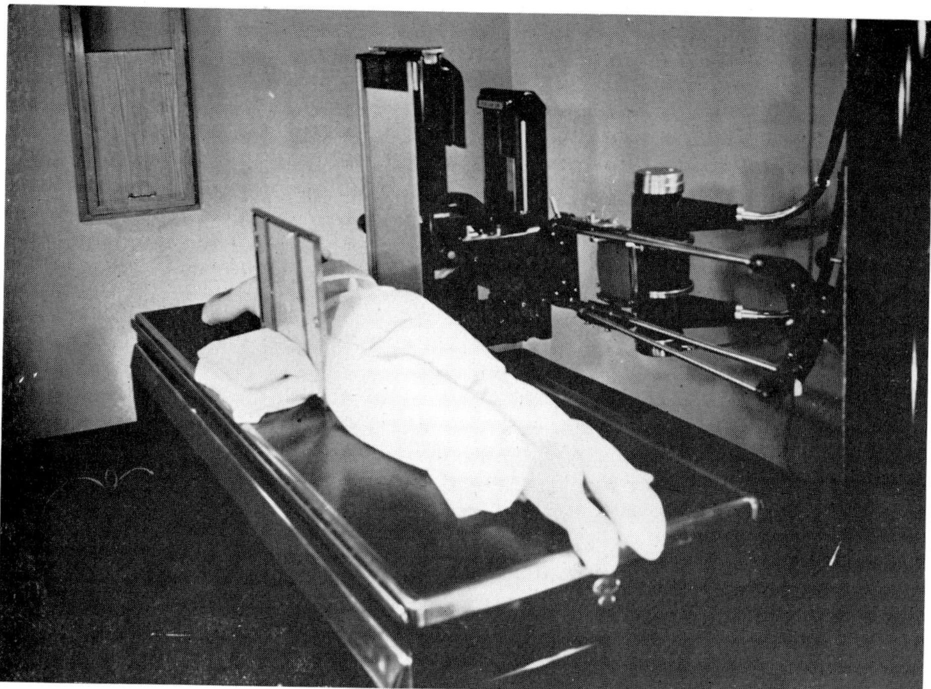

FIG. 624.—LUMBAR RADIOGRAPHY, LATERAL PROJECTION, PRONE

After collecting the oil at the desired level, a grid-front cassette is placed at the patient's side and held by sandbags. The x-ray tube is placed at the side of the table at the level of the patient's spine. A cone or diaphragm to limit the x-ray beam will improve the quality of radiographs made in this manner, and will reduce radiation dosage to the patient.

interpretation difficult. The authors are not familiar with the use of extremely large quantities of Pantopaque, 30 cc. or more, as advocated by some radiologists. After the injection of Pantopaque is completed, the stylet is replaced, and a sterile gauze dressing is wrapped around the exposed portion of the spinal needle and secured with an elastic band.

Fluoroscopic and radiographic examination. The patient is examined in the prone position. The feet are placed firmly against the footrest of the fluoroscopic table so that the patient may bear weight when the table is tilted upright. An adjustable lock incorporated in the fluoroscopic screen arm must be used to fix the lowest level to which the screen may be moved toward the patient. This will make certain that the fluoroscopic screen, in its motion in the dark, will not strike the needle and push it forward.

Tilting of the fluoroscopic table should be slow, since Pantopaque usually flows rapidly in the spinal subarachnoid space. Gradual tilting will maintain the oil as a single radiopaque column. The foot of the table is lowered until the oil is pooled in the sacral cul-de-sac (fig. 623). By rotating the patient, all surfaces of the opaque column can be viewed easily. The entire lumbosacral subarachnoid space thus may be thoroughly investigated by tilting the fluoroscopic table to various angles between vertical and horizontal.

The spinal subarachnoid space as high as the first cervical segment may be examined by making the Pantopaque flow cephalad. When the radiopaque oil reaches the upper lumbar region, the patient's head should be placed straight, with only the chin resting on the table, and the neck hyperextended (see below). Spot films are made in the anteroposterior direction and lateral views with the patient in the prone position are made with the horizontal x-ray beam and with a grid-front cassette placed on the side of the patient (fig. 624).

In performing *lumbar myelography*, it is best to start by placing the patient in an almost erect position in order to bring the oil as low down as it would possibly go. A spot film is exposed. The table is then tilted down and when the center of the oil column is situated behind the L5–S1 interspace, another spot film is exposed. Care should be taken not to expose the film when either the caudal end or the cephalic end of the oil column are over the L5–S1 disc space, but rather the center of the oil column should be at the interspace. At this point, two oblique views are also made by rotating the patient about 30 to 40° to the right and to the left. Again the oil column should be centered at the L5–S1 disc space, which may require slight tilting of the table in order to adjust the center of the oil column when the patient is turned to either side. After this space has been thoroughly examined, the table is tilted downward a little further until the center of the oil column is at the L4–5 disc space. The same care should be taken not to try to straddle the oil so that it covers two spaces, for this usually results in an improper picture of both interspaces. Immediately thereafter, oblique right and left views of the L4–5 interspace are then made. The table is then tilted further and the center of the oil column is brought to the L3–4 intervertebral disc space and a spot film exposed at this time; further tilting will bring the oil to L2–3 and another spot film is made. At this time the flow of oil should be continued cephalad until it reaches at least the midthoracic region. It is our belief that no lumbar myelogram can be considered complete unless the oil has been observed fluoroscopically to reach the level of the midthoracic region. An occasionally high lesion is overlooked on myelography because of failure to do this and because clinically the patient's neurologic history and findings were not typical of a thoracic lesion. The patient is now brought back to the semierect position and lateral films with the patient in the prone position are taken to cover the L5–S1, L4–5, and the L3–4 disc spaces. Other views may be taken if required. Sometimes, if there is a question of whether or not the failure of satisfactory filling of a root axilla or sleeve is abnormal, the taking of right and left lateral decubitus films with the horizontal x-ray beam and a grid-front cassette is advisable (fig. 625). It is expected that in the lateral decubitus position the root axillae and sleeves should fill if they are fillable. Failure to fill in this position is usually due to an abnormal condition. If only 6 cc. of Pantopaque are used and the spinal canal is congenitally very wide, the oil tends to break up in droplets. In these cases it is necessary to add another 6 to 9 cc. of Pantopaque in order to perform a satisfactory lumbar examination.

In examining *the thoracic region*, 12 cc. of Pantopaque are recommended. The oil tends to break up in droplets as it is moved cephalad when the level of approximately the 9th or 8th thoracic vertebrae is reached. In order to keep the Pantopaque column together as long as possible, it is recommended that the table be tilted very slowly, and that the patient be asked to take deep breaths to prevent his executing an unintentional Valsalva maneuver. In this manner the oil column is kept together as long as possible and sometimes a satisfactory picture can be obtained with the spot device up to the level of the 8th thoracic vertebra and occasionally higher. However, once the oil column begins to break up in droplets it is more advantageous to tilt the table rapidly an additional 15 to 20° to collect the oil in the cervical region. When doing so, it is necessary to elevate the chin off the table top, that is, to hyperextend the head by using the fluoroscopist's gloved left hand on the patient's forehead to insure that hyperextension is being maintained. When enough oil has collected in the cervical region, the table is tilted to a horizontal position; following this, the patient's chin is again placed on the pad, and the patient is advised not to turn the head. It is usually possible to bring the oil in a caudad direction by tilting the table slowly, and maintaining a solid oil column down to about T5. Satisfactory spot films can be taken at this time. Below T5 the column of oil usually

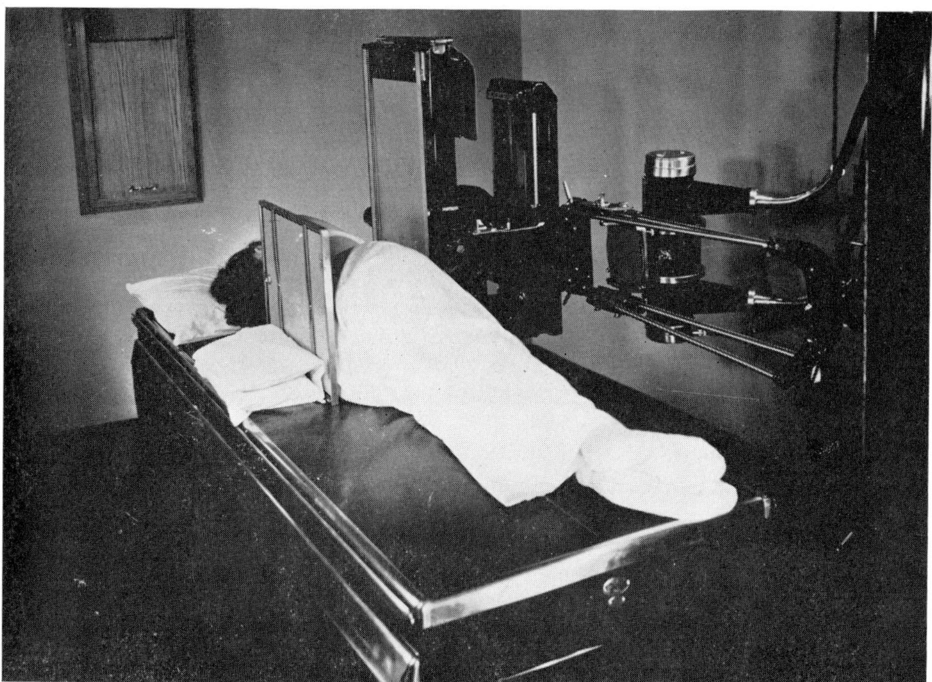

FIG. 625.—LUMBAR RADIOGRAPHY, FRONTAL PROJECTION, LATERAL DECUBITUS
The patient is turned onto the left (or right) side. A grid-front cassette is placed behind (or in front of) the patient. The radiographic tube is at the side of the table at the level of the vertebral column. A cone or limiting diaphragm may be used, as for the lateral projection, which will improve radiographic detail and reduce radiation exposure.

begins to break in droplets leaving a gap of about 3 to 4 vertebrae where spot films with a solid oil column are not usually obtained. Of course, the presence of a complete block or a partial block will facilitate visualization of any area in the thoracic region by the slowing of the flow that this causes. It is sometimes possible to visualize this area with a solid oil column by, again, bringing the oil down from the cervical region while compressing the jugular veins with a blood pressure cuff. The cuff is inflated to about 30 to 40 mm. of mercury, which results in an elongation of the oil column in many instances (Decker, 1960). In the thoracic region it is necessary to obtain lateral views of the Pantopaque column in the prone position with the overhead tube in all cases suspected of having disc herniation. Spot films of the thoracic region must always be made whether something is seen fluoroscopically or not. This is necessary because vascular anomalies of the spinal cord are most frequent in the thoracic region and they usually cannot be seen adequately on the fluoroscopic screen. Therefore, filming is essential. It is possible that the taking of movie films of the flow of oil through the thoracic region would be of help in studying this area more satisfactorily, but it should be said also that a false sense of security may be gained if the prone lateral views are not made. Sometimes, thoracic disc protrusions are clinically significant when they are very small due to the fact that the subarachnoid space in the thoracic region is rather narrow and the cord has little room to move around. Therefore, a small disc protrusion may press on the anterior aspect of the cord because this structure is against the posterior margins of the vertebral bodies, owing to the kyphotic curve normally present in this region of the spine. However, in most of these cases, a slight delay in passage of the oil through the area of a protruded disc is encountered, and sometimes a partial block is present. The obtaining of lateral prone films in the thoracic region is difficult but can be performed by bringing the oil cephalad slowly until it begins to break in droplets, at about T8. At this point, the room lights are turned on and the overhead x-ray tube and the grid-front cassette are centered to the area of interest, and when all is ready, the table is tilted rapidly an additional 15°. After a pause of about 10 seconds, a lateral film is exposed. This film will usually show the relationship of the central portion of the subarachnoid space to the posterior vertebral margin, even if the column of oil is quite narrow in its transverse diameter. The same maneuver may be repeated upon bringing the oil from the cervical region, thereby getting a satisfactory coverage of the entire thoracic region in the prone position. It has been our custom to place the patient in a lateral decubitus position and under fluoroscopic control to center the oil to the thoracic region. This is easy to accomplish. If the patient is turned slightly toward a prone position from the lateral, it is possible to take vertical beam lateral as well as horizontal beam anteroposterior films with the patient lying both on the left and on the right side. In this manner small, laterally-placed lesions may be shown. In the prone position they may be overlooked because of the thinness of the oil column in the thoracic region (since the oil runs in the central portion of the subarachnoid space). In examining the thoracic region, it is usually necessary to place a lead marker over the thoracic region possibly in two different places in order to identify the spot films. A large film is exposed in the frontal projection which will identify the levels at which the lead markers are.

In examining the *cervical subarachnoid space*, it is necessary to collect all of the Pantopaque in this region. Usually 9 cc. are employed. The table should be tilted slowly to keep the oil collected until it has reached the level of about T8, when it begins to break up in droplets. The patient should be made to take deep breaths to help maintain the column of oil together. When the oil begins to break in droplets, the table is tilted rapidly an additional 15 to 20° to have all the oil pass together as rapidly as possible into the cervical region. It is necessary to hyperextend the patient's head by holding the patient's forehead with the chin lifted off the table, using the fluoroscopist's gloved left hand. This would insure that the extended position will be maintained during this initial period. All of the oil, in normal cases, would collect in the upper cervical region and foramen magnum region. When all of the oil has passed cephalad the table is brought to the horizontal position and the chin is placed on the table, usually on a small pad, at the same time that the patient is instructed not to turn the head to either side. The best position for examination of the cervical spine is one in which the clivus follows a line which is the cephalic continuation of the posterior margin of the cervical vertebral bodies (fig. 626). According to Malis, this is achieved by flexing the neck on the trunk and, at the same time, extending the head on the neck. If the patient has a flat chest, a pillow may have to be placed under the chest; if the patient has a large chest, a thicker pad must be placed under the patient's chin. This position should be checked before beginning fluoroscopy and a film may be exposed to ascertain that the correct position for cervical myelography has been achieved. Once the oil is in the cervical region, several spot films are made by tilting the table up and down slightly in the anteroposterior projection using the spot device. The taking of several spot films in the straight anteroposterior position is strongly recommended at the same time that the table is tilted slightly up and down two or three times to insure that a small defect involving the root is persistent and not due to insufficient filling in a given position. Because in the cervical region it is necessary to rely on small defects for diagnosis of root compression by myelography, it is necessary to expose films; reliance on fluoroscopy alone is considered a poor technique.

In examining the area of the *foramen magnum* it is our custom first to examine this region in the oblique projection, while oblique films are not used to examine the

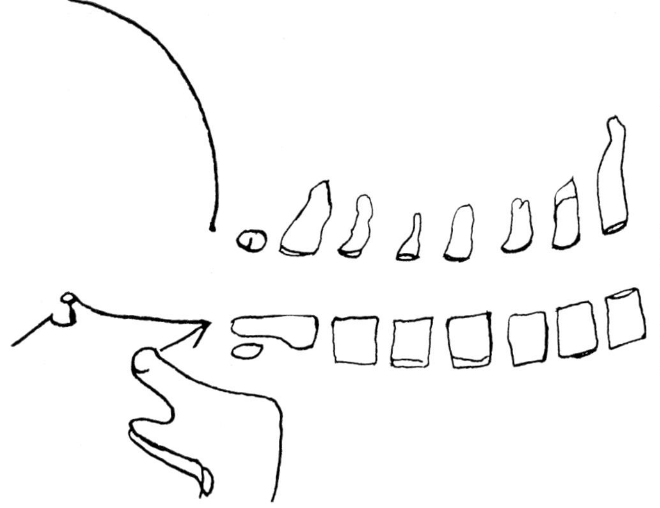

Fig. 626.—Correct Position for Myelographic Examination of Upper Cervical Spine and Foramen Magnum Region

The aim is to place the clivus on the same line with the anterior margin of the cervical vertebral canal (posterior margin of vertebral bodies). In this way the oil would run past the foramen magnum with greater ease.

mid and lower cervical region. The foramen magnum region is examined by turning the head to one side first with the head of the table tilted upwards slightly to prevent passage into the foramen magnum before we are ready for it. The table is then tilted slowly, head down, and when the oil column begins to penetrate the foramen magnum, it will be seen to describe a curve concave toward the patient's face. This happens as the oil is passing over the transverse ligament behind the odontoid process. When the curve has been completed, films are exposed using the spot device. Immediately after the film is exposed (usually double the exposure of that used in the lower cervical region is required), the head is straightened, as before, and the chin placed back on the pad. The table is then brought up so that the head is above the horizontal again, and the head is turned to the opposite side. The same maneuver is then repeated. If the head is turned to the side excessively, the oil column will have a tendency to divide into droplets, and some of the oil may pass laterally by falling off the clivus. Therefore, the head should be turned only 45° to 60° to either side. This maneuver permits us to outline the anterolateral gutter of the subarachnoid space in the region of the foramen magnum on each side. To examine the central portion, the table is simply tilted with the head in the correct position for cervical myelography (fig. 626) and the oil column will pass over the odontoid process and onto the clivus. If the head is maintained in the extended position, the column of oil will not pass beyond the membrane of Lilliquist and can be brought back down without any significant residual in the cephalic subarachnoid space. As the oil column passes through the foramen magnum it will present a slight area of narrowing over the transverse ligament behind the odontoid process. If the patient were to flex the head while the column of oil is over the clivus, the Pantopaque would immediately pass over the dorsum sellae and accumulate in the suprasellar cisterns and in the *cisterna fossae sylvii.* For this reason, it would be advantageous, if one is not sure of the patient's cooperation, to fill the foramen magnum region without filling any other area. Therefore, our technique of examination of the foramen magnum region consists of the outlining of this area with Pantopaque, as explained above, followed immediately, or on another day, by examination with air which will satisfactorily depict the dorsal side of the subarachnoid space.

In the cervical region as well as in the foramen magnum area, it is necessary to take prone lateral views. A minimum of three lateral views is required to outline the entire area, including the foramen magnum. If the foramen magnum region is not being examined, only two lateral views are made. The first lateral film of the cervical region is made with the oil extending from C2 to C7, and with the shoulders as far caudad as possible. The second lateral view is made by placing the arm away from the x-ray tube over the patient's head (swimmer's position). The oil is centered over the lower cervical and upper thoracic region for this film. In the usual film made with both shoulders down, the C6–7 and C7–T1 disc spaces are usually obscured whereas, in the swimmer's position, they are well shown. The central beam should be placed about 3 inches above the shoulder to insure that the shadow of the shoulder is going to be thrown caudad and will not overlie the disc spaces in which we are interested. The third lateral view is made only when we are interested in the region of the foramen magnum. In such cases, the swimmer's position film may be omitted.

It is only occasionally that lateral decubitus films using the horizontal x-ray beam are necessary. The authors have found these to be advantageous when the patient has so much pain and muscle spasm that he is unable to extend the head. When the patient is unable to place the cervical spine in extension, it is not possible to pool the oil effectively over the areas in which we are interested, and therefore, it becomes necessary to place the patient in the decubitus lateral position to show the site of disc herniation. In these cases, the excessive pain is usually associated with acute disc herniations.

Care should be taken in extending the patient's head during fluoroscopy because, being in the dark, it is not possible to note the patient's status. In some patients, extension of the head may result in embarrassment of respiration due to interference with movement of the diaphragm if they have an obstructing lesion in the midcervical region. For this reason, it is recommended very strongly that whenever a difficult cervical myelogram is to be performed, the maneuver of extending the head and placing the patient in the correct position for myelography be done ahead of time with the light on, and even a film may be exposed to give sufficient time to ascertain the fact that the patient is indeed capable of maintaining an extended head position without respiratory embarrassment. At least one instance of respiratory arrest has been seen by us in a young patient with an intramedullary tumor. Fortunately, the condition was diagnosed rapidly and intubation was carried out followed by surgical intervention. For lesions in the foramen magnum, extension of the head usually does not result in any additional compression on the medulla, whereas flexion of the head, as for pneumoencephalography, may result in compression of vital centers.

If obstruction to the flow of radiopaque oil is encountered at any level, lateral as well as frontal prone roentgenograms should be made. It cannot be emphasized strongly enough that the omission of prone lateral roentgenograms may result in an unsatisfactory and nondiagnostic examination and will considerably reduce the accuracy of the procedure. When a block is present, the maximum tilt of the table should be used to ascertain the fact that the oil column is indeed against the highest possible point of passage. It is not uncommon to find that the oil column will stop at a certain distance from the obstruction, and if at this point roentgenograms are made, the level of the lesion, as outlined by oil, will be lower than the actual level, and the myelographic diagnosis of the type of lesion cannot be made. This is a common source of error which can be avoided by using a maximum tilt to expose both the frontal and the lateral films. A very high protein level in the cerebrospinal fluid, of the order of over 1000 mg. per 100 ml., is one of the causes of a slow flow of contrast material in a cephalad direction which may produce a false block at a lower level than the actual lesion.

In performing cervical myelography, it is rather common to see that in patients with cervical spondylosis and a relative constriction of the subarachnoid space owing to ventral ridges, as well as osteoarthritic changes in the apophyseal joints with thickening of the ligaments, the presence of a block to the cephalad flow of Pantopaque may be encountered in the lower cervical region. Even if the table is tilted further, it is not possible to get the oil to pass this level.

(*Revised 1963*)

Yet, when the table is dropped to a horizontal position, and the head gently turned slightly to one side and then to the other, the oil will be seen to pass upward without any difficulty. This is due to two factors. In the first place, the patient may, unknowingly, perform a Valsalva maneuver, and in the second place, there is an increased pooling of blood in the epidural plexus with the patient in a pronounced Trendelenburg position. When the patient relaxes and the normal content of blood in the venous epidural plexus is restored by the horizontal position, the oil will then pass cephalad without difficulty. It may be necessary to turn the head slightly to one side or the other to obtain this effect. Therefore, a cervical block which is seen only in the Trendelenburg position and which is not confirmed by more films made with the horizontal and vertical beams after the patient is placed in a horizontal position, cannot be considered as a true block, as explained above.

It is often helpful to both the radiologist and the neurosurgeon to place a marker at the level of a pathologic process at the time of fluoroscopy, so that accurate relocation of the lesion can be carried out at a later date. This is particularly important for thoracic lesions. A lead number attached to a piece of adhesive tape may be placed on the patient's skin at the level of the lesion. The position of the lead marker in relation to bony landmarks and the myelographic deformity can then be checked fluoroscopically, and recorded on a large film made in the posteroanterior projection with the overhead tube. If the marker is found to be in the correct position, indigo carmine, or a similar dye may be injected into the skin and subcutaneous tissues and even into the muscles, where it is believed that the skin may move a considerable distance over the bony structures when the patient is placed in another position.

When excruciating pain is induced by necessary movements, opiates—administered by parenteral injection and sometimes even intravenously—are useful to allow proper positioning of the patient on the fluoroscopic table. In patients afflicted with spastic paralysis, the administration by infusion of an antispasmodic drug of the curare type may facilitate fluoroscopic examination. Care should be taken to continue the infusion until Pantopaque removal has been accomplished.

Further examination 24 and 48 hours after the primary procedure may be of diagnostic value in some instances when an obstruction to the caudad flow of Pantopaque is found, and some oil remains in the subarachnoid space after completion of the examination. Frontal and lateral films made with the patient erect will determine whether or not oil passes caudad to the obstruction after an interval of time, and in this way the lateral or inferior margin of a tumor may be delineated. Any re-examination should be done at an early date after the original, however, since the oil occasionally escapes from the lumbar subarachnoid space through the needle hole in the meninges.

Removal of Pantopaque. It is our custom to remove as much Pantopaque as possible at the end of the examination. It is felt that the smaller the amount of Pantopaque remaining in the canal, the better; if a very small quantity, 1 cc. or less, is left within the canal, most authors agree that this is of no consequence (Garland and Morrissey, 1940). If a complete obstruction to the flow of Pantopaque is present, it may be desirable to leave the oil rather than reduce cerebrospinal fluid pressure further. Considerable diminution of cerebrospinal fluid pressure below an obstruction may increase the pressure of a tumor on the spinal cord.

For Pantopaque removal, the table is tilted until the radiopaque medium is observed fluoroscopically to be collected around the tip of the needle. Careful positioning of the oil at the needle tip greatly facilitates its removal. The needle should be advanced to the ventral wall of the subarachnoid space because Pantopaque gravitates to this part of the canal with the patient in the prone position. If the needle is in the center of the subarachnoid space, the deepest oil collection is created beneath the needle when the patient is prone. If the needle tip is to the right or to the left of the midline, a deeper collection occurs about the needle

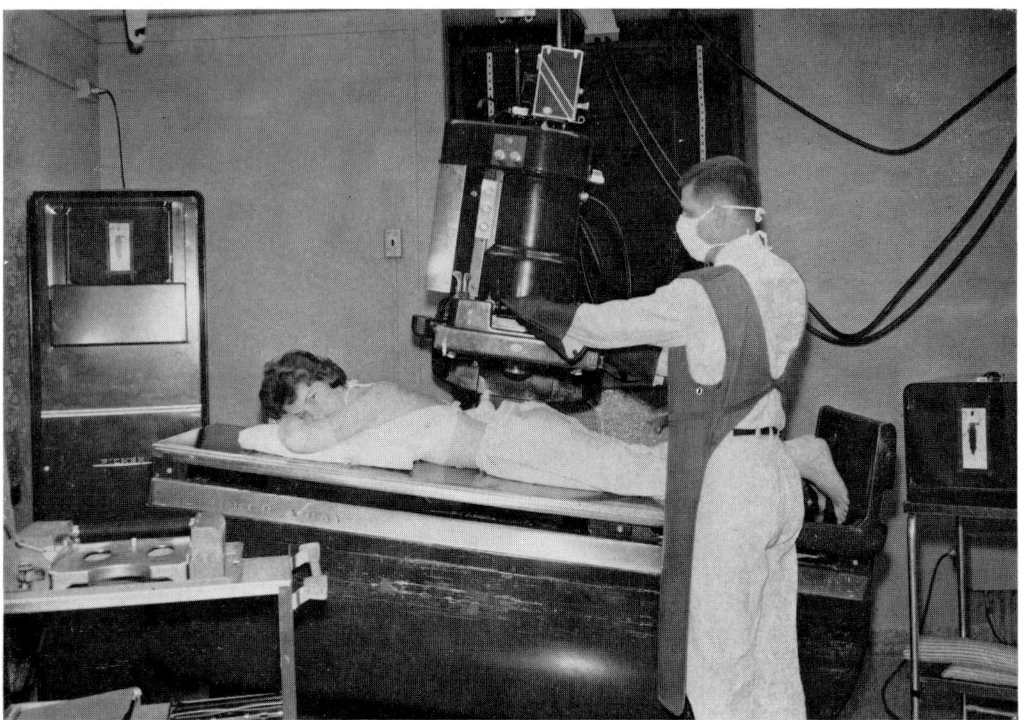

FIG. 627.—FLUOROSCOPIC SETUP FOR MYELOGRAPHY WITH THE USE OF TELEVISION MONITORS
Two television monitors are used, as illustrated, for easier inspection in the various positions of tilt from the erect to the Trendelenburg positions.

tip when the patient is rotated to the right or to the left anterior oblique position. As much as possible of the opaque medium is aspirated by means of an empty sterile syringe attached to the needle. If spinal nerve roots are pulled against the needle tip during the aspiration of Pantopaque, the patient will experience radicular pain. A small syringe of 2 cc. size or a syringe without Luer lock attachment does not create as great suction as the larger syringe. Minor changes in the depth of the tip and the direction of the bevel may avoid nerve root injury. Finally, the rapid injection of a small quantity of air may dislodge a nerve root at the needle tip when other methods have failed.

The remaining Pantopaque, after the initial withdrawal, should be recollected at intervals at the needle tip under fluoroscopic guidance. To accomplish this, the position of the patient may be changed by tilting the fluoroscopic table, or the ventral lumbar curve may be increased by placing pillows under the patient's chest and hips. A slight oblique rotation of the patient again may be helpful, as an attempt is made to withdraw the last cubic centimeter of Pantopaque.

The removal of Pantopaque can be effected most easily at the L5–S1 level. There is no objection to making the second puncture at this level to remove the oil if great difficulty is encountered at the level above. At L5–S1, the operator has the greatest effect of gravity to collect the oil at the needle, and the fewest nerve roots are found.

Small quantities of Pantopaque (less than 1 cc.) remaining in the subarachnoid space after the examination probably are of no consequence, as explained above, and it might be more advantageous to leave a small amount of Pantopaque than to cause trauma by insisting upon the removal of the last drop when technical difficulties are encountered. When removal of Pantopaque has been completed, the spinal needle is

(Revised 1963)

withdrawn and a dry sterile dressing is applied to the site of puncture. The patient is permitted to move from the fluoroscopic table to the stretcher. Thereafter, the same precaution should be taken as following a simple lumbar puncture. In general it is our custom to advise the patient to lie in bed for 24 hours, which tends to minimize the occurrence of post-lumbar puncture headache.

Care should be exercised not to expose the patient to an excessive amount of radiation during the examination. Myelography is best carried out utilizing image intensification and television monitors (fig. 627); this not only minimizes radiation, but allows the use of subdued lighting during the procedure, which is important during instrumentation and helpful for positioning.

Low density Pantopaque. Because 30 per cent Pantopaque is excessively dense for certain clinical problems, we have been interested in the development of a less opaque medium which would not obscure the shadow of the spinal cord and nerve roots. Such a substance containing 15 per cent iodine has been prepared for us by the manufacturer, through dilution of ordinary Pantopaque with a noniodinated phenylundecylic ester. Animal experiments have revealed this contrast material to have the same biological properties as ordinary Pantopaque. Clinical usage over the last year has borne out the theoretical advantages of "light" Pantopaque.

MYELOGRAPHIC ANATOMY

Lumbosacral region. In the frontal projection, the width of the subarachnoid oil column varies from 15 to 25 mm. on the average. When the lower vertebral canal is large, as frequently occurs with spina bifida or where epidural areolar tissue is scanty, the width of the subarachnoid space may be 3 cm. or more. The width of the lumbar subarachnoid space decreases rapidly as it extends caudad with the result that at L5 the arachnoid sac fills only the central half of the vertebral canal, while at L1 the width is three-quarters of the interpediculate distance. At its lower end, the subarachnoid space is continuous with the cul-de-sac in the sacral canal which tapers evenly and terminates usually at the level of S2 (fig. 628).

A symmetrical flare in the lateral borders of the radiopaque column is visible opposite the vertebral pedicles at each level, which are the axillary pouches of the nerve roots. When the patient is rotated to the anterior oblique position the nerve roots sheaths, or axillary pouches, are projected in profile (fig. 629). In most instances, only the axillary pouch is visible and the root itself is beyond the lateral margin of this axillary pouch (fig. 630). In some instances, Pantopaque fills the lateral aspect, that is, the space between the root and the lateral surface of the subarachnoid space, and projects caudally for a certain distance (fig. 631).

(Revised 1963)

In this case, it is possible to visualize the actual root as a radiolucent line for as far as the oil extends caudally. Sometimes the nerve root sheath is more capacious, and more oil is seen to separate from the main column. In these cases, the nerve roots may actually be obscured by the excessive amount of Pantopaque, and we may speak of capacious root sleeves. Sometimes a cystlike collection of Pantopaque forms in this region, and we may refer to this as cystic dilatation of the root sleeves (fig. 632).

The root that is lateral to the axillary pouch is the one that is to emerge beneath the adjacent pedicle. This is above the intervertebral disc space and is usually not affected by protrusions or herniations of intervertebral discs. It must be kept in mind that due to the fact that no oil is present between the root and the lateral margin of the lumbosacral subarachnoid space, the root itself is not visualized (fig. 630). Only when there is a capacious root sleeve is the root itself visible. As explained in the diagram in Figures 620 and 630, the root that traverses the L5–S1 disc space is the S1 root; the L5 root exits above the L5–S1 intervertebral disc space. This explains how the S1 root is compressed by herniations or protrusions of the L5–S1 intervertebral disc, and similarly, how the L5 root is compressed by protrusions and herniations of the L4–5 disc.

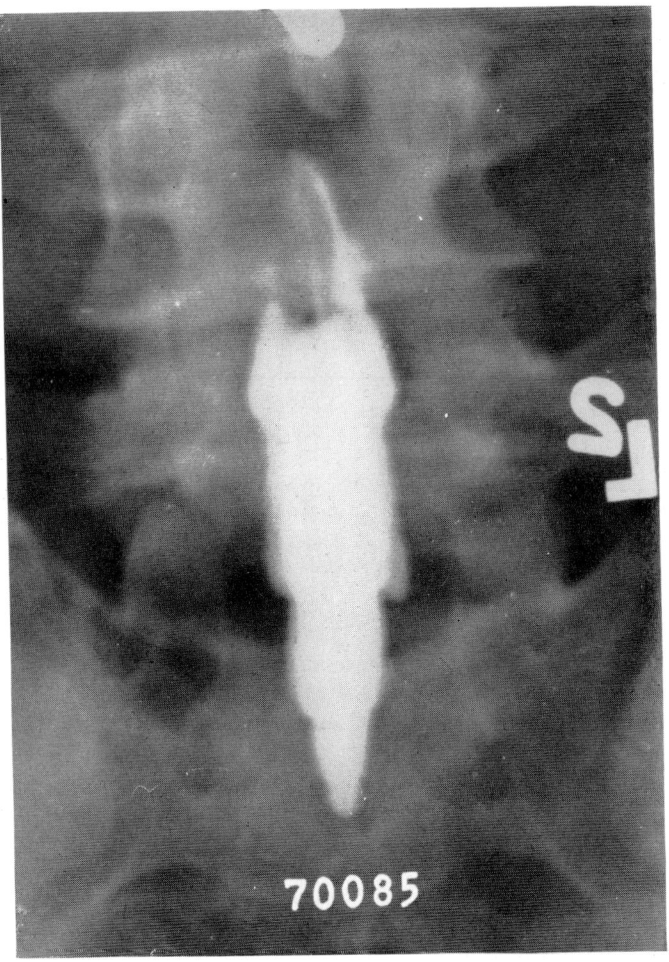

Fig. 628.—Normal Pantopaque Myelogram (Lumbosacral, Frontal View)

A spot film was made with the patient tilted to a semierect position on the fluoroscopic table. The column of oil tapers down to the lumbosacral cul-de-sac. The axillary pouches are usually fairly symmetrical but very often are not entirely symmetrical in the frontal projection in normal cases. Whether these asymmetries are to be regarded as abnormal depends on other factors, including the appearance in the oblique projections, and the distance from the oil column to the medial margins of the pedicles.

Usually the root shadows are not visualized through the column of Pantopaque because Pantopaque is too dense. It is possible to see them laterally when there is oil lateral to the root as explained above. Also, it is possible to see root shadows when there is edema of the roots with an increase in their size or, in certain cases, extravasation of cerebrospinal fluid into the dorsal subdural space, which tends to compress all of the roots ventrad.

In the lateral myelogram, made with the patient prone, or in an upright lateral film made after the injection of a large quantity of opaque material into the subarachnoid space, a tangential view of the anterior margin of the opaque column is obtained (fig. 633). The ventral margin of the subarachnoid space is smooth and either slightly curved or flat, depending on the alignment of the lumbar vertebrae.

The subarachnoid oil column usually is

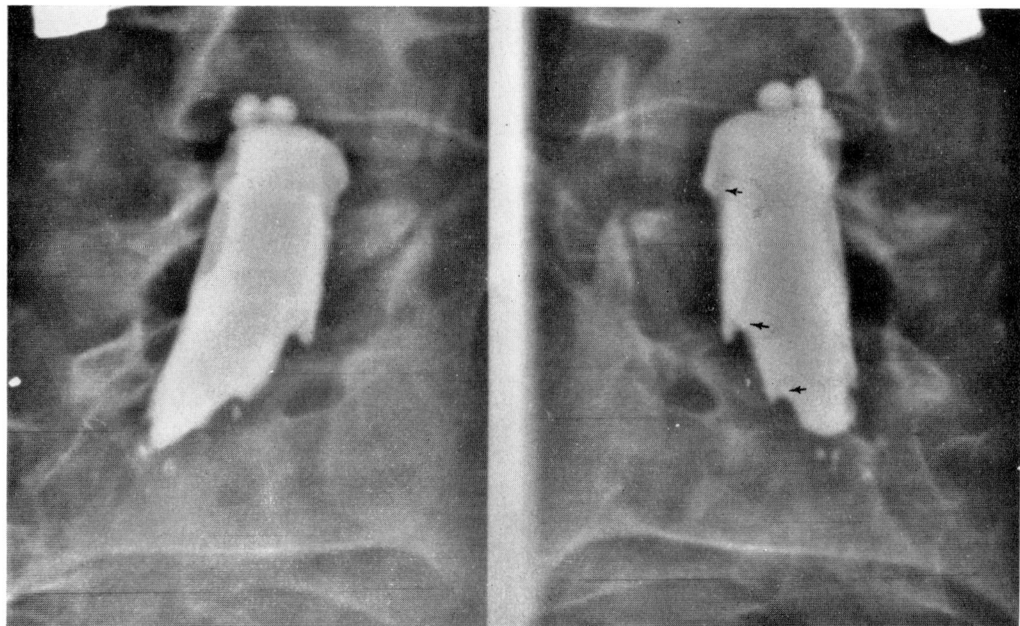

Fig. 629.—Oblique Views of a Normal Lumbar Myelogram

Only the axillary pouches of the nerve roots ordinarily are visible in oblique myelograms. The distance from the highest point (axilla) of each of a pair of pouches to the main column of oil (*arrows*) usually is symmetrical when the left side is compared with the right.

separated from the vertebrae and intervertebral disc by epidural soft tissue of varying thickness, which appears as a radiolucent zone between the Pantopaque and the posterior margins of the vertebrae. Sometimes the epidural soft tissue space is rather thick, measuring as much as 5 mm., whereas at other times, the oil column is practically against the posterior margins of the vertebral bodies and the discs. The epidural soft tissue space enlarges toward the lumbosacral region and decreases as it reaches the upper lumbar level. Because the epidural soft tissue space is made up of the epidural venous plexus which contains a variable amount of blood, and semiliquid areolar tissue, its thickness varies with the position of the patient. In the erect position, the epidural space is thinner as outlined by Pantopaque than in the horizontal position. This is evidently related to hydrostatic pressure of the column of cerebrospinal fluid and the added higher specific gravity of Pantopaque (fig. 633). The epidural soft tissue space is sometimes very large at the lumbosacral junction, so much so that the portion of the spinal canal occupied by the column of Pantopaque may be no more than 20 per cent of the cross sectional area. For this reason, it is possible to have a relatively large herniation of the disc at L5–S1 without producing any defect in the oil column.

In films made with the lower back in extension, or with the patient standing, the anterior border of the arachnoid sac may appear to be in contact with the posterior margins of the vertebral bodies, and a shallow indentation of the radiopaque column may be present behind an intervertebral disc. In fact, if the patient has a very thin epidural space, an indentation will be present behind each intervertebral disc which is normal because the upper and lower margins of the vertebral bodies usually protrude slightly due to the normally concave configuration of each segment posteriorly. The intervertebral discs extend at least to the vertebral margins and, therefore, they often

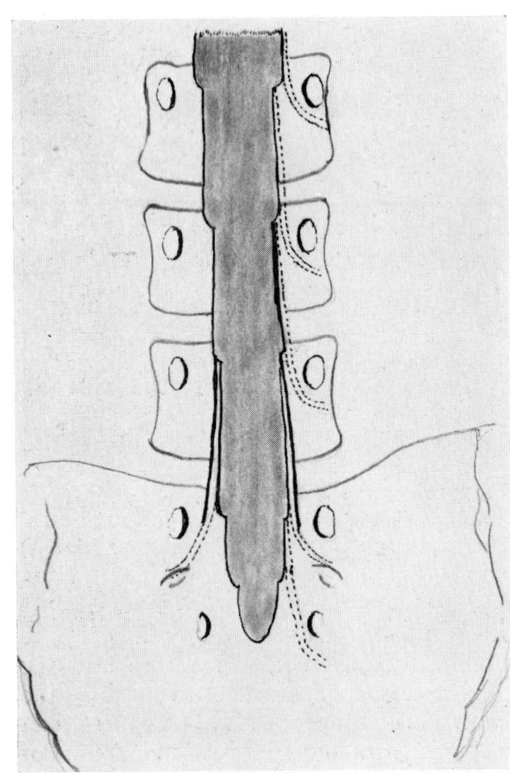

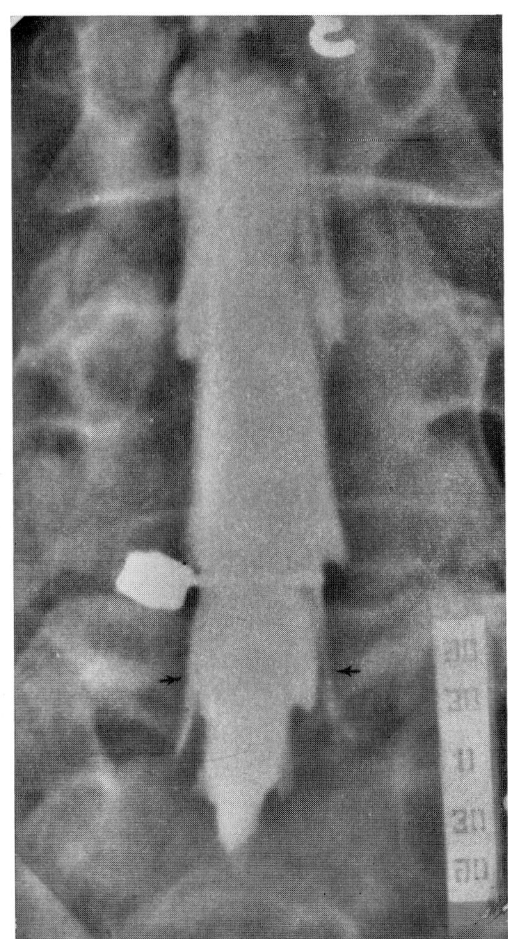

Fig. 630 Fig. 631

Fig. 630.—Diagram Explaining the Relationships of the Roots to the Axillary Pouches in Normal Lumbar Myelography

The exiting root is against the lateral aspect of the Pantopaque column, and usually there is no oil lateral to this root, as explained in the text. Occasionally, some oil is seen lateral to the root, and in these cases the entire root shadow can be followed. See Fig. 631, the myelogram from which the drawing was made.

Fig. 631.—Normal Lumbar Myelogram

At the lower level on each side (*arrows*) Pantopaque is seen lateral to the root shadow, whereas at the levels above the needle, no Pantopaque is seen lateral to the nerve root which exits at the lateral margin of each axillary pouch.

protrude slightly (fig. 633). This is a normal appearance. With flexion of the spine the dural sac and its contents are drawn taut, with the result that the ventral margin of the subarachnoid sac does not project ventrally behind the intervertebral body and the normal prominence of each intervertebral disc is de-emphasized. The same occurs when the epidural soft tissue space smooths out this surface. The dorsal margin of the subarachnoid space is not visualized in the lumbar region when the thickness of the oil column is less than the depth of the subarachnoid space, since the Pantopaque occupies the most ventral portion of the arachnoid sac with the patient in the prone

(*Revised 1963*)

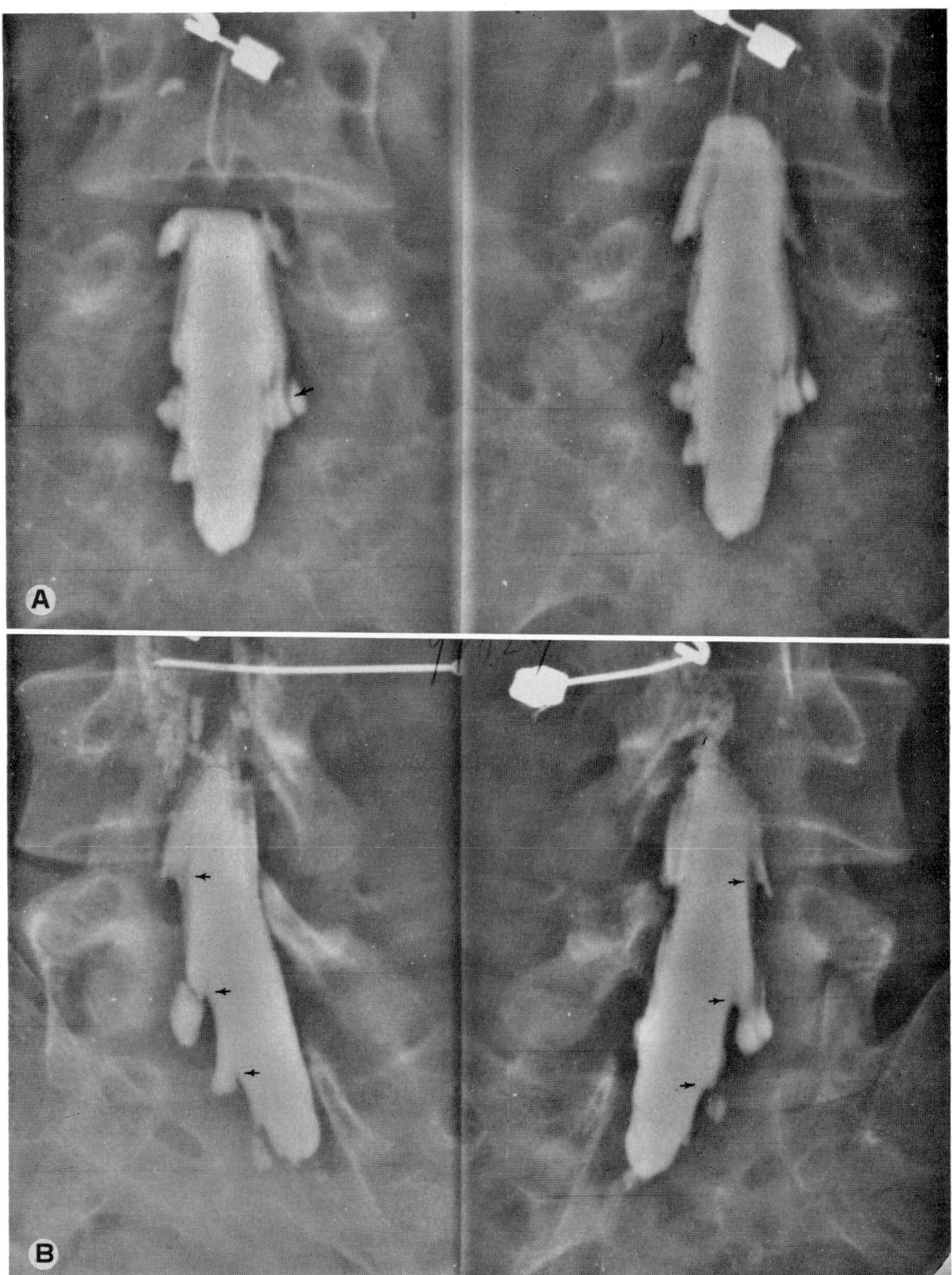

Fig. 632.—Capacious Root Sleeves in Normal Lumbar Myelogram

In the frontal projection, the exact anatomical configuration cannot be made out because of the enlarged root sleeves (A). On the left side, the S1 root can be seen crossing the dilated root sleeve with Pantopaque medial as well as lateral to it (*arrow*). The oblique projections (B) demonstrate the enlarged root sleeves to better advantage. The distances between the highest points of the axillary pouches and the main oil column remain symmetrical when the right side is compared with the left (*arrows*).

(*Revised 1963*)

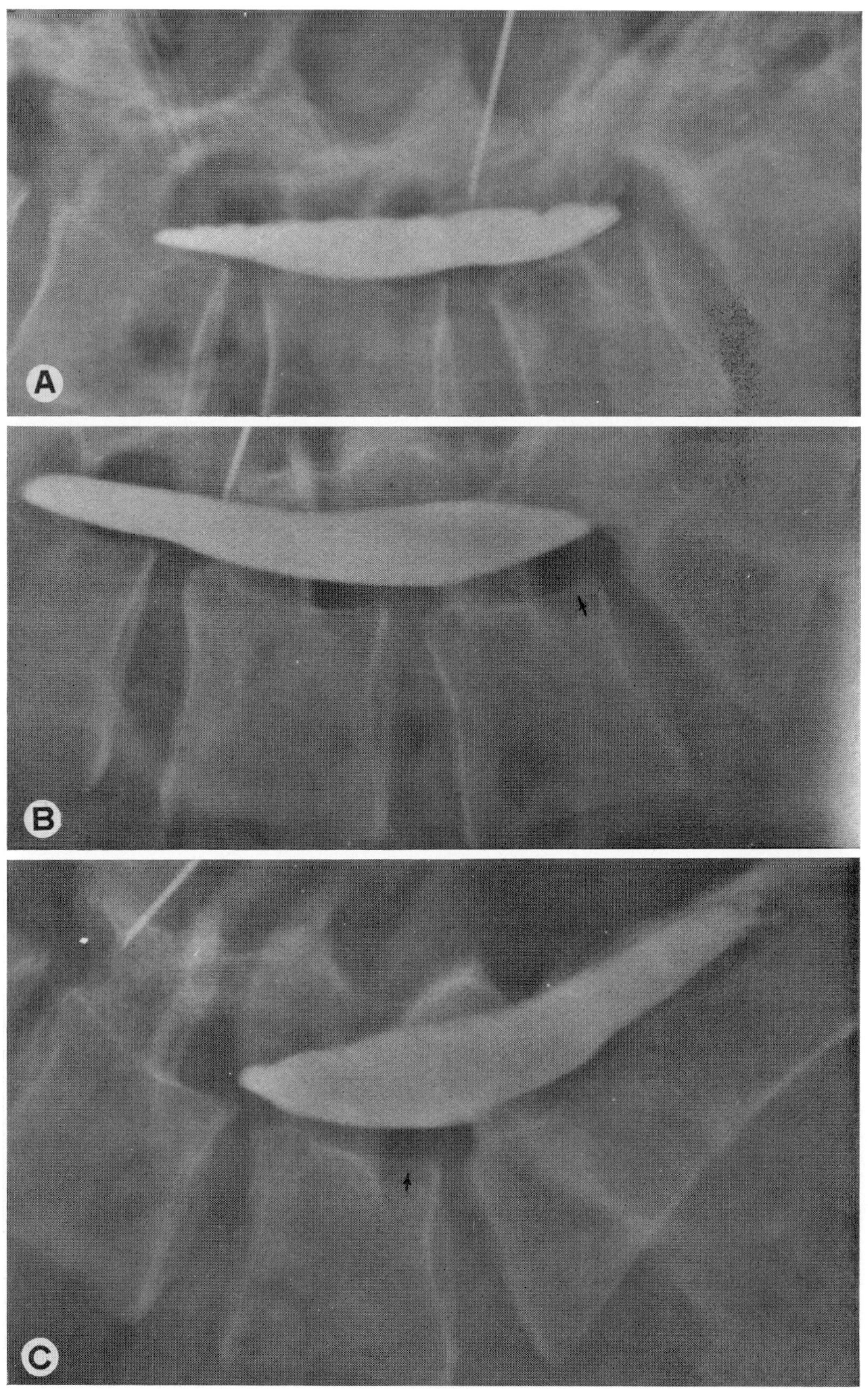

Fig. 633

(Revised 1963)

position. Lateral views with the patient in the lateral recumbent position are of little value since the Pantopaque forms a long thin column along the lateral wall of the vertebral canal well away from the midsagittal plane. Frontal films, on the other hand, made with the horizontal ray with the patient in the lateral decubitus position, may demonstrate irregularities of the lateral margin of the subarachnoid contour and of the nerve roots which cannot be demonstrated in other views (fig. 696).

The axillary pouches which produce the symmetrical widening of the oil column in prone position are seen in the mid and lower lumbar regions but are often not visualized in the upper lumbar or thoracic regions. This is simply due to the fact that the level of the Pantopaque column, which only outlines the ventral aspect of the canal, does not reach the opening of the root sleeve. However, all of the axillary pouches, including those in the thoracic region, can be shown when the patient lies in the lateral decubitus position and a horizontal beam x-ray film is exposed.

The height of the cul-de-sac is variable. In some patients, it may reach caudad to S3 whereas, at other times, the cul-de-sac ends at the upper margin of S1. Usually, the cul-de-sac tapers not only in the transverse diameter but also in its anteroposterior diameter and it is directed backward away from the ventral surface of the spinal canal (fig. 634). This normal anatomical configuration should be kept in mind when it is necessary to differentiate a short cul-de-sac from a constriction at the lower margin of the subarachnoid space produced by an epidural mass lesion.

In the *thoracic region*, the opacified subarachnoid space usually appears as a band which measures about 15 mm. in width in the frontal projection (fig. 635). At T1 the subarachnoid width is greater, but caudad to T2 the space narrows gradually and the caliber is smallest at T9. Further caudad the arachnoid sac expands rapidly, corresponding to the lumbar enlargement of the spinal cord, and often exceeds 20 mm. in width at T12. In relation to the interpediculate measurements, the arachnoid sac occupies seven-eighths of the vertebral canal in the upper thoracic area and three-fourths of the space in the lower thoracic region. Occasionally, slight convexity of the lateral subarachnoid margin is seen adjacent to each vertebral pedicle, beneath which the nerve roots pass through the intervertebral foramen, but as explained above, this symmetrical widening at the root exit level is often not seen in the thoracic region because of incomplete filling; the column of Pantopaque is too thin in its anteroposterior diameter and does not reach the level of root exit.

The central portion of the oil column is reduced in density by the thoracic spinal cord which appears as a smooth grey band occupying the middle half of the vertebral canal, provided there is sufficient Pantopaque (fig. 636). Satisfactory lateral views of the normal thoracic subarachnoid space are difficult to obtain with the patient prone. Here, as in the lumbar region, the anterior margin of the subarachnoid oil column is smooth and concave ventrally corresponding to the dorsal curve of the thoracic spine. A radiolucent linear shadow is seen often in the central portion of the canal due to the anterior spinal vessels. Sometimes the radicular arteries which enter the spine accompanying the nerve roots are seen to join the anterior spinal artery (fig. 636).

Irregularities of the radiopaque column in the thoracic area and high lumbar region normally are common. A smooth unilateral

---

FIG. 633.—LATERAL PRONE FILMS OF NORMAL LUMBAR MYELOGRAMS

In (A) there is practically no ventral epidural space. In these cases, the Pantopaque column is slightly displaced dorsad at each disc level. In (B) there is a moderate ventral epidural space which becomes wider as it approaches the lumbosacral junction. Near the lower margin of L5 the ventral epidural space measures between 6 and 7 mm. in thickness. This film was made with the patient in the horizontal position. In (C), a film of the same patient as (B) made in the semierect position, the ventral epidural space behind L5 has become much smaller (*arrow*); it measures only a maximum of 4 mm. The ventral epidural space becomes smaller as the patient assumes the erect position.

(Revised 1963)

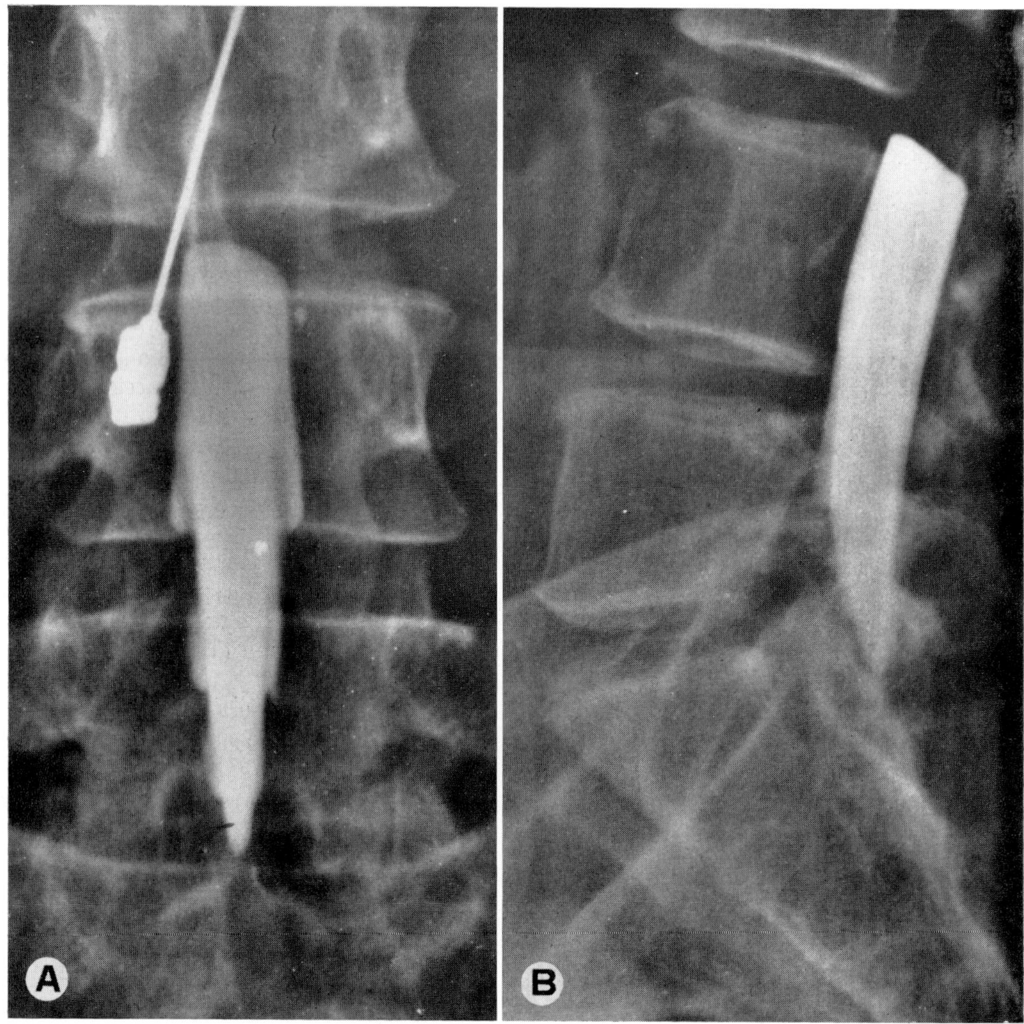

FIG. 634.—NORMAL MYELOGRAM OF PATIENT WITH A SHORT LUMBOSACRAL CUL-DE-SAC
The lateral erect film (B) reveals that the bottom of the oil column is no lower than the upper margin of the first sacral vertebra. The oil tapers dorsad and the ventral epidural space increases gradually. In these cases, it is usually impossible to rule out a disc herniation at the L5-S1 level. The anteroposterior projection (A) shows the tapering of the oil column in the transverse direction as well.

concavity or an hourglass configuration of the oil column may be produced as the elongated shallow column passes over a normal intervertebral disc prominence. Because of the marked thinness of the oil column in its anteroposterior diameter, any small indentation on the ventral aspect may produce a large defect. For this reason, care should be taken in diagnosing significant protrusions of the thoracic intervertebral discs, particularly in the mid and lower portion from T6 through L1. Lateral indentations are usually of no significance because of their frequency. On the other hand, if a ventral protrusion of the intervertebral disc can be demonstrated in lateral prone views, this may be more significant. The majority of the irregularities noted in the thoracic region are inconstant and cannot be reproduced on repeated passages of the oil, or they disappear when sufficient oil is collected to produce a column several millimeters

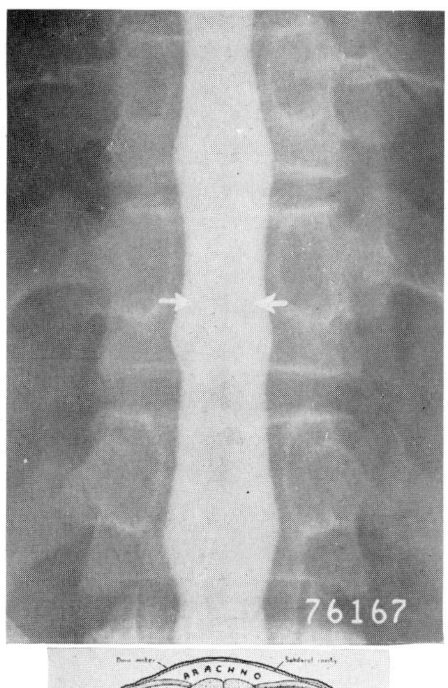

FIG. 635.—NORMAL PANTOPAQUE MYELOGRAM (THORACIC, FRONTAL VIEW)

A spot film was made with the head of the table tilted below the horizontal. The spinal cord appears as a broad band of diminished density in the center of the opaque oil column (*arrows*).

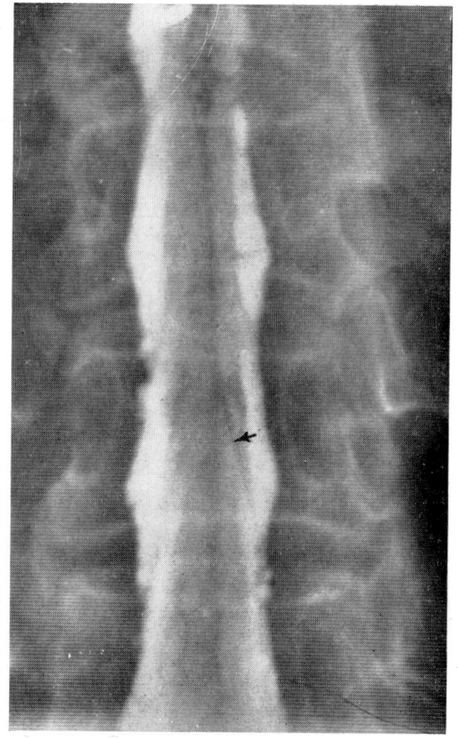

FIG. 636.—NORMAL THORACIC MYELOGRAM

The spinal cord is seen as a radiolucent band within the spinal subarachnoid space. The anterior spinal vessels are seen as a radiolucent line near the center of the spinal cord. A radicular artery (*arrow*) is seen entering to join the anterior spinal vessels.

in depth. All thoracic irregularities which are not accompanied by some degree of obstruction to the flow of radiopaque material should be considered of doubtful pathologic significance, with the exception of varicose veins and vascular malformations (fig. 637).

The *normal cervical myelogram* discloses a large subarachnoid space which, in frontal projection, may measure up to 30 mm. in width. The subarachnoid width is seven-eighths of the interpediculate distance throughout the cervical area. Along the lateral margins are symmetrical short, almost triangular outpouchings which are the arachnoid sheaths of the cervical nerve roots. Frequently rather broad bands of diminished density, which are the large cervical nerve roots, can be seen passing obliquely downward and lateralward in the arachnoid sheath, obliterating the apex of the triangle. If well exposed films are available, it will be seen that the shadows of the roots can be continued medially by a series of lines which form a fanlike configuration that represents the rootlets as they arise from the anterior aspect of the cord to form the anterior roots (fig. 638). There are both ventral and dorsal rootlets which can be shown on the myelogram but, because the column of oil is usually not thick enough to outline the dorsal side of the spinal cord, only the ventral rootlets become visible.

The cervical spinal cord can be seen clearly in properly exposed films, occupying the central two-thirds of the cervical subarachnoid space. In the upper cervical region, the

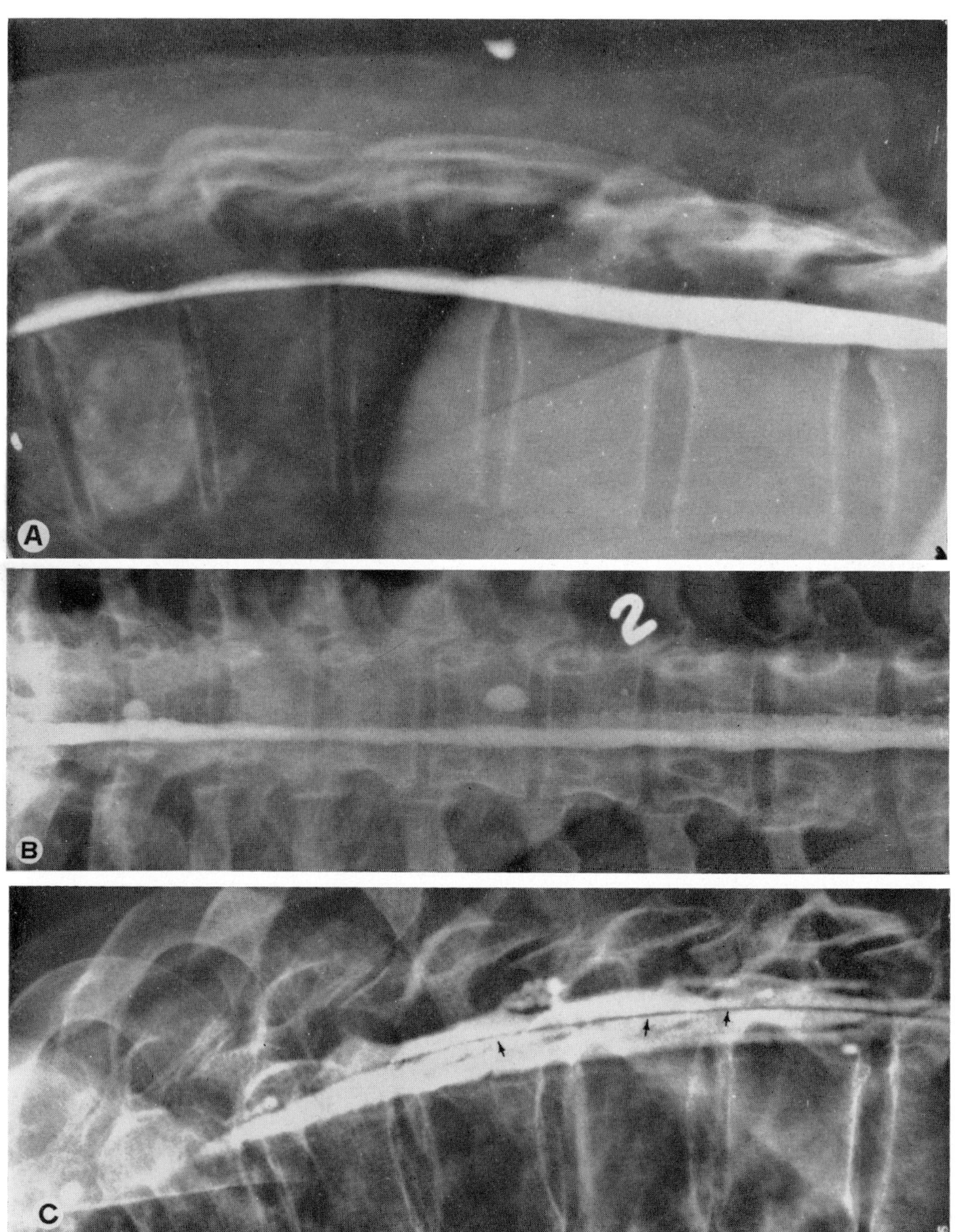

FIG. 637.—LATERAL FILM, PRONE (THORACIC MYELOGRAM, NORMAL)

It is possible to obtain lateral prone radiographs during thoracic myelography by using variations of the technique as described in the text. The film (A) demonstrates the extreme thinness of the oil column in the thoracic region, and thus any defect in the ventral surface of the canal produced by slight irregularities of the disc surfaces, or of the ligaments, will produce sizable defects in the anteroposterior view. Also, the ventral epidural space is very thin.

(*Revised 1963*)

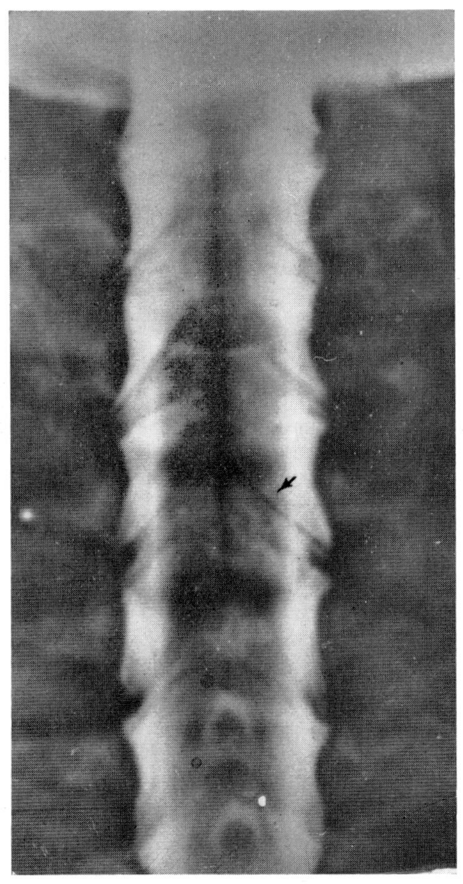

Fig. 638.—Anteroposterior View, Normal Cervical Myelogram

The spinal cord is a radiolucent band occupying approximately two-thirds of the diameter of the subarachnoid Pantopaque oil column. The sites of exit of the roots are marked by slight protrusions of the lateral margin of the oil column, and the ventral rootlets can be followed medially at most levels. A radiolucent line produced by the anterior spinal vessels is seen running up and down the center of the spinal cord shadow. A radicular artery is seen to join the anterior spinal artery (*arrow*).

spinal cord is smaller than at the level of the cervical enlargement. The width of the spinal cord is approximately one-half the interpediculate distance except at the level of the maximum cervical enlargement at C5, where the spinal cord occupies almost two-thirds of the vertebral canal. Efforts have been made to determine the normal width of the spinal cord by other methods. We feel that the method that relates the width of the spinal cord to the total width of the subarachnoid space or to the interpediculate distance, or to both, is more accurate, owing to the varying magnification that occurs during myelography and spot filming; at one time the screen may be close to the head whereas at another time the screen may be far away from the head of the patient. Usually, the spinal cord occupies almost exactly two-thirds of the width of the subarachnoid space measured from C4 through C7 or, as explained above, other measurements may be used. The cord normally becomes thinner at C3 and above. Cramer and Hudson (1659) found that using the spot films in a series of patients at the Neurological Institute, the maximum width of the cord was 20 mm. Above this level, the cord was usually found to be enlarged.

Along the center of the cord, a radiolucent line is almost always clearly seen which represents the anterior spinal vessels; the shadow is probably produced by the anterior spinal artery. Radicular arteries are seen to enter the spinal canal accompanying the roots and to join the anterior spinal artery. They can be recognized because they extend to the midline and join the shadow of the anterior spinal vessels, whereas the rootlets stop before reaching the midline (fig. 638).

In lateral projection, with the patient prone, both the ventral portion of the sub-

---

(B) and (C) illustrate the decubitus position, anteroposterior and lateral views. With the patient lying on the side, it is possible to fill this portion of the subarachnoid space (B). In this way, small defects on the lateral aspect, at the root exit level, can be seen. Lateral radiographs with the vertical beam also can be made (C). In this position, the ventral surface of the oil column is slightly separated from the posterior margin of the vertebral bodies, and therefore, small ventral defects will go undetected. The shadows of the dentate ligaments are often visible as a sharp radiolucent line traversing the center of the oil column (*arrows*).

(*Revised 1963*)

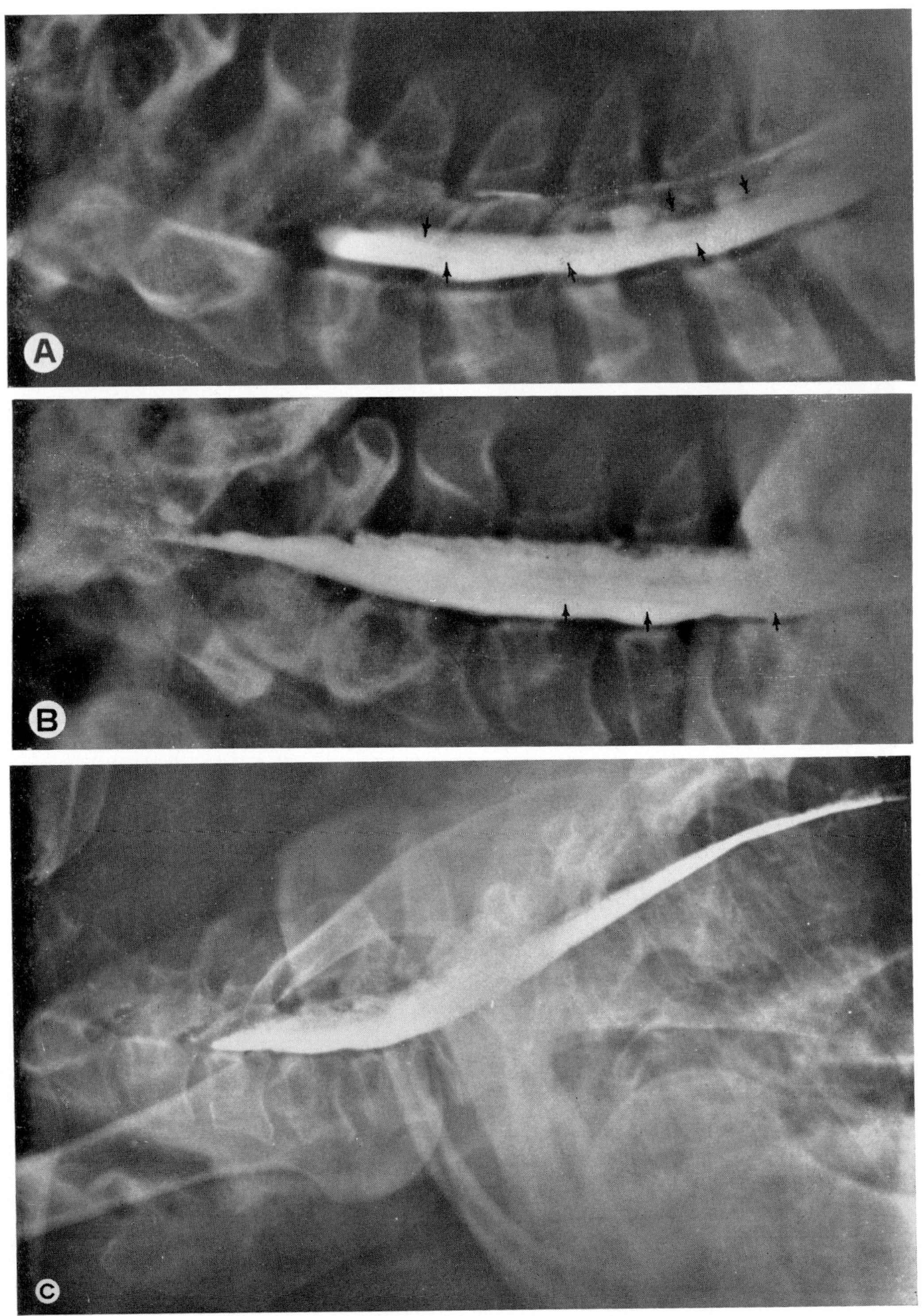

Fig. 639

(*Revised 1963*)

arachnoid space and the ventral margin of the cervical spinal cord are clearly delineated (fig. 639). Usually the spinal cord is approximately 3 mm. from the ventral surface of the oil column. On frequent occasions, the oil collection is of sufficient depth to outline the dorsal surface of the spinal cord also. With the neck in hyperextension, the spinal cord occupies the dorsal portion of the subarachnoid space, and an oil collection of 3 to 5 mm. in thickness is present ventral to the spinal cord. The ventral subarachnoid surface, seen tangentially in lateral view, is smooth and convex, corresponding to the ventral curve of the cervical spine. The density of the Pantopaque column sometimes makes it slightly difficult to identify the anterior margin of the spinal cord. However, in films that are sufficiently well exposed, there is usually no difficulty. Care should be taken not to confuse the shadow of the dentate ligaments with the anterior margin of the spinal cord. The shadow of the dentate ligaments is usually extremely well shown when the oil is both on the ventral and dorsal aspects of the site of attachment of this ligament (figs. 637C and 639). At other times, only the ventral side of this ligament is shown. The ventral surface of the spinal cord is usually outlined by a radiolucent line which appears to be slightly more radiolucent than the immediately adjacent portion of the cord. It is probable that this radiolucent line is produced by the anterior rootlets as well as the anterior spinal vessels added to the shadow of the cord itself. This added radiolucency identifies the anterior margin of the cord in cases where there is doubt about whether the dentate ligaments actually represent the anterior cord margin or whether this is at a lower level in the column of oil. In the anteroposterior view of the cervical myelogram, the root shadows and their corresponding sleeves are usually quite symmetrical when the right is compared with the left. The distances between the roots is also symmetrical. Occasionally, inequality in these distances is noted when the right side is compared with the left, and in these cases the possibility of abnormal tension on

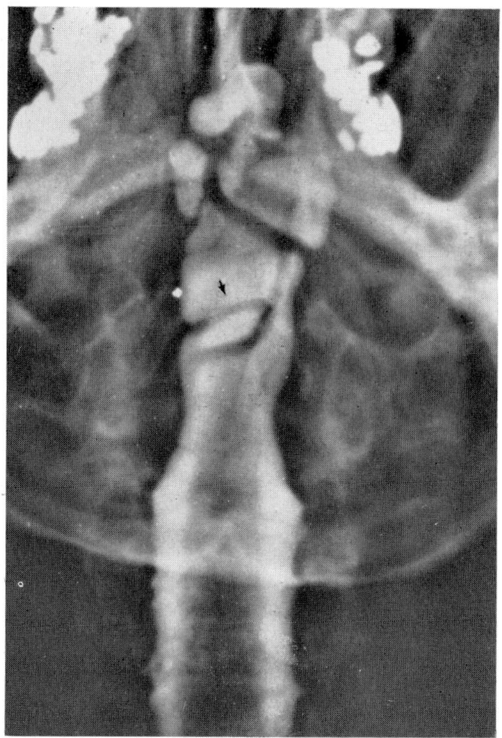

Fig. 640.—Normal Myelogram, Foramen Magnum Region, Anteroposterior Projection

The shadow of the spinal cord becomes slightly thinner as it extends upward. There is slight narrowing of the transverse diameter of the oil column as it passes over the odontoid process due to the ventral elevation produced by the transverse ligament. The vertebral arteries and the large posterior inferior cerebellar artery (*arrow*) can be seen.

Fig. 639.—Normal Lateral Cervical Myelogram, Prone Position

The shadow of the spinal cord dips into the ventral oil column to a distance of about 3 mm. from the vertebral surface. A sharp, straight upper margin is usually visible which is formed by the dentate ligaments (*two upper arrows in* (A)) and not by the anterior margin of the cord which is ventral to it. In (A) there is a small amount of Pantopaque dorsal to the cord, but in (B) the posterior portion of the cord is not outlined. The dorsal rootlets are visible in (B); the ventral surface of the cord is demarcated by a thin radiolucent line (*arrows*). (C) represents a lateral cervical myelogram made in swimmer's position with elevation of the arm which is away from the x-ray tube over the head.

(Revised 1963)

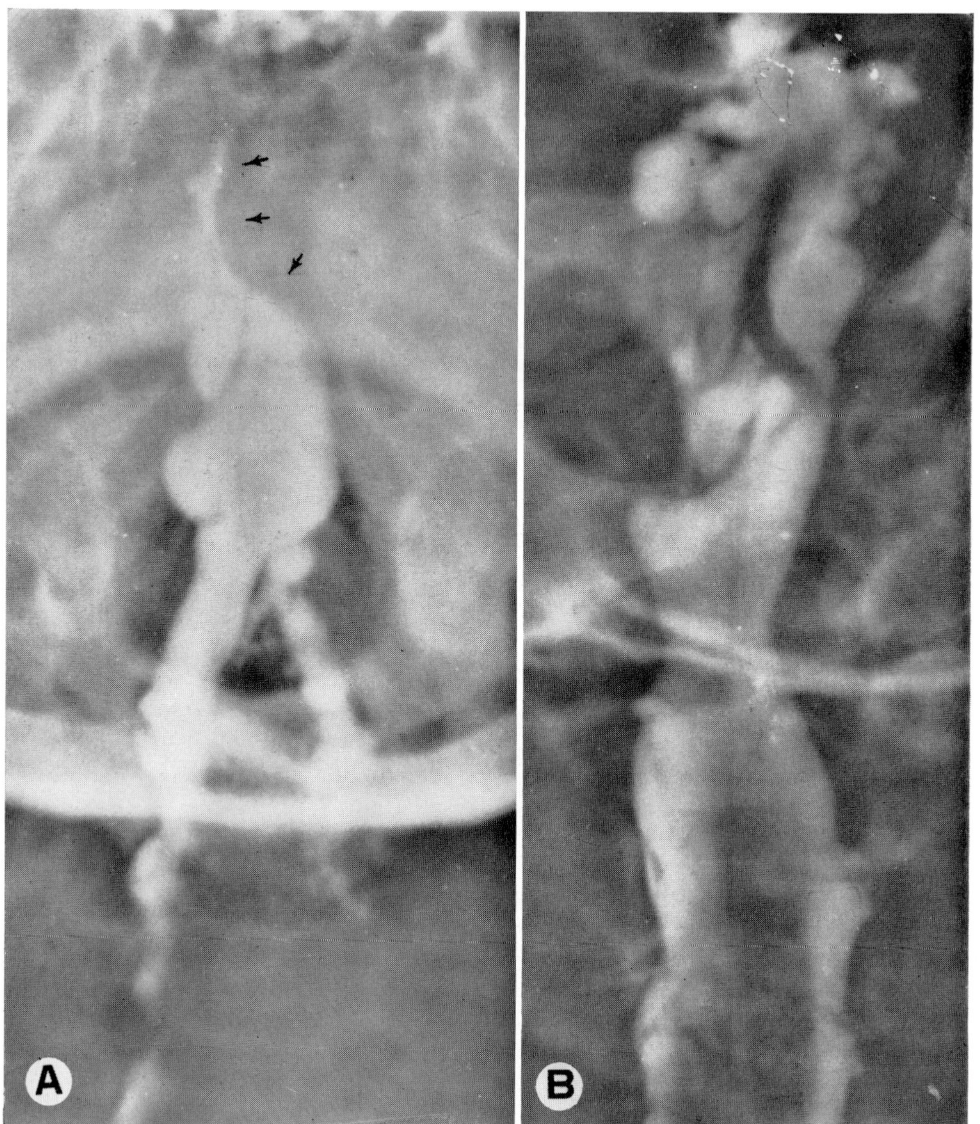

FIG. 641.—NORMAL ANTEROPOSTERIOR MYELOGRAM, FORAMEN MAGNUM REGION

In (A) the oil column stops and has a contour suggestive of a tumor (*arrows*). Later, with more filling of this area, it is seen that the appearance is caused by the margins of the vertebral and basilar arteries (B); this becomes clear when oil is seen on both sides of the vessels.

the dura should be suspected. Asymmetry of the distances between the cervical roots may be produced by scoliosis.

The *high cervical myelogram* is extremely important. In the lateral projection, the column of oil is seen to separate slightly from the dorsal aspect of the cervical vertebrae as it goes over the odontoid process because the transverse ligament is interposed between the oil and the odontoid process. In some instances, the ventral surface of the oil column will actually describe a gentle concave curve at this point, but at other times, the entire outline of the ventral surface of the oil column is perfectly smooth without this indentation. When the

(*Revised 1963*)

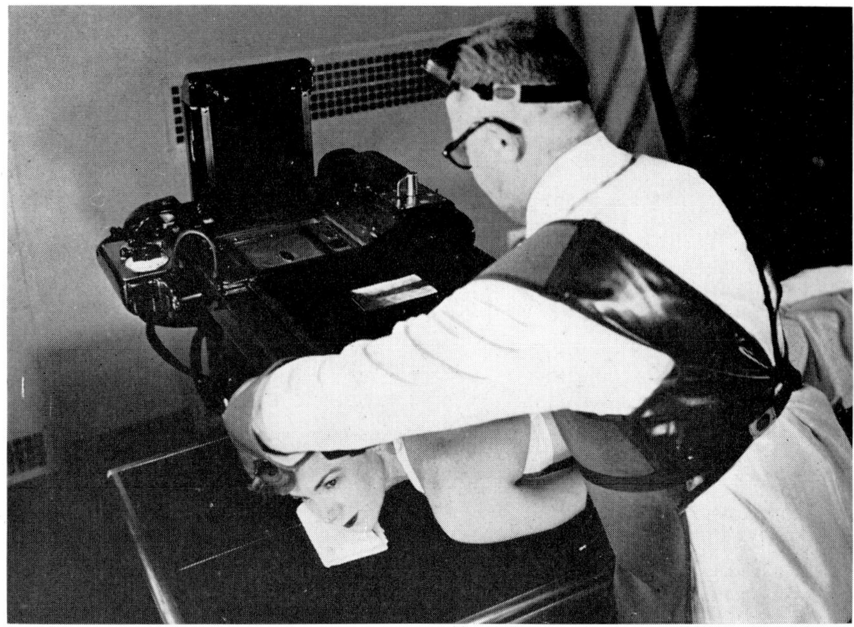

Fig. 642.—High Cervical Fluoroscopy

Investigation may be carried to the foramen magnum without tilting the table from the horizontal position, or by tilting it only slightly. The radiopaque oil flows cephalad on turning the head to a semi-lateral position under fluoroscopic guidance as explained in the text.

column of oil penetrates the skull it is seen to rest over the dorsal surface of the clivus from which it is separated by a very thin epidural space.

In the anteroposterior projection, the high cervical myelogram will usually show the shadow of the spinal cord to become thinner and the entire column of oil may become slightly narrower behind the odontoid process (fig. 640). Higher up, the oil column expands over the clivus. The exact configuration is somewhat dependent upon the shape of the clivus. In this region, the shadows of the vertebral arteries and of the basilar artery are clearly visualized. Branches of these arteries are also visible in some instances (fig. 640). Care should be taken not to diagnose defects such as may be produced by tumors in cases where the column of oil stops at one side of a vertebral artery and does not pass over to the other side to outline the entire vessel. In these cases a concave configuration with a sharp cut-off often is produced. The location in the typical position for the vertebral vessels is diagnostic (fig. 641). As previously stated, as long as the head is not turned to either side and is not flexed, it is possible to maintain the oil column on the clivus without fear of having it spill over the rest of the subarachnoid space. Some techniques have been introduced, however (Mones and Werman, 1959), to demonstrate the subarachnoid spaces and the cerebellopontine angles on both sides. This technique has not been employed at the Neurological Institute.

The oblique views of the foramen magnum will demonstrate the oil outline of the anterolateral gutter of the foramen magnum region on each side. A shadow with a concave margin directed toward the face is produced by the odontoid process and the transverse ligament (figs. 642 and 643).

As previously mentioned, the dorsal side of the foramen magnum cannot be adequately demonstrated by Pantopaque myelography unless the patient is placed in the supine position, but we prefer to inject air following the removal of the Pantopaque

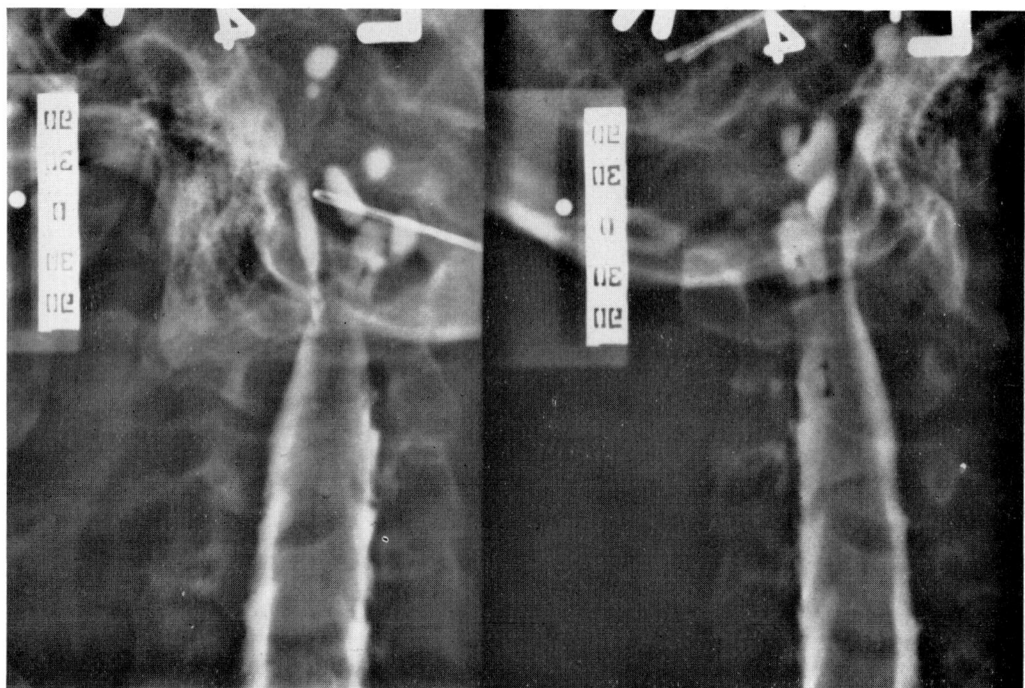

FIG. 643.—RIGHT AND LEFT OBLIQUE VIEWS OF THE FORAMEN MAGNUM
Upon passing through the foramen magnum region, the Pantopaque column describes a smooth curve which is concave towards the patient's face, produced by the transverse ligament. When there is less oil in this region, the curvature is more pronounced.

to outline the dorsal side of the cervical subarachnoid space and the foramen magnum region, as explained in the second dealing with techniques.

TECHNICAL ERRORS

Unsatisfactory myelograms occur more than twice as frequently among patients who have had previous lumbar punctures than among those patients who do not have diagnostic punctures prior to myelography. Presumably, a diagnostic spinal tap is frequently followed by extravasation of cerebrospinal fluid into extra-arachnoidal spaces; partial collapse of the subarachnoid space follows formation of a subdural hydroma. Normally the subdural space is quite narrow and contains only a very small amount of fluid which serves to moisten the opposed surface of the arachnoid and dural membranes. After the meninges are pierced by a needle, fluid may pass out of the subarachnoid space to dissect the arachnoid from the dura and create a large fluid-filled subdural space. When the second puncture for myelography is attempted, fluid may be obtained from the subdural space or even from the extradural space, which may lead the operator to believe that the tip of the needle is in the correct position in the subarachnoid space. At least a week should be allowed to elapse between a diagnostic lumbar puncture and myelography, to permit the absorption of extravasated fluid and the disappearance of swelling due to trauma produced by the needle. It is possible, also, for an extra-arachnoidal injection to occur when the bevel of the needle is not entirely subarachnoid in position in the absence of previous extravasation of cerebrospinal fluid. This occurs most commonly when the needle tip

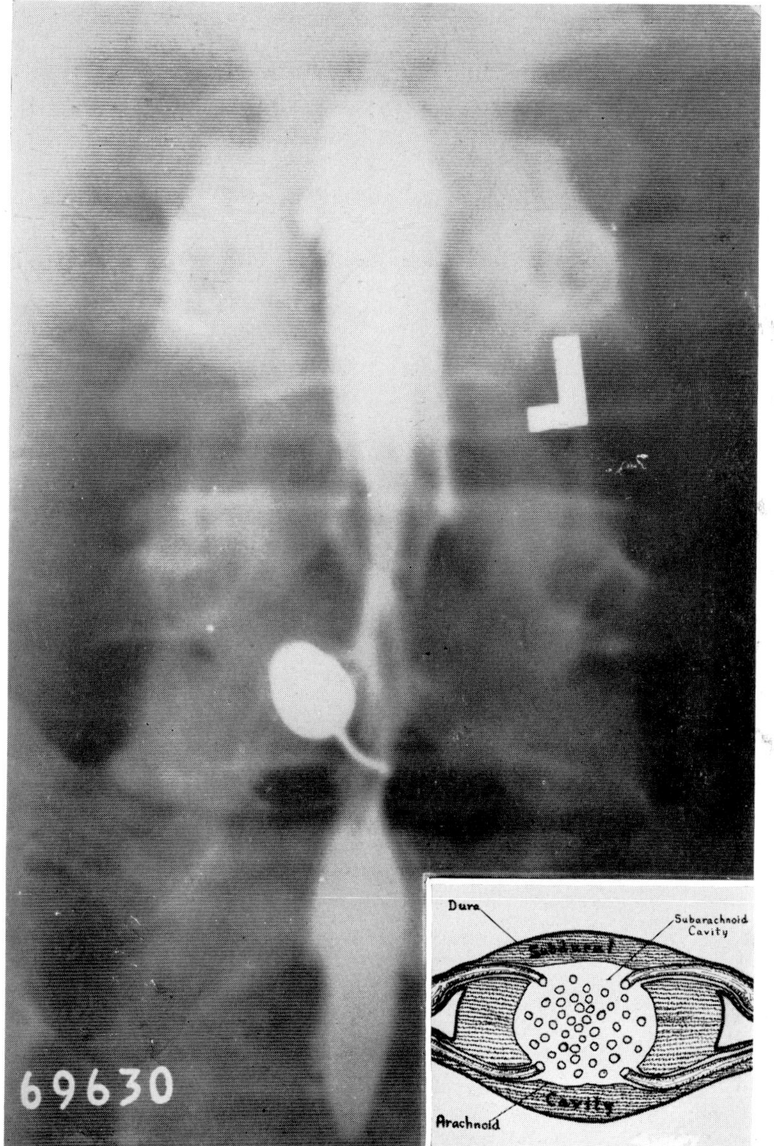

Fig. 644.—Extravasation of Cerebrospinal Fluid

After repeated punctures, Pantopaque was injected into a subarachnoid space which is narrowed symmetrically. Laminectomy following the myelogram failed to disclose a pathologic process. The deformity is the result of cerebrospinal fluid in the subdural and epidural spaces, compressing the arachnoid sac which is outlined by the radiopaque oil.

is too superficial, too deep, or too far lateral in the vertebral canal.

When a successful subarachnoid Pantopaque injection is made soon after a diagnostic lumbar puncture, a constriction of the subarachnoid outline may be seen at the site of previous puncture. In certain respects this is similar to the deformity produced by an extradural tumor which constricts the dural sac (fig. 644). At other times, all of the fluid may be collected on the dorsal side of the canal and may constrict the subarachnoid space in the anteroposterior plane, thus causing the root sha-

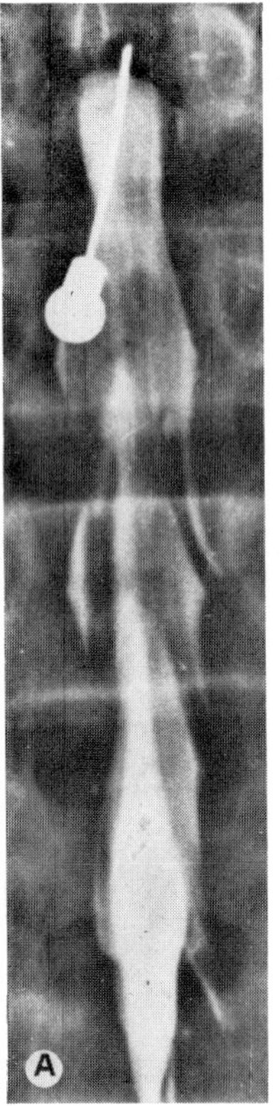

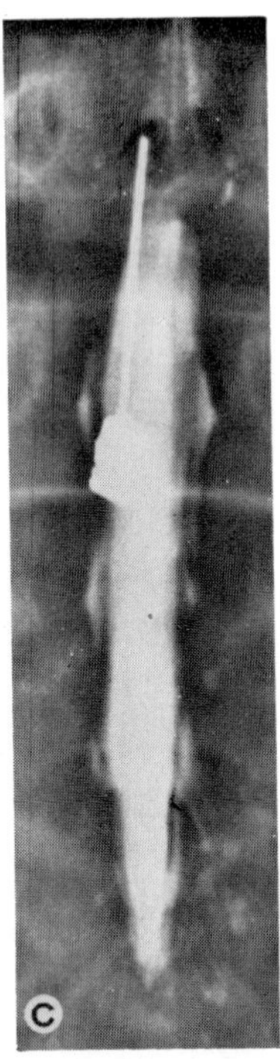

Fig. 645.—Extravasation of Cerebrospinal Fluid in Dorsal Subdural Space Compressing Subarachnoid Space Ventrally

In the original anteroposterior film (A) there is an appearance suggestive of marked swelling of the roots, an appearance which has been described in hypertrophic neuropathy. In the lateral projection (B) it is noted that the oil column is thin, and there is an apparent long indentation on the dorsal side. Re-examination was performed three months later and at this time the appearance in the frontal and in the lateral projection has returned almost to normal ((C) and (D)).

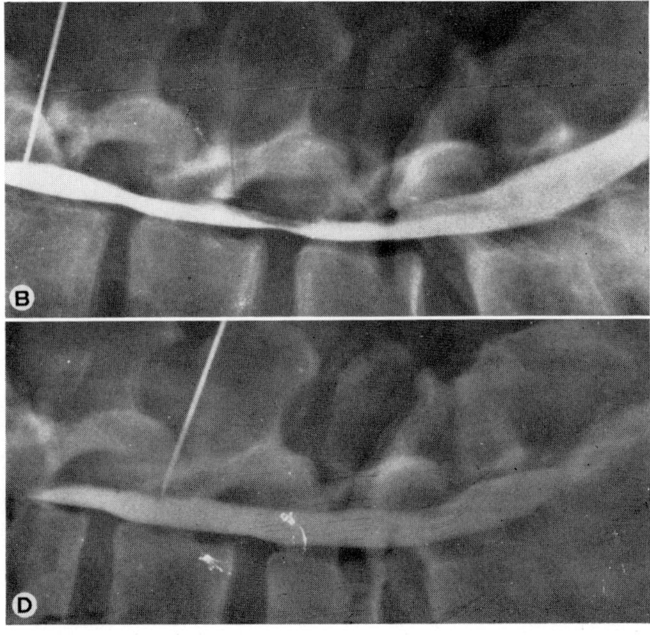

dows to be depicted prominently when actually they are normal (fig. 645).

The subdural injection is the most common technical complication of myelography. A time-consuming procedure is carried out, the opaque oil often cannot be removed, and little or no information of diagnostic value for the patient is gained. The radiopaque material, which occupies an abnormally wide subdural space, is disposed in a cufflike manner around the periphery of the subarachnoid sac. Most often the greater part of the Pantopaque is dorsal in position and a broad thin sheath of oil extends anteriorly on each side of the vertebral canal. The radiopaque substance at first is contained in an enlarged subdural compartment of relatively short length. The effect of gravity on the radiopaque material, with change in the position of the patient, may produce further dissection of the arachnoid from the dura with elongation of the widened subdural space in either a cephalic or caudal direction. At fluoroscopy an irregular distribution of Pantopaque is observed, rather than the usual homogeneous column of opaque material. The opaque oil moves slowly, and movement usually is induced only after tilting the patient to a greater angle than usual. The Pantopaque is observed fluoroscopically to trail in streaks behind the main column, and it cannot be recollected completely on returning the patient to the original position. The Pantopaque usually has sharp angles at the upper and lower margins and the usual shape of the lumbosacral cul-de-sac cannot be seen when the patient is placed in the erect position.

In the frontal myelogram, the major portion of the Pantopaque may appear to be in a continuous column but numerous scattered small collections of oil are present above and below the main body of oil. The lateral view, with the patient prone, is diagnostic of a subdural injection since the oil does not gravitate to the ventral part of the subarachnoid space, although it remains within the confines of the dural sac (fig. 646). Whenever a subdural injection is encountered, it is advisable to remove as much of the oil as possible and to perform another myelogram at a later time.

The injection of Pantopaque into the epidural space is an uncommon error at myelography. This may occur either after an extradural extravasation of cerebrospinal fluid or when a needle placed in the subarachnoid space is dislodged before the opaque oil is injected. Epidural Pantopaque diffuses rapidly in the areolar tissue. At the first fluoroscopic observation the Pantopaque will be widely scattered throughout the lumbar vertebral canal in an irregular manner. Often the opaque oil is observed extending through the intervertebral foramina into the paraspinal soft tissues along the course of the spinal nerves (fig. 647). The presence of Pantopaque in the extradural space and in paraspinal tissues is not uncommonly observed on the day after a satisfactory myelogram, when all of the oil has not been removed following the examination. Presumably the opaque oil escapes through the needle defect in a manner similar to the extravasation of cerebrospinal fluid following a simple lumbar puncture.

It is not possible for epidural oil to flow cephalad for any distance, whereas the subdural oil will maintain itself in a fairly complete column when the patient is tilted in a Trendelenburg position. The subdural oil can reach the cervical region of the spinal canal and will usually be arrested at the foramen magnum. In these cases, if the operator is not familiar with the appearance of subdural oil, there may be some difficulty in differentiating subdural from subarachnoid oil injection. Usually, in the cervical region, the shadow of the spinal cord is not visible in the anteroposterior films and the root shadows do not have their usual normal configuration. Moreover, in lateral prone position, the oil is likely to be entirely dorsal, or at least partly dorsal, in position which is rarely seen with the oil in the subarachnoid space.

The admission of Pantopaque into the cranial cavity is to be avoided, ordinarily. As described above, however, some Pantopaque must pass into the subarachnoid

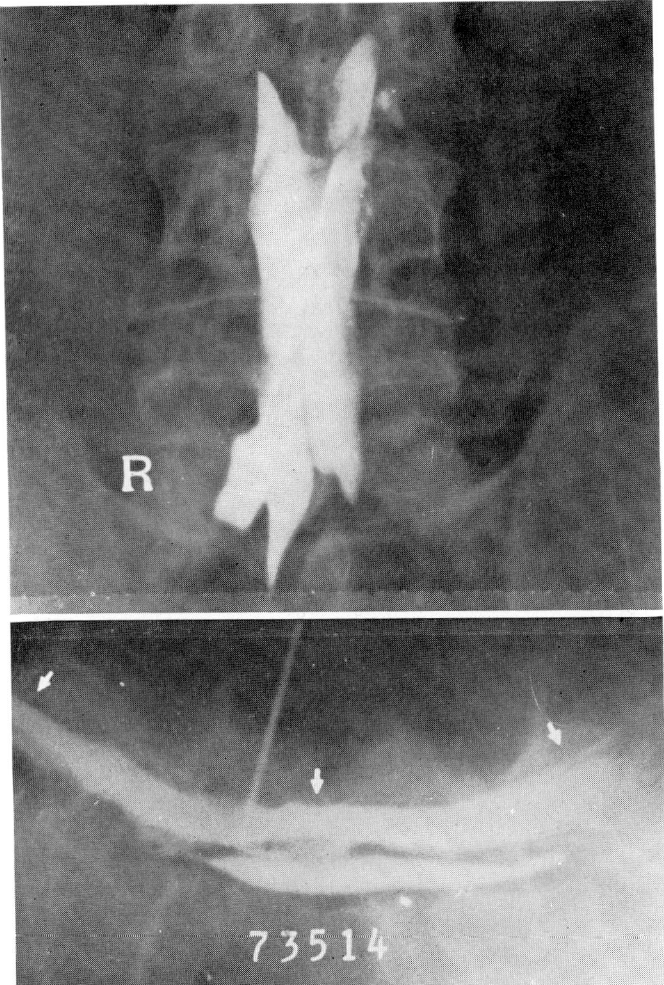

Fig. 646.—Subdural Pantopaque

The needle was inserted to the left of the midline. In the frontal projection, the oil collection is dichotomous, while in the lateral view, the major portion of the radiopaque oil is dorsal (*arrows*) rather than in the usual dependent ventral position.

cisterns to investigate thoroughly the region of the atlanto-occipital junction. This should be done slowly and if possible the oil should not be allowed to pass beyond the cisterna magna. Pantopaque usually will descend from the cisterna magna into the spinal subarachnoid space without difficulty if the patient is tilted upright promptly. When oil is retained in the subarachnoid cisterns, it may be disseminated into the cerebellar subarachnoid spaces. A moderate meningeal reaction with headache, stiff neck, temperature elevation to 102°F., and pleocytosis may occur occasionally, but usually symptoms and fever disappear within 48 hours. Late sequelae of the lodging of Pantopaque in the cranial subarachnoid space are uncommon, if indeed they occur at all. By following the steps previously described in studying the foramen magnum, it is usually possible to avoid dissemination of an undesirable amount of Pantopaque in the cranial subarachnoid space, but the retention of a few droplets of Pantopaque is the rule, following a thorough examination of the foramen magnum.

(*Revised 1963*)

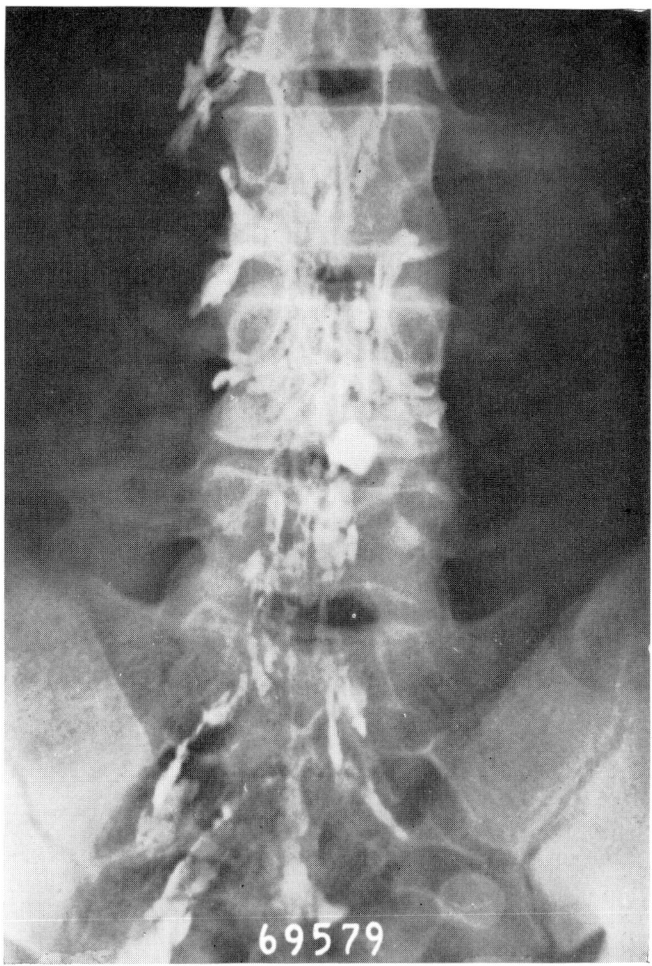

FIG. 647.—EXTRADURAL PANTOPAQUE

The radiopaque oil appears as irregular shadows of increased density in the extradural areolar tissue. Streaks of Pantopaque extend through the intervertebral foramina and lie along nerve pathways well outside of the vertebral column.

Myelography with Nonoleic Radiopaque Media

Myelography with Thorotrast. Prior to the discovery of Pantopaque a number of investigators who were unwilling to use Lipiodol because of its latent effects and who were dissatisfied with the degree of contrast afforded by gas, utilized a colloidal suspension of thorium dioxide as a contrast medium. Thorotrast affords good radiopacity (fig. 648) and the water-miscible substance enters the finer ramifications of the subarachnoid sac. The method was never accepted generally because of the radioactivity of thorium. When Thorotrast is used, cerebrospinal fluid drainage, with the intravenous injection of hypertonic saline solution, is recommended for the removal of the material at the completion of the examination (Nosik, 1943, 1944).

Myelography with Abrodil. The use of water-soluble organic compounds containing iodine for myelography has been popularized in Europe because the substances are absorbed into the bloodstream from the subarachnoid space, thus obviating the neces-

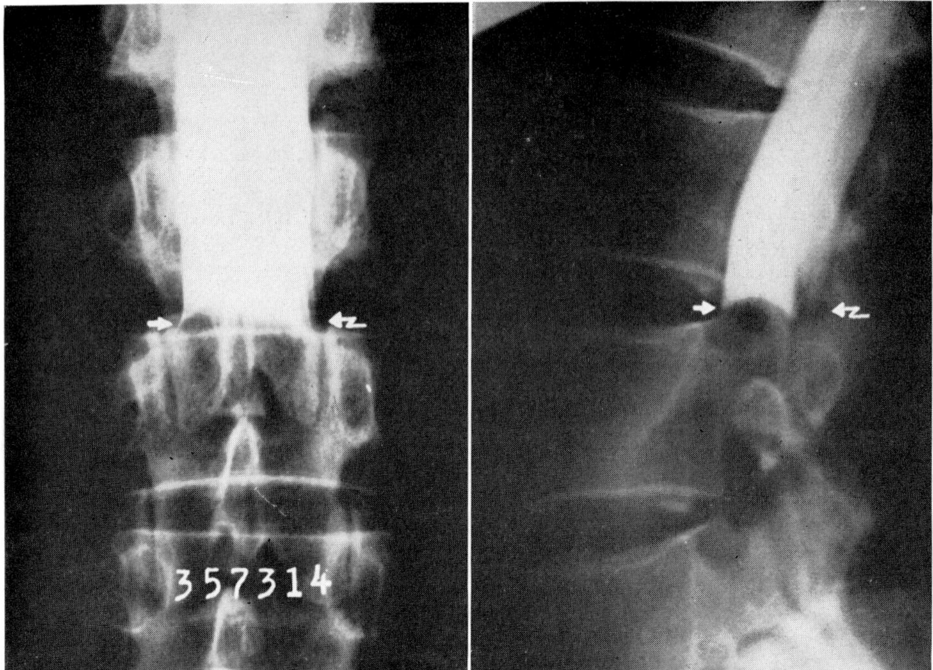

FIG. 648.—THOROTRAST MYELOGRAM (MENINGIOMA AT L3)
The superior surface of an intradural tumor (*straight arrows*) is defined by the contrast material. The displaced cauda equina roots (*wavy arrows*) are well demonstrated by the colloidal suspension of high radiopacity.

sity of removal of the opaque material by the operator, and the retention of unremovable residues. Usually a 20 per cent solution of Abrodil (Skiodan) is employed, 10 cc. being a satisfactory quantity to outline the lumbosacral subarachnoid space.

As with colloidal suspensions, the water-soluble radiopaque material has the advantage of demonstrating clearly the small reflections of the arachnoid sac and, in addition, the cauda equina roots themselves (fig. 649). With careful positioning, gravitational control of the position of the Abrodil can be maintained, since the opaque medium is slightly heavier than cerebrospinal fluid. Films made with the horizontal beam, therefore, have diagnostic value as well as those made in the ordinary manner with the vertical x-ray beam.

Unfortunately, these substances are extremely irritating to the neural tissues and to the meninges, and the introduction of the opaque material must always be preceded by good spinal anesthesia. If the spina anesthesia is not satisfactory or if the Abrodil is allowed to pass cephalad to, or above, the level of the anesthesia, severe pain and frequently shock may result because of the irritative nature of the contrast material (Lindblom, 1950). For this reason, the use of Abrodil is ordinarily limited to radiography of the lumbosacral region. The occurrence of headache and stiff neck for several days after the examination also denotes meningeal irritation at a higher level. The occasional occurrence of latent radicular pain and muscular spasm in the lower extremities, and the rare occurrence of paraplegia and sphincteric disturbances, indicate the irritative effect of the water-soluble contrast substances on nervous tissues.

Complications of Myelography

Myelography with Pantopaque is followed by surprisingly few side reactions aside from

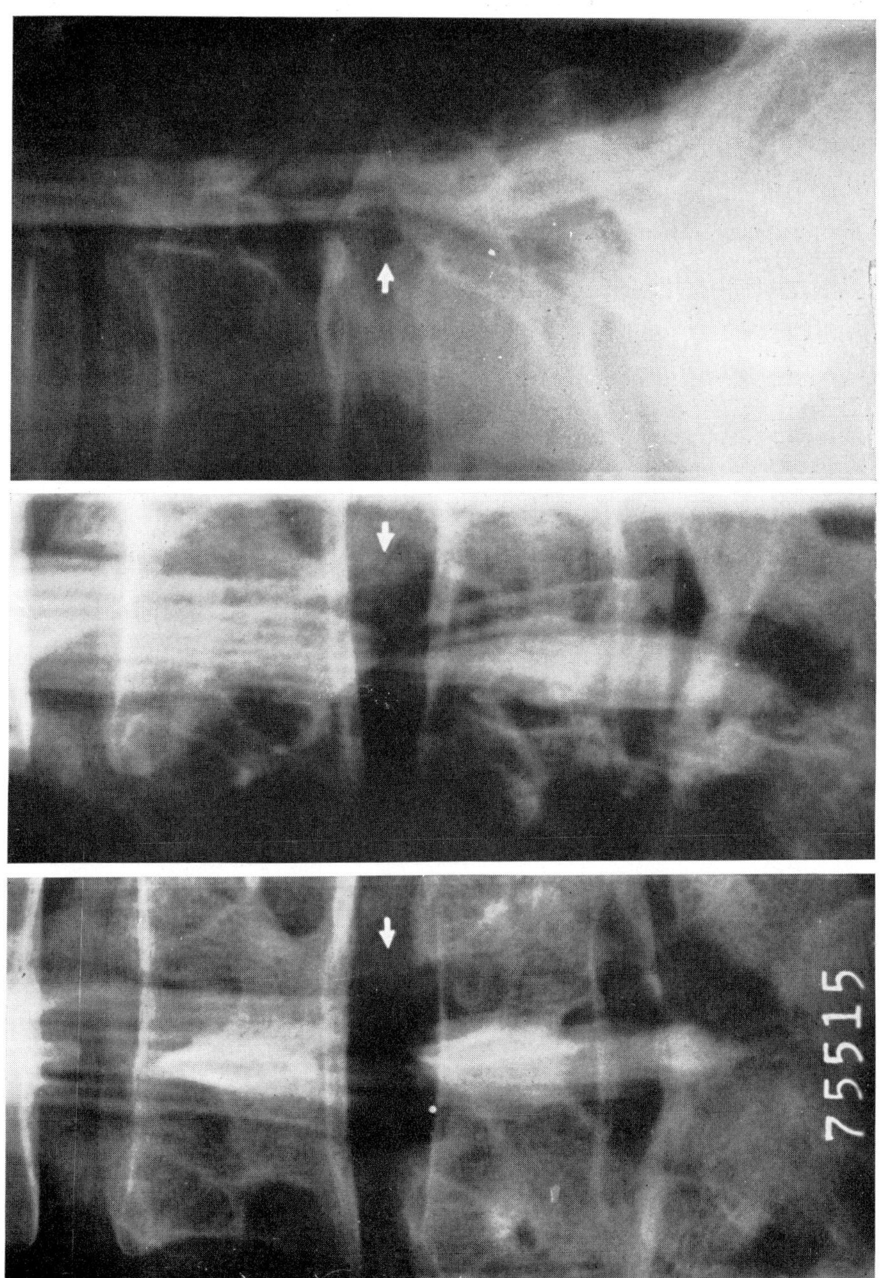

FIG. 649.—ABRODIL MYELOGRAM (HERNIATED DISC, L4-5)

A deformity of the water-soluble column of contrast material by a ventrolateral mass (*arrows*) at L4-5 is clearly depicted in frontal, oblique, and lateral projections. (Courtesy of Dr. Sigfred Arnell.)

those usually associated with spinal punctures. Some patients will complain of radicular pain in both legs for several days or weeks following myelography, but this is usually not severe. Occasionally, some patients will show elevation of temperature and an aseptic meningeal reaction which may be associated with chemical impurities of the Pantopaque with, perhaps, some free iodine present. Several of these reactions were seen approximately 8 years ago at the Neurological Institute, but in the last several years no cerebrospinal meningitic reactions have been observed.

Precautions should be taken to avoid the introduction of infection into the subarachnoid space. It is our custom to wear a cap and mask whenever a spinal puncture is to be performed to carry out either myelography or pneumoencephalography, because it is felt that the resistance of the subarachnoid space to infection is relatively low and aseptic precautions tend to minimize the possibilities of infection. When epidural injection of contrast material takes place, either directly or following extravasation through the needle puncture when the oil was in the subarachnoid space, it is followed by the passage of oil along the nerve roots into the plexus and sometimes it follows the nerves into the thigh. This is ordinarily asymptomatic.

Pantopaque may become encysted in the subarachnoid space after being divided into small droplets. In this case, the material will not move with changes in posture. It is possible that traumatic taps which may in themselves produce adhesions due to the presence of blood in the subarachnoid space, may lead to loculation of the oil. In the cranial subarachnoid space, Pantopaque usually becomes encysted and immobile.

Pantopaque is absorbed from the subarachnoid space at a rate of approximately 1 cc. every two years. It is absorbed much more rapidly when it is in the epidural space.

It is possible that some patients may actually be sensitive to Pantopaque which may lead to the formation of adhesions around the residues of this substance in the subarachnoid space. When the patient has a history of allergy to iodine, it may be advisable to perform an intradermal test by injecting 0.1 cc. of Pantopaque. A reaction may be called positive if a papule of 1 cm. in diameter is formed and persists. In the presence of a positive skin test, it is probably not advisable to perform Pantopaque myelography. In these cases, it is preferable to perform air myelography if an examination is necessary. Discography, unfortunately, also must be performed with iodinated radiopaque agents, and for that reason it would not be advocated if the patient may be sensitive to the substance.

It is likely that any reactions to myelography related to the Pantopaque itself must be inconsequential because in several countries, including England, the material usually is not removed following myelography; it is obvious, therefore, that if the presence of Pantopaque in the subarachnoid space were a source of irritation and untoward reactions, that this practice would not have been continued. As explained above, however, inasmuch as Pantopaque represents a foreign substance, it is preferable, in our opinion, to remove as much of it as possible.

Additional Techniques of Examination

Discography

Radiography of the nucleus pulposus following its opacification with contrast substances has been advocated by Lindblom (1950) and has been practiced with enthusiasm in many localities. The procedure is used chiefly to study the lower lumbar region. A preliminary lateral film of the lumbosacral spine is made with a metal marker attached to the midline of the lower back so that an accurate measurement of the distance from the skin to the center of the intervertebral disc in the midsagittal plane can be determined. Two needles of suitable length and caliber, usually an 18-gauge needle and 26-gauge needle, are selected and

(Revised 1963)

it is made certain that the smaller needle can pass through the lumen of the larger needle without difficulty. The length of the inner needle must be at least 2 cm. longer than that of the outer needle so that it can pass beyond the tip of the outer needle. Ordinary puncture of the subarachnoid space is then performed, with care taken to pass the needle as nearly in the midline as possible and to have the long axis of the needle directed toward the center of the intervertebral space. The insertion of the needle may be checked by fluoroscopic observation as desired at intervals during its passage. Ordinarily, both the L4–5 and L5–S1 intervertebral spaces are investigated, and if no abnormality is found, Lindblom (1950) recommends examination of the L3–4 intervertebral space. When the dural and arachnoid sacs have been pierced, the stylette is withdrawn and a small sample of cerebrospinal fluid can be removed if desired. The needle is then passed as far as possible with ease toward the ventral aspect of the vertebral canal. The smaller needle is then passed through the lumen of the larger needle and advanced to a depth previously calculated to insure the needle tip being in the center of the intervertebral space where the nucleus pulposus should be encountered.

Following nuclear puncture, the stylette of the smaller needle is withdrawn and 1 to 2 cc. of an opaque organic compound of iodine are injected into the nucleus pulposus. When a herniation is present, the patient's radicular pain may be reproduced or aggravated by injection of the opaque material under pressure into the diseased nucleus. The injection of radiopaque material may be painful and for this reason it might be desirable to mix it with small amounts of procaine. Radiographs should be made as soon as possible after the injection of the nucleus pulposus in frontal and lateral, and if desired, in oblique projections. In the normal discogram, the nucleus pulposus is outlined as an oval space outlined with contrast material. The exact shape of the nucleus pulposus varies, but it usually does not reach the edge of the intervertebral disc. If the shadow reaches the edge of the intervertebral disc, a rupture of the annulus fibrosus may exist.

When a defect in the annulus fibrosus is present, varying quantities of the opaque material may be demonstrated passing from the intervertebral space into the ventral portion of the vertebral canal. The rupture is not necessarily toward the ventral side of the canal and may be lateral or even anterior. In some patients with disc protrusion, the lateral projection may demonstrate a semilunar collection of Diodrast directly behind the intervertebral space which simulates calcification occurring in a degenerated herniated disc. With large disc extrusions, collections of the radiopaque material may be seen over a considerable area in the ventral part of the vertebral epidural space. A degenerated intervertebral disc which is not herniated will usually reveal an irregular cavity divided into two portions and with ragged margins instead of the usual oval smooth normal nucleus pulposus.

Discography has disadvantages. It requires multiple lumbar punctures and intermittent fluoroscopic control, although this may be done with films and, to increase speed, Polaroid films may be used. The possibility that needle puncture of the intervertebral disc, particularly of the nucleus pulposus, may induce degenerative changes leading to disc disease at a later date cannot be dismissed.

While discography demonstrates very clearly the position and contour of the nucleus that is injected, it seems highly probable that the offending pathologic process will be overlooked in many instances when this method alone is employed, even in cases where abnormal nuclei are demonstrated at L4–5 and L5–S1. The importance of thoroughly investigating the full length of the subarachnoid space with opaque material has been repeatedly emphasized by Camp (1938, 1950).

Recently, in one year alone, three neoplasms of the cauda equina were disclosed by myelography at the Neurological Institute in patients in whom the symptoms and neurologic findings were indistinguishable from those usually associated with intervertebral disc herniations.

Discography has the further disadvantage of not actually demonstrating the relationship of disc herniation to the nerve roots unless myelography is performed simultaneously. Horwitz (1943) has emphasized the frequent occurrence of herniated intervertebral discs as an incidental finding in anatomic material. Perhaps the greatest value of nuclear puncture is not the radiologic aspect at all but the reproduction of the patient's chief pain which can be done by injecting the nucleus with saline. This is necessary in view of the frequent occurrence of asymptomatic degenerative disc disease.

It may be found desirable to restrict the use of discography to patients in whom anatomic variations, such as a subarachnoid space of small caliber associated with a large epidural fat space, make it impossible to determine from myelography whether herniation is present. The procedure may be of extraordinary value where technical errors of myelography occur with unsatisfactory examination by ordinary myelographic methods. Careful consideration of all of these factors has deterred most radiologists and neurosurgeons from the widespread use of discography.

In general, it may be said that if the procedure of discography is carried out, it indicates that the diagnosis of herniated intervertebral disc has already been made, and it is only a matter of localizing the offending herniated disc, whereas we look upon myelography as a procedure that not only will localize the herniated intervertebral discs but will also rule in or out the presence of a neoplasm in the subarachnoid space or in the epidural space, not only in the lumbar region but also in the lower thoracic region, which often gives a symptomatology indistinguishable from a lumbar root syndrome.

For the latter reason the authors do not recommend myelography with the use of water-soluble contrast media since the examination must be limited to the lumbar region, and more than one case examined in this manner has come to our attention where Pantopaque myelography performed shortly thereafter demonstrated an intra-arachnoidal tumor at the level of the 12th thoracic vertebra which had not been seen with the water-soluble contrast material. It is for this reason that the authors feel that Pantopaque myelography is the best all around method of examination of the spinal subarachnoid space. Under certain circumstances, as explained under "Technique," air myelography is found to be helpful as a complementary procedure.

Discography may also be used in the cervical spine and the same objections raised in the lumbar region may be raised in the cervical region. Degenerated intervertebral discs, particularly at C5–6 and C6–7 and also at C4–5, are extremely common in the later decades of life, and a discogram will almost invariably show an abnormal disc at these levels. The advocates of this method in the cervical region argue that the reproduction of pain referable to the area at the time of the injection of the contrast material indicates that the correct intervertebral disc is being injected. However, if a complete examination were to be performed, it would be necessary to inject as many as five cervical intervertebral discs up to C3–4 which is a frequent site of disc herniation.

Scintillography

This designation applies to the injection of a radioactive substance, such as radioiodinated serum albumin, into the spinal canal. The material will mix with the cerebrospinal fluid and will ascend to demonstrate the lower level of a block. This is the only use of this method; the authors do not feel that scintillography would be satisfactory to diagnose intervertebral disc disease or other intraspinal lesions not associated with a block to the flow of cerebrospinal fluid.

Intraosseous Venography

The use of intraosseous venography after injecting one of the lumbar spinous processes has been advocated by Schobinger, Krueger, and Sobel (1961). It is possible to diagnose by this method the presence of intervertebral disc herniations and some intraspinal tumors, particularly the epidural tumors.

(Revised 1963)

The intervertebral disc herniations produce a displacement of the epidural plexus and, if they are very large, they could produce a complete block to the flow of contrast substance. The epidural neoplasms always produce a complete block to the flow of contrast substance through the epidural plexus which is helpful in some cases in which myelography may as yet not show any deformity. However, this method, like discography, is limited in scope in that it does not reveal the intra-arachnoidal spaces and, any lesion, intramedullary or intradural and extramedullary, may go undetected. Intraosseous venography may also be employed in the cervical region.

Developmental Abnormalities

Meningocele

A meningocele is an out-pocketing of leptomeninges through a developmental defect in the dura mater. The arches of one or more vertebrae and the spinal muscles and ligaments frequently are involved in the malformation, with the result that the meningeal sac is covered only by a thin layer of skin. A meningocele may be simple, filled with cerebrospinal fluid, or complex, containing elements of the spinal cord or cauda equina (meningomyelocele) in addition to the fluid. The cavity of the sac is continuous with the subarachnoid space through a narrow neck. The deformities occur most frequently at the end of the spinal axis in the lumbosacral region and in the suboccipital area.

In plain spine radiographs made in frontal projection, maldevelopment of the laminae, usually, bilateral, of one or more vertebral segments is demonstrated. The vertebral canal is wide and the pedicles are separated to a considerable degree and in some instances the pedicles appear flattened. In lateral projection aplasia or hypoplasia of the spinous processes is demonstrated and displaced rudiments of the vertebral arches may be present in the region of the retrospinal soft tissues (fig. 650). In films made with soft tissue technique, a sessile or pedunculated extraneous shadow of water density may be present which represents the meningocele itself. Deposits of fat are commonly found in association with meningoceles, particularly those in the lumbar and lumbosacral regions. Sometimes the spinal canal may be considerably widened when the subarachnoid space is actually narrow. The remainder of the space is occupied by excessive fatty tissue.

(Revised 1963)

Anterior sacral meningoceles are characterized by the presence of a defect in the anterior aspect of the sacrum with absence of bone involving one or more sacral vertebral bodies (fig. 651). Myelography usually demonstrates these meningoceles very

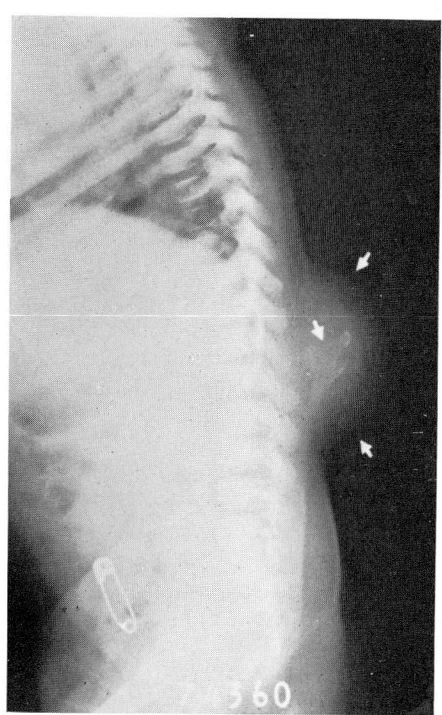

FIG. 650.—MENINGOCELE

A saccular extraneous mass in the midline of the lower back is depicted in profile (*right arrows*). Deformity of the underlying bone structures is apparent and a displaced rudiment of the vertebral arch lies in the retrospinal soft tissues (*left middle arrow*).

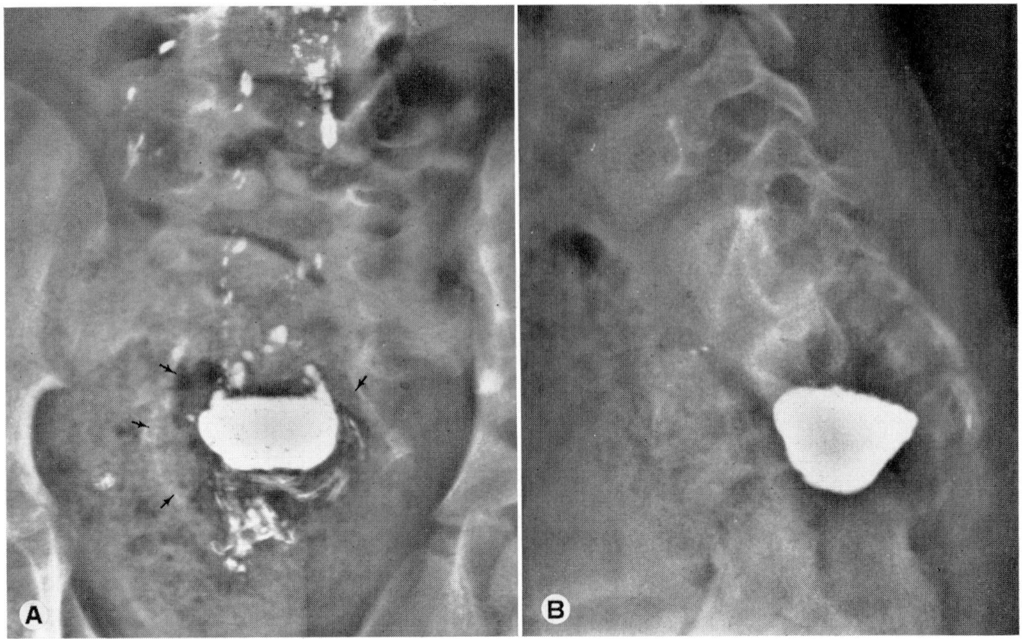

FIG. 651.—ANTERIOR SACRAL MENINGOCELE

The frontal projection (A) demonstrates a large collection of Pantopaque in the sacral region. The edges of the widened canal in this region can be seen (*arrows*). There is also an increase in the width of the interpediculate distance in the lumbosacral region. The lateral projection (B), taken in the erect position, demonstrates the collection of Pantopaque anterior to the sacrum at the level of the 3d and 4th sacral segments.

clearly. They are important because a mass may be felt on rectal examination which could be misdiagnosed leading to an infection of the sac and meningitis if the pouch is opened by the anterior route. The rectum may be displaced laterally or laterally and forward by the anterior sacral meningoceles. The diagnosis can be made by rectal examination because of the increase in the firmness of the mass produced by the performance of a Valsalva maneuver when the child cries or by jugular compression. The communication of the meningocele with the subarachnoid space may be very narrow, and it may take time to fill. When a meningocele is suspected, it is advantageous to leave the oil in the spinal canal, keep the patient in a semisitting supine position, and repeat the examination several hours or a day later to ascertain the fact that there is no communication between the subarachnoid space and a suspected meningocele.

Occult meningoceles may be demonstrated at myelography. The outpocketings usually are small and are encountered most frequently in the sacrum just caudad to the usual point of termination of the subarachnoid space at S2 (fig. 652). Small lateral out-pocketings of the subarachnoid space are frequently demonstrated at myelography which actually are no more than anatomic variations in the meningeal reflections of the spinal nerve roots. They represent capacious root sleeves or, if they have a narrow communication with the subarachnoid space, a *true root meningocele* is present. The latter entity is important because, like other meningoceles, they may grow with the passage of time and produce local erosions of the sacrum (fig. 653). The occult meningoceles in the sacral cul-de-sac also produce erosion of the pedicles and adjacent portions of the sacrum, which are often demonstrated by laminography in the lateral projection (fig. 654). It is important to realize that in these instances we are

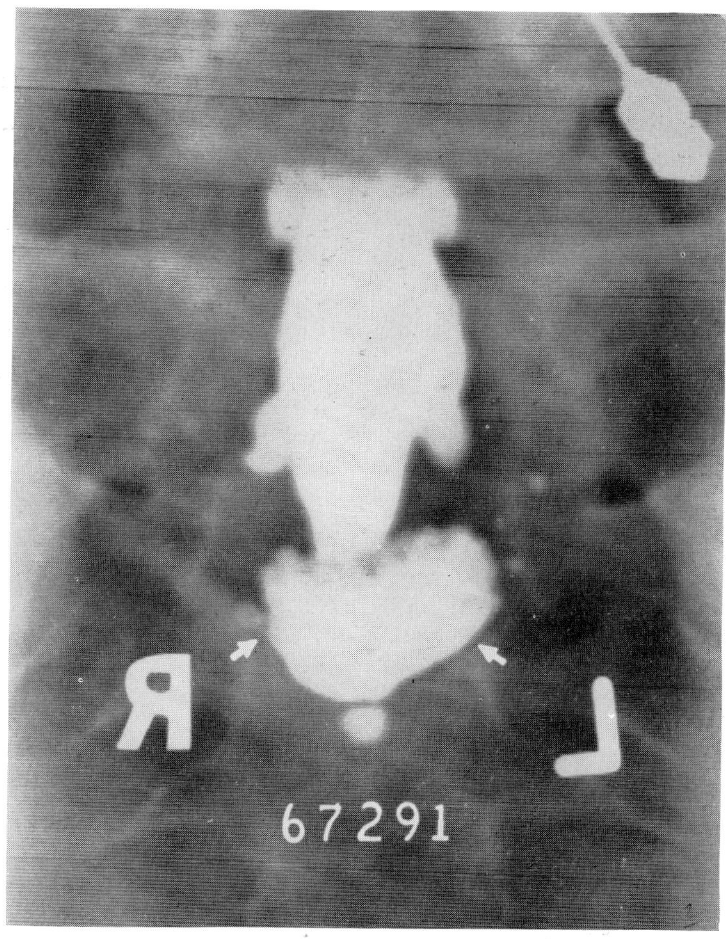

FIG. 652.—MENINGOCELE (OCCULT)

A large meningeal outpouching (*arrows*) from the sacral cul-de-sac communicates by a large stoma with the subarachnoid space. At fluoroscopy the meningocele could be filled and emptied at will by tilting the fluoroscopic table.

dealing with a true entity, inasmuch as the communication of the sac with the subarachnoid space is narrow and there is a tendency for growth. Often the fluid within these cysts has a high protein content which also tends to make them grow with the passage of time. Tarlov described the perineural cysts which are a different entity from the one discussed in the above paragraph. Characteristically, the perineural cyst arises in the perineural space, but may invade the nerve and become surrounded by nerve fibers. The cyst does not communicate with the subarachnoid space, according to Tarlov (1953).

(Revised 1963)

Large *lateral meningoceles* are encountered occasionally which may be mistaken for paraspinal neoplasms in plain spine radiographs, particularly in the thoracic region, but their communication with the subarachnoid space is readily demonstrated at myelography. In the thoracic region, the lateral meningoceles may occur in patients with neurofibromatosis. They may be seen on plain roentgenograms of the chest outlined by the air-containing lung, and at fluoroscopy, observation of a change in size of the mass when the patient executes the Valsalva maneuver (expiration against a closed glottis) and a Mueller experiment

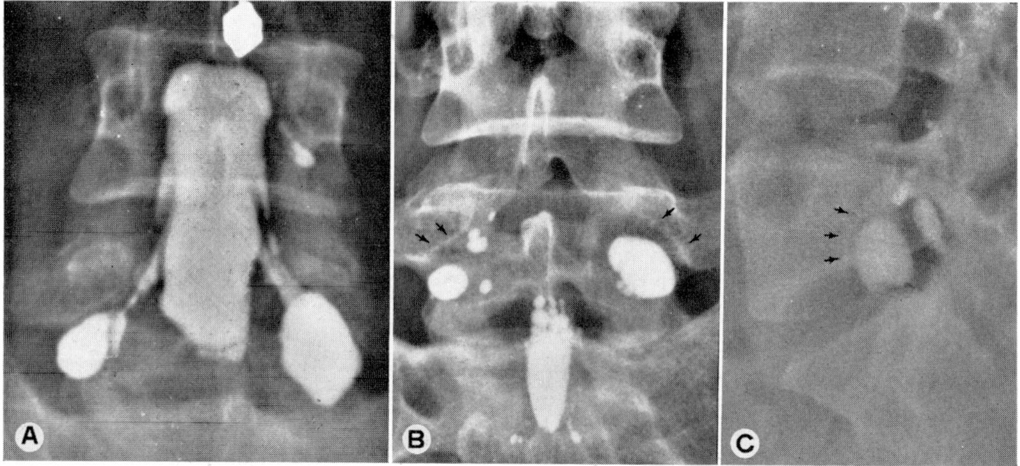

FIG. 653.—LUMBAR ROOT CYSTS (ROOT MENINGOCELES)

The Pantopaque myelogram (A) reveals evidence of large dilatations which evidently connect with the root sleeves. On the right side, there is a radiolucent line which probably represents the root situated against the medial wall of the pouch. A plain film made in the frontal projection (B) discloses an area of erosion on the inferior aspect of the pedicle on the left side which is outlined by the residual Pantopaque within the root cyst (*arrows*). The lateral projection (C) shows that the erosion extends to involve the vertebral body on its posteroinferior aspect (*arrows*).

(inspiration against a closed glottis) may be of diagnostic value.

Small root meningoceles may be frequently observed in the cervical region and are usually of no clinical significance. Sometimes they are fairly large and produce slight erosion of the corresponding pedicle.

Diverticula of the subarachnoid space are not rare in the thoracic region. They represent isolation of a small area of the subarachnoid space by an adhesion, usually on the dorsal side of the canal. They are demonstrated when the patient is placed in the supine position and are usually of no clinical significance.

The lateral thoracic meningoceles are best demonstrated by the injection of air while placing the side of the meningocele uppermost. Anteroposterior films with the patient lying on the opposite side of the meningocele will demonstrate a fluid level and the filling of the mass with gas.

Postoperative meningoceles may occur when an area of the dura remains open. The arachnoid then herniates through the opening in the dura and a meningocele is formed which may tend to grow with the passage of time. Huge meningocele cavities have been seen following improper closure of the lumbar dural sac.

Arnold-Chiari Malformation

The deformity consists of a caudal extension of portions of the cerebellum and brain stem through the foramen magnum into the cervical portion of the vertebral canal. The lesions resemble foraminal herniation of the posterior fossa structures usually occurring with cerebellar tumor, although in Arnold-Chiari deformities, the caudal misplacement of intracranial structures may involve chiefly or entirely the brain stem, and impaction may not be present (Penfield and Coburn, 1938). Spina bifida or meningocele is frequently coexistent with Arnold-Chiari deformities, and in such an event, a causal relationship may be implicated. Abnormal fixation of the spinal cord or spinal nerve roots at the site of the meningocele presumably prevents normal cephalic migration of the spinal cord with growth of the vertebral column.

Plain roentgenograms of the cervical spine may disclose no abnormality, but in some cases they may show an unusually wide

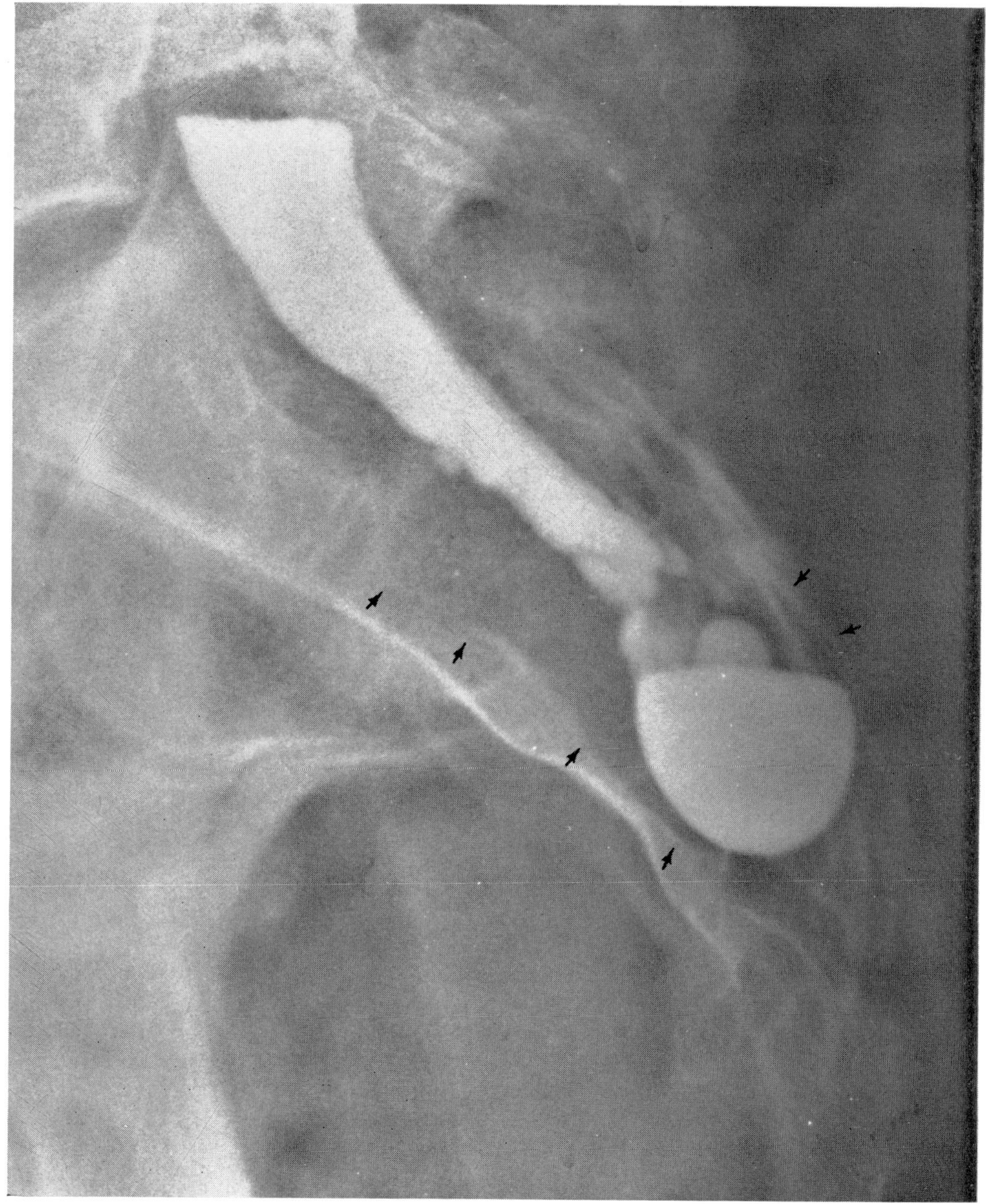

FIG. 654.—OCCULT SACRAL MENINGOCELE PRODUCING EROSION OF SACRAL CANAL
A wide area of thinning of the sacral vertebral bodies is seen due to enlargement by erosion of the sacral canal secondary to transmitted pulsations of the meningocele (*arrows*). There may be an associated lipoma.

foramen magnum and the upper cervical vertebrae may be unfused. Normally the arches of the upper cervical vertebrae are unfused in infancy, so that enlargement of the cervical vertebrae, vertebral canals and other pressure deformities cannot be detected by plain film methods at this age. Examination of other portions of the spine

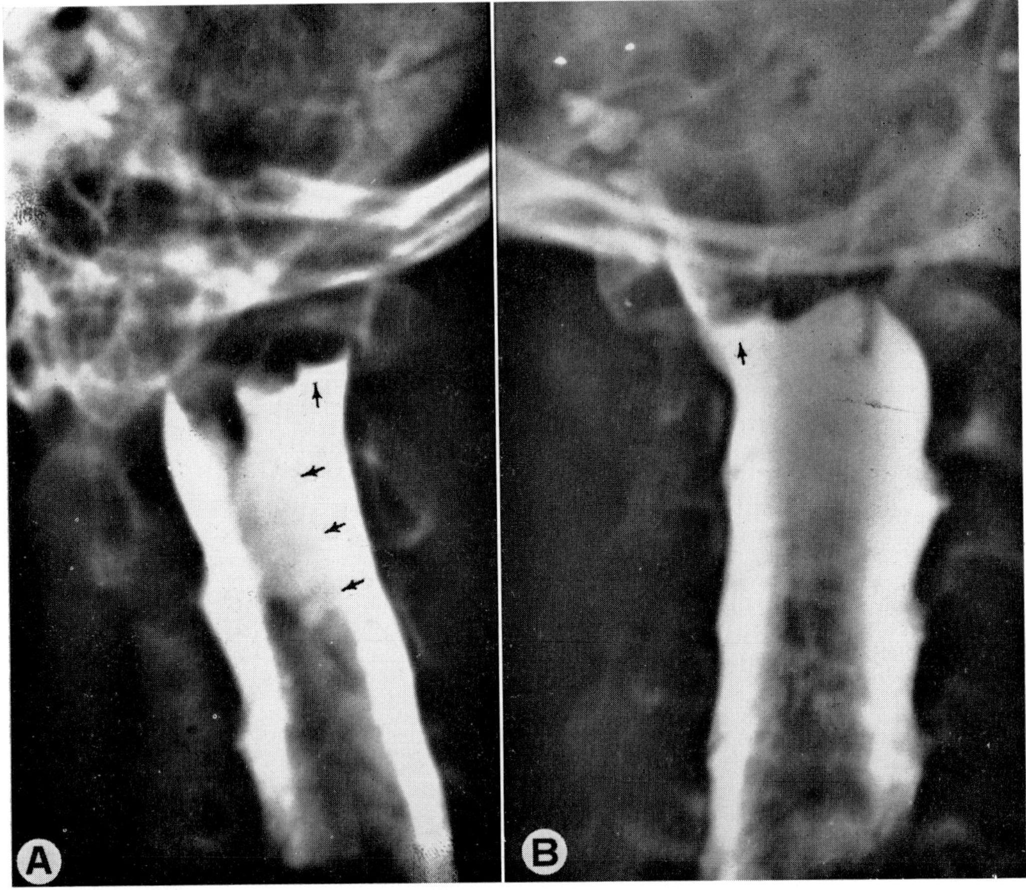

FIG. 655.—ARNOLD-CHIARI MALFORMATION PRODUCING DORSALLY PLACED SYMMETRICAL DEFECT AND BLOCK TO PANTOPAQUE FLOW

Both oblique views of the foramen magnum (A) and (B) demonstrate a dorsally placed defect which is symmetrical in position, and forward displacement of the spinal cord (*arrows*).

may reveal a meningocele. Skull films may disclose megacephalus resulting from hydrocephalus that is caused by obstruction to the egress of fluid from the caudal end of the 4th ventricle. The importance of examining the cervical spine at ventriculography in hydrocephalic infants in order to detect the presence of Arnold-Chiari deformity has been emphasized by Marks and Livingston (1949). Where congenital deformities do not preclude lumbar puncture, myelography is of diagnostic value. The diagnosis may be established by demonstrating an obstruction in the upper or mid portion of the cervical area in upright lateral views of the cervical spine made after the instillation of 3 to 5 cc. of gas by the lumbar route, that is, by means of pneumoencephalography as explained under foramen magnum "Herniations" (p. 1.255). However, the diagnosis may also be made easily by pantopaque myelography through the demonstration of obstruction of the Pantopaque with concave symmetrical deformity on the dorsolateral aspect on both sides (fig. 655). The shadow of the spinal cord is displaced ventrally and can also be shown by Pantopaque myelography. Some characteristic features of the Arnold-Chiari malformation emphasized by Liliequist (1960) have been mentioned previously.

Extradural Cyst

Benign cystlike, fluid-filled sacs may be found in the midthoracic region during

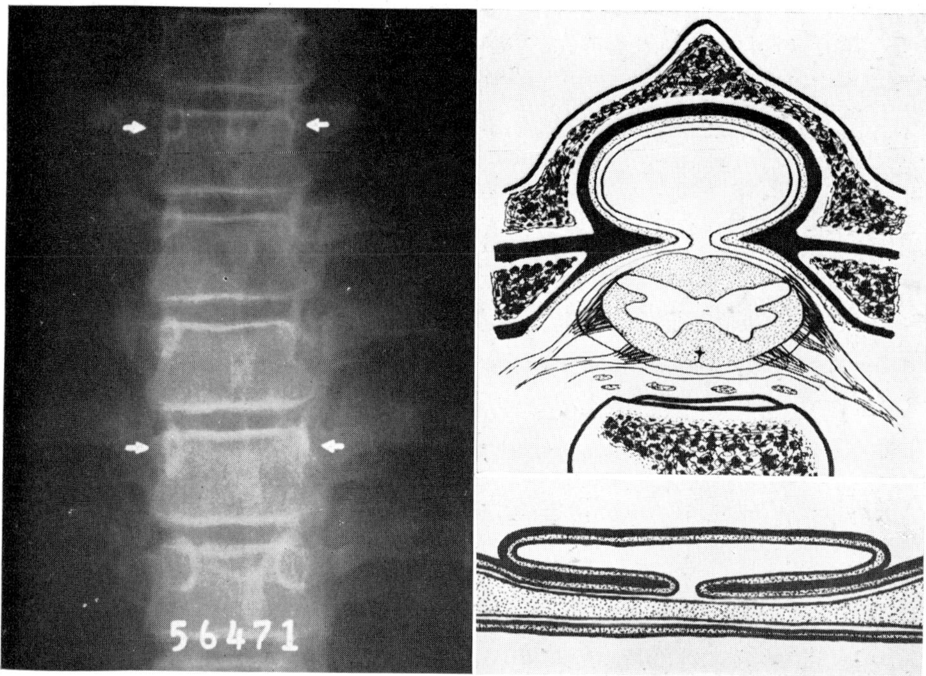

FIG. 656.—EXTRADURAL CYST, T4 to T7

The vertebral canal is widened in the frontal view (*arrows*). A cystlike structure lay extradurally along the dorsal aspect of the spinal cord, but it communicated with the subarachnoid space by a stalk. (Sketch shows the relation of the cyst to the meninges.)

adolescence. Occasionally idiopathic cysts may be found intradurally (Elsberg, Dyke, and Brewer, 1934). The occurrence of these cysts early in life and exclusively in the thoracic area together with the frequent occurrence of true meningocele in this region, may be more than coincidence. Indeed, some of the lesions are not cysts at all but are called meningoceles (fig. 656), with the cavity of the extradural membranous sac continuous with the subarachnoid space by a narrow neck.

In plain roentgenograms of the spine, a fusiform enlargement of the vertebral canal at the site of the lesion may be demonstrable. The pedicles of two or three consecutive midthoracic vertebrae may be separated to an abnormal degree, and the medial borders of the pedicles may appear flat. The laminae are often thinned and the posterior margins of the vertebral bodies may have an increase in normal concavity which indicate that the vertebral canal is abnormally large in depth.

(*Revised 1963*)

The enlargement in depth as well as the enlargement in width, as shown by interpedicular measurements, is gradual over the several segments involved, and at the center of the fusiform enlargement of the vertebral canal, the diameter may be increased from 0.5 to 1 cm. above normal. A narrow cleft between the laminae and hypoplasia of the spinous process, occasionally seen at the level of the center of the lesion, may indicate the congenital nature of the process. This lesion is quite rare; not a single case has been seen at the Neurological Institute in the last ten years.

Diastematomyelia

Diastematomyelia is a sagittal division or pseudoduplication of a segment of the spinal cord, which may be associated with a congenital anomaly of the vertebral column in which an osseous or fibrocartilaginous septum transfixes the spinal cord at the point of diastasis. The septum, which is attached anteriorly to one or more vertebral bodies and posteriorly to the dura, passes through the spinal cord and fixes it in low anatomic position, so that Arnold-Chiari deformity may result. Diastematomyelia most frequently occurs in the lower thoracic and in the upper lumbar regions. Characteristic roentgenographic changes have been described by Neuhauser, Wittenborg, and Dehlinger (1950). Plain spine roentgenograms often show, in frontal projection, widening of the vertebral canal which may extend longitudinally for as many as six vertebral segments. The interpedicular distance is increased in a fusiform manner over these segments. Numerous developmental abnormalities of the vertebral bodies and arches may be present in association with the widening of the vertebral canal (fig. 657). The pedicles, bodies, and laminae of the vertebrae show no evidence of bone atrophy, such as is usually present when the canal is enlarged as the result of an expanding lesion; that is, the pedicles are round although the interpedicular distance is widened and the posterior aspect of the vertebral bodies is not excavated. When the septum dividing the spinal cord is ossified, roentgenograms in the frontal projection may demonstrate a linear shadow of calcium density of approximately 1.0 to 1.5 cm. in size, in the midsagittal plane of the vertebral canal. This may be best demonstrated by laminagraphy. In lateral view, calcification may be seen in the anterior portion of the septum behind the vertebral bodies, or occasionally, in the

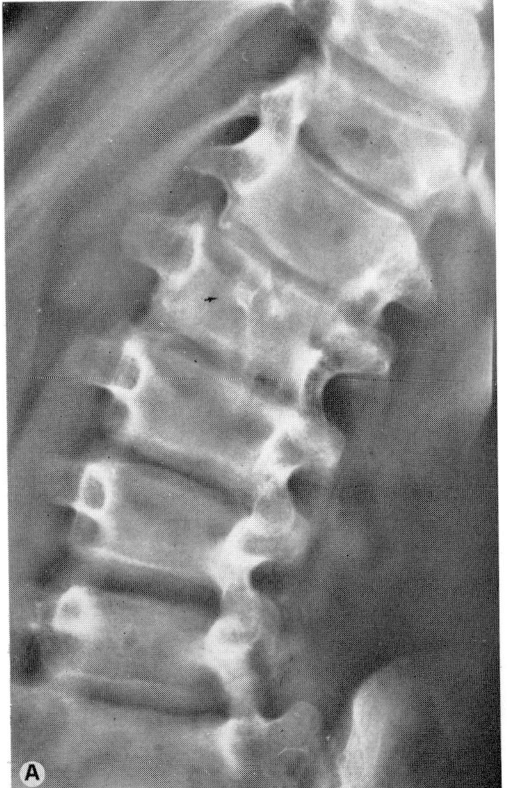

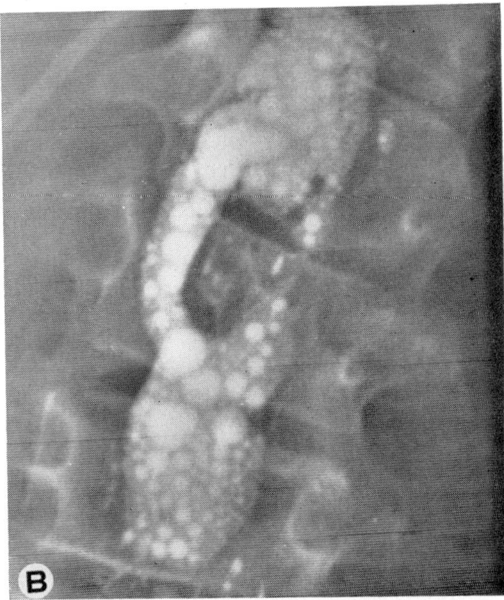

FIG. 657.—DIASTEMATOMYELIA

The laminagram made in the anteroposterior projection (A) demonstrates a large bony spicule (*arrow*) situated in the middle, between the two pedicles of the second lumbar vertebra. Other vertebral anomalies are seen above. The myelogram (B) demonstrates the central filling defect which is typical of diastematomyelia.

(*Revised 1963*)

posterior portion of the septum near the laminae. Here again, laminagraphy may be of use.

Myelography will demonstrate the cleft in the spinal cord and its relationship to the sagittal septum, even in those instances where the septum is cartilaginous or insufficiently ossified to be visible in plain spine roentgenograms. The septum produces an elongated filling defect in the central portion of the radiopaque column or, when the septum is small, only a tiny rounded filling defect may be demonstrable (fig. 657). In the case in which an ossified spicule is present, a linear calcium shadow may be demonstrated within the central zone of defective filling in the myelogram.

Other Vertebral Abnormalities

Spina bifida, at several levels, is such a common radiologic observation in examinations of the vertebral column that many radiologists regard it as of no clinical significance. Failure of fusion of the vertebral arch at C1, S1 and in the lower sacral region is of no clinical significance.

Nevertheless, spina bifida is a dysraphic malformation, and as such it may be a component of a complex abnormality of the nervous and skeletal systems (Lichtenstein, 1949). The true nature of vertebral bifidism is most sharply emphasized in meningoceles and with congenital spinal cord tumors, such as the dermoid. Whenever a spinal cord lesion is found in association with spina bifida, especially at an unusual level, the possibility that the vertebral cleft may be more of a coincidental finding should be considered.

Anterior spina bifida is not rare; it may be associated with a butterfly vertebra or it may be seen in an otherwise normally shaped vertebral body. The presence of anterior spina bifida has been recognized in cases associated with abnormalities of the gastrointestinal tract, particularly duplications and sometimes with cardiovascular abnormalities.

Klippel-Feil malformation. This condition is the result of a congenital synostosis or failure of segmentation of two vertebrae and is most commonly seen in the upper

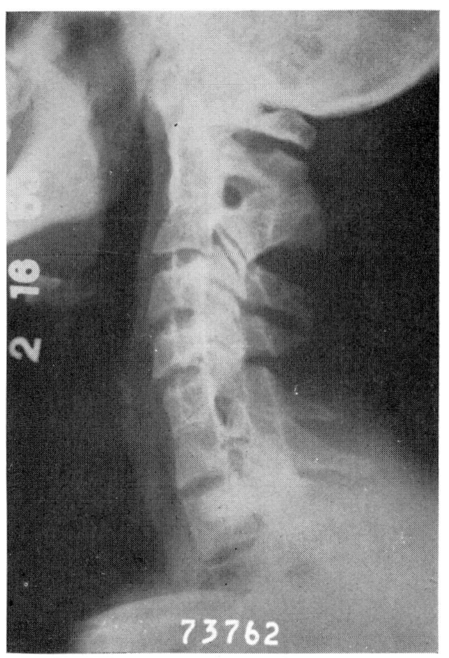

FIG. 658.—KLIPPEL-FEIL MALFORMATION (DOUBLE)

Failure of segmentation of the vertebral bodies and arches at C2-3 and C6-7 has occurred. The normal cervical ventral curvature is reduced. Brevicollis is not apparent.

cervical region (fig. 658). Usually the arches as well as the bodies of the involved vertebrae are joined, which is helpful in differentiating the malformations from vertebral fusion following an inflammatory process. In addition, the vertebral bodies at the site of the rudimentary disc space are narrower in their anteroposterior diameters than at the other end of the vertebral body, where they are separated from the adjacent vertebrae by normal discs. This latter finding is very helpful in differentiating congenital from acquired fusion when the arches are not fused.

Spondylolisthesis

This is a deformity of the vertebral column that is produced by forward displacement of one segment in relation to another, most commonly L5 on S1. The displacement results from stress on a vertebra in which one or more congenital malformations of the vertebral arch are present. The point of failure of fusion of the vertebral arch usually can be demonstrated in plain film radiographs, especially in films made in oblique projection. A fibrous rather than an osseous union occurs in the interarticular portion of the vertebral arch, often bilaterally. The body, pedicles, and supra-articular processes of the vertebra move forward, but the spinous process, laminae, and infra-articular processes remain in normal position.

The defect in the pars interarticularis is usually referred to as spondylolysis. Of neurologic importance is the result of narrowing of the intervertebral foramen which occurs. The spinal nerve root may be compressed and may produce sciatic syndrome,

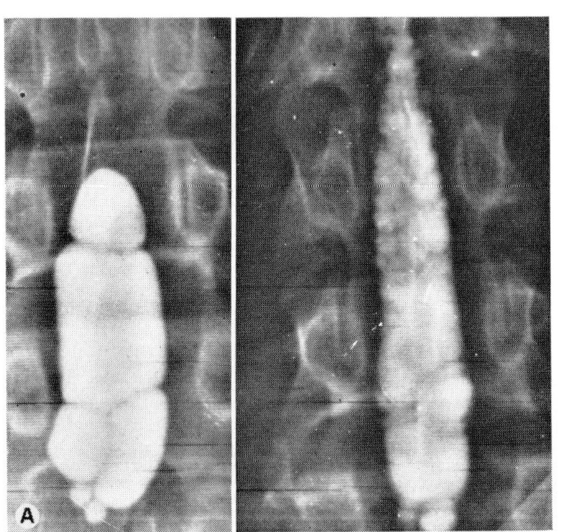

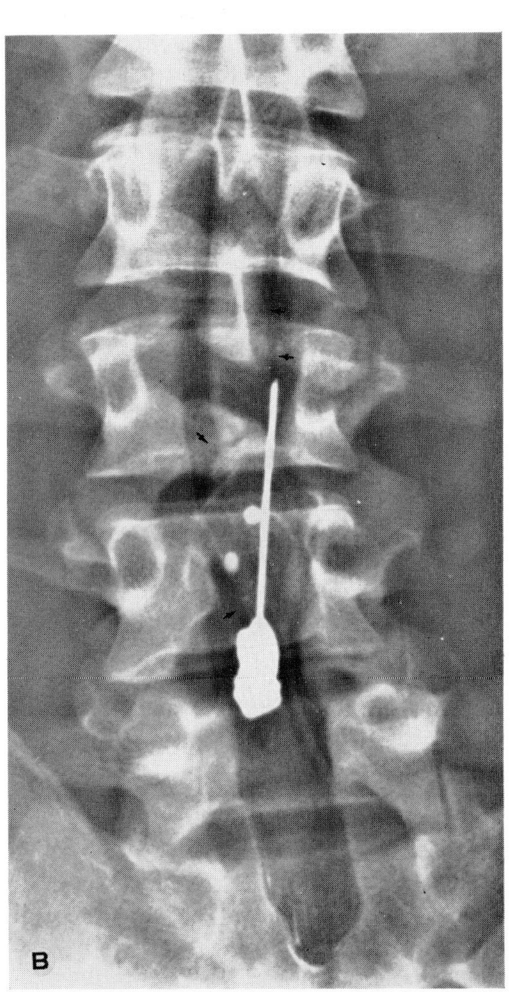

Fig. 659.—Multiple Anomalies of Lumbosacral Spine with a Low Position of the Lower End of the Spinal Cord

The Pantopaque myelogram (A) did not show the shadow of the spinal cord. This is common in patients with a wide canal, such as is the case in multiple congenital anomalies of the spine. The reason is that the column of oil does not reach the level of the spinal cord which actually lies above the column of Pantopaque in the prone position. The air myelogram (B), performed immediately after the Pantopaque myelogram, demonstrates that the spinal cord extends down to the lower margin of L4 (*arrows*). It is seen that the needle is just at the lateral margin of the spinal cord, and without sufficient care, it could easily injure this structure.

(Revised 1963)

which clinically may be indistinguishable from that caused by herniation of the intervertebral disc. Even after the demonstration of spondylolisthesis in plain spine films, myelography may usually determine the presence or absence of associated disc herniation, especially if surgical fusion of the spine is contemplated. Myelography usually demonstrates a triangular soft tissue space at the site of the spondylolisthesis and usually without any additional bulging of the corresponding intervertebral disc. In addition there is, in the frontal projection, a bilateral notch which is produced by the posterior elements of the vertebra above.

Spondylolisthesis may occur without the presence of congenital defects in the pars interarticularis. It may be the result of changes in the apophyseal joints, with disappearance of the cartilage and degenerative changes in the subarticular bone, which permit a considerable degree of forward movement of the vertebra. The term "false spondylolisthesis" has been applied to the deformity which is present. However, it may preferably be called spondylolisthesis without spondylolysis. The term "degenerative spondylolisthesis" may also be used because it results from disease of the apophyseal joints.

Multiple anomalies of the lumbosacral spine are common in which a combination of hemivertebra with marked scoliosis, wide spina bifida, wide interpedicular distances, and block-vertebra (failure of segmentation) are seen. Neurologic findings in these cases are often encountered if a careful neurologic examination is carried out, although most of these patients show no significant neurologic deficit. When symptoms are present, one frequently encounters an anomalous position of the lower end of the spinal cord which may extend down to possibly the fourth or the fifth lumbar and sometimes as low as the sacrum. It is for this reason that great care should be exercised in inserting the needle for lumbar puncture in any patient who has multiple lumbar spinal anomalies. It is our custom to advance the needle very slowly and to stop as soon as cerebrospinal fluid is obtained. After the Pantopaque myelogram, which may demonstrate a meningocele or only a congenitally wide spinal canal, air is injected through the same needle to demonstrate the spinal cord (fig. 659). Often, the cord cannot be visualized with Pantopaque because it is actually suspended in the cerebrospinal fluid above the Pantopaque. If a larger amount of Pantopaque is used, it will usually result in obscuration of the cord shadow.

Inflammatory Lesions

Suppurative inflammation within the substance of the spinal cord itself is a rare occurrence. Intramedullary pyogenic abscess, however, has been reported (Woltman and Adson, 1926), as have gumma and tuberculoma. As with their thecal counterparts, purulent meningitis, tuberculous meningitis, and meningovascular lues, radiologic examination plays little or no part in diagnosis. Chronic intradural and extradural inflammatory processes may, on the other hand, be dependent upon roentgenologic findings for an accurate diagnosis.

Chronic Adhesive Arachnoiditis

Arachnoidal adhesions occur most frequently in the thoracic and lower cervical portions of the vertebral canal. Fibrous bands between the pia and arachnoid may be a sequela of acute meningitis or may follow trauma and surgical procedures on the spinal cord. In some instances, adhesions occur in association with tumors and degenerative diseases of the spinal cord. The introduction of foreign materials into the spinal subarachnoid space, such as antibiotics, radiopaque substances, and anesthetic agents, may be followed months or years later by the onset of spinal cord symptoms resulting from chronic adhesive arachnoiditis. Important work which establishes beyond reasonable doubt a causal relationship between spinal anesthesia and chronic

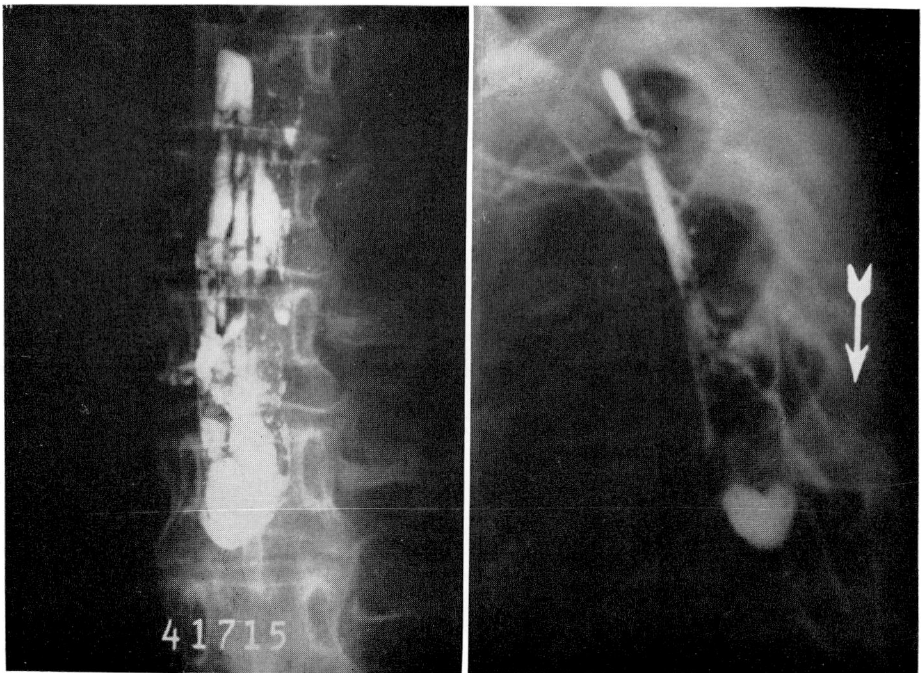

FIG. 660.—ADHESIVE ARACHNOIDITIS, T4 TO T7
An obstruction to the caudad flow of the radiopaque oil is present in the midthoracic region. For several segments above the complete obstruction, which is at T7, there are irregular pocketed collections of opaque material. The patient's symptoms began following meningitis, which was treated by the intrathecal injection of specific serum.

adhesive arachnoiditis, especially in the use of high, prolonged, or continuous spinal anesthesia, is reported by Kennedy, Effron, and Perry (1950). These authors state that high concentration of anesthetic agents may result in grave spinal cord paralyses. The frequent occurrence of arachnoidal adhesions in the midthoracic region is explained by Williams (1950) as resulting from the lowest point of the spine often falling in this area when the patient is supine during anesthesia.

Leptomeningeal adhesions develop slowly and gradually and increase in extent. The arachnoid is thickened. The bands that extend between the arachnoid and pia and which also connect the arachnoid and dura may be delicate or dense. Closed cavities containing fluid may be formed; these are leptomeningeal cysts. The fibrous bands and cysts may distort and compress into the spinal cord or spinal nerve roots, or they may interfere with the blood supply.

Myelography serves to establish the correct diagnosis in almost all instances where chronic adhesive arachnoiditis exists. A partial or complete obstruction to the passage of opaque material usually is found at fluoroscopy. Ordinarily there is not one point but numerous points over several vertebral segments at which the radiopaque material will be delayed, deviated from its normal course, or retained in small pockets. If the radiopaque column passes the involved area, residues of contrast material in linear, rounded, irregular forms may remain scattered throughout the abnormal zone. Such multiple reproducible deformities in the myelogram, which extend for a considerable longitudinal distance and which are not accompanied by a filling defect to suggest tumor, usually are indicative of chronic inflammatory disease (fig. 660). It is perhaps worthy of mention that a subdural injection of radiopaque material may cause a somewhat similar appearance at fluoroscopy and in frontal myelograms. A technical error of instillation is usually recognized at the beginning of the fluoroscopic examination and the subdural position of the radiopaque material can be identified by a lateral film made with the patient prone (fig. 646). The typical configuration of a block produced by arachnoiditis is one in which the special configuration usually produced by a tumor cannot be seen. The oil column does not show "cupping" in either the frontal or the lateral roentgenograms, or the oil column may be split before stopping. Most frequently the dome of the advancing column of Pantopaque is rounded instead of concave, as is seen in tumors. The most characteristic appearance of a block produced by adhesions is, therefore, the absence of the usual signs of neoplasms which will be described below.

Parasitic infestation is a rare cause of chronic leptomeningitis in the United States but is not rare in many countries throughout the world, particularly in Eastern Europe, Asia, and South America. Generally speaking, however, animal parasites are a common cause of nervous system disease. The nervous system is said to be involved in 80 per cent of patients with cysticercosis (Dixon and Hargreaves, 1944) where man acts as the intermediate host for *Taenia solium*, and neural involvement is frequent with hydatid disease (Dew, 1928). The larval cysts of *Taenia solium* and *Taenia echinococcus* are more apt to occur in the brain than in the spinal cord, and in cysticercosis the leptomeninges are more often involved than the parenchyma. Primary hydatid cysts are single and form more frequently in the spinal epidural space than within the dural sac (Rogers and Tudhope, 1938). *Cysticerci cellolosae* may be present in large numbers in the chorioid plexus, and it is thought that in this manner they reach the cerebrospinal fluid, in which they circulate, and then they gravitate to the lower spinal subarachnoid space.

Thick arachnoidal adhesions are observed most frequently about the base of the brain and the cauda equina. Plain spine roentgenographs of the patient whose myelogram is demonstrated in Figure 661 disclosed enlargement of the vertebral canal from L1 to S1, which lead to a mistaken diagnosis of a giant tumor of the cauda equina. In the frontal projection, the pedicles of all of the vertebrae were observed to be flattened and concave medially, and the interpediculate measurements were increased above normal. In lateral view, exaggeration of the concavity of the dorsal margins of the vertebral bodies was demonstrated, and the vertebral laminae were thinned. These changes are indicative of a slowly expanding lesion of the vertebral canal; they are explained in cysticercosis by the fact that the larval cysts enlarge with age and vary from 1 mm. in diameter when young up to 3 cm. or more in diameter when quite old.

In the myelogram, a large number of filling defects in the contrast outline of the lumbosacral subarachnoid space are shown and some lesions are present in the large nerve root sheaths. The lesions vary considerably in size and present a rounded configuration in both frontal and lateral views, indicating their spherical form. Of diagnostic importance is the dorsal position of the cysts in the lateral film with the patient prone, since the cysts show considerable mobility and rise to the surface of the dependent radiopaque medium.

Epidural Infections

The majority of infections of the spinal epidural space are pyogenic or tuberculous in origin. While a host of organisms may act as etiologic agents, the staphylococcus is indicated most often in nontuberculous infections in this area. The organisms may enter by direct extension from an inflammatory process in the paraspinal tissues, such as a perinephric abscess, or septic metastasis may occur from a distant focus of infection. Evidence has been collected by Browder and Meyers (1937) to support the belief that a hematogenous spread of infection directly to the epidural space is a rare occurrence and more commonly metastatic vertebral osteomyelitis occurs first, with the infection subsequently spreading into the spinal epidural space. Certainly, this is the more common sequence of events with tuberculosis.

Nontuberculous epidural infections are

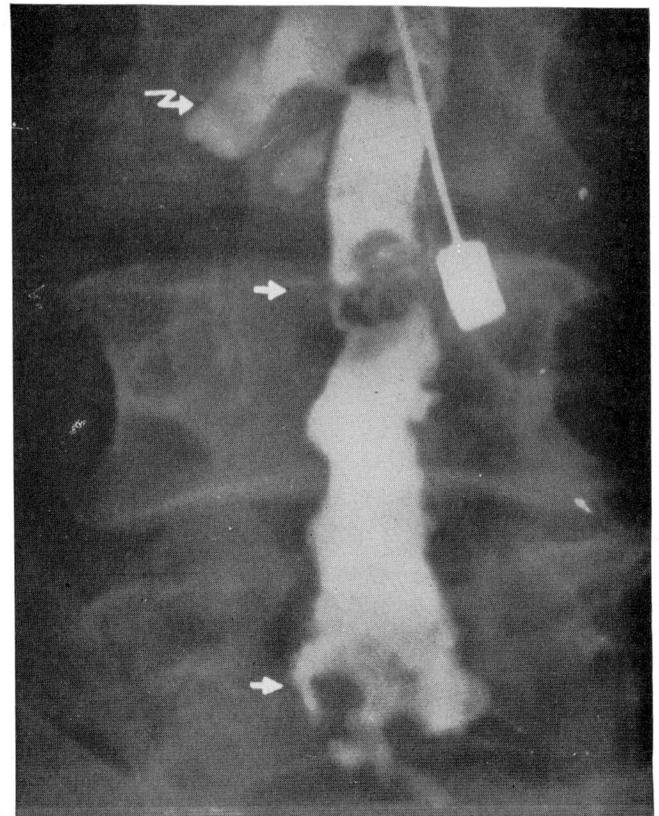

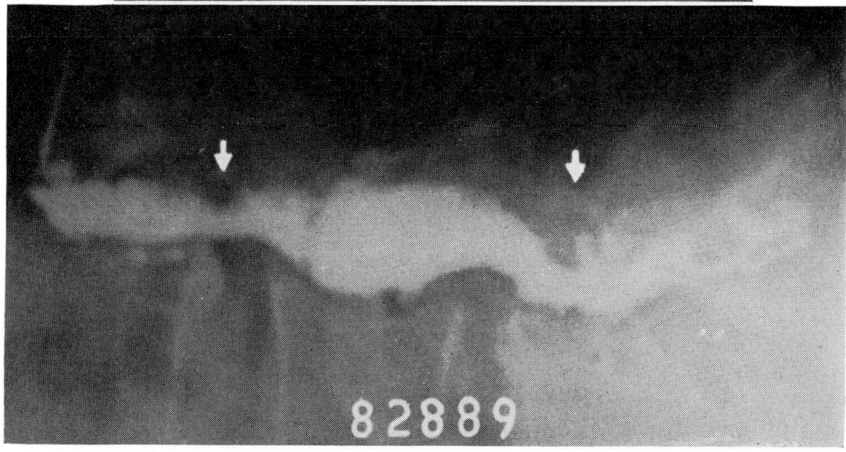

Fig. 661.—Cysticercosis

Spherical masses of variable size are outlined in the frontal projection, including two small cysts in the nerve root sheath at L3 (*wavy arrow*). In the lateral view the cysts are situated dorsally floating on the heavy oil (*straight arrows*).

not always accompanied by frank suppuration and formation of epidural abscess. Some infections produce a more chronic inflammatory lesion, usually designated as spinal epidural granuloma. All grades of reaction are encountered between abscess formation and production of granulation tissue, depending on the more fulminating or more

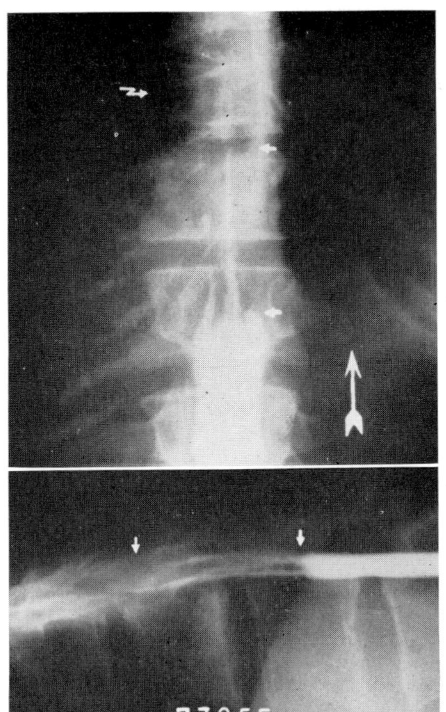

FIG. 662.—EPIDURAL ABSCESS T10 TO L1
The cephalad flow of Pantopaque is delayed at L1. A small amount of radiopaque material passes as high as T11 in the constricted subarachnoid space (*straight arrows*). The osteolytic changes of T11 result from tuberculosis (*wavy arrow*).

chronic nature of the infection. In tuberculosis, also, the epidural infection may take the form either of a cold abscess or masses of granulation tissue.

In plain spine radiographs, evidence of vertebral infection, which is probably the most frequent source of epidural inflammation, is more often seen with tuberculosis than with pyogenic processes. Characteristically, tuberculosis produces destruction in the contiguous portions of adjacent vertebrae without a striking marginal reaction of the cancellous bone. Marked narrowing of the intervertebral disc space is often present. When extra-osseous extension of the tuberculous process occurs, associated laterally convex paraspinal shadows usually are visible in the radiograph, particularly in the thoracic region. The posterior counterpart of the paraspinal mass is not seen in plain spine films, but it is an epidural cold abscess.

(*Revised 1963*)

A rather similar roentgenographic appearance may be produced by nontuberculous infections but certain differences between pyogenic osteomyelitis and vertebral tuberculosis may be observed in radiographs in a high percentage of cases (Phemister, 1924). Beveling of the vertebral edges associated with only moderate narrowing of the intervertebral space are prominent features of suppurative infections. An absence of the bone plate and a well defined margin of cancellous bone, often with a zone of increased density adjacent to the intervertebral space, are suggestive of pyogenic osteomyelitis. Pyogenic infection begins more frequently in the vertebral arch than does tuberculosis, and this may be correlated with the more frequent occurrence of spinal epidural abscess along the posterior and lateral aspect of the dural sac than in the ventral epidural space (Browder and Meyers, 1937). In serial radiographs, the faster tempo of pyogenic infections may be manifested by a more active progression of the destructive phase and earlier appearance of bone repair than with tuberculosis. With antibiotic therapy, an almost diagnostic acceleration of the healing phase in the involved bone is disclosed in pyogenic infections.

At myelography, the contrast outline of the subarachnoid space may have a unique appearance (fig. 662). A partial obstruction to the passage of radiopaque material may be encountered at some distance, often several vertebral segments, before the level of a known destructive lesion of bone is reached. Beyond the point of delay, the opaque column is markedly narrowed. It appears as a thin, linear shadow on each side of the spinal cord in frontal and lateral projections up to the point where complete obstruction occurs, which is usually near the site of origin of the infection in the bone. The appearance is that of an epidural mass which produces absolute narrowing of the transverse or the anteroposterior diameter of the spinal subarachnoid space or both, as outlined by oil. This cannot actually be differentiated from any other epidural type of lesion without other manifestations of bone involvement or the clinical history of possible infection. See under "Extradural Lesions," page 1.888.

Traumatic Disorders

A description of the various types of fractures of the vertebrae will not be included here; only a discussion of injuries that cause neurologic signs of compression of the roots and spinal cord will be given.

The presence and extent of spinal cord damage that accompanies vertebral fracture and dislocation can be readily established by neurologic examination. Furthermore, it is usually undesirable to carry out any cumbersome fluoroscopic or radiographic examination which might result in further injury to the spinal cord. The plain film examinations, particularly in the cervical region, should include only anteroposterior and lateral views made without having the patient turn his head. Emphasis is placed on the demonstration of possible dislocations at the cervicothoracic junction, which is usually obscured by the shoulders. Therefore, no radiographic examination of the cervical spine can be considered complete unless this area has been demonstrated. Pulling the shoulders down may be helpful, and lateral views may be obtained by elevating one arm, the arm away from the tube, and taking a lateral view by centering the central x-ray beam approximately 3 inches above the shoulder with the patient in the supine position. The prone position is preferable, but it should not be assumed if it is thought that the symptoms of cord or root compression may be aggravated by such a maneuver.

The conservative type of management of spinal cord injuries used by most neurosurgeons, which generally consists of immobilization on the Stryker frame in a position to shorten the neural axis, cranial traction for cervical spine injury, proper management of sphincteric disturbances, and meticulous nursing care, generally requires little from the radiologist. Once the diagnosis of vertebral fracture or dislocation has been established, further radiographic examination has its greatest role in evaluating the efficacy of treatment, such as traction, and checking the progress of healing. These examinations usually can be carried out in a satisfactory manner at the patient's bedside with portable apparatus.

In highly selective cases, myelography may be performed prior to surgical decompression to visualize the soft tissue derangement which occurs as a result of fracture-dislocation of a vertebral body. Dislocation usually produces an obstruction to the passage of radiopaque material into the subarachnoid space. In frontal projection, the head of the oil column usually is transverse in configuration, while in the lateral view the oil column tapers posteriorly to a point of occlusion (fig. 663). When the ventral pressure on the dural sac and its contents is the result of a displaced bone fragment, the obstruction of the oil column will appear near the midportion of the posteriorly dislocated fragment of the compressed vertebral body, rather than at the level of the intervertebral disc space.

It is not uncommon to find, in patients who are quadriparetic following cervical spinal injury, that the myelogram is entirely normal. In these cases, it is probable that the intervertebral disc herniated and struck the cord, producing severe damage, but then returned to the intervertebral space and so myelography revealed no abnormality. In these instances, the neurologic symptoms indicate that the paralysis was observed immediately after the injury and did not progress any further.

Depressed laminar fractures constitute a small group of spinal injuries which most frequently are treated by open reduction (Pool, 1951). Such injuries usually are the result of a direct blow to the vertebral column with the result that comminuted fractures of the vertebral arch are driven into the vertebral canal. The injury may be caused by a fall on a sharp object, violent compression against protruding objects,

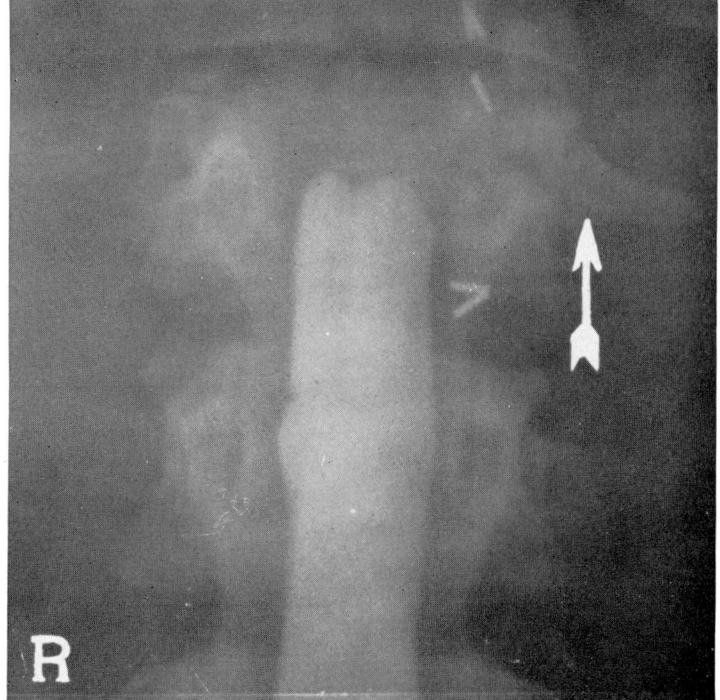

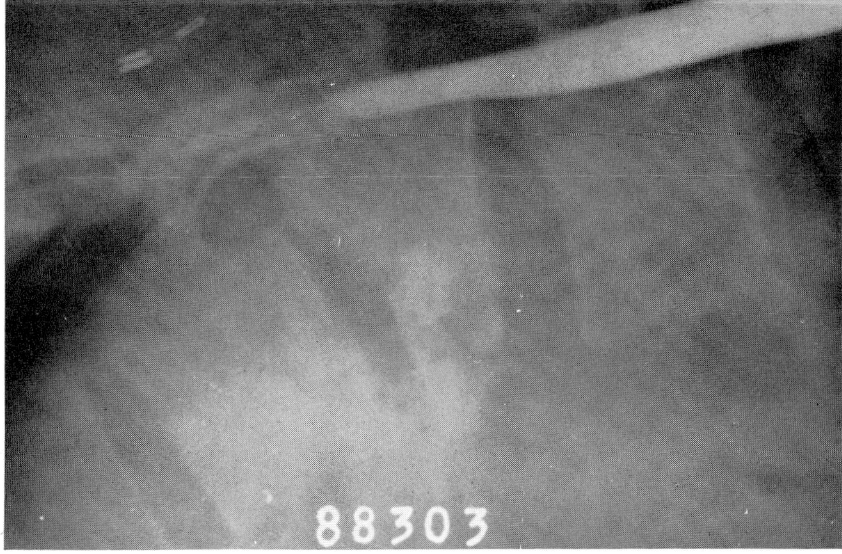

FIG. 663.—FRACTURE DISLOCATION, L1

The body of the first lumbar vertebra is collapsed as a result of compression fracture two months previously. The main posterior fragment of bone is displaced backward into the vertebral canal. An obstruction to the cephalad flow of radiopaque medium is present behind the body of L1 resulting from compression and angulation of the dural sac from the ventral side. (Silver clips were inserted at the time of an operation that was designed to produce a decompression of the spinal cord.)

(Revised 1963)

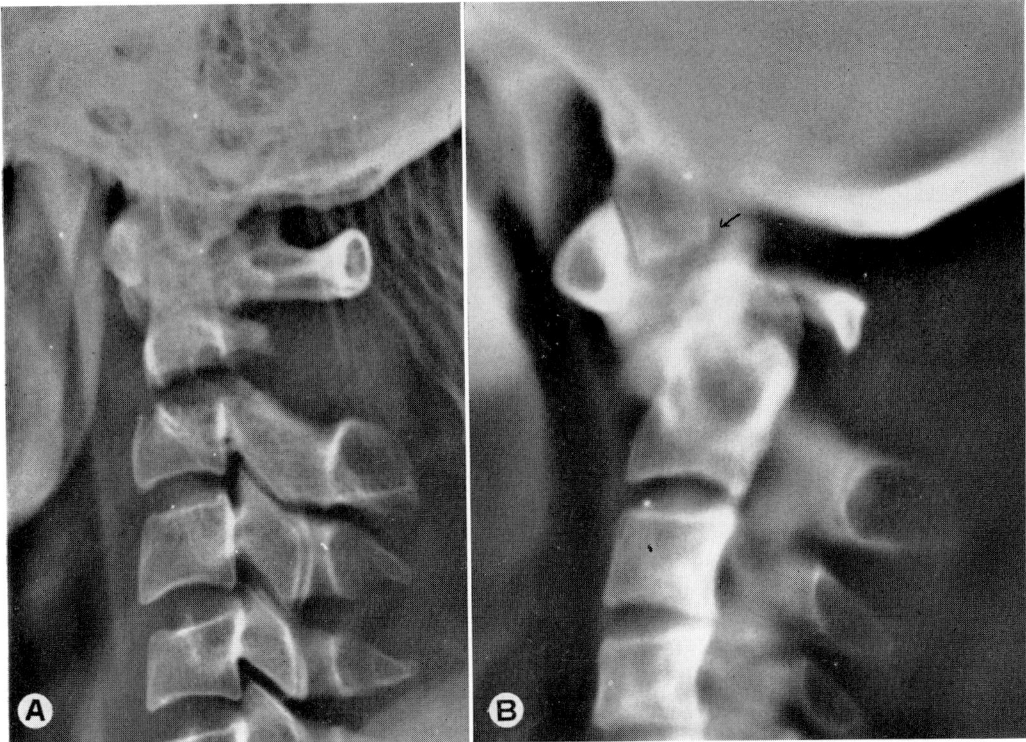

FIG. 664.—FRACTURE AND CONGENITAL ANOMALY OF ODONTOID PROCESS

(A) represents a fracture of the odontoid which usually occurs just below the base of this structure. The edges are ragged. (B) is a laminagram of an ununited odontoid process which shows a smooth upper margin of C2 and occurs at the base of the dens.

vehicular accidents, and gunshot wounds. The Queckenstedt test may be used for the detection of spinal cord compression and as a guide to whether extensive radiologic examination and surgery should be performed. Stereoscopic roentgenograms in frontal projection may disclose a fragment of lamina projecting into the vertebral canal, or even detached and displaced into the canal. Laminograms may be of the greatest value in determining whether, and to what degree, the vertebral canal is encroached on by fracture fragments.

Because of the tendency of missiles to ricochet, the longitudinal extent of spinal injuries resulting from *gunshot wounds* is not always readily detected. Hinkel and Nichols (1946) made a valuable contribution to the evaluation of such injuries by describing the findings at myelography performed at one to two weeks after the injury had occurred. In patients whose recovery of function has been slight, or whose recovery has become arrested, especially in wounds of the dorsolumbar area, myelography often proves useful. The examination may disclose an extradural mass compressing the spinal cord or cauda equina which may be a hematoma, depressed fragment of bone, or a metallic fragment remaining in the vertebral canal. Cervical decompression can result in marked improvement in patients in whom irreparable neural damage by contusion or laceration previously was thought to exist.

Intervertebral disc herniations may result from acute trauma, with or without associated fracture of the vertebra. The latent effects of trauma may also be manifested in disc degeneration and herniation. Osteoarthritic proliferative changes associated with and following fracture repair may result in sessile exostosis at the vertebral margin.

(Revised 1963)

The lesions usually encroach on the intervertebral canal from the ventral aspect or on the intervertebral foramen, and myelography is a satisfactory method of detecting their presence and evaluating the extent of spinal cord or nerve root compression which may result. Intervertebral disc disease is more extensively dealt with elsewhere (p. 1.892).

Lesions of the odontoid process may be traumatic or congenital. Fractures of the odontoid process may occur usually at the base, extending slightly below the visible lower margin of the odontoid process (fig. 664). On the other hand, congenital anomalies, that is, failure of fusion of the odontoid process is also common, and this should not be confused with fractures, which require a different therapeutic approach (Schlesinger and Taveras, 1958). Fractures usually have ragged edges at the sites of traumatic separation, whereas congenital failure of fusion is associated with a smooth margin. Either fracture or congenital failure of fusion results in dislocations of the odontoid process and compression of the spinal cord between the upper margin of the posterior aspect of the body of the second cervical vertebra and the posterior arch of the atlas. Compression occurs with the head in flexion and disappears with the head in extension. This is one reason why the taking of flexion and extension views routinely is not recommended, particularly where there has been a spinal injury. These films should always be taken after the absence of odontoid lesion has been ascertained.

Dislocation of the odontoid below the transverse ligament occurs in cases of congenitally hypoplastic odontoid processes.

In performing myelography in patients who have a spinal fracture with kyphosis, it is not uncommon to find that the oil does not flow properly up to the area of the fracture. This may be produced by adhesions in this region in the subarachnoid space as a result of the trauma. Sometimes it is due to the fact that insufficient tilt of the table is used. By placing the patient in the prone oblique position or in the lateral decubitus position, the oil may pass the area quite freely. This maneuver may be employed any time that there is an exaggerated kyphotic curve in the thoracic region.

Neoplastic and Other Diseases of the Spinal Cord, Nerve Roots, and Meninges

Tumors of the spinal cord and its membranes are similar in type to those found in the cranial cavity. There is, however, considerable difference in the frequency of occurrence of the various types of tumors in the two areas. This is readily understood when the relative quantity of medullary tissue to spinal meninges is compared to the mass of the brain in relation to its covering. Fifty per cent of the neoplasms affecting the spinal cord arise from its enveloping structures and are about equally divided between meningioma and neurinoma. Gliomas, on the other hand, account for only 10 per cent of spinal cord lesions. The mass of the cord is one-seventh that of the brain, where gliomas account for more than one-half of all primary tumors.

Involvement of the spinal cord by metastatic tumors from other organs occurs more frequently than cerebral metastases. Two-thirds of all spinal metastases originate either in the lung or breasts.

A difference in behavior of metastatic tumors of the spinal cord as compared with those of the brain is also of interest. Intracranial metastases are almost always intracerebral, while metastases to the spinal cord are usually epidural and rarely extend to the meninges to invade the spinal cord itself.

Roentgenologically, tumors of the spinal cord and its membranes produce changes in the adjacent vertebrae and soft tissues, which indicate their location, in approximately 15 per cent of cases. In this way, spinal cord tumors behave differently from brain tumors. Localizing changes in adjacent bony structures are observed infrequently with brain tumors, and changes of generalized pressure occur in bony structures at a

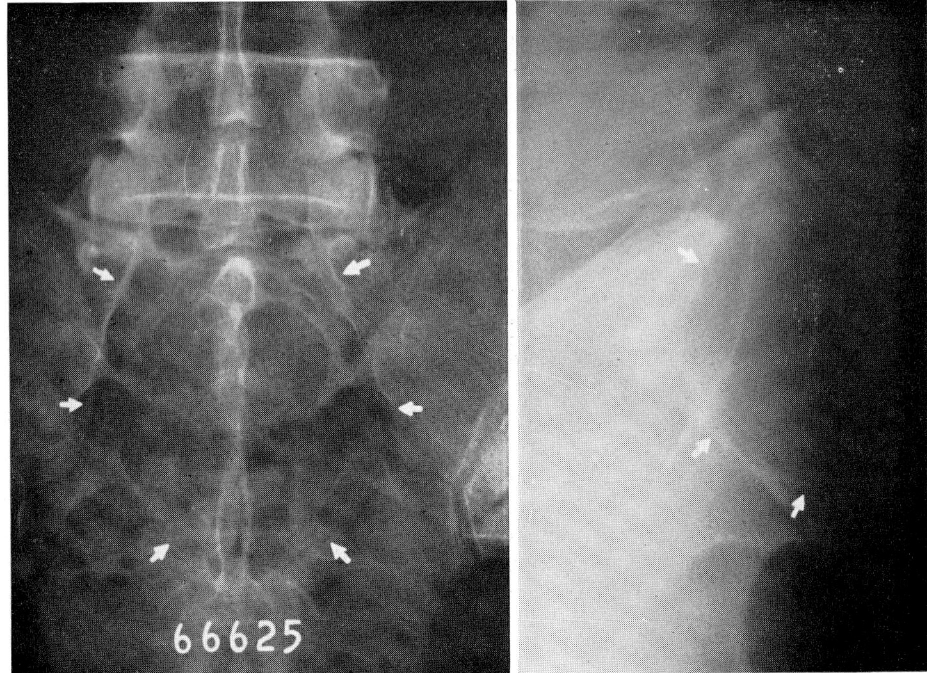

FIG. 665.—EPENDYMOMA OF THE FILUM TERMINALE

The sacral canal is expanded (*arrows*) in both frontal and lateral projections. The margins of the enlarged canal are smooth. Expansion is symmetrical with a fusiform dilatation extending from S1 to S3.

distance from the lesion. In plain spine roentgenograms, one or more of three fundamental changes in adjacent portions of the vertebral column may denote the presence of tumor:

1. Enlargement of the vertebral canal as manifested by flattening or concavity of the medial margins of the pedicles with increase in the interpediculate distance, scalloping of the posterior margins of the vertebral body, and thinning of the lamina, all the result of atrophy of the bone by the pulsating pressure of the tumor (figs. 665, 666, and 667).

2. Enlargement of the intervertebral foramen, which results from an isthmus of tumor in the foramen joining the medial masses of the dumbbell-shaped tumor which lies partially within and partially without the vertebral canal (figs. 668 and 669).

3. Calcification within the tumor in the vertebral canal (fig. 670).

The relative incidence of intraspinal tumors is shown in Table VIII (p. 1.870).

In addition to the characteristic changes caused by primary spinal cord tumor, metastatic neoplasms may produce abnormalities in plain spine roentgenograms. The spinal cord is frequently affected by an extension of a malignant metastasis from the vertebra to the epidural space, and in such instances, osteolytic or osteoblastic changes in the adjacent vertebrae may be apparent. An extraneous paraspinal shadow may result from a retropleural or retroperitoneal tumor which frequently, although not necessarily, extends through one or more intervertebral foramina to invade the epidural tissues. Metastatic epidural tumors usually affect the spinal cord by compression rather than invasion through the meninges. Tumors arising in the spinal cord do not invade the surrounding bone.

By myelography, the spinal cord tumor usually can be classified in one of three categories—intramedullary, extramedullary intradural, or extradural. The majority of intramedullary tumors are gliomas which

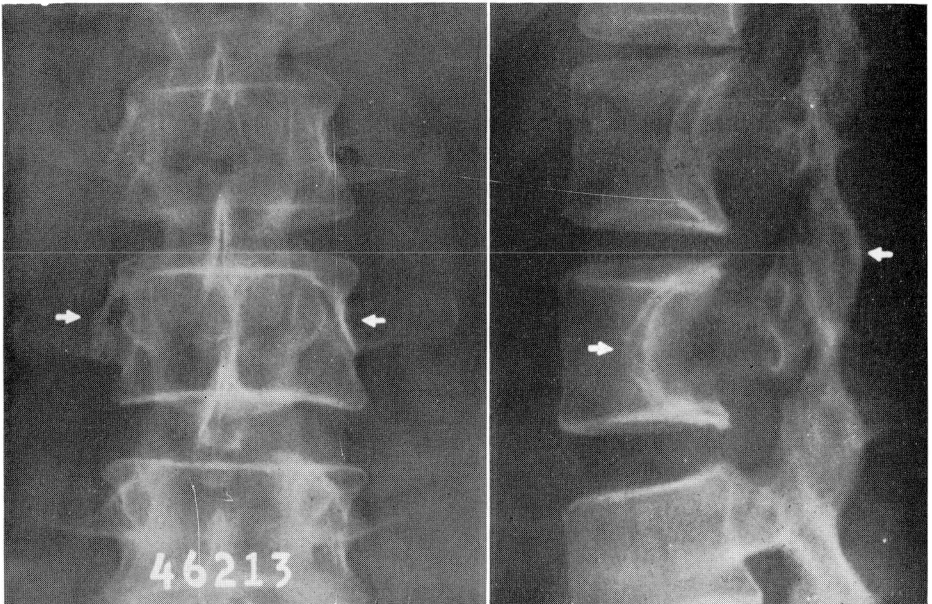

FIG. 666.—EPENDYMOMA, L1, 2, and 3

The thoracolumbar canal is symmetrically expanded (*arrows*) in both frontal and lateral projections. In the lateral view, the enlargement results in scalloping of the posterior margins of the vertebral bodies and thinning of the laminae. Even erosion of the vertebrae with sharply defined bone margins occurs because the tumor is intradural and slowly growing. The intervertebral fibrocartilage is spared because of its elasticity.

expand the spinal cord in all directions until the spinal subarachnoid space is obliterated and the dural sac is distended. An obstruction to the flow of the contrast medium, either partial or complete, is found in the majority of cases. The shadow of the spinal cord is enlarged, most often in a fusiform manner, at the level of the neoplasm. Extramedullary intradural tumors, the majority of which are encapsulated neurinomas or meningiomas lying in the intrathecal spaces are distinguishable by myelography. A margin of the tumor is delineated sharply by the contrast material which is in close contact with the neoplastic mass. The spinal cord or cauda equina is displaced and compressed by the tumor. Narrow spaces often are present between the tumor and the spinal cord through which varying amounts of contrast medium may pass to outline the neoplasm on more than one side, so that the longitudinal extent of the tumor frequently can be well defined. Tumors of the epidural space, which envelop and compress

(Revised 1963)

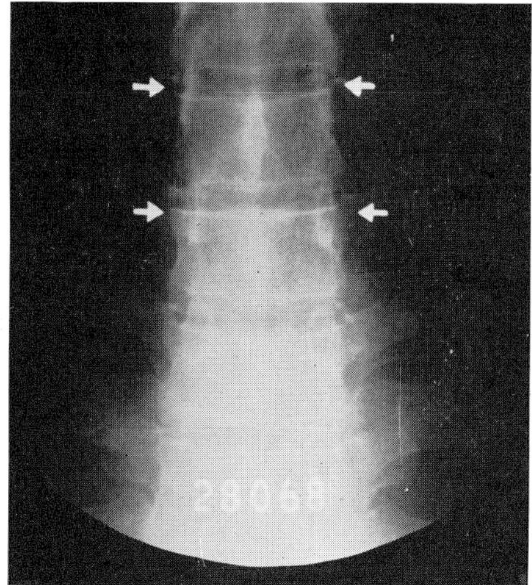

FIG. 667.—LIPOMA, T5, 6, AND 7

Thinning of the pedicles and an increase in the interpediculate distances, centered at T6 is demonstrated. The widened midthoracic vertebral canal has a fusiform configuration in the frontal projection. Such changes in the thoracic area are usually the result of either a lipoma or an extradural cyst.

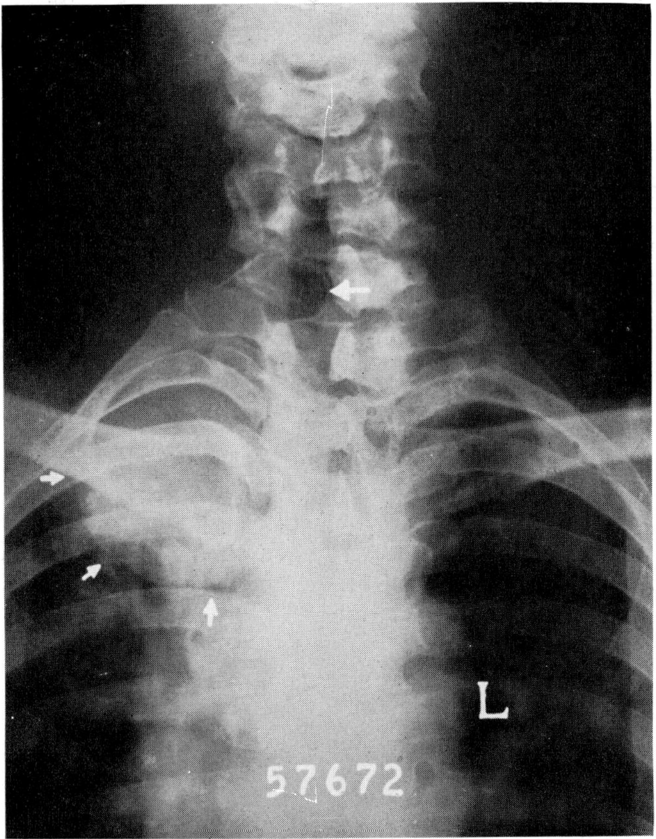

FIG. 668.—DUMBBELL NEURINOMA, C7-T1

The tumor has expanded an intervertebral foramen (*upper arrow*) and has extended into the right upper thorax. The large intrathoracic component of the tumor lies extrapleurally at the lung apex (*small arrows*).

the dural sac, narrow or obliterate the subarachnoid space outlined by radiopaque medium. At the site of the tumor, the column of contrast material usually is narrowed conically by degrees, rather than abruptly, because the dura is interposed between the opaque medium and the neoplasm. If the greater part of the tumor is on one side of the vertebral canal, the dural sac may be angulated and the radiopaque column narrowed abruptly.

Intramedullary Lesions

Gliomas of the spinal cord. These are classified microscopically, in the vast majority of instances, as *ependymoma* or *astrocytoma*. Occasionally oligodendrogliomas, spongioblastoma, medulloblastoma, and rarely gliomas of other histologic types may be encountered (Kernohan, Woltman, and Adson, 1933). Ependymomas, which comprise 70 per cent of the group, originate most frequently in the region of the conus medullaris, where normally, in proportion to the mass of surrounding neural tissue, there is more ependymal tissue in the walls of the terminal ventricle of the central canal than elsewhere in the nervous system. An ependymoma may extend along the filum terminale for a remarkable distance, and in some instances, the lumbosacral portion of the subarachnoid space may fill with tumor throughout its entire length. Because of the great size of some of these tumors, they have been referred to as *giant tumors* of the cauda equina.

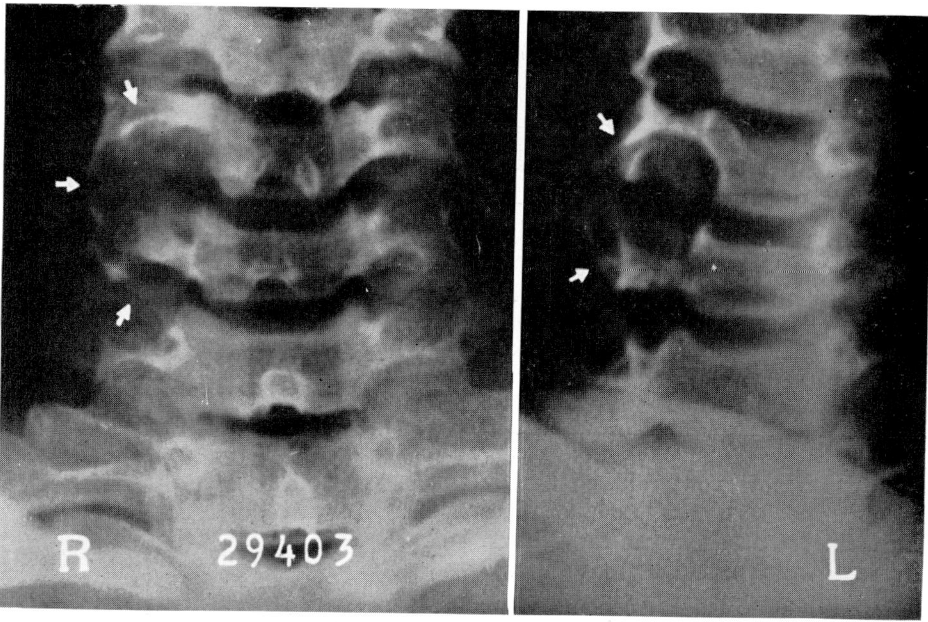

FIG. 669.—DUMBBELL NEURINOMA C5-6

An intervertebral foramen is enlarged markedly (*arrows*) by the growth of an encapsulated tumor arising intradurally along the course of the nerve root. The posterior oblique film shows the enlarged intervertebral foramen *en face*.

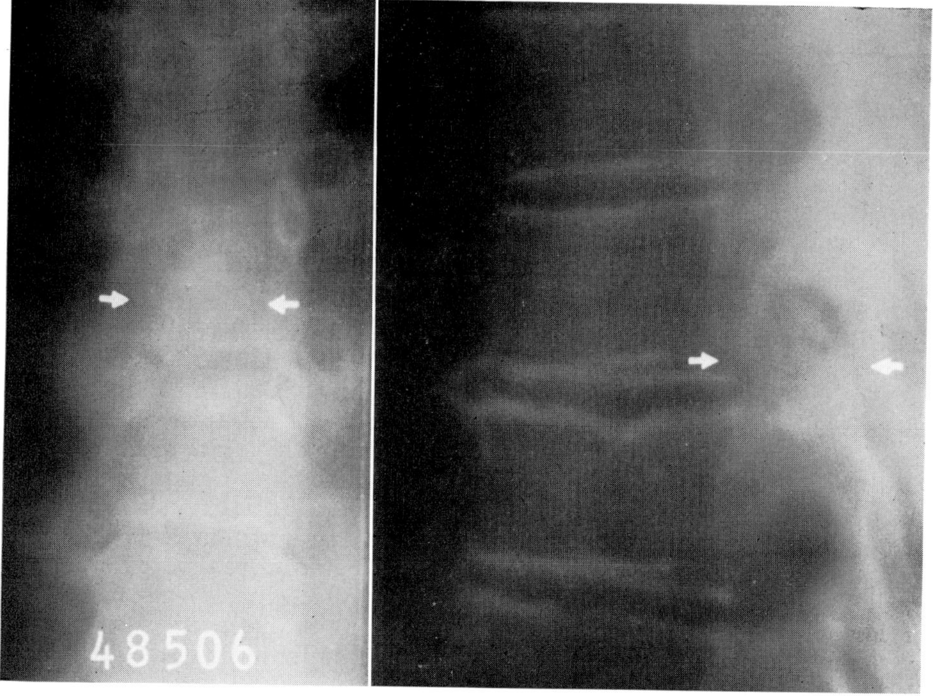

FIG. 670.—MENINGIOMA T6

An oval psammomatous tumor is shown in the vertebral canal (*arrows*). The calcification is irregular, yet the boundaries of the tumor are well defined. The fact that the tumor is not in contact with bone or the intervertebral fibrocartilage is noteworthy.

(*Revised 1963*)

TABLE VIII

RELATIVE INCIDENCE OF BRAIN AND SPINAL CORD TUMORS OF VARIOUS TYPES IN PERCENTAGE (WOLF)

Tumor	Brain	Spinal Cord
Neurinoma	10	26
Metastatic from other organs	10	25
Meningioma	15	24
Glioma	50	10
Metastatic from brain	—	4
Hemangioblastoma	4	3
Congenital tumors (dermoids, etc.)	5	2
Others	6	6

Because of the slow growth of the majority of the spinal cord gliomas, bone changes in plain spine roentgenograms may occur. Ependymomas, in particular, may expand the thoracolumbar portion of the vertebral canal for the length of five or six vertebral segments, with pressure atrophy of the medial portion of the pedicles and increase in the interpediculate measurements. Scalloping of the posterior margins of the vertebral bodies and thinning of the laminae often are demonstrated in the lateral views (fig. 666).

At myelography, gliomas of the spinal cord occurring in the cervical and thoracic areas cause a fusiform enlargement of the spinal cord shadow (fig. 671) which may be large enough to cause a partial obstruction to the passage of the contrast material (fig. 672). Gliomas of the conus, when large, obliterate the entire subarachnoid space, and when radiopaque material is introduced below the lesion, a smooth inferior tumor surface may be demonstrated by the head of the radiopaque column (fig. 673). In other instances, gliomas of the cauda equina grow irregularly along the spinal nerve roots (fig. 674), and the tumor surface may be uneven.

Angiomas, of the neoplastic variety, occur in the form of *hemangioblastomas*, which are similar histologically to the tumors commonly encountered in the cerebellum (Lindau, 1930). Primary hemangioblastoma of the spinal cord usually is solitary and occurs most frequently in the cervical and thoracic

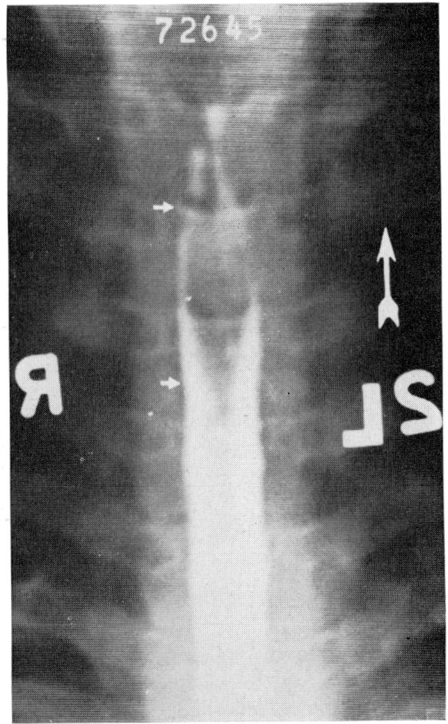

FIG. 671.—GLIOMA, T4-5
The thoracic spinal cord is enlarged symmetrically. In frontal projection the portion expanded by an intramedullary tumor appears as a fusiform enlargement of the band of diminished density which represents the thoracic cord (*arrows*).

regions. The tumors may present at the surface of the spinal cord and extend into the subarachnoid space. Rarely do they extend in the subarachnoid space to other parts of the spinal cord (Wyburn-Mason, 1944; Wood *et al.*, 1953).

Ordinarily no abnormalities are demonstrated in plain spine roentgenograms; angiomas of the spinal cord do not induce vertebral changes. Cavernous hemangioma of the vertebra usually is not associated with a vascular abnormality of the meninges and spinal cord, although large epidural veins may sometimes be associated. Myelography may disclose enlargement of the spinal cord and in instances where the tumor presents on the spinal cord surface, a filling defect or obstruction of the subarachnoid space may be demonstrated. Increased

(Revised 1963)

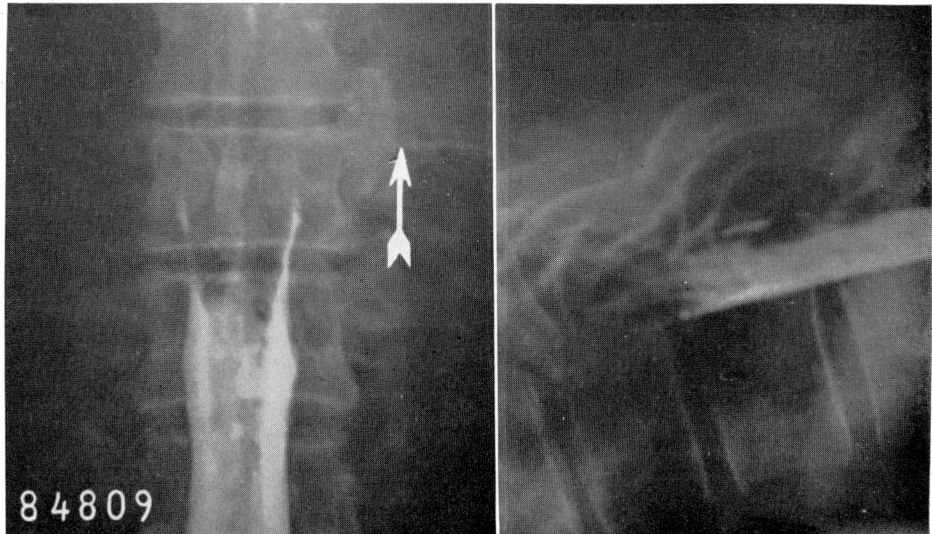

FIG. 672.—GLIOMA (ASTROCYTOMA) T9

The lower thoracic spinal cord is expanded to fill completely the dural sac. Pantopaque entering the recess between the tumor and the arachnoid membrane tapers away from the midline, which indicates that the expanding lesion is intramedullary.

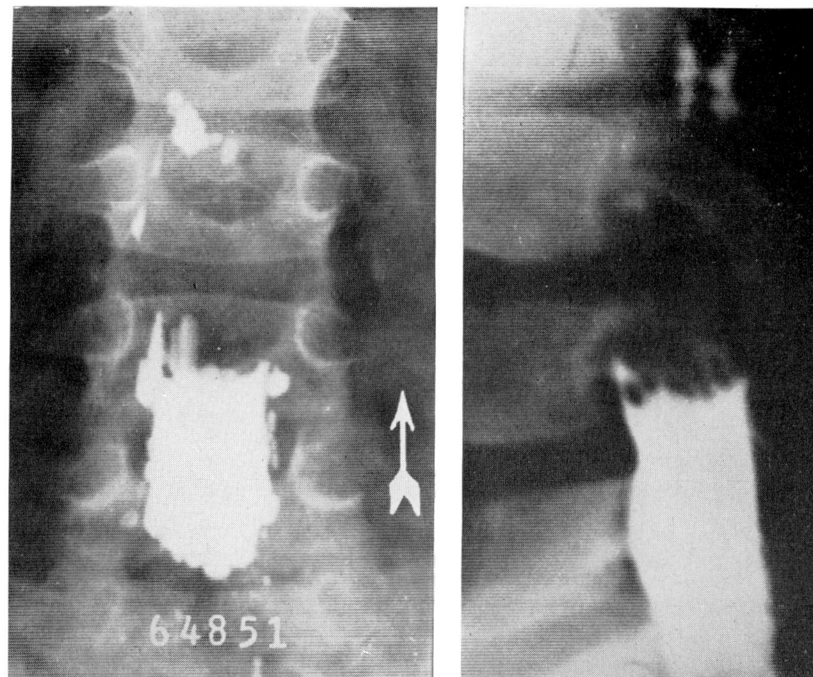

FIG. 673.—ASTROCYTOMA L4

The head of the radiopaque oil column appears concave both in prone frontal view and in a lateral film made with the patient lying on his right side. The lower margin of the intradural tumor causes a semilunar indentation of the head of the oil column.

(Revised 1963)

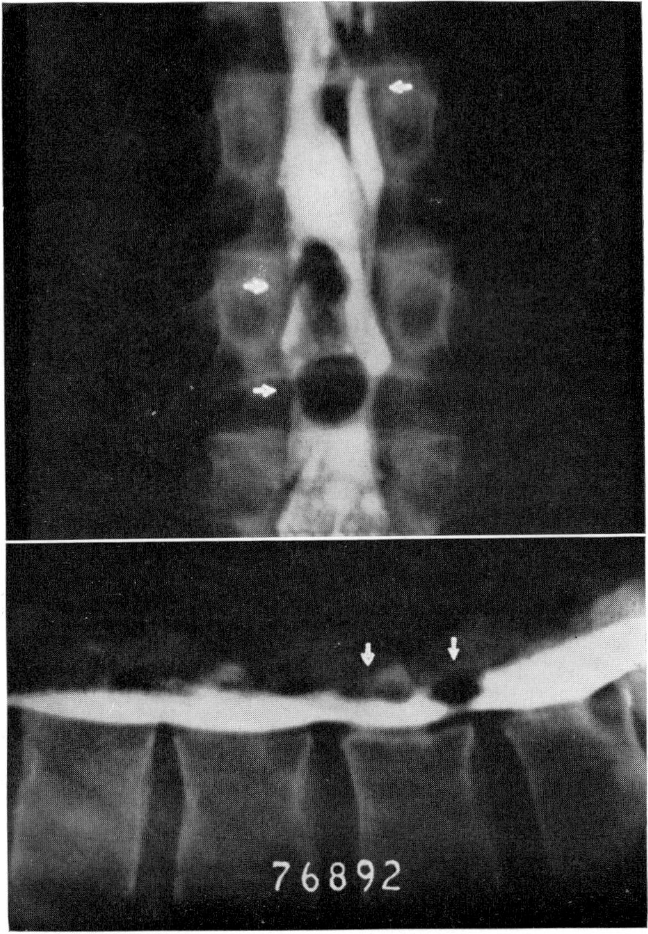

FIG. 674.—EPENDYMOMA (RECURRENT), L2-3

Three rounded filling defects in the radiopaque outline of the lumbar subarachnoid space are visible in the frontal view (*arrows*). Two of the masses produce dorsal impressions on the Pantopaque column in lateral projection (*arrows*). Myelography was performed because pain and weakness of the lower extremities recurred five years after the surgical removal of an ependymoma of the cauda equina.

vascularity and varicose veins frequently occur in the vicinity of a spinal cord tumor. Usually these changes are the result of obstruction of the venous drainage by the tumor, and they should not be considered as primary vascular lesions until every effort has been made to exclude a neoplasm. In the case of hemangioblastomas, it is difficult to see the actual neoplasm because the accompanying enlarged vessels are very large and may obscure the tumor nodules. For further details see below.

Rare intramedullary tumors include neurinoma, fibroma, lipoma, dermoid, and teratoma (Ingraham, 1938). Although these tumors arise from tissue not normally present in the spinal cord, they may be found on occasion as a result of embryonal inclusion. Radiologically, these tumors appear the same as other expanding lesions of the spinal cord. Dermoids may be associated with dysraphic abnormalities of the vertebra and soft tissues of the back.

Vascular abnormalities of the spinal cord. Enlarged vessels in the spinal cord are commonly encountered in association with intramedullary lesions (fig. 675). These vessels are usually tortuous and in some

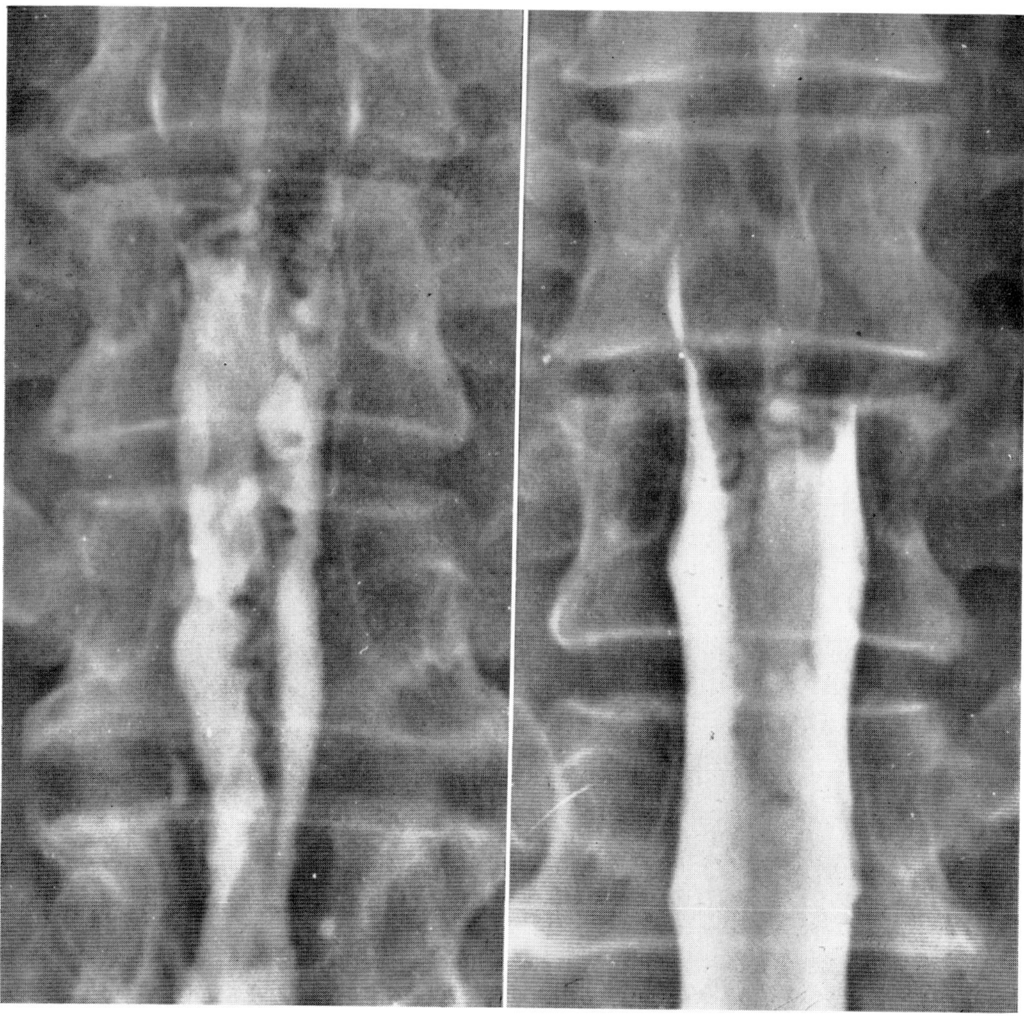

Fig. 675.—Enlarged Vessels in Patient with Intramedullary Tumor
There is a fusiform widening of the spinal cord. Below the area of the tumor, and at the level of the tumor, there are convoluted radiolucent shadows representing enlarged vessels, probably veins.

instances fairly numerous. At other times only one or two enlarged, tortuous vessels can be seen which represent usually enlarged veins. Localized dilatation of spinal vessels may result also from chronic adhesive arachnoiditis and may be seen in cases of narrowing of the vertebral canal by non-neoplastic processes, such as ruptured intervertebral disc, producing a high degree of obstruction. In some instances, in the cervical region a large herniation of the intervertebral disc which is not producing a block may be accompanied by enlarged vessels.

(Revised 1963)

The vascular malformations of the cord can be classified in several ways.

1. *Arteriovenous malformations.* In this type of abnormality the blood passes rapidly from the arteries to the veins, and the veins are seen to contain arterial blood upon surgical inspection of the lesion. Out of 16 cases seen at the Neurological Institute and operated upon, 6 were of this type (Taveras and Dalton, 1961). This type of lesion tends to occur most frequently in the thoracic region and less frequently in the cervical region. They are usually more prominent

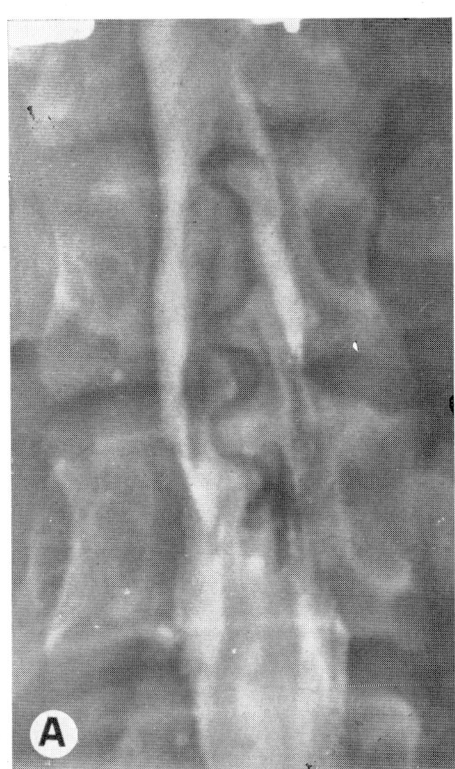

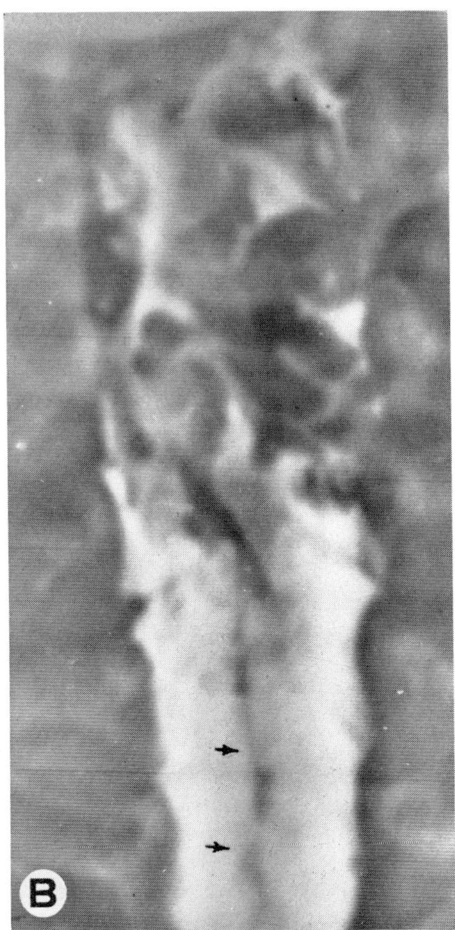

FIG. 676.—VASCULAR MALFORMATION OF THE SPINAL CORD

In the case shown in (A), the lesion is in the lower thoracic region and is accompanied by a very slight widening of the spinal cord shadow as shown on the myelogram. In (B), the lesion is in the cervical region and consists of an extremely large area of involvement with unusually marked dilatation of vessels. The anterior spinal vessels are also enlarged below the lesion (*arrows*) and extend for a considerable distance.

on the dorsal side of the spinal cord than on the ventral surface. For this reason, it is possible to overlook the lesions, when they are small, by myelography with Pantopaque even when films are made. This is one indication for the removal of the needle and the placing of the patient in the supine position to outline the dorsal surface of the thoracic and cervical spinal cord. *At myelography,* numerous enlarged vessels are seen usually extending over several vertebral segments. The size of the vessels, which are usually markedly convoluted, is much greater than that which is seen in association with spinal cord neoplasms, arachnoiditis, and some herniated discs (fig. 676). The diagnosis is usually obvious because of the large size of these lesions. Some instances are seen where the increased vascularity extends over a very large area from the lumbar to the cervical region.

2. *Venous angiomas.* In this case we may speak of true varices of the spinal cord. At inspection during surgical intervention, the vessels are enlarged and they all contain venous blood. The lesions are much more

frequent in men than in women and it is possible that this particular type of vascular abnormality is similar to varicose veins of the lower extremities. Instances in which there is a great length of the enlarged vessels possibly may be examples of varicosities. Nine of the sixteen cases reported by Taveras and Dalton were classified as "venous anomalies" on surgical inspection.

3. *Arterial angiomas.* Arterial angiomas here, as elsewhere in the central nervous system, are very rarely encountered because they usually cause the blood to pass extremely rapidly through them and into the veins; the latter then become arterialized. It is probable that this designation is due to an error in the interpretation of the histological appearance because the veins have become arterialized, owing to the continued increased pressure through an arteriovenous malformation.

4. *Saccular aneurysms.* This is a rare entity and has been described in cases of coarctation of the aorta (Wyburn-Mason, 1944).

5. *Cavernous angiomas of the spinal cord.* These angiomas have a histological appearance similar to cavernous angiomas elsewhere. They partially replace the cord tissue, sparing many of the fibers, and for this reason may not lead to any significant neurologic findings until an episode of hemorrhage will lead to hematomyelia. In one instance of a centrally located hemangioma of the cord which bled, the myelogram revealed a normal cord without any widening and with normal anterior spinal vessels. Surgical intervention did not reveal any evidence of hematomyelia. The patient died, and autopsy disclosed a central hemorrhage within the cord in a cavernous angioma. In another instance, the angioma was demonstrated (fig. 593).

For the sake of completeness, it may be useful to mention here the so-called *epidural varices*, found in the lumbar region during disc operations. This used to be a frequent finding described at operation for intervertebral discs in years past, which was evidently due to the presence of dilated veins in the epidural space, probably associated with faulty positioning of the patient, with poor venous return, and consequent congestion of the epidural plexus leading to considerable hemorrhage at the time of operation. In the last six years at the Neurological Institute not a single case of epidural varices in the lumbar region has been described in over a thousand operations for lumbar herniated intervertebral discs.

On the other hand, *epidural angiomas* may be encountered, particularly in the thoracic and lower cervical regions, which may lead to spontaneous epidural hemorrhages. Clinically, the history is that of a sudden hemorrhage producing acute pain and neurologic findings indicative of cord compression. Myelography demonstrates an epidural lesion, and the diagnosis may be suggested because of the combination of an epidural lesion with the clinical findings of sudden onset.

The vascular malformations of the spinal cord cannot be diagnosed by plain films and can only be suspected or diagnosed by myelography. Because the convoluted radiolucent shadows are not usually clearly visible at fluoroscopy, it is indispensable to obtain adequate spot film coverage of the entire spinal canal at least in the anteroposterior projection when performing myelography. It is not sufficient to describe the absence of a block during a barium enema to rule out disease of the colon, and it is not possible to rule out disease of the intraspinal contents by fluoroscopy alone. Many neurologic syndromes suggestive of disease of the spinal cord go undiagnosed clinically because of our inadequate means of diagnosis at the moment. Myelography is a fairly sensitive method to diagnose spinal cord disease and, when performed carefully, our accuracy improves.

Syringomyelia. Intramedullary gliosis with degenerative excavation (syringomyelia), which usually begins about the central canal, occurs most commonly in the cervical region. The gliosis is irregular in distribution and pathologically, the lesions frequently have a serpentine form which extends longitudinally for a considerable distance in the spinal cord. The fluid-filled cavities vary in size from the microscopic to those several centimeters in diameter.

When large cavities develop, the spinal cord becomes enlarged and soft, but the cavity may develop without producing enlargement of the spinal cord, or at least atrophy or shrinkage occurs at a later date so that there is no gross enlargement of the outside diameter of the cord.

Syringomyelia ordinarily is a disease of the early part of life, in which event it may be considered as a developmental malformation or myelodysplasia. Some pathologists, on the contrary, regard the process as a benign neoplasia of glial tissue in which ependymal cells play a prominent part. Syringomyelia frequently is found in association with congenital anomalies, congenital diseases, and intramedullary tumors. The lesion is rarely associated with extramedullary neoplasm. Syringomyelia may result from disturbances of the circulation of the spinal cord either caused by vascular occlusion or by embarrassment of the circulation such as may be produced by extrinsic pressure.

At myelography, the spinal cord frequently appears normal or slightly atrophic, when the changes are microscopic. Characteristically, when gross cysts are present, the myelographic findings resemble those of an intramedullary spinal cord tumor. The spinal cord may be expanded in a fusiform manner or uniformly expanded so that in both frontal and lateral projections, the shadow of the cord is increased in diameter (fig. 677). The spinal cord may fill the arachnoid sac over many segments and obliterate almost completely the subarachnoid space. The radiopaque material is distributed in narrow streaks at the circumference of the subarachnoid space, and it is necessary to make certain that a subdural injection of the contrast substance has not taken place because the appearance resembles subdural injection. Rarely, localized cystlike collections of fluid are present which may present on one surface of the spinal cord and project beyond it into the subarachnoid space, with the result that the myelographic deformity resembles that associated with an extramedullary intradural tumor.

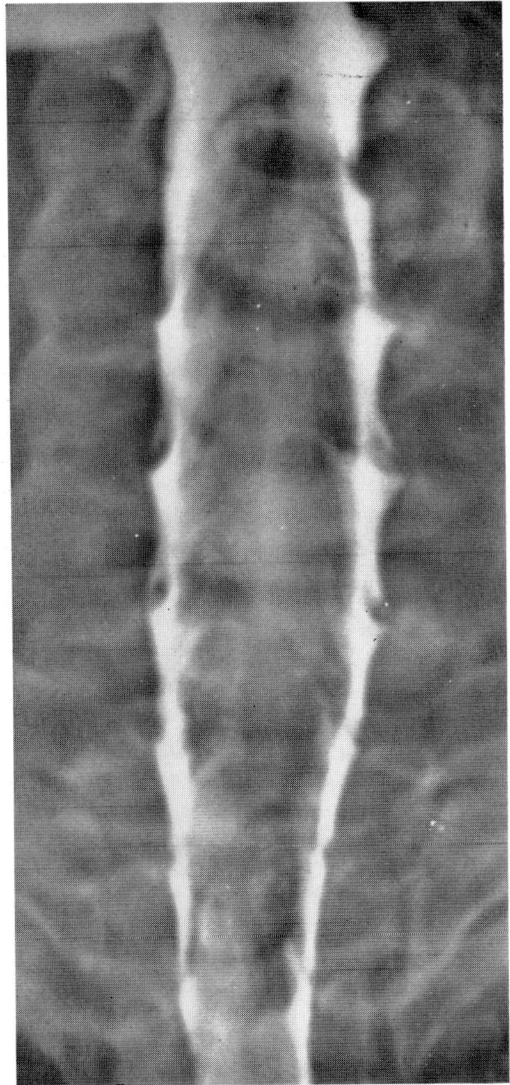

FIG. 677.—SYRINGOMYELIA WITH EXPANSION OF THE SPINAL CORD

There is marked uniform widening of the spinal cord extending from the upper cervical region to the lower thoracic region. Enlargement over such a great length is seen more often in patients with hydromyelia than syringomyelia.

Hydromyelia. This is a simple dilatation of the central canal of the spinal cord analogous to hydrocephalus. The whole or only a part of the spinal cord may be affected. Hydromyelia may be developmental, resulting from delayed closure of the neural tube, or it may be found in association with a variety of other lesions. The central canal is filled with clear fluid, and the spinal cord may be

(*Revised 1963*)

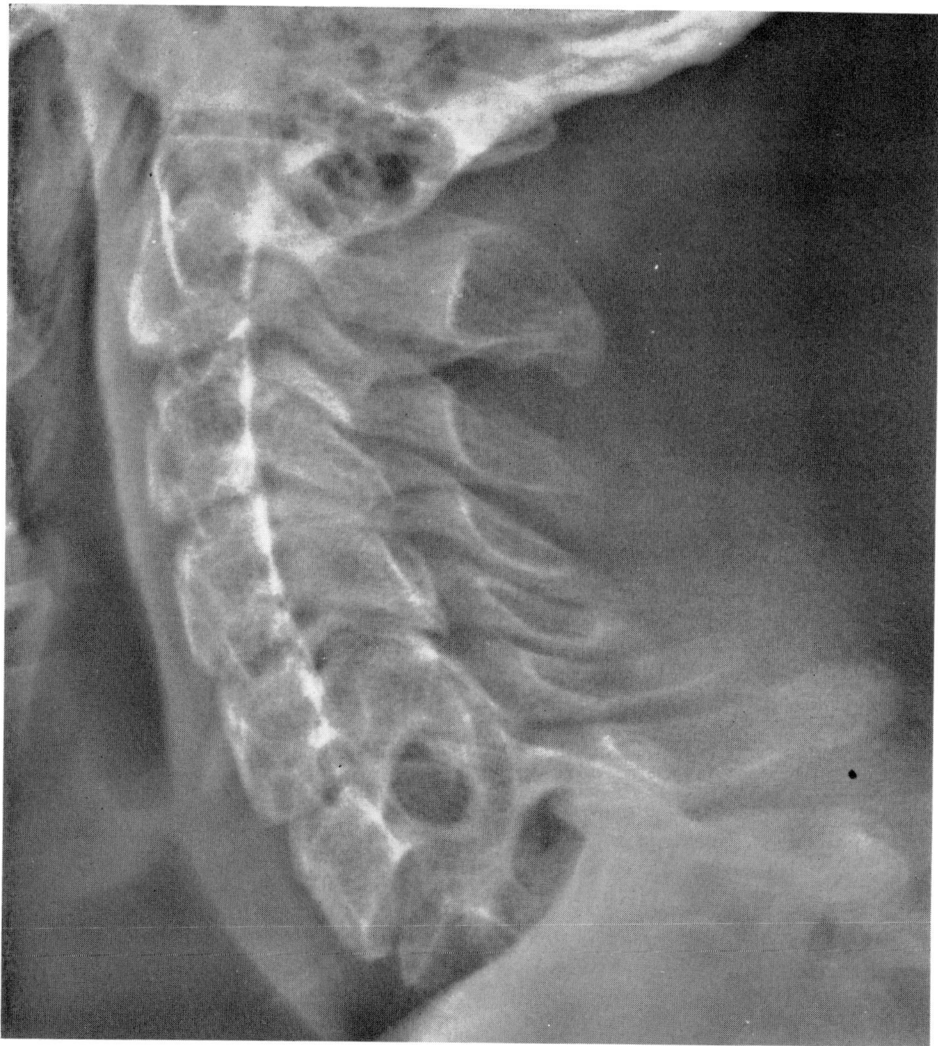

Fig. 678.—Wide Anteroposterior Diameter of Cervical Canal in Patient with Syringomyelia

There is a wide anteroposterior diameter of the canal which measures a minimum of 25 mm. and there is a relative increase in the height of the vertebral bodies in comparison with their anteroposterior diameter. There is also an upper dorsal kyphosis with increased lordotic curve of the cervical region.

enlarged throughout its length. The myelographic findings may vary. With the patient upright, the spinal cord may appear small and atrophic. In the horizontal or Trendelenburg position, the spinal cord may appear markedly widened when outlined by Pantopaque, as in Figure 677. Occasionally, the central canal of the spinal cord may communicate openly at the medullary junction, with the result that Pantopaque may enter and outline the central canal.

(Revised 1963)

Plain film findings are sometimes seen in patients with hydromyelia as well as syringomyelia associated with cord enlargement. The plain film findings consist usually of an increased lordotic curve of the cervical region and an increase in the width of the anteroposterior diameter of the spinal canal. The vertebral bodies are narrow in their anteroposterior diameter and are relatively high (fig. 678). The increased lordosis may be secondary to muscle weakness.

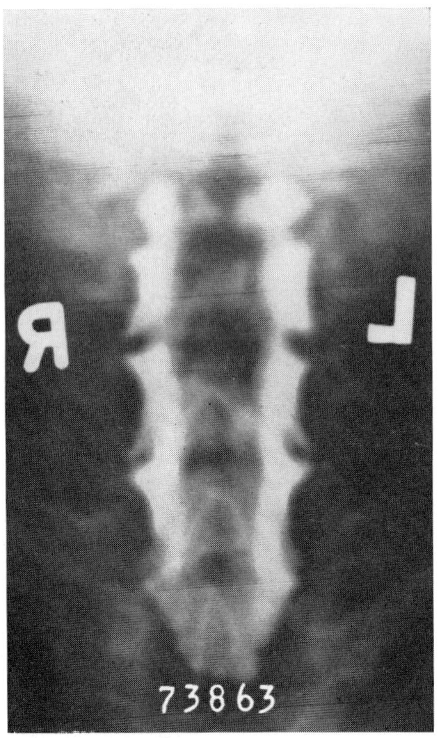

FIG. 679.—SPINAL CORD ATROPHY
The width of the spinal cord is less than 50 per cent of the diameter of the subarachnoid space at C5, 6 and 7, which is below average in this region. The collections of Pantopaque beside the spinal cord are considerably wider than usual.

Spinal cord atrophy. Moderately severe or marked spinal cord atrophy, regardless of the etiology, may be demonstrated by myelography. The lesion is most frequently demonstrated myelographically in the cervical region with Pantopaque myelography, but it may also be seen in the thoracic region. Air myelography, however, is more satisfactory to demonstrate cord atrophy in the thoracic region. The width of the spinal cord can be measured accurately in frontal myelograms. The measurements obtained for any particular patient may be compared with the average, normal measurement, or the relative width of the spinal cord to the interpediculate distance, as measured on the same film, may be determined. Throughout the greater part of the cervical and thoracic areas, the width of the spinal cord is approximately one-half the width of the vertebral canal, as determined by measuring the distance between the most medial portions of the vertebral pedicles (see p. 1.806). When the width of the spinal cord is reduced considerably below the average, a roentgen diagnosis of spinal cord atrophy is justified (fig. 679). The width of the spinal cord is best determined by outlining the subarachnoid space with radiopaque medium. An unusually wide collection of radiopaque material occurs on each side of the atrophic spinal cord. The thickness of the spinal cord in the cervical region frequently can be satisfactorily estimated by gas myelography, as explained above. When laminagraphy is used in combination with gas myelography, artifacts may be produced which suggest cord atrophy when the spinal cord is not exactly parallel to the plane of the laminagraphic cut. Local areas of cord thinning should not be diagnosed as cord atrophy, unless confirmed by more than one film, including also stereoscopic lateral views.

Atrophy of the spinal cord may be the result of degenerative disease, vascular occlusion, prolonged compression, or postradiation myelitis.

Extramedullary Intradural Lesions

Meningiomas. The tumors, which are thought to arise from nidi of arachnoid cells implanted in the dura mater, are encountered most frequently in the thoracic region in female patients over the age of 40 years. Together with neurinomas, they form the vast majority of extramedullary intradural tumors and constitute between 60 and 70 per cent of all primary neoplasms of the vertebral canal. Meningiomas are firm growths which discretely compress and displace the spinal cord. Usually meningiomas are adherent to the dura over a broad surface.

Unfortunately, plain spine film changes resulting from meningiomas are demonstrable in less than 10 per cent of cases. Evidence of erosion of bone from pressure usually is slight, and only a single pedicle may be involved. Mere thinning of the cortical bone that forms the medial margin of the pedicle may be present. A relative, rather than an actual, abnormal increase in interpediculate measurements may be demonstrated, which makes roentgen diagnosis uncertain.

On rare occasions, *psammomatous meningiomas* contain sufficient calcium to be directly demonstrable in plain spine roentgenograms. The visible calcification appears as an ovoid irregular shadow in the vertebral canal, which results from the conglomeration of a multitude of small lime deposits in psammoma bodies of the tumor (fig. 670). Sometimes the anteroposterior and lateral views may not demonstrate the calcification, whereas a lateral laminagram may show them well. Whenever a macroscopic deposit of calcium is present within the vertebral canal, the likelihood of a meningioma is strongly suspected (Gray, 1942). Degenerative calcium plaques that occur in the dorsal portion of the spinal meninges are frequently encountered at necropsy. These calcifications are probably too thin to be visible through the surrounding bony structures in the majority of instances, since they do not give rise to problems in differential diagnosis for meningioma. Calcified herniated intervertebral discs, which rarely occur in the thoracic region, must be considered in the differential diagnosis. Calcification with meningioma is most often seen in the center of the vertebral canal and is not necessarily at the level of the intervertebral disc space. Calcified intervertebral discs are lenticular in contour, more homogeneously calcified than meningioma, and based along the intervertebral space. Calcific degeneration in the intervertebral disc space with thinning of the disc space at the level of the herniation may be present.

Neurinomas. These, which are called also schwannomas and neurilemomas, presumably arise from the nerve sheath cells of Schwann. The tumors are encountered in almost equal frequency in the cervical, thoracic, and lumbar areas. Neurinomas occur equally often in men and women, and, on the average, patients with neurinomas are younger than those who harbor meningiomas. While meningiomas and neurinomas occasionally may be confused even on gross inspection, neurinomas differ from meningiomas in that they are soft in consistency, often cystic, and usually do not make as deep an impression in the spinal cord as meningiomas. Neurinomas usually are attached to the posterior nerve roots and rarely are adherent to the dura. As a rule, nerve sheath tumors are smoother and larger than meningiomas and may be multiple.

(Revised 1963)

Bone changes in plain spine radiographs are caused four times as often by neurinomas as by meningiomas, but it should be emphasized that plain film changes are found in only advanced cases. Enlargement of the vertebral canal, erosion of pedicles, increase in interpediculate distances, scalloping of the posterior margins of the vertebral bodies, and thinning of laminae are changes frequently encountered. As contrasted with meningioma, atrophy of bone, when present, is usually more clearly defined and more extensive, two vertebrae often being affected. Neurinomas of the cauda equina, may attain a tremendous size, extending throughout the entire length of the lumbar subarachnoid space. The nerve sheath tumors, as well as ependymomas, are referred to as "giant tumors" of the cauda equina under such circumstances. In plain spine radiographs, the changes caused by giant ependymomas and giant neurinomas of the cauda equina may be indistinguishable. More marked atrophy of the pedicles and laminae has been observed with neurinomas than with ependymomas in advanced cases, but statistically, ependymomas more commonly produce the diffuse areas of bone erosion and thinning of several segments than neurinomas.

Certain specific roentgen changes in plain spine films may be of diagnostic value for differentiation of meningioma and neurinoma. Neurinomas do not calcify, while meningiomas of the psammomatous type may contain grossly visible accumulations of calcium. Neurinomas, while remaining encapsulated, may extend out of the vertebral canal with the spinal nerve root and grow also in the paraspinal area. Such dumbbell neurinomas usually enlarge the intervertebral foramen (fig. 669), which is strong evidence for the diagnosis of neurinoma. A rounded soft tissue mass demonstrated in the paraspinal area, in association with

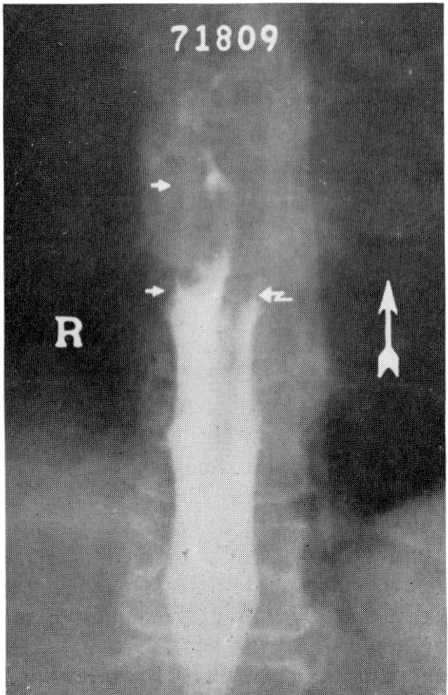

FIG. 680.—MENINGIOMA, T7
The oval tumor (*arrows*) in the right side of the subarachnoid space attached laterally to the meninges, is sharply outlined by Pantopaque. The spinal cord is displaced to the left and it is compressed (*wavy arrow*).

enlargement of the vertebral canal, also is strong evidence in favor of neurinoma and unfavorable for the diagnosis of a tumor of any other type.

In some instances, the extravertebral part of a neurinoma is extremely large, frequently many times the size of its intraspinal component (fig. 668). The extravertebral portion of the tumor, when it is large, can be depicted in plain roentgenograms of the cervical and lumbosacral areas as an extraneous soft tissue mass which may displace normal structures. In the thoracic region, small paraspinal masses may be demonstrable because they are outlined by contact with air-containing lung. Large tumors occurring in the thoracic region may erode the posterior ends of one or more ribs, and the intercostal space between two affected ribs may be widened appreciably.

At myelography, the extramedullary and intradural tumors are easy to distinguish. They produce a sharply circumscribed defect in the oil column with or without complete block to the flow of Pantopaque. The upper margin of the defect may be cuplike, usually concave upward because the oil is usually arrested below the level of the tumor. The spinal cord is always displaced from its normal position. If the tumor is laterally placed, the cord will be displaced sideways against the opposite margin of the vertebral canal (fig. 680). If the tumor is situated ventrally, it will displace the spinal cord dorsally and, vice versa if dorsally situated it will displace the spinal cord ventrally (figs. 681 and 682). If the tumor is situated exactly in the midline, either ventral or dorsal, the myelographic picture will be that of a centrally placed defect which suggests the lower half of a fusiform widening produced by an intramedullary tumor. This mistake is easily avoided by taking a lateral prone film which will show the shadow of the spinal cord displaced either dorsally or ventrally, whichever is the case (figs. 681 and 682). The importance of taking two radiographs at right angles to each other, usually a spot anteroposterior film and a lateral prone film, cannot be overemphasized. If the tumor is ventrolateral or dorsolateral in location, the spinal cord would be displaced lateralward as well as ventrad or dorsad.

Displacement is not a feature of the *intramedullary tumors* which are centered to the spinal canal both in the anteroposterior and in the lateral prone films (fig. 672). The latter is the most important single distinguishing diagnostic point in differentiating between intramedullary and extramedullary intradural lesions. It is only rarely that an intramedullary tumor is situated sufficiently to one side of the organ to produce an exophytic mass that will displace the cord itself.

The cord is usually compressed and thinned out almost to a ribbon in the area adjacent to the intradural extramedullary neoplasms. In patients with tumors located below the lower end of the spinal cord, frontal myelograms show the outline of spinal nerve roots displaced lateralward by the neoplasm and lateral projections may

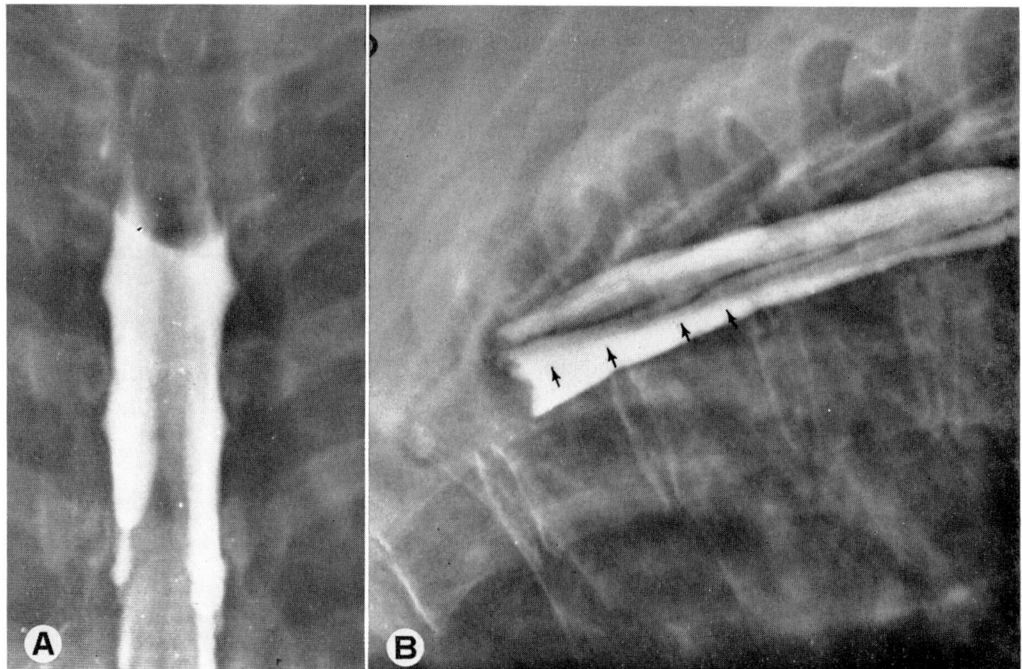

FIG. 681.—VENTRALLY PLACED EXTRAMEDULLARY AND INTRADURAL NEOPLASM (MENINGIOMA)
In the frontal projection (A), the defect is situated in the center of the canal and might suggest an intramedullary tumor. The lateral projection (B), however, shows that the spinal cord is displaced dorsally. A triangle of Pantopaque is seen on the ventral side (*arrows*) with a radiolucent band representing the cord on the dorsal side.

show ventral or dorsal displacement of the cauda equina roots. Where the spinal cord is present, a triangle of Pantopaque is formed on the side where the tumor is located. It is not uncommon to find two radiolucent defects at the upper margin of the Pantopaque where the block occurs. The tumor is situated where the triangular configuration of the Pantopaque shadow is present, and the cord is on the other side (figs. 681 and 682). Intradural, extramedullary tumors in the region of the foramen magnum are usually meningiomas, commonly ventrally placed; rarely are they dorsal to the spinal cord. The cord is usually displaced laterally or dorsally or both. Care should be taken to pass the oil through the foramen magnum and over the clivus (fig. 681C, D, and E). If air is injected immediately after Pantopaque myelography, the dorsal aspect of the lesion may be seen in some cases. The position of the spinal cord can be demonstrated by this method (fig. 681F). Air myelography is superior to Pantopaque in demonstration of dorsally placed masses, but these can also be demonstrated with radiopaque substances if there is a block at the foramen magnum. Some of the cases of dorsally placed masses in the region of the foramen magnum may be herniated tonsils, such as may be seen in the Arnold-Chiari malformation (fig. 655).

Neurofibromatosis. Neurofibromas are nerve sheath tumors which principally differ from neurinomas in that nerve fibers are found passing through them. The histologic appearance of a neurofibroma, otherwise is much like that of an ordinary nerve sheath tumor, although the connective tissue fiber content is high and the pattern somewhat irregular. Neurofibromas are found most commonly in cases of von Recklinghausen's disease where the tumors are multiple. In neurofibromatosis the nerve sheath tumors

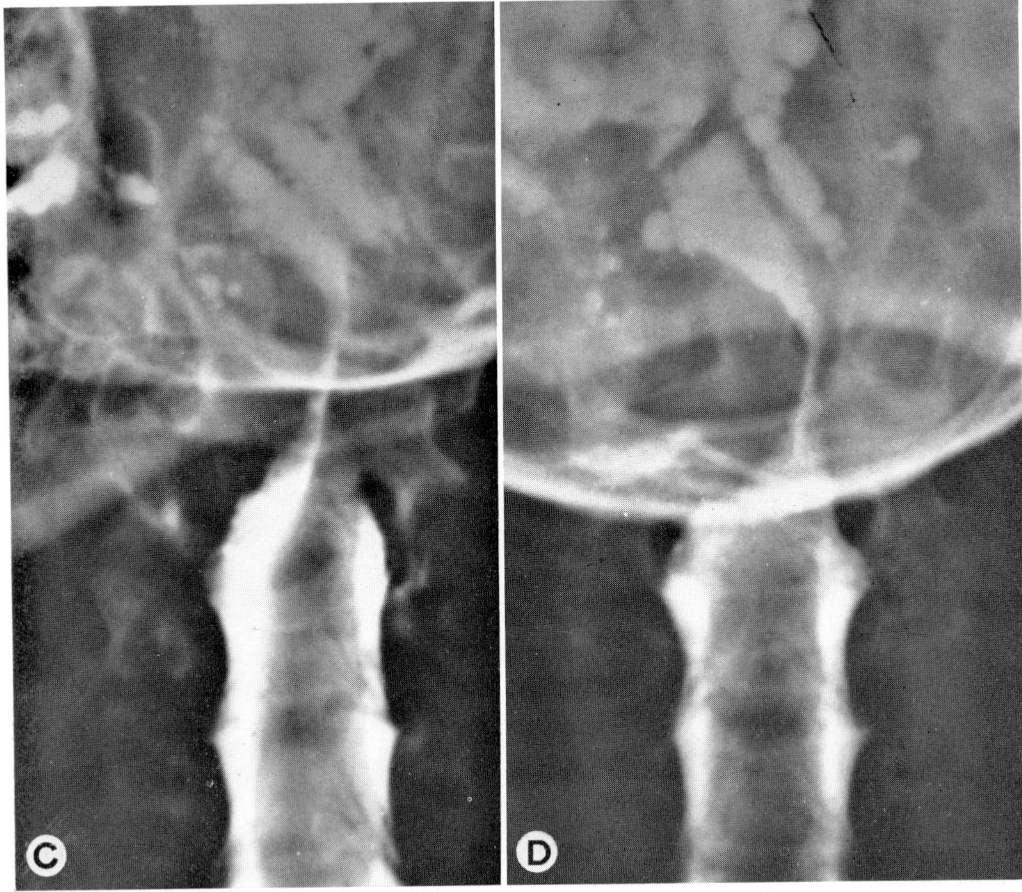

FIG. 681 (*Cont.*).—FORAMEN MAGNUM MENINGIOMA

In the oblique projection (C) of the foramen magnum an indentation is noted which is concave toward the face, similar to that normally observed at C1; however, the indentation is deeper and broader than usual. In the frontal projection (D), unilateral defect can be seen in the region of the entrance of the Pantopaque into the skull. The lateral projection (E) demonstrates only an excessively elevated appearance of the Pantopaque oil column in the region of the foramen magnum; this is to be expected with a unilaterally placed mass.

may occur in association with a neoplasm of some other type. Congenital malformations within and outside of the central nervous system may be encountered.

Vertebral changes, resulting from pressure by the tumors, are not observed as frequently in neurofibromatosis as with a single neurinoma. When neurofibromas arise intrathecally from spinal nerve roots in von Recklinghausen's disease, there is often a multitude of small tumors, bilaterally placed, which may be found over great lengths of the spinal cord. Usually none of the tumors is sufficiently large to erode the bone. Congenital malformations of one or more segments of the vertebral column may be present which should not be mistaken for atrophy of bone resulting from pressure by the tumors. Separate bilateral paraspinal masses which result from two large tumors of dumbbell shape, may be observed in rare instances in plain spine radiographs, which warrants the diagnosis of multiple neurofibromata.

Myelography will establish the presence of multiple neurofibromas arising from the

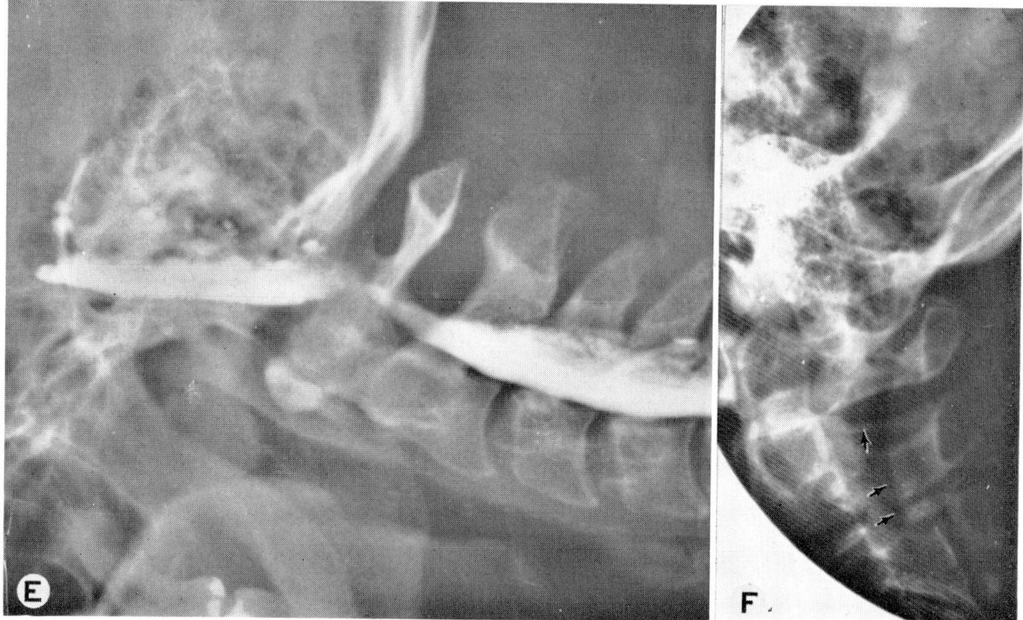

Fig. 681 (*Cont.*).—Ventrally Placed Tumor Displacing the Spinal Cord Dorsally (Meningioma)

(F) The tumor is faintly visualized (*upper arrow*). The spinal cord is displaced dorsally (*lower arrows*) and it is markedly flattened and pressed against the posterior arch of the atlas.

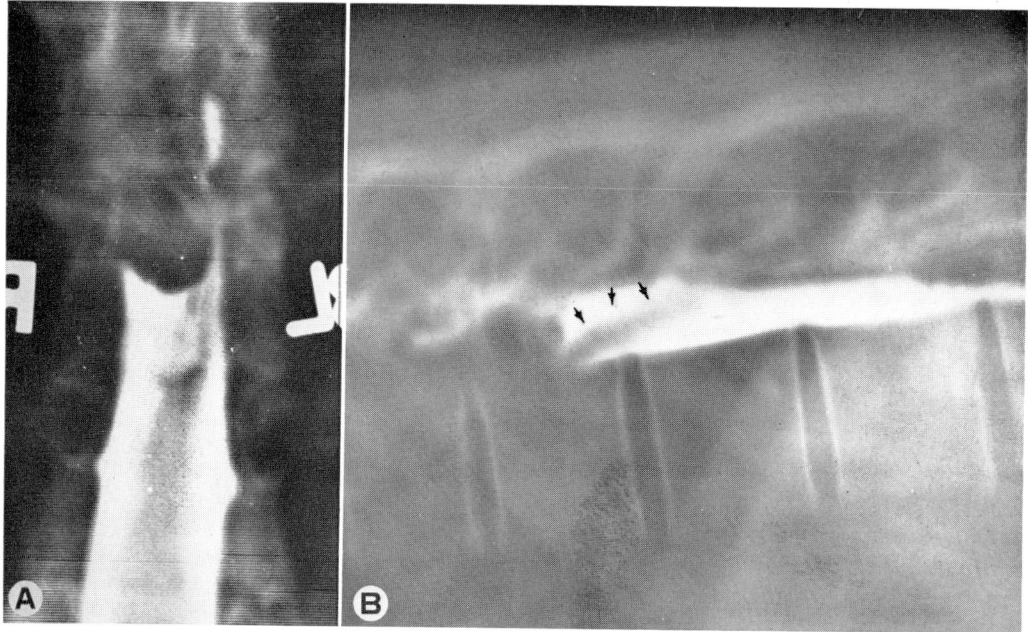

Fig. 682.—Dorsally Placed Extramedullary and Intradural Tumor (Meningioma)

As in the preceding figure, the defect in the frontal projection is situated in the center of the canal, and might be mistaken for an intramedullary tumor (A). In the lateral prone film (B), the radiolucent shadow of the spinal cord is displaced ventrally, and a triangle of Pantopaque is seen on the dorsal side, the side of the tumor (*arrows*).

(*Revised 1963*)

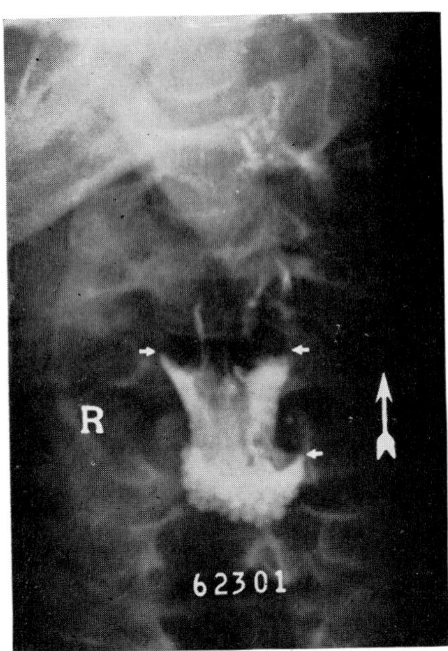

FIG. 683.—VON RECKLINGHAUSEN'S DISEASE
On each side of the oil column, concavities are present which represent the margins of multiple neurofibromas (*arrows*). The spinal cord is in the midline, and it is compressed between bilateral tumors.

spinal nerve roots in von Recklinghausen's disease. Several tumors may be found, widely scattered in the subarachnoid space, in which event changes in the myelogram at each individual level of involvement are similar to those found in solitary neurinoma. The more typical change, however, is the presence of a multitude of small tumors which cause filling defects of various size in the contrast outline of the subarachnoid space. The filling defects characteristically are bilateral and symmetrically situated in the lateral portions of the subarachnoid cavity where the tumors are attached to the spinal nerve roots (fig. 683). When multiple symmetrical tumors are present on each side of the spinal cord, the outline of the spinal cord in the myelogram is not displaced in any one direction, but it may be compressed centrally between the laterally situated tumors.

Dermoid and epidermoid tumors. These constitute a small percentage of new growths involving the spinal cord. The majority of the tumors are extramedullary and intradural and are well encapsulated lesions of the subarachnoid space. Some of the tumors are adherent to the medial surface of the spinal cord and occasionally they may occur within the substance of the spinal cord as intramedullary tumors. Only rarely are such tumors extradural in location (Gross, 1934). Spinal epidermoids, like similar congenital tumors occurring elsewhere in the body, are composed of epidermal elements while the dermoids contain tissue of the corium, or dermis, as well. Tumors of each type occur with about equal frequency. The tumors may be located in any part of the subarachnoid space from the upper cervical region to the sacrum. A rather high incidence of the lesions is found in the region of the conus medullaris and cauda equina. An epidermoid is smooth, white, and soft because of its cystic interior, which is filled with white, caseous, and crumbly desquamated, keratinized epithelium. The dermoid differs from the epidermoid in that the central cyst also contains hair.

Ordinarily dermoids and epidermoids cause no demonstrable changes in plain spine radiographs. Rarely the tumors may cause atrophy of the vertebral pedicles and laminae and an increase in the interpediculate measurements (Naffziger and Jones, 1935). The tumors do not extend outside of the vertebral canal and do not contain calcium. At myelography, the tumors cannot be differentiated from neurinomas since ordinarily the lesions are well encapsulated, and discretely outlined by the contrast material in the subarachnoid space. There is an obstruction to the flow of the contrast material, which is usually incomplete, and the spinal cord or cauda equina is displaced by the tumor (fig. 684). The presence of other congenital anomalies, such as spina bifida, pilonidal sinus, an area of hypertrichosis, telangiectasis, and subcutaneous lipoma, may suggest the possibility of an epidermoid or dermoid of the spinal cord. In children, the presence of a small, draining sinus in the midline should always suggest the possibility of an intrathecal epidermoid.

(Revised 1963)

Lipomas. These form a small group of tumors which, for some unknown reason, involve almost exclusively the lower cervical and upper thoracic portions of the spinal cord. The majority of tumors reported are extramedullary and intradural although several intramedullary lipomas and a number of extradural lipomas have been recorded (Stookey, 1927). The tumors are encountered in patients in the first or second decade of life. The lesion extends over a number of vertebral segments and evidence of enlargement of the vertebral canal may be seen in three or more vertebrae in plain spine roentgenograms (fig. 667). This is of diagnostic importance because, aside from the large tumors of the cauda equina and the congenital cysts, which also occur in the thoracic region in young individuals, it is unusual for a tumor to affect more than two vertebrae in its growth. The tumors do not contain sufficient adult fat to be radiologically demonstrable because of diminished density, as may occur with intracerebral lipomas. At myelography, a tumor with extramedullary intradural characteristics is encountered most often or a fusiform expansion of the spinal cord is demonstrated if the tumor is intramedullary.

Metastatic gliomas. Metastatic gliomas of the spinal cord extend by way of the cerebrospinal fluid circulation from primary tumors of the brain. Cairns and Russell (1931) emphasize the fact that many types of primary intracerebral tumors, both supratentorial and infratentorial, may give rise to spinal cord metastases. The brain tumors which most frequently give rise to spinal implants are glioblastoma multiforme, medulloblastoma, and ependymoma. Of the three, medulloblastoma is the most common, in our experience. In one instance, a patient with a hemangioblastoma of the cerebellum who had a recurrence appeared to have developed implants in the lumbar region (Wood *et al.*, 1953). The metastatic lesions usually are multiple, may occur at any level of the spinal cord or cauda equina, and most commonly appear as nodular masses firmly attached to the spinal cord surface usually on the dorsal side. Sometimes a sheath of tumor on the dorsal side of the spinal cord is found which could be overlooked on myelography.

(*Revised 1963*)

Plain spine radiographs disclose no abnormality of the bony structures or soft tissues probably because the majority of the lesions are rapidly growing. At myelography, multiple round or oval filling defects in the contrast outline of the subarachnoid space are demonstrated because of nodular neoplastic masses on the surface of the spinal cord (figs. 685 and 686). The lesions may vary in size from the minute up to two or more cm. in diameter. The larger masses frequently cause an obstruction, more often incomplete, to the flow of the radiopaque material in the subarachnoid space. Im-

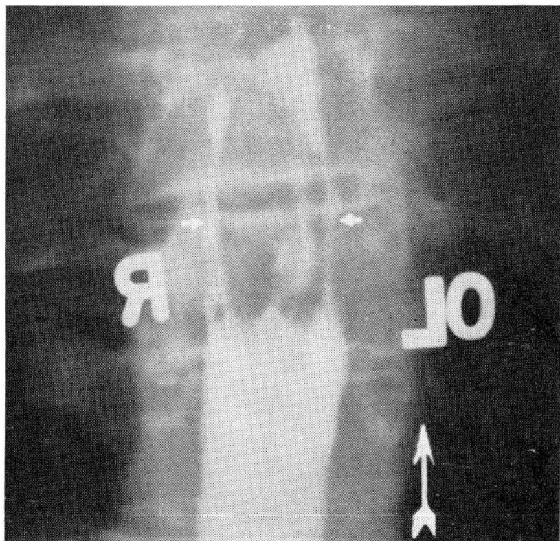

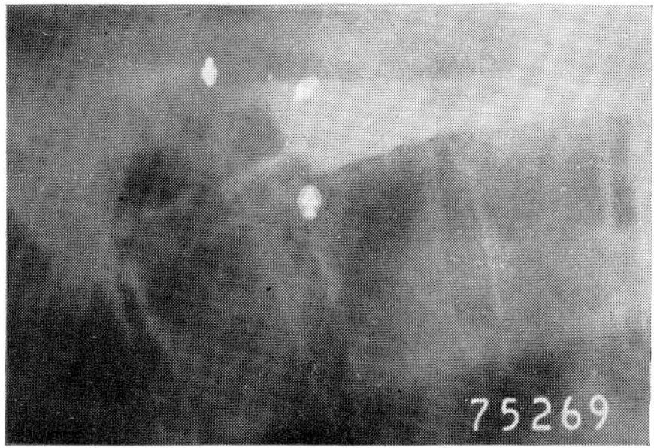

FIG. 684.—EPIDERMOID T8

In frontal view (A), the shadow of a dorsal midline tumor and the spinal cord are continuous (*arrows*), with the result that a fusiform enlargement of the cord, which occurs with intramedullary tumors, is simulated. The lateral film (B) shows that the spinal cord is displaced ventrally by the tumor (*arrows*). The widening of the spinal cord depicted in the frontal view is the result of compression and flattening of the cord.

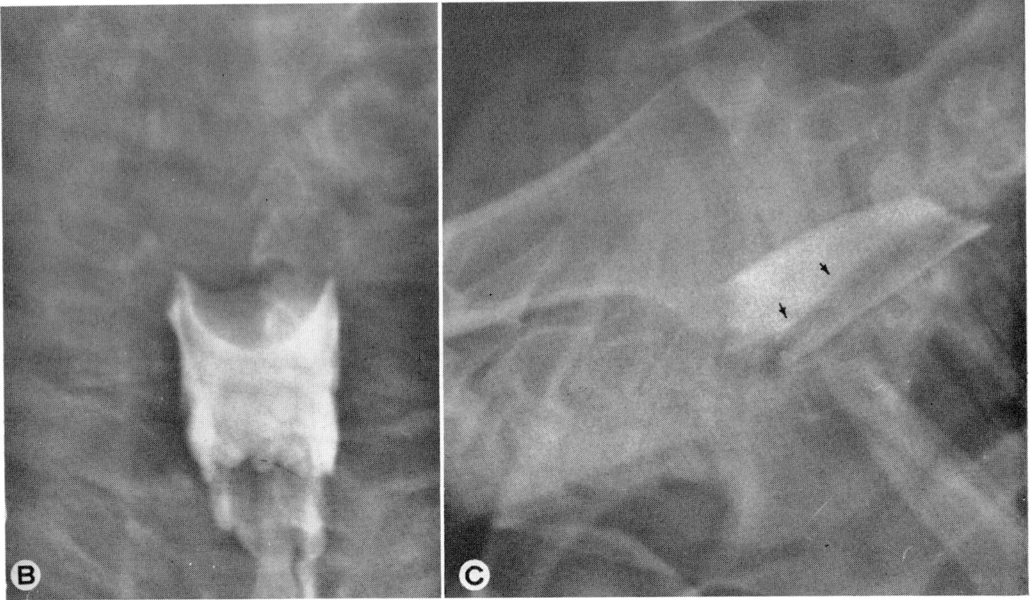

FIG. 684 (*Cont.*).—CONGENITAL INTRADURAL EXTRAMEDULLARY CYST

The patient was a 22-year-old girl; the frontal myelogram (C) shows a centrally placed but sharply circumscribed cuplike shadow indicative of an intradural mass. The shadow of the spinal cord is widened. The lateral projection (D) demonstrates marked ventral displacement of the spinal cord (*arrows*). These cysts are considered by some to be teratomatous in origin (Hoefnagel *et al.*).

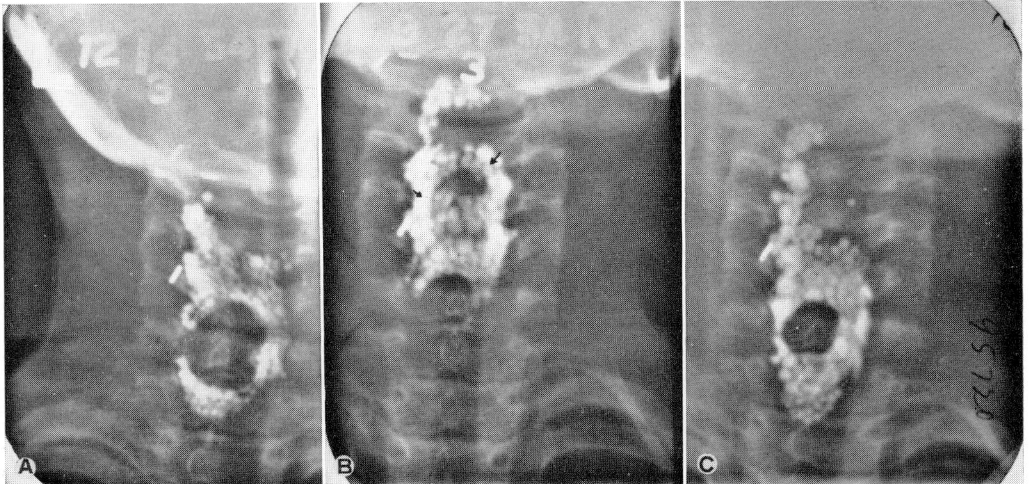

FIG. 685.—METASTATIC MEDULLOBLASTOMA TO THE CERVICAL SPINAL CORD

The initial examination shows a large nodular shadow in the cervical region. (A); similar shadows were demonstrated in other areas of the cord. Another radiolucency is faintly visualized cephalad to the first (B). A second myelogram (C), performed after the administration of radiation therapy, shows a decrease in size of the rounded defects, but not complete disappearance of the metastatic implants.

(Revised 1963)

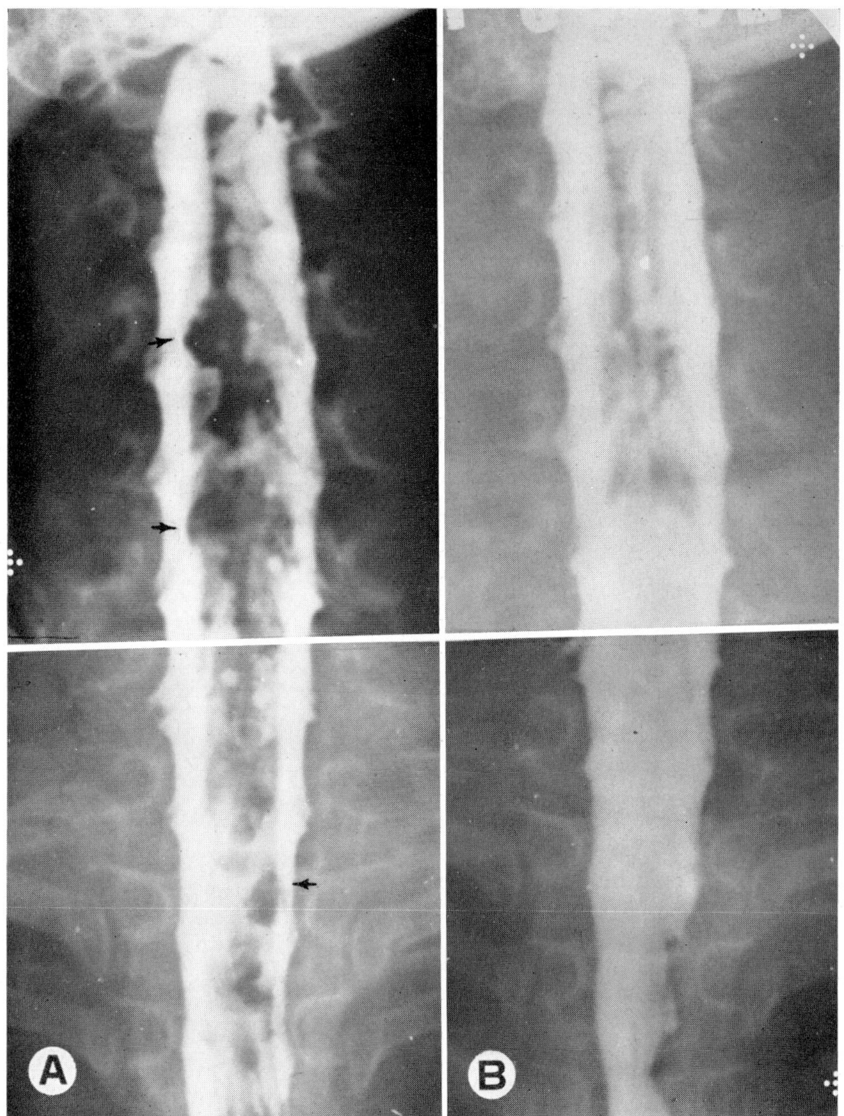

FIG. 686.—METASTATIC GLIOBLASTOMA OF THE SPINAL CORD
SHOWING RESPONSE TO RADIATION THERAPY

Myelograms (A) made nine months after incomplete removal of the intracranial tumor, disclose multiple, well defined, rounded filling defects in the Pantopaque outline of the subarachnoid space resulting from implantation of metastases upon the spinal cord (*arrows*). Myelography performed nineteen days later (B) reveals that the metastatic masses disappeared following the administration of 1000 r in air through fields directed toward the posterior aspect of the cervical and upper thoracic spine.

plants are sometimes not demarcated sharply from the outline of the spinal cord in the myelogram because the tumors characteristically invade the cord, with the result that the shadows blend. At other times they are very sharply outlined. In the majority of instances, the spinal cord is not displaced, which may be explained by the presence of multiple lesions on all sides of the cord which prevent gross movement in any one direction. The roots of the cauda equina, on the contrary, may be displaced and distorted to a considerable degree as they pass among the multiple neoplastic masses. In cases of metastatic medulloblastoma, the Pantopaque may be left in place in the canal and re-examination performed following radiation therapy to demonstrate effects of treatment as well as the possibility of future recurrence of the lesions (figs. 685 and 686).

Among the extramedullary intradural lesions should also be included arachnoiditis, arachnoidal adhesions and cysticerocosis (see under "Inflammatory Lesions," p. 1.857).

Extradural Lesions

The principal extradural lesions are: (1) primary neoplasms, (2) vertebral neoplasms that produce compression of the intradural contents, (3) abscesses and granulomas, (4) herniated intervertebral discs, (5) spondylosis, Paget's disease, and other conditions causing compression of the spinal cord or nerve roots.

Extradural Tumors

Extradural neoplasms of both benign and malignant character are encountered, although the vast majority are malignant. This situation differs from that of neoplasms occurring in the intradural extramedullary compartment, which are almost all benign. The malignant neoplasms may be primary within the vertebral canal or may metastasize from elsewhere. Primary extradural tumors, benign and malignant, may arise from the dura, from nerve roots external to the dura, from connective tissue, fat, blood vessels, lymphatic tissues, and other tissues resident in the epidural space.

Benign extradural tumors include meningiomas, neurinomas, fibromas, lipomas, dermoids or epidermoids, and vascular lesions. Benign tumors are encountered infrequently, however, in proportion to the occurrence of their intradural counterparts, and usually they have an intradural component that can be diagnosed as such by myelography. Except for the neurinomas, specific changes characteristic of the type of lesion present are not observed on the plain films. Erosion, with loss of well defined margins, of various portions of the vertebrae found in the vertebral canal may result from local pressure by the tumor. Extradural neurinomas frequently extend through one or more intervertebral foramina, which may be enlarged, and the lesions may be continuous with a large mass in the paraspinal region. Extradural meningiomas are much less common but may produce local erosion of vertebral pedicles, laminae, or bodies similar to that seen with intrathecal meningiomas. The extradural lipomas are composed of mature fat, which differs little from the areolar tissue of the epidural space. The lesions frequently are associated with spina bifida or some other anomaly of the vertebral column, as explained under congenital anomalies.

At myelography, benign extradural tumors cause an indentation of one margin of the opacified subarachnoid space. The indentation usually extends over one or two vertebral segments, depending on the size of the tumor. The greatest indentation of the radiopaque oil column is usually at the center of the defect with the caliber of the subarachnoid space returning by degrees toward normal above and below the lesion. The over-all appearance of the deformity simulates a triangle which is wide based laterally, ventrally, or dorsally. When the tumors are of sufficient size, the dural sac may be compressed and the subarachnoid space collapsed, with the result that the contrast outline of the subarachnoid cavity tapers to a point of complete obstruction (fig. 687). In some instances, the subarachnoid space is abruptly collapsed without tapering as a result of angulation of the dural sac and the spinal cord by tumor. These tumors are usually intradural as well as extradural, and less commonly they are strictly extradural, except in neurofibromatosis. Among the benign extradural masses should be included acute epidural hematomas resulting from hemorrhage from epidural angiomas. The clinical history is

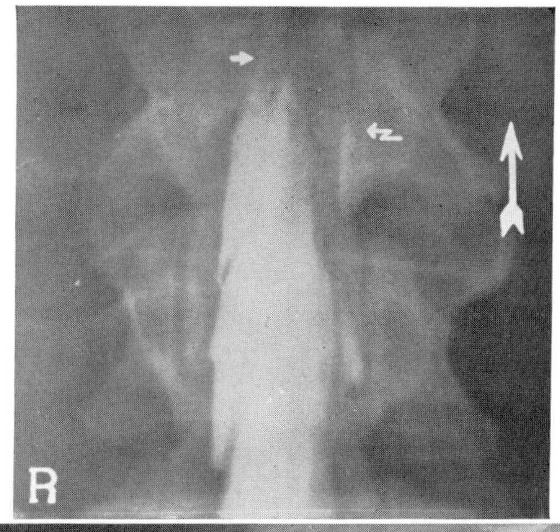

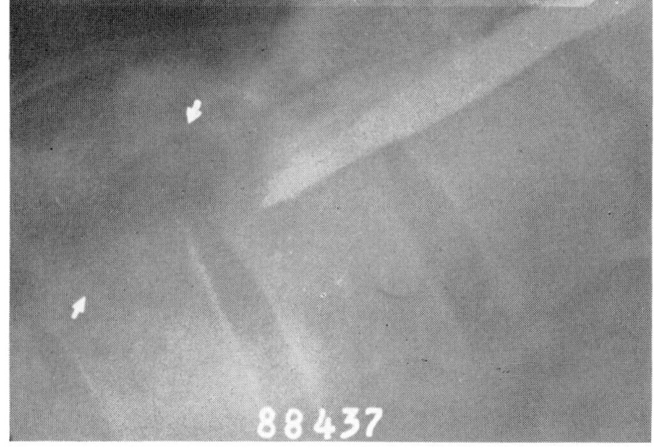

FIG. 687.—EXTRADURAL NEURINOMA T12 AND L1

In the frontal view the head of the radiopaque oil column tapers toward the left side to a point of obstruction at T12-L1 (*straight arrow*). The lower spinal cord and the higher cauda equina roots are displaced to the left, and they are compressed against the lateral wall of the vertebral canal (*wavy arrow*). The lateral film discloses that the obstruction to the cephalad passage of Pantopaque is at the inferior margin of a markedly enlarged intervertebral foramen (*arrows*). At operation, a neurinoma, wholly extradural, was found with a 4 cm. diameter extension through the T12-L1 intervertebral foramen.

usually that of an acute episode of back pain followed by signs of spinal cord compression.

Primary malignant epidural tumors most commonly are of lymphatic origin. Approximately 5 per cent of patients with lymphosarcoma, Hodgkin's disease, and leukemia originally present themselves because of symptoms resulting from involvement of the spinal cord and spinal nerve roots. Sarcomas originating in the vertebral canal from other than lymphatic tissues occur infrequently.

Extradural *sarcoma* ordinarily does not produce bony changes visible in plain spine roentgenograms. If the lesion has extended through one or more intervertebral foramina into the paraspinal soft tissues, a lateral convexity of the paraspinal shadow may be demonstrable. At myelography, a sweeping indentation of the radiopaque subarachnoid outline is demonstrated which is similar, in general, to the deformity encountered with benign extradural lesions. The deformity from malignant disease usually is more extensive and smoother in contour (fig. 688). Statistically, however, malignant lesions are much more common,

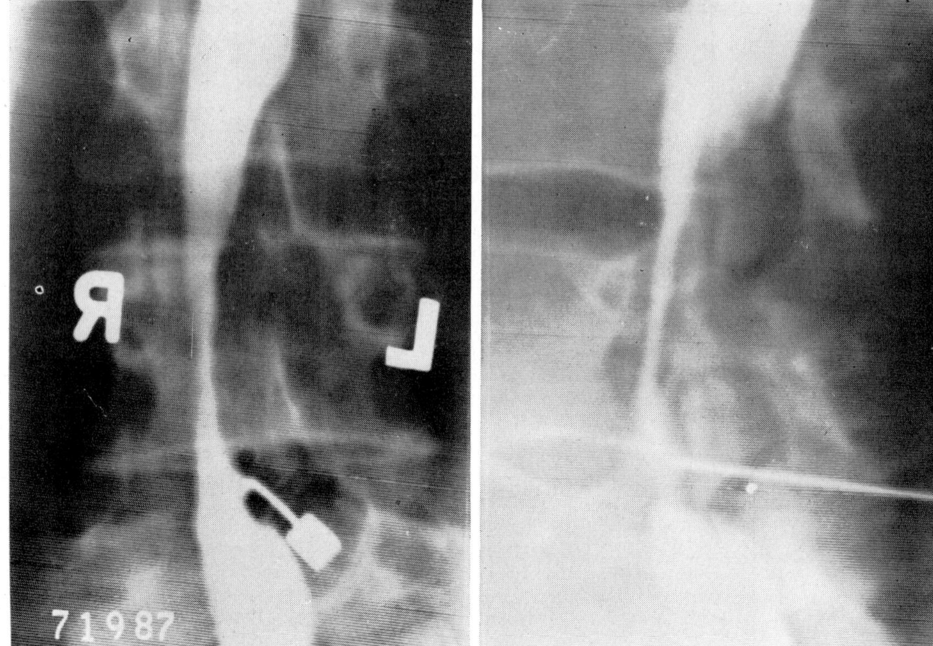

FIG. 688.—LYMPHOSARCOMA, L4

A sweeping deformity of the left dorsal aspect of the subarachnoid space is demonstrated. An extensive smooth, graded indentation of the radiopaque column suggests a large extradural mass, the most characteristic feature being the diminution in the diameter of the oil column.

particularly in the absence of any intradural component, and therefore, the diagnosis can usually be made accurately of a malignant extradural tumor. Frequently malignant masses encroach on the dorsal sac from more than one side, since the malignant neoplasm tends to encircle the dura. When the dural sac is surrounded by tumor, the contrast outline of the subarachnoid space is attenuated to a point of complete obstruction, and at this point the myelographic outline of the spinal cord may be visibly compressed. Deformities of the subarachnoid space usually are more abrupt at spinal cord levels since the dural sac may be angulated against the spinal cord by the tumor. Caudad to L1, elongated sweeping deformities of the radiopaque column may be present without complete collapse of the subarachnoid space. It may be difficult at times to differentiate an intramedullary tumor causing a block from an extradural encircling lesion in the thoracic area. If the head of the Pantopaque column at the block is carefully scrutinized, however, it will be noted that the right and left edges, or the dorsal and ventral edges, whichever is the case, will be displaced medially, toward the shadow of the cord. This is the opposite of intramedullary tumors causing a block which actually produce a slight widening of the column of Pantopaque at the point of the block (fig. 672). This may be an important differential diagnosis to make because in certain cases the neoplastic infiltration of the epidural tissues is so slight that it is actually microscopic and cannot be seen by the surgeon at the operating table without histologic examination. The myelographic appearance prior to operation in these cases would indicate that one is dealing with an extradural, and not an intramedullary lesion; correct diagnosis may prevent unnecessarily extensive exploration, opening of the dura, and needling of the spinal cord. This is one type of case where *intraosseous venography* may be of help in differentiating between an intramedullary and an extradural lesion because the extradural lesions usually produce a block to the upward venous flow.

Metastatic tumors of the epidural space may be either sarcomas or carcinomas. The majority of metastatic sarcomas are of the lymphoma group and frequently extend to the epidural space from the retropleural and retroperitoneal lymph nodes by way of the intravertebral foramina. With such lesions, paraspinal masses frequently may be observed in plain spine roentgenograms. Osteolytic or osteoblastic changes in one or more vertebrae are visible in about 20 per cent of patients with either lymphosarcoma or Hodgkin's disease. Osteogenic sarcoma may invade the epidural space from the vertebrae as may any primary or metastatic sarcoma of the spinal column. Osteolytic and osteoblastic changes may be observed in the vertebrae in plain spine radiographs and an adjacent paraspinal soft tissue tumor frequently is demonstrable, which indicates extraosseous extension of the neoplasm. At myelography the appearance of the deformity produced by metastatic sarcoma is no different from that produced by primary epidural malignant neoplasm, unless there is a pathologic vertebral fracture, which may result in an abrupt angulation and compression of the radiopaque column.

The vast majority of metastatic carcinomas of the epidural space originate either in the breast or the lung. Extradural carcinoma most commonly is a secondary extension from an involved vertebra, especially with metastasis from the breast. Metastatic carcinoma from the breast may produce osteolytic, osteoblastic, or mixed reactions in the involved vertebrae. Pathologic fracture of one or more vertebrae frequently is demonstrable in plain spine roentgenograms. Extension of bronchogenic carcinoma into the epidural space through the intervertebral foramina does occur with or without involvement of the vertebrae themselves. The vertebral change resulting from involvement by bronchogenic carcinoma is osteolysis. Often there is destruction of one-half of one or more vertebral bodies, the ipsilateral portions of the vertebral arches and the posterior portions of the adjacent ribs. A paravertebral soft tissue mass may be

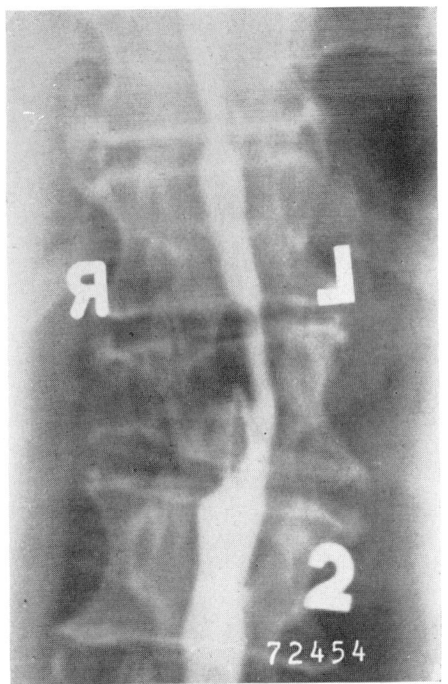

Fig. 689.—Metastatic Carcinoma, L-1 (Originating in the Breast)

A pathologic fracture of the body of L1 has occurred on the right side as a result of bone destruction by an osteolytic metastasis. Neoplastic tissue, which has extended into the epidural space, deforms the subarachnoid oil column on its lateral aspect.

visible in the involved area, or the lung carcinoma may be demonstrated in plain spine radiographs.

When the tumor encroaches on the epidural space from one side, the subarachnoid radiopaque column at myelography is indented and narrowed unilaterally. If there is unilateral collapse of one vertebra, lateral angulation of the subarachnoid oil column occurs at this level (fig. 689). Where extensive extradural growths occur, which cloak the dural sac, the arachnoid cavity is narrowed gradually to a point of obstruction beyond which the spinal cord itself is compressed. If the dural sac is encircled evenly, the spinal cord will remain in normal position (fig. 690). But when the major portion of epidural growth is on one side of the vertebral canal, contralateral displacement

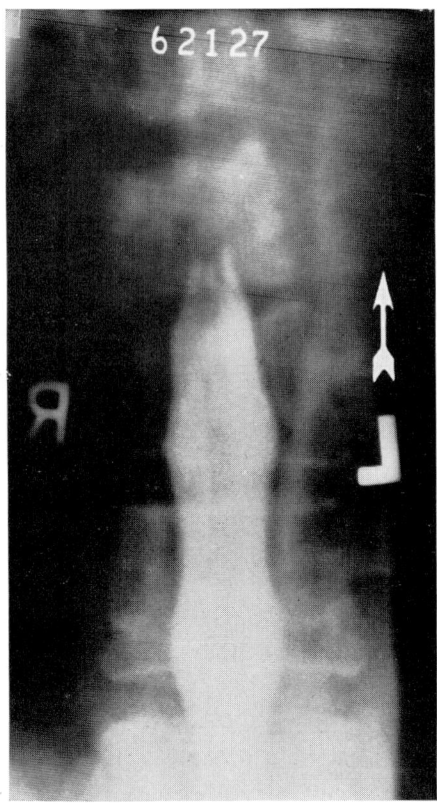

FIG. 690.—METASTATIC CARCINOMA, T9 (ORIGINATING IN THE BREAST)

The bodies of T8, 9 and 10 are involved by mixed osteolytic and osteoblastic metastases. An obstruction to the cephalad flow of Pantopaque results from neoplastic tissue filling the epidural space at T9 and constricting the dural sac by encirclement. The lateral margins of the radiopaque oil column taper toward the spinal cord, which remains in the midline.

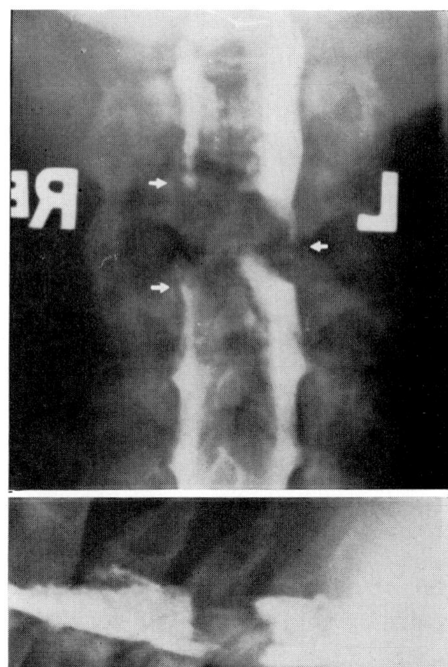

FIG. 691.—METASTATIC CARCINOMA, C4-5 (ORIGINATING IN THE LUNG)

A solitary intradural mass is present, the superior and inferior margins of which are well defined by Pantopaque. The left side of the subarachnoid space is widened as a result of displacement in the cervical spinal cord toward the right (*arrows*).

and compression of the spinal cord are demonstrable.

Extradural sarcoma, either primary or metastatic, does not extend through the dural membrane. Metastatic carcinoma, also, remains outside of the dural sac, as a rule. An exception is an occasional pulmonary carcinoma which may invade the dura and present on its internal surface, or even invade the spinal cord. In one such instance, a solitary tumor was demonstrated in the lateral portion of the subarachnoid space in the cervical region (fig. 691). The margins of the filling defect produced in the subarachnoid oil column are well defined and smooth. The spinal cord is displaced and compressed by the tumor against the contralateral side of the vertebral canal in a manner usually associated with benign tumors of the intrathecal spaces.

Intervertebral Disc Disease

Certain lesions of the vertebral column are of importance only, or primarily, because they involve the nervous system. Herniation of an intervertebral disc and osteoarthritis of the spine account for the majority of the complaints for which radiographic examination of this part of the body is carried out. A number of other lesions, belonging primarily in the category of diseases of the osseous system, such as osteitis deformans, hemangioma, and giant cell tumor, may have their chief clinical importance in neurologic involvement. Even malignant tumors which originate in vertebrae or which extensively involve the spinal column by metastases may manifest themselves only by compression of the spinal cord. The latter group of lesions is discussed in the section dealing with metastatic tumors of the epidural space. It is not the purpose of this chapter to describe individually each of the diseases of bone which may involve secondarily the spinal cord and spinal nerve roots. All of these lesions belong in the group of epidural lesions which, by virtue of their frequency, constitute by far the most frequent type of lesion encountered in the spinal canal which causes compression of nerve structures. As explained above in the description of intraspinal neoplasms, benign tumors are much more frequently encountered proportionately in the intradural extramedullary group, whereas the malignant tumors occur much more frequently in the epidural space, and benign tumors are uncommon in this space. However, other types of epidural lesions that compress nerve tissue, which are not neoplastic, abound in the epidural space as attested by the great frequency of herniated and protruding intervertebral discs.

Rupture of the intervertebral disc. Although fibrocartilaginous masses in the ventral portion of the vertebral canal which compress the spinal cord or nerve roots were recognized and successfully removed by surgery as early as 1909, the true nature of the lesions was first explained by Mixter and Barr in 1934. It is now generally agreed that trauma, single or repeated, exerted on a disc which has been weakened by degenerative changes, produces a rupture of the nucleus pulposus through the annulus fibrosus and protrusion or extrusion of intervertebral disc material into the vertebral canal.

Disc degeneration is a phenomenon of aging from normal wear and tear. It may occur in younger people who have instability of the vertebral column because of anatomic variations or congenital defects. The process is thought to begin with an exaggerated desiccation of the disc which is a normal tendency with advancing age. The nucleus pulposus becomes inelastic, then soft, following which fissures and erosions of the cartilaginous plate of the vertebrae occur. Fibrous tissue and blood vessels extend through the bone plates from the vertebrae into the intervertebral disc resulting in fibrosis, vascularization, and atrophy of the fibrocartilage. When the inelasticity of the disc is thus reduced by early or advanced degeneration, unusual forces applied to the spine may result in herniation of the intervertebral fibrocartilage into the vertebral canal and through the posterior longitudinal ligament. Occasionally, severe trauma will result in a rupture of an apparently healthy disc.

Herniation of the intervertebral disc may occur in any direction. Under pressure, the elastic nucleus pulposus becomes flattened and broadened, so that the resistant annulus fibrosus is displaced outward at the periphery. The lesions that are of clinical importance, however, are those which extend posteriorly or posterolaterally and compress the spinal cord or spinal nerve roots. Posterior ruptures most commonly result from force exerted on the spine in flexion (Bradford and Spurling, 1945).

Lumbar disc protrusions and herniations. Disc herniations occur most frequently in the lower lumbar and lower cervical regions. The intervertebral discs at L4–5 and L5–S1 are involved with almost equal frequency, while the L3–4 disc is less frequently subject to rupture. In the cervical region herniation of the disc at C5–6 or C6–7 most often is encountered. The more frequent occurrence of disc herniations at these levels is explained both by the strong force applied with the spine in flexion and the anatomic size and shape of the discs in these areas. The nucleus pulposus is especially well developed in the lumbar region. The intervertebral fibrocartilages in the lumbar and cervical regions are thicker in front than behind, which contributes to the ventral convexity of these portions of the vertebral column. In the thoracic region, the discs are nearly uniform in thickness and the dorsal convexity in this part of the spinal column results almost entirely from the shape of the vertebral bodies. Normally, the intervertebral discs increase progressively in thickness from T12 to L5, and to a less marked degree there is a relative increase in thickness of the cervical discs from C2 to C7. The lower cervical and lower lumbar portions of the spine have a relatively large proportion of the intervertebral disc material of the entire vertebral column, with the result that there is much greater freedom of movement here than elsewhere.

Plain spine roentgenograms may disclose few abnormalities as the result of a posterior intervertebral disc herniation. A common finding, however, is alteration of alignment of the vertebrae in the involved area. The ventral curve is usually reduced and may be absent in the cervical and lumbar region. Occasionally, the normal ventral curvature is reversed so that a slight dorsal angulation or convexity is present, usually maximum at the level of the lesion. Lateral angulation or scoliosis of the spine may be visible in frontal films. When lateral angulation is centered at one intervertebral level, it is strongly suggestive of intervertebral disc disease. This type of angulation should be differentiated from rotary scoliosis which is common in the lumbar region and is usually not associated with local disc disease. Rotary scoliosis is commonly of unknown origin or it may be associated with multiple disc disease.

The changes in vertebral curvature are the result of muscle spasm, which is an attempt, occurring by reflex, to shorten the course of the spinal nerve root involved and thereby reduce the tension on it.

Thinning of an intervertebral space is rarely present in acute disc herniation but is often observed as a result of degeneration of a disc without herniation. Since disc degeneration predisposes to rupture, however, narrowing of an intervertebral space may be interpreted as suggestive of a herniated disc if it is found at the appropriate level and when clinical examination discloses evidence of spinal cord or nerve root compression. The degree of disc thinning observed may be slight and may be detected only by comparison with the intervertebral spaces above and below. Marked narrowing of one disc space in the lumbar region is

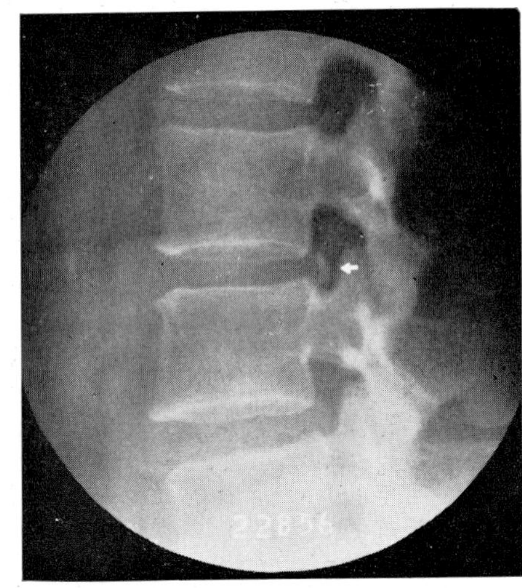

FIG. 692.—HERNIATED INTERVERTEBRAL DISC L3-4
Calcium deposited at the periphery of a herniated fibrocartilage appears as a ventrally concave, curvilinear shadow posterior to the intervertebral disc space. Calcium deposition suggests long-standing disease.

suggestive of herniation at that level, but by itself does not justify a diagnosis of this condition because simple disc degeneration or other diseases, *e.g.*, tuberculosis, may be responsible for the same appearance. It is also not rare to find that there is marked disc narrowing whereas myelography reveals no evidence of any disc protrusion. This might be the result of a primary degeneration of the disc without herniation or, perhaps, the herniation is entirely anterolateral in position where myelography would not show it. Anterolateral herniation would not compress the nerve roots, and therefore, would produce no neurologic findings, but it may be a cause of back pain.

Calcification within the vertebral canal dorsal to an intervertebral space may be seen occasionally when advanced degenerative changes have occurred in the herniated portion of the disc. Ordinarily, the calcification is crescentic in shape, concave ventrally with the greatest dorsal convexity behind the center of the intervertebral disc space (fig. 692). The calcification may extend 0.5 cm. or more behind the posterior margin of the contiguous vertebral bodies at the level of the lesion. While these calcium

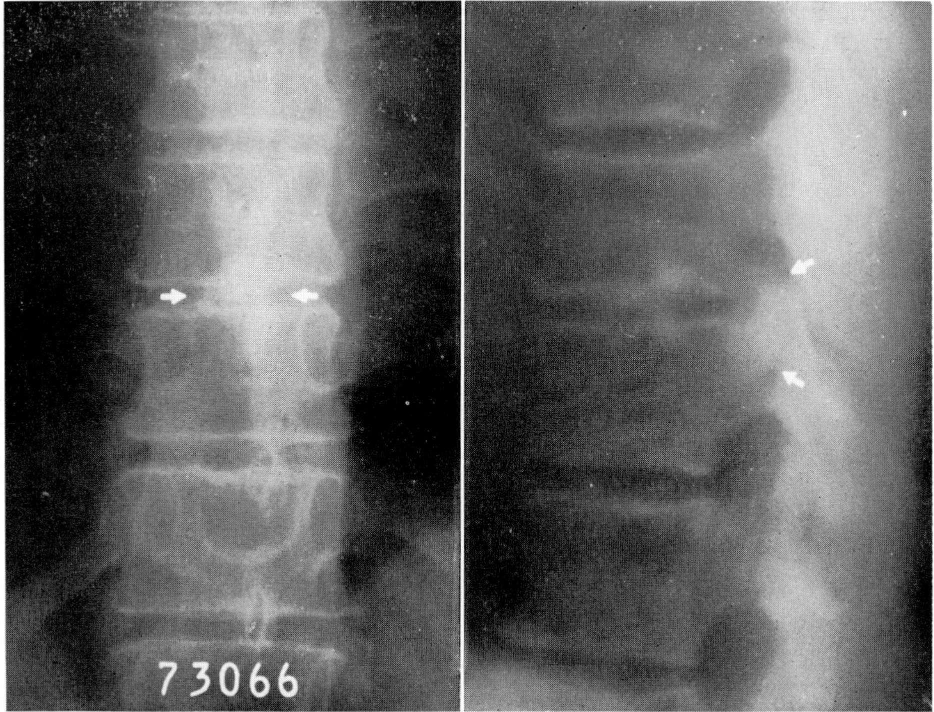

FIG. 693.—HERNIATED INTERVERTEBRAL DISC, T10-11
A herniated thoracic intervertebral disc has undergone homogeneous calcification (*arrows*). The mass is kidney shaped with its concave surface adjacent to the intervertebral disc space.

shadows are curvilinear, some calcifications may be rounded or oval in configuration, and occasionally lenticular, but almost always the center of the calcification is at the level of the middle of the intervertebral space. The size and shape of the calcification may suggest that the entire nucleus has been extruded and calcified. The undisplaced portion of the disc, which remains in the intervertebral space, frequently shows evidence of calcific degeneration when the herniated portion is calcified (fig. 693). Radiographically demonstrable calcium deposits in the intervertebral space are commonplace without disc herniation, especially in the thoracic region. Occasionally, the entire nucleus is calcified in a homogeneous manner, although more often linear and irregular scattered calcification in the fibrocartilage is demonstrated. Hypertrophic spurs projecting into the vertebral canal at the level of a herniated disc are the result of osteoarthritis associated with the disc degeneration rather than the result of the herniation per se (Hadley, 1951). However, whenever osteophytes are seen arising from the margins of the vertebrae, it may be concluded that the disc extends to the level of the apex of the osteophyte. It is possible, however, with herniated discs of long standing, in which further thinning of the intervertebral disc occurs, that localized osteoarthritis may develop more rapidly and to a greater degree than in other portions of the same spine (Oppenheimer, 1937). Reversal of the cervical vertebral curve may make it difficult to obtain face-on views of the intervertebral foramina in oblique projection with the result that several foramina may appear unduly narrowed in the routine oblique views, making it necessary to obtain additional oblique views using a greater and a lesser degree of rotation. The importance of osteoarthritis, either localized at the level of the lesion or diffuse, is of more prognostic than diagnostic significance. Hypertrophic changes denote degeneration and chronicity, and in such individuals, technical difficulties in surgical removal of the disc may be encountered, with incomplete relief or early recurrence of symptoms.

In some clinics, frontal films with the patient bending to the right and left and lateral views in flexion and extension are used in an attempt to detect and localize disc herniations. These maneuvers depend on muscle spasm (effects of which are often seen in ordinary radiographs) to prevent movement of the spine in a direction which increases the tension upon a compressed nerve root. There are other factors, both voluntary and involuntary, which affect the pliancy of the spine, and the results of the bending experiments frequently are inconclusive. Absence of compression of a disc with lateral bending is suggestive, however, of disc disease. Changes in width of the intervertebral space often may be demonstrated to best advantage in frontal films made with the patient prone.

The changes occurring in plain spine roentgenograms, aside from calcification within the vertebral canal, constitute indirect evidence of disc rupture since they do not depict the offending lesion. A diagnosis of posterior herniation of an intervertebral disc cannot be made justifiably unless a soft tissue mass in the vertebral canal continuous with the soft tissue shadow of the intervertebral space is demonstrated, which usually requires contrast methods. The actual demonstration of compression of the spinal cord or spinal nerve roots by the extraneous mass is a valuable part of any examination. Demonstration of disc protrusion alone is not enough, since the frequent occurrence of asymptomatic protruded discs is well known (Horwitz, 1943; McRae, 1956). For accurate diagnosis, it is essential that the morphologic changes present be depicted by the most accurate procedures available and that an objective correlation of the roentgen and clinical findings be made. The great number of procedures using contrast media which have been devised bespeak the importance of the problem and the lack of a completely satisfactory method of roentgen diagnosis.

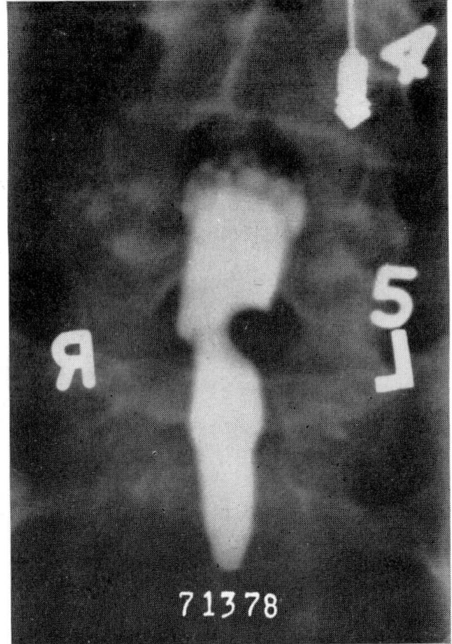

Fig. 694.—Herniated Disc, L5-S1
A smooth indentation of the lateral margin of the subarachnoid oil column is present. The left root sheath is not filled with Pantopaque at the L5-S1 level.

Myelography with radiopaque oil is generally accepted as the most satisfactory roentgen method for the diagnosis of intervertebral disc herniation at the present time. The procedure, as ordinarily executed, includes fluoroscopic examination and the liberal use of spot films so that a radiographic record of the morphology of the subarachnoid space well above and below the suspected level of the pathologic process can be obtained. The use of the horizontal x-ray beam from a tube at the side of the table usually is restricted to radiography because the width of the torso impairs fluoroscopic visualization of the radiopaque column in the lateral projection.

In frontal myelograms, a herniated intervertebral disc may cause deformity of the contrast outline of the central subarachnoid space or defective filling of a nerve root sheath. In the lumbar region, the herniated disc may produce a rounded indentation of the lateral aspect of the subarachnoid oil column which may vary from a shallow

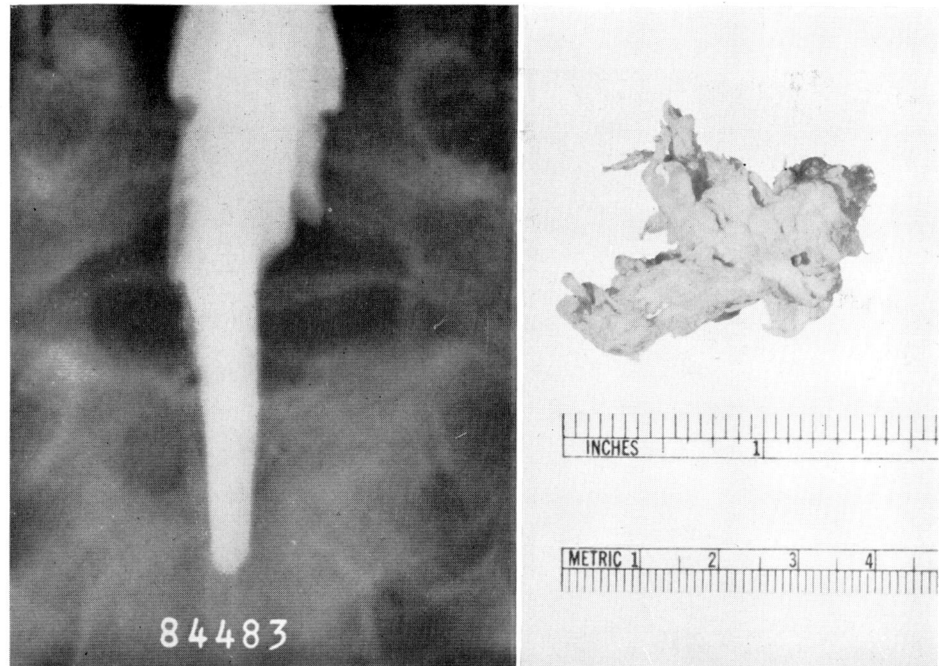

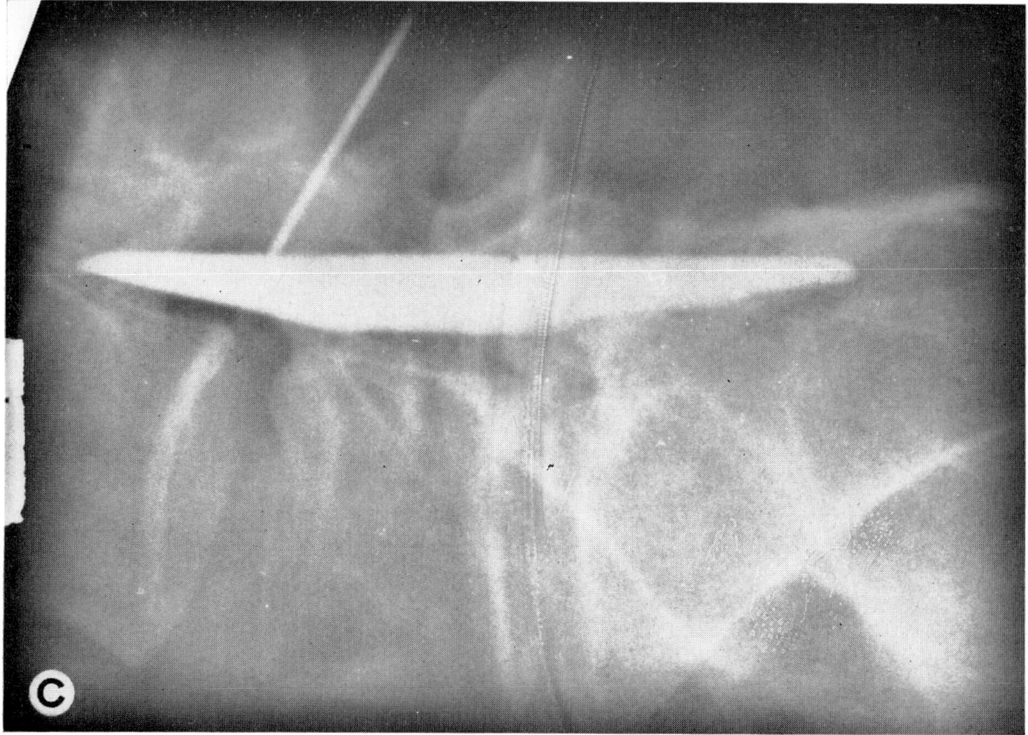

Fig. 695.—Herniated Disc L5-S1

A large lateral filling defect in the frontal myelogram is present behind the L5-S1 intervertebral space on the left side. A photograph of the gross specimen, which consisted of a single large extruded piece of disc material, is shown in the upper panel (A and B). The lateral prone projection (C) (*lower panel*) shows no definite defect at L5-Sl, the level of the herniated disc. This is because even though this is a large disc herniation, it is laterally placed. There is, however, some slight general flattening of the contour of the oil column which is not diagnostic in itself.

(*Revised 1963*)

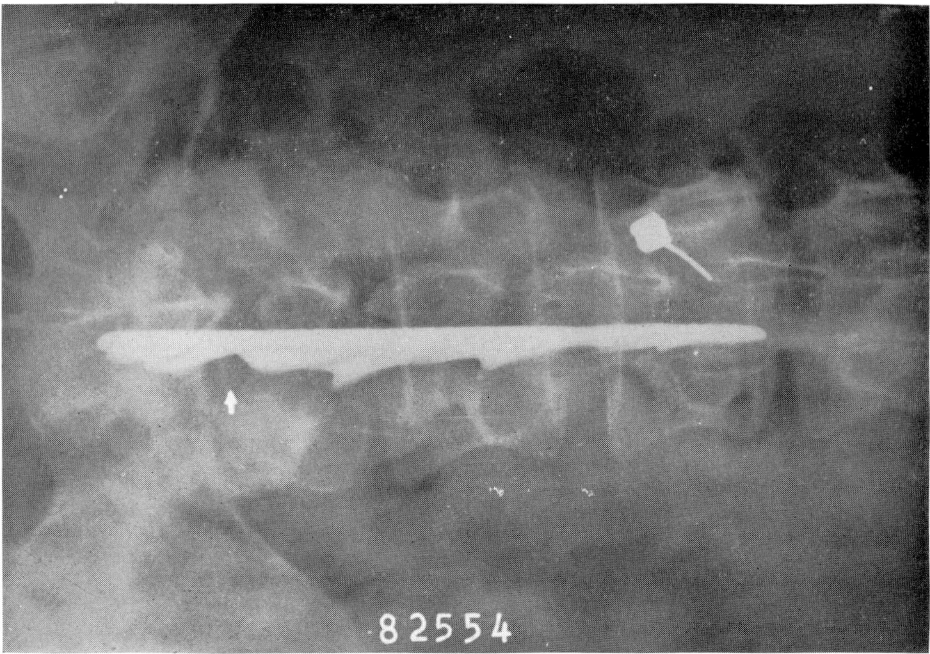

FIG. 996.—HERNIATED DISC, L5-S1

A frontal film, made with the patient on the left side, discloses a triangular indentation (*arrow*) of the lateral aspect of the Pantopaque oil column. No deformity was shown in other projections which might indicate the presence of a ruptured intervertebral disc.

impression to a deep incisura which extends half the distance across the vertebral canal (fig. 694). The indentation usually is smooth in contour with the deepest portion of the notch directed transversely toward the center of the vertebral canal. With large extruded intervertebral discs, the indentation may be more irregular. At L5–S1 the herniation may produce a shelflike deformity of the lateral margin of the radiopaque oil column (fig. 695). The nerve root sheath may be incompletely filled or it may not fill at all. In the lumbar region, deformity of the nerve root sheath usually is seen to best advantage in films made with the patient in the anterior oblique position. Occasionally a deformity will be demonstrable only in frontal films made with the patient in lateral decubitus position, where the terminal portion of the nerve root sheath is outlined to best advantage by the dependent radiopaque oil (fig. 696). Rotation of the patient a few degrees toward the ventral side from the straight lateral decubitus position may depict the nerve root sheath more prominently in some individuals. The lateral decubitus position is used routinely in our departments whenever there is a question whether or not the lack of filling of a root sleeve, or lack of clear visualization of the axillary pouch of a root, is a significant and constant finding. If it does not fill in this position it may be stated that there is indeed a local deformity which prevents the filling of the axillary pouch. Both sides should usually be taken, that is, one with the patient lying on the right side and one with the patient lying on the left side.

The lateral myelogram, made with the patient prone, usually will demonstrate the subarachnoid deformity produced by a herniated lumbar intervertebral disc in profile (figs. 697 and 698). Herniations which are laterally situated may be obscured in this view. From the lateral projection, the mass resulting in deformity of the subarachnoid space can be assumed to be a

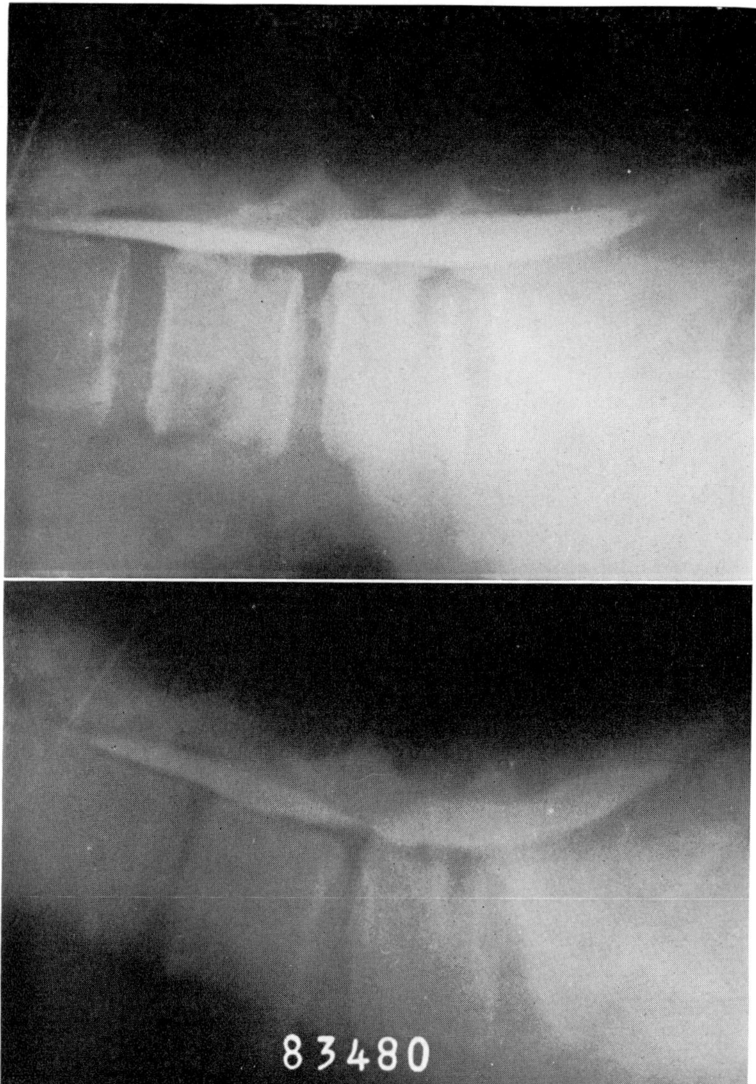

FIG. 697.—HERNIATED DISC L4-5 (LATERAL PROJECTION IN FLEXION AND EXTENSION)
The upper film, made with a sandbag beneath the abdomen to produce flexion, discloses a shallow ventral indentation of the Pantopaque column at L4-5. The lower film, made with a pillow beneath the chest to produce hyperextension, reveals a more conspicuous defect.

ruptured disc if the lesion is in the ventral part of the vertebral canal and at the level of an intervertebral space. When there is a significant ventral indentation on the oil column, it may be stated that the corresponding intervertebral disc is protruding into the spinal canal. Whether it has actually herniated and is lying partly free under the posterior common ligament cannot be stated from the myelogram. On the other hand, if there is a lateral defect seen in the anteroposterior film only on one side this is usually due to a unilateral herniation of the nucleus pulposus. It should be remembered that the lateral herniations not accompanied by protrusions of the midline portion of the disc may not cause any ventral indentation on the oil column (fig. 695C). Sometimes a

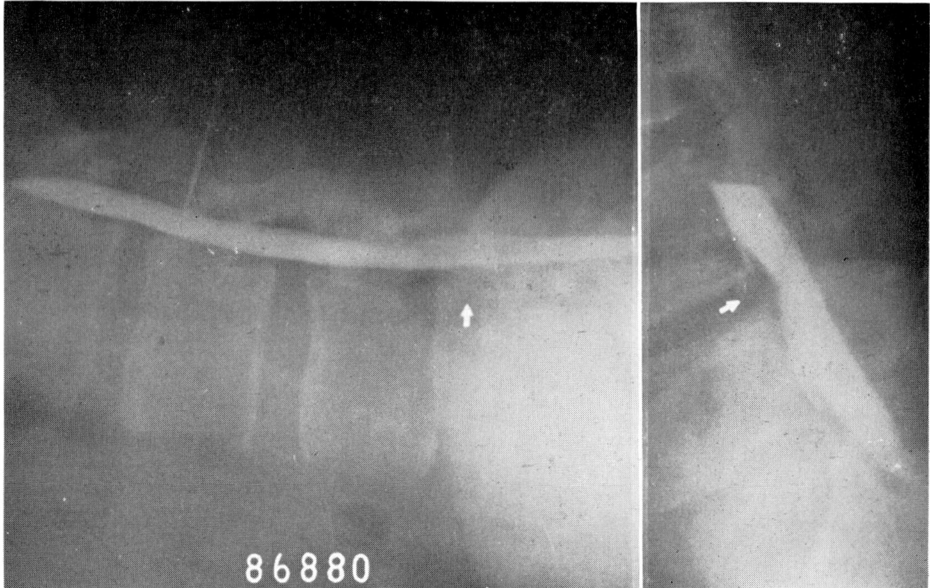

Fig. 698.—Herniated Disc, L4-5, Lateral Projection, Prone and Standing

The ventral defect from a protruding intervertebral disc may become more conspicuous in the erect as compared to the recumbent position. The reason may be that there is normally a decrease in the size of the ventral epidural space occurring when the individual assumes the erect position. This tends to push the anterior surface of the Pantopaque column closer to the vertebral bodies above and below the disc, thereby emphasizing the concave defect. Also, the disc may protrude further in the erect position.

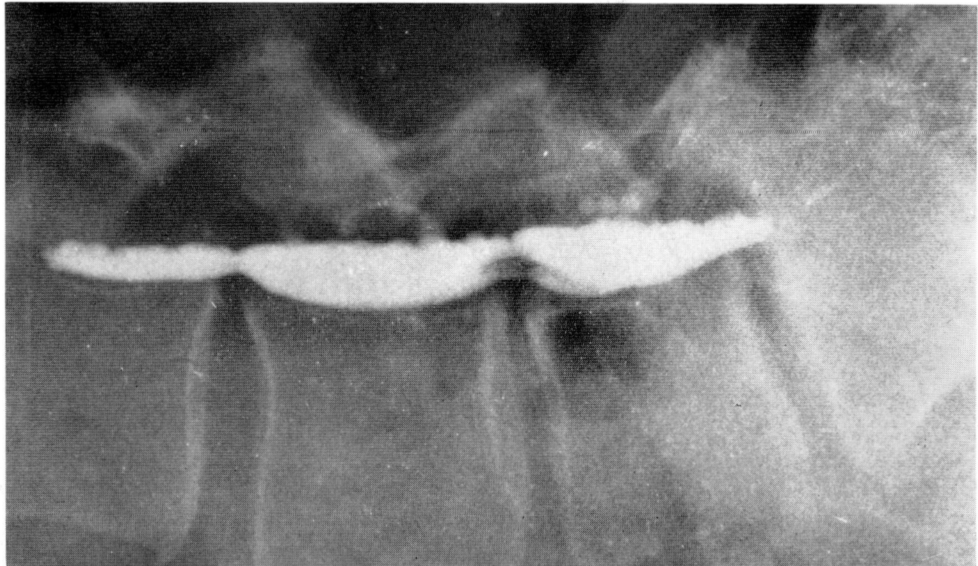

Fig. 699.—Lumbar Myelogram, Lateral View, Prone, Demonstrating Double Contour of Ventral Aspect of Oil Column

A unilateral lifting of the oil column produces a double contour of the oil which should be looked for in lateral prone films. A double contour is frequently obscured because ordinary Pantopaque is very dense.

(Revised 1963)

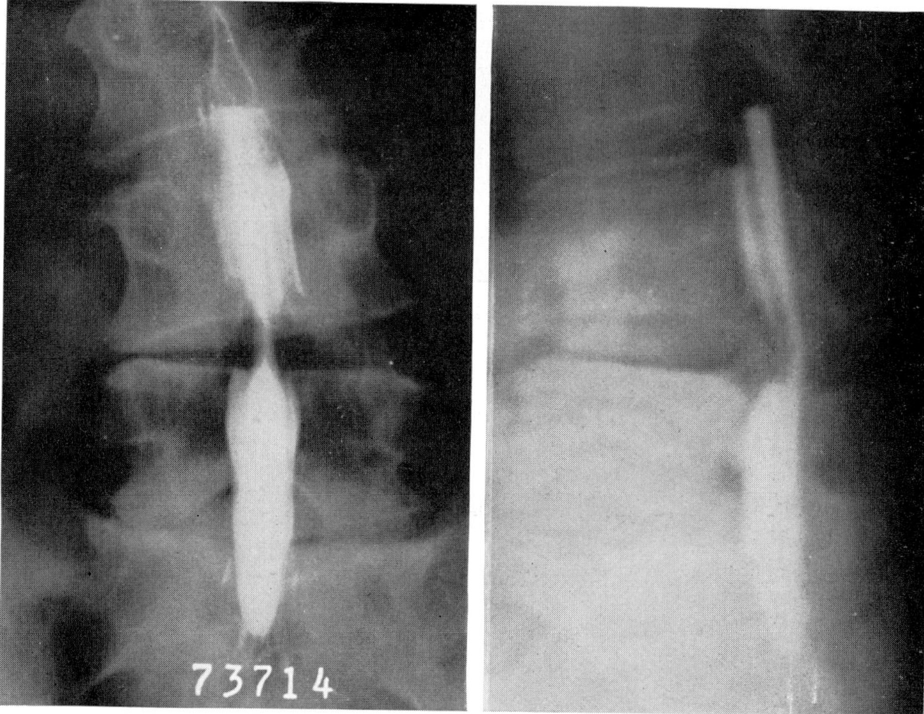

FIG. 700.—HERNIATED DISC, L4-5

In the frontal projection, an hourglass deformity of the Pantopaque column is present, resulting from a large fibrocartilaginous herniation. In the lateral view, with the patient standing, there is a ventral indentation of the column directly behind the intervertebral space.

double contour is seen behind the disc where the radiopaque oil is against the posterior margin of the normal intervertebral disc on one side and displaced dorsally on the other side (fig. 699).

In a small percentage of patients, the herniated intervertebral disc is of sufficient size, even in the lumbar region where no spinal cord exists, to cause a partial or complete obstruction of the subarachnoid space. Obstruction is more often incomplete than complete and is observed most frequently with large midline herniations. The neural sac is compressed between the large herniated disc in the ventral part of the vertebral canal and thickened ligamenta flavum posteriorly, with the result that only a narrow subarachnoid channel remains for the passage of the spinal nerve roots and the radiopaque medium. In frontal projection an hourglass deformity of the radiopaque oil column then is seen (fig. 700). The radiopaque column is of normal caliber above and below the herniation and the normal portions are connected by isthmus of radiopaque material which is in the midline. In the lateral film, the radiopaque column is greatly deformed on its ventral aspect by a large domelike mass behind the intervertebral space. A shallow dorsal indentation of the subarachnoid oil column may result from thickening of the ligamenta flavum. The narrowed subarachnoid channel is situated in the dorsal portion of the vertebral canal. With large disc herniations even the narrow channel over the dome of the herniated disc is occluded. The end of the radiopaque column in frontal projection then is transverse in configuration at the point of obstruction. In lateral projection, the column is observed to taper posteriorly to a point where it is obliterated directly behind the intervertebral space (fig. 701). Large herniated lumbar discs must always

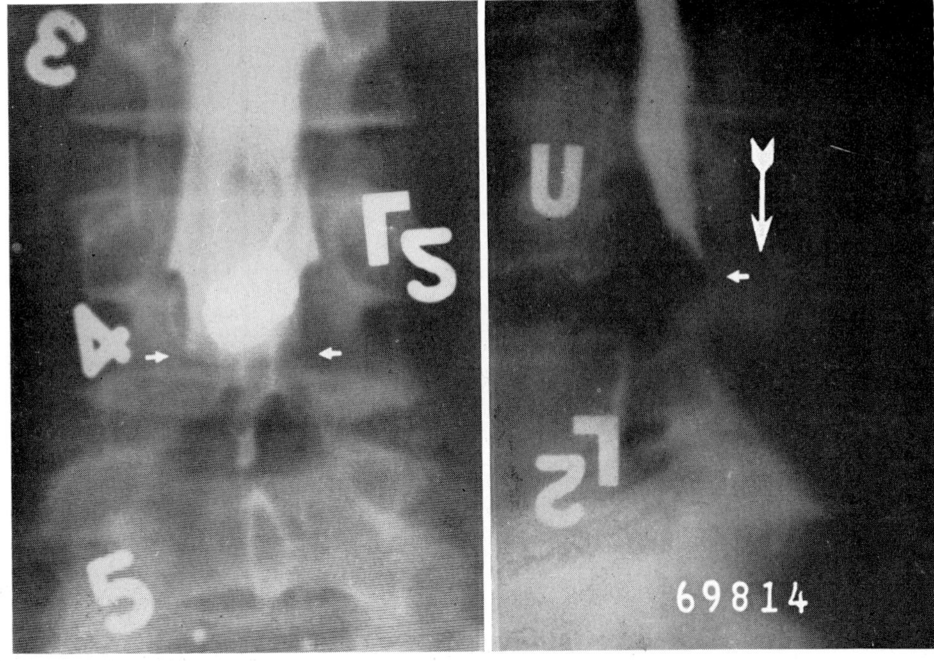

A

Fig. 701.—Herniated Disc, L4-5

The upright films (A) show an obstruction to the caudad flow of Pantopaque. In the frontal view, the lower margin of the radiopaque oil column is transverse in configuration (*arrows*), while in the lateral projection the column tapers posteriorly (*arrow*) behind the intervertebral space.

be differentiated from epidural tumors. The clear demonstration in the lateral projection that the lesion is entirely ventral in relation to the subarachnoid space and that it is centered directly behind an intervertebral space is presumptive evidence that the pathologic process is a herniated intervertebral disc.

Correlation between the myelographic findings with the actual presence of disc herniation is excellent at the L4–5 disc space. That is, a considerable percentage of disc herniations at this level will be seen on a good myelogram, and the absence of myelographic findings of disc herniation is very infrequent. It is probable that almost 98 per cent of herniated intervertebral discs at the L4–5 level can be diagnosed by myelography. On the other hand, as explained under "Myelographic Anatomy," at L5–S1 there is a considerable amount of epidural fat and epidural plexus which occupies most of the available space in this region, particularly in some individuals. It will be noted upon looking at the lateral projection that in some individuals, the column of oil is against the posterior margin of the sacrum and it is likely that any disc herniation or protrusion at L5–S1 will be visualized in these individuals. More frequently, however, the subarachnoid space, as outlined by Pantopaque, tapers toward the lower end and gets so narrow both in the anteroposterior and in the lateral plane that it may only occupy 20 per cent or even less of the cross-sectional space at this level. Under these circumstances, disc herniations at L5–S1 will produce no visible deformities of the oil column.

Some valuable help may be obtained in diagnosing L5–S1 disc abnormalities by careful attention to detail. In the first place, the axillary pouch of the root may be asymmetrical; it may be smaller on one side than the other, and the abnormal side will be that where the axillary pouch is smaller. It is our custom to compare the

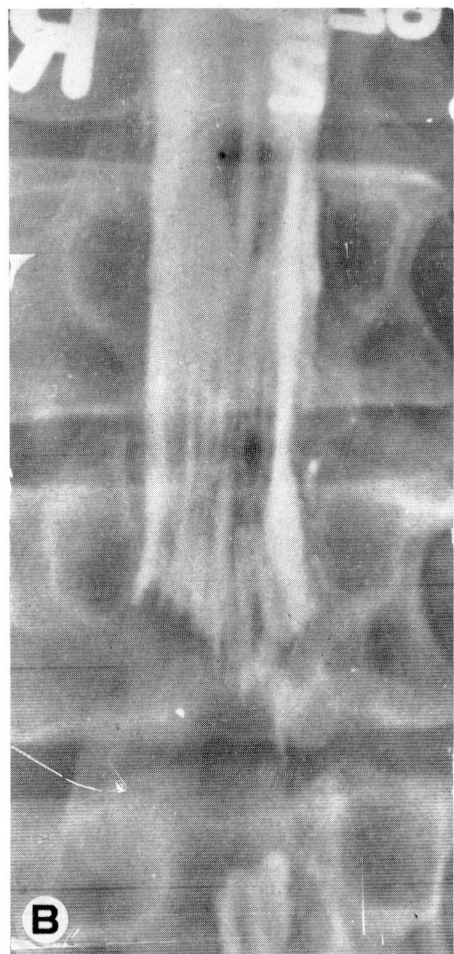

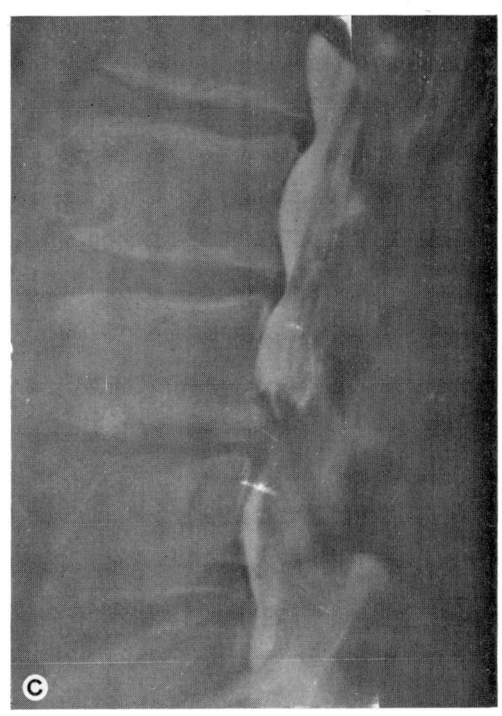

FIG. 701 (*Cont.*).—ALMOST COMPLETE BLOCK TO THE FLOW OF PANTOPAQUE PRODUCED BY HERNIATED INTERVERTEBRAL DISC

The root shadows often become very prominent in cases where there are myelographic blocks produced by herniated discs or a combination of discs and osteoarthritis, and ligamentous thickening. This is partly produced by diffuse swelling of the roots and partly produced by crowding of the roots into a small area due to displacement; the roots then become more visible. The column often acquires a paintbrush configuration such as is seen in this instance. (B) frontal view, (C) lateral view.

distance from the axillary pouch of the S2 root to the axillary pouch of the S1 root on one side with that of the other side in the oblique projections. Normally this distance should be almost identical on both sides when it is measured up to the axilla (figs. 629 and 632), and in cases where there is elevation of an axilla, this is usually indicative of a disc herniation on that side (fig. 702). Another finding which is helpful is that of lateral displacement of the cul-de-sac. The distance from the lateral margin of the oil column to the pedicle of the first sacral vertebra should be approximately equal on both sides. When there is displacement of the oil column to one side or the other in the absence of scoliosis, this displacement should be interpreted as probably due to a disc herniation that is causing no actual deformity of the oil column (fig. 703). In the presence of scoliosis, the margin of the oil column is closer to the convex side in its

(*Revised 1963*)

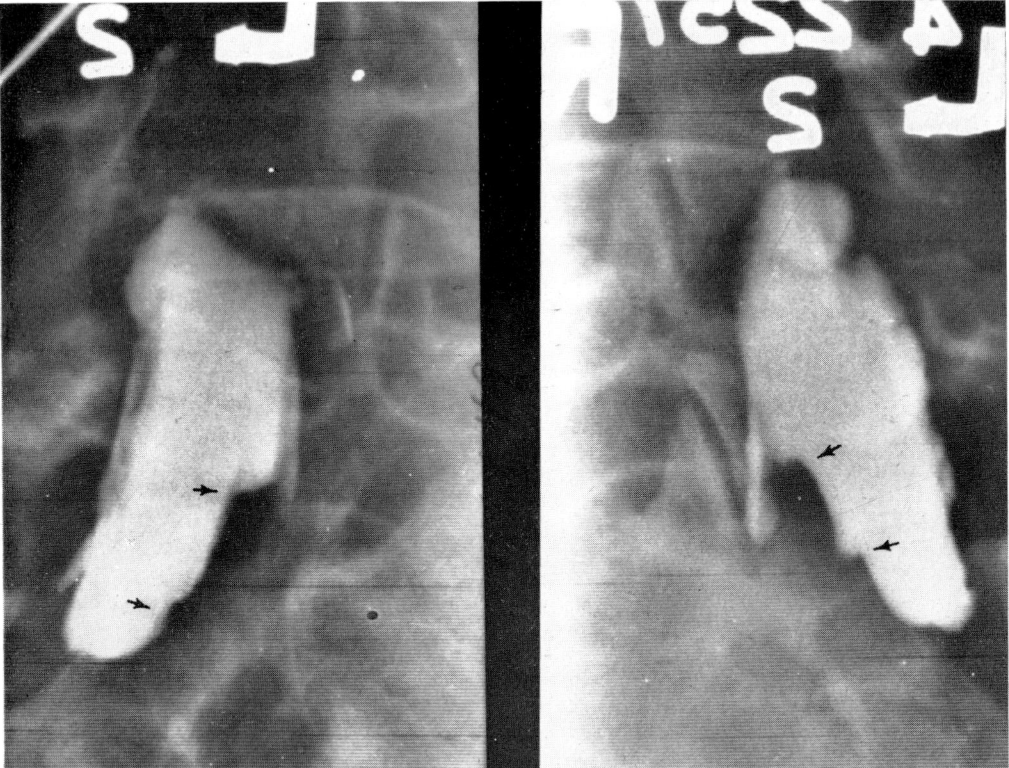

FIG. 702.—HERNIATED INTERVERTEBRAL DISC, EXHIBITING ONLY ASYMMETRICAL ROOTS

There is a difference in the distances between the axillary pouches when the right is compared with the left. On the left side, the axilla has been elevated in comparison to the right and this was interpreted as being due to a herniated intervertebral disc at L5-S1 on the left side. This was confirmed upon surgical intervention.

lower portion, and under these circumstances, the off-center position is not significant.

At the L5–S1 disc space, attention should be paid to minor deviations from the normal. There should be normally a smooth convex configuration to the ventral surface of the oil column. If there is a flattening of the oil column at this level, even though there is as yet no real concave indentation, the flattening should be interpreted as probably due to a protruding intervertebral disc. This, of course, is only important in the cases where there is a large ventral, epidural space. Obviously, if the epidural space is very small, then a ventral protrusion would be seen. In fact, care should be taken not to "overdiagnose" disc protrusions at all levels in the patients who have a narrow epidural space, because the slightest degree of bulging of the intervertebral disc will produce a ventral indentation which is not necessarily a pathologic finding (fig. 633). In interpreting whether a ventral indentation is or is not significant, it is important to compare the distance from the ventral surface of the oil column to the calculated posterior margin of the disc, and to compare this distance to that seen behind the posterior margin of the vertebral bodies above and below. When there is elevation of the oil produced by a protruding intervertebral disc, there is a gradual increase in the distance between the ventral surface of the oil column and the posterior margin of the vertebral bodies as the oil approaches the intervertebral disc (fig. 704). This indicates that the dura has been stretched and is

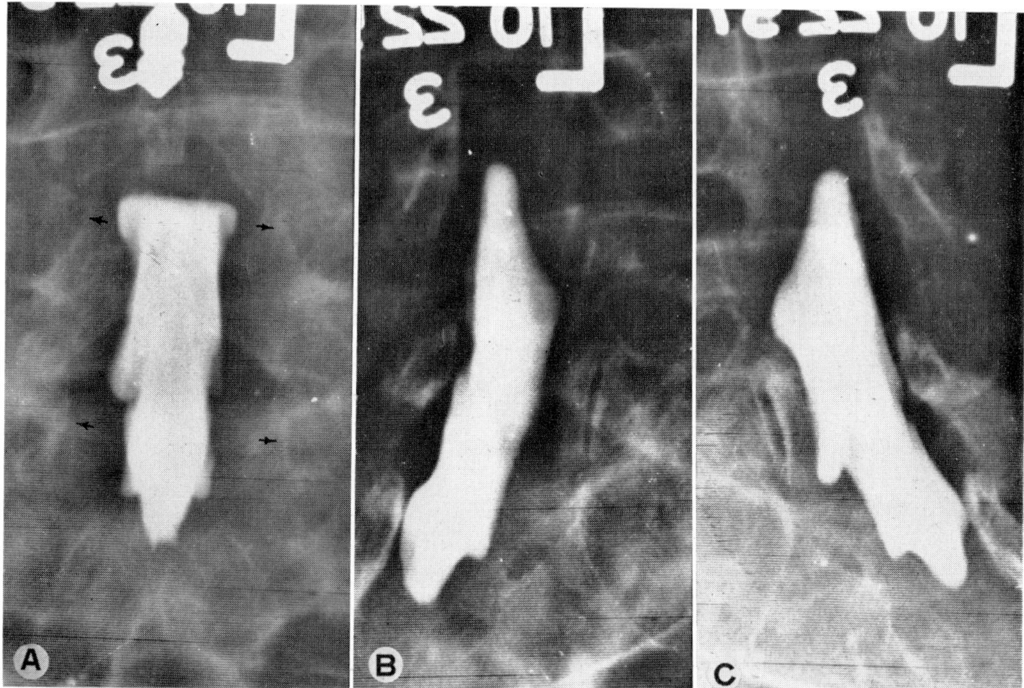

FIG. 703.—HERNIATED INTERVERTEBRAL DISC, LUMBAR, CAUSING ASYMMETRICAL ROOTS AND INCREASE IN DISTANCE FROM OIL COLUMN TO PEDICLE

The frontal film (A) shows that the distance from the lateral margin of the oil column to the pedicle is increased on the left side as compared to the right. The axillary pouch on the left is not well filled. The oblique projections (B and C) both of the right and the left side illustrate that the root is not anomalous (or in a more medial and anterior position than usual), but that the axillary pouch is actually partly obliterated and, therefore, in the oblique projection is not visible.

elevated tentlike, thus diverging gradually from the posterior margin of the vertebral body.

In fact, the tentlike deformity of the dura in the lumbar region as well as elsewhere in the spinal canal indicates an acute or a subacute type of condition where the dura has been stretched and is taut. On the other hand, protrusions of intervertebral discs secondary to longstanding degeneration, and osteoarthritic ridges usually produce indentations on the oil column that are sharply delimited and localized to the protruding intervertebral disc (fig. 705). This indicates a slowly growing, longstanding condition where the dura has become elongated and no longer produces the tentlike deformity.

Herniation of intervertebral discs at the L3–4 level is much less common than in the lower two interspaces. However, slight disc protrusions at this level or slight bulging of the intervertebral disc are common findings at L3–4. Also, it is not uncommon to see slight disc protrusion at L2–3 and at L1–2. The very slight disc bulging at the high levels produce very large defects in the lateral aspect of the oil column. *The size of a myelographic defect in anteroposterior views is dependent on the thickness of the oil column in its anteroposterior diameter and the size of the protruding mass.* It, therefore, follows that a paper-thin oil column will show a large indentation produced by a very small elevation of the floor of the spinal canal, and likewise, a large protrusion of the floor is required to produce a deformity if the oil column is thick. It is not uncommon to see at L4–5, or particularly at L5–S1, a very minor abnormality which is interpreted as a

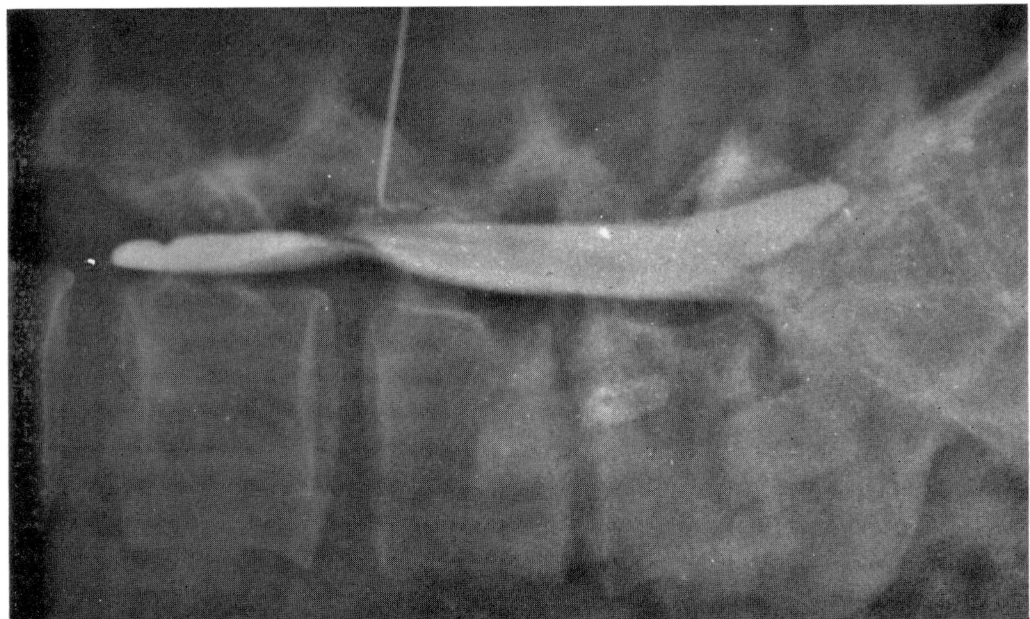

Fig. 704.—Gradual Separation of Oil Column from Vertebral Margins Due to Disc Herniation

There is a tentlike configuration of the ventral margin of the oil column which indicates that the dura is stretched and has been separated from the vertebral margins. The apex of the tent is at the disc space. Smaller degrees of deformity with this configuration should be also noted. The patient had previously had an interbody fusion at L4-5 and at L5-S1 and this time the disc herniated above the level of the fusion.

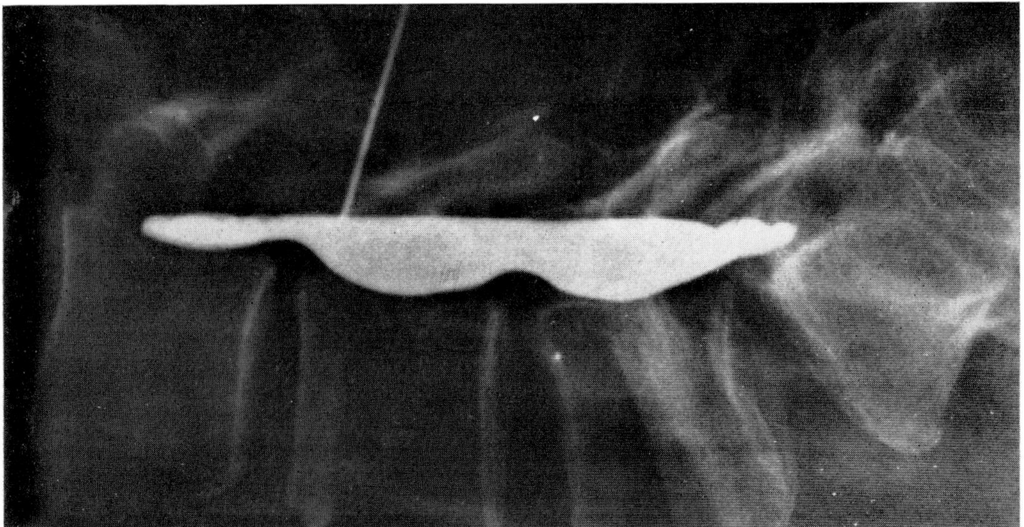

Fig. 705.—Multiple Protrusions of Intervertebral Discs, Chronic

There are sharp elevations of the ventral surface of the oil column at L3-4 and also at L4-5 without significant tenting; that is, the oil column remains close to the posterior margin of the vertebral bodies almost until it reaches the disc level. This indicates a long-standing type of protrusion seen in degenerative disease and in osteoarthritic ridges.

(Revised 1963)

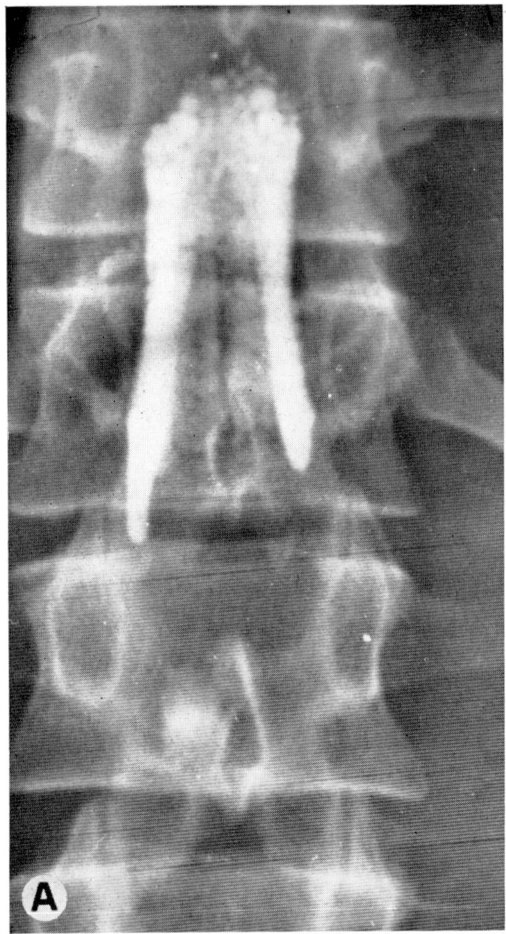

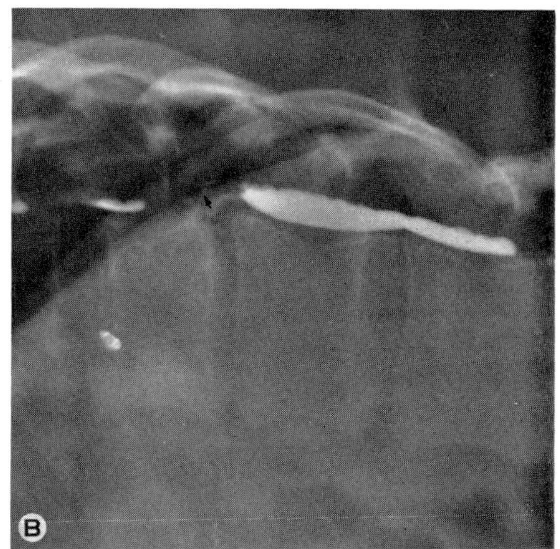

Fig. 706.—Herniated Intervertebral Disc at T12-L1

In the frontal projection (A) there is a gradual increase in the width of the spinal cord which has its maximum width at the T12-L1 disc space. The anterior spinal vessels are prominent. This increase in width is decidedly abnormal since usually the shadow of the conus is not appreciably different from the adjacent spinal cord in the lumbar myelograms. There is also narrowing of the T12-L1 disc space as compared to the others. The lateral projection (B) demonstrates an interruption of the oil column at this point, and only a small amount of Pantopaque can be seen behind the T12-L1 disc space which is displaced dorsally (*arrow*). Satisfactory lateral views are often difficult to obtain in high disc herniations due to segmentation of the oil column.

herniated intervertebral disc on the myelogram and yet, in the same case, a large defect may be seen at L2–3 which will be considered insignificant and passed up. This requires an explanation. The explanation lies in the fact stated above, namely that the oil column is very thin in its anteroposterior diameter when it is allowed to run up cephalad to outline the upper lumbar region. Because the oil column is so thin, a very slight degree of elevation of the ventral surface of the canal will produce a large defect in the oil column. On the other hand, at L4–5 and L5–S1 where the column is thickest, a larger elevation of the ventral or lateral aspects of the oil column is required to produce a defect. Therefore, at the high level, the size of a defect has to be evaluated in relation to the thickness of the oil column as seen in the lateral projection. It is very common to demonstrate a large defect in the lateral aspect at the higher lumbar and lower thoracic levels, and the film made with the horizontal x-ray beam demonstrates only a minute elevation of the floor of the canal. If it is desired to evaluate the significance of the lateral indentation of the oil column at the upper levels, the patient may be placed in the lateral decubitus position as explained above, and a horizontal beam anteroposterior film is made. This will usually show the upper root sleeves, and no actual lateral defect will be demonstrated in most instances. Still the question remains as to when is a visible defect in the upper lumbar area significant. It is our custom to refer to significant defects at the upper levels when a ventral indentation of at least a few millimeters can be demonstrated in the lateral projection and when this, of course, corresponds to the clinical findings. Adding more Pantopaque may be helpful. Unfortunately, the herniations of intervertebral discs at the upper lumbar levels often produce atypical clinical syndromes. Herniations at T12-L1 may produce symptoms and signs of a conus medullary lesion simulating an intramedullary tumor. The lesion may even be confused with an intramedullary tumor at myelography if a satisfactory prone lateral view is not made (fig. 706).

Multiple disc protrusions. It is not uncommon to find a patient who presents multiple protrusions of the intervertebral discs. Most often multiple disc protrusions are encountered in older individuals and are secondary to degeneration; when encountered in a younger individual, it is probable that the multiple protruding discs are representative of ruptured discs. When a disc degenerates, it becomes wider and broader and it bulges all the way around and thus it will protrude not only dorsally, where it will produce a myelographic defect, but also anteriorly and laterally, where it will provoke the formation of osteophytes by stimulation of the osteoblasts. It is our custom, in the presence of multiple disc protrusions, to conclude that the largest one is probably the more significant of the group. Of course, the neurologic findings are of paramount importance in deciding, if an operation is

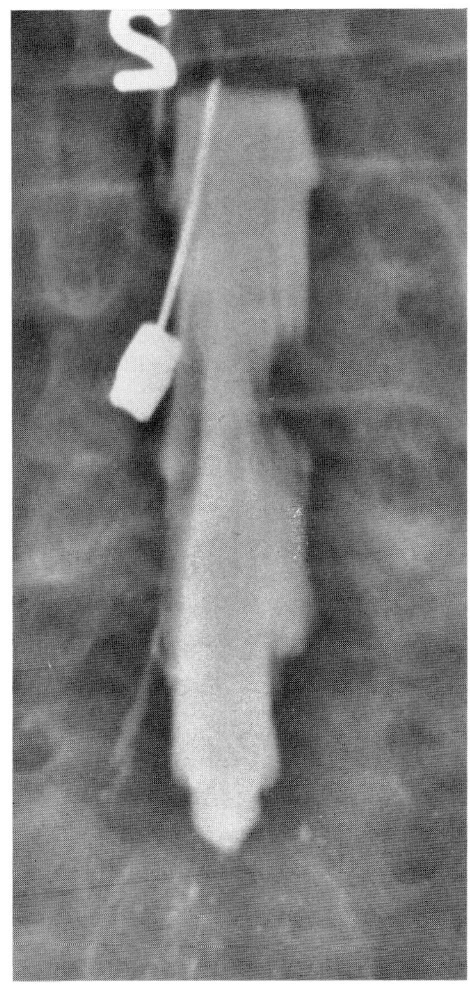

Fig. 707.—Herniated Intervertebral Disc at L4-5 With Defect at Level Below

There is a clear-cut myelographic defect at L4-5 indicative of a herniated intervertebral disc. At L5-S1 there is also a slight defect on the left side, the same side as the herniation above. In these cases, it is difficult to decide whether the defect below is due to the displacement of the roots and the congestion and edema in the epidural space occurring as a result of the adjacent herniation (distance from oil to pedicles is increased on left side as compared to the right). Myelographically it is not possible to distinguish between the above condition and another herniated or protruding disc at the level below. Therefore, exploration is usually recommended in these cases if surgical intervention is to be performed, inasmuch as the adjacent defect is on the same side as the herniation.

(Revised 1963)

to be performed, at which level inspection of a disc is indicated, since it is not feasible to remove all of the protruding discs.

Adjacent defects. Another problem in myelography is the presence of a defect in the lateral aspect of the oil column at a level above or below a herniated intervertebral disc which is large and clearly shown on myelography (fig. 707). In these cases, if the defect is on the same side, it is not possible to tell whether the defect present may be due to another disc herniation at the level above or whether it is secondary to the displacement of the oil column and of the root at the level below. For this reason, it is usually recommended that both interspaces be explored at the time of surgery. These appearances are usually encountered at L4–5 when there is an L5–S1 disc on the same side or vice versa and, usually, it is the custom of most surgeons to explore both of these spaces when a herniated disc is encountered and, particularly, if there is a question on the myelogram.

Edema of the roots. It is not uncommon to observe what is usually referred to as "swollen roots" in myelograms in the presence of herniated intervertebral discs. It is usually found at the operating table that these roots are actually edematous and that the edema is secondary to the compression. However, sometimes edematous roots are found and no evidence of root compression is demonstrated on the myelogram. In these cases, we have to assume that there is either a mechanical compression of the root at a point outside of the reach of the myelogram, or there is a condition which is causing the swelling of the root other than mechanical compression. This is one of the myelographic problems which requires further study. It is not uncommon to find that there is a swollen root at the level above or below a demonstrated herniation on the myelogram. It is difficult to explain the finding and, usually, it is disregarded on the myelogram unless it is accompanied by a deformity of the oil column. The term "hypertrophic neuropathy" has been applied to those cases in which multiple swollen roots are encountered. This diagnosis has not been made myelographically at the Neurological Institute in the last several years. Cases have been encountered, however, where technical difficulties, namely extravasation of cerebrospinal fluid on the dorsal side of the subdural space, caused compression of the subarachnoid space, and produced crowding of the roots ventrally, the thinning of the oil column, thereby, bringing out the shadows of the roots much more clearly. In one instance, it was possible to show a disappearance of the "swollen roots" on repeat myelography, at which time there were no technical difficulties (fig. 645).

Narrow spinal canal. Some patients have a congenitally narrow spinal canal; both in the anteroposterior and in the transverse diameters. This is usually diagnosed from plain films of the spine by a short interpediculate distance. Often a narrow interpediculate width receives little attention when the spine films are examined, whereas an increase in the interpediculate distance is usually observed and commented upon by the radiologist. In the cases that have a narrow spinal canal, a slight degree of protrusion or herniation of the intervertebral discs will produce signs of multiple root compression or severe signs of single root compression when the degree of protrusion into the spinal canal is rather small. This results from the fact that these patients have little available space (fig. 708). The myelogram, not uncommonly, shows complete or incomplete block to the flow of Pantopaque at more than one level, and the lateral myelogram films made in the prone position show only a slight degree of protrusion. In these cases, one is often puzzled to explain the large defects and the presence of a block in the presence of only minor dorsal deviation of the oil column. The explanation lies in the congenital narrowing of the spinal canal which causes a simple disc to produce multiple signs of root compression often suggestive of a spinal cord tumor (Schlesinger and Taveras, 1953). The interpediculate distances at the levels of L3 and L4 will often fall at the 23 and 24 mm. level instead of around 26 to 30 mm., which is a more common range encountered. Less space is present for the roots to move within the dural sac (fig. 709).

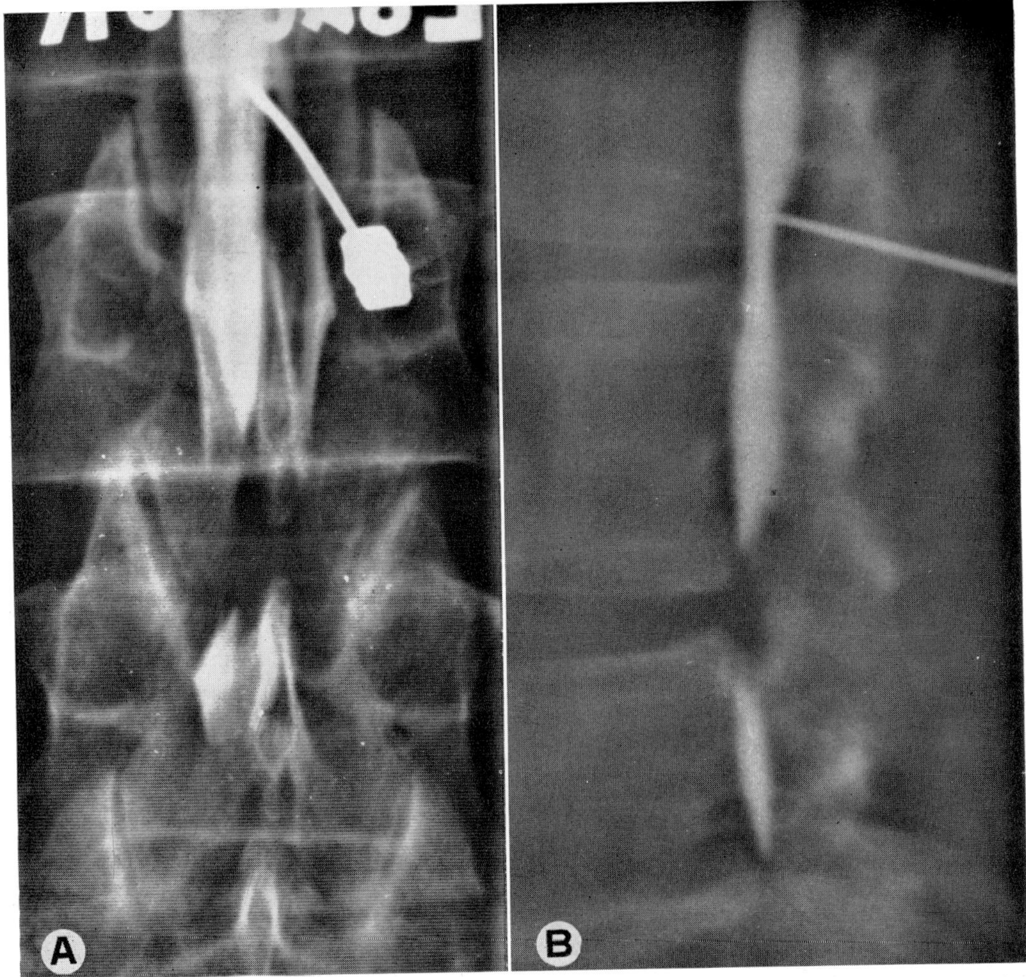

FIG. 708.—PARTIAL AND COMPLETE BLOCK IN LUMBAR MYELOGRAM ASSOCIATED WITH CONGENITALLY NARROW SPINAL CANAL

In the frontal projection (A), there is noted partial block at the level of L3-4 and complete block at L4-5. The oil did not go down beyond this point. In the lateral projection (B), there is only interruption of the oil shadow near the disc spaces with very little lifting away from the ventral surface of the canal. The interpediculate distance in this patient is of the order of 23 mm. or less at L3, L4, and L5. The canal was very narrow in its anteroposterior diameter as well. There is no significant osteophyte formation around the margins of the vertebral bodies. The patient had a paraparesis secondary to multiple root involvement.

Large "asymptomatic" defects. It is often commented that a patient may have symptoms on one side where a very small defect is encountered at one of the two most common interspaces in the myelogram, whereas a much larger defect is encountered on the opposite side at the same or another level where the patient does not complain of symptoms. In our experience, the usual explanation is that if the past history is reviewed carefully, the patient will indicate that there were symptoms on the opposite side at one time, which later disappeared. Sometimes there are residual neurologic findings which may be demonstrated and, at other times, if the fragment of this material has become extruded, it may be lying in a position where it is not significantly

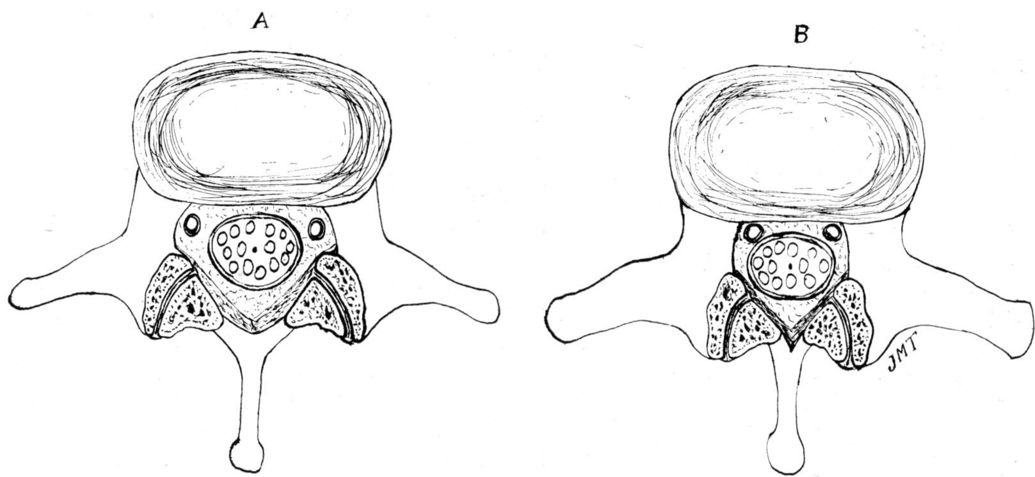

FIG. 709.—CONFIGURATION OF THE SPINAL CANAL AND RELATION OF SPINAL ROOT TO DURAL SAC IN INDIVIDUALS WITH NORMAL AND NARROW SPINAL CANAL

(A) Usual relationships in patient with normal spinal canal. (B) Relationship in patient with narrow spinal canal. The root is often underneath instead of lateral to the dural sac. The bones are more massive, and when approached through the interlaminar space, the first thing that the surgeon may see is the dural sac rather than the root.

compressing the root any longer. At other times, the root has become elongated; it has adapted to the deformity and is no longer symptomatic. This fact emphasizes the importance of myelography or a procedure capable of demonstrating an asymptomatic lesion, at times even larger than the symptomatic one; often it will be deemed advisable to remove the former at operation.

Cervical disc protrusions and herniations. Cervical and thoracic herniated intervertebral discs may encroach on the spinal cord as well as on nerve roots. Stookey (1928) called attention to three clinical states which result from ventral cartilagenous masses in the cervical region; the syndrome of bilateral ventral pressure on the spinal cord, the syndrome of unilateral ventral pressure on the spinal cord, and the syndrome of nerve root pressure. Likewise, in the myelogram, central disc herniation or posterolateral herniation may be demonstrated.

Despite these well known facts, clinical errors in differentiating between degenerative diseases of the spinal cord (especially amyotrophic lateral sclerosis and multiple sclerosis) and compression of the spinal cord are relatively common, as re-emphasized by Bucy, Heimburger, and Oberhill (1948). Myelography is a satisfactory method of making the distinction between degenerative disc disease and herniated disc. It is recommended that myelography be performed before the diagnosis of a hopeless condition is assigned to the patient whenever the clinical findings are in any way atypical.

The intervertebral disc, including the nucleus pulposus, is smaller in the cervical region than in the lumbar area, and the herniations encountered are much smaller. On the average, the herniated masses are approximately 0.5 cm. in diameter, although lesions as large as 1.5 cm. in diameter may occur. The spinal cord occupies a large part of the arachnoid sac, and the ventral epidural space is thinner there than in the lumbar area. Lesions of small size, therefore, readily produce clinical symptoms or signs, and the morphologic changes are easily demonstrated at myelography. A small ventral extradural mass may compress the spinal cord and even cause an obstruction to the passage of radiopaque material in the subarachnoid space.

In the cervical myelogram, the most common deformity, which is the result of

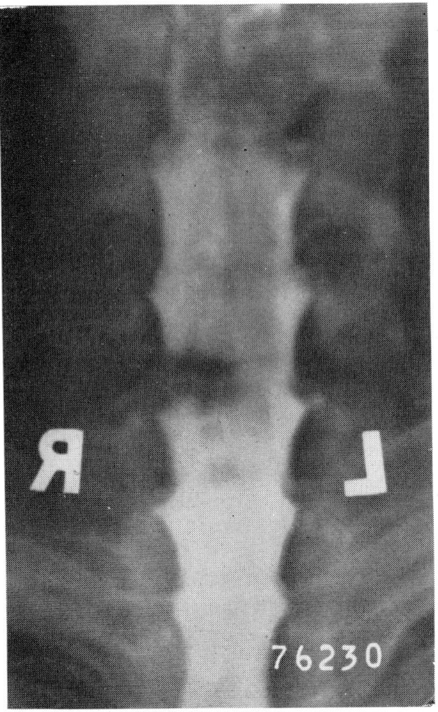

FIG. 710.—HERNIATED DISC, C6-7
A smooth filling defect is present in the right half of the Pantopaque column directly behind the intervertebral space. The corresponding nerve root sheath is occluded.

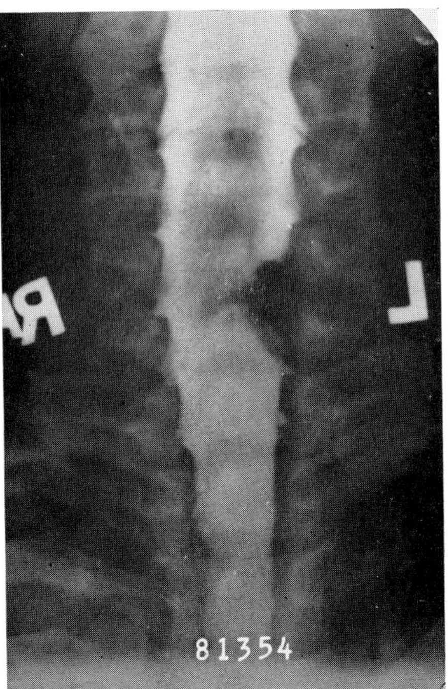

FIG. 711.—HERNIATED DISC, C6-7
The frontal myelogram discloses an irregular concave defect in the Pantopaque column which extends from the midportion of C6 to the lower margin of C7 on the left side. The nerve root sheath is obliterated at C6-7 and the sheath at C7-T1 is distorted. The spinal cord is displaced slightly toward the right.

anterolateral disc herniation, is defective filling or obliteration of a nerve root sheath. In other instances, the lateral margin of the subarachnoid oil column is indented and the notch may reach as far as the midline (fig. 710). The impression may be rounded and smooth or triangular and slightly irregular in contour. The base of the dome-like or pyramidal mass is centered laterally at the level of the occluded nerve root sheath which overlies the herniated disc. In some instances, the lesion is of sufficient size to displace the spinal cord laterally (fig. 711). In lateral projection, the herniated discs which compress the nerve roots alone may cause little or no visible ventral indentation of the opaque oil column, since the Pantopaque in the normal half of the subarachnoid space is frequently of sufficient thickness to obscure the lesion.

Herniated discs situated centrally and large lesions placed laterally in the ventral portion of the cervical vertebral canal frequently compress the spinal cord as well as interfere with the filling of the nerve root sheath. In the frontal myelogram, the outline of the spinal cord may appear wider than normal because it is compressed from its ventral aspect (fig. 712). Elevation and compression of the spinal cord by a ventral mass frequently exert tension on the cervical nerve roots, and defective filling of the nerve root sheath may occur bilaterally at the level of the lesion. A partial or complete obstruction to the passage of the Pantopaque in the subarachnoid space may also be found. The head of the radiopaque column at the point of obstruction is transverse in configuration (fig. 713). The straight edge of the oil column is depicted frequently across the shadow of the intervertebral space. Usually the shadow of the spinal cord

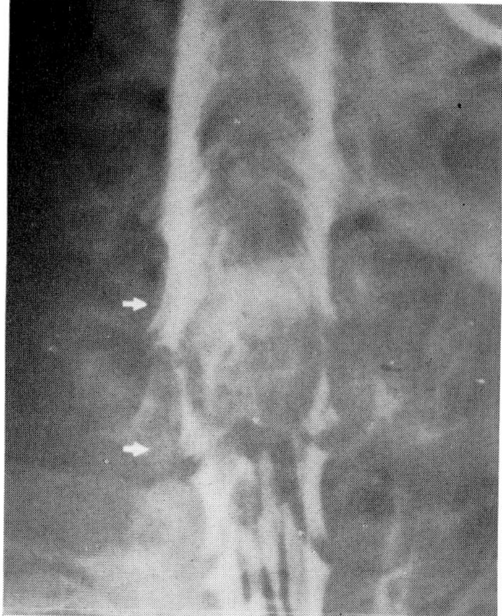

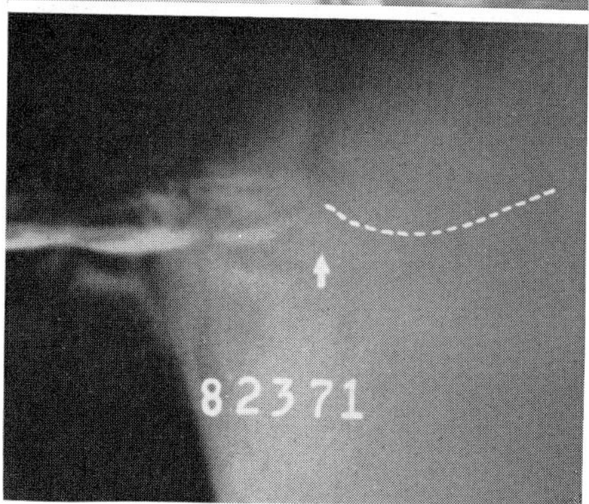

FIG. 712.—HERNIATED DISC, C6-7
(CORD COMPRESSION TYPE)

In frontal projection, localized widening of the spinal cord is shown (*arrows*). The lateral view reveals that the deformity results from posterior displacement and flattening of the spinal cord by a ventral epidural mass (*arrow*). (The broken line traces the ventral aspect of the subarachnoid space caudal to the lesion.)

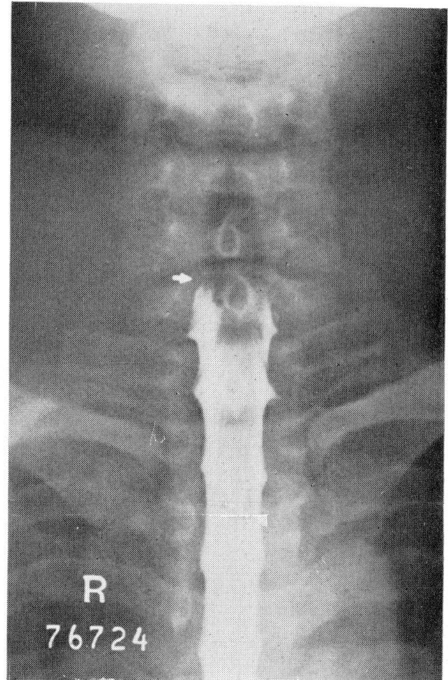

FIG. 713.—HERNIATED DISC, C6-7
(CORD COMPRESSION TYPE)

An obstruction to the cephalad flow of Pantopaque is present and the head of the radiopaque oil column is transverse in configuration. The spinal cord is displaced to the left (*arrow*), as well as posteriorly, with the result that the Pantopaque-filled, subarachnoid space is wider on the right side.

becomes slightly wider immediately before the complete block, indicating that it has been flattened so that its transverse diameter increases. At the same time, if there is disc material lateral to the block, the oil column will be displaced away from the pedicle.

In lateral projection, the central and paracentral disc herniations are viewed tangentially. The portion of the subarachnoid space ventral to the spinal cord is occluded. The maximum dorsal deviation of the oil column usually is demonstrable directly behind the intervertebral space. The spinal cord is displaced dorsally and compressed, and any radiopaque material which passes beyond the lesion moves dorsally or laterally around the spinal cord. Frequently, no opaque material is seen to extend beyond the obstruction. In such instances, the head of the radiopaque column tapers sharply toward the dorsal aspect of the vertebral canal to a point of complete obstruction.

Not all herniated intervertebral discs are clear-cut in the myelogram, and for this reason, it is necessary to make multiple exposures of the cervical region. In the first place, it is not possible to differentiate in many cases between a small herniated disc and an osteoarthritic spur which produces

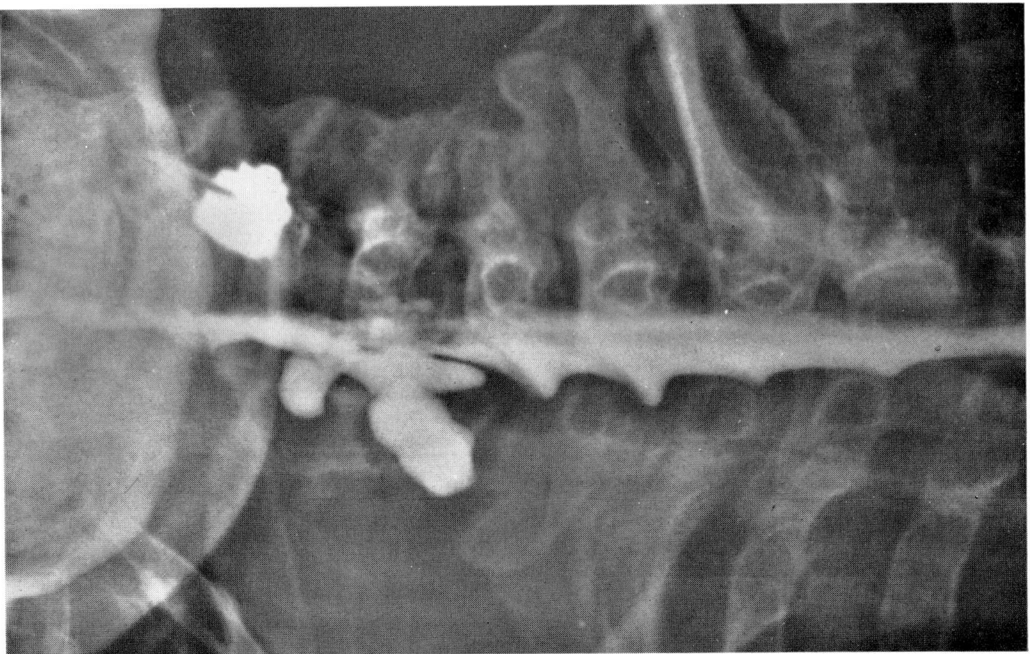

FIG. 714.—AVULSION OF BRACHIAL PLEXUS WITH POST-TRAUMATIC MENINGOCELE
With the patient lying in lateral decubitus position, two large irregular outpouchings are seen which are secondary to the tear of the dura at the site where the root was avulsed. With the passage of time, these root meningoceles produce erosion of the adjacent pedicles.

widening of a root shadow. To be considered significant, widening of the root shadow should be demonstrated in several films. It is possible to have one film show a root sleeve incompletely filled, whereas another one made with slightly different tilting of the table will show good filling. It is our custom to take six different spot films of the cervical region, in straight anteroposterior projection, using slightly different tilts of the table but without turning the head. Oblique views of the lower cervical region are not taken routinely because they are usually found not to add any additional information.

Not uncommonly, there is a great deal of spasm of the cervical muscles due to pain in acute disc herniations which prevents the patient from being able to extend the head and assume the usual cervical myelographic position. In these cases, it is extremely difficult to pool the oil in the cervical area with the patient in the prone position. Under these circumstances, it may be necessary to give the patient an increased amount of sedation in order that the examination may be performed adequately. In some cases the spasm is so great that it will not relax even with heavy sedation. In these instances, it is possible to obtain satisfactory examinations with the patient lying on one side, having the oil ascend to the cervical region with only a slight degree of tilt of the table thus outlining the site of disc herniation by taking horizontal anteroposterior films.

As previously mentioned, at least two lateral views are made in the cervical region, one to include the mid and upper level extending at least to the C2–3 disc space and another one in the swimmer's position with the arm away from the x-ray tube elevated and the head end of the table a little higher so as to bring the oil caudad to outline the first two thoracic disc spaces.

Avulsion of brachial plexus has a typical myelographic configuration; at the site of tearing of the dura, an outpouching of Pantopaque takes place due to the bulging of the arachnoid membrane secondary to the post-traumatic meningocele (fig. 714).

Herniated thoracic discs. Herniated thoracic intervertebral discs occur rarely and account for approximately 0.5 per cent of all disc ruptures; when they do occur, they are usually located in the mid and lower thoracic zones. Calcification in a herniated thoracic disc occurs relatively more often than in the cervical and lumbar areas. Myelography may be useful to differentiate a thoracic disc herniation from a psammomatous meningioma. The majority of meningiomas are intradural and at myelography present the usual appearance of an extramedullary tumor of the intrathecal cavity. Herniated thoracic discs are ventral to the dura. While in frontal projection the flattening and widening of the thoracic spinal cord shadow that occurs might be caused by a meningioma, it is readily seen in lateral projection that the entire subarachnoid oil column is displaced dorsally by the lesion. When a herniated thoracic disc is not calcified, it cannot be differentiated satisfactorily from an extradural tumor.

Because of the relatively narrow subarachnoid space in the thoracic region, most of which is occupied by the spinal cord, relatively small disc protrusions and herniations in the thoracic region may cause an incomplete and even a complete block to the flow of contrast substance. Even relatively small discs that only cause a halt in the upward or downward flow of Pantopaque are capable of producing a severe neurologic deficit. This is because the cord is normally very close to the anterior margin of the subarachnoid space, that is, to the posterior margin of the vertebral bodies, due to the normal kyphotic curve of the thoracic spine. Particularly with the individual in the erect or prone position, the spinal cord is immediately or almost immediately against the posterior margin of the vertebral bodies because the epidural space is usually very small in the thoracic region and there is very little cushioning effect. It is important for this reason to look for minor deviations from the normal. A temporary halt in the cephalad or caudad flow of Pantopaque should be given attention, and an effort made to obtain prone lateral views. This may be difficult to accomplish but, as explained before under technique, this can be obtained in all cases if sufficient time and thought is given to the individual situation. Small *lateral defects* are common in the thoracic region and are usually insignificant. They are sometimes due to a conglomeration of epidural veins, and at other times, they are due to slight bulging of the intervertebral disc occurring on one side. However, unless a midline elevation of the oil column in prone lateral views is demonstrated or there is partial block to the flow of Pantopaque, they should not be regarded as significant.

(Revised 1963)

Thoracic disc herniations are often seen in relatively young individuals who present irregularities of the upper and lower margins of the vertebral bodies; that is, in individuals who present signs that we associate with juvenile osteochondrosis or Scheuermann's disease. The increased kyphotic curve in any individual places an added mechanical disadvantage in the presence of disc protrusion in the thoracic region because, under these circumstances, a smaller disc protrusion is capable of producing significant compression of the spinal cord. It is probable that cinemyelography will be able to help us in increasing our accuracy in the diagnosis of thoracic protruding and herniated intervertebral discs, in those cases where only a slight halt of the contrast substance takes place. Nevertheless, we still have to rely on the taking of satisfactory prone lateral films. A deviation of 2 to 3 mm. dorsad behind the intervertebral disc in the thoracic region is considered as probably significant. The vertical beam lateral views made with the patient in the right and left decubitus positions may give a false sense of security and should not be considered as a complete substitute for the prone lateral views. The lateral views made with the patient lying on the side should be made by turning the patient slightly ventrad so as to bring the level of the oil closer to the center of the subarachnoid space. As can be seen by glancing at Figure 637, the level of the oil does not reach the midline of the subarachnoid space when the patient lies on the side because the column of oil is spread over a very long segment.

Thoracic disc herniations producing par-

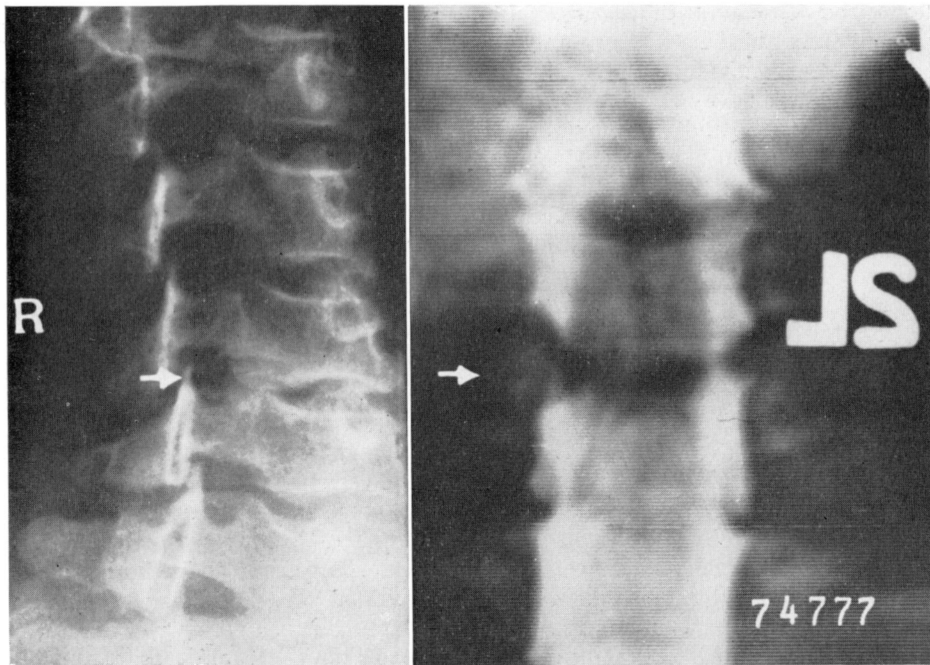

Fig. 715.—Osteoarthritis, C5-6 (Root Compression Type)

The plain spine roentgenogram made in posterior oblique projection discloses localized foraminal narrowing by hypertrophic spurs (*arrow*). A triangular filling defect is present in the myelogram and the nerve root sheath is not filled (*arrow*).

tial or complete block to the flow of Pantopaque may be confused with intramedullary tumors if proper lateral views are not made because of the widening of the spinal cord shadow, due to flattening, which takes place (fig. 706).

Vertebral Osteoarthritis

Cervical osteoarthritis (spondylosis). Osteoarthritis of the vertebral column is commonly seen; it is a natural process of aging. Rarely is a patient beyond middle age seen in whom osteoarthritis of the vertebral column is not demonstrable. In the vast majority of instances, osteoarthritis of the spine does not give rise to neurologic symptoms. Occasionally, however, unusually large osteophytes project into the vertebral canal or narrow an intervertebral foramen to such a degree that spinal cord or nerve root compression occurs. Neurologic symptoms, which may be attributed to osteoarthritis, arise most frequently in the cervical area (Mettier and Capp, 1941; Bailey and Casamajor, 1911). Radicular pain, when present, may be severe, as exemplified by the patients in whom left arm pain may be misinterpreted as a manifestation of angina pectoris.

It is impossible from the radiologic examination of the vertebral column alone to evaluate the full significance of osteoarthritis. The lesions which encroach on the vertebral canal and which narrow the intervertebral foramina, especially in the cervical region, are noteworthy but the roentgen findings must be correlated closely with the patient's symptoms and neurologic disturbances. Osteoarthritis demonstrable in plain films of the spine is frequently used to explain a radicular syndrome, or even a simple neuralgia, when actually a herniated intervertebral disc or spinal cord tumor is the cause of the patient's distress.

When thorough radiologic evaluation of the significance of osteoarthritic changes is desirable, in terms of encroachment on the spinal cord or spinal nerve roots, myelogra-

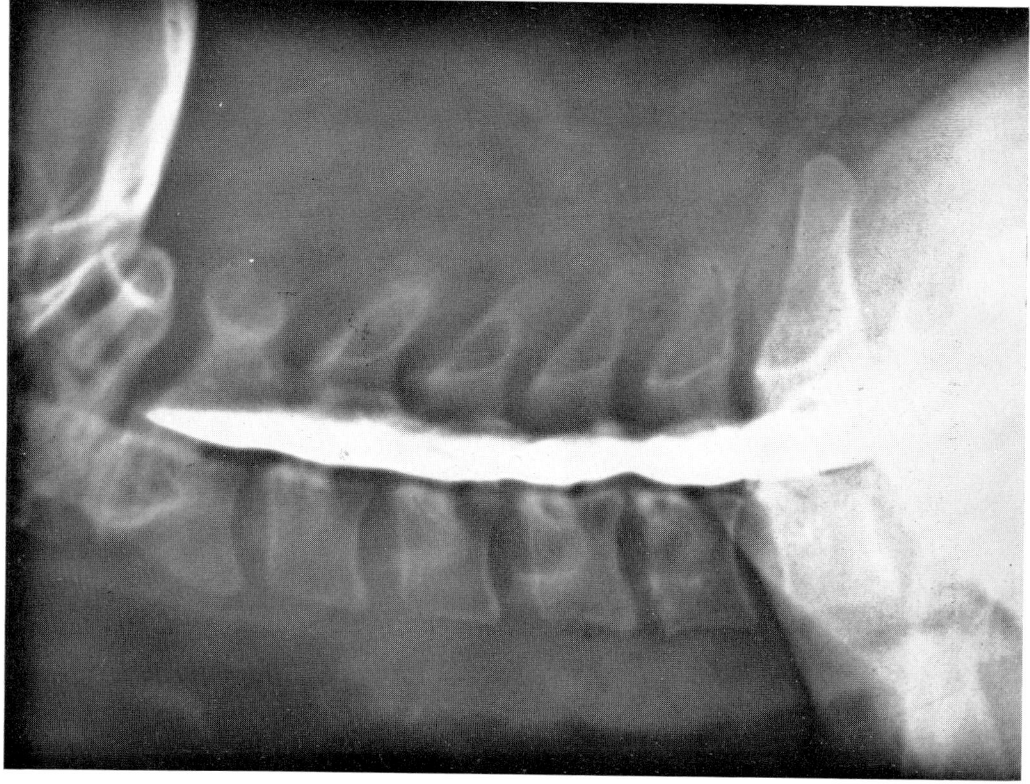

Fig. 716.—Small Cervical Osteoarthritic Ridge Producing Ventral Indentation on the Oil Column

This ventral indentation does not reach the level of the spinal cord, and in the anteroposterior projection it was not seen to produce any lateral defects. Therefore, this is believed to be a nonsignificant finding.

phy is the most satisfactory method of completing the examination. Myelographic deformities produced by osteoarthritic spurs are not dissimilar to those produced by herniated intervertebral discs. Compression of one or more nerve root sheaths, lateral or ventral encroachment on the main subarachnoid oil column, and, in the cervical region, partial or complete obstruction to the passage of radiopaque material in the subarachnoid space may be encountered. In most instances, the deformities produced by osteoarthritis alone are smaller in size and are more angular than herniated disc deformities, which frequently are large and rounded (fig. 715). An important difference is the frequent occurrence of multiple filling defects resulting from osteoarthritis, which emphasizes the diffuse degenerative nature of the process.

(Revised 1963)

Myelographic irregularities produced by osteoarthritis are considered significant only when compression of spinal nerve roots or the spinal cord can be demonstrated radiographically. Multiple irregularities of the ventral aspect of the radiopaque column are frequently demonstrable in the lateral myelogram as a result of ordinary osteoarthritis of the spine. Ventral indentation alone is not considered as significant unless, as occurs in the cervical region, spurs are sufficiently large to obliterate the ventral subarachnoid space and reach the anterior surface of the spinal cord (fig. 716). This rule must not be overlooked. In fact, when there is significant cord compression by a

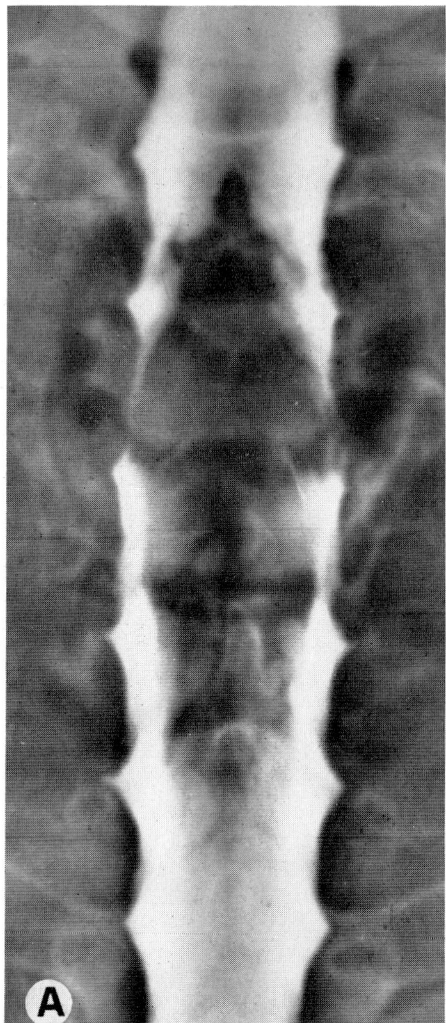

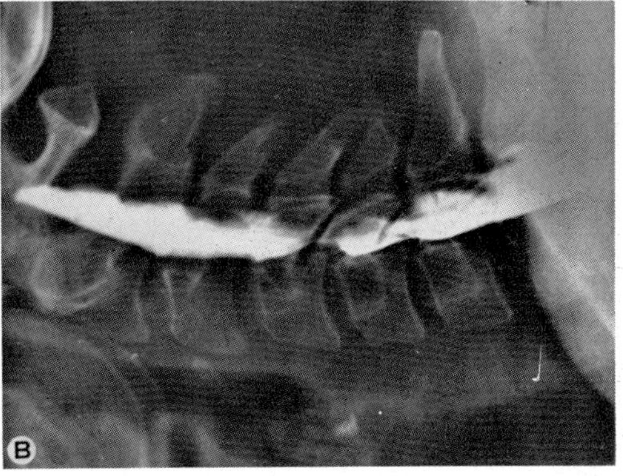

FIG. 717.—PROTRUDING INTERVERTEBRAL DISC AND INTRAMEDULLARY SPINAL CORD TUMOR COEXISTING IN CERVICAL REGION

The lateral projection (B) demonstrates a fairly sizable ventral indentation at C4-5. In the frontal projection (A), there is a fusiform widening of the spinal cord which, however, extends over a much longer area than might be expected from flattening of the cord secondary to ventral compression by a disc. Compare with Fig. 712.

ventral ridge, there is a fusiform widening of the transverse diameter of the spinal cord behind the corresponding disc space. In the lateral projection, the oil is seen to reach the level of the spinal cord, and sufficient oil should be brought up to the cervical region to demonstrate this fact clearly. Otherwise, errors in diagnosis will be made by attributing an unusual degree of significance to a small unimportant osteoarthritic ridge. Cases have been seen of intramedullary tumors of the spinal cord misdiagnosed as ostearthritic ridges, or herniated discs, that were considered insignificant. In tumors, the widened segment of the spinal cord is much longer than the area of fusiform widening usually seen with localized cord compression (fig. 717).

The most significant factor in the production of compression of the spinal cord

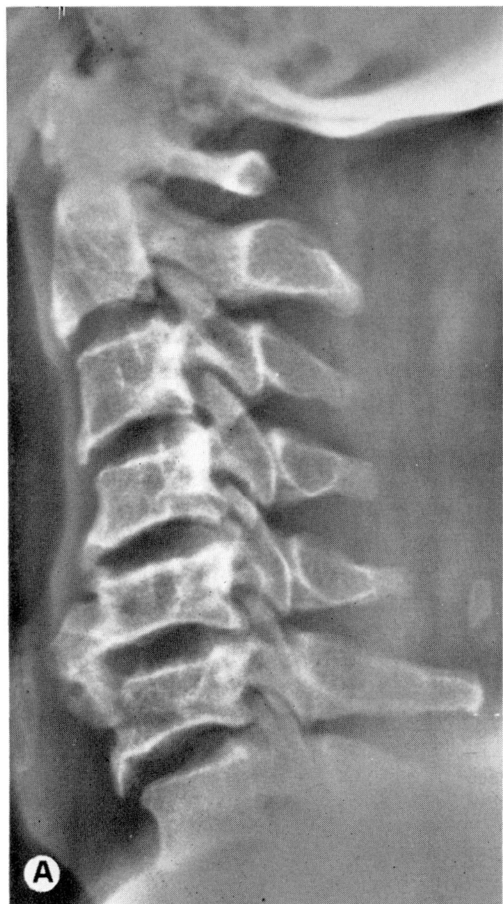

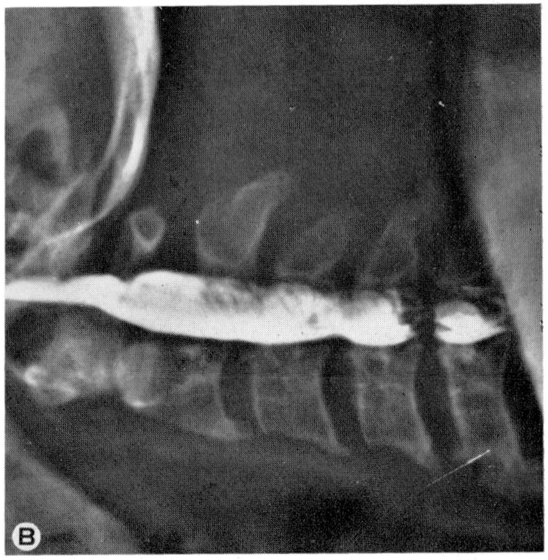

FIG. 718.—CONGENITALLY NARROW SPINAL CANAL IN CERVICAL REGION WITH SEVERE NEUROLOGIC DISTURBANCES

The plain film lateral view (A) discloses a narrow spinal canal which at C4, C5, and C6 only measures 11 to 12 mm. in anteroposterior diameter. A mild degree of posterior osteophyte formation is present. In the prone lateral myelogram (B), only relatively small ventral indentations are present at C4-5 and at C5-6. The patient had a moderate paraparesis and, at the time of admission, was actually unable to walk. Following surgical decompression, the symptoms improved considerably.

by osteoarthritic ridges is perhaps the width of the spinal canal in its anteroposterior diameter. This is variable in normal individuals, and measurements of 13 to 20 mm. in anteroposterior diameter are encountered in the cervical spine measured from the posterior margin of the vertebral bodies to the anterior margin of the spinous processes. Measurements under 13 mm. are often encountered in patients who have neurologic signs secondary to spondylosis with compression of the spinal cord. In a survey of this subject performed by Pallis, Jones, and Spillane (1954), it was found that the most significant factor that seemed to predispose the patient to the production of symptoms was the congenitally narrow spinal canal. Investigation of patients admitted to a general hospital to services other than neurology showed, on careful neurologic examination, the presence of frequent neurologic deficits of root compression in some cases, and cord compression in others, that were not sufficiently severe to bring the patients in this older age group to the neurologic service. It was found that the patients that presented signs of cord compression were those with the smaller anteroposterior diameter of the vertebral bodies. The same has been true in the experience of the authors; the case shown in figure 718 demonstrates this fact. It is interesting to note that, in these cases, the myelogram may show only a relatively small osteoarthritic ridge but, because of the small canal, it is sufficient to cause damaging cord compression. It is still argued whether the symptoms are strictly produced by cord compression from the osteoarthritic ridges accompanied by the protruding disc that always accompanies the osteophytes, or whether the cord degenerates as a result of continued long-standing compression. It is felt that in the initial stages, the symptoms are produced by cord compression and may not be too severe and so, in an older patient, it is disregarded as related to old age by the patient and the patient's family. Later, when the symptoms become aggravated with the passage of time, the patient may seek medical help; when a myelogram is performed, cord atrophy may be demonstrated (fig. 679). Under these circumstances, surgical intervention and decompression of the spinal cord would be foolish, inasmuch as the cord is no longer compressed. Surgical intervention is only advisable when compression of the spinal cord is actually demonstrated.

On plain film examinations, an osteoarthritic ridge may be considered as significant when it encroaches on 25 to 30 per cent of the anteroposterior diameter of the vertebral canal at the same level. In a patient with a 13 mm. or less anteroposterior spinal diameter, an osteoarthritic ridge measuring 3 mm. is highly significant, whereas in a patient with an anteroposterior diameter of 18 mm., a ridge of this size may not be significant.

A factor to consider is the possibility that the visible ridge is not in the central portion of the canal but is only on one or both sides and is superimposed. To ascertain that the ridge is indeed in the central portion of the spinal canal, lateral laminagrams of the cervical spine are required. Stereoscopic views may also be of help, but laminagraphy is superior.

In trying to determine spinal cord compression, well exposed lateral views are necessary with sufficient oil in this region. As noted in "Myelographic Anatomy," the anterior margin of the spinal cord is about 5 mm. ventral to the shadow of the dentate ligaments which are usually identified with ease when there is sufficient filling. The anterior margin of the cord is identified by an extra line of density which, as mentioned previously, may be produced by the anterior spinal vessels and the anterior rootlets of the cervical nerve roots superimposed upon the shadow of the anterior margin of the cord itself (fig. 639). This helps in identifying the anterior margin of the cord and will be shown to be displaced dorsad when there is a ventral protrusion produced by either an osteoarthritic ridge or herniated intervertebral disc.

The evaluation of root compression by osteoarthritic spurs is more difficult. As can be easily understood, if there is elevation of the ventral aspect of the root sleeve by any process, the myelogram, which usually outlines only the ventral aspect of the root sleeve, will demonstrate widening of the root shadow (fig. 719). Widening of the root shadow may be due to compression of the root at the same level, but this is not necessarily so, for as explained above, if the floor of the foramen is elevated, as by small spurs, the elevation of the arachnoid membrane at the same point may also cause widening of the root shadow on the myelogram. It is a matter of degree, and it is likely that if there is marked increase in width of the root shadow, there is a significant degree of root compression, whereas if the root shadow is only slightly widened, it may not be significant. However, the authors have seen many cases where the root shadow is only slightly widened and yet clinically the symptoms are localized to that particular root, and surgical intervention may demonstrate a small herniated disc or a spur at that level with improvement of the patient's neurologic signs following surgical intervention. Of course, the root may be compressed outside the subarachnoid space in the intervertebral foramen, and the small myelographic defect was only the beginning

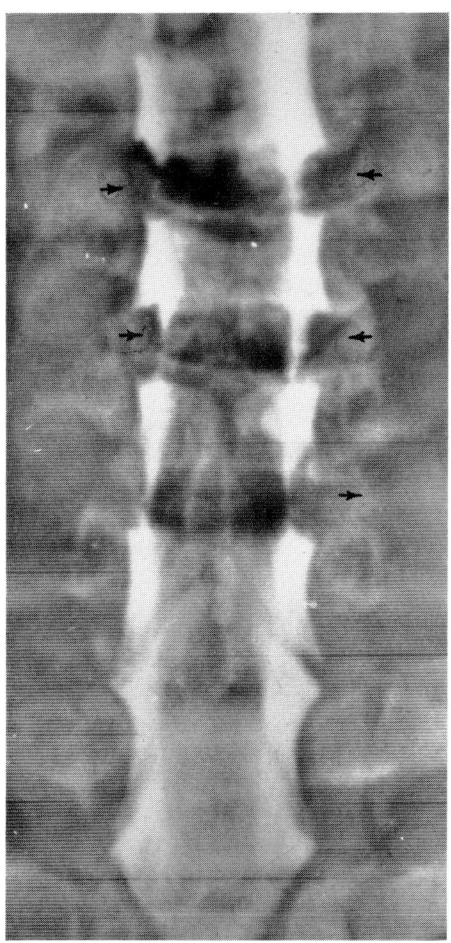

FIG. 719.—MULTIPLE ROOT SHADOW WIDENING ASSOCIATED WITH OSTEOARTHRITIS

There is widening of the root shadow on both sides at the level indicated by *arrows*. While this may indicate actual root compression at the time of the myelogram, it is not necessarily symptomatic, and the root may well have accommodated to the elevation of the ventral aspect of the root sleeve produced by osteoarthritic spurs.

of a larger spur which compressed the root further laterally.

If the lateral margin of the Pantopaque column is displaced medially, away from the adjacent pedicle, it indicates tenting of the dura. This associated finding increases the likelihood that the root widening is clinically significant (fig. 720).

An intervertebral foramen may be encroached upon by spurs. This is an extremely common finding in older individuals. It is common to find large spurs projecting into intervertebral foramina without radicular signs of root compression being present clinically. Although the presence of encroachment upon the intervertebral foramen by a spur does not mean that the patient must have radicular signs of root compression at that time, intermittent signs of root compression are not uncommon in these patients and the appearance of symptoms may be precipitated by a sharp movement, a slight degree of trauma, or simply sleeping in an improper position. It is, therefore, very important not to dismiss these findings at a given time but simply to look upon them as having developed so slowly that the root has been able to adapt to the deformity—to the extra curve that it must make to go around the obstacle—and that another factor is required to trigger the appearance of symptoms. The same may be true of the multiple "root widening" which is seen on the myelographic films in these patients. Of course, the presence of widening of the root shadow in the myelogram is slightly more significant than the presence of an osteoarthritic spur, but it is common to find them in patients who have no signs of root compression at those levels (fig. 719). It might be mentioned at this point that osteoarthritic spurs may also arise from the margins of the articular facets; these protrude on the posterolateral aspect of the root and intervertebral foramen. In the myelogram, they produce lateral defects that are situated just above the root instead of at the root, as is usually the case with osteoarthritic spurs arising on the posterolateral aspect of the disc margins.

A helpful consideration for diagnosis is that herniated intervertebral discs are situated underneath the root and produce a concentric widening of the shadow of this structure; osteoarthritis spurs often are situated slightly above the root and may displace the root downward, thus, producing more deformity of the upper aspect of the root shadow than the lower. The difference occurs because the osteoarthritic spurs may arise from the most lateral margin of the vertebral body which, as is well known, in the cervical region turns upward forming a lip (erroneously referred to as joints of Luschka). Likewise, if the osteophyte arises from the articular facet, the defect is well above the root and is easily identifiable.

Position is important in the production of symptoms in cervical spondylosis. With the patient's head extended, the cord is in the most favorable position to avoid ventral compression. On the other hand, with the head in flexion, the cord will come closer to the ventral surface of the spinal canal and compression can occur with greater ease. This is particularly to be considered in relation to the patient's sleeping habits in the supine position, possibly on a high pillow.

The myelogram is performed with the head extended, in the most favorable position, and flexion may be tried during myelography, at least to a slight degree, compatible with the oil remaining in the cervical region without running into the cephalic portion of the subarachnoid space. This maneuver may demonstrate a greater degree of interference with the flow of Pantopaque than with the head in extension.

An interesting phenomenon often seen in patients with osteoarthritis or spondylosis is that a complete block to the cephalad flow of Pantopaque will be encountered with the patient in the Trendelenburg position. As explained previously, the obstruction probably is due to the fact that the patient is straining at the time, even when asked not to do so, and at the same time, a reversal of the venous flow will increase the quantity of blood in the epidural plexus in the Trendelenburg position. When the patient is brought back to the horizontal position, the oil will be seen to pass slowly upward above the block, and it is then demonstrated that there was only a partial difficulty in the passage of oil through the area and not a complete block. Therefore, the taking of spot films only in the Trendelenburg position in the presence of a block may be misleading; on the contrary, it is advisable to take films with the head in horizontal or almost horizontal position using the slight variations in tilt of the table as explained earlier. Sometimes, when the obstruction is more complete, the turning of the head to one side or the other will permit passage of some of the oil cephalad, thus enabling us to outline the upper as well as the lower margin of the lesion.

Thickening of the ligamentum flavum and osteoarthritis of the apophyseal joints. Thickening of the spinal ligaments, in particular the ligamentum flavum, along each dorsolateral aspect of the vertebral canal, usually occurs in conjunction with other spinal lesions, especially herniation of the intervertebral disc. At the same time, there is hypertrophic osteoarthritic involvement of the apophyseal joints. Thickening of the ligamentum flavum occasionally may occur alone but then it is of doubtful clinical significance. While grossly the ligaments appear enlarged, suggesting hypertrophy, histologic examination shows that the increase in size is the result of mild edema, swelling, and degeneration of the elastic fibers, and an increase in the quantity of interstitial connective tissue. The process is not one of compensatory hypertrophy associated with disc rupture or other abnormality of the vertebral column, but rather a degenerative process with resulting fibrosis. Therefore, the change is more correctly termed thickening of the ligamentum flavum than hypertrophy (Dockerty and Love, 1940).

The ligamentum flavum is situated dorsolaterally and connects the laminae of successive vertebrae. Although each lateral portion of every ligament bounds an intervertebral foramen posteriorly, it is doubtful that thickening is ever sufficiently extensive to narrow significantly the intervertebral foramen. Ligamentous thickening does, however, impede the posterior displacement of the dural sac by a large ventral mass, such as a herniated intervertebral disc. Therefore, it can contribute to further compression of the root when a ventral mass displaces it backward. The ligamentum flavum contributes to the hourglass deformity of the subarachnoid space seen with unusually large central disc herniations (fig. 700).

Thickening of the ligamentum flavum produces a radiolucent band on the dorsal

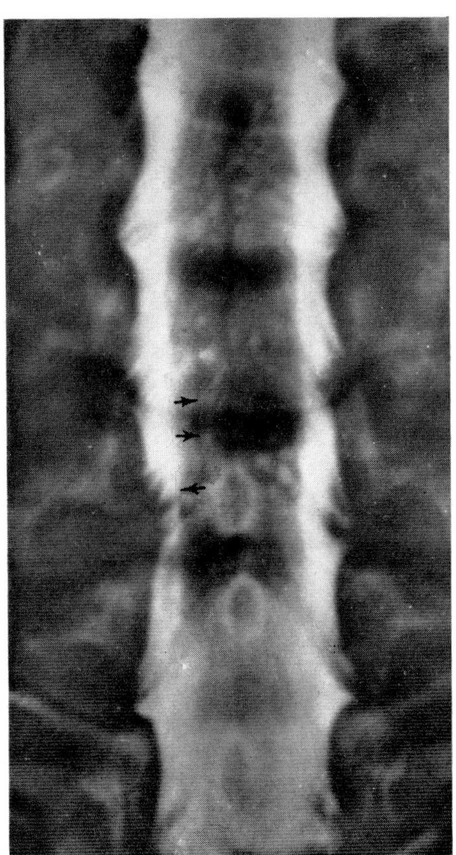

FIG. 720.—SINGLE ROOT LESION AT C6-7 ON THE RIGHT SIDE PRODUCING DISPLACEMENT OF LATERAL MARGIN OF OIL COLUMN

There is a gradual, tentlike displacement of the lateral margin of the oil column away from the pedicles centered at the root shadow which is itself slightly elevated (*arrows*). This is produced by tenting of the dura and is usually associated with acute disc herniation but is usually not present in osteoarthritic spurs because the dura has had time to accommodate to the deformity. In addition to the shadow of the anterior spinal artery, there are other vascular shadows on the cord (*two arrows*) which represent engorged veins. Prominent vessels on the cord are often seen in association with acute disc herniations.

side of the subarachnoid space, the anterior margin of which is seen to extend from above downward and from the dorsal to the ventral side in lumbar myelograms.

Other Non-neoplastic Vertebral Lesions

Charcot's disease. Neurotrophic arthropathies may occur in the lower thoracic and lumbar portions of the vertebral column as a result of tabes dorsalis or syringomyelia. The bone and joint changes basically resemble those of osteoarthritis and the course is similar inasmuch as repeated trauma plays a major role in their development. In tabetic arthropathy, the eburnation of bone and the proliferative changes at the margins of the vertebral bodies are more extensive than those seen in ordinary osteoarthritis. The loss of sensory modality which protects the joints from injury, or from excessive use after injury, is thought by some authorities to be responsible for fragmentation of the hypertrophied margins of the vertebrae and extensive degeneration of the intervertebral discs at multiple levels. On the contrary, there is little evidence to support the notion that the bones of patients with tabes are exposed to excessive trauma. Another explanation is that neurotrophic disease affects the vertebrae directly through a disturbance of bone metabolism. The posterior and posterolateral bony excrescenses and disc protrusions eventually may impinge on motor fibers of the cauda equina supplying the lower extremities and may cause sphincteric disturbances, which further complicate the neurologic disturbances of tabes dorsalis.

Occasionally, surgical intervention for relief of cauda equina compression is necessary. In such instances, it may be desirable to carry out myelography to determine the point at which maximum deformity of the subarachnoid space is present. The myelogram shows marked generalized narrowing of the subarachnoid space as a result of bony proliferation, disc protrusion, and thickening of the ligaments of the vertebral canal. Bilateral constriction of the subarachnoid oil column is shown at multiple intervertebral levels in the frontal myelogram, and in the lateral view, ventral encroachment on the subarachnoid space outlined by contrast material is demonstrated. Frequently, the encroachment is sufficiently extensive to cause a partial or complete occlusion of the arachnoid sac at one or more intervertebral levels.

Paget's disease. Monostotic or polyostotic osteitis deformans may occur in the

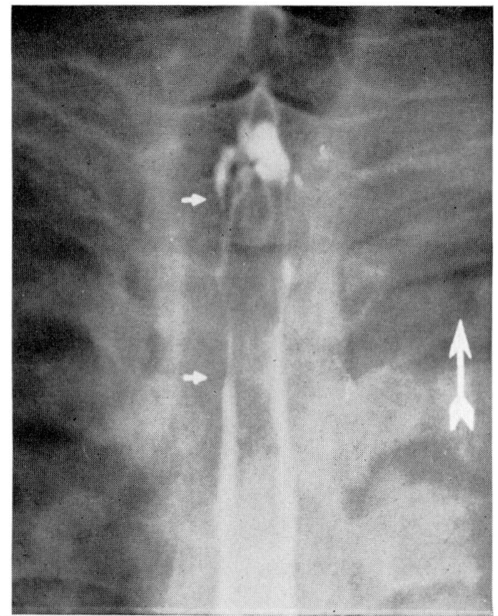

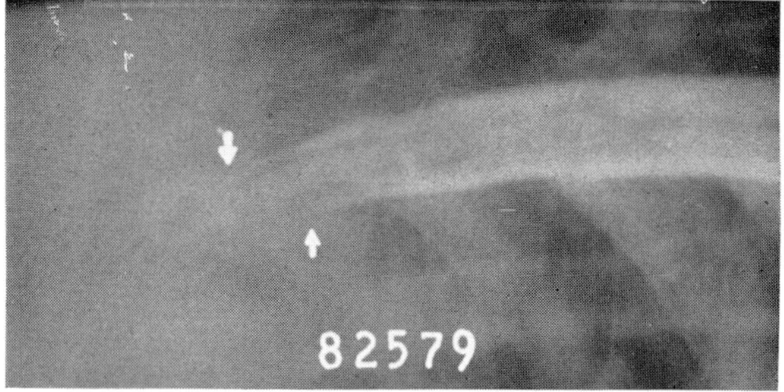

FIG. 721.—PAGET'S DISEASE, T3, 4, AND 5
The radiopaque oil column becomes narrowed on both sides from the midportion of the body of T3 to T5. Tapering of the opaque column toward the spinal cord in frontal and lateral views (*arrows*) denotes that the lesion is encircling the dural sac.

vertebral column. The changes usually observed are the result of a combined destructive and reparative process. The reparative process more often predominates presumably because of weight-bearing and stress on the spinal column. The changes are most frequently observed in the vertebral body but often the vertebral arch also is involved.

The changes in bony architecture resulting from Paget's disease of the vertebra are not unlike those observed in other bones. The longitudinal trabeculae of the vertebral body are increased in thickness and density, and the trabecular spaces undergo irregular widening. In some instances, there is marked sclerosis with loss of trabecular detail, and oval areas of diminished density which vary in size are scattered throughout the vertebrae. The most prominent reparative change occurs about the periphery of the vertebral body. The vertebra frequently is increased in width and reduced in height, especially in the central portion, because of compression of the abnormally soft bone. Convex masses of partially calcified osteoid tissue frequently project beyond the vertebral body and displace the paraspinal shadow. This change is best observed in frontal films of the thoracic spine. The vertebral pedicles also may be enlarged in Paget's disease. The combination of flattening of the vertebral body and proliferation of osteoid tissue on all sides of the vertebra, with or without enlargement of the pedicles, may cause significant constriction of the vertebral canal and intervertebral foramina resulting in compression of the spinal cord and nerve roots (Schwarz and Reback, 1939).

Dorsal bowing of the posterior surface of the vertebral body is demonstrable in plain spine roentgenograms in the lateral projection. The osteoid tissue, which extends posteriorly beyond the margins of the bone, usually cannot be appreciated from plain film examination. Encroachment on the vertebral canal frequently occurs at more than one vertebral level. Myelography is useful to determine the extent to which a subarachnoid space is narrowed.

The myelographic deformities of Paget's disease resemble those which occur with extradural tumor in which neoplastic tissue extends into the vertebral canal from a vertebra. The subarachnoid oil column is compressed from one or more sides (fig. 721), most often from the ventral aspect. The radiopaque column tapers dorsally to a point of partial or complete obliteration behind the *center* of the deformed vertebral body. With lesions cephalad to the lumbar spine, the shadow of the spinal cord is visibly displaced posteriorly in the lateral myelogram, and in frontal projection it may appear widened by compression. If an acute compression deformity of a vertebral body has occurred, the arachnoid sac containing the spinal cord may be markedly displaced dorsally and sharply angulated. In such instances, a complete obstruction to the passage of radiopaque material in the subarachnoid space is usually encountered. The head of the radiopaque column undergoes an abrupt bilateral medial tapering in frontal projection in association with an acute tapering of the oil column ventral to the spinal cord in lateral view. Ordinarily, the intervertebral discs remain intact and the maximum deformity is seen at the level of the center of the vertebral body. On rare occasions, osteogenic sarcoma may develop in a vertebra affected by Paget's disease, and areas of true osteolytis then may become demonstrable in the involved segments.

Vertebral Tumors

Benign tumors. *Hemangioma* and *giant cell tumor* are two benign lesions of the vertebral column which occasionally are associated with neurologic symptoms.

Cavernous hemangioma most commonly involves the vertebrae in the lower thoracic or lumbar area. When first seen, the process may involve only a part of the vertebra, often a quadrant of the vertebral body or a pedicle, or the entire body, and both pedicles may be affected. The vertebra involved is not denser than the adjacent segments on the radiograph. The longitudinal trabeculae are increased in density and thickness, while the more delicate transverse trabeculae disappear, with the result that the internal portion of the vertebra appears striated. The trabecular spaces are widened but the increase in width occurs in a fairly regular manner with essentially no peripheral reaction in the bone, as contrasted to Paget's disease. The pedicles seen *en face* in the frontal film appear spongy as a result of the alternating thickened trabeculae and widened trabecular spaces (Bucy and Capp, 1930). In the majority of instances, cavernous hemangioma of the spinal column does not cause symptoms. It is worthy of mention that Paget's disease and some slowly growing malignant neoplasms, including myeloma and chordoma, may simulate the appearance of cavernous hemangioma in roentgenograms. Neurologic symptoms, when present, result from simultaneous involvement of the meninges and the spinal cord or from pathologic vertebral fractures with compression of the spinal cord (Bailey and Bucy, 1929). Back pain produced by hemangiomas of the vertebrae is not an uncommon occurrence.

Giant cell tumor is rare in the vertebral column. It may often be of the type which is now usually called aneurysmal bone cyst. Marked expansion of the vertebral body and vertebral arch may narrow the vertebral canal and intervertebral foramina at the level of the lesion. When the pedicles are expanded, the interpediculate measurements may be reduced. Nevertheless, encroachment on nervous system structures occurs rarely unless the tumor extends beyond the confines of the bony cortex or a pathologic fracture of the vertebra takes place.

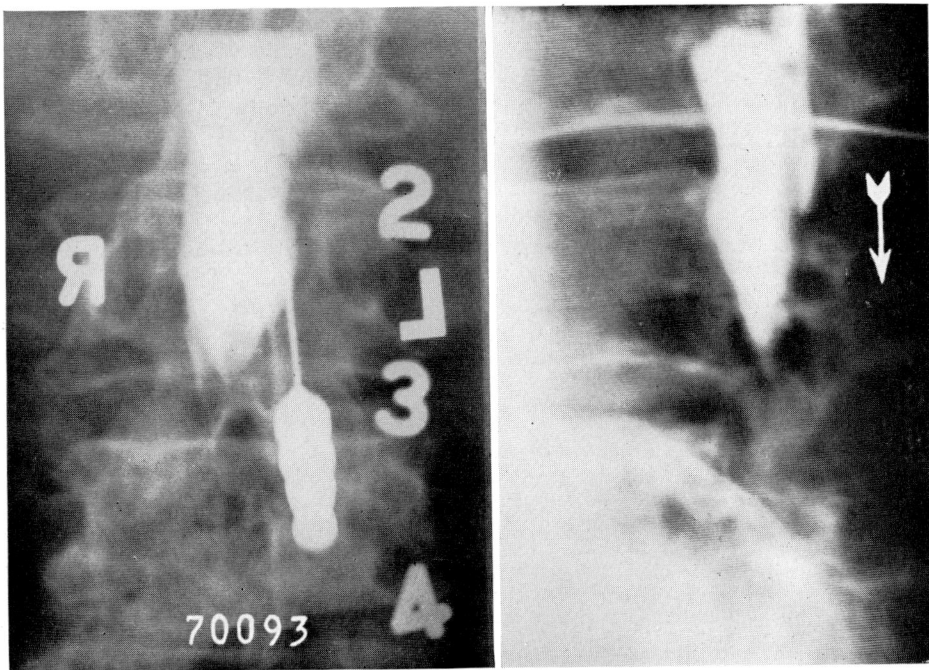

FIG. 722.—CHORDOMA, L4

Films made with the patient erect disclose an obstruction to the caudad flow of Pantopaque at the level of the L3-4 intervertebral space. The lower end of the opaque column is conic because the tumor envelopes the dural sac. The tumor has produced a mixed osteolytic and osteoblastic reaction in the body of L4.

Malignant tumors. Chordoma is a malignant tumor which arises almost exclusively within the axial skeleton. The neoplasms take origin in remnants of the notochord and, therefore, may be found at any point from the skull to the coccyx. The majority of lesions are encountered at the ends of the axial skeleton and are either cranial or sacral coccygeal. A lesser number is reported as occurring at various vertebral levels, chiefly in the upper cervical region.

Chordomas are neoplasms of relatively low malignancy and may grow locally for long periods of time, involving the spinal cord and spinal nerve roots in one area. Initially, the growths are encapsulated but later they break through the capsule and invade the adjacent bone and soft tissues. Metastasis occurs only from those tumors which arise in the sacral coccygeal area and is said to occur in from 5 to 10 per cent of cases. For some unknown reason, those which originate elsewhere apparently do not metastasize. Bone destruction resulting from infiltration by tumor is the predominant manifestation of chordoma in plain spine radiographs. The vertebral body first is involved, following which the arch may be invaded. Bone expansion often occurs early, following which extraosseous extension of the tumor may take place in any direction with the result that a paraspinal mass is demonstrable lateral or anterior to the involved vertebra. Calcium shadows, which represent either fragments of sequestrated bone or a degenerative change in the tumor may be visible in the paraspinal mass. An osteoblastic reaction in association with bone destruction occurs in a small percentage of patients with vertebral chordoma (Wood and Himadi, 1950). Two, or sometimes three, successive vertebrae characteristically are involved and the intervening intervertebral discs invaded.

Posterior extension of the tumor into the vertebral canal may result in compression of the spinal cord or cauda equina, with an obstruction of the subarachnoid space. At myelography, the subarachnoid radiopaque column tapers gradually to a point of obstruction in the manner ordinarily seen with epidural masses compressing the spinal cord (fig. 722). Myelography is valuable only to determine the limit of epidural extension of the tumor, when surgical decompression is to be performed, since the tumor can be detected, localized, and, on occasion, correctly identified from plain spine roentgenograms.

Sources of Errors in Diagnosis by Myelography

Sources of error and the limitations of myelography for the diagnosis of disc herniations should be recognized. Herniations which most frequently avoid detection at myelography occur at the L5–S1 interspace. At the lumbosacral junction, considerable anatomic narrowing of the subarachnoid space is present prior to its termination at S2. In frontal projection, the width of the subarachnoid radiopaque column at S1 is, on the average, smaller than that noted at L4–5 and frequently occupies less than half the caliber of the column at L1. Some of these facts have been discussed in dealing with lumbar disc herniations.

In the lateral view, dorsal tapering of the ventral margin of the subarachnoid space frequently begins behind the body of L5. At L5–S1 intervertebral level, there may be a normal space of considerable thickness between the anterior aspect of the radiopaque column and the posterior margin of the sacrum. Herniated L5–S1 discs which extend into the sacral canal in the ventral epidural fat may be of considerable size without deforming the anterior aspect of the radiopaque oil column. When an anatomic variation is present, with termination of the sacral cul-de-sac at the level of S1 (short cul-de-sac), the possibility of failing to demonstrate a herniation of the L5–S1 disc is enhanced.

More cephalad, in the lumbar region, the most common causes of error at myelography are anatomic variations (1) in the caliber of the subarachnoid space, or (2) in the quantity of epidural areolar tissue between the arachnoid sac and the walls of the vertebral canal. When the subarachnoid space is of small caliber, possibly less than 1.5 cm.– and uniformly separated from the margins of the vertebrae by a wide, clear zone of soft tissue–disc lesions, especially protrusions, may be imbedded in the areolar tissue without causing an indentation of the lateral or ventral aspect of the main oil column at myelography. Defective filling of the arachnoid sheath of the nerve roots also is absent if the roots are compressed lateral to the short arachnoid encasements.

On the contrary, a patient with a large subarachnoid space, in whom there is little soft tissue between the ventral and lateral margins of the subarachnoid oil column and the vertebral column, may have shallow irregularities in the Pantopaque column at myelography which are not the result of disc herniation. Normally, there is a slight posterior bulge of the intervertebral disc beyond the level of the posterior margins of the contiguous vertebrae. The bulge becomes more prominent with advancing age as ordinary degenerative changes progress. An erroneous impression of single or, more often, multiple posterior disc herniations may be gained at myelography when the subarachnoid caliber is greater than average. In the lateral myelogram, the degree of posterior extension of normal discs may be used as a base line for comparison with indentation of the radiopaque column at an intervertebral level where disc herniation is suspected.

Another hazard for the correct diagnosis of ruptured intervertebral disc is the reduction of the normal disc indentation of the radiopaque column created when the normal ventral lumbar curve is lost, or when flexion is produced by placing a pillow beneath the abdomen of the prone patient. It is possible that even herniated discs demonstrated by myelography in the neutral position, or in hyperextension, may appear to recede or become flattened when the vertebral column is in flexion (fig. 697). Neurosurgeons are familiar with the maneuver of extending the spine at the operating table to make lesions more conspicuous when they are difficult to identify in flexion. A discussion on the recognition of extra-arachnoidal injections of Pantopaque is given on page 1.836.

REFERENCES

Albright, F., Butler, A. M., Hampton, A. O., and Smith, P.: Syndrome characterized by osteitis fibrosa disseminata, areas of pigmentation and endocrine dysfunction, with precocious puberty in females; report of five cases. New England J. Med., 216:727, 1937.

Albright, F., and Reifenstein, E. C., Jr.: The Parathyroid Glands and Metabolic Bone Disease. Baltimore, Maryland, The Williams & Wilkins Company, 1948.

Alexander, W. G.: Report of a case of so-called "marble bones" with a review of the literature and a translation of an article. Am. J. Roentgenol., 10:280, 1923.

Amplatz, K., and Harner, R.: A new subclavian artery catheterization technique. Preliminary report. Radiology, 78:963, 1962.

Andersen, P. E.: The lenticulo-striate arteries and their diagnostic value. A preliminary report. Acta radiol., 50:84, 1958.

Aoyagi, T., and Kyunō, K.: Über die endothelialen Zellzapfen in der Dura mater cerebri und ihre Lokalisation in derselben, nebst ihrer Beziehung zur Geschwulstbildung in der Dura mater. Neurologia, 11:1, 1912.

Arnell, S.: Myelography with water-soluble contrast with special regard to the normal roentgen picture. Acta radiol. Supp., 75:70, 1948.

Azambuja, N., Arana, I. R., Sande, M. T., and Garcia, G. A.: Central ventriculography. Acta neurol. latinoam., 2:58, 1956.

Azambuja, N., Barrios, R. R., and Garcia, E.: Charges in CSF pressure during pneumoencephalography. Presented at the VI Symposium Neuroradiologicum. Rome, 1961.

Azambuja, N., Lindgren, E., and Sjögren, S. E.: Tentorial herniations. I. Anatomy. Acta radiol., 46:215, 1956; III. Angiography. Acta radiol., 46:232, 1956.

Bailey, P., and Bucy, P. C.: Cavernous hemangioma of the vertebrae. J.A.M.A., 92:1748, 1929.

Bailey, P., and Casamajor, L.: Osteo-arthritis of the spine as a cause of compression of the spinal cord and its roots, with reports of five cases. J. Nerv. & Ment. Dis., 38:588, 1911.

Baker, A. B.: An Outline of Neuropathology, Ed. 3, Minneapolis, Minnesota, University of Minnesota Press, 1943.

Baker, H. L., Jr.: A new approach to percutaneous subclavian angiography. Proc. Staff Meet. Mayo Clin., 35:169, 1960.

Baker, H. L., Jr.: Cerebral arteriography: technics and results. Proc. Staff Meet. Mayo Clin., 35: 482, 1960.

Baker, H. L., Jr.: Intracerebral hemorrhage masquerading as a neoplasm. A difficult neuroradiologic problem. Radiology, 78:914, 1962.

Baker, T. W., and Shelden, W. D.: Coarctation of the aorta with intermittent leakage of a congenital cerebral aneurysm. Am. J. M. Sc., 191: 626, 1936.

Balado, M., and Carillo, R.: Estudio comparativo de los modernos procedimientos de diagnóstico neuroquirúrgico resultados de la yodoventriculografía. Semana méd., 42:717, 1935.

Baldwin, M., and Bailey, P. (editors): International Colloquium on Temporal Lobe Epilepsy. Springfield, Illinois, Charles C Thomas, 1958.

Barbieri, P. L., and Verdecchia, G. C.: Vertebral arteriography by percutaneous puncture of the subclavian artery. Acta radiol., 48:444, 1957.

Barnett, D. J.: Radiologic aspects of craniopharyngiomas. Radiology, 72:14, 1959.

Bassett, R. C., Rogers, J. S., Cherry, G. R., and Gruzhit, C.: The effect of contrast media on the blood-brain-barrier. J. Neurosurg., 10:38, 1953.

Begg, A. C.: Radiographic demonstration of the "hypoglossal artery." A rare type of persistent anomalous carotid-basilar anastomosis. Clin. Radiol., 12:187, 1961.

Berk, M. E.: Chemodectoma of the glomus intravagale: A case report and review. Clin. Radiol., 12:219, 1961.

Berkwitz, N. J., and Rigler, L. G.: Tuberous sclerosis diagnosed with cerebral pneumography. A.M.A. Arch. Neurol. & Psychiat., 34:833, 1935.

Bernasconi, V., and Casinari, V.: Caratteritische angiografiche dei meningiomi del tentorio, Radiol. Med., 43:1015, 1957.

Borden, W. C.: The Use of the Röntgen Ray by the Medical Department of the United States

Army in the War with Spain (1898). Washington, D. C., Government Printing Office, 1900.

Bossi, R., and Pisani, C.: Collateral cerebral circulation through the ophthalmic artery and its efficiency in internal carotid occlusion. Brit. J. Radiol., 28:462, 1955.

Bradford, F. K., and Spurling, R. G.: The Intervertebral Disc. Springfield, Illinois, Charles C Thomas, 1945, p. 58.

Bray, P. F., Carter, S., and Taveras, J. M.: Brainstem tumors in children. Neurology, 8:1, 1958.

Brierley, J. B.: The prolonged and distant effects of experimental brain injury on cerebral blood vessels as demonstrated by radioactive indicators. J. Neurol., Neurosurg. & Psychiat., 19:202, 1956.

Broadridge, A. T., and Leslie, E. V.: Cerebral angiographic contrast media. A comparison of Hypaque 45% and Urografin 60% and an assessment of the relative clinical toxicity of Urografin 60%, Hypaque 45%, Diaginol 25%, and Diodone 35% in carotid arteriography. Brit. J. Radiol., 31:556, 1958.

Broman, T., Forssman, B., and Olsson, O.: Further experimental investigations of injuries from contrast media in cerebral angiography. Summation of various injurious factors. Acta radiol., 34:135, 1950.

Broman, T., and Olsson, O.: Experimental study of contrast media for cerebral angiography with reference to possible injurious effects on the cerebral blood vessels. Acta radiol., 31:321, 1949.

Browder, J., and Hollister, N. R.: Air encephalography and ventriculography as diagnostic aids in craniocerebral trauma. In: Trauma of the Central Nervous System. Proceedings of the Association of Research in Nervous and Mental Disease, Vol. 24, Chap. 16. Baltimore, The Williams & Wilkins Company, 1945, p. 421.

Browder, J., and Meyers, R.: Infections of the spinal epidural space: an aspect of vertebral osteomyelitis. Am. J. Surg., 37:4, 1937.

Bucy, P. C.: Hydrocephalus. In: Brenneman's Practice of Pediatrics. Hagerstown, Maryland, W. F. Prior Company, 1939, Vol. 4, Chap. 3, p. 1.

Bucy, P. C., and Capp, C. S.: Primary hemangioma of bone. With special reference to roentgenologic diagnosis. Am. J. Roentgenol., 23:1, 1930.

Bucy, P. C., Heimburger, R. F., and Oberhill, H. R.: Compression of the cervical spinal cord by herniated intervertebral discs. J. Neurosurg., 5:471, 1948.

Bull, J. W. D.: The normal variations in the position of the optic recess of the third ventricle. Acta radiol., 46:72, 1956.

Bull, J. W. D.: The volume of the cerebral ventricles. Neurology, 11:1, 1961.

Bull, J. W. D., Nixon, W. L. B., and Pratt, R. T. C.: The radiological criteria and familial occurrence of primary basilar impression. Brain, 78:Part 2, 229, 1955.

Bull, J. W. D., Nixon, W. L. B., Pratt, R. T. C., and Robinson, P. K.: Paget's disease of the skull and secondary basilar impression. Brain, 82: 10, 1959. (Abstract: Radiology, 75:654, 1960.)

Caffey, J.: Multiple fractures in the long bones of infants suffering from chronic subdural hematoma. Am. J. Roentgenol., 56:163, 1946.

Caffey, J.: On accessory ossicles of the supraoccipital bone. Some newly recognized roentgen fractures of the normal infantile skull. Am. J. Roentgenol, 70:401, 1953.

Caffey, J.: Pediatric X-Ray Diagnosis, Ed. 4, Chicago, Year Book Medical Publishers, Inc., 1961.

Cairns, H., and Russell, D. S.: Intracranial and spinal metastases in gliomas of the brain. Brain, 54: 377, 1931.

Camp, J. D.: The normal and pathologic anatomy of the sella turcica as revealed at necropsy. Radiology, 1:65, 1923.

Camp, J. D.: II. The normal and pathologic anatomy of the sella turcica as revealed by roentgenograms. Am. J. Roentgenol., 12:143, 1924.

Camp, J. D.: The significance of osseous changes in the roentgenographic diagnosis of tumors of the spinal cord and associated soft tissues. Radiology, 22:295, 1934.

Camp, J. D.: Multiple tumors within the spinal canal. Am. J. Roentgenol., 36:775, 1936.

Camp, J. D.: The roentgenologic localization of tumors affecting the spinal cord. Am. J. Roentgenol., 40:540, 1938.

Camp, J. D.: Roentgenologic observations concerning erosion of the sella turcica. Radiology, 53:666, 1949.

Camp, J. D.: Contrast myelography past and present. Radiology, 54: 477, 1950.

Camp, J. D.: Significance of intracranial calcification in the roentgenologic diagnosis of intracranial neoplasms. Radiology, 55:659, 1950.

Camp, J. D., and Cilley, E. I. L.: The significance of asymmetry of the pori acustici as an aid in diagnosis of eighth nerve tumors. Am. J. Roentgenol., 41:713, 1939.

Camp, J. D., and Nash, L. A.: Developmental thinness of the parietal bones. Radiology, 42:42, 1944.

Carpenter, M. B., Noback, C. R., and Moss, M. L.: The anterior choroidal artery. Its origins, course, distribution, and variations. A.M.A. Arch. Neurol. & Psychiat., 71:714, 1954.

Carton, C. A.: Cerebral Angiography in the Management of Head Trauma. Springfield, Illinois, Charles C Thomas, 1959.

Chamberlain, W. E., and Stauffer, H. M.: A new device for stereoscopic cerebral and cardiac angiography. Trans. Coll. Phys. Phila., 19: 148, 1951.

Chamberlain, W. E., and Young, B. R.: The diagnosis of intervertebral disk protrusion by intraspinal injection of air; air myelography. J.A.M.A., 113:2022, 1939.

Chase, N. E., and Taveras, J. M.: Cerebral angiography in the diagnosis of suprasellar tumors. Am. J. Roentgenol., 84:154, 1961.

Chase, N. E., and Taveras, J. M.: Carotid angiography in the diagnosis of extradural parasellar tumor. Acta radiol., 1:214, 1963.

Chase, N. E., and Taveras, J. M.: Temporal tumors studied by serial angiography—A review of 150 cases. Acta radiol., 1:225, 1963.

Childe, A. E.: Localized thinning and enlargement of the cranium with special reference to the middle fossa. Am. J. Roentgenol., 70:1, 1953.

Childe, A. E.: The roentgen-ray diagnosis of diseases of the skull and intracranial contents. Additional considerations. In: Golden's Diagnostic Roentgenology, Vol. I, Laurence L. Robbins, Editor. Baltimore, The Williams & Wilkins Company, 1961, p. 34 BO.

Childe, A. E., and Penfield, W.: Anatomic and pneumographic studies of the temporal horn with a further note on pneumographic analysis of the cerebral ventricles. A.M.A. Arch. Neurol. & Psychiat., 37:1021, 1937.

Childe, A. E., and Penfield, W.: The role of x-ray in the study of local atrophic lesions of the brain. Am. J. Psychiat., 101:30, 1944.

Coblentz, R. G.: Cerebellar subdural hematoma in infant 2 weeks old with secondary hydrocephalus. Operation with recovery. Surgery, 8:771, 1940.

Coddon, D. R., and Krieger, H. P.: Circumstances surrounding complications of cerebral angiography. Analysis of 546 consecutive cerebral angiograms. Am. J. Med., 25:580, 1958.

Coppoletta, J. M., and Wolbach, S. B.: Body length and organ weights of infants and children. A study of the body length and normal weights of the more important organs of the body between birth and twelve years of age. Am. J. Path., 9:55, 1933.

Courville, C. B.: Pathology of the Central Nervous System, Ed. 1, Mountain View, California, Pacific Press Publishing Association, 1937.

Courville, C. B.: Pathology of the Central Nervous System, Ed. 2, Mountain View, California, Pacific Press Publishing Association, 1945.

Courville, C. B.: Pathology of the Central Nervous System, Ed. 3, Mountain View, California, Pacific Press Publishing Association, 1950.

Courville, C. B., and Abbott, K. H.: The angioblastic group of meningiomas. A study of thirteen verified cases. Bull. Los Angeles Neurol. Soc., 5:47, 1941.

Craig, W. McK., and Gogela, L. J.: Meningioma of the optic foramen as a cause of slowly progressive blindness. Report of three cases. J. Neurosurg., 7:44, 1950.

Craig, W. McK., and Kernohan, J. W.: Tumors of the fourth ventricle. J.A.M.A., 111:2370, 1938.

Cramer, F., and Hudson, F.: Myelographically demonstrated cervical intervertebral discs, coexisting with tumors. Tr. Am. Neurol. A., 81: 171, 1956.

Crawford, E. S., De Bakey, M. E., Fields, W. S., Cooley, D. A., and Morris, G. C., Jr.: Surgical treatment of atherosclerotic occlusive lesions in patients with cerebral arterial insufficiency. Circulation, 20:168, 1959.

Crawford, J. V., and Russell, D. S.: Cryptic arteriovenous and venous hamartomas of the brain. J. Neurol. Neurosurg. & Psychiat., 19:1, 1956.

Crawford, T.: The pathological effects of cerebral arteriography. J. Neurol. Neurosurg. & Psychiat., 19:217, 1956.

Crosby, R. M. N., and Dennis, J. M.: Subdural collections of fluid in infants and children. I. Visualization of the capsule with thorium dioxide. Am. J. Roentgenol., 76:507, 1956.

Cruveilhier, J.: Anatomie Pathologique du Corps Humain. Paris, J. B. Baillière & Fils, 1829.

Cruveilhier, J.: Traité d'Anatomie Pathologique Générale. Paris, J. B. Baillière & Fils, 1856.

Cummins, F. M., Taveras, J. M., and Schlesinger, E. B.: Treatment of gliomas of the third ventricle and pinealomas; with special reference to the value of radiotherapy. Neurology, 10: 1031, 1960.

Curran, E. J.: Variations in the posterior horn of the lateral ventricle with notes on their development, and suggestions as to their clinical significance. Boston Med. and Surg. J., 161: 777, 1909.

Currarino, G., Neuhauser, E. B. D., Reyersbach, G. C., and Sobel, E. H.: Hypophosphatasia. Am. J. Roentgenol., 78:392, 1957.

Cushing, H.: The Pituitary Body and Its Disorders. Philadelphia, J. B. Lippincott Company, 1912.

Cushing, H.: The meningiomas (dural endotheliomas): Their source, and favoured seats of origin. Brain, 45:282, 1922.

Cushing, H.: Experiences with orbito-ethmoidal osteomata having intracranial complications. With the report of four cases. Surg. Gynec. & Obst., 44:721, 1927.

Cushing, H.: The basophil adenomas of the pituitary body and their clinical manifestations (pituitary basophilism). Bull. Johns Hopkins Hosp., 50:137, 1932.

Cushing, H.: Intracranial Tumours. Springfield, Illinois, Charles C Thomas, 1932, p. 8.

Cushing, H., and Bailey, P.: Tumors arising from the blood-vessels of the brain. Springfield, Illinois, Charles C Thomas, 1928, p. 211.

Cushing, H., and Eisenhardt, L.: Meningiomas. Springfield, Illinois, Charles C Thomas, 1938, p. 76.

Dandy, W. E.: Ventriculography following the injection of air into the cerebral ventricles. Ann. Surg., 68:5, 1918.

Dandy, W. E.: Röntgenography of the brain after the injection of air into the spinal canal. Ann. Surg., 70:397, 1919.

Dandy, W. E.: The diagnosis and treatment of hydrocephalus due to occlusions of the foramina of Magendie and Luschka. Surg. Gynec. & Obst., 32:112, 1921.

Dandy, W. E.: Carotid-cavernous aneurysms (pulsating exophthalmus). Zentralbl. Neurochir., 2:77, 1937.

Dandy, W. E.: Intracranial Arterial Aneurysms. Ithaca, New York, Comstock, 1944.

Dandy, W. E.: Surgery of the brain. In: Lewis' Practice of Surgery, Vol. 12. Hagerstown, Maryland, W. F. Prior Company, Inc., 1945.

Davidoff, L. M.: Coarctation of the walls of the lateral angles of the lateral cerebral ventricles. J. Neurosurg., 3:250, 1946.

Davidoff, L. M., and Dyke, C. G.: An improved method of encephalography. Bull. Neurol. Inst. New York, 2:75, 1932.

Davidoff, L. M., and Dyke, C. G.: Agenesis of the corpus callosum, its diagnosis by encephalography; report of three cases. Am. J. Roentgenol., 32:1, 1934.

Davidoff, L. M., and Dyke, C. G.: Relapsing juvenile chronic subdural hematoma. A clinical and roentgenographic study. Bull. Neurol. Inst. New York, 7:95, 1938.

Davidoff, L. M., and Dyke, C. G.: The Normal Encephalogram, Ed. 3, Philadelphia, Lea & Febiger, 1951.

Davidoff, L. M., and Epstein, B. S.: The Abnormal Pneumoencephalogram. Philadelphia, Lea and Febiger, 1950.

Davidoff, L. M., and Gass, H.: Convolutional markings in the skull roentgenograms of patients with headache. Am. J. Roentgenol., 61:317, 1949.

Davis, J. B.: Thesaurus Craniorum. London, 1867.

Davis, L.: The Principles of Neurological Surgery, Ed. 2, Philadelphia, Lea & Febiger, 1942, p. 106.

DeBakey, M. E., Crawford, E. S., and Fields, W. S.: Surgical treatment of patients with cerebral arterial insufficiency associated with extracranial arterial occlusive lesions. Proceedings of International Conference on Vascular Diseases of the Brain. Neurology, 11:145, 1961.

Decker, K.: Der Spasmus der A. carotis interna. Acta radiol., 46:351, 1956.

Decker, K. (ed.): Klinische Neuroradiologie. Thieme, Stuttgart, 1960.

Deery, E. M.: Note on calcification in pituitary adenomas. Endocrinology, 13:455, 1929.

Dew, H. R.: Hydatid Disease. Sydney, Australasian Med. Pub. Co., Ltd., 1928, p. 380.

Di Chiro, G.: The width (third dimension) of the sella turcica. Am. J. Roentgenol., 84:26, 1960.

Di Chiro, G.: Ophthalmic arteriography. Radiology, 77:948, 1961.

Di Chiro, G.: An Atlas of Detailed Normal Pneumoencephalographic Anatomy. Springfield, Illinois, Charles C Thomas, 1961.

Di Chiro, G., and Nelson, K. B.: The volume of the sella turcica. Am. J. Roentgenol., 87:989, 1962.

Dimant, S., Moxon, C. P., and Lewtas, N. A.: Cerebral angiography in a neurosurgical service. Brit. Med. J., 2:10, 1956.

Dixon, H. B. F., and Hargreaves, W. H.: Cysticercosis (*Taenia solium*). A further ten years' clinical study, covering 284 cases. Quart. J. Med., 13:107, 1944.

Dockerty, M. B., and Love, J. G.: Thickening and fibrosis (so-called hypertrophy) of the ligamentum flavum: A pathologic study of fifty cases. Proc. Staff Meet. Mayo Clin., 15:161, 1940.

Dyke, C. G.: Indirect signs of brain tumor as noted in routine roentgen examinations; displacement of pineal shadow. A survey of 3000 consecutive skull examinations. Am. J. Roentgenol., 23:598, 1930.

Dyke, C. G.: A pathognomonic encephalographic sign of subdural hematoma. Bull. Neurol. Inst. New York, 5:135, 1936.

Dyke, C. G.: The roentgen-ray diagnosis of diseases of skull and intracranial contents. In: Diagnostic Roentgenology. Ross Golden, Editor. New York, Thomas Nelson, 1941.

Dyke, C. G.: The roentgen ray diagnosis of diseases

of the spinal cord, meninges, and vertebrae. In C. A. Elsberg: Surgical Diseases of the Spinal Cord, Membranes, and Nerve Roots. New York, P. B. Hoeber, Inc., 1941, p. 42.

Dyke, C. G.: Acquired subtentorial pressure diverticulum of a cerebral lateral ventricle. Radiology, 39:167, 1942.

Dyke, C. G., and Davidoff, L. M.: The significance of abnormally shaped subarachnoid cisterns as seen in encephalogram: correlation with clinical cases. Am. J. Roentgenol., 32:743, 1934.

Dyke, C. G., and Davidoff, L. M.: Pneumo-encephalographic appearance of hemangioblastoma of the cerebellum. Am. J. Roentgenol., 44:1, 1940.

Dyke, C. G., Davidoff, L. M., and Masson, C. B.: Cerebral hemiatrophy with homolateral hypertrophy of the skull and sinuses. Surg. Gynec. & Obst., 57:588, 1933.

Dyke, C. G., Elsberg, C. A., and Davidoff, L. M.: Enlargment of the defect in the air shadow normally produced by the choroid plexus; its occurrence after ventricular puncture. Am. J. Roentgenol., 33:736, 1935.

Eaton, L. McK., Camp, J. D., and Love, J. C.: Symmetrical cerebral calcification, particularly of the basal ganglia, demonstrable roentgenographically. Calcification of the finer cerebral blood vessels. Arch. Neurol. & Psychiat., 41:921, 1939.

Ecker, A. D.: Spasm of the internal carotid artery. J. Neurosurg., 2:479, 1945.

Ecker, A. D.: The Normal Cerebral Angiogram. Springfield, Illinois, Charles C Thomas, 1951.

Ecker, A., and Riemenschneider, P. A.: Angiographic Localization of Intracranial Masses. Springfield, Illinois, Charles C Thomas, 1955.

Elsberg, C. A.: Diagnosis and Treatment of Surgical Diseases of the Spinal Cord and Its Membranes. Philadelphia, W. B. Saunders Co., 1916, p. 34.

Elsberg, C. A.: Surgical Diseases of the Spinal Cord, Membranes, and Nerve Roots. New York, P. B. Hoeber, Inc., 1941, p. 208.

Elsberg, C. A., and Dyke, C. G.: The diagnosis and localization of tumors of the spinal cord by means of measurements made on the x-ray films of the vertebrae, and the correlation of clinical and x-ray findings. Bull. Neurol. Inst. New York, 3:359, 1934.

Elsberg, C. A., Dyke, C. G., and Brewer, E. D.: The symptoms and diagnosis of extradural cysts. Bull. Neurol. Inst. New York, 3:395, 1934.

Elvidge, A. R.: The cerebral vessels studied by angiography. Res. Pub. A. Nerv. & Mental Dis., 18:110, 1938.

Engels, E. P.: Roentgenographic demonstration of a hypophysical subarachnoid space. Am. J. Roentgenol., 80:1001, 1958.

Epstein, B. S., and Davidoff, L. M.: The roentgenologic diagnosis of dilatations of the spinal cord veins. Am. J. Roentgenol., 49:476, 1943.

Ethelberg, S., and Vaernet, K.: The angiographic configuration of intracerebral metastatic tumors. Radiology, 61:39, 1953.

Etter, L. E.: Atlas of Roentgen Anatomy of the Skull. Springfield, Illinois, Charles C Thomas, 1955.

Fields, W. S., Crawford, E. S., and DeBakey, M. E.: Surgical considerations in cerebral arterial insufficiency. Neurology, 8:801, 1958.

Fischer, E.: Die Lageabweichungen der vorderen Hirnarterie im Gefässbild. Zentralbl. Neurochir 3:300, 1938.

Fischgold, H., David, M., and Brégeat, P.: La Tomographie de la Base du Crâne en Neurochirurgie et Neuro-ophtalmologie. Paris, Masson & Cie., 1952.

Fisher, M.: Occlusion of the carotid arteries. Further experiences. A.M.A. Arch. Neurol. & Psychiat., 72:187, 1954.

Fletcher, T. M., Taveras, J. M., and Pool, J. L.: Cerebral vasospasm in angiography for intracranial aneurysms. Incidence and significance in one hundred consecutive angiograms. A.M.A. Arch Neurol., 1:38, July, 1959.

Flippen, J. H., Jr.: Cranio-facial dysostosis of Crouzon. Report of a case in which the malformation occurred in four generations. Pediatrics, 5:90, 1950.

Flügel, F. E.: Die Encephalographie als neurologische Untersuchungsmethode. Kritische Bearbeitung von 603 encephalographischen Untersuchungen von 506 Kranken. Ergebn. inn. Med. u. Kinderh., 44:327, 1932.

Fowler, E. P., and Swenson, P. C.: Petrositis: A roentgenologic and pathologic correlation. Am. J. Roentgenol., 41:317, 1939.

Fray, W. W.: A roentgenological study of pineal orientation. Am. J. Roentgenol., 39:899, 1938.

French, L.: Tumors—Intracranial & cranial. In: Pediatric Neurosurgery, I. J. Jackson and R. K. Thompson, Editors. Oxford, Blackwell Scientific Publications, 1959.

Friedmann, G., Krenkel, W., and Tönnis, W.: Angiographie oder Pneumographie? Vergleichende Untersuchung bei 670 supratentoriellen Tumoren. Fortschr. Röntgenstr., 96:181, 1962.

Frøvig, A. G., and Koppang, K.: Cerebral complications following percutaneous carotid angiography with contrast media of the Diodrast group. Acta psychiat. et neurol. scandinav., 28:339, 1953.

Frugoni, P., Nori, A., Galligioni, F., and Giammusso, V.: A particular angiographic sign in meningiomas of the tentorium: The artery of Bernasconi and Cassinari. Neurochirurgia, 2:142, 1960.

Galloway, J. R., and Greitz, T.: The medial and lateral choroid arteries: An anatomic and roentgenographic study. Acta radiol., 53:353, 1960.

Gardner, W. J.: The therapeutic effects of encephalography. Pennsylvania M. J., 33:126, 1929.

Garland, L. H., and Morrissey, E. J.: Intracranial collections of iodized oil following lumbar myelography. Surg. Gynec. & Obst., 70:196, 1940.

Gensini, G. G., and Ecker, A.: Percutaneous aortocerebral angiography. Radiology, 75:885, 1960.

Geyelin, H. R., and Penfield, W.: Cerebral calcification epilepsy; endarteritis calcificans cerebri. A.M.A. Arch. Neurol. & Psychiat., 21:1020, 1929.

Giraud, M., Bret, P., Anjou, A., Chollat, L., and Feuillade, C.: Exploration radiographique et tomographique du canal déchiré postérieur normal et pathologique. Ann. Radiol. (Paris) 4: 543, 1961.

Gladstone, R. J., and Wakeley, C. P. G.: The Pineal Organ. London, Baillière, Tindall and Cox, 1940, p. 467.

Globus, J. H., and Doshay, L. J.: Venous dilatations and other intraspinal vessel alterations, including true angiomata with signs and symptoms of cord compression. A report of four cases with a review of the literature. Surg. Gynec. & Obst., 48:345, 1929.

Goldensohn, E. S.: Temporal lobe epilepsy: neurologic and electrical studies. Bull. New York Acad. Med., 38:653, 1962.

Gordon, M. B., and Bell, A. L.: A roentgenographic study of the sella turcica in normal children. N. Y. State J. Med., 22:54, 1922.

Gordon-Shaw, C.: Two cases of reduplication of the arteria cerebri posterior. J. Anat. and Physiol., 44:244, 1910.

Gould, P. L., Peyton, W. T., and French, L. A.: Vertebral angiography by retrograde injection of the brachial artery. J. Neurosurg., 12: 369, 1955.

Grantham, E. G., and Smolik, E. A.: Calcified intracerebral hematoma. Ann. Surg., 115:465, 1942.

Gray, E. D.: Calcification and ossification of spinal tumours. Brit. J. Radiol., 15:365, 1942.

(Revised 1963)

Gray, H.: Anatomy of the Human Body. Philadelphia, Lea & Febiger, 1959, p. 633.

Greitz, T.: A radiologic study of the brain circulation by rapid serial angiography of the carotid artery. Acta radiol., Supp. No. 140, 1956.

Gross, S. W.: Concerning intraspinal dermoids and epidermoids, with report of a case. J. Nerv. & Ment. Dis., 80:274, 1934.

Gurdjian, E. S., Lindner, D. W., Hardy, W. G., and Thomas, L. M.: Incidence of surgically treatable lesions in cases studied angiographically. Proceedings of International Conference on Vascular Diseases of the Brain. Neurology, 11:150, 1961.

Gurdjian, E. S., Lindner, D. W., Hardy, W. G., and Thomas, L. M.: Arteriography. In: C. H. Millikan, Chairman, Cerebral Vascular Diseases, 3d Princeton Conference. New York, Grune & Stratton, 1961, p. 200.

Gurdjian, E. S., Lindner, D. W., Hardy, W. G., and Webster, J. E.: Cerebrovascular disease. An analysis of 600 cases. Neurology, 10:372, 1960.

Gurdjian, E. S., Webster, J. E., and Lissner, H. R.: The mechanism of skull fracture. J. Neurosurg., 7:106, 1950.

Gurdjian, E. S., Webster, J. E., and Lissner, H. R.: Observations on prediction of fracture site in head injury. Radiology, 60:226, 1953.

Haas, L.: Erfahrungen auf dem Gebiete der radiologischen Selladiagnostik. Fortschr. Geb. Roentgenstrahlen, 33:419 and 469, 1925.

Hadley, L. A.: Subluxation of the apophyseal articulations with bony impingement as a cause of back pain. Am. J. Roentgenol., 33: 209, 1935.

Hadley, L. A.: Pathologic conditions of the spine: Painful disturbances of the intervertebral foramina. J.A.M.A., 110:275, 1938.

Hadley, L. A.: Intervertebral joint subluxation, bony impingement and foramen encroachment with nerve root changes. Am. J. Roentgenol., 65:377, 1951.

Hamby, W. B.: Intracranial Aneurysms. Springfield, Illinois, Charles C Thomas, 1952.

Hamil, J.: Personal communication, 1961.

Hampton, A. O., and Robinson, J. M.: The roentgenographic demonstration of rupture of the intervertebral disc into the spinal canal after the injection of lipiodol. Am. J. Roentgenol., 36:782, 1936.

Hardman, J.: The angioarchitecture of the glioblastoma multiforme type of tumour and its bearing on angiography. Lisboa méd., 15: 329, 1938.

Hare, H. F., Silveus, E., and Smedal, M. I.:

Roentgenologic diagnosis of pituitary tumors. Radiology, 52:193, 1949.

Hassler, O., and Saltzman, G. F.: Angiographic and histologic changes in infundibular widening of the posterior communicating artery. Acta radiol., 1:321, 1963.

Hinck, V. C., Hopkins, C. E., and Savara, B. H.: Diagnostic criteria of basilar impression. Radiology, 76:572, 1961.

Hinkel, C. L., and Nichols, R. L.: Opaque myelography in penetrating wounds of the spinal canal. Am. J. Roentgenol., 55:689, 1946.

Hobæk, A.: Fibrous dysplasia—fibro-osteoma—Osteoma of the facial bones and the skull. Acta radiol., 36:97, 1951.

Hodes, P. J., Campoy, F., Riggs, H. E., and Bly, P.: Cerebral angiography. Fundamentals in anatomy and physiology. Am. J. Roentgenol., 70:61, 1953.

Hoefnagel, D., Benirschke, K., and Duarte, J.: Teratomatous cysts within the vertebral canal. Observations on the occurrence of sex chromatin. J. Neurol. Neurosurg. Psychiat., 25:159, 1962.

Hoessly, G. F., and Olivecrona, H.: Report on 280 cases of verified parasagittal meningioma. J. Neurosurg., 12:614, 1955.

Holman, C. B.: The application of closed-circuit television in diagnostic roentgenology. Proc. Mayo Clin., 38:67, 1963.

Holman, C. B., Olive, I., and Svien, H. J.: Roentgenologic features of neurofibromas involving the Gasserian ganglion. Am. J. Roentgenol., 86:148, 1961.

Holt, J. F., and Dickerson, W. W.: The osseous lesions of tuberous sclerosis. Radiology, 58:1, 1952.

Holt, W. L., Jr., and Pearson, G. B.: The encephalographic diagnosis of chronic bilateral subdural hematoma. Tr. Am. Neurol. A., 62:162, 1936.

Horrax, G.: The role of pinealomas in the causation of diabetes insipidus. Ann. Surg., 126: 725, 1947.

Horrax, G., and Wyatt, J. P.: Ectopic pinealomas in the chiasmal region; report of three cases. J. Neurosurg., 4:309, 1947.

Horwitz, N. H., and Dunsmore, R. H.: Some factors influencing the nonvisualization of the internal carotid artery by angiography. J. Neurosurg., 13:155, 1956.

Horwitz, T.: The diagnosis of posterior protrusion of the intervertebral disc. With special reference to (1) its differentiation from certain degenerative lesions of the disc and its related structures and (2) the interpretation of contrast myelography. Am. J. Roentgenol., 49: 199, 1943.

Housepian, E. M., and Pool, J. L.: A systematic analysis of intracranial aneurysms from the autopsy file of the Presbyterian Hospital, 1914 to 1956. J. Neuropath. & Exper. Neurol., 17: 409, 1958.

Hughson, W.: Meningeal relations of hypophysis cerebri. Anat. Rec., 23:21, 1922.

Hunter, C. R., and Mayfield, F. H.: The oblique view in cerebral angiography. J. Neurosurg., 12:79, 1955.

Hurxthal, L. M.: Pituitary tumor. S. Clin. North America, 1947, p. 530.

Ingraham, F. D.: Intraspinal tumors in infancy and childhood. Am. J. Surg., 39:342, 1938.

Ingraham, F. D., and Matson, D. D.: Subdural hematoma in infancy. J. Pediat., 24:1, 1944.

Ingraham, F. D., and Matson, D. D.: Neurosurgery of Infancy and Childhood. Springfield, Illinois, Charles C Thomas, 1954.

Irwin, G. L.: Roentgen determination of the time of closure of the spheno-occipital synchondrosis. Radiology, 75:450, 1960.

Jefferson, A., and Sheldon, P.: Transtentorial herniation of the brain as revealed by the displacement of arteries. Acta radiol., 46:480, 1956.

Jefferson, G.: Extrasellar extensions of pituitary adenomas: President's address. Proc. Royal Soc. Med., 33:433, 1940.

Jefferson, G.: Trigeminal neurinomas with some remarks on malignant invasion of the Gasserian ganglion. In: Clinical Neurosurgery: Proceedings of the Congress of Neurological Surgeons, 1953. Baltimore, The Williams & Wilkins Company, 1955, p. 11.

Jefferson, G.: The Trigeminal Neurinomas. In: Selected Papers. Springfield, Illinois, Charles C Thomas, 1960, p. 500.

Jirout, J.: Encefalografie. Praze, Lékařské Knihfupectví a Nakladatelství, 1948 (Quoted by Robertson, 1957).

Johnson, R. T., and Yates, P. O.: Clinico-pathological aspects of pressure changes at the tentorium. Acta radiol., 46:242, 1956.

Kågström, E., Lindgren, P., and Törnell, G.: Circulatory disturbances during cerebral angiography. An experimental evaluation of certain contrast media. Acta radiol., 54:3, 1960.

Kahn, E., Lion, E. G., and Zimmerman, H. M.: Cerebral cortical calcification simulating Pick's disease. Am. J. Psychiat., 95:1027, 1939.

Kaplan, A. D., and Walker, A. E.: Complications of cerebral angiography. Neurology, 4:643, 1954.

Kaplan, H. A.: Vascular supply of the base of the brain. In: Pathogenesis and Treatment of Parkinsonism. W. S. Fields, Editor. Houston Neurological Society, 6th Annual Scientific Meeting. Springfield, Illinois, Charles C Thomas, 1958, p. 135.

Kaplan, H. A.: The transcerebral venous system. A.M.A. Arch. Neurol., 1:148, 1959.

Kasabach, H. H., and Dyke, C. G.: Osteoporosis circumscripta of the skull as a form of osteitis deformans. Am. J. Roentgenol., 28:192, 1932.

Kaufmann, J.: Dissertatio de tumore capitis fungoso post cariem cranii exorto. Helmstad, 6 Dec. 1743. In: Haller's Disputationes chirurgicae selectae, Lausanne, 1:45, 1755.

Kearns, T. P., Salassa, R. M., Kernohan, J. W., and MacCarty, C. S.: Ocular manifestations of pituitary tumor in Cushing's syndrome. A.M.A. Arch. Ophth., 62:242, 1959.

Keith, A: The pineal eye. In J. I. Kitay and M. D. Altschule: The Pineal Gland. Cambridge, Massachusetts, Harvard University Press, 1954.

Kennedy, F.: Retrobulbar neuritis as an exact diagnostic sign of certain tumors and abscesses in the frontal lobes. Am. J. M. Sc., 142:355, 1911.

Kennedy, F., Effron, A. S., and Perry, G.: The grave spinal cord paralyses caused by spinal anesthesia. Surg. Gynec. & Obst., 91:385, 1950.

Kerman, W. Z., Perlstein, M. A., and Levinson, A.: Bacillus pyocyaneus meningitis following pneumoencephalography. A.M.A. J. Dis. Child., 65:912, 1943.

Kernohan, J. W., Woltman, H. W., and Adson, A. W.: Intramedullary tumors of the spinal cord. A review of fifty-one cases, with an attempt at histological classification. A.M.A. Arch. Neurol. & Psychiat., 25:679, 1931.

Kernohan, J. W., Woltman, H. W., and Adson, A. W.: Gliomas arising from the region of the cauda equina. Clinical, surgical and histologic considerations. A.M.A. Arch. Neurol. & Psychiat., 29:287, 1933.

Key, A., and Retzius, G.: Studien in der Anatomie des Nervensystems und des Bindegewebes, v. I. Stockholm, Samsons Wallin, 1875.

Keyes, J. E. L.: Observations on four thousand optic foramina in human skulls of known origin. A.M.A. Arch. Ophth., 13:538, 1935.

King, A. B., and Gould, D. M.: Symmetrical calcification in the cerebellum. Am. J. Roentgenol., 67:562, 1952.

King, A. B., and Otenasek, F. J.: Air embolism occurring during encephalography; report of two cases. J. Neurosurg., 5:577, 1948.

(Revised 1963)

King, T. T., and Couch, R. S. C.: The diagnosis of cerebral hydatid disease. Clin. Radiol., 12: 190, 1961.

Kitay, J. I., and Altschule, M. D.: The Pineal Gland. A Review of the Physiologic Literature. Cambridge, Massachusetts, Harvard Univeristy Press, 1954, p. vii.

Klotz, O.: Studies on calcareous degeneration. I. The process of pathological calcification. J. Exper. Med., 7:633, 1905.

Knisely, M. H., Warner, L., and Harding, F.: Antemortem settling. Microscopic observations and analyses of the settling of agglutinated blood-cell masses to the lower sides of vessels during life; a contribution to the biophysics of disease. Angiology, 11:535, 1960.

Krayenbühl, H., and Richter, H. R.: Die zerebrale Angiographie. Stuttgart, Thieme, 1952.

Krayenbühl, H., and Yasargil, M. G.: Die vaskulären Erkrankungen im Gebiet der Arteria Vertebralis und Arteria Basialis. Stuttgart, Thieme, 1957.

Kuhn, R. A.: The revolution produced by cerebral angiography in management of the patient with "stroke." J. M. Soc. New Jersey, 56:68, 1959.

Kuhn, R. A.: Brachial cerebral angiography. J. Neurosurg., 17:955, 1960.

Laine, E., Delandtsheer, J. M., Galibert, P., and Delandtsheer-Arnott, G.: Phlebography in tumors of hemispheres and central grey matter. Acta radiol., 46:203, 1956.

Last, R. J., and Tompsett, D. H.: Casts of the cerebral ventricles. Brit. J. Surg., 40:525, 1953.

Leeds, N. E., and Seamen, W. B.: Fibrous dysplasia of the skull and its differential diagnosis. A clinical and roentgenographic study of 46 cases. Radiology, 78:570, 1962.

Leeds, N. E., and Taveras, J. M.: Diagnostic value of changes in local circulation time in frontal and parietal tumors. Acta radiol., 1: 332, 1963.

Liber, A. F., and Lisa, J. R.: Stromal tumors of choroid plexus. Am. J. Clin. Path., 10:710, 1940.

Lichtenstein, B. W.: A Textbook of Neuropathology. Philadelphia, W. B. Saunders Co., 1949, p. 321.

Liliequist, B.: The anatomy of the subarachnoid cisterns. Acta radiol., 46:61, 1956.

Liliequist, B.: The subarachnoid cisterns. An anatomic and roentgenologic study. Acta radiol., Supplement 185, 1959.

Liliequist, B.: Encephalography in the Arnold-Chiari malformation. Acta radiol., 53:17, 1960.

Liliequist, B.: Encephalographic changes in the axial pressure cone syndrome. Acta. radiol., 54:369, 1960.

Lima, P. M. de A. Cerebral Angiography. New York, Oxford University Press, 1950.

Lin, P. M., Mokrohisky, J. F., Stauffer, H. M., and Scott, M.: Importance of the deep cerebral veins in cerebral angiography, with special emphasis on the orientation of the foramen of Monro through visualization of the "venous angle" of the brain. J. Neurosurg., 12:256, 1955.

Lindau, A.: Studien über Kleinhirncysten. Acta path. et microbiol. scandinav., Suppl. 1:93, 1926.

Lindau, A.: Zur Frage der Angiomatosis retinae und ihrer Hirnkomplikationen. Acta ophth., 4:193, 1927.

Lindau, A.: Discussion on vascular tumours of the brain and spinal cord. Proc. Roy. Soc. Med., 24:363, 1930.

Lindblom, K.: A roentgenographic study of the vascular channels of the skull, with special reference to intracranial tumors and arterio-venous aneurysms. Acta radiol., Supplement 30, 1936.

Lindblom, K.: Complications of myelography by abrodil. Acta radiol., 28:69, 1947.

Lindblom, K.: Technique and results in myelography and disc puncture. Acta radiol., 34:321, 1950.

Lindén, L.: Effect of stellate ganglion block on cerebral circulation in cerebrovascular accidents. Acta med. scandinav., Supp. 301, 1955.

Lindgren, E.: Eine enzephalographische Formvariante des Seitenventrikels. Acta radiol., 22:722, 1941.

Lindgren, E.: Das Röntgenbild bei Tumoren des Ganglion Gasseri. Acta chir. scandinav., 85: 181, 1941.

Lindgren, E.: The normal temporal horn and its deformities by tumours in the middle cerebral fossa. Proc. Roy. Soc. Med., 40:859, 1947.

Lindgren, E.: A pneumographic study of the temporal horn, with special reference to tumours in the temporal region. Acta radiol., Supplement 69, 1948.

Lindgren, E.: Some aspects of the techniques of encephalography. Acta radiol., 31:161, 1949.

Lindgren, E.: Percutaneous angiography of the vertebral artery. Acta radiol., 33:389, 1950.

Lindgren, E.: Encephalographic examination of tumours in the posterior fossa. Acta radiol., 34:331, 1950.

Lindgren, E.: Röntgenologie. In: Handbuch der Neurochirugie. Bd. II. Hrsgb. von Olivecrona und Tönnis, Berlin, Springer, 1954.

Lindgren, E.: Radiologic examination of the brain and spinal cord. Acta radiol., Supplement 151, 1957.

List, C. F., Holt, J. F., and Everett, M.: Lipoma of the corpus callosum. A clinicopathologic study. Am. J. Roentgenol., 55:125, 1946.

Locke, C. E., Jr.: Internal intracranial arterio-venous aneurysm or pulsating exophthalmus. Ann. Surg., 80:1 and 272, 1924.

Löfgren, F. O.: Vertebral angiography in the diagnosis of hydrocephalus and differentiation between stenosis of the aqueduct and cerebellar tumour. Acta radiol., 46:186, 1956.

Löfgren, F. O.: Vertebral angiography in the diagnosis of tumours in the pineal region. Acta radiol., 50:108, 1958.

Loman, J., and Myerson, A.: Visualization of the cerebral vessels by direct intracarotid injection of thorium dioxide (Thorotrast). Am. J. Roentgenol., 35:188, 1936.

Lombardi, G.: The occipital vertebra. Am. J. Roentgenol., 86:260, 1961.

Lombardi, G., Cecchini, A., and De Donato, E.: L'artère ophthalmique dans les méningiomes péri-orbitaires. Ann. Radiol., 3:165, 1960.

Lorber, J.: Intracranial calcification following tuberculous meningitis in children. Am. Rev. Tuberc., 78:38, 1958.

Lorenz, R.: Differentialdiagnose der arteriographisch darstellbaren, intrakraniellen Geschwültste: Glioblastom, Meningeom, Sarkom. Zentralbl. Neurochir., 5:30, 1940.

Louis, A.: Mémoire sur les tumeurs fongueuses de la dure-mère. Mém. Acad. roy. chir. Paris, 5:1, 1774.

Lowman, R. M., Shapiro, R., and Collins, L. C.: The significance of the widened septum pellucidum. Am. J. Roentgenol., 59:177, 1948.

Luckett, W. H.: Air in the ventricles of the brain following a fracture of the skull; report of a case. Surg. Gynec. & Obst., 17:237, 1913.

Lysholm, E., Ebenius, B., and Sahlstedt, H.: Das Ventrikulogramm, I. Teil. Röntgentechnik. Acta radiol., Supplement 24, 1935.

MacCarty, W. C., Jr., and Russell, D. G.: Tuberous sclerosis. Report of a case with ependymoma. Radiology, 71:833, Dec. 1958.

McDonald, C. A., and Korb, M.: Intracranial aneurysms. A.M.A. Arch. Neurol. & Psychiat., 42:298, 1939.

McGregor, M.: The significance of certain measurements of the skull in diagnosis of basilar impression. Brit. J. Radiol. 21:171, 1948.

McGuire, T. H., Greenwood, J., Jr., and Newton,

B. L.: Bilateral angioma of choroid plexus; case report. J. Neurosurg., 11:428, 1954.

McKhann, C. F.: Lead poisoning in children; The cerebral manifestations. A.M.A. Arch. Neurol. & Psychiat., 27:294, 1932.

McRae, D. L.: Occipitalization of the atlas. Am. J. Roentgenol., 70:23, 1953.

McRae, D. L.: Asymptomatic intervertebral disc protrusions. Acta radiol., 46:9, 1956.

McRae, D. L.: Facial epilepsy: correlation of the pathological and radiological findings. Radiology, 50:439, 1948.

McRae, D. L., and Elliott, A. W.: Radiological aspects of cerebellar astrocytomas and medulloblastomas. Acta radiol., 50:52, 1958.

McRae, D. L., and Valentino, V. Pneumographic findings in angioma of the brain. Acta radiol., 50:18, 1958.

Mahmoud, M. El S.: The sella in health and disease. Brit. J. Radiol., Supp. No. 8, 1958.

Malbin, M.: Mobile calcified choroid plexuses. Radiology, 51:383, 1948.

Malis, L. I.: The myelographic examination of the foramen magnum. Radiology, 70:196, 1958.

Margolis, G., Odon, G. L., Woodhall, B., and Bloor, B. M.: The role of small angiomatous malformations in the production of intracerebral hematomas. J. Neurosurg., 8:564, 1951.

Marie, P.: Sur deux cas d'acromégalie; hypertrophie singulière non congénitale des extrémités supérieures, inférieures et céphalique. Rev. de méd., 6: 297, 1886.

Marks, J. H., and Livingston, K. E.: The cervical subarachnoid space, with particular reference to syringomyelia and the Arnold Chiari deformity. Radiology, 52:63, 1949.

Martin, P., and Cushing, H.: Primary gliomas of the chiasm and optic nerves in their intracranial portion. A.M.A. Arch. Ophth., 52:209, 1923.

Martin, M. J., Sayre, G. P., and Whisnant, J. P.: Incidence of occlusive vascular disease in the extracranial arteries contributing to the cerebral circulation. Tr. Am. Neurol. A., 85: 103, 1960.

Martin, M. J., Whisnant, J. P., and Sayre, G. P.: Occlusive vascular disease in the extracranial cerebral circulation. A.M.A. Arch. Neurol., 3:530, 1960.

Martland, H. S.: Spontaneous subarachnoid hemorrhage and congenital "Berry" aneurysms of the circle of Willis. Am. J. Surg., 43: 10, 1939.

Mascherpa, F., and Valentino, V.: Intracranial Calcification. Springfield, Illinois, Charles C Thomas, 1959.

Maslowski, H. A.: Vertebral angiography. Percutaneous lateral atlanto-occipital method. Brit. J. Surg., 43:1, 1955.

Mason, M. S., and Raaf, J.: Physiological alterations and clinical effects of urea-induced diuresis. J. Neurosurg., 18:645, 1961.

Matson, D. D., and Crofton, F. D. L.: Papilloma of the choroid plexus in childhood. J. Neurosurg., 17:1002, 1960.

Matsubara, T., and Nomura, T.: Emulsified iodized oil ventriculography. Am. J. Roentgenol., 84:48, 1960.

Matthias, R. C.: A composite representation of a lateral radiograph of the skull, and a drawing of the brain and the cerebral ventricles. M. Radiog. & Photog., 28:76, 1952.

Merrill, V.: Atlas of Roentgenographic Positions. St. Louis, C. V. Mosby Company, 1949, p. 358.

Merrill, V.: Atlas of Roentgenographic Positions, Vol. Two, Ed. 2, St. Louis, Missouri, C. V. Mosby Company, 1959.

Mettier, S. R., and Capp, C. S.: Neurological symptoms and clinical findings in patients with cervical degenerative arthritis. Ann. Int. Med., 14:1315, 1941.

Meyer, A.: Das Verhalten des Blutdrucks bei der Encephalographie. Klin. Wchnschr., 11:1873, 1932.

Millikan, C. H.: A classification and outline of cerebrovascular diseases. Introduction. Neurology 8:401, 1958.

Mitchell, N., and Angrist, A.: Intracranial aneurysms—a report of thirty-six cases. Ann. Int. Med., 19:909, 1943.

Mixter, W. J., and Barr, J. S.: Rupture of the intervertebral disc with involvement of the spinal canal. New England J. Med., 211:210, 1934.

Mokrohisky, J. F., Paul, R. E., Lin, P. M., and Stauffer, M.: The diagnostic importance of normal variants in deep cerebral phlebography. With special emphasis on the true and false "venous angles of the brain" and evaluation of venous angle measurements. Radiology, 67:34, 1956.

Mones, R.: Vertebral angiography. An analysis of 106 cases. Radiology, 76:230, 1961.

Mones, R., and Werman, R.: Pantopaque myeloencephalography. Radiology, 72:803, 1959.

Moniz, E.: L'Angiographie Cerebrale. Paris, Masson et Cie., 1934.

Moniz, E., Lima, A., and de Lacerda, R.: Hémiplégies par thrombose de la carotide interne. Presse Méd., 45:977, 1937.

Monro, A.: Observations on the structure and functions of the nervous system. Edinburgh, Creech, 1783.

Moore, M. T.: The Morgagni-Stewart-Morel syndrome. Report of a case with pneumoencephalographic findings. A.M.A. Arch. Int. Med., 73:7, 1944.

Moore, S.: Metabolic craniopathy. Am. J. Roentgenol., 35:30, 1936.

Moore, S.: Hyperostosis Cranii. Springfield, Illinois, Charles C Thomas, 1955.

Morello, A., and Cooper, I. S.: Arteriographic anatomy of the anterior choroidal artery. Am. J. Roentgenol., 73:748, 1955.

Moss, M. L.: The pathogenesis of premature cranial synostosis in man. Acta Anat., 37:351, 1959.

Mount, L. A.: Surgical treatment of craniostenosis with long term follow-up. Personal communication, 1961.

Mount, L. A., and Taveras, J. M.: Cerebral angiographic studies following surgical treatment of intracranial aneurysms. Angiographic evaluation of results. Acta radiol., 46:333, 1956.

Mount, L. A., and Taveras, J. M.: Arteriographic demonstration of the collateral circulation of the cerebral hemispheres. A.M.A. Arch. Neurol. & Psychiat., 78:235, 1957.

Mount, L. A., and Taveras, J. M.: Further observations of the significance of the collateral circulation of the brain as demonstrated arteriographically. Tr. Am. Neurol. A., 1960, p. 109.

Mueller, J.: Über den feinern Bau und die Formen der krankhaften Geschwülste. Berlin, Reimer, 1838.

Murtagh, F., Chamberlain, W. E., Scott, M., and Wycis, H. T.: Cervical air myelography. Am. J. Roentgenol., 74:1, 1955.

Naffziger, H. C., and Jones, O. W., Jr.: Dermoid tumors of the spinal cord. Report of four cases, with observations on a clinical test for the differentiation of the source of radicular pain. A.M.A. Arch. Neurol. & Psychiat., 33: 941, 1935.

Nellhaus, G., and Chutorian, A.: Narcosis for Neuroradiologic Procedures in Children, in press.

Netsky, M. G., and Lapresle, J.: The first account of a meningioma. Bull. Hist. Med., 30:465, 1956.

Neuhauser, E. B. D., Wittenborg, M. H., and Dehlinger, K.: Diastematomyelia. Transfixation of the cord or cauda equina with congenital anomalies of the spine. Radiology, 54:659, 1950.

Newton, T. H.: The axillary artery approach to arteriography of the aorta and its branches. Am. J. Roentgenol., 89:275, 1963.

Niemeyer, P.: Discussion on "Supratentorial Angiomas." Ier Congrès International de Neurochirurgie. Rapports et discussions. Brussels, Editions "Acta Medica Belgica," 1957, p. 252.

Norman, O.: Angiographic differentiation between acute and chronic subdural and extradural haematomas. Acta radiol., 46:371, 1956.

Northfield, D.W.C., and Russell, D. S.: The fate of thorium dioxide (Thorotrast) in cerebral arteriography. Lancet, 1:377, 1937 (Feb. 13).

Nosik, W. A.: Intraspinal Thorotrast. Am. J. Roentgenol., 49:214, 1943.

Nosik, W. A.: Roentgenography: Thorotrast myelography. In: O. Glasser: Medical Physics. V. 1. Chicago, Year Book Publishers, Inc., 1944, pp. 1323, 1324.

Nylin, G.: Application of blood flow measurements to future investigation. In C. H. Millikan, Chairman, Cerebral Vascular Diseases, 3d Princeton Conference, New York, Grune & Stratton, 1961, p. 67.

Obici, G., and Bollici, P.: Applicazione dei raggi x alla diagnosi di sede dei corpi estranei della testa e dei tumori intracranici. Riv. di. Patol. Nerv., 2:433, 1897.

Obrador, S.: Clinical aspects of cerebral cysticercosis. A.M.A. Arch. Neurol. and Psychiat., 50:457, 1948.

Olsson, O.: Vertebral angiography in the diagnosis of acoustic nerve tumours. Acta radiol., 39: 265, 1953.

Olsson, O.: Vertebral angiography in cerebellar haemangioma. Acta radiol., 40:9, 1953.

Olsson, O.: Vertebral angiography. Acta radiol., 40:103, 1953.

Oppenheimer, A.: Diseases affecting the intervertebral foramina. Radiology, 28:582, 1937.

Ostertag, B.: Die anbestimmte Lokalisation gebundenen Konkremente des Zentralnervensystems und ihre Beziehung zur "Verkalkung intracerebraler Gefässe" beigewissen endokrinen Erkrankungen. Virchows Arch. path. Anat., 275:828, 1930.

Padget, D. H.: The circle of Willis, its embryology and anatomy. In: W. E. Dandy: Intracranial Arterial Aneurysms. Ithaca, New York, Comstock, 1944, p. 67

Pallis, C., Jones, A. M., and Spillane, J. D.: Cervical spondylosis; incidence and implications. Brain, 77:274, 1954.

Pancoast, H. K., Pendergrass, E. P., and Schaeffer, J. P.: The Head and Neck in Roentgen Diagnosis. Springfield, Illinois, Charles C Thomas, 1940.

Parsonage, M. J., and Turner, J. W. A.: Neuralgic

amyotrophy; the shoulder-girdle syndrome. Lancet, 1:973, 1948.

Pendergrass, E. P., Schaeffer, J. P., and Hodes, P. J.: The Head and Neck in Roentgen Diagnosis. Springfield, Illinois, Charles C Thomas, 1956.

Penfield, W.: Chronic meningeal (post-traumatic) headache and its specific treatment by lumbar air insufflation; encephalography. Surg. Gynec. & Obst., 45:747, 1927.

Penfield, W., and Coburn, D. F.: Arnold-Chiari malformation and its operative treatment. A.M.A. Arch. Neurol. & Psychiat., 40:328, 1938.

Penfield, W., and Erickson, T. C.: Cranial Roentgenography. Springfield, Illinois, Charles C Thomas, 1941, p. 362.

Pepper, O. H. P., and Pendergrass, E. P.: Hereditary occurrence of enlarged parietal foramina; their diagnostic importance. Am. J. Roentgenol., 35:1, 1936.

Peterman, A. F., Hayles, A. B., Dockerty, M. B., and Love, J. G.: Encephalotrigeminal angiomatosis (Sturge-Weber disease). A clinical study of thirty-five cases. J.A.M.A., 167:2169, 1958.

Peyton, W. T., and Peterson, H. O.: Congenital deformities in the region of the foramen magnum: Basilar impression. Radiology, 38:131, 1942.

Phemister, D. B.: The effect of pressure on articular surfaces in pyogenic and tuberculous arthritides and its bearing on treatment. Ann. Surg., 80:481, 1924.

Plater, F.: Observationum in hominis affectibus plerisque, corpori et animo, functionum laesione, dolore, aliave molestia et vitio incommodantibus, libri tres. Basileae, (Impensis) Ludovici König, 1614.

Pool, J. L.: The Neurosurgical Treatment of Traumatic Paraplegia. Springfield, Illinois, Charles C Thomas, 1951, p. 41.

Poser, C. M., and Taveras, J. M.: Cerebral angiography in encephalo-trigeminal angiomatosis. Radiology 68:327, 1957.

Potter, J. M.: Angiomatous malformations of the brain: their nature and prognosis. Ann. Roy. Coll. Surgeons, England, 16:227, 1955.

Potts, D. G.: Variations of the circle of Willis associated with intracranial aneurysms. Thesis for the Degree of Doctor of Medicine, New Zealand, 1960.

Potts, D. G., and Taveras, J. M.: The differential diagnosis of space-occupying lesions around the thalamus by cerebral angiography. Acta radiol, 1:373, 1963.

(Revised 1963)

Pousner, H.: Personal Communication to the author, 1961.

Pribram, H. F. W.: Angiographic appearances in acute intracranial hypertension. Neurology, 11:10, 1961.

Pygott, F., and Hutton, C. F.: Vertebral arteriography by percutaneous brachial artery catheterisation. Brit. J. Radiol., 32:114, 1959.

Radner, S.: Vertebral angiography by catheterization. A new method employed in 221 cases. Acta radiol., Supp. 87, 1951.

Ramos, M., and Mount, L. A.: Carotid cavernous fistula with signs on contralateral side. Case report. J. Neurosurg., 10:178, 1953.

Rasmussen, A. T.: A quantitative study of the human hypophysis cerebri, or pituitary body. Endocrinology, 8:509, 1924.

Raynor, R. B., and Ross, G.: Arteriography and vasospasm. The effects of intracarotid contrast media on vasospasm. J. Neurosurg., 17:1055, 1960.

Remak, R. von: Ein Beitrag zur Entwicklungsgeschichte der krebshaften Geschwülste. Deutsche Klin. 6:70, 1854.

Retzius, G. M.: Das Menschenhirn. Stockholm, Norstedt, 1892.

Rice, R. P., and Holman, C. B.: The roentgenographic manifestations of tumors of the glomus jugulare (Chemodectoma). Am. J. Roentgenol., 89:1201, 1963.

Riggs, H. E.: Anomalies of circle of Willis. Tr. Philadelphia Neurol. Soc., Dec. 1937.

Riggs, H. E.: In Hodes *et al.* (1953) *q.v.*

Riggs, H. E., and Griffiths, J. O.: Anomalies of the circle of Willis in persons with nervous and mental disorders. A.M.A. Arch. Neurol. Psychiat., 39:1352, 1938.

Riggs, H. E., and Rupp, C.: Miliary aneurysms: relation of anomalies of the circle of Willis to formation of aneurysms. A.M.A. Arch. Neurol. & Psychiat., 49:615, 1943.

Ring, B. A.: Variations in the striate and other cerebral veins affecting measurements of the "venous angle." Acta radiol., 52:433, 1959.

Robertson, E. G.: Encephalography. Melbourne, Macmillan and Co., 1941.

Robertson, E. G.: Further Studies in Encephalography. Melbourne, Macmillan and Co., 1946.

Robertson, E. G.: Pneumoencephalography. Springfield, Illinois, Charles C Thomas, 1957.

Rogers, J. S. Y., and Tudhope, G. R.: Hydatid cyst of the spinal canal successfully treated by operation. Arch. Dis. Childhood, 13:269, 1938.

Rowbotham, G. F.: The hyperostoses in relation with the meningiomas. Brit. J. Surg., 26:593, 1939.

Ruggiero, G.: L'Encephalographie Fractionnée. Paris, Masson & Cie., 1957.

Ruggiero, G.: Technique Neuroradiologique. Paris, Masson & Cie., 1959.

Russell, D. S.: The pathology of spontaneous intracranial haemorrhage. Proc. Roy. Soc. Med., 47:689, 1954.

Russell, D. S., and Rubinstein, L. J.: Pathology of Tumors of the Nervous System. London, Edward Arnold, Ltd., 1959.

Sahlstedt, H.: Writing in Lysholm's Das Ventrikulogramm, I. Teil. Acta radiol., Supplement, 24:1935.

Sahs, A. L.: Intracranial aneurysms and polycystic kidney. A.M.A. Arch. Neurol. & Psychiat., 63:524, 1950.

Salassa, R. M., Kearns, T. P., Kernohan, J. W., Sprague, R. G., and MacCarty, C. S.: Pituitary tumors in patients with Cushing's syndrome. J. Clin. Endocrinol., 19:1523, 1959.

Saltman, G.-F.: Angiographic demonstration of the posterior communicating and posterior cerebral arteries. I. Normal angiography. Acta radiol., 51:1, 1959; II. Pathologic angiography. Acta radiol., 52:114, 1959.

Sanford, H., and Doub, H. P.: Epidurography. A method of roentgenologic visualization of protruded intervertebral disks. Radiology, 36: 712, 1941.

Scarff, J. E.: Nonobstructive hydrocephalus. Treatment by endoscopic cauterization of the choroid plexus. Long term results. J. Neurosurg., 9:164, 1952.

Schechter, M. M., and de Gutiérrez-Mahoney, C. G.: Autotomography. Showing the normal and abnormal mid-line ventricular structures and basal cisterns. Brit. J. Radiol., 35:438, 1962.

Schechter, M. M., and Jing, B.-S.: Improved visualization of the ventricular system with the technic of autotomography. Radiology, 74:593, 1960.

Scheinberg, L., and Yahr, M. D.: The unsatisfactory pneumoencephalogram. Tr. Am. Neurol. A., 80:221, 1955.

Schlesinger, B.: The insulo-opercular arteries of the brain, with special reference to angiography of striothalamic tumors. Am. J. Roentgenol., 70:555, 1953.

Schlesinger, E. B., and Taveras, J. M.: Factors in the production of "cauda equina" syndromes in lumbar discs. Tr. Am. Neurol. A., 78:263, 1953.

Schlesinger, E. B., and Taveras, J. M.: Lesions of the odontoid and their management. Am. J. Surg., 95:641, April 1958.

Schmitz, A. L., and Haveson, S. B.: The roentgen diagnosis of eighth nerve tumors. Radiology, 75:531, 1960.

Schobinger, R. A., Krueger, E. G., and Sobel, G. L.: Comparison of intraosseous vertebral venography and Pantopaque myelography in the diagnosis of surgical conditions of the lumber spine and nerve roots. Radiology, 77: 376, 1961.

Schreiber, F.: Intracranial pressure: The correlation of choked disc and roentgenologic pressure signs. Am. J. Roentgenol., 23:607, 1930.

Schüller, A.: Röntgen-Diagnostik der Erkrankungen des Kopfes. Wien, Hölder, 1912.

Schüller, A.: Roentgen Diagnosis of Diseases of the Head. Tr. F. F. Stocking. St. Louis, C. V. Mosby Co., 1918.

Schunk, H., and Maryuama, Y.: Two vascular grooves of the external table of the skull which simulate fractures. Acta radiol., 54:186, 1960.

Schwarz, G. A., and Reback, S.: Compression of the spinal cord in osteitis deformans (Paget's disease) of the vertebrae. Am. J. Roentgenol., 42: 345, 1939.

Seldinger, S. I.: Catheter replacement of the needle in percutaneous arteriography. A new technique. Acta radiol., 39:368, 1953.

Shapiro, R. and Janzen, A. H.: The Normal Skull—A Roentgen Study. New York, Paul B. Hoeber, 1960.

Sheldon, P.: A special needle for percutaneous vertebral angiography. Brit. J. Radiol., 29: 231, 1956.

Shimidzu, K.: Beiträge zur Arteriographie des Gehirnseinfache percutane Methode. Arch. klin. Chir., 188:295, 1937.

Sicard, J. A., and Forestier, J.: Méthode générale d'exploration radiologique par l'huile iodée (Lipiodol). Bull. et mém. Soc. méd. hôp. Paris, 46:463, 1922.

Siekert, R. G.: Diagnosis and classification of focal ischemic cerebrovascular disease. Proc. Staff Meet. Mayo Clin., 35:473, 1960.

Silverman, F. N.: Roentgen standards for size of the pituitary fossa from infancy through adolescence. Am. J. Roentgenol., 78:451, 1957.

Simmons, D. R., Peyton, W. T.: Premature closure of the cranial sutures. J. Pediat., 31:528, 1947.

Sjögren, S. E.: Percutaneous vertebral angiography. Acta radiol., 40:113, 1953.

Sjögren, S. E.: The anterior choroidal artery. Acta radiol., 46:143, 1956.

Slosberg, P., and Bornstein, M.: Pneumoencephalography with minimal withdrawal of cerebrospinal fluid. Tr. Am. Neurol. A., 80:223, 1955.

Sokoloff, L.: Aspects of cerebral circulator physiology of relevance to cerebrovascular disease. Proceedings of International Conference on

Vascular Diseases of the Brain. Neurology, 11:34, 1961.
Sosman, M. C.: Radiology as aid in diagnosis of skull and intracranial lesions. Radiology, 9: 396, 1927.
Sosman, M. C., and Putnam, T. J.: Roentgenological aspects of brain tumors—meningiomas. Am. J. Roentgenol., 13:1, 1925.
Sosman, M. C., and Vogt, E. C.: Aneurysms of the internal carotid artery and circle of Willis, from a roentgenological viewpoint. Am. J. Roentgenol., 15:122, 1926.
Stattin, S.: Meningeal vessels of the internal carotid artery and their angiographic significance. Acta radiol., 55:329, 1961.
Stauffer, H. M., Murtagh, F., Mokrohisky, J. F., and Paul, R. E., Jr.: Biplane stereoscopic cerebral angiography. Acta radiol., 46:262, 1956.
Stauffer, H. M., Snow, L. B., and Adams, A. B.: Roentgenologic recognition of habenular calcification as distinct from calcification in the pineal body. Its application in cerebral localization. Am. J. Roentgenol., 70:83, 1953.
Stein, B. M., McCormick, W., Rodriguez, J. N., and Taveras, J. M.: Incidence and significance of occlusive vascular disease of the extracranial arteries as demonstrated by postmortem angiography. Tr. Am. Neurol. A., 86:60, 1961.
Stein, B. M., McCormick, W. F., Rodriguez, J. N., and Taveras, J. M.: Postmortem angiography of cerebral vascular system. Arch. Neurol., 7:545, 1962.
Steinberg, I., and Evans, J. A.: Technique of intravenous carotid and vertebral arteriography. Am. J. Roentgenol., 85: 1138, 1961.
Steinberg, I., Finby, N., and Evans, J. A.: A safe and practical intravenous method for abdominal aortography, peripheral arteriography, and cerebral angiography. Am. J. Roentgenol., 82:758, 1959.
Steinberg, H., and Waldron, B. R.: Idiopathic hypoparathyroidism: an analysis of fifty-two cases, including the report of a new case. Medicine, 31:133, 1952.
Stenvers, H. W.: Roentgenology of the os petrosum. Arch. Radiology and Electrotherapy, 22:97, 1917.
Stookey, B.: Intradural spinal lipoma. A report of a case and symptoms for ten years in a child aged eleven, review of the literature. A.M.A. Arch. Neurol. & Psychiat., 18:16, 1927.
Stookey, B.: Compression of the spinal cord due to ventral extradural cervical chondromas. Diagnosis and surgical treatment. A.M.A. Arch. Neurol. & Psychiat., 20:275, 1928.

(Revised 1963)

Strain, W. H., Plati, J. T., and Warren, S. L.: Iodinated organic compounds as contrast media for radiographic diagnosis. I. Iodinated aracyl esters. J. Am. Chem. Soc., 64:1436, 1942.
Sugar, O.: Discussion of "Use and Limitations of Angiography." Proceedings of International Conference on Vascular Diseases of the Brain. Neurology 11:91, 1961.
Sugar, O., Holden, L. B., and Powell, C. B.: Vertebral angiography. Am. J. Roentgenol., 61:166, 1949.
Sutton, D.: The radiological assessment of the normal aqueduct and fourth ventricle. Brit. J. Radiol., 23:208, 1950.
Sutton, D.: Radiologic aspects of pontine gliomata. Acta radiol., 40:234, 1953.
Svien, H. J., Olive, I., and Angulo-Rivero, P.: The fate of patients who have cerebral arteriovenous anomalies without definitive surgical treatments. J. Neurosurg., 13:381, 1956.
Swann, G. F.: Vertebral arteriography using the Sheldon needle and modifications of it. Brit. J. Radiol., 31:23, 1958.
Sweet, W. H., and Bennett, H. S.: Changes in internal carotid pressure during carotid and jugular occlusion and their clinical significance. J. Neurosurg., 5:178, 1948.
Swift, G. W.: Variations in cerebroventricular studies. S. Clin. North America, 4:1285, 1924.
Taggart, J. K., Jr., and Walker, A. E.: Congenital atresia of the foramens of Luschka and Magendie. A.M.A. Arch. Neurol. & Psychiat., 48:583, 1942.
Tarlov, I. M.: Sacral nerve-root cysts. Springfield, Illinois, Charles C Thomas, 1953.
Taveras, J. M.: The roentgen diagnosis of intracranial incisural space occupying lesions. Am. J. Roentgenol., 84:52, 1960.
Taveras, J. M.: Angiographic observations in occlusive cerebrovascular disease. Neurology, 11:86, 1961.
Taveras, J. M., and Dalton, C. J.: Myelographic aspects of vascular malformations of the spinal cord. Trans. (IX International Congress of Radiology, Munich, 1959) Stuttgart, Thieme, 1961, p. 453.
Taveras, J. M., Mount, L. A., and Friedenberg, R. M.: Arteriographic demonstration of external-internal carotid anastomosis through the ophthalmic arteries. Radiology, 63:525, 1954.
Taveras, J. M., Mount, L. A. and Wood, E. H.: The value of radiation therapy in the management of glioma of the optic nerves and chiasm. Radiology, 66:518, 1956.
Taveras, J. M., and Poser, C. M.: Roentgenologic

aspects of cerebral angiography in children. Am. J. Roentgenol., 82:371, 1959.

Taylor, E. H., and Haughton, W. S.: Some recent researches on the topography of the convolutions and fissures of the brain. Tr. Roy. Acad., Ireland, 18:511, 1900.

Testut, L., and Latarjet, A.: Tratado de Anatomia Humana, Vol. II. Barcelona, Salvat, 1930, p. 275.

Theander, G.: Arteriographic demonstration of stationary arterial waves. Acta radiol., 53:417, 1960.

Thibaut, A.: Symétrie du crâne normal chez les adolescents et les adultes. Acta radiol., 55:433, 1961.

Todd, T. W., and Lyon, D. W., Jr.: Endocranial suture closure, its progress and age relationship. Am. J. Phys. Anthropol. 7:325, 1924; 8: 23, 149, 1925.

Tönnis, W., and Schiefer, W.: Zur Frage des Wachstums arteriovenöser Angiome. Zentralbl. Neurochirurgie 15: 145, 1955.

Tönnis, W., and Schiefer, W.: Zirkulationsstörungen des Gehirns im Serienangiogram. Berlin, Springer, 1959.

Torkildsen, A.: Carotid angiography. With special reference to the diagnosis of cerebral gliomas. Acta psychiat. et neurol. Scandinav., Supp. 55, 1949.

Traub, S. P.: Roentgenology of Intracranial Meningiomas. Springfield, Illinois, Charles C Thomas, 1961.

Turnbull, I.: Agenesis of the internal carotid artery. Neurology, 12:588, 1962.

Twining, E. W.: Radiology of the third and fourth ventricles. Part I (p. 385) and Part II (p. 569). Brit. J. Radiol., 12, 1939.

Udvarhelyi, G. B., Wlater, W., and Schiefer, W.: Die Gefassstruktur des Glioblastoma multiforme in angiographischer und histologischer Darstellung. Acta neurochir., 4:109, 1955.

Utterback, R. A., and Haymaker, W.: Fatal complications from the use of Diodrast for cerebral and thyroid angiography. A clinico-pathological report of four cases. J. Nerv. & Ment. Dis., 116:739, 1952.

Vallebona, A.: Study of a method of microradiography. Liguria Medica, No. 12, 1928.

Vallebona, A.: Una modalità di tecnica per la dissociazione radiografica delle ombre applicata allo studio del cranio. Radiol. med., 17:1090, 1930.

Vander Eecken, H.: Discussion of "Collateral Circulation of the Brain." Proceedings of International Conference on Vascular Diseases of the Brain. Neurology, 11:16, 1961.

Vander Eecken, H. M., and Adams, R. D.: The anatomy and functional significance of the meningeal arterial anastomoses of the human brain. J. Neuropath. & Exper. Neurol., 12:132, 1953.

van der Plaats, G. J.: La technique d'agrandissement radiologique. J. belge radiol., 33:89, 1950.

Van Wyk, J. J., and Grumbach, M. M.: Syndrome of precocious menstruation and galactorrhea in juvenile hypothyroidism: an example of hormonal overlap in pituitary feedback. J. Pediat., 57:416, 1960.

Vastine, J. H., and Kinney, K. K.: The pineal shadow as aid in the localization of brain tumors. Am. J. Roentgenol., 17:320, 1927.

Virchow, R.: Die krankhaften Geschwülste. Berlin, A. Hirschwald, 1864.

Wagman, A. D., Weiss, E. K., and Riggs, H. E.: Hyperplasia of the skull associated with intraosseous meningioma in the absence of gross tumor. J. Neuropath. & Exper. Neurol., 19: 111, 1960.

Walker, A. E.: A case of congenital atresia of the foramina of Luschka and Magendie: surgical cure. J. Neuropath. & Exper. Neurol., 3:368, 1944.

Weatherall, M.: The pharmacological actions of some contrast media and a comparison of their merits. Brit. J. Radiol., 15:129, 1942.

Webster, J. E., Gurdjian, E. S., Lindner, D. W., and Hardy, W. G.: Proximal occlusion of the anterior cerebral artery. A.M.A. Arch. Neurol., 2:19, 1960.

Weed, L. H.: A note on calcification in cerebral neoplasms. A.M.A. Arch. Neurol. & Psychiat., 6: 190, 1914.

Weiner, I. H., Azzato, N. M., and Mendelsohn, R. A.: Cerebral angiography. A new technique; catheterization of the common carotid artery via the superficial temporal artery. J. Neurosurg., 15:618, 1958.

Welcker, H.: Untersuchungen über Wachsthum und Bau des menschlichen Schädels. Leipzig, W. Engelmann, 1862.

Wells, C. E. C., Spillane, J. D., and Bligh, A. S.: The cervical spinal canal in syringomyelia. Brain, 82:23, 1959; Abstract in Radiology, 75: 657, 1960.

Wells, H. G.: Calcification and ossification. Harvey Lectures, 6:102, 1910–1911.

Wermer, P.: Genetic aspects of adenomatosis of endocrine glands. Am. J. Med. 16:363, 1954.

Wickbom, I.: Angiographic determination of tumour pathology. Acta radiol., 40:529, 1953.

Wickbom, I., and Bartley, O. Arterial "spasm" in peripheral arteriography using the catheter method. Acta radiol., 47:433, 1957.

Williams, H., Schulze, W. H., Rothchild, H. B., Brown, A. S., and Smith, F. R., Jr.: Lead poisoning from the burning of battery casings. J.A.M.A., 100:1485, 1933.

Williams, J. M.: Discussion of paper by Kennedy, F., Effron, A. S., and Perry, G.: The grave spinal cord paralyses caused by spinal anesthesia. Tr. Am. Neurol. A., 1950, p. 23.

Willis, T.: Two Discourses Concerning the Soul of the Brutes, in his Practice of Physick, Being the Whole Works of That Renowned and Famous Physician, Containing These Eleven Several Treatises. London, T. Dring, C. Harper, & J. Leigh, 1684.

Wislocki, G. B.: The meningeal relations of the hypophysis cerebri. II. An embryological study of the meninges and blood vessels of the human hypophysis. Am. J. Anat., 61:95, 1937.

Wolf, A.: Tumors of the spinal cord, nerve roots, and membranes. In: C. A. Elsberg: Surgical Diseases of the Spinal Cord, Membranes, and Nerve Roots. New York, P. B. Hoeber, Inc., 1941, p. 231.

Wolf, B. S., Newman, C. M., and Schlesinger, B.: The diagnostic value of the deep cerebral veins in cerebral angiography. Radiology, 64:161, 1955.

Woltman, H. W., and Adson, A. W.: Abscess of spinal cord: Report of a case with functional recovery after operation. Brain, 49:193, 1926.

Wood, E. H.: Angiographic identification of the ruptured lesion in patients with multiple cerebral aneurysms. J. Neurosurg., in press.

Wood, E. H., Jr.: Some roentgenological and pathological aspects of calcification of the choroid plexus. Am. J. Roentgenol., 52:388, 1944.

Wood, E. H., Jr.: An Atlas of Myelography. American Registry of Pathology, Washington, D. C., 1948, p. 111.

Wood, E. H., Jr.: The diagnostic significance of change in position of metallic foreign bodies in brain abscess. Am. J. Roentgenol., 59:52, 1948.

Wood, E. H., Jr.: The diagnosis of spinal meningiomas and schwannomas by myelography. Am. J. Roentgenol., 61:683, 1949.

(Revised 1963)

Wood, E. H., and Bream, C. A.: Enlargement radiography without special apparatus other than a very fine focal spot tube. North Carolina M. J., 15:69, 1954.

Wood, E. H., and Farmer, T. W.: Cerebral infarction simulating brain tumor. Radiology, 69:693, 1957.

Wood, E. H., Jr., and Himadi, G. M.: Chordomas: A roentgenologic study of sixteen cases previously unreported. Radiology, 54:706, 1950.

Wood, E. H., Taveras, J. M., and Pool, J. L.: Myelographic demonstration of spinal cord metastases from primary brain tumors. Am. J. Roentgenol., 69:221, Feb. 1953.

World Federation of Neurology. Problem Commission of Neuroradiology. Study meeting on projections and nomenclature. Brit. J. Radiol., 35:501, 1962.

Worm, O.: Controversias Medicas. Copenhagen, 1634.

Wyatt, G. M., and Carey, B. W., Jr.: Congenital neurosyphilis; report of a case with unusual encephalographic changes. Am. J. Roentgenol., 41:779, 1939.

Wyburn-Mason, R.: The Vascular Abnormalities and Tumours of the Spinal Cord and Its Membranes. St. Louis, C. V. Mosby Co., 1944, p. 60.

Yakovlev, P. I., and Guthrie, R. H.: Congenital ectodermoses (neurocutaneous syndromes) in epileptic patients. A.M.A. Arch. Neurol. & Psychiat., 26:1145, 1931.

Zellweger, H.: Die Cisterna interventricularis und ihre klinische Bedeutung. Helvet. paediat. acta., 6:484, 1951.

Ziedses des Plantes, B. G.: Planigraphie en subtractie. Röntgenographische Differentiatiemethoden. Thesis, 1934.

Ziedses des Plantes, B. G.: Subtraktion. Eine röntgenographische Methode zur separaten Abbildung bestimmter Teile des Objekts. Fortschr. Geb. Röntgenstrahlen, 52:69, 1935.

Ziedses des Plantes, B. G.: Examen du troisième et du quatrième ventricule au moyen de petites quantités d'air. Acta radiol., 34:399, 1950.

INDEX

B

D

E

J

K

L

Q

R

S

5 5 3 7 3

8112818
3 1378 00811 2818